Pediatric Dentistry

SEVENTH EDITION

Pediatric Dentistry

INFANCY THROUGH ADOLESCENCE

ARTHUR J. NOWAK, DMD
Professor Emeritus
Departments of Pediatric Dentistry and Pediatrics
Colleges of Dentistry and Medicine
The University of Iowa
Iowa City, Iowa

Martha H. Wells, DMD, MS
Member, St. Jude Faculty
Chief of Dentistry, Surgery Department
Division of Dentistry
St. Jude Children's Research Hospital
Memphis, Tennessee

Matthew K. Geneser, DDS
Clinical Professor
Department of Pediatric Dentistry
University of Iowa College of Dentistry
Iowa City, Iowa

John R. Christensen, DDS, MS
Adjunct Associate Professor
School of Dentistry
University of North Carolina at Chapel Hill
Chapel Hill, North Carolina
Private Practice
Durham, North Carolina

Janice A. Townsend, DDS, MS
Department of Dentistry
Nationwide Children's Hospital;
Adjunct Professor
Division of Pediatric Dentistry
The Ohio State University
Columbus, Ohio

ELSEVIER

Elsevier
3251 Riverport Lane
St. Louis, Missouri 63043

PEDIATRIC DENTISTRY: INFANCY THROUGH ADOLESCENCE,
SEVENTH EDITION
ISBN: 978-0-443-24617-3

Senior Content Strategist: Kelly Skelton
Senior Content Development Specialist: Rishabh Gupta
Publishing Services Manager: Deepthi Unni
Book Specialist: Kamatchi Madhavan
Designer: Brian Salisbury

Printed in India
Thomson Press India Private Ltd,
18/35, Delhi-Mathura Road, Faridabad-121007, Haryana

Last digit is the print number: 9 8 7 6 5 4 3 2 1

Contributors

Bhavini Acharya, BDS, MPH
Associate Professor
Pediatric Dentistry
University of Texas Houston School of Dentistry
Houston, Texas

Marvellous A. Akinlotan, BDS, PhD
Clinical Assistant Professor
Pediatric Dentistry
Texas A&M University College of Dentistry
Dallas, Texas

Alexander Alcaraz, DMD
Department Co-Chair
Department of Pediatric Dentistry and Orthodontics
Herman Ostrow School of Dentistry of USC
Los Angeles, California;
Program Director
Department of Pediatric Dentistry and Orthodontics
Herman Ostrow School of Dentistry of USC
Los Angeles, California

Veerasathpurush Allareddy, BDS, MBA, MHA, PhD, MMSc
Professor and Head of Department of Orthodontics
University of Illinois Chicago College of Dentistry
Chicago, Illinois

Sahar M. Alrayyes, DDS, MS
Clinical Professor
Department of Pediatric Dentistry
University of Illinois at Chicago College of Dentistry
Chicago, Illinois

Erik B. Anderson, BS, DDS
Oral and Maxillofacial Radiologist
Assistant Professor
Uniformed Services University
San Antonio, Texas

Paul Andrews, BSc, DDS, Dip Pedo, MSc, FRCD
Assistant Professor
Pediatric Dentistry
University of Toronto
Toronto, Ontario, Canada

David M. Avenetti, DDS, MSD, MPH
Associate Professor and Department Head
Department of Pediatric Dentistry
University of Illinois Chicago College of Dentistry
Chicago, Illinois

Ehsan N. Azadani, DDS, MS
Associate Professor
Division of Pediatric Dentistry
The Ohio State University College of Dentistry
Columbus, Ohio;
Attending Pediatric Dentist
Department of Dentistry
Nationwide Children's Hospital
Columbus, Ohio

Joel H. Berg, DDS, MS
Professor Emeritus
Pediatric Dentistry
University of Washington
Glendale, AZ

R. John Brewer, EMT-P
Pittsburgh Institute of Dentistry
Pittsburgh, Pennsylvania

Erin Ealba Bumann, DDS, PhD, MS
Associate Professor
Oral and Craniofacial Sciences
University of Missouri-Kansas City
Kansas City, Missouri

Dan Burch, DDS
Clinical Professor
Director, Pediatric Dentistry Residency
Chair and Chief of Dental Medicine
St. Christopher's Hospital for Children
Philadelphia, Pennsylvania

M. Gentry Byrd, DDS, MPH
Private Practice
Pediatric Dentistry
Duke Street Pediatric Dentistry
Durham, North Carolina;
Assistant Consulting Professor
Department of Surgery
Duke University
Durham, North Carolina;
Adjunct Assistant Professor
Pediatric Dentistry and Public Health
University of North Carolina at Chapel Hill Adams School of Dentistry
Chapel Hill, North Carolina

Erica Caffrey, DDS
Clinical Assistant Professor
Department of Pediatric Dentistry and Orthodontics
University of Maryland School of Dentistry
Baltimore, Maryland

Paul S. Casamassimo, DDS, MS
Professor Emeritus
Pediatric Dentistry
The Ohio State University College of Dentistry
Columbus, Ohio;
Attending Dentist
Department of Dentistry
Nationwide Children's Hospital
Columbus, Ohio

Zafer C. Cehreli, DDS, PhD
Professor
Pediatric Dentistry
Istanbul Health and Technology University
Istanbul, Turkey

John R. Christensen, DDS, MS
Adjunct Associate Professor
School of Dentistry
University of North Carolina at Chapel Hill
Chapel Hill, North Carolina
Private Practice
Durham, North Carolina

Matthew R. Cooke, DDS, MD, MPH
Professor and Program Director
Department of Pediatric Dentistry
University of Florida
Gainesville, Florida

Jennifer L. Cully, DMD, MEd
Chief and Director of Research
Division of Oral Health
Children's National Hospital
Washington, District of Columbia;
Associate Professor
Department of Pediatrics
George Washington University
Washington, District of Columbia

Marcio A. da Fonseca, DDS, MS
Emeritus Professor
Pediatric Dentistry
University of Illinois Chicago College of Dentistry
Chicago, Illinois;
Visiting Professor
Pediatric Dentistry
Chulalongkorn University
Bangkok, Thailand

Vineet Dhar, BDS, MDS, PhD
Clinical Professor and Chair, Assistant Dean of Postgraduate and Professional Studies
Orthodontics and Pediatric Dentistry
University of Maryland School of Dentistry
Baltimore, Maryland

Keri Discepolo, DDS, MPH
Clinical Associate Professor
Pediatric Dentistry
Boston University
Boston, Massachusetts

Kevin J. Donly, BS, DDS, MS
Professor and Chair Emeritus
Developmental Dentistry
UT Health San Antonio
San Antonio, Texas

Clarice Law Eyre, DMD, MS
Associate Professor and Chair
Pediatric Dentistry and Community Oral Health
University of Tennessee Health Sciences Center
Memphis, Tennessee

Henry Fields, BA, DDS, MS, MSD
Emeritus Professor
Orthodontics
The Ohio State University College of Dentistry
Columbus, Ohio;
Chief, Section of Orthodontics
Dentistry
Nationwide Children's Hospital
Columbus, Ohio

Catherine M. Flaitz, DDS, MS
Professor and Chair, Oral & Maxillofacial Pathology
Diagnostic Sciences
University of Colorado School of Dental Medicine
Aurora, Colorado;
Consultant, Oral & Maxillofacial Pathology
Pediatric Dentistry
Children's Hospital Colorado
Aurora, Colorado

Chelsea Fosse, DMD, MPH
Vice President
Research and Policy Center
American Academy of Pediatric Dentistry
Chicago, Illinois

Matthew K. Geneser, DDS
Clinical Professor
Department of Pediatric Dentistry
University of Iowa College of Dentistry
Iowa City, Iowa

Manuel R. Gomez, DDS, FICD
Clinical Associate Professor and Graduate Program Director
Department of Endodontics
University of Iowa College of Dentistry
Iowa City, Iowa

Elizabeth S. Gosnell, DMD, MS
Professor
University of Cincinnati College of Medicine
Cincinnati, Ohio;
Division Director
Pediatric Dentistry and Orthodontics
Cincinnati Children's Hospital Medical Center
Cincinnati, Ohio

Amy R. Greenwood, PharmD
Clinical Assistant Professor
Department of Oral Pathology, Radiology and Medicine
University of Iowa College of Dentistry and Dental Clinics
Iowa City, Iowa;
Clinical Assistant Professor
Department of Pharmacy Practice and Science
University of Iowa College of Pharmacy
Iowa City, Iowa

Ann L. Griffen, DDS, MS
Professor and Chair
Biosciences
The Ohio State University College of Dentistry
Columbus, Ohio;
Professor
Pediatric Dentistry
The Ohio State University College of Dentistry
Columbus, Ohio

Erin L. Gross, DDS, PhD, MS
Associate Professor-Clinical
Division of Pediatric Dentistry
The Ohio State University College of Dentistry
Columbus, Ohio

Christel M. Haberland, DDS, MS
Staff Oral Pathologist
Oral Pathology
Ohio ENT and Allergy Physicians
Westerville, Ohio

Kerrod B. Hallett, MDSc, MPH
Clinical Associate Professor
Dentistry
Royal Australasian College of Dental Surgeons
Sydney, Australia

Kimberly J. Hammersmith, DDS, MPH, MS
Program Director, Advanced Education in Pediatric Dentistry
Department of Dentistry
Nationwide Children's Hospital
Columbus, Ohio;
Associate Professor
Division of Pediatric Dentistry
The Ohio State University College of Dentistry
Columbus, Ohio

Gideon Holan, Clinical Associated Professor (Emeritus)
Volunteer
Department of Pediatric Dentistry
The Hebrew University - Hadassah School of Dental Medicine
Jerusalem, Israel

Catherine Hong, BDS, Cert (Oral Medicine), MS (Pediatric Dentistry)
Associate Professor
Discipline of Orthodontics and Paediatric Dentistry
Faculty of Dentistry, National University of Singapore
Singapore

Cody C. Hughes, DMD, MSD
Pediatric Dentist
Pediatrics
Valley Pediatric Dental and Orthodontics
Mesquite, Nevada;
Honorary Faculty
Advanced Education in Pediatric Dentistry
UNLV School of Dental Medicine
Las Vegas, Nevada

Pollyanne Iben, DDS
Clinical Assistant Professor
Department of Pediatric Dentistry
University of Iowa College of Dentistry
Iowa City, Iowa

Michael A. Ignelzi Jr., DDS, PhD
Adjunct Professor
Department of Pediatric Dentistry
University of North Carolina at Chapel Hill Adams School of Dentistry
Chapel Hill, North Carolina;
Founding Partner
Lake Jeanette Orthodontics & Pediatric Dentistry
Greensboro, North Carolina

Janice G. Jackson, DMD
Professor and Program Director
Pediatric Dentistry
University of Alabama
Birmingham, Alabama

Faris Z. Jamjoom, BDS, MS, DMSc, FRCDC
Associate Professor
Department of Restorative and Prosthetic Dental Sciences
King Saud bin Abdulaziz University for Health Sciences
Riyadh, Saudi Arabia;
Assistant Consultant
Prosthodontics Division, King Abdulaziz Medical City
Ministry of National Guard - Health Affairs
Riyadh, Saudi Arabia

Jayakumar Jayaraman, BDS, MDS, FDSRCS, MS, PhD
Pediatric Dentist
Private Dental Practice
Richmond Pediatric Dentistry & Orthodontics
Richmond, Virginia

Michael Kanellis, DDS, MS
Professor
Department of Pediatric Dentistry
University of Iowa College of Dentistry
Iowa City, IA

Lisa Knobloch, DDS, MS
Professor
Department of Restorative Sciences and Prosthodontics
The Ohio State University College of Dentistry
Columbus, Ohio

Evelina Kratunova, BDS, MDS, DChDent, FFD
Associate Professor
Department of Pediatric Dentistry
College of Dentistry, University of Illinois Chicago
Chicago, Illinois

David K. Langford, DDS, MDS, BSChE
Assistant Professor
Department of Pediatric Dentistry and Community Oral Health
University of Mississippi Medical Center / Batson Children's Hospital

Kecia S. Leary, DDS, MS
Associate Dean of Clinics
Clinical Professor
Department of Pediatric Dentistry
University of Iowa College of Dentistry
Iowa City, IA

Jessica Y. Lee, DDS, MPH, PhD
Distinguished Professor
Pediatric Dentistry
University of North Carolina at Chapel Hill Adams School of Dentistry
Chapel Hill, North Carolina

Kyulim Lee, DMD, MS, PhD
Assistant Professor
Pediatric Dentistry
The Ohio State University College of Dentistry
Columbus, Ohio;
Assistant Professor
Dentistry
Nationwide Children's Hospital
Columbus, Ohio

Sonny Long
Associate Adjunct Professor
Department of Pediatric Dentistry
UNC School of Dentistry
Chapel Hill, North Carolina;
Private Practice: Laxer Long and Savage Pediatric Dentistry and Orthodontics
Charlotte and Monroe, North Carolina

Teresa A. Marshall, PhD, RD/LD
Professor
Department of Preventive and Community Dentistry
University of Iowa College of Dentistry
Iowa City, IA

Dennis J. McTigue, BS, DDS, MS
Professor Emeritus
Pediatric Dentistry
The Ohio State University College of Dentistry
Columbus, Ohio

Jessica A. Meeske, DDS, MS
Private Practice
Senior partner
Pediatric Dental Specialists of Greater Nebraska
Hastings, Nebraska

Anna H. Messner, MD
Professor
Otolaryngology/Head & Neck Surgery
Baylor College of Medicine
Houston, Texas

Beau D. Meyer, DDS, MPH
Associate Professor
Pediatric Dentistry
The Ohio State University College of Dentistry
Columbus, Ohio

Amy B. Miers, DDS, MS
Clinical Assistant Professor
Department of Pediatric Dentistry
University of Iowa College of Dentistry
Iowa City, IA

Stephen Craig Mills, BS, DDS
Private Practice of Pediatric Dentistry
Scarborough, Maine

Travis Nelson, DDS, MSD, MPH
Associate Professor and Chair
Department of Pediatric Dentistry
University of Washington School of Dentistry
Seattle, Washington

Allegra Nottoli, DDS, MPH
Resident
Pediatric Dentistry and Dental Public Health
University of North Carolina at Chapel Hill Adams School of Dentistry
Chapel Hill, North Carolina;
Pediatric Dentist
Private Practice
Los Angeles, California

Arthur J. Nowak, DMD
Professor Emeritus
Departments of Pediatric Dentistry and Pediatrics
Colleges of Dentistry and Medicine
The University of Iowa
Iowa City, Iowa

Heesoo Oh, DDS, PhD, MSD
Chair and Professor
Orthodontics
University of the Pacific Arthur A. Dugoni School of Dentistry
San Francisco, California

Diana Ram, DMD
Associate Professor
Pediatric Dentistry
The Hebrew University - Hadassah School of Medicine
Jerusalem, Israel

Cameron L. Randall, PhD
Assistant Professor
Department of Oral Health Sciences
University of Washington School of Dentistry
Seattle, Washington

Nina Ray, DDS
Clinical Associate Professor
Pediatric Dentistry
Texas A&M University College of Dentistry
Dallas, Texas

Steve K. Rayes, DDS, MS
Owner, Just Kids Pediatric Dentistry, PLC
Pediatric Dentistry
Just Kids Pediatric Dentistry
Norwich, Vermont

Shaun Rotenberg, DMD, MS
Assistant Professor
Periodontology
The Ohio State University College of Dentistry
Columbus, Ohio;
Private Practice
Steiner, Rotenberg, & Lindsey LLC
Columbus, Ohio;
Periodontist
Dentistry
Nationwide Children's Hospital
Columbus, Ohio

Patrick T. Ruck, DDS
Assistant Professor
Pediatric Dentistry
Cincinnati Children's Hospital Medical Center
Cincinnati, Ohio

Elise W. Sarvas, DDS, MSD, MPH
Consultant
Dental Specialties
Mayo Clinic
Rochester, Minnesota;
Consultant
Pediatric and Adolescent Medicine
Mayo Clinic
Rochester, Minnesota

Caroline Sawicki, DDS, PhD
Assistant Professor
Pediatric Dentistry and Dental Public Health
University of North Carolina at Chapel Hill Adams School of Dentistry
Chapel Hill, North Carolina

Scott B. Schwartz, DDS, MPH
Associate Professor
Department of Pediatrics
University of Cincinnati - College of Medicine
Cincinnati, Ohio;
Associate Professor
Division of Pediatric Dentistry and Orthodontics
Cincinnati Children's Hospital Medical Center
Cincinnati, Ohio

Poojan Shrestha, BDS, MSc, PhD
Associate Professor
Department of Pediatric Dentistry and Dental Public Health
University of North Carolina at Chapel Hill Adams School of Dentistry
Chapel Hill, North Carolina

Miguel A. Simancas-Pallares, DDS, MS, MSc
Associate Professor and Predoctoral Program Director in Pediatric Dentistry
Department of Pediatric Dentistry and Dental Public Health
University of North Carolina at Chapel Hill Adams School of Dentistry
Chapel Hill, North Carolina

Sujatha Sivaraman, BDS, DMD, MPH
Pediatric Dental Director
Pediatric Dentistry
Compass Health
Columbia, Missouri;
Associate Director
Advanced Education in Pediatric Dentistry
NYU Langone
Columbia, Missouri

Rebecca L. Slayton, MS, DDS, PhD
Professor Emerita
Pediatric Dentistry
University of Iowa College of Dentistry
Hardeeville, SC

Mary Austin Smith, DDS, MS
Pediatric Dentist
Department of Surgery
St. Jude Children's Research Hospital
Memphis, Tennessee

Andrew Spadinger, DDS
Pediatric Dentist
Private Practice
Children's Dentistry & Orthodontics
Bridgeport, Connecticut

Brian J. Specht, MD
Assistant Professor
Department of Anesthesiology
University of North Carolina Hospitals
Chapel Hill, North Carolina

Thomas R. Stark, DDS
Professor
Pediatric Dentistry
Uniformed Services University Postgraduate Dental College
Bethesda, Maryland

Heidi M. Steinkamp, DDS, PhD, MS
Assistant Professor and Graduate Program Director
Department of Pediatric Dentistry
University of Iowa College of Dentistry
Iowa City, IA

Kevin G. Stephenson, PhD
Assistant Professor
Pediatrics
The Ohio State University College of Dentistry
Columbus, Ohio;
Neurodevelopmental Psychologist
Psychology
Nationwide Children's Hospital
Columbus, Ohio

Natalie M. Stinton, DMD
Chair : Department of Oral Medicine & Maxillofacial Surgery
Program Director: Pediatric Dental Residency
Assistant Professor: Pediatric Dentistry
Geisinger Health System
Danville, PA

Thomas Tanbonliong, DDS
Professor and Program Director
Pediatric Dentistry
University of Washington School of Dentistry
Seattle, Washington

Anupama R. Tate, DMD, MPH
Director of Faculty Development & Advocacy
Division Oral Health
Children's National Hospital
Washington, District of Columbia;
Associate Professor
Department of Pediatrics
George Washington University School of Medicine and Health Sciences
Washington, District of Columbia

Sarat Thikkurissy, DDS, MS
Professor
Division of Pediatric Dentistry & Division of Bone Marrow Transplant and Immune Deficiency
Cincinnati Children's Hospital
Cincinnati, Ohio

Janice A. Townsend, DDS, MS
Department of Dentistry
Nationwide Children's Hospital;
Adjunct Professor
Division of Pediatric Dentistry
The Ohio State University
Columbus, Ohio

John H. Unkel, MD, DDS, MPA
Medical and Residency Director
Pediatrics and Pediatric Dentistry
Bon Secour Mercy Health
Richmond, Virginia

Mark Veazie, DDS, MPH
Clinical Assistant Professor
Pediatric Dentistry
NYU College of Dentistry
New York, New York

Craig V. Vinall, DDS, MDS
Distinguished Professor and Program Director
Department of Pediatric Dentistry and Community Oral Health
The University of Tennessee Health Science Center
Memphis, Tennessee

William F. Waggoner, DDS, MS
Private Practice
Las Vegas, Nevada

Jillian A. Wallen, BDS, MS
Professor and Dean
Creighton University School of Dentistry
Omaha, Nebraska

John Warren, DDS, MS
Professor
Department of Preventive and Community Dentistry
University of Iowa College of Dentistry
Iowa City, IA

Jessica Webb, DDS, MSD, MA, MSRT
Affiliate Assistant Professor
Department of Pediatric Dentistry
University of Washington
Seattle, Washington

Karin Weber-Gasparoni, DDS, MS, PHD
Professor and Chair
Department of Pediatric Dentistry
University of Iowa College of Dentistry
Iowa City, Iowa

Martha H. Wells, DMD, MS
Member, St. Jude Faculty
Chief of Dentistry, Surgery Department
Division of Dentistry
St. Jude Children's Research Hospital
Memphis, Tennessee

A. Jeffrey Wood, DDS
Professor and Chair Emeritus
Pediatric Dentistry
University of the Pacific Arthur A. Dugoni School of Dentistry
San Francisco, California

J. Timothy Wright, DDS, MS
Professor
Pediatric Dentistry and Dental Public Health
University of North Carolina at Chapel Hill Adams School of Dentistry
Chapel Hill, North Carolina;
Editor in Chief
Journal of the American Dental Association
American Dental Association
Chicago, Illinois

Juan F. Yepes, DDS, MD, MPH, MS, DrPH
Professor
Pediatric Dentistry and Associate Dean
Indiana University School of Dentistry
Indianapolis, Indiana;
Visiting Professor
Pediatric Dentistry
CES University
Medellin, Antioquia, Colombia

Audrey Jung-Sun Yoon, DDS
Clinical Professor
Sleep Medicine Division, Department of Psychiatry and Behavioral Science
Stanford University
Redwood City, California;
Assistant Clinical Professor
Orthodontics
University of the Pacific Arthur A. Dugoni School of Dentistry, San Francisco
San Francisco, California

Foreword

Since the early 1970s, pediatric dentistry has witnessed an explosion of scientific interest and inquiry. This rapid advancement necessitated the evolution of textbooks to capture critical elements of the specialty for the contemporary reader. Dr. Arthur Nowak, a visionary leader in the field, long recognized the need for such resources. Under his editorial leadership, this textbook has become a trusted foundation for students, residents, and clinicians around the world.

The release of the 7th edition is especially timely, as scientific advances have multiplied since the last edition in 2019. Long-standing paradigms—such as those related to caries management, fluoride effectiveness, oral-systemic health relationships, pediatric pharmacology and dental materials—require reevaluation considering current evidence-based science. To achieve the best possible clinical outcomes for the children we serve, it is essential that we remain grounded in current science. Nothing less is acceptable.

The 7th edition of *Pediatric Dentistry: Infancy Through Adolescence* meets this moment with the latest innovations and insights in pediatric dentistry. New and updated chapters bring this edition to the forefront of pediatric dentistry as an art and a science. The dental community of general practitioners as well as specialists will find that this text has captured the most important areas of contemporary clinical practice that are so vital in today's evolving and ever more complex healthcare delivery system. For those early in their dental careers, including dental students and pediatric dentistry residents, this textbook offers an invaluable reference to arm them for the many challenges and decisions they will encounter as providers. For seasoned specialists, this text places them on the cutting edge of pediatric oral healthcare.

The current edition brings together the most prominent thought leaders in dentistry and medicine, building on over the three decades of contributors—many pioneers in their specialty. The editors have sought out those most knowledgeable and thoughtful in the oral healthcare of children and their wisdom and knowledge lie within this text.

It indeed is my honor to provide this foreword to the 7th edition. I'm very supportive of this remarkable textbook and those who have dedicated their lives to shining a bright light on the critical knowledge and skills necessary to provide optimal oral health to all children. My deepest respect goes to Dr. Arthur J. Nowak and his associate editors—Drs. John R. Christensen, Matthew K. Geneser, Janice A. Townsend, and Martha H. Wells—in bringing forth an impactful and timely resource to the field of pediatric dentistry and the entire dental profession.

John Rutkauskas, DDS, MBA, CAE
Chief Executive Officer
American Academy of Pediatric Dentistry
American Academy of Pediatric Dentistry Foundation
Chicago, Illinois

Preface

We live in a world of change. New information is constantly being reported. With the explosion of the Internet into every office, home, and pocket, we are inundated with information on new discoveries, new drugs, and new procedures. In addition, generative AI is accelerating knowledge and advancing research and clinical practice. Time-honored treatments will be challenged and be replaced with new evidence-based possibilities. And so, it is in pediatric dentistry.

Since the 2019 edition, our understanding of the importance of oral health and systemic health has grown: children can develop and grow without cavities; the caries process is preventable; early stress in the mother's and infant's lives can have profound effects on the child's growth, development, and behavior; common risk factors have been identified that lead to cavities; we know more about the contribution of genetics to susceptibility or resistance to dental caries; infant oral health is embraced by most primary care providers, dentists, and parents; the importance of caries risk assessment early in the baby's life during the well-baby visits by primary care providers is now understood; fluoride content of community waters continues but is being questioned by Federal agencies; fluoride varnish applications have become standard practice; use of esthetic crowns to restore badly destroyed primary teeth is now a common treatment; use of medicinal agents to arrest the caries process is common; new treatments for vital and necrotic primary pulps are available; retention of traumatized teeth has been extended; regenerative endodontic techniques for luxated teeth with open apices hold promise; and adolescent health, risky behaviors including smoking/vaping, bullying, and suicide, and transition from pediatric to adult dental supervision have become a part of our practice.

This seventh edition is intended for all audiences, from the undergraduate dental student to residents in training, and, finally, to seasoned practitioners. In addition, those in the allied health professions will find the text an excellent reference for understanding the oral health needs of all children.

With this edition, we introduce a new associate editor and 44 authors to continue the work contributed by 57 colleagues in the first six editions. Their enthusiasm and creativity were greatly appreciated by the senior and associate editors.

The support this textbook receives is greatly appreciated. The text is recognized by educational programs throughout the world. All chapters have been comprehensively reviewed and updated with evidence-based references and guideline-supported recommendations.

Thirty-seven years ago, the first edition of the textbook was designed around developmental stages of childhood, whereby most textbooks were disease oriented. This format highlighted the dramatic changes in the patients we treat as they develop from infancy through adolescence. With the seventh edition we have developed a hybrid model that maintains the developmental stages of childhood in addition to 38 topic-specific chapters with in-depth understanding of the topics.

What else is new? The text continues to be available electronically through the Elsevier eBooks+ platform. Many chapters are accompanied by case studies and videos to enhance the learning experience. There are dedicated chapters on "hot topics" in pediatric dentistry including management of tethered oral tissues, replacing missing teeth in children, obstructive sleep apnea, managing avulsed young permanent teeth, managing pediatric pain, behavioral guidance both pharmacologic and nonpharmacologic and caring for children with special healthcare needs.

The foundation for a lifetime of good oral health is established early in the child's life, even before a child is born. We hope this new edition of *Pediatric Dentistry: Infancy Through Adolescence* will provide you with information and tools to provide optimal oral healthcare for all your pediatric patients.

I would like to acknowledge the following individuals from Elsevier who helped produce this edition: Kelly Skelton, Brian Salisbury, Rishabh Gupta, and Kamatchi Madhavan.

As senior editor, I appreciate the contributions of the associate editors, who accepted their assignments and worked tirelessly addressing author questions and meeting deadlines. Your expertise and friendship are greatly appreciated.

Finally, we acknowledge the contributions of the late Jimmy R. Pinkham, whose insight for a textbook based on the developmental stages of childhood was the foundation for the initial edition and following six editions.

Arthur J. Nowak

Contents

Video Contents

PART 1

Dynamics of Change

1 Importance of Pediatric Dentistry

PAUL S. CASAMASSIMO

CHAPTER OUTLINE

Since the last edition of this textbook, the world has seen a pandemic and its consequences,[1] public questioning of the scientific basis of immunization and fluoride therapy,[2] and recognition that addressing social determinants of health and their management fall within the clinician's responsibility as a health provider.[3] The pediatric dentist's responsibility to educate and advocate for a childhood free of pain and dental disease for all children regardless of nationality, ethnicity, or socioeconomic background remains critical in the care paradigm, with ever-increasing numbers of children being born into poverty.[4] Fortunately, science and technology have improved our ability to care for these children. This chapter attempts to place the changes affecting the oral health of children into a clearer picture for the general practitioner and pediatric dental specialist and create a broader concept of the dental home to best serve the interests of children.

Table 1.1 provides a timeline that depicts the evolution of dentistry for children. The historic mission of pediatric dentistry was threefold: stop the advance of early childhood caries (ECC) with restoration, pulp therapy, and extraction; establish prevention to stop recurrence of disease; and develop a regular care seeker to help ensure oral health into adulthood. In truth, the mission differed little from that for adults. It was not until the turn of the last century that the dental profession recognized the continuing epidemic of ECC and its disparate effect on the poor and underserved minority communities and a broader view of pediatric dentistry began to emerge.[5] Overlaying this continued epidemic was a changing social matrix that altered traditional doctor-directed care into a more complex mosaic, still accounting for management of dental caries but within a more complicated set of expectations and conditions.[6] Parents, society, the media, other professionals, and a host of environmental and scientific variables emerged to challenge traditional approaches to the tripartite mission of pediatric dentistry.[7] In Table 1.2, we attempt to lay out these changes, using the multidimensional model of Fisher-Owens et al.[8]

The remainder of this chapter explains how these new variables impact the delivery of care to children and preview much of what will follow in more detail in this text on current therapies used in pediatric dentistry.

Prevention and Diagnosis

For decades, our preventive arsenal remained the same, with a four-part message of drink fluoridated water, brush teeth with fluoridated dentifrice, eat wisely (which meant low sugar intake), and see a dentist twice a year. We have moved from a general blanket preventive message to one that is keyed to the individual child and the family's characteristics based on caries risk assessment (CRA); better diagnosis of caries; and an ever-increasing choice of preventive agents, including fluoride varnish and silver diamine fluoride (SDF).[9] Digital radiography and other electronic diagnostic tools offer better assessment of caries progression, adding to our ability to more individually manage this disease in person-centered care.[10] Application of artificial intelligence (AI) to caries diagnosis, especially in imaging interpretation, will likely complement CRA to make accuracy better and minimize low-value care that is often applied to patients indiscriminately due to vague caries susceptibility. Dental sealants have withstood critical review and achieved universal acceptance as a caries-preventive technique promising a significant reduction in the lifelong caries experience of many Americans.[11] Also gaining wider acceptance is CRA, which promises to be a useful chairside diagnostic aid also supporting individualized, patient-centered care. More research is needed to achieve the sensitivity and specificity of a truly useful clinical tool. When CRA is matched with early intervention, the promise of a "cavity-free generation" may finally be realized.[12]

Behavior Guidance

Along with advances in dental science are changes in how children and families engage the dental profession in oral healthcare. Long-standing beliefs on how best to manage a child's in-office behavior and communicate with families have been reassessed as society changes and the value of oral health, acceptance of advice

TABLE 1.1 Milestones in Dentistry for Children in the United States

1900	Few children are treated in dental offices. Little or no instruction in the care of "baby teeth" is given in the 50 dental schools in the United States.
1924	First comprehensive textbook on dentistry for children is published.
1926	The Gies Report on dental education notes that only 5 of 43 dental schools in the United States have facilities especially designed for treating children.
1927	After almost a decade of frustration to organize a professional group to promote dentistry for children, the American Society for the Promotion of Dentistry for Children is established at the meeting of the American Dental Association (ADA) in Detroit.
1932	A report of the American Society for the Promotion of Dentistry for Children stated that in 1928, 15 dental schools provided no clinical experience with children, and 22 schools had no didactic information in pediatric dentistry.
1935	Six graduate programs and eight postgraduate programs exist in pedodontics.
1940	The American Society for the Promotion of Dentistry for Children changes its name to the American Society of Dentistry for Children.
1941	Children's Dental Health Day is observed in Cleveland, Ohio, and Children's Dental Health Week is observed in Akron, Ohio.
1942	The effectiveness of topical fluoride applications at preventing caries is described. The Council on Dental Education recommends that all dental schools have pedodontics as part of their curriculum.
1945	First artificial water fluoridation plant is opened in Grand Rapids, Michigan.
1947	The American Academy of Pedodontics is formed. (To a large degree, the start of the Academy was prompted by the need for a more scientifically focused organization concerned with the dental health of children.)
1948	The American Board of Pedodontics, a credentialing body to certify candidates in the practice of dentistry for children, is formally recognized by the Council on Dental Education of the ADA.
1949	The first full week of February is designated National Children's Dental Health Week.
1955	The acid-etch technique is described.
1960	Eighteen graduate programs and 17 postgraduate programs in pedodontics exist.
1964	Crest becomes the first ADA-approved fluoridated toothpaste.
1974	The International Workshop on Fluorides and Dental Caries Reductions recommends that appropriate fluoride supplementation begin as soon after birth as possible. (This recommendation was later modified by authorities to start at 6 months of age.)
1976	*Dentistry for the Handicapped Patient* is the first textbook dedicated to special patients.
1981	February is designated National Children's Dental Health Month.
1983	A Consensus Development Conference held at the National Institutes of Dental Health endorses the effectiveness and usefulness of sealants.
1984	The American Academy of Pedodontics changes its name to the American Academy of Pediatric Dentistry (AAPD).
1986	AAPD endorses the age of the first professional visit at the time of the eruption of the first tooth and no later than 12 months of age.
1987	AAPD participates in CDC panel developing "The Selection of Patients for X-Ray Examination."
1991	AAPD adopts Periodicity of Examination, Preventive Dental Services, Anticipatory Guidance/Counseling, and Oral Treatment for Infants, Children, and Adolescents.
1995	A new definition is adopted for the specialty of pediatric dentistry by the ADA's House of Delegates: *Pediatric dentistry* is an age-defined specialty that provides both primary and comprehensive preventive and therapeutic oral healthcare for infants and children through adolescence, including those with special healthcare needs.
2001	AAPD adopts "Policy on the Dental Home."
2003	The AAP establishes "Policy Statement on Oral Health Risk Assessment Timing and Establishment of a Dental Home," and issuance of this policy statement will be manifested in several outcomes, including the need to identify effective means for rapid screening in pediatricians' offices, and the mechanisms for swift referral and intervention for high-risk children.
2004	AAPD Leadership Institute partners with Kellogg School of Management at Northwestern University to provide educational activities important for leadership development.
2011	The AAPD establishes the Pediatric Oral Health Research and Policy Center to inform and advance research and policy analysis to promote optimal oral healthcare for children.
2017	Pediatric Dentistry MATCH results show 676 applicants for 408 positions, which exceeds all other specialties.
2021	NIDCR publishes "Oral Health in America: Advances and Challenges on Status of Oral Health of Americans."
2023	84 CODA-Accredited Pediatric Dentistry Advanced Education Programs
2024	Patient shielding during radiography is no longer recommended, American Academy of Oral and Maxillofacial Radiology. Community water fluoridation is challenged at the federal level.

AAP, American Academy of Pediatrics; *CDC*, Centers for Disease Control and Prevention; *CODA*, Commission on Dental Accreditation; *NIDCR*, National Institute of Dental and Craniofacial Research.

TABLE 1.2 A Cross-Millennium View of the Changing Character of Pediatric Dentistry

Traditional Elements of Pediatric Oral Care for Children	Current and Future Directions and Their Drivers
Prevention	
• Diagnosis with traditional radiography and caries diagnostics	• Digital radiography and electronic caries detection aided by artificial intelligence
• A preventive arsenal composed largely of fluoride options including water fluoridation, fluoride dentifrice, office fluoride, fluoride supplements, and at home over-the-counter (OTC) fluoride rinses	• Prevention continues to emphasize most traditional modalities but now includes silver diamine fluoride (SDF), and a caries risk paradigm to the application of fluoride and other techniques, discontinuing supplementation
• Dental sealants to prevent occlusal and pit and fissure caries selectively applied	• Dental sealants now evidence-based and accepted universally as a primary preventive technique and has therapeutic implications
• Caries risk assessment not considered essential to provision of preventive services	• Caries risk assessment now considered integral to preventive therapeutic plans and compensation for preventive services
• Restorative and surgical intervention considered the optimal treatment	• Minimally invasive dentistry using nonsurgical techniques enters the care paradigm integrated into traditional treatment
Behavioral Guidance	
• Simplistic application of communicative and more advanced techniques based on chairside behaviors and special needs with dentist directing choice	• More sophisticated application of techniques with attention to chairside and other aspects of behavior with a strong parental advisement component
• Parental separation from clinical aspects of care	• Recognition of the changing parental attitudes toward restraint, pharmacologic management, and parental presence
• All children managed with the same paradigm and hierarchy of behavior techniques without regard to systemic, emotional, and other mitigating factors	• Recognition of the effects of poverty and culture on child behavior from toxic stress and adverse childhood experiences (ACEs)
• Pain and anxiety addressed primarily as preoperative treatment need	• Greater understanding and subsequent management of pain and anxiety as factors in care avoidance, social and developmental behaviors, and intraoperative outcomes during dental treatment
• Largely office-based nonpharmacologic management of behavior	• Newer models of advanced behavior guidance using sedation, general anesthesia in-office with dental and medical anesthesiologists and surgery centers
• Simplistic vision of behavior in the dental office based on traditional family structure, majority social characteristics, and middle-class value system	• Recognition of the contribution of culture, poverty, and other nontraditional factors on behavior in the dental office
Treatment of ECC	
• Simplistic armamentarium of composite, amalgam, stainless steel crowns	• Fuller integration of preveneered crowns, zirconia crowns, resin infiltration
• Pulpotomy as a preferred therapy using formocresol, ferric sulfate	• Pulp therapy with fuller range of options, including indirect techniques, mineral trioxide aggregate (MTA)
• Emphasis on immediate and primary tooth lifespan success in choice of materials and techniques	• Addition of safety and toxicity concerns in choices of restorative care
• Definitive treatment (restoration or extraction) in most cases of ECC	• Consideration of a range of treatment options including deferral of treatment, use of fluoride, and other caries-static agents like SDF teamed with more frequent interventions
Dental Diseases Emphasis	
• Dental caries as the preeminent singular driver of care for children	• Greater recognition of esthetic concerns (fluorosis, tooth whiteness) in pediatric dentistry • Emergence of new conditions such as molar-incisal hypomineralization (MIH) and dental erosion as treatment considerations
Systemic Disease and Conditions and Oral Health	
• Traditional disease entities occurring in predictable patterns allowing application of consistent management	• New disease entities such as obesity and its management considerations; other eating disorders; increase in autism spectrum
• Predictable dental outcomes based on disease progression in special needs patients	• Lifespan elongation with complications of end-organ damage, effects of new medication, and growing technology dependence to support life and function

TABLE 1.2 A Cross-Millennium View of the Changing Character of Pediatric Dentistry—cont'd

Traditional Elements of Pediatric Oral Care for Children	Current and Future Directions and Their Drivers
Practice Considerations	
• Paper-based records and office management	• Digitalization of records, billing, imaging, and laboratory procedures
• Simplistic safety orientation (OSHA, NIOSH, CDC)	• Office safety including risk mitigation, growing concerns about radiation exposure with introduction of CBCT and other digital advances; HIPAA changes, waterline management
• Global dental consent procedures	• Changing consent requirements based on procedures
• Regional and training-based care patterns	• Emergence of evidence-based guidelines for pediatric dental care

CBCT, Cone-beam computed tomography; *CDC,* Centers for Disease Control and Prevention; *ECC,* early childhood caries; *HIPAA,* Health Insurance Portability and Accountability Act of 1996; *NIOSH,* National Institute for Occupational Safety and Health; *OSHA,* Occupational Safety and Health Administration.

and trust of health professionals, and parental involvement in direct provision of care evolve. No doubt, the generational changes that affect both providers and parents have made interaction with children at chairside more challenging.[13,14] Similarly, concentration of ECC in the poor and minority child populations and emergence of cultural subgroups needing care have complicated a simple traditional hierarchical approach to child behavior.[15,16] The application of basic behavior guidance techniques advocated by the American Academy of Pediatric Dentistry (AAPD) now must be meshed with our deeper understanding of adverse childhood experiences (ACEs) in the lives of those most affected with dental caries and, even more simply, the cultural overlays that, for example, limit touch and gender interactions in a clinical setting.[17] Parents want to be present during treatment and will seek providers who will commit to that practice.[18] Compliance with out-of-office professional advice has also been affected by social media and the Internet. Misinformation in healthcare will likely grow and challenge acceptance of professional advice, question validity of proven science, and add ineffective and potentially dangerous popular alternative approaches to prevention of disease.

Pharmacologic management of behavior continues to be a major consideration in pediatric dental care but has also seen dramatic change. Sedation deaths have prompted new guidelines, better training, better patient monitoring, and, of course, greater scrutiny of how this service is delivered.[19,20] Drugs such as chloral hydrate, long a staple of pediatric sedation, have largely been replaced by medications thought to be safer and reversible.[21] General anesthesia for dental treatment has seen a dramatic increase, in part due to the epidemic of ECC. In spite of that pharmacologic option as the top choice of parents, it too is challenged by cost, availability of surgical sites, and growing research on possible effects of anesthetics on early brain development.[22] Also driving changes in behavior guidance is a greater recognition of the role of pain in behavior, both chairside and in care seeking.[23] We more often confront a very young child who has been in pain from dental caries for many days, challenging the simple notion that pain control is confined to administration of local anesthesia.[24]

The science and clinical translation of anxiety, pain, and pharmacologic behavior guidance will likely continue. Our tools will also change as we add more powerful local anesthetics and intranasally administered local anesthesia, and as reversal agents like phentolamine sodium gain acceptance.[25,26] Subsequent chapters in this text address both long-standing and new approaches to management of pain, anxiety, and chairside behavior.

Treatment Options

The treatment of ECC continues to change with the science of materials and understanding of biology of the oral cavity and teeth. Today, clinicians can approach pulpal therapy with more choices and better outcomes. Mineral trioxide aggregate (MTA) and bioactive glass stand to revolutionize both permanent and primary teeth pulpal therapy.[27] Indirect pulp caps with various agents, including traditional calcium hydroxide and more recent glass ionomer cements, have challenged traditional thinking that a primary tooth with a large carious lesion is doomed to invasive pulp therapy.[28,29] Traumatic injuries now benefit from larger and longer studies that direct clinicians to better outcomes. Autotransplantation is an accepted alternative for hopeless permanent teeth due to caries or trauma.[30,31] Advances in regeneration techniques can now add vitality to immature teeth that traditionally had a poor long-term prognosis and may lead to full tooth regeneration in the future, along with other systemic therapies.[32]

Restorative choices for primary teeth continue to increase. The strip crown, long a stalwart of anterior primary tooth restoration, has been joined by the preveneered stainless steel crown. Zirconia crowns, offering better esthetics, strength, and technique ease, have gained favor, especially for posterior primary teeth.[33] The open-faced stainless steel crown has joined its less esthetic stainless steel crown in the annals of pediatric history. Bioactive restorative materials may lead to a class of restorative materials with intrinsic reparative abilities.[34]

Perhaps the most exciting advance in care of ECC, especially for very young children, is the expansion of our thinking about treatment urgency, restoration longevity, and adjunctive nonrestorative care. Restoration or extraction once dominated treatment of ECC, and application was often immediate, with accompanying use of behavioral techniques to accomplish care. Today, clinicians can reliably use nonrestorative techniques to stop ECC's advance, such as fluoride varnish and SDF, and avoid a costly general anesthetic that too often is just a precursor to another in the future.[35,36] A Hall technique crown can also be reliably and safely placed to stop caries and restore function, requiring minimal cooperation by the child.[37] The advances in treatment of ECC have made care safer, more effective, and more palatable to many families.

Dental Disease Emphasis and Systemic Disease

ECC has long been and remains the driver of attendance in a dental home, but other conditions have emerged as considerations in pediatric dental care, such as fluorosis, esthetic challenges, and management of molar-incisor hypomineralization.[38] Dental erosion has moved from an isolated condition suggestive of an eating disorder to a more widespread condition in children.[39] These conditions join inherited disorders of the dentition, such as amelogenesis imperfecta, dentinogenesis imperfecta, ectodermal dysplasia, intrinsic staining, and tooth number irregularities, as important intersection points in childhood oral assessment.

Systemic diseases and developmental disabilities affecting children fall into the purview of dentists caring for children by default. Caring for children with special needs requires a working knowledge of medical, functional, and social programming aspects of the lives of these children. Medical advances have prolonged life in many conditions but brought into play technology dependence, such as cerebral shunts and implanted devices, and organ effects from drugs, surgery, or the continued onslaught of the original condition. Care of these children requires the dentist to understand the disease, its treatment, and the effects on oral physiology and function, but more so today, the social and programmatic aspects of the lives of these children.[40] Although pediatric dentists continue to take the lead in caring for the very young with special needs, the intent of our healthcare system is to transition them to adult care as their dental needs grow outside the usual concerns of pediatric dentistry.[41,42]

Contemporary Practice and Care of Children

As dental practice moves along the path of growing sophistication and digitalization, those areas addressing care of children follow. Paper-based offices are an anachronism, and movement to the full electronic office means systems that can track caries risk, health histories, referrals, and serial disease manifestations and treatment. Dental models, radiographs, and analyses of the developing dentition are now electronic files.[43] As treatment techniques advance using lasers and other approaches, consent procedures for children become more complicated, especially with changing family structures. Office design, toys, and other aspects of dental offices have special considerations when children are a part of the patient family. Teledentistry offers the advantages of improved access, diminished costs to families, and better triage of urgent and emergency care and environmental benefits of reduced travel.[44]

The concern of parents about safety of their children requires more detailed attention to protective considerations, regulations, and office environment. Basic infection control remains a keystone of patient safety, but waterline safety, chemicals in dental materials, and radiation have emerged as special considerations in the dental care of children.[45] A growing area is interprofessional care, which suggests that dentists treating children need to heed obesity, immunizations, and other areas not necessarily considered in the realm of dentistry. Child abuse continues to be a required safety consideration for those treating children.

This Edition

Many of these topics are dealt with in depth in this latest edition. New chapters on nutrition and dietary management, care of children with special healthcare needs, child abuse and neglect, temporomandibular disorders, management of missing teeth, obstructive sleep apnea, and managing tethered oral tissues have been added to address the changing nature of oral healthcare for children. New online content has been added to enhance the understanding of basic principles and to address advanced topics in pediatric dentistry. The textbook format moves to a hybrid model by retaining its developmental view of pediatric dentistry and adding dedicated chapters on challenging topics, validating changing science, including the benefits of early intervention and new age-related conditions and treatments. Welcome to this seventh edition!

Visit eBooks.Health.Elsevier.com to see full list of references.

2

Craniofacial Growth—Conception Through Adolescence

ARTHUR J. NOWAK

CHAPTER OUTLINE

Physical, Craniofacial, and Dental Changes: From Birth Through Adolescence

Growth and Development: Birth to 3 Years

No year is more dramatic in terms of growth than the first year of life, during which most children undergo a 50% increase in length and almost a 200% increase in weight. Toward the end of the first year of life, the growth rate slows. After the first birthday, the growth rate stabilizes, and the height and weight increments of the child remain relatively predictable all the way to adolescence.

There are no accurate predictors of the child's final height before age 3 years. However, at age 3, correlations between the child's height and weight at maturity are strong. The process of a newborn changing into an adult is one of elongation. The legs, at first shorter than the trunk, become longer. In addition, the length of the child's trunk, compared with the breadth, becomes considerably greater.

As the body changes and matures, the infant is afforded increasingly sophisticated postural and locomotive actions. eTable 2.1 shows some of the physical and cognitive developmental hallmarks of a child during the first 18 months of life.

By age 2 years, a child has the gross motor skills to run, climb, walk up and down steps, and kick a ball. Fine motor skills allow them to stack blocks (up to six), make parallel crayon strokes, and turn the pages of a book one page at a time. eTable 2.2 shows a variety of motor skills and the mean age at which they are acquired.

The nervous system of the child grows dramatically from birth until age 3 years. By the end of the second year the child's brain has already attained 75% of its adult weight.[1]

Craniofacial Growth and Development

At birth, the bony face and skull show little differentiation among individuals. Newborns have tiny mouths and virtually no chins. Their faces are small, although their eyes, compared with the small face, are exceedingly large. The forehead and top of the head are relatively large. It is difficult to imagine the diversity of individual looks that will develop over the course of childhood and adolescence from such similar infant faces (eFig. 2.1).

The maxilla of the newborn is very low frontally and relatively small. By the age of 9 months, the jaw has become considerably wider and higher. There is also a remarkable increase in size of the maxillary sinus. At birth, the bones that compose the cranium are not fused and are separated by six membrane-filled gaps called *fontanels* (eFig. 2.2). These gaps completely close by ossification within 2 years of birth.

The face of the newborn appears broad and flat. The lower jaw appears underdeveloped and receded. The overall broadness of the face results from the lack of vertical growth, which is yet to commence. The horizontal dimensions are more nearly adult-like. According to Ranly,[2] the upper face height of the newborn is only 43% of adult height. Similarly, the total face height of the newborn is only 40% of adult face height. This demonstrates that the most striking and complex growth of the head is associated with the face. After an initial spurt during the first 3 years, the rate of increase of these dimensions slows. It remains steady until the adult size is reached. The cranium of the infant, as represented by cranial width and length, is closer to adult size than any other part of the head. This can be explained by the development of the brain, which by the eighth month of intrauterine life has all of the nerve cells it will ever have. The growth of the cranial vault is complete before that of the maxilla, and maxillary growth is complete before mandibular growth. This is an example of the cephalocaudal growth gradient, which indicates that the cranial structures are closer to their adult size during infancy and childhood than other body parts.[3] Symphyseal growth increases the width of the mandible. By the second year, the symphysis is closed and growth becomes localized in the mandible and in the nasomaxillary complex. An enormous metamorphosis has taken place, but many more changes need to occur before the child's adult appearance is realized.

Dental Changes

The primary teeth begin to form at 6 weeks in utero, and the enamel of all of the primary teeth is usually completed by the first year of age (eFigs. 2.3 and 2.4). The first primary teeth to erupt are the primary mandibular central incisors at 6 months of age, and all of the primary teeth generally erupt by age 2.

The first permanent molar is the first tooth to show germ formation, which occurs at age 3½ to 4 months in utero. It is followed by the central and lateral incisors, which demonstrate formation at 5 to 5½ months in utero. The canines are the only other permanent teeth that begin formation before birth, at 5½ to 6 months in utero. The first and second premolars and the second and third molars demonstrate germ formation after birth.

At birth, the only permanent teeth that show a trace of hard tissue formation are the first permanent molars.[4] With the exception of the third molars, all permanent teeth demonstrate hard tissue formation by 3 years of age (eTable 2.3).[5]

Growth and Development: 3 to 6 Years

By the third birthday the average boy is 39 inches tall and weighs about 35 pounds, whereas the average girl is 38.6 inches tall and weighs nearly a pound less. Growth slows during the preschool years, and children gain approximately 5 pounds and 3 inches in height each year. More important than a child's weight or height during this time is the maintenance of their rate of growth. Children who are tall or heavy at age 2 years are very likely to remain tall or heavy at age 5 years, and children who are short or light at age 2 years are very likely to be short or light at age 5 years.[1] Similar to the growth of younger children, body elongation continues to be apparent during the preschool years. Head growth seems slow, whereas limb growth seems extremely rapid. Trunk growth can be regarded as intermediate, and the protuberant, pudgy abdomen of the toddling 2-year-old child gradually disappears between the ages of 3 and 4 years.

A variety of other body changes take place during these years. Both the heart rate and the respiration rate slow down, and blood pressure rises. Because of a change in the rate of the growth of the muscular system around age 4, approximately 75% of a child's acquired weight during the fifth year of development is the result of muscle acquisition.[2] The cartilage in the skeletal system is being increasingly replaced by bone, and all the bones of the body become more calcified and harder.

Craniofacial Growth and Development

The head and face continue to grow during the period from ages 3 to 6. However, eFig. 2.5 shows that the percentage of increase in facial growth becomes greater than cranial growth around age 3.[3] This change has important effects on a child's craniofacial structures and appearance. Preschoolers' faces become larger, wider, longer, and more detailed compared with the faces of newborns. During this stage of life, one begins to see the effects of the impending eruption of permanent teeth.[4]

Vann and colleagues[5] reported the results of a study reviewing cephalometric analysis of the primary dentition in 4-year-old children. They compared 17 cephalometric norms from a sample of 32 White children of North American ancestry with those of adults. There were no statistical differences between males and females. The investigators drew the following conclusions based on information given in eTable 2.4:

1. The primary incisors are more upright than the permanent incisors (compare UI-SN and UI-F in eTable 2.4).
2. The similarity of angle SNA in children (82.9 degrees) and adults (82.0 degrees) supports the concept that the nasion and point A move forward in relation to the sella, so that angle SNA is no different in preschool children and adults.
3. Angles SNB and SNPg in children measure 78.1 and 77.4 degrees, respectively, whereas in adults they measure 80.0 and 83.0 degrees. The ANB angle is greater in children (4.9 degrees) than in adults (2.0 degrees).

The soft tissue prominence of the nose and, to some extent, the mandible continues to increase consistently with some reduction in overall facial convexity (eFig. 2.6).[5] It is hard to judge the underlying skeletal configuration based on the soft tissue in this age group. Vertically, there is a lowering of the palatal vault with sutural growth and apposition on the oral side of the palate and resorption on the nasal side. There is an even greater lowering of the lowest point of the chin, but the mandibular plane (lower border of the mandible) stays parallel to its original orientation. This occurs because condylar growth exceeds the vertical maxillary growth, which prevents opening of the mandibular plane angle.

There is also considerable growth in the transverse direction during this time (eFig. 2.7).[5] Transverse growth comes to an end earlier than growth in other dimensions, so attention to problems in this dimension is important. Transverse maxillary growth during this period is largely the result of midpalatal sutural changes, whereas the growth of the body and angles of the mandible are the result of apposition and resorption.

Posterior maxillary and mandibular growth (sutural growth in the maxilla and endochondral growth in the mandible) help to accommodate the emerging permanent first molars. There is some appositional growth at the dentoalveolar ridges as the permanent anterior teeth erupt. Consistent with eruption of the new permanent teeth is the continued eruption of the primary teeth. Often the magnitude of this vertical change is unappreciated. It is also obvious that the permanent anterior teeth will occupy a more anterior and protrusive position in the face.

Dental Changes

eTable 2.5 presents a chronology of the human dentition. This table demonstrates that the entire primary dentition has erupted and completed root development by 3 years of age. This is a relatively stable period for the primary dentition. Changes in the dental arches will occur with the eruption of the permanent teeth, but during this period, there is little change in primary incisor spacing, intercanine distance, or arch width. Arch length decreases slightly when posterior spaces close before eruption of the permanent molars.[6] Although the primary dentition is stable, this is a significant period of time for the development of the crowns of the permanent dentition (eFig. 2.8), which will erupt soon. Resorption of the roots of the primary incisors will begin for most children during the end of this period.

When the permanent dentition erupts, some obvious differences in morphology between it and the primary dentition will become apparent (eFig. 2.9). *Wheeler's Dental Anatomy and Physiology*[7] described the following essential differences:

1. The crowns of primary anterior teeth are wider mesiodistally in comparison with their cervicoincisal length than are the crowns of the permanent teeth.
2. The roots of the primary anterior teeth are narrower mesiodistally. Narrow roots with wide crowns present a morphologic appearance at the cervical third of the crown and root that differs markedly from that of the permanent anterior teeth. When the teeth are examined from the mesial or distal aspects, a similar situation in the root and crown measurement at the cervix is observed. The cervical ridge of enamel at the cervical third of the crown, labially and lingually, is much more prominent in the primary teeth than in the permanent teeth.
3. The crowns and roots of the primary molars are more slender mesiodistally at the cervical third than those of the permanent molars.

4. The cervical ridge buccally on the primary molars is much more pronounced, especially on both the maxillary and mandibular first molars.
5. The roots of the primary molars are relatively more slender and longer than the roots of the permanent molars. They also flare more apically, extending beyond the projected outlines of the crowns. This flaring allows room between the roots for the development of permanent tooth crowns before it is time for the primary molars to lose their anchorage.
6. The buccal and lingual surfaces of the primary molars are flatter above the cervical curvatures than those of the permanent molars.
7. The primary teeth are usually lighter in color than the permanent teeth.

Growth and Development: 6 to 12 Years

The median (50th percentile) weight and height of 6-year-old boys in the United States are 47.5 pounds and 45.5 inches, respectively, whereas the same medians for girls are 46 pounds and 45 inches. By the time children reach age 12 years, boys will weigh 90 pounds and be 59 inches tall, and girls will weigh 90.25 pounds and be 59.5 inches tall. This is a time of substantial continuous growth.[1]

During the period between the ages of 6 and 10 years, boys as a group are generally slightly taller than girls until around age 10 years. From age 10 years to around age 15 years, girls are slightly taller than boys. From a weight standpoint, boys are slightly heavier than girls until around age 11 years, when girls overtake boys in weight for a brief time. Although it is generally assumed that girls are a couple of years ahead of boys in their sexual and general maturation, this may be an overstatement due to the observability of the changes taking place. The real difference is about 1 year. This is because height and breast development are considered the main markers of female development compared with penis, scrotum, and height development in males. Nonetheless, the pregrowth spurt in males is steady and creates a larger platform upon which to launch the more robust, later spurt compared with the pattern in females. This accounts for the larger terminal size of males, in general, to females.

Other growth and developmental changes that are noteworthy during these years are further increases in blood pressure, continuing decreases in the pulse rate, increased mineralization of the skeleton, and increases in muscular tissue. In addition, the lymphatic tissues reach a peak of development during these years, to the point where they exceed the amounts found in adults.

Craniofacial Growth and Development

The period from ages 6 through 12 years represents a continuous progression of the growth in the head and neck. From ages 5 to 10 years neural and cranial growth are found to be almost entirely complete (eFig. 2.10). During this same age span, the maxilla and mandible (see eFig. 2.10) grow at a faster rate than the cranium.

Using the Bolton standards for illustrative purposes,[2] nasal projection and increased mandibular prominence are demonstrated (eFig. 2.11). The nasal cartilage and mandibular condyle continue to grow by endochondral bone formation for some time. The female mandibular growth spurt is most likely completed during this time period, whereas the mandibular growth spurt in males is yet to come. Growth modification can therefore be considered in this age group. Changes in cranial base length caused by endochondral bone formation at the sphenooccipital synchondrosis cease in early adolescence, but some appositional changes continue to occur at the basion and nasion. Vertically, there is a continued lowering of the palatal vault with sutural growth and apposition on the oral side of the palate and resorption on the nasal side as the intramembranous process of bone formation continues. Vertical facial growth is also complemented by dentoalveolar growth as the permanent teeth erupt and the alveolar ridges develop.

In the transverse plane, there is continued growth at the midpalatal suture. Most transverse palatal sutural growth is completed for females during this period when the first bridging of the suture occurs. Transverse appositional widening of the alveolar ridge occurs with eruption of the permanent teeth. Widening of the anterior arch accompanies lateral incisor eruption and is followed by width increases in the canines and premolars (eFig. 2.12).

The implications of these changes are that anteroposterior growth modification for class III problems should be attempted during this time. It seems there is more total facial change in this age group than in older patients.[3] For class II problems, growth modification can be attempted now or during early adolescence with equivalent results. Transverse changes should be completed using lingual arch-type appliances or rapid palatal expansion if greater forces are necessary to interrupt the stable midpalatal suture late in this age group. Vertical growth will continue in the face through late adolescence.

Dental Changes

Early during this period most children experience the eruption of all four first permanent molars and the exfoliation of the mandibular and maxillary primary central and lateral incisors. The permanent incisors erupt between the ages of 6 and 7 years (see eTable 2.5). However, it is not unusual for the maxillary permanent lateral incisors to erupt later than age 7 years in some children. Eruption of the anterior teeth should be carefully and easily observed by the practitioner for developmental and esthetic reasons.

Except for third molars, all of the permanent teeth usually have erupted by the end of the 12th year. Permanent tooth enamel formation is complete by age 8 years. In the mandibular arch (except for the first permanent molar), molars erupt in immediate succession, that is, centrals, laterals, canines, first and second premolars, and second permanent molars from 6 to 7 years through 11 to 13 years of age. The same sequence takes place in the maxillary arch except for the maxillary canine, which usually erupts after one or both premolars and at about the same time as or before the eruption of the second permanent molars (eFig. 2.13).

The mandibular central incisor roots are complete by age 9 or 10 years. The roots of the four first permanent molars, the maxillary central incisors, and the mandibular lateral incisors are usually complete by age 10 years. The roots of the maxillary lateral incisors are complete by age 11 years.[4]

Because the position of the dental lamina of the permanent teeth is located to the lingual side of all of the primary teeth (except for the dental lamina coming off the second primary molars for the three permanent molars), the anterior teeth develop in their vault or crypt lingual to and near the apex of the primary incisors. When the roots begin to form on the permanent teeth, the permanent teeth start to migrate to the oral cavity. Generally, they follow a pattern such that they come across the primary root, resorbing it and erupting slightly lingual to the location sustained by the primary tooth (eFig. 2.14). Ultimately the permanent teeth are usually angulated more buccally compared with their primary predecessors (eFig. 2.15). The developing premolars develop between the roots of the primary molars and continue to erupt in a slightly buccal position.

It is normal to find diastemas between the primary incisors. This helps provide space for the larger permanent incisors. The permanent canine in the maxillary arch is usually the last permanent tooth to erupt mesial to the first permanent molar. As the permanent canine begins to erupt, it migrates down the distal root surface of the maxillary lateral incisor and ultimately moves the crowns of the incisors mesially and will close moderate to small diastemas. This period of development has been called the "ugly duckling stage" (eFig. 2.16).[5]

Most of the eruption problems occur during this time period, and the clinician should be checking for these at each examination. Ectopic eruption of permanent first molars, ectopic eruption of lateral incisors due to positioning or crowding, ectopic canine eruption, and transpositions all can be traced to this period of development. Obviously monitoring and intervention in these conditions are crucial to a normally developing dentition. By the end of this period, most of the residual space resulting from either idiopathic spacing or leeway spacing has closed. Further eruption and drift occur in response to continued growth.

Growth and Development: Adolescence

Adolescence in some societies is a very short transitional period that marks the arrival of a child to full citizenship within their respective tribe and culture. No longer children but not quite adults, adolescents confront a combination of physical and mental health issues that may result in long-term problems in adulthood, ranging from obesity to hypertension, substance abuse, and depression.

Critical to the definition of adolescence, regardless of culture, and to the understanding of the adolescent physically is the concept of puberty. Puberty is the landmark in physical development when an individual becomes capable of sexual reproduction. In common law, this has been established historically in our society as age 14 years for boys and age 12 years for girls. The advent of puberty is paralleled by the development of genital tissue and secondary sexual characteristics, such as the development of hair in the genital area.

It is also a time when there is an increase in the mass of muscles, a redistribution of body fat, and an increase in the rate of skeletal growth. A growth spurt is associated with this time of life. This growth spurt follows two different forms, depending on sex. It appears earlier in females than in males. The average onset in males is 2 years later than that in females. The fact that males experience their growth spurt later than females and therefore have a longer maturation period before the growth period is one of the reasons why the height of males generally exceeds the height of females. The earlier growth spurt of females also accounts for the period of time during which mean height of a group of young female adolescents may exceed that of males. It is also important to realize that in females menarche serves as a signal that growth is ending, but for males no such marker exists. The magnitude of the velocity of change during the growth spurt also differs between the sexes. In 1975, Tanner and colleagues[1] concluded that the growth spurt in females peaks at a 9-cm change per year at age 12 years, and that in males it peaks at just over 10 cm at age 14 years.

Craniofacial Growth and Development

During and after adolescence, continued changes in the skeletal growth of the face and skull take place because the facial sutures are still open and viable[2] and mandibular growth can potentially continue. These changes not only cause variation and individuality in facial appearance[3] but also affect the dental structures. The continued changes make a final and unchanging dentition and occlusion a difficult concept to imagine, much less attain. There is a slow increase in facial height accompanied by an increase in prognathism in males.[4,5]

Profile changes occur as changes in specific locations take place. The brow area becomes larger as a result of pneumatization of the frontal sinuses and apposition on the glabella.[6] Also, appositional changes during adolescence and early adult life in the frontal bone area and brow result in this area becoming more prominent.[4] In adolescence, the nose and chin also become more prominent. The tip of the nasal bone lies well ahead of the basal bone of the premaxilla. Soft tissue changes also contribute to the growth in the length of the nose and can affect the harmony existing between the nose, lips, and chin. The mandible shows a greater prognathism than the maxilla because of the circumpubertal growth spurt, which has more effect on the mandible than on the maxilla, especially in males. The chin also becomes more prominent due to local bone deposition. Lip prominence is reduced by these changes in adjacent structures.

Underlying maxillary changes also occur. The maxillary sinuses, which have expanded laterally and vertically since birth, occupy the space left by the permanent teeth as they erupt. By puberty, the sinuses are usually fully developed, although they may continue to enlarge. Considerable individual variation in the size of the maxillary sinuses occurs, and they often lack symmetry. Lowering of the palatal vault continues because of remodeling. Björk[7] concluded that sutural growth as well as appositional growth of the maxilla contributed significantly to the increase in the height of the maxillary body (eFig. 2.17). This can be an example of sexual dimorphism in skeletal growth (see eTable 2.5). Vertical maxillary facial growth is often greater in females. Because the mandible does not continue to grow as much in females, marked vertical changes in the maxilla can result in downward and backward positioning of the mandible and an increase in facial convexity (eFig. 2.18).[4]

Mandibular growth contributes more than profile changes. This growth may be sufficient to provide room for the third molars. In many cases growth is inadequate, and these molars become impacted (eFig. 2.19). The marked mesial inclination of the posterior permanent teeth diminishes somewhat as the mandible completes its growth from under the maxilla, and the lower incisors tend to become upright. Often this is accompanied by crowding of the lower incisors.[2]

Late mandibular growth imparts an increase in the vertical height of the mandibular ramus, which becomes more upright. The elongation of the ramus accommodates the massive vertical expansion of the nasal region and the lowering of the palate, which is accompanied by dental eruption. Usually, maxillary growth and mandibular growth are compatible and coordinated. If they are not, significant orthodontic problems may result. Particularly in males, there may be late anterior growth that is undesirable.[4]

Dental Changes

All permanent teeth generally have erupted by age 12 years, except possibly the four second molars, which may erupt as late as age 13 years, and the third molars, which usually erupt between the ages of 17 and 21 years.

The roots of all teeth are considered to have been completed by age 16 years except for those of the third molars, which can achieve completion as late as age 25 years.

Visit eBooks.Health.Elsevier.com to see full list of references.

3

Cognitive, Emotional, and Social Development—Infancy to Age 3

ERIN L. GROSS

CHAPTER OUTLINE

Cognitive Changes

Cognitive development occurs rapidly during the first years of life. It is known that infants can smell, see, hear, and experience sensations of pain, touch, and changes in body position from the first day of life, but newborn behaviors are instinctual. At 2 months they begin to explore their world more purposefully using their senses to develop an understanding of cause and effect.[1] Mussen and coworkers[2] noted that there are four major areas of cognitive development that occur during the first year of a child's life. The first is *perception.* Even very young infants can perceive movement, facial relationships, and color. The second major cognitive area is the *recognition* of information. Infants create mental representations of things they have previously encountered. They then recognize certain stimuli, such as a face, by comparing it with what they already know. The third major cognitive area is the ability to *categorize.* Children group things together by way of shape, color, and use as early as 1 year of age. Enhancement of *memory* is the fourth area of cognitive development noted in the first year of life. At age 6 months and older, the ability to recall past experiences appears obvious. At this age, most children can recall events and use the information gained from that event to help them form a reaction to new situations.

There are several learning theories that try to explain how individuals acquire knowledge.[3] Two theories of particular interest in pediatric dentistry are behaviorism and cognitivism. An example of behaviorism is operant conditioning, which says that behaviors that are reinforced or rewarded are more likely to occur again. When a baby smiles and is rewarded by their parent's smile, the baby will smile again to get the same response. The cognitive development theory of Jean Piaget[4] says that children learn from birth to age 2 years from their interactions with objects in their environment. He called this the sensorimotor stage, and during this stage children learn object permanence and causality. Children develop object permanence around 6 months when they know that objects continue to exist even when they are no longer perceived. As they continue to learn, they come to understand that events have causes. Piaget used the term *circular reaction* (primary, secondary, and tertiary) to describe the development of causality. A primary circular reaction describes recreating an already known satisfying action, such as thumb-sucking. A secondary circular reaction is the recreation of an accidentally discovered cause and effect. Tertiary circular reactions involve experimentation, and, as one might guess, such behaviors often exasperate the child's parents. Children enter the Piaget preoperational stage at age 2 and begin to use symbols to represent other things. The preoperational stage will continue until age 7. Although some parts of Piagetian theory have been shown to be inaccurate, it remains extremely useful to researchers, clinicians, parents, and other observers of infants because Piaget based his conclusions on observations of his own children's behavior. The behaviors he witnessed are common among children.

Language development is slow at first. Importantly, infants and toddlers can understand more than they can express themselves. At age 1 children say only one or two words, but by age 2 they should say at least 50 words.[5] By age 3 their speech is becoming clear, though it may still be hard for people who do not know them well to understand,[6] and they begin to ask "how" and "why" questions.

Emotional and Social Changes

Emotional and social development also occur rapidly during the first years of life. There are many human emotions, such as shame, guilt, anger, joy, fear, and sadness. Emotions can be discerned by observing behavioral reactions (crying), measuring physiologic responses (increased heart rate), or having a person tell you how they feel ("I'm depressed"). The latter two methods of discernment are of little or no value in determining the emotional state of very young children, so adults assign whatever emotion they believe the child should feel in a particular situation. If a young child spills milk, one parent may interpret the child's crying as frustration over their mistake, whereas the other parent interprets it as sadness about having nothing else to drink.

At age 2 months infants display their first social smile, which is the first major social behavior that is not crying. With this smile, and the smile of their parent in return, the infant is learning a new way to express themselves. The most important social interaction to occur during the first year of life is the development of strong and secure attachments to nurturing and caring adults. Ainsworth[7] concluded that children who have a strong relationship with their primary caregivers could use that relationship as a place from which to venture into wider social circles by exploration. Conversely, children with poorly developed relationships with their caregivers are not able to undertake such exploration because they lack a sense of security.

At age 9 months many infants develop a fear of strangers, although its intensity varies from child to child. At the same time, they are developing a fear of separation from their parents. Some children do not develop this separation anxiety until they are 15 or 18 months old. The basis for the onset of this fear is probably the development of object permanence. When the child remembers the parent even when the parent is not present, separation becomes distressful. For many children their separation anxiety is declining by the time they are 3 years old.

As children get slightly older, they begin to test boundaries. Two-year-olds are sometimes described as being in their "terrible twos." Parents can be frustrated by rapid and unexpected changes in their child's behavior, but children at this age have not acquired internal control of their emotions yet. They may be resistant to change and use the word "no!" any time they want. Temper tantrums are normal and are best ignored. Physical punishment is usually contraindicated and can actually make a misbehaving child behave worse.

Developmental Surveillance

In 2022 the American Academy of Pediatrics (AAP) and the Centers for Disease Control and Prevention (CDC) published new developmental surveillance checklists.[8] The authors made several improvements to the previous CDC checklists. A notable change was that the checklists now represent milestones that most children (≥75%) should have reached, making it easier for families and their doctors to identify children who may be at risk for delays, prompting additional developmental screening. The evidence-informed milestones are now across 12 checklists based on the age of pediatrician health surveillance visits. Each checklist is divided into four domains: social-emotional milestones, language and communication milestones, cognitive milestones, and motor milestones. Using the checklists, developmental concerns can be identified early, referrals to specialists can be made, and necessary interventions can begin.

Screen Time for Infants and Toddlers

Achieving developmental milestones is critical and pediatricians share strategies that parents can use to set their children up for success in all four domains. Because children learn so much from their interactions with the world around them and the people in it, time spent on screens can hinder their language and social-emotional development. The AAP has created Media Use Guidelines for children of all ages, including infants and young children.[9] Children under age 2 should have very limited media use and only with an adult. At age 2, as language skill is increasing, children may benefit from live video chatting, but screen use should still be less than 1 hour per day. When used appropriately, there is also benefit to screen time. Children with better-quality screen use, like watching educational programming and co-viewing with caregivers, have been shown to have stronger language skills.[10]

Visit eBooks.Health.Elsevier.com to see full list of references.

4

Cognitive, Emotional, and Social Development—Ages 3 to 6 years

POLLYANNE IBEN

CHAPTER OUTLINE

The Spanish flu pandemic began in 1918 and lasted through the end of World War I in 1920. An estimated 50 million people died as a result of this infectious global outbreak. Almost 100 years later, another deadly virus, COVID-19, caused nearly 3 million deaths and substantial morbidity worldwide. Both viral outbreaks resulted in abrupt disruptions to daily life and affecting children's physical and mental health, and the cognitive, social, and emotional development of young people everywhere.[1] Prolonged isolation and the absence of structured learning environments during the COVID-19 pandemic significantly affected children's psychosocial well-being.[2]

The US Centers for Disease Control and Prevention (CDC) defines adverse childhood experiences (ACEs) as "potentially traumatic events that occur in childhood, such as violence, abuse, and growing up in a family with mental health or substance use problems." The COVID-19 pandemic was also considered to be an ACE due to the tremendous loss of life during the pandemic.[3]

The pandemic introduced the concept of death to many young children. Toddlers cannot fully grasp the notion of death and its meaning, but they do recognize that something in their environment is different. The understanding of death changes as children age. Those in the 4- to 6-year range start to realize that their parents may not live forever, and this can produce feelings of anxiety and fear.[4]

Children who lost a parent, grandparent, or special caregiver during the pandemic faced a plethora of mental health and behavioral issues including prolonged grief, social withdrawal, anxiety, depression, fear of the dark, abandonment, and contemplation of the possibility that they themselves may die.

Manifestations of these fears presented in many ways. Some children refused to be left alone even for short periods of time or be hesitant to partake in typical everyday events like going to school or the grocery store. Some children turned to excessive physicality in the form of temper tantrums and clingy behavior to deal with the reality of their confusing and frightening circumstances. The weight of parental loss is especially heavy for children who have already experienced some other type of adversity before the pandemic, such as poverty or an unstable home life.

Most youngsters who have suffered an ACE display resilience over time. However, the grief and recovery process after an ACE takes time. Long-term consequences may include difficulties in school, impaired social relationships, and emotional disturbances.[5] Supportive interventions, such as therapy and counseling, have been found to be crucial in helping these children process their grief.[6]

Some parents who were negatively affected by the COVID-19 pandemic and its consequences suffered from parental burnout, a condition characterized by emotional exhaustion and distancing from one's children. During the pandemic, parental burnout was exacerbated due to increased stressors like lockdowns, school closures, and economic challenges. Parents who viewed their children as being difficult or challenging were more likely to engage in violent behaviors, which further intensified negative behavior in their children.[7] Targeted interventions that address parental stress and burnout necessary to reduce the incidence of violence toward children and promote healthier parent-child relationships, not only in times of crisis like the COVID-19 pandemic, but in everyday life as well.[8]

The COVID-19 pandemic disrupted early childhood education and care (ECEC) programs, leading to significant socio-emotional consequences for young children. Children missed critical social interactions, routines, and developmental opportunities provided by ECEC settings, which negatively affected their emotional well-being. Parents reported increased tantrums, anxiety, and boredom in children during lockdowns, highlighting the essential role of ECEC in socio-emotional development.[9]

There is a strong association between social isolation and increased levels of anxiety and depression among children and adolescents. Isolation may lead to elevated cortisol levels, which negatively affect cognitive development. Healthcare professionals were instrumental both during and after the pandemic in helping mitigate the long-term effects of social isolation on this extremely vulnerable population.[10]

Screen Time

In 1973, engineers Dr. Martin Cooper and John F. Mitchell made history when they demonstrated the first ever handheld mobile phone call. The groundbreaking experimental call was made on the Motorola brand DynaTAC phone. In 1983, this device became the first commercially available handheld cellular mobile phone in the world and changed human communication forever.

In 2022 the world's population was estimated to be approximately 8 billion. In that same year there were more mobile phone subscriptions than people on the planet, and the number of cell phones is likely to rise in coming decades.[11]

During the COVID pandemic screen time usage rose by 52% compared with prepandemic levels. Increases were reported across all screen platforms including educational, social media, and recreational means. This rise in screen time was driven by lockdowns, school closures, and increased online learning, all of which precipitated concerns about the long-term negative effects of screen time on the physical and mental health of young users including increased anxiety, depression, and behavioral issues. Encouraging a healthy balance between recreational screen time and other activities like physical exercise, creative playtime, and fostering family involvement is vital to help families develop healthier post-pandemic screen habits.[12,13]

Parental involvement is crucial to successfully manage screen time. Parents are encouraged to set screen time limits, remove screens from children's bedrooms, and encourage alternative activities like physical exercise or social interactions. It is also advised that parents co-view programs with their children, diligently scrutinize screen content, and limit exposure to primarily high-quality educational content. Although screen time can offer educational benefits when managed correctly, excessive use, especially without proper content oversight, can pose risks to children's overall development. Parents, educators, and healthcare professionals need to adopt strategies to reduce screen time and foster healthier habits in children.[14]

The popularity of digital games has increased over the years as graphics and storylines improve. Game-based learning promotes cognitive skills, such as critical thinking, problem solving, and imaginative play, which are essential for creativity development. Well-designed educational games can help children enhance their knowledge transfer, build a positive attitude toward learning, and engage more deeply in creative processes and growth. Additionally, these games offer opportunities for children to develop emotionally and socially by engaging in collaborative problem solving and exploration. Digital game-based learning can significantly contribute to a child's creative growth, offering new ways to integrate digital learning with cognitive and emotional development in early childhood education. Aligning game content with educational goals may ensure that the games not only entertain but also contribute meaningfully to the development of creativity and other core skills.[15]

Screen time influences the development of young children both positively and negatively in several critical areas. When managed properly, digital devices can offer educational value, but excessive use poses significant risks to development, especially for children under the age of 8.

In terms of cognitive development consequences, excessive screen exposure can impair attention span, memory, and executive functioning, despite potential benefits from educational programs designed to engage young minds. These negative effects are particularly noticeable in cases where children engage with passive content for prolonged periods, leading to reduced mental stimulation.

Language development may also be detrimentally affected. Screens limit face-to-face interactions, which are crucial for developing vocabulary and conversational skills. Children who spend significant time with digital devices often have delayed speech development and fewer opportunities to practice social communication.

Screen time effects on children's physical development is linked to decreases in physical activity, which contributes to health issues like obesity and poor motor skills. Additionally, extended screen use interferes with sleep patterns, further exacerbating these physical health problems.

Social and emotional development may also be affected. Children with high screen exposure may have increased anxiety, trouble regulating emotions, and underdeveloped interpersonal communication skills. This can result in negative behavioral issues, a reduced ability to develop empathy, and ineffective social skills.

Regulating screen time according to age-appropriate guidelines is critical. Children under 2 years of age should not have any screen exposure time. Children in the 3 to 5 age range should only be exposed to screens for fewer than 60 minutes. The maximum suggested screen time for 6- to 8-year-olds is 60 minutes. Parents are encouraged to explore alternative activities to screen time, such as physical play, reading, and direct interaction with caregivers to ensure their child's balanced development.

Although screens can provide educational benefits, it is very important for parents to be involved in screen management to support healthy cognitive, physical, and socio-emotional growth.[16]

Some parents use mobile devices as a calming tool for young children. However, for those with higher temperamental reactivity, this may lead to increased emotional reactivity and potentially poorer development of executive functioning. These children may miss out on learning important self-regulation skills as mobile devices are used as a substitute for other emotion-calming strategies.

Digital devices are a quick fix for managing children's emotions. However, this practice could lead to long-term challenges in their emotional regulation and behavior. Pediatric health professionals are encouraged to help parents explore alternative methods for soothing children that support their emotional growth and self-regulation abilities.[17]

Parenting Styles

There are four primary parenting styles—authoritarian, authoritative, permissive, and uninvolved—and their distinct effect on child development, highlighting the role of cultural, socioeconomic, and family dynamics in shaping these approaches.

1. **Authoritarian parenting** is characterized by strict rule enforcement with limited flexibility and minimal nurturing. Children in authoritarian households often follow rules out of fear of punishment rather than understanding, which can lead to outward compliance but may also foster issues such as aggression, social challenges, and low self-esteem.
2. **Authoritative parenting** is considered the most beneficial style. It combines nurturing support with clear, reasonable expectations. Authoritative parents use discipline as a teaching tool rather than punishment, fostering a supportive environment where children participate in decision-making. This approach is associated with positive outcomes in social skills, academic success, emotional regulation, and self-confidence.
3. **Permissive parenting** features a nurturing approach with few expectations or rules. These parents often assume a friendlike role, allowing their children considerable freedom to make choices, even in areas like diet, bedtime, and media use. Although permissive parenting may lead to high self-esteem

and social skills, it can also result in impulsivity, poor self-regulation, and health concerns related to a lack of moderation.

4. **Uninvolved parenting** involves minimal engagement or emotional investment in the child's life beyond meeting basic needs. Children raised in uninvolved households often become self-reliant out of necessity but may struggle with emotional regulation, social skills, and academic performance due to a lack of parental support.

Understanding these styles is crucial for clinicians working with children.[18]

Different parenting styles profoundly affect children's anxiety and behavior in the dental treatment setting. Parenting styles have a significant effect on dental anxiety and behavior in preschool-aged children with no prior dental experiences or dental phobia. However, for school-aged children with dental experience, the relationship is less pronounced. Parenting styles, particularly in early childhood, play a critical role in shaping a child's dental behavior, especially when they have limited dental exposure. Nurturing or disciplinary approaches taken by parents can either alleviate or exacerbate children's fear and anxiety in dental settings. This knowledge could be crucial for pediatric dentists and parents alike, as understanding these associations helps create more positive dental experiences for young children.[19]

Pediatric dentists vary on their views of allowing parents in the treatment area. The use of the Parental Presence or Absence (PPA) technique, along with nonpharmacologic interventions like tell-show-do, may improve children's behavior during dental treatment. Parental presence can have calming effects on children; however, it may occasionally exacerbate behavior depending on the treatment session.[20]

Shifts in US parenting styles have influenced pediatric dental practices. More permissive and protective parenting styles have led to increased challenges in managing child behavior during dental visits, emphasizing the importance of tailored behavioral management techniques in modern pediatric dentistry.[21] Children with authoritative parents show more positive behavior in the dental setting.

Not surprisingly, parenting styles affect the behavioral and emotional development of preschool children. Positive, supportive parenting is linked to increased prosocial behavior in children, whereas more authoritarian, permissive, and coercive parenting styles are associated with a rise in conduct issues, hyperactivity, and emotional maladjustment.

The early years are critical for social and emotional development, and the way parents interact with their children significantly influences these outcomes. Preschoolers are particularly sensitive to their home environment, and warm, supportive relationships between parents and children can reduce the likelihood of behavioral disorders such as anxiety, attention-deficit/hyperactivity disorder (ADHD), and oppositional defiant disorder (ODD). Parenting styles are key in shaping a child's ability to adapt and function in social settings. There continues to be a need for parental guidance programs that encourage positive, nurturing parenting to support healthy development in young children.[22]

Visit eBooks.Health.Elsevier.com to see full list of references.

5

Cognitive, Emotional, and Social Development—Ages 6 to 12 Years

KIMBERLY J. HAMMERSMITH AND KEVIN G. STEPHENSON

CHAPTER OUTLINE

Cognitive Changes

Between ages 6 and 12 years, a child's cognitive acquisitions, adjustments, and sophisticated changes are many. Mental capacity and attention span grow extensively. Children are curious about their world. They master basic math, reading, and writing skills during this period, with evidence for distinct learning profiles,[1–4] although learning trajectories can be highly individualistic and even fluid within a child over time.[4]

Historically, a child has become literate during these school-age years of 6 to 12. With the advent of technology such as tablets and smartphones, children are now technologically sophisticated even sooner. By age 12, most children have accomplished an appropriate approach to grammar and syntax and can produce increasingly sophisticated oral and written communications.

Developmental psychologist Jean Piaget proposed four major periods of intellectual development[5]:

1. *Sensorimotor:* Birth to 18 months
2. *Preoperational:* 18 months to 7 years
3. *Concrete operations:* 7 to 12 years
4. *Formal operations:* 12 years and onward

This chapter equates roughly with Piaget's third major developmental stage of cognition. The concrete operations stage involves logical and sophisticated changes in the child's mental abilities. For instance, a 5-year-old may be able to walk "two blocks down, one block right to the second white house" to get to a friend's house, but the same 5-year-old could not draw this route on a piece of paper. However, by age 7 or 8, the child could portray the route on a self-drawn map. In other words, mental representations of actions become a child's cognitive abilities during these years. For the dentist, it is helpful to design discussions based on the child's mental representation ability.

Between ages 7 and 12, children acquire the ability to understand the constancies between length, mass, number, and weight despite external differences. Relativity also emerges in the child's evaluation system. To the 4-year-old, the word *dark* means black. The 10-year-old can talk about a "dark" green car. By age 12, mind and mental prowess have matured, and real as well as theoretical or abstract information can be assimilated as evidenced by continued development of the prefrontal cortex.[6]

Egocentrism has traditionally been thought to decrease during childhood as they realize that others have their own thoughts, but recent research shows continued egocentrism throughout adulthood, although it has less effect on decision making in adults, perhaps due to development of other cognitive processes such as inhibitory control.[7] In addition to development of perspective-taking skills, continued development of the concept of self matures during this time of life. Self-concept is multifaceted and can include, for example, self-esteem, self-compassion, mindsets, and self-perceived ability.[8]

Emotional Changes

The period from 6 to 12 years is when the child advances toward accepting societal norms of behavior. Crying, tantrums, and other rages will, in normal children, diminish as possible modes to express frustration. Whereas the preschooler needs and perhaps demands immediate rewards and satisfaction, the child in the transitional years masters the emotional ability to delay gratification. This awareness of delay is reinforced by the child's schooling, and increasingly the child is guided toward the appropriate investment of their time in worthwhile activities. Homework, household chores, caring for pets, and extracurricular activities such as scouting, team sports, dance, and music lessons are some behaviors expected of this age group, which were almost impossible during the preschool years. These activities also improve outcomes in a variety of academic, social, and emotional areas.[9,10]

There is also a process of emotional development and, subsequently, emotional control. Throughout this period, children form emotional concepts, starting with basic (e.g., anger, fear, joy) and progressing to more complex (e.g., relief, embarrassment). As children learn the concepts of these emotions, they start to recognize the internal cues of how they experience them. Concurrently, children learn additional ways to process and modulate their external expression of emotion. Much of this is done by modeling parents. The ability of parents to talk about and regulate their own emotions in developmentally appropriate ways around their children can greatly affect their own children's development of emotion regulation skills, including being able to identify emotions.[11]

Another emotional refinement that should develop between ages 6 and 12 is the ability to use life's tasks to effectively stave off boredom. Previously, the preschooler immersed their mind in an activity until all their energy and attention were spent. Then, at the point of burnout, the preschooler looked to parents or other attendants to find something else for them to do. In this transitional period, however, the need for adults to direct the child's attention rapidly recedes, and by age 12, a child usually has a ledger of wants and desires, a sense of the time that should be spent in their pursuit, and an ability to set priorities for which wants and desires should come first or last. The advent of tablets and smartphones, as well as overprotective parenting, are threatening these abilities for children to counter their boredom.[12]

Unquestionably, for most children, the importance of body image will become most dramatic during adolescence, but it emerges as an emotional feature earlier.[13] Whereas the 6-year-old usually cares little about having ketchup on their face or mud on their pants, the 12-year-old may agonize over a blemish or wearing unstylish clothes. Body appearance and awareness and emphasis during these years has dental ramifications. A 6-year-old may be indifferent to the appearance of hypomineralized incisors or a malocclusion. By age 12, such conditions may account for a loss of self-esteem due to negative peer social judgments.[14] Although there certainly are exceptions, most children ages 6 to 12 find overall emotional satisfaction only when they are accepted socially by their peers. Lack of acceptance, outright ostracism, teasing, and bullying can certainly be very damaging emotionally.[15]

During these years, with the help of parents, teachers, role models, and other significant individuals, it is important for the child to become emotionally resilient. The abilities to handle and recover from humiliation, frustration, loss, and disappointment should at least begin to emerge during these years. If they do not, then adolescence may become tumultuous years.[16]

Children between ages 6 and 11 have a higher prevalence of behavior problems than groups both younger and older, with males having a higher prevalence than females.[17] About 10% of children ages 6 to 11 have had an attention-deficit/hyperactivity disorder (ADHD) diagnosis and 69% of those are taking ADHD medication.[18] Although 2.3% of children ages 6 to 11 have had a diagnosis of depression,[17] this prevalence is increasing[19] and no gender differences in depression are noted until age 12.[20] Children with anxiety equals 8.6% in this age group, with no differences between males and females.[17]

Social Changes

These years are clearly more complicated socially than the earlier years due to expansion of the child's social environment, demands of school, discovering and exploring a sense of self, and increasing importance of peers. These years see children intensifying their focus on and pursuance of existing interests and competencies while minimizing or eliminating others.

Children in middle childhood spend most of their time in school, an extrafamilial world, where interaction with other children and teachers may reinforce social responses learned at home, provide new ones, and even discourage others. In school, children are expected to control themselves, cultivate good work habits, sit quietly for long periods of time, and comply with rules and expectations for personal conduct set by adults.[21] Perhaps surprisingly, most children anticipate school positively and remain enthusiastic about their experiences there.[22]

Middle childhood is usually a period of positive emotional growth and development, but as children try new things and receive failure feedback, this period also can be fraught with declining self-confidence, motivation, mental health, and involvement in extracurricular activities,[21] a trend that continues through adolescence. Children may shy away from new activities; however, if they can see that they can become competent with practice and development, supportive adults can help children manage their frustrations.[21]

Gender Identity

Children at this age are exploring their new sense of self, including their perception of gender identity and gender congruence, from as early as ages 3 to 5, with an average age of by 8.5 years for those who later identified as transgender.[23] Children develop a sexual orientation as they mature, along with many other sexual developmental milestones.[24] Transgender youth are more visible due to support via social media, although they are at higher risk of experiencing social challenges including other's lack of understanding, rejection, isolation, victimization, and discrimination. Education of the public, advocacy, and safe schools can help transgender youth.[23]

Peers, Friendships, and Bullying

The peer group that a child joins also can be a powerful socializing force.[25] Early parent-child attachment is significantly related to the strength of peer relationships in school-aged children.[26] Sometimes the values of the peer group are antithetical to those of the teacher and parents. This presents a conflict for the child who may risk reprimand from authoritative adults or ridicule or rejection from peers upon conforming to one or the other's expectations. Parents must understand these conflicts and how socially influential peer pressure can be during middle childhood. It is also important to note that the child who eagerly accepts a peer value that disappoints their parents may in fact be doing so to gain acceptance and nurturing that are not provided sufficiently at home.[27]

Also marking the middle childhood years are increasingly stronger, more stable, and more meaningful friendships. Generally, friendships are made with children of the same gender.[28] However, girls tend to start branching out to mixed- or opposite-sex peers during the middle childhood years, whereas boys tend to wait until early adolescence. Additionally, adult supervision is critical in mixed-sex peer groups as supervised time leads to better school performance, whereas unsupervised time leads to increased problem behaviors.[29] Friends at this age level, as a rule, also share similar socioeconomic status, race, intelligence, behaviors, maturity, and interests.[30,31] At the same time, it is important to recognize that as closer bonds and friendships are defined, social cruelty and bullying also increase. Children in grades 3 to 6 show a range of strategies for peer influence including various prosocial and coercive strategies as well as a combination of the two.[32]

Bullying is the intentional and repeated behavior of someone causing another person harm or discomfort. In person, bullying can take physical or word form, or it can be more subtle. Cyberbullying takes place through electronic technology including text messaging, email, and social media. Generally, the bullied child does nothing to cause the bullying and has difficulty defending themselves.[33] An estimated 1 in 5 "tweens" (between the ages of 9 and 12) have been exposed to cyberbullying, either as a victim, bully, or witness. Rates of cyberbullying are increasing over time, whereas face-to-face bullying is showing an opposite trend.[34] The frequency of bullying also seems to be worse among late childhood compared with later adolescence,[34] and there is a wealth of research highlighting the negative outcomes including emotional distress and disease, substance use, and psychosocial problems.[35] As children approach adolescence, the transition can invite increased risk of behavioral, emotional, and mental health problems through cyberbullying.[36] Therefore in response to increasing prevalence of mental health symptoms, depression, and suicides, the Surgeon General highlighted that while technology allows new communities, better resource delivery, and access to information, it can have harmful effects such as reinforcing ideas of hate, exclusion, and bullying.[37]

Smartphones, Internet, and Social Media

Cell phone use has a major influence on the behavior of 6- to 12-year-olds and their interactions with siblings, peers, parents, and teachers. Their obsession with social media has produced more negative outcomes than positive ones. The arrival of smartphones and the expansion of broadband Internet encourage virality of social media, and the front-facing camera has led to drastic changes in social media and gaming addiction contributing to a mental health crisis among youth.[38] Children between ages 8 and 12 spend almost 5 hours daily in front of a screen for nonschool activities. Video watching doubled from 2015 to 2019, and TV watching decreased.[39]

Most parents of children under the age of 12 are concerned their children have too much screen time. Smartphone ownership has increased in the past decade and increases with each year of a child's age. By age 11, more than half of children have their own smartphone, which increases to more than two-thirds by age 12. Although males enjoy gaming more than females, females enjoy music, reading, and social media more than males.[39] Research that includes asking youth themselves about their screen time indicates that screen usage increases in late childhood and that child screen time is underestimated by parents.[40] Parents are concerned about online predators and their child accessing violent or sexually explicit content. Some check the call records and messages on smartphones used by children in this age range or use their device as a location tracker.[41] Most parents of this age group limit their child's screen time and revoke the smartphone or Internet privileges as punishment.[41]

Despite age 13 being the minimum for joining most platforms, almost half of children ages 8 to 12 use social media. Social media can provide connection and positive communities, information access, the opportunity for self-expression, and also encouragement for struggling individuals to seek help. There is not enough evidence to determine whether social media is safe for children, and although there is a potential for benefit, there are indicators of mental health harm. More easily than before, children can access inappropriate and harmful content, which may seem normalized through delivery on social media platforms. Social media also drives social comparison, which may compromise self-image, expose users to hate-based content, and allow predatory and threatening behavior from strangers. Social media depends on user engagement, and engagement drives addiction-like behaviors and self-control difficulties in children. Among other organizations including the American Academy of Pediatrics and the American Psychological Association, the Surgeon General recommends limiting time spent using social media.[42]

Behavioral, emotional, and mental health problems may be exacerbated by new technologies, including social media, if not used properly.[43] The rise in problems parallels the rise in digital technology use and the two are linked only with weak correlations.[44,45] Nevertheless, children choose who to "like" and "follow" on social media, although built-in algorithms also affect what social media content the child will experience. Family background, home environment, neurologic development, intellectual development, maturity, strengths, vulnerabilities, and understanding of risk may all affect how the information is received and processed by a child.[46] Therefore the beneficial or harmful effects of social media vary by child, by age, and by sex.

Some children can form social connections that would not be possible without digital communication tools. Additionally, social media use may even increase the amount of offline time spent with friends, although this is less likely for socially anxious children who may use digital interactions to avoid in-person interactions.[47]

With the dramatic changes in screen time and smartphone usage, there has been an increased interest in understanding the developmental effects of this use of technology. To date, amount of screen time has not been associated with clear differences in neurocognitive brain development.[48] However, there are significant effects with behavioral and emotional outcomes. Higher social media use in females ages 11 to 13 leads to decreased life satisfaction ratings; however, for males, the period of decreased life satisfaction comes later (14 to 15 years).[49] For children ages 9 to 10, increased screen time has been associated with poorer outcomes in academic performance and sleep. Children with more screen time are also more likely to have poorer mental health. The size of the effects are modest, so more research is needed.[50] Regarding specific behavioral disorders, higher screen usage has been associated with increased rates of both conduct disorder and oppositional defiant disorder, with greater than 4 hours combined screen time per day associated with the highest prevalences of both disorders, although there is not enough evidence to determine the causal direction of the relationship.[51] On a positive side, screen time may be associated with improvements in the quality of peer relationships at this age.[50]

Effects of Parenting

One of the most well-known models of parenting includes four primary parenting styles: authoritative, permissive, authoritarian, and neglectful.[52] Authoritative parenting, characterized by firm limits, yet nurturing and responsive, has consistently been associated with the strongest developmental benefits including emotional skills (self-esteem, resilience) and academic achievement. In contrast, an authoritarian parenting style involves extreme rigidness, perhaps unrealistic expectations, and limited warmth. This parenting style, along with permissive and neglectful parenting, have been linked with poorer developmental outcomes, including poorer emotional functioning, poorer school performance, and increased behavioral challenges.[52] Parenting practices can also shape development of the child brain and cognitive functioning such as emotional arousal and regulation, processing of rewards, inhibition, and social-emotional functioning.[53]

More recently there has been increased attention on another parenting style, overprotective or "helicopter" parenting. Overprotective parenting involves constant micromanaging, supervising, consoling, and sheltering of children, controlling their social sphere, preventing them from taking on responsibilities or acting independently. As a result, and ironically considering an overprotective parent's intention, children can grow up to lack resilience, patience, and the practice to become proactive or independent adolescents or adults.[54] Overprotective parenting may also be connected with increased internalizing symptoms, such as anxiety and depression, both in childhood and into adulthood.[55,56] In fact, Canadian pediatricians feel strongly that children need "risky play," which they liken to preventative medicine for mental health. Although overprotective parents may avoid unstructured, child-directed play for fear of injury, this activity aids in social-emotional development and teaches children problem solving, risk-taking, managing fear, and autonomy, versus parent-led play, which leads to more injuries in the future.[57]

Knowing the potential impact of positive parenting styles on child development, teaching parents effective parenting practices is essential. Healthy parenting principles and strategies are also applicable to online activities.[44] Luckily, many evidence-based training programs exist, such as the Positive Parenting Program (Triple P), which has decades of evidence of both short- and long-term benefits,[58] and programs to promote positive parenting are not limited to specialist centers and can be successfully implemented in primary care settings.[59]

COVID-19 Pandemic Effects

The COVID-19 pandemic had profound effects on children in middle childhood with the shutdown of schools leading to both short-term loss of education and long-term effects on children's education, including estimated reduced life expectancy.[60] School closures can be common during emergency situations, with the COVID-19 pandemic being the most widespread event in recent years. School closures during the pandemic had a negative effect on learning, either through the loss of acquired knowledge, lack of learning new information, increased rates of future dropout, and worsening of existing educational disparities within marginalized groups.[61] There are other less obvious effects as well ranging from increased underreporting of child maltreatment[62] to downstream consequences such as reduced projected lifetime earnings and welfare losses.[63]

Emotional distress during the COVID-19 pandemic was significantly higher than prepandemic levels, including elevated levels of anxiety, depression, irritability, and traumatic stress. Those students with prolonged virtual or hybrid schooling were also worse off emotionally compared with their peers that returned to in-person schooling.[64] There were also physical effects of school closures during the COVID-19 pandemic. Moderate exercise (and reduced screen time) is related to better emotional health,[65] yet during the pandemic, school-aged children, on average, had decreased physical activity, increased sedentary lifestyle, and less participation in organized sports, particularly for those who were in virtual or hybrid versus in-person schooling.[64]

Problematic Media Exposure

Because a small percentage of children are already using tobacco products in middle school, tobacco prevention messaging should start early.[66] Exposure to advertisements of e-cigarettes in childhood can reduce the perception of harm, which might make children more likely to use in adolescence.[67] This period is truly a formative time and the influence of marketing campaigns can contribute to eating habits and childhood obesity[68] and shape perceptions of products (for good or for bad) into adulthood.[69] Caregivers should also be mindful of media content that children consume. Although not ubiquitous, school-aged children who frequently consume media (e.g., music, video games, videos) with violent themes or relational aggression experience an increased risk of serious violent behaviors[70] and relational (social) aggression.[71] Extreme care also should be taken in protecting children from sexual media as it is becoming more and more prevalent and can lead to distorted views of healthy sexual activity and lack of knowledge of responsible practices.[72]

Summary

The period from ages 6 through 12 years is probably the most dynamic period for cognitive, emotional, and social changes in a child's growth. Any dentist's intervention during this time is undertaken on a rapidly changing social and emotional substructure and understanding these changes is critical to achieve good outcomes.

Visit eBooks.Health.Elsevier.com to see full list of references.

6

Cognitive, Emotional and Social Development—Adolescence

KECIA S. LEARY

CHAPTER OUTLINE

Cognitive Changes

The adolescent time period is defined as approximately 11 to 21 years old, maybe even older. This time period coalesces with the initiation of puberty, a key period of growth and development because it marks the transition from childhood to adult and changes in physical development. The literature describes roughly three to possibly even four periods; early adolescence (ages 11 to 14), middle adolescence (ages 15 to 17), late adolescence (ages 18 to 21), and early adulthood (ages 22 to 25).[1] From a cognitive standpoint Piaget discussed adolescents moving from Concrete Operational functions to the Formal Operations stage in their development, and by middle to late adolescence they are capable of extremely sophisticated intellectual tasks. High ability abstract thinking allows the adolescent to deal with complex and difficult vocational and educational challenges. Formal operational thinking and the ability to store information in the memory after perceiving it are hallmarks of the maturation of cognitive ability in adolescents. However, at this stage in development there may be more of a focus on the short-term rather than long-term outcomes.[1]

There are three concepts in the psychosocial development of adolescents: to establish autonomy, develop identity, and develop the ability for future orientation.[2] The early adolescent becomes economically and emotionally independent from their family structure meaning they may have decreased interest in family activities/parental involvement and increased interest in their peer group, especially their same-sex peer group.[2] Due to these changes and the need for independence, it is not uncommon for the adolescent to change clothes, cars, hairstyles, tastes in music, and identification with certain people or groups. These reflect the early adolescent's need to develop their own sense of identity. They are trying to find the "right fit." In middle adolescence the peer group may become more mixed-sex and the adolescent may begin experimentation in dating and sexual experiences. This is the period that family conflict is likely to be at its peak as independence continues to broaden.[2] The late adolescent has developed a separate identity from their parents as well as moving from their peers to adult status. With this development, the late adolescent has developed the cognitive maturity to develop realistic goals and are refining their moral, religious, and sexual values.[2] The adolescent is using social norms from many different groups, such as parents, peers, or the larger culture, to help make decisions.[1]

The change in cognitive development will play a role in how an oral health provider can communicate with a patient. In the earlier phase, concrete thinker information is very black and white. Providing anticipatory guidance responds better to simple straightforward consequences: you eat sugar, you get cavities. In the later adolescence, the more abstract thinker, with more experience, the more problem-solving skills; for instance, if you eat certain kinds of sugar you can get cavities.[3] Counseling the early abstract thinker may actually take more time because they need to unwind all of the information provided.[4] This is a large period of cognitive development where changes are focused on deductive reasoning, social cognition, thinking about thinking, and executive functioning.[5]

During this time of cognitive change, it is important to recognize that adolescents are attempting to create autonomy over their own medical and oral health while still requiring a parent or legal guardian to consent for many healthcare procedures. This can create some discomfort as adolescents may have more knowledge over their medical history than the parent/guardian does, especially when it comes to sensitive topics such as tobacco, drug use, or pregnancy. According to the American Academy of Pediatrics

(AAP), it is important to give the adolescent private time with their healthcare providers to ensure confidentiality and recognize that there may be some topics—such as sexually transmitted infections (STIs), pregnancy, or even mental health—that cannot, in some states, be disclosed without the adolescent's permission. Providing care during adolescence will help transition healthcare to adulthood.[6] Although, able to make decisions, it is important that the adult parent and care provider provide all the relevant information including short-term and long-term consequences to decision making.[1]

In summary, during this time of cognitive change it is important to help develop healthy habits to enter adulthood. By mid to late adolescence, most young people are capable of formal operational thinking, and can, both in and out of school, master subject material that is extensive, difficult, and abstract. These measures of cognitive development correlate with age and experience. Adolescents are able to plan effectively, have increased reasoning ability, and are able to exhibit inhibitory control. These aspects of brain maturation continue to develop even after adolescence is over into early adulthood.

Emotional Changes

The very rapid and dramatic changes that occur in adolescents may be paralleled by many emotional circumstances. The self-confidence and personal identity of an adolescent may be compromised if their feelings about body image are negative. In 1984, Mussen and colleagues[7] noted that the following issues create the possibility of misinterpretation and anxiety for this age group:

- Being attractive or unattractive
- Being loved or unloved
- Being strong or weak
- Being masculine or feminine

For females, the onset of menstruation may present circumstances that can be anxiety provoking. This is not necessarily the rule, but the chances of anxiety rise if there is a prevailing negative reaction to the menstrual process by family and peers, if the child is showered with sympathy, or if there is considerable pain before and during menses. Reassurance that menstruation is a normal bodily function sometimes accompanied with emotional swings due to hormonal fluctuations may alleviate the adolescent's anxiety.

For males, puberty is a period where there can be a growth spurt, they develop facial and body hair, and they develop romantic and sexual interests. As these physical characteristics develop, there may be social pressures to fit into the social norm of gender. Males who do not fit these traditional roles may demonstrate signs of aggression. There are many factors that play a role in these views including parents, peers, and their own self-view.[8]

The advent of puberty and the hormones associated with puberty lead to sexual feelings and urges as well as the emotion of love. The timing of this process, its nature and magnitude, and the choice of what to do about these feelings and urges is handled differently from one adolescent to another. Family guidance, the adolescent's own values, the values of peers, and the value system of the person that the adolescent first loves are just a few of the factors that ultimately predict how they will deal with these new feelings.

Social Changes

Adolescence represents the final transition socially from childhood to adulthood. Characteristic behaviors of adolescence can include self-consciousness, mood changes, risk taking, and finding their peers; these events help establish stable adults.[9] Adolescence is a time to learn and develop new skills. When it is over, if everything proceeded as it should, the emerging young adult will be able to establish and maintain loving and sexual relationships with a partner, be independent of the parents, be capable of working with peers, and be self-directed. There is no other period in human development distinguished by psychosocial changes of the same magnitude as those experienced during adolescence.

Peers are important social agents in large technologic societies, where children of the same age group are often kept together. It can be argued that as relationships and dependencies on parents start to decline, the importance of peers escalates. This shift in relationships contributes to the development of intimacy by increasing comfort with peers and encouraging openness and self-disclosure with others. Increasingly, the adolescent may find that it is difficult to share secrets, thoughts, and fantasies with their parents. In these situations, the close friend becomes the adolescent's confidant. The superficial sharing of activities with friends that sufficed during childhood is replaced during adolescence by concern, loyalty, reliability, and respect between adolescent friends.

Risk taking is an important, and also difficult, aspect of adolescent development. Although sometimes seen as a negative, it can also be positive. Appropriate risk taking is developed throughout life.[9]

As adolescents develop, emotional regulation will occur; the early adolescent is more sensitive to rejection compared with older adolescents. Despite the obvious value of peers, there are peer relationships that are not so fortunate for the involved adolescent. For example, to avoid rejection or ridicule from peers, an adolescent may experiment with drugs, participate in criminal acts, or defy authority.

Another important social change in the adolescent is an increase in the size and range of acquaintances. Children younger than adolescents tend to limit their friends to those of their neighborhood, school, and perhaps religious groups. Adolescents, on the other hand, may have individual friends, belong to a circle of friends, and can identify with larger groups such as those in extracurricular activities like music, theater, sports, or "friends" from social media. An adolescent's ability to sustain relationships with many of these groups indicates good social skills and is a sign that the socialization process is going well.

There are few adolescents who are not preoccupied with acceptance by peers. The following qualities in an adolescent seem to correlate with social acceptance by peers:

- Friendly, likes other people
- Energetic and enthusiastic
- Flexible and forgiving
- Laughs, good sense of humor
- Outgoing
- Self-confident but not conceited
- Appears natural
- Tolerant of the shortcomings of others
- Shows leadership qualities
- Others feel good when this person is around

The adolescent who gets along with their peer group seems to relate successfully to adults. Those who do not achieve peer acceptance seem to have more difficulty with adults and grow up to have a variety of social and emotional difficulties.[10] Some of the issues facing adolescents will be discussed.

Bullying

Bullying in youth is an intentional negative behavior that typically occurs repeatedly and where there is an imbalance of power, with a more powerful person or group attacking a less powerful one.[11] Bullying is defined as having three elements: aggressive or deliberately harmful behavior (1) between peers that is (2) repeated and over time and (3) involves an imbalance of power, for example, related to physical strength or popularity, making it difficult for the victims to defend themselves.[12]

Behavior falls into four categories: direct-physical (e.g., assault, theft), direct-verbal (e.g., threats, insults, name-calling), indirect-relational (e.g., social exclusion, spreading rumors), and cyberbullying. Cross-sectional findings indicate that there is an increased risk of suicidal ideation and/or suicide attempts associated with bullying behavior and cyberbullying.[13] Nineteen percent of students report being bullied at school, and 16% report being electronically bullied.[14]

Bullying can be a predictor for future mental health problems. Studies have shown that bullying behavior in childhood or adolescence is a predictor of antisocial behavior and antisocial personality disorder (PD) in adulthood. Studies have focused on three groups: those who were victims, those who were bullies, and those who were both victims and bullies (bully/victims). Children and adolescents involved in bullying behavior had the worst outcomes when they were both bullies and victims, leading to depression, anxiety, and suicidality (suicidality only among males) as adults.[15,16] More recently, it was found that female victims of bullying have an almost fourfold likelihood of developing a PD later in life compared with adolescents with no involvement in bullying behavior. Female adolescents diagnosed with anxiety disorder during adolescence had more than a threefold risk of developing a PD during late adolescence or early adulthood.[17]

Pediatric dentists can identify a range of health conditions that affect not only adolescents' functioning and opportunities, but also the quality of their adult lives. Assessment for adolescents with psychopathology, other signs of emotional distress, or unusual chronic complaints should also include screening for participation in bullying as victims or bullies.

Mental Health and Emotional Well-Being

Mental health disorders can be attributed to diagnoses such as attention-deficit/hyperactivity disorder (ADHD), depression, or anxiety problems.[18] According to the National Survey of Children's Health, there is a prevalence that 16.5% of children suffer from at least one mental health disorder.[18] Mental health is associated with many characteristics including gender, socioeconomic status, indigenous identity, immigrant status, race, disability, and sexual orientation.[19] However, since the COVID-19 pandemic, mental health has been a bigger concern among the adolescent groups. In Canadian females and males the gap in negative self-perceived mental health increased during the pandemic. This is especially a concern for adolescents that suffer from adverse childhood experiences (ACEs).[20] Due to the increase in mental health concerns in adolescents and the limited number of mental health providers, many adolescents may find themselves "boarding" in the emergency department to wait for available inpatient mental healthcare.[21] Mental health challenges can lead to other negative outcomes.

Suicide among young people continues to be a serious problem. It is the second leading cause of death for people 15 to 24 years old.[22] For some teens, suicide may appear to be a solution to their problems and stress due to depression and suicidal feelings.[22] Suicide rates may have increased due to the stresses and anger levels induced by electronic media and a reluctance to use antidepressant medication. Fewer antidepressants have been prescribed since 2004 when the US Food and Drug Administration (FDA) required black box warning labels on antidepressants to warn healthcare providers of increased risks of suicidal thinking and behavior among children and adolescents being treated with such medications.[23]

In 2017, 6241 suicides occurred in people 15 to 24 years old; 5016 were male and 1225 were female.[24] The 2017 suicide rate averaged 11.8 per 100,000, up from previous studies.[24] Since the COVID-19 pandemic, there has been a significant amount of information about mental health in the adolescent and how to identify and treat mental health concerns.[21]

Suicide is especially high among teens because of the severe stressors of adolescence and the immaturity of the adolescent brain.[25] Any attempt to categorize adolescence is destined to fall woefully short of the complexity of today's reality. The best we can do as pediatric dentists is to keep pace with the emerging scientific evidence and assimilate that information with our own experiences and foundational knowledge. The goal of this approach goes beyond the mere exercise of intellectual curiosity; it reaches for an understanding of the world of the next adolescent who sits in your dental chair.

The AAP updated its guidelines for screening patients for suicidal thoughts, identifying risks factors for suicide, and assisting at-risk young people.[23] The AAP recommends that pediatricians look for risk factors linked to teen suicide, which include a history of physical or sexual abuse, mood disorders, substance use, and teens who identify as lesbian, gay, or bisexual.

Additionally, according to the American Foundation for Suicide Prevention (AFSP), the nation's largest suicide prevention network, because the risk of suicide is heightened by a convergence of multiple risk factors, screening for these risks is the first critically important step in preventing suicide death.

As oral health professionals it is our professional responsibility to help identify those adolescents who may be at higher risk for suicide. Positive youth development suggests that a good interpersonal relationship between the adolescent patient and the pediatric dentist may influence an improvement in the adolescent's oral health and at the same time, serve as a good role model. Because dental health professionals frequently encounter adolescents in their practices over time and in their communities, we may have several opportunities to observe changes in behavior and to ask appropriate questions to identify adolescents at high risk for psychological problems. Referral should be made when the treatment needs are beyond the treating dentist's scope of practice, and consultation with nondental professionals or a team approach may be indicated.[26]

The first step in identifying adolescents at risk is a thorough medical history that includes both systemic conditions and behavioral issues. Routine history taking should include questions about mood disorders, antidepressant medications, school problems, and stressful life events. Asking open-ended questions may elicit more than a "yes" or a "no" response. If the adolescent appears to be sad at the dental appointment, allow your responses to reflect the patient's mood. This approach may allow the adolescent to feel understood, and a dialogue may follow. Adolescents at risk for suicide can be identified through direct questioning or screening by self-report accompanied by knowledge of the risk factors. Ask questions such as the following: Are you feeling sad or depressed, are you thinking about hurting or killing yourself, and have you ever thought about hurting or killing yourself? It is important for the pediatric dentist to maintain a nonjudgmental and open approach in questioning the adolescent. These questions provide assurance that somebody is willing to talk about their problems.

A second step in identification occurs while performing the comprehensive oral examination. Be alert to teens whose appearances and/or behaviors are beyond normal self-expression. Signs that may be indicative of inner turmoil include self-injury and increased risk-taking behavior. Extensive body art and/or branding are some examples of risky behaviors that may manifest during adolescence. Regularly weigh your patient at recall examinations. A significant increase or decrease in weight or appetite could be a characteristic of depression or eating disorders (EDs). Ask if the patient is experiencing any energy loss, sleep problems, or lack of interest in daily activities. Adolescents in crisis may exhibit one or more of these behaviors, and the dental health professional should be aware of these indicators.

Finally, familiarize yourself with local, state, and national resources for treatment of psychopathology and suicide prevention. Advocate and participate in a multipronged and multidisciplinary approach to mental healthcare. A list of telephone numbers of mental health agencies, family and children services, and intervention agencies should be available in the dental office for possible referral of your adolescent patients and their parents. It is important to provide information about the national crisis hotline in the United States, launched in 2022, called the 988 Suicide & Crisis Lifeline. It provides resources for evidence-based mental health response in a crisis. Severe moodiness in a teenager may not be something that will be outgrown; it may be a behavior that requires our recognition and appropriate referral for proper intervention.

Gender Identity

Along with sexual activity, sexual identity develops and may solidify during adolescence. Gender identity and subsequent discussions with the patient are relatively recent to medical and dental providers. In 1983, the AAP issued its first report on sexual minority teens and then made revisions in 1993 and 2004.[27] Since that time the AAP has broadened their view on providing care to adolescents including "ensuring comprehensive care and support for transgender and gender-diverse children and adolescents." This policy statement was adopted in 2018 and reaffirmed in 2023.[28] Since the last update, research on this subject has expanded with numerous publications about lesbian, gay, bisexual, transgender, and questioning (LGBTQ+) youth. In 2011, the Institute of Medicine published a report documenting the health of the individuals who identify as LGBTQ+.[29] They stated that being a member of this group of adolescents is not, itself, a risky behavior. In addition, sexual minority youth should not be considered abnormal.[29]

Typically, a young person's sexual orientation emerges before or early in adolescence.[30] In fact, many teens are in conflict with their sexual attractions, and some may refer to themselves as "questioning."[30] In the United States, the exact prevalence of adolescent homosexuality and same-sex experiences is unknown. A study of 9th to 12th graders from Massachusetts reported 3% as gay, lesbian, or bisexual and another 1% reported as "questioning."[31] In the National Survey of Family Growth, 13.4% of females and 4.0% of males self-reported having sex with someone of the same gender.[32] So, the pediatrician and the pediatric dentist need to be cognizant that some of the concerns their patients may have are regarding their sexual orientation. Over the years, the pediatric dentist develops lasting relationships with their patients, and these patients may be comfortable in discussing their concerns with the pediatric dentist. The dentist should be able to provide current and nonjudgmental information in a confidential manner. In addition, the dental professional should assist the adolescent with the names of other healthcare professionals and agencies for possible referral. Pediatric healthcare providers are important in facilitating a healthy transition from adolescence to adulthood, so the pediatric dentist needs to be knowledgeable about the issues facing sexual and gender minority in youth. Many adolescent patients may also be facing depression, anxiety, posttraumatic stress disorder (PTSD), EDs, autism spectrum disorder, and bipolar disorder.[33] Adolescents who are transgender report suicidal ideation (74.7%), exhibit self-harm (55.7%), and had more suicide attempts (30.4%).[33] Over half of these students also report school victimization.[33]

Healthcare issues and disparities exist among LGBTQ+ teens, and unfortunately, many of the public health systems have ignored them. From a psychological standpoint, the disclosing of one's sexual orientation may result in significant stress for the adolescent and their families. The family may reject or disapprove this disclosure, resulting in a lack of social support from families and friends. Some sexual minority and gender minority youth may experience physical or emotional abuse; therefore as mandated reporters, pediatric dentists need to be aware of the probable root cause of the abuse and the perpetrator.

Seventy-five percent of the adolescents that identify as transgender live in rural areas or small cities.[34] The process of gender affirmation includes five key components: social affirmation, puberty blockers, cross-sex hormone therapy, gender-affirming surgeries, and legal affirmation.[28] Two areas of gender affirmation that the pediatric dentist should be familiar with for providing direct patient care are social and legal affirmation. Social affirmation includes recognizing gender pronouns, gender identity in name, and using the restrooms and other facilities that are specific to the preferred gender. Many adolescents may begin their expression of gender identity by engaging in the process of socially using a gender different than one assigned at birth. Legal affirmation includes changing gender and name on legal documents. In both cases, the patient record should reflect what the patient desires. Both of these affirmations are reversible and do not require medical intervention.

By making minor modifications in the health record including providing separate sections for "sex at birth" and "gender identity" as well as "legal name" and "chosen name," asking how patients would like to be addressed, and avoiding making assumptions about gender the pediatric dentist can become more knowledgeable and sensitive to the adolescents medical and dental needs.[35]

Nutrition and Physical Fitness

Nutrition and physical fitness in the adolescent patient are important at this developmental stage, because the habits that develop in adolescence may continue over a lifetime.[36] Concerns come into play when an adolescent has an obsession with food, and these obsessions are starting at ages more consistent with the early adolescent, about age 12.[37] Social media presence has demonstrated that there may be increased risk of body dissatisfaction. Disordered eating can be a result of social media pressures and challenging schedules. Prevalence of EDs over a lifetime are 8.4% for females and 2.2% for males.[38] Even though studies continually demonstrate a higher prevalence of females with EDs, the trajectories are the same between males and females.[37] These can include loss of control of eating, feeling overweight, and attributing the food to other symptoms.[37] These symptoms can include the following conditions: anorexia, limiting all food and caloric intake; bulimia, secretive bouts of overeating followed by self-induced vomiting or purging; and extreme physical fitness and use of diet drugs.

Oral effects of EDs include reduced salivary flow and erosion of teeth for both bulimia and anorexia nervosa. Soft tissue manifestations can include dry lips, angular cheilitis, erythema of the palate and lips, palatal ulcers, coated tongue, and a yellow-orange palate. These could be due to vomiting episodes or self-injurious behaviors.[39] Due to these concerns, it is important to council the adolescent patient about a healthy weight for any body and refer patients that may be exhibiting signs of disordered eating.

Physical fitness is a key lifetime experience. This can promote overall good adult coping skills with physical activity, mental health, and opportunities to engage with other individuals. There is a continued professionalization of youth sports, which leads to overuse injury, overtraining, and burnout in adolescent athletes.[40]

As pediatric dentists it is important to recognize that patients may be benefiting from some of the opportunities from increased nutrition and physical activity, but there can be detriments. As oral health professionals, we can recommend healthy habits and the use of sports mouthguards. We can also encourage the input of other healthcare professionals including physical therapists, mental healthcare providers, and school/team trainers to our patients if there are concerns.

Risky Behaviors

During the adolescent years there are many factors at play in making choices. First, is the idea of self-identity. As discussed earlier many adolescents are "trying on" new lifestyles. There is the shunning of the family and increase of friends as a resource. This in turn can lead to more risky behaviors. Being aware of the risks may still fail because the adolescent is just beginning to understand cause and effect.[2] Risks are not always negative; however, this section will discuss potentially risky behaviors in the adolescent because they are more likely to take risks.[41]

Tobacco and Nicotine Products

Tobacco products are any products that deliver nicotine to the brain. Today tobacco products include e-cigarettes, cigarettes, cigars, smokeless tobacco, hookahs, pipe tobacco, heated tobacco products, and nicotine "tobacco-free" items. Over the past 20 years the number of adolescents smoking has decreased. However, there has been an increase of individuals using electronic nicotine delivery systems (ENDS). These are e-cigarettes or vaping. The use of tobacco products by adolescents is widespread and may not only result in chronic systemic effects but also contribute to oral soft tissue damage. In addition to oral malodor and stained teeth, adolescents who smoke experience impaired gingival health and delayed wound healing. Cigarette smoking is also a significant contributing factor for the development and subsequent life-threatening effects caused by oral, pharyngeal, and laryngeal carcinomas.

E-cigarettes have a battery, a heating element, and a container to hold a solution that includes nicotine (sometimes flavored like candy). These devices have names such as e-cigs, e-hookahs, mods, pods, vapes, vape pens, tank systems, and electronic nicotine delivery systems. They may also be referred to as their brand names and are unique because they may resemble everyday items like USB drives and are easy to conceal and carry. The system heats the e-liquid or e-juice and creates a fine mist that is inhaled and exhaled, much like a traditional cigarette. The misconception is that the use of the electronic device will help an individual quit using traditional tobacco products.

Currently, the use of e-cigarettes and vaporizers is replacing the traditional cigarette. A survey of US students over the years indicated the changes in adolescent tobacco use. Students are more likely to use e-cigarettes (25.1% to 32.6%) than traditional cigarettes (30.0% to 22.2%) for frequent tobacco users.[42] The authors reported that its use is driven by the belief that e-cigarettes are less harmful.[43] Many adolescents surveyed believed that e-cigarettes were a harmless form of entertainment and were unaware that they could contribute to nicotine addiction. The dentist should be concerned that this type of tobacco use may serve as a gateway to smoking cigarettes because the products are similar. The e-cigarette market is now facing the same regulatory pressure that cigarettes did. This has included limiting the sale and advertisement of these devices. There is little oversight for safety in the manufacturing of these products, which could account for some of the heavy metals such as lead and zinc that have been detected in some e-cigarettes.

E-cigarettes may be preferred due to their colors and flavors and their extensive marketing campaigns.[44] However, the reality is that those that choose to use e-cigarettes may be at higher risk of dental caries, white spot lesions, and gingivitis, all of which can lead to tooth loss.[45] This is different than traditional cigarette use that may demonstrate an increase in tooth loss alone.

Another adolescent smoking trend is the rising use of smoking cigars (3.5% of current users).[42] Health officials believe several factors are responsible for this upswing. Unlike cigarettes, cigars are promoted with candy, chocolate, and fruit flavors. Cigars are taxed less and can be sold in single lots, unlike cigarettes that must be sold in packs of 20 and are more expensive. Smokeless tobacco users also account for 6.0% of tobacco users.[42]

The use of tobacco products is not just the person using the products but also the environmental tobacco smoke (ETS), also referred to as secondhand and thirdhand smoke. Secondhand smoke is the smoke emitted from a product when exhaled and then inhaled by a person that does not smoke. Thirdhand smoke is the smoke that is absorbed onto layers thereby exposing someone to tobacco long after the use of the product has ceased. Examples of this are the smoke residue that is left on clothes, in houses, or in the car. These examples lead to overall tobacco exposure and the direct use of tobacco products.[46]

Sexual Activity

Many adolescents engage in sexual activity that may directly or indirectly affect their oral health. These adolescent sexual behaviors include a range of activities from kissing and fondling to oral, anal, and vaginal sex. The most recent Youth Risk Behavior Survey of US high school students reports:

- 32% had sexual intercourse.
- 21% are currently sexually active.

- 52% used a condom the last time they had sex.
- 33% use hormonal birth control.[14]

Risky sexual behaviors place adolescents at risk for unplanned pregnancies and STIs, including HIV, gonorrhea, and syphilis. Certain behaviors place the adolescent at higher risk for developing STIs. These include (1) ever having sex, (2) having four or more lifetime sexual partners, and (3) being sexually active. Protective factors include (1) using a condom during last sexual intercourse, (2) using effective hormonal birth control, and (3) being tested for HIV or other STIs.[14] Adolescents contract STIs at a higher rate than adults because of sexual risk taking and possible barriers to healthcare access.[47] During a teen's dental examination, sexually active adolescents may present with herpes simplex virus (HSV)-2 lesions in the oral and perioral regions. According to a recent national survey, more than two-thirds of US teenagers have engaged in oral sex, including nearly 25% who have never experienced intercourse.[48] Consequently, STIs are spreading faster among teens than any other age group. In addition, females are more likely than males to contract HSV-2 from a single act of unprotected sex.[48] Palliative treatment is recommended and may include analgesics (e.g., acetaminophen) and antiviral medications (e.g., acyclovir) to alleviate the symptoms. Recurrent herpes labialis may be treated with topical penciclovir cream for vesicular perioral lesions.[49] The cream may have a small, favorable effect on the duration of symptoms if applied at the onset of the infection. However, many patients will choose to treat the condition at home with topical treatment. Thus it is important for the pediatric dentist to address the adolescent's sexual activity and use this opportunity to discuss risk reduction as a component of the overall medical history.

It is also an opportunity for the oral healthcare provider to provide information and counseling on prevention of STIs including human papillomavirus (HPV). The US immunization schedule has recommended the HPV vaccine for more than 20 years. This vaccine can help prevent the transmission of HPV strains 6, 11, 16, and 18. These strains are linked to both cervical cancer and genital warts. These cancers can be seen in adulthood as oral lesions, so the recommendation of this vaccine is within the oral healthcare providers scope of training. The Current Dental Terminology provides codes for vaccine administration by the oral health provider and for immunization counseling.[50]

By building a trusting relationship with the adolescent over time, the dentist may be able to obtain an honest, detailed health history to ascertain the teen's sexual activity. Because sexuality is an expected stage in the development of adolescents and young adults, pediatric dentists have a professional responsibility to be knowledgeable in initial screening and management/referral of common sexual health issues. The dental health professional's ability to listen to adolescents' concerns and to help them access necessary community resources will allow the dentist to serve their teenage patients effectively.

Social Media and Internet Use

Social media has become a part of the daily life of adolescents. [51] These platforms are changing rapidly. According to the Surgeon General's Report of Social Media and Youth Mental Health, there is not enough evidence to determine whether social media is safe for children and adolescents. Over 77% of youth report using social media several times a day.[52] Early adolescence is when identities of sense and self-worth are forming and the adolescent is the most susceptible to social pressures and peers.[9]

When evaluating the research on social media and mental health in adolescents the focus of a positive relationship seems to be rare.[53] The scientific content in these studies includes potential risk of harm from content and excessive/problematic use.[52] There are some known evidence gaps including the differences between social versus digital interactions, harm to mental health/well-being, what content/intensity creates the most harms, beneficial effects, and the mental health aspects of social media.[52]

Cyberbullying is a part of the social media concerns. Cyberbullying occurs when technology is used to demean, inflect harm, or cause pain to another person. Any means of electronic devices can be used including social media, videos/computer games, discussion boards, or even text messaging on mobile devices. Adolescents that suffer from bullying in any capacity suffer from higher rates of suicidal ideation and behaviors.[16] However, adolescents that suffer from cyberbullying encounter educational harm, anxiety, low self-esteem, antisocial behavior, and depression.[54] It is important to recognize that traditional bullying and cyberbullying are closely related.

As pediatric dentists, we can support research that gains understanding for the use of social media and support parents/caregivers as they help students. It is important to look at social media through the lens of "harm reduction." This means that there is a recognition that social media is not going away, but that adolescents need to be given the tools to establish boundaries and education about the positives and negatives of social media.

Teen Dating Violence and Human Trafficking

Teen dating violence (TDV) is a form of intimate partner violence (IPV), and according to the CDC, it can include a variety of behaviors including physical violence, sexual violence, psychological aggression, and stalking.[55] According to the Youth Risk Behavior Survey in 2019, 1 in 12 teens experienced physical dating violence and 1 in 12 experienced sexual dating violence.[14] TDV can happen in person and also virtually. TDV is not just limited to one gender or one group of people: the global prevalence is 34.1% of girls and 26.7% of boys experience some sort of TDV.[56]

Some teens are more at risk than others for TDV and this can include those with early sexual debut, substance use including alcohol and cannabis, and acceptance of violence before the TDV.[57,58] Other studies also indicate that low self-esteem, holding traditional gender stereotypes, and having poor conflict resolution can also be risk factors for TDV.[57] Positive predictors in this field are that there is social support from parents and teachers can help limit TDV.[56] COVID-19 may have decreased the experiences of TDV from 7.5% to 5.52% during the first part of the pandemic, but it is unknown if these drops have been sustained.[58]

According to the Trafficking Victims Protection Act of 2000, human trafficking is federally criminalized and is defined as the recruitment and exploitation of people in the sex industry, labor, or services by means of force, fraud, and coercion. Since 2000, the US Justice Department and many states have provided statutes on modern day slave trafficking. However, there are still issues with human trafficking, especially among some teen groups. Teens at risk include those with antisocial romantic relationships, as they are 1.3 times more likely to experience human trafficking experiences.[59] Running away from home, witnessing violence in the home, having ACEs, identifying as LGBTQ+, and poverty are also predictors for human trafficking.[60,61]

Dental professionals have identified that they are not always comfortable providing IPV screenings, and less than one-half of providers believe that this should be part of the examination.[61] However, nonaccidental trauma is more likely to occur to the maxilla and upper face.[62] Those facing some sort of violence often delay getting care for more than a week. Trauma to maxillary teeth can also be indicators to this type of violence. As oral health professionals, female providers are more likely than their male counterparts to discuss IPV and ask questions about safety at home or in a relationship.[61] Patients may be more willing to confide in some providers over others.[63] Anytime there is a delay in seeking care, it is important to separate the adolescent from the adult or care provider who brings them in for treatment, to ask open-ended questions, and to inquire about safety and living situations.[63] All states require that if there are questions about trauma or possible abuse that it be reported to state authorities, it is not the oral health providers responsibility to investigate, but to report. As healthcare providers it is important to treat all patients the same, offering uniform education and resources to combat IPV and human trafficking.[64]

Drug and Alcohol Use

Adolescence is a time of experimentation that can include drug and alcohol use and misuse. The substances misused in the adolescent can include, but are not limited to, alcohol, inhalants, opiates, amphetamines, cocaine, marijuana, barbiturates, benzodiazepines, hallucinogens, and anabolic steroids. Even though some of these substances may be legal, like opioids for pain or amphetamines for ADHD, when not taking them for their intended use or misusing the medications, a substance use disorder (SUD) may develop.

Over the past several years some drugs have decreased in their use, like alcohol.[14] The rate of students who report drinking alcohol has decreased from 35% to 22% However, for others there has been an increase in their use, like marijuana. Currently 17% report using marijuana, and it was 16% in the previous report.[14] According to the National Conference for State Legislatures in 2024, 24 states, two territories, and the District of Columbia have legalized the use of marijuana for either recreational use, medical use, or both. Even though marijuana use may be regulated by the state and require individuals to be 21 to purchase the products, there is more access to this drug than in the past for adolescents.

When an adolescent has an SUD, there are several cognitive and behavioral manifestations that may happen depending on the drug. Behaviors that are uncharacteristic of the patient or do not match the situation should be closely monitored. There are also perioral and oral signs that can include a variety of symptoms, such as sores around the lips and mouth, lip licking, bruxism, trismus, neglected/poor oral health, dental caries, and leukoplakia.[65] SUD can also coexist with other psychiatric conditions such as depression, anxiety, ADHD, oppositional defiant disorder (ODD), conduct disorder, bipolar disorder, PTSD, and others.[66]

As dentists our position is not to treat the disorder, but to be aware of SUD and the potential for SUD. It is important to take an accurate medical history and realize that the parent/guardian may not be aware of the use of substances at this age. There are specific state laws and regulations regarding the disclosure of such conditions to the legal guardian, and so it is best to consult a professional regarding specific questions. However, as medical professionals it is important to know and be able to refer to the appropriate providers in the community. SUD affects treatment recommendations including using sedative medications or prescribing pain relievers postoperatively. It has been well documented that the best pain relief for many dental procedures at this age includes a combination of acetaminophen and ibuprofen.[67] This is to reduce the potentiality of developing an addiction to habit-forming pain relievers.

Summary

Adolescence is the transitional period between puberty and maturity associated with accelerated physical growth and dynamic hormonal changes, contradictions in self-awareness, and the conflicting demands of modern society. Adolescent dental patients have distinct oral needs that require enhanced understanding by dental professionals to provide high-quality dental services to this age group.

Acknowledgments

Jamie Kremsreiter Elizalde, PhD, NCSP, Clinical Associate Professor, UIHC Department of Psychiatry, for her help to organize concepts of adolescent development.

Also please correct to Clinical Associate Professor, UIHC Department of Psychiatry.

Visit eBooks.Health.Elsevier.com to see full list of references.

7

Principles of Anatomy and Physiology for the Pediatric Dentist

JOHN H. UNKEL AND BRIAN J. SPECHT

CHAPTER OUTLINE

Introduction

Anatomy is the structure of the body, and physiology is the function of the body. Pediatric anatomy and physiology differ from adults. Children's organs must grow in size and physiologically develop function to correspond with structure. Although the change in size from a child to an adult is obvious, the change in function of organ systems is important to the pediatric provider. The focus of the chapter will be on systems and structures that directly pertain to the practice of pediatric dentistry. Initially the discussion will address the head and neck, followed by discussion of nervous (brain and cranial nerves), respiratory, and cardiovascular systems.

Head and Neck

The head is relatively large compared with the torso at birth. At birth the head is 25% of its adult size. Head circumference increases by 50% at 6 months of age, and 10 cm during the first year and 2 to 3 cm during the second year, at which time it approximates three-quarters of the adult size. The cranium only increases 6 cm between age 3 and adulthood.[1–3]

Bone formation and ossification occur via two distinct mechanisms: intramembranous ossification and endochondral ossification. Intramembranous ossification occurs by mesenchymal cells differentiating into osteoblasts, which lay down a matrix that eventually forms bone[4,5] such as the cranium. Endochondral ossification occurs by mesenchymal cells undergoing chondrogenesis to form cartilage, which becomes bone such as in the cranial base and long bones.[5,6]

The mesenchyme of the neurocranium is arranged in a capsular membrane surrounding the growing brain. Two layers form the membrane: (1) the ectomeninx, the outer layer forming the dura mater, and (2) the endomeninx forming the pia mater and arachnoid. The ectomeninx also ossifies becoming the calvaria, while the ectomeninx on the floor of the brain chondrifies becoming the cranial base. Ossification of the calvaria intramembranous bones depends on the development of the brain, without which (anencephaly) bone is not laid down. The ectomeninx ossification leads to formation of the frontal, parietal, petrous temporal, and occipital bones. The lacrimal, nasal, zygomatic, maxillary, and mandibular facial bones are derived from the neural crest. The membranous mesenchyme covering bone becomes periosteum.[2]

Ossification begins in the sixth to eighth week in utero but is not complete until after birth. Four significant fontanelles (anterior, anterolateral, posterior, and posterolateral) and four significant sutures (metopic, sagittal, lambdoidal, and coronal) separate the cranial bones at birth. The sutures and fontanelles permit flexibility of the head to pass through the birth canal. The order of closure of the fontanelles is approximately as follows: (1) posterior 2 months, (2) anterolateral 3 months, and (3) anterior and posterolateral approaching the child's second birthday. Growth of the calvarian bones is by sutural growth, surface apposition/resorption, and the enlarging brain. The bones enlarge at the sutures primarily by accretion as a toddler and later by surface apposition. The contraction of facial muscles accounts for modulation of the mastoid process, pterygoids, temporal and nuchal lines of the cranium, coronoid process, and angle of the mandible. In addition to the enlarging brain, altered intracranial pressure due to hydrocephalus or reduced brain size due to microcephaly can change the shape of the calvaria.[2]

The facial portion of the infant head is smaller than the cranium by a ratio of 1:8. The forehead of the infant is high and slightly bulbous because of the frontal lobe of the brain. The larger skull-to-face proportion is visible to approximately age 7. Growth of the face occurs in bursts related to respiratory requirements and tooth-jaw development. This burst occurs during the first 6 months, the 3rd to 4th years, and the 7th to 11th years during childhood and puberty. The initial facial growth spurt occurs with the vertical growth of the nasal cavity.[3]

The neck vertebrae are primarily cartilaginous in the infant, which is slowly replaced with bone. The neck ligaments are weaker than the adult. The articular facets connecting the vertebrae are shallow, and the cervical vertebrae are more anteriorly located and wedged. The dentocentral synchondrosis between the odontoid process and C2 is not fused. In addition, increased water content of the intervertebral disks and weak cervical paraspinal musculature all contribute to uncontrolled and passive cervical spine movement. The base of the cranium occipital condyles, C1, and C2 move in unison during neck flexion and extension of the infant and in some children can result in pseudosubluxation and/or physiologic anterior displacement in C2 to C3 of more than 3 mm.[3,7] In a full-term infant, the neck is short and extremely flexible, which allows the chin to reach the level of the second rib permitting obstruction of the upper airway.[1] Given these anatomical and developmental differences between infants, children, and adults, proper head position for procedures involving sedation or anesthesia is vital. Maintaining head and neck extension during procedures allows for reduced risk of airway compromise.[7] The maturation of the spine is a continuous process approximately reaching adulthood around 8 to 9 years old.[8]

Nervous System

The nervous system interacts with the other bodily systems through its various divisions. The two main divisions consist of the central nervous system (CNS) and peripheral nervous system (PNS). The CNS consists of the brain and spinal cord, and the PNS consists of the sensory receptors, sensory and motor nerves, and ganglia outside the CNS. The focus of this section will be the brain in the CNS and cranial nerves in the PNS.

Embryologically the nervous system begins with the development of the neural tube. In utero the neural plate develops by day 19 and by neurulation closes into a tube by day 22. The anterior portion (cephalad end) closes at day 26, and the distal portion (caudal end) closes at day 28. Developmental defects at the cephalad end may result in anencephaly or an encephalocele. At the caudal spinal end, developmental defects may result in spina bifida. At approximately the fourth week, the neural tube differentiates into the three brain vesicles of the CNS: prosencephalon (forebrain), mesencephalon (midbrain), and rhombencephalon (hindbrain). These further divide and eventually lead to the following: prosencephalon becomes thalamus, hypothalamus, and cerebrum; mesencephalon becomes midbrain; and rhombencephalon becomes pons, cerebellum, medulla oblongata, and spinal cord. The PNS develops from neural crest cells adjacent to the neural tube around 4 weeks. Neural crest cells lead to the formation of the ganglia of the cranial nerves.[9,10]

The cells of the nervous system differentiate into neurons and support cells for the neurons. Neurons consist of dendrites (receive information), cell bodies (encircle the nucleus and produce proteins), and axons (forward information to other neurons and muscles). Supporting glial cells consist of astrocytes (supply substances to neurons, secrete factors, and produce neurotransmitters), oligodendrocytes in the CNS, and Schwann cells in the PNS, which produce myelin. Microglial cells roam for debris after an injury. Nerve cell connections via axons remodel in response to stimuli, and, at birth, one-fourth of all neural cells exist with the spinal cord. By age 1, the development of the CNS is almost complete with the spinal cord at the first lumbar vertebrae. By age 3, the dendritic expansion and myelinization continue to occur.[1,11] Neurogenesis continues until approximately 10 years of age until the brain reaches the adult size.

The autonomic nervous system orchestrates the involuntary responses to maintain bodily equilibrium by its two components: the sympathetic nervous system (excitation) and the parasympathetic nervous system (inhibition). The sympathetic system influences the body's "fight-or-flight" mechanisms in response to stress by releasing norepinephrine and epinephrine, which in turn raise blood pressure and release glucose. The sympathetic system may take up to 6 months to complete after birth. The parasympathetic system regulates the body at rest and during sleep by releasing acetylcholine; its cardiovascular components are functional at birth.[1,10] The delayed maturity of the CNS in infants and children has a direct relationship to medications used for sedation and anesthesia. In general, infants and children are more sensitive to most medications used for sedation, hypnosis, and pain control because of increased brain and CNS immaturity compared with adults.[12]

Brain

The brain can be divided into four anatomical subdivisions: cerebrum (cortex, hemispheres, and basal ganglia), diencephalon (thalamus, epithalamus, and hypothalamus), cerebellum, and brain stem. There are two cerebral hemispheres in the cerebrum, each containing four lobes: frontal, temporal, parietal, and occipital. The frontal lobe contains four general areas: (1) prefrontal cortex, which addresses critical thinking and other cognitive functions, (2) premotor area, which plays roles in imitation learning and arranging and then triggers motor movement, (3) primary motor area, which is responsible for motor movements and areas of the body requiring more complex movement, and (4) Broca's area only found in the left hemisphere, which permits generation of speech- and language-associated movements. The parietal lobe is responsible for receiving and integrating sensory information from smell, taste, sight, hearing, touch, pain, and temperature. Once sensory information is received, the construction of a mental map is made to create a visual image of the surrounding environment. The temporal lobe has two general areas: auditory area, which processes auditory information and creates a memory of sounds, and Wernicke's area, which is associated with speech recollection (phonologic retrieval and comprehension). The occipital lobe receives visual information from the retina of the eye. It assists with distinguishing and processing distance and depth perception, memory, motion, and color. The basal ganglia connect the thalamus to the primary motor area permitting voluntary motor control and learning. The ganglia connect to the limbic system participating in formation of behaviors, emotions, and habits.[10]

The cerebral tissue consumes 80% of the intracranial space, cerebrospinal fluid (CSF) consumes 10%, and blood consumes the remainder. The CSF is produced in the choroid plexus in the walls of the ventricles and fills the ventricles and arachnoid spaces of brain and spinal cord. Its function in children less than 2 years old is not thoroughly understood. In adults, it provides buoyancy and protection for supporting the brain, delivers nutrients, eliminates waste products, assists with homeostasis monitoring pH and ionic composition, and, lastly, repairs the CNS. The flow of the CSF moves through four ventricles, initially from the two lateral ventricles through the foramen of Monroe to the third ventricle, then through the aqueduct of Sylvius to the fourth ventricle, after which it flows into the spinal arachnoid space via the foramens of

Magendie and Luschka. The CSF volume in infants begins as 40 mL and increases to 150 mL later in childhood, which equates to the adult volume. Half the CSF in infants is in the spinal subarachnoid space as opposed to adults where it is reduced to 25%.[13]

The diencephalon contains the thalamus, epithalamus, and hypothalamus. The thalamus is primarily a relay station moving sensory information to the cerebral cortex from the spinal cord and forwarding motor instructions to the brain stem and spinal cord. The epithalamus connects the limbic system to other areas of the brain. It contains the pineal gland for melatonin production affecting circadian rhythms (i.e., sleep cycles and awake periods). Finally, the hypothalamus connects with the limbic system and is associated with the pituitary gland to address hunger, thirst, and blood pressure via hormone release.[10]

The cerebellum addresses motor control through monitoring and regulation assisting with balance and movement. It ensures movement is timed correctly, specific to intention, and coordinated.[10]

The brain stem connects the cerebrum and cerebellum to the spinal cord and matures around 1 year of age. It consists of four components: (1) midbrain, (2) pons, (3) medulla oblongata, and (4) reticular formation. The brain stem houses 10 of the 12 cranial nerve nuclei giving rise to their respective nerves. It plays a role in facial movement and sensation and monitors autonomic functions preserving homeostasis. The midbrain is the home of nuclei for cranial nerves III and IV. It is involved with visual movement and auditory processing, assists the basal ganglia regulating movement, and is involved with reward pathways and pain suppression. The midbrain coordinates sensory information from the spinal cord to the cortex and motor information from the cortex to the spinal cord. Cranial nerves arising from the pons include V, VI, VII, and VIII, which contribute to facial and eye movement, sensation, and hearing. The pons is involved with respiratory effort and rhythm. The pons connects the cerebrum with the cerebellum, thus participating in motor control, balance, and posture. The medulla connects the pons to the spinal cord and plays an essential role in cardiovascular and respiratory functions. It is the origin of cranial nerves IX through XII and provides sensation and movement to the mouth, throat, and neck. The reticular formation is an archaic network connecting the spinal cord via the brain stem to the diencephalon and permitting superior and inferior signaling of sensory and motor information. It contains the reticular activating system and uses a process called ***habituation*** to eliminate meaningless stimuli. The reticular formation also assists with autonomic regulation of cardiovascular and respiratory function, reflexes to pain perception and adjustment, taste, and sleep-wake periods.[10,14]

The limbic system is located beneath the temporal lobes, consists of the amygdala and hippocampus, and interacts with the hypothalamus. The system processes and regulates emotion and memory. It employes cognitive information to coordinate physiologic responses. It is associated with the autonomic and endocrine system and plays a role in the stress reactions. The amygdala plays a significant role in attaching memories to emotions, creating long-term retention of the experiences. The hippocampus is located inside the temporal lobes and plays a role in neurogenesis (i.e., generating new neurons). It also plays a role in memory by transforming a recent memory into long-term memories. The hippocampus is involved with special memory formation, and it navigates and assists the hypothalamic and pituitary responses when the body encounters a stressful situation.[10]

The cerebral blood flow (CBF) to the brain is delivered by the two vertebral arteries, which become the basilar artery, and the internal carotid arteries, which give rise to the circle of Willis and its branches. There are multiple mechanisms that regulate cerebral circulation: metabolism, partial pressure of arterial carbon dioxide ($PaCO_2$), partial pressure of arterial oxygen (PaO_2), blood viscosity, and cerebral autoregulation. Increased $PaCO_2$ results in blood vessel dilatation and increased CBF. Decreased $PaCO_2$ results in blood vessel constriction and decreased CBF. This vasoreactivity is more pronounced in children than adults. PaO_2 has less of an effect on CBF than $PaCO_2$. Blood viscosity is affected by hematocrit and decreased hematocrit (e.g., anemia results in increased CBF to adjust for low oxygen tension).[13]

The cerebral metabolic rate of oxygen ($CMRO_2$) and cerebral glucose level (CMR_{glu}) are greater in children than adults. Increasing myelination and synaptogenesis in children 8 years of age and younger appears to be the reason. The increased $CMRO_2$ and CMR_{glu} may be related to changes in blood flow–metabolism coupling with change in age. The primary control of cerebral circulation under normal conditions may be the relationship of CBF with $CMRO_2$ and cerebral metabolism. At rest, $CMRO_2$ correlates directly with CBF; however, during periods of increased CNS activity or altered oxygenation and ventilation, CBF increases relative to oxygen extraction from the blood. The blood flow–metabolism coupling is affected by multiple mediators such as nitric oxide (vasodilation) and hypothermia.[13] In addition to the complexity of CBF related to $PaCO_2$, O_2, and $CMRO_2$, blood flow to the brain requires adequate mean arterial pressure (MAP) in order to supply a consistent amount of blood to the brain. In adults, CBF autoregulation occurs with MAP between 60 and 150 mm Hg, and there is evidence that the lower threshold in infants and children is as low as an MAP of 40 mm Hg.[12]

The blood-brain barrier is incomplete in infants allowing passage of large molecules such as proteins. The barrier lies between the cerebral capillary blood flow and the CSF and consists of endothelial cells of the choroid plexus and cerebral capillaries. Endothelial cells line the capillaries assisted by astrocytes, which modify their permeability. At birth, proteins, lipid soluble substances, CO_2, O_2, and water cross the barrier, whereas larger substances such as proteins and cholesterol cannot cross after the barrier matures around 4 months of age. The function of the mature barrier is to limit diffusion of harmful substances and toxins, preventing loss of CNS neurotransmitters into the systemic circulation and maintaining homeostasis for survival of neurons.[10,11]

Understanding the clinical relevance of the maturing brain is useful to help reduce the risk of unwanted side effects from procedural sedation and anesthesia, such as nausea and vomiting. There are well-established risk factors for nausea and vomiting in pediatrics relevant to dental procedures and surgeries such as: age greater than 3, length of procedure (>30 minutes), previous personal or family history of nausea and vomiting, opioid use for pain control, and nitrous oxide use for the procedure.[15] For patients at high risk, it is important to avoid such triggers and may be useful to treat with antiemetics to decrease the incidence of nausea and vomiting. Antiemetic medications target several different receptors, and the more common medications used for high-risk pediatric patients include anticholinergics, antihistamines, serotonin receptor antagonists, and corticosteroids.

Cranial Nerves

There are 12 (I through XII) cranial nerves (Table 7.1): 10 are part of the PNS, whereas the olfactory (I) and optic (II) nerves are fiber tracts directly from the brain.

TABLE 7.1 Cranial Nerves

Cranial Nerves	Function	Origin	Destination
Olfactory (I)	Sense of smell	Olfactory bulb	Olfactory cortex
Optic (II)	Vision	Retina	Visual cortex
Oculomotor (III)	Eye movement, pupil constriction	Midbrain	Eye muscles
Trochlear (IV)	Eye movement (superior oblique muscle)	Midbrain	Superior oblique muscle
Trigeminal (V)	Sensation in face, chewing	Pons	Face, jaw muscles
Abducens (VI)	Eye movement (lateral rectus muscle)	Pons	Lateral rectus muscle
Facial (VII)	Facial expressions, taste (anterior ⅔ of tongue)	Pons	Facial muscles, tongue
Vestibulocochlear (VIII)	Hearing, balance	Inner ear	Auditory cortex, cerebellum
Glossopharyngeal (IX)	Taste (posterior ⅓ of tongue), swallowing	Medulla oblongata	Tongue, pharynx
Vagus (X)	Autonomic functions, taste	Medulla oblongata	Thoracic and abdominal organs
Accessory (XI)	Shoulder and neck muscles	Medulla oblongata, spinal cord	Sternocleidomastoid, trapezius muscles
Hypoglossal (XII)	Tongue movement	Medulla oblongata	Tongue muscles

Olfactory Nerve (I). CN I is a sensory nerve providing the sense of smell that extends from the nasal olfactory nerve fibers through the cribriform plate of the ethmoid bone to the olfactory bulb and brain.[16]

Optic and Oculomotor Nerves (II and III). CN II is a special somatic afferent nerve that provides vision. A visual field is the area seen by the eye when the individual focuses on a distant object or point. The total visual field is divided into nasal (closest to the nose) and lateral temporal fields. Fields are further divided into upper and lower quadrants. The total visual field of both eyes has overlapping binocular vision centrally and monocular vision laterally. Reactivity to a stimulus involves the optic nerve and its connection to the Edinger Westfall nucleus and parasympathetic fibers of CN III in the midbrain, which subsequently activate the iris sphincter and ciliary muscles leading to pupillary constriction.[14,16]

Oculomotor, Trochlear, and Abducens Nerves (III, IV, and VI). CN III, IV, and VI are efferent nerves for extraocular eye movement. CN III activates the three rectus (medial, superior, and inferior) muscles, which adduct, elevate, and depress the globe, as well as the inferior oblique muscle that elevates and abducts the globe. Lastly, the nerve elevates the upper eyelid via the levator palpebrae muscle. CN IV leaves the brain stem and innervates the superior oblique muscle, which intorts and moves the eye down. This nerve travels around the midbrain and is the only cranial nerve to exit posteriorly. CN VI departs the brain stem and innervates the lateral rectus muscle and abducts the eye toward the lateral side of the face.[14,16]

Trigeminal Nerve (V). This nerve contains both motor and sensory fibers and has three branches: ophthalmic V-1, maxillary V-2, and mandibular V-3. The efferent V-3 branch innervates and provides motor ability to the muscles of mastication (temporalis, masseter, and pterygoids), the tensor tympani, mylohyoid, and anterior digastric. The somatic efferent branches of V1-3 provide sensation to the skin of the upper, middle, and lower face, mucosa of the mouth, nose and frontal and maxillary sinuses, and lacrimal glands. The V-1 is responsible for the corneal reflex.[16] A clinically significant complication that can be seen with CN V stimulation and/or manipulation is sudden reflex bradycardia or asystole. This can occur with stimulation of any of the sensory branches of CN V (ophthalmic, maxillary, mandibular) during dental procedures or surgeries.[17]

Facial Nerve (VII). CN VII is a complex motor and sensory nerve with sensory, special sensory, parasympathetic properties and motor function. Somatic afferent fibers provide sensation by innervating the posterior surface of the auricle and external auditory canal. Visceral afferent and efferent fibers provide sensation to the soft palate and pharyngeal wall and stimulate submandibular and sublingual saliva and lacrimal tear release. The special visceral afferent and efferent fibers innervate the muscles of facial expression, platysma, stapedius, stylohyoid, and digastric muscles, and fibers of the chorda tympani, which provides taste in the anterior two-thirds of the tongue. The facial nerve innervates the upper facial muscles (forehead) ipsilaterally and the lower face by the contralateral nerve.[16]

Vestibulocochlear Nerve (VIII). CN VIII is a sensory nerve with two portions: vestibular and cochlear. The vestibular portion maintains equilibrium, balance, and orientation in space, whereas the cochlear portion is for hearing. Hearing is crucial for language development, especially during the first three years of life. The posterior cochlear nucleus interprets high-frequency sound, and the anterior cochlear nucleus interprets low-frequency sound.[14]

Glossopharyngeal and Vagus Nerves (IX and X). CN IX is primarily a sensory nerve, whereas CN X has sensory components but is primarily motor in the head and neck. CN IX provides sensation to the external ear, auditory canal, tympanic membrane, posterior tongue, and pharynx, which can lead to a gag reflex. The nerve also innervates the carotid sinus baroreceptors and carotid body chemoreceptors, which monitor blood pressure and blood pH, PO_2, and PCO_2. The posterior taste buds detect bitter substances and are innervated by the special visceral efferent component. The production of saliva is performed by parasympathetic innervation of the nerve. Motor innervation to the uvula, pharynx, larynx (gag reflex), and esophagus is performed by CN X. Parasympathetic activities in the neck, heart, lungs, and abdomen are performed by CN X.[16]

Accessory Nerve (XI). CN XI originates from the medulla and the upper cervical spinal cord to C5. Thus it is a visceral motor nerve of both cranial and spinal nerve roots that innervates the sternocleidomastoid and trapezius muscles. This nerve permits flexion of the neck, elevation of the shoulders, and rotation of the head contralaterally.[14,16]

Hypoglossal Nerve (XII). CN XII permits tongue movement. This innervates muscles of the tongue and extrinsic muscles (genioglossus, styloglossus, and hyoglossus). The tongue receives innervation from both hemispheres of the brain. The genioglossus, however, is innervated only by the contralateral side.[14,16]

Respiratory System

The placenta provides oxygen from the mother to the fetus and serves as the gas-exchange surface; thus this is the component to deliver oxygen as lung respiration is not occurring. Oxygenated blood leaves the placenta through the umbilical vein passing into the ductus venous and then into the inferior vena cava on its way to the right atrium. Deoxygenated blood enters the umbilical arteries from the iliac arteries and returns to the placenta. The lungs have very low blood flow because respiration is not yet occurring.

Formation of the respiratory tract begins around 22 days in utero with the development of the trachea, lungs, bronchi, and alveoli. The developmental process is divided into five stages: embryonic, pseudoglandular, canalicular, saccular, and alveolar. Complete maturation of the lungs occurs around age 8. The embryonic stage occurs between 3 and 6 weeks. The primitive foregut endoderm gives rise to the respiratory diverticulum posterior to the pharynx. After elongation, the endoderm becomes the trachea and esophagus. The caudal end of the trachea bifurcates into the branchial buds beginning morphogenesis for development of the bronchopulmonary segment of the mature lung. The pseudoglandular stage occurs between 5 and 17 weeks. At this stage tertiary bronchial buds continue morphogenesis to form the initial 20 generations of the respiratory airways. This stage ends with the development of the terminal bronchioles. The canalicular stage occurs between 16 and 25 weeks. At this stage formation of the acinus is composed of respiratory bronchioles. The bronchioles have three to six alveolar ducts. The saccular stage lasts from 24 weeks to birth. Saccules develop as clusters of growing airspaces enlarging the gas-exchange surface of the developing lungs. Capillaries enter the thin saccule walls constructed of type I pneumocytes forming the blood-air barrier by sharing a basement membrane. Surfactant production, needed to reduce surface tension of alveoli, begins at 24 weeks' gestation and is sufficient at approximately 32 weeks to prevent collapse of the alveoli (atelectasis). During the alveolar stage, the sacculi increase in size and develop into alveoli after septation. The alveoli increase in both number and size until age 8.[18]

There are anatomical differences in the respiratory systems between the child and the adult. Neonates prefer breathing through their nose, and the narrow nasal passages are prone to blockage by secretions. As mentioned, the head and occiput of the infant and child are larger relative to body size, compared with adults, which can complicate patient positioning. Additionally, the tongue is larger in children in relation to the oral cavity, and many children have enlarged tonsils (Fig. 7.1) that can cause clinically significant airway and respiratory issues. In the neck, the larynx is positioned higher and more anterior at the level of C3 to C4 versus lower in the adult (C4 to C6), and the epiglottis is stiff, long, and U shaped. It is traditionally believed the larynx is funnel shaped and that the narrowest part of the upper airway is the cricoid cartilage. This has been recently challenged stating the larynx is cylindrical and contains the narrowest portion of the upper airway at the glottis, as in the adult population. The cricoid cartilage is the narrowest solid portion of the upper airway.[1] In the chest, the carina of the child is slightly higher at T3 to T4 versus at T4 to T5 in adults. The carina is the point of bifurcation of the trachea into the left bronchus and straighter, wider, and shorter right bronchus leading to the lungs. The diameter of the lower airways in infants and children is narrower than adults, which, when subjected to inflammation, mucus collection, edema, and bronchospasm, can result in obstruction (Fig. 7.2). The chest wall is more compliant with horizontal ribs and through the first year of life has a low percentage of slow-twitch, fatigue-resistant, type I muscle fibers.

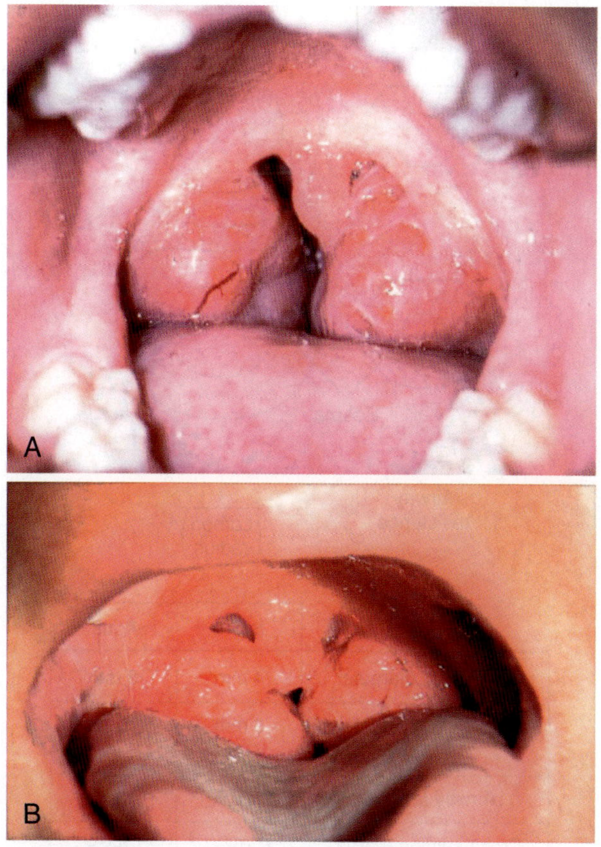

• **Fig. 7.1** (A–B) Enlarged tonsils. (Courtesy Mark Saxen, DDS, PhD)

Breathing occurs through a cycle of inspiratory and expiratory events. Inspiration is initiated when the diaphragm contracts creating an increase in thoracic and lung volume. This creates negative intrathoracic pressure pulling air into the lungs because of the creation of a pressure gradient between the atmosphere and the alveoli. Expiration is normally passive via the elastic recoil of the lungs and chest wall with assistance of some sustained contraction of the diaphragm and upper airway muscles and narrowing of the glottis. Ventilation can be enhanced during exercise by abdominal, upper airway, chest accessory, and intercostal muscles.[19,20]

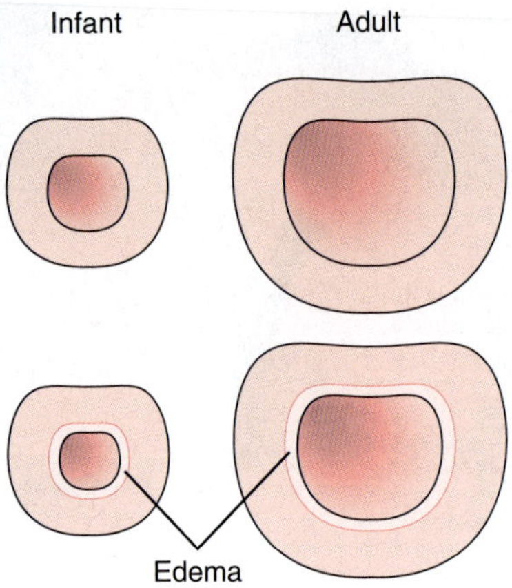

Airway resistance or $R \propto \dfrac{1}{\left(\text{Lumen radius}\right)^4}$

	Infant	Adult
Airway diameter	4 mm	8 mm
Airway diameter with edema	3 mm	7 mm
Airway resistance	↑ 16 x	↑ 3 x
Cross-sectional area	↓ 75%	↓ 44%

• **Fig. 7.2** Airway Narrowing Differences. (Redrawn from King C, Rappaport LD. Emergent endotracheal intubation. In: King C, Henretig FM, eds. *Textbook of Pediatric Emergency Procedures*. 2nd ed. Philadelphia: Lippincott Williams & Wilkins; 2008. Modified from Cote CJ, Todres ID. The pediatric airway. In: Cote CJ, Ryan JF, Todres ID, et al, eds. *A Practice of Anesthesia for Infants and Children*. 2nd ed. Philadelphia: WB Saunders: 1993.)

TABLE 7.2 Vital Signs by Age

Age	Heart Rate (beats/min)	Blood Pressure[b] (mm Hg)	Respiratory Rate[c] (breaths/min)
Premature	120–205[a]	60–76/31–45	40–70
Neonate	100–205[a]	67–84/35–53	35–55
Infant	100–180	72–104/37–56	30–53
Toddler	98–140	86–106/42–63	22–37
Preschooler	80–120	89–112/46–72	20–29
School-aged child	75–118	97–120/57–80	18–25
Adolescent	60–100	110–131/64–83	12–20

Normal Vital Signs According to Age

[a]In sleep, heart rates may be significantly lower, but if perfusion is maintained, no intervention is required.

[b]A blood pressure cuff should cover approximately two-thirds of the arm; too small a cuff yields spuriously high pressure readings, and too large a cuff yields spuriously low pressure readings. Values are systolic/diastolic and assume 50th percentile for height for children 1 year and older.

[c]The respiratory rate is expected to increase in the presence of fever and stress.

Modified from Hazinski MF. Children are different. In: Hazinski MF, ed. *Nursing Care of the Critically Ill Child.* 3rd ed. Mosby; 2013:1-18.

Breathing is controlled by neural and chemoreceptor interaction. Respiratory neurons are located in the medulla, reticular formation, and pons. The medulla has the dorsal respiratory group (DRG) and ventral respiratory group (VRG) neurons. The DRG uses cranial nerves IX and X to drive rhythmic breathing and is primarily involved during inspiration. The nerves of afferent fibers consist of mechanoreceptors from the airway (including the lungs), heart, and peripheral arterial chemoreceptors. The DRG also provides inspiratory drive to the phrenic nerve and potentially intercostal motor neurons. The VRG is responsible for active expiration during periods of high activity (e.g., exercise). The pons contains both inspiratory and expiratory neurons. The respiratory neurons in the pons are termed the pontine respiratory group or pneumotaxic center, which inhibits inspiration to a degree, and the apneustic center, which stimulates inspiration via apneusis (apnea with deep prolonged inspiration) or by apneustic breathing (slow rhythmic breathing with an increase in inspiratory retention).[19,20] Importantly, respiratory rate (breaths/min) differs greatly based on age (Table 7.2): neonate (50 ± 10); 6 months (30 ± 5); 12 months to 3 years (24 ± 6); 5 years (23 ± 5); 9 years (20 ± 5); 12 years (18 ± 5); adult (12 ± 3).[21]

The central chemoreceptors in the medulla and peripheral chemoreceptors participate in alveolar ventilation by monitoring pH or PO_2 and PCO_2. The central receptors located on the ventrolateral medulla are sensitive to CO_2 via changes in the hydrogen ion concentration (pH) in the CSF. Increases in the PCO_2 (decreased pH) cause increased ventilation, which eliminates CO_2 and returns the CSF pH to the normal range. The peripheral chemoreceptors (carotid and aortic bodies) are located at the bifurcation of the common carotid artery and around the aortic arch. Sensory nerve fibers travel from the carotid arch body to the brain stem via the glossopharyngeal nerve and from aortic bodies through the vagus nerve. These bodies are sensitive to low levels of arterial oxygen ($PaO_2 < 60$ mm Hg). This low oxygen level is called hypoxemia and stimulates an increase in breathing (with the exception of newborns and premature infants). Individuals with elevated arterial CO_2 levels caused by chronic diseases resulting in hypercapnia are reliant on the peripheral receptor response to low PaO_2 to provide the drive to breathe.[19,20]

Total lung capacity (TLC) is the maximum volume the lungs can hold. The TLC is divided into various components (Fig. 7.3).

Sustained respiratory muscle tension makes the thorax stiffer in infants and young children by several mechanisms maintaining functional residual capacity (FRC). Thus the FRC in infants is dynamically determined and therefore is not a fixed amount. Lung volumes are related to body size, which is relatively constant in healthy school-aged children to adulthood. Patients with asthma/chronic obstructive lung disease or restrictive lung disease (e.g., fibrosis) have decreased forced expiratory volume relative to healthy individual. The forced expiratory volume in 1 second (FEV1 test) can be measured by spirometry. Those with obstructive lung diseases have decreased FEV1/FVC as opposed to those who have increased FEV1/FVC in restrictive lung disease.[19,20]

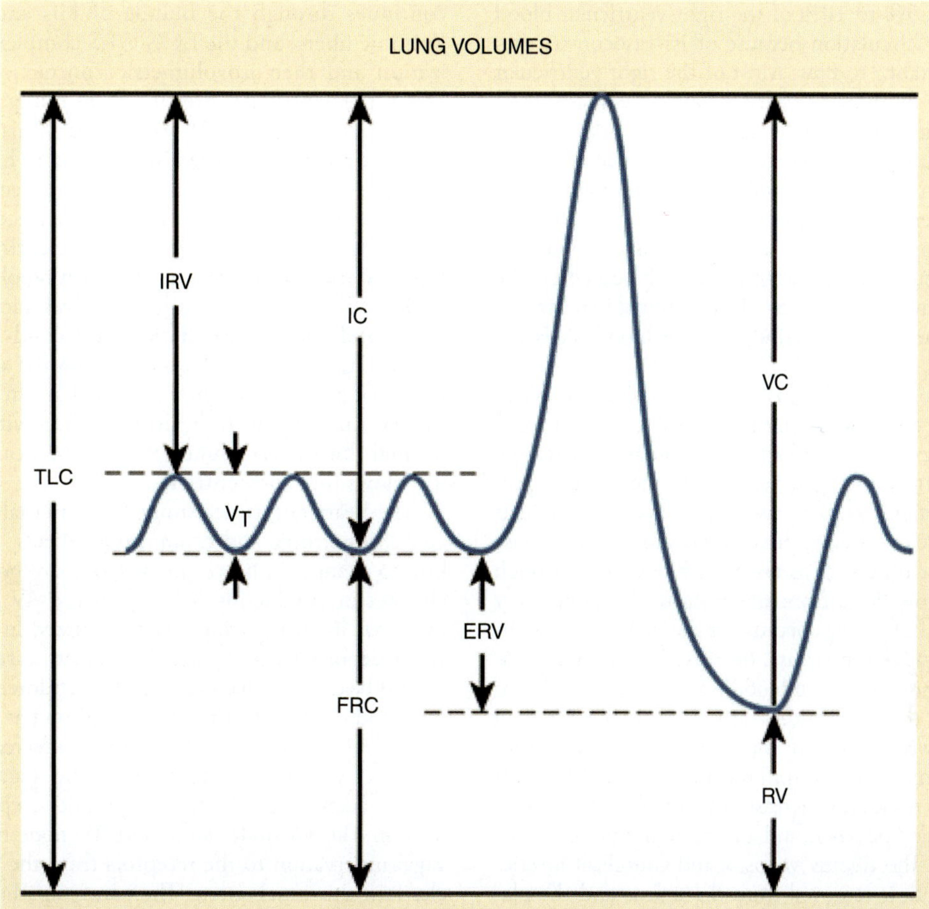

• **Fig. 7.3** Respiratory Physiology. Expiratory Reserve Volume (ERV) = volume expired after expiration of tidal volume; Functional Residual Capacity (FRC) = ERV + RV, the amount that remains in lungs after normal expiration of tidal volume and in an upright position is approximately 50% of TLC in healthy children and young adults; Inspiratory Capacity = TV + IRV; Inspiratory Reserve Volume (IRV) = volume inspired beyond the tidal volume; Reserve Volume = Volume remaining in lungs after the amount that can be expired and in healthy children is approximately 25% of total lung capacity (TLC); Tidal Volume (TV) = volume of air expired and inspired with each normal breath; Vital Capacity/Forced Vital Capacity (FVC) = IRV+TV + ERV, the amount of air forcibly expired and inspired. (From Motoyama EK, Finder JD. *Smith's Anesthesia for Infants and Children*. 2021:28-77.e12. Copyright 2022.)

Cardiovascular System

The heart is the first organ to develop and become functional. The heart forms from mesoderm at about 18 to 19 days after fertilization. It initially begins as cardiogenic cords and then develops into tubes called the *endocardial tubes.* The tubes then fuse into a single tube, which at about day 22 differentiates into the truncus arteriosus, sinus venosus, primitive atrium, ventricle, superior and inferior vena cava, base aorta, and bulbus cordis. At 4 weeks the heart begins pumping blood through vessels. Septa inside the heart develop around 4 to 7 weeks dividing the heart into separate ventricles and atria. The semilunar and atrioventricular valves form between 5 and 9 weeks.[22,23]

In utero, the placenta provides oxygen to the fetus as the lungs are not performing functional gas exchange, and therefore the majority of blood is shunted away from the high-resistance pulmonary circulation. The objective of the fetal circulation is then to receive oxygenated blood from the placenta, move the oxygen systemically to the tissues, and return carbon dioxide and waste products to the placenta. The placenta is not as efficient as the lungs in exchange of gases, so the umbilical vein receives less oxygen from the mother compared with the pulmonary veins after birth of the child. The umbilical vein delivers half the blood to the liver via the portal vein, and the remaining half passes through the ductus venosus to the inferior vena cava under high pressure. The portal vein is smaller, and blood primarily flows to the right lobe of the liver before moving on to the inferior vena cava, whereas the left lobe receives blood from the ductus venosus. The blood flow through the ductus is adjusted by a sphincter around the junction with the umbilical vein. During uterine contractions the vein sphincter can divert more blood to the liver so as not to overload the heart with blood. The inferior vena cava after attachment of the ductus venosus is a mixture of oxygenated blood from the placenta and deoxygenated blood from the fetal lower systemic circulation.[23,24]

Upon reaching the right atrium, oxygenated inferior vena cava blood is primarily diverted through the foramen ovale to the left atrium. Superior vena cava blood generally flows to the right ventricle. Only about 5% to 10% of the right ventricular blood enters the pulmonary circulation because of its vasoconstriction resulting in high resistance to flow. Most of the right ventricular blood passes from the pulmonary artery through the ductus arteriosus to the aorta. The right ventricle has a higher workload than the left ventricle in utero. The patent ductus arteriosus (PDA) attaches to the aorta proximal or distal to the subclavian artery. Blood from the left ventricle is approximately 65% to 70% saturated with oxygen upon reaching the aorta. The aortic blood then feeds the systemic circulation. About 65% of the blood enters the placenta after leaving the aorta by way of the internal iliac arteries to the umbilical arteries. The remainder of the blood feeds the fetal tissues.[23,24]

A transition in blood flow begins around the time of birth. Pulmonary vascular resistance decreases with a concomitant increase in chest wall expansion and an increase in arterial oxygen. Blood flow increases from the right ventricle to the lungs as pulmonary vascular resistance is now lower than systemic vascular resistance. The increase in systemic vascular resistance and decrease in pulmonary vascular resistance reverses the blood flow through the PDA, so blood now flows from the aorta to the pulmonary artery. Eventually the PDA closes because of the increase in vascular oxygen tension, bradykinin release, decrease in placental prostaglandins (PGE1), and decrease in blood flow through the PDA. The ductus becomes the ligamentum arteriosum. The foramen ovale begins to close when the valve is pressed against the septum secundum as the volume of blood from the lungs to the left atrium and systemic vascular resistance increases. It has been shown that up to 30% of the general pediatric and adult population has a patent foramen ovale.[25] The ductus venosus and umbilical arteries close when the placenta is removed from the uterus and the placenta no longer supplies blood flow through the umbilical vein. The left ventricle wall begins to thicken after the low-resistance placental vascular bed is removed from the circulation, and it now must move blood through the entire systemic circulation with increased vascular resistance rather than just the upper body. Consequently, because of high neonate metabolic demands and increased systemic vascular resistance after birth, the stroke volume (SV) and heart rate increase and thus increase the cardiac output (CO). The CO (corrected for body weight) declines after birth (350 mL/kg/min) over the first few months to 150 mL/kg/min and continues gradually declining, approaching that of an adult (75 mL/kg/min). Fetal hemoglobin production begins to decline (70% to 80%) as full-term birth approaches and by 6 months postpartum declines to less than 5%.[23,24]

The location of the pediatric heart changes with age. The newborn heart lays more horizontal with the apex at the fourth intercostal space, consumes approximately 40% of the lungs fields, and consumes a higher ratio of body mass. Over time with the increase in lung volume, the apex is depressed to the fifth intercostal space.[26]

Cardiac physiology of the child depends on the cardiac cycle (rate and rhythm) and CO (preload, contractility, and afterload). The heart rhythm is detected by the electrocardiogram (ECG). The electrical path through the heart begins at the sinoatrial (SA) node located in the right atrium near the vena cava entrance. Inward current allows discharge to occur, which is represented by the P wave on the ECG. The electrical current passes through the atria allowing depolarization and contraction. The ECG PR interval is the duration from the initiation of atrial depolarization/contraction to the initiation of depolarization at the atrioventricular (AV) node. The current then continues through the bundle of His and branches into the Purkinje fibers, and the ECG QRS complex represents depolarization and then isovolumetric contraction of the ventricles. When the ventricular pressure from filling becomes larger than the atrial pressure, the AV valves close. This is the first sound on auscultation and is labeled S_1. Eventually, because of ventricular contraction, the ventricular pressure exceeds that of the aorta and pulmonary artery, and blood is ejected into the vessels. Finally, the QT interval represents the entire depolarization and repolarization of the ventricles. Upon repolarization of the ventricles (T wave) the semilunar valves (aortic and pulmonic) close, and, upon auscultation, a second heart sound (S_2) is heard. During ventricular contraction the atria are filling, when the atrial pressure becomes greater than the ventricular pressure the AV valves open. In healthy children with thin chest walls, a normal third heart sound (S_3) may be heard as the blood rapidly flows into the ventricles.[27]

The heart rate is determined by internal and external factors and chronotropic and dromotropic effects. Chronotropic effects lead to changes in heart rate, whereas dromotropic effects lead to changes in conduction velocity in the AV node. Internally the heart has its own pacing system initiated in the SA node, which varies depolarization by age. In infants heart rate ranges from 70 to 160 beats/min, decreases in older children to 70 to 110 beats/min, and declines further into adulthood at 60 to 100 beats/min (Table 7.2). Externally the heart is affected by the autonomic nervous system and hormones. The parasympathetic system releases acetylcholine at the muscarinic receptors to slow depolarization. The SA node, atria, and AV node have parasympathetic vagal innervation to the receptors from the medulla. The ventricles lack this innervation. The parasympathetic negative chronotropic effect decreases heart rate by reducing the speed of phase 4 depolarization, so there are fewer action potentials per unit time. The negative dromotropic effects reduce conduction velocity from the atria through the AV node to increase the PR interval. The sympathetic accelerator nerve (cardiosplanchnic nerves) originating in the cervical ganglion of the sympathetic trunk of the sympathetic system release norepinephrine, which acts on the B1 receptors and acts during times of stress or activity. Positive chronotropic effects increase heart rate by elevating the rate of phase 4 depolarization and lead to more depolarizations per unit time, and positive dromotropic effects increase the conduction velocity via the AV node, thus reducing the PR interval. Norepinephrine and epinephrine released from sympathetic postganglionic fibers and the adrenal glands act on the SA node to increase heart rate. Thyroid hormones (T_3 and T_4) can increase the heart rate. T_3 may have a unique genomic effect where it directly binds to the cardiomyocyte nucleus, which regulates transcription to exert its effect.[26–28]

Blood pressure is determined by the formula: CO multiplied by systemic vascular resistance. CO is the amount of blood the heart pumps in 1 minute, which is crucial for delivering oxygen and nutrients to tissues and removing waste products. The formula for cardiac output is $CO = SV \times HR$, where SV stands for stroke volume (the amount of blood pumped with each heartbeat) and HR stands for heart rate (the number of heartbeats per minute) (see Table 7.3).

SV is defined as the volume of blood ejected from a ventricle with each beat. It is determined by the equation SV = end-diastolic volume − end-systolic volume and consists of three components: preload, contractility, and afterload. Preload is the end-diastolic volume and is correlated with right atrial pressure. Contractility is

TABLE 7.3 Pediatric Cardiovascular Definitions

Term	Definition	Formula
Blood pressure (BP)	The force exerted by circulating blood on the walls of blood vessels.	BP = CO × SVR
Cardiac output (CO)	The volume of blood ejected from the heart in 1 minute. Essential for tissue perfusion, delivering oxygen and nutrients, and carrying waste products to excretion sites.	CO = SV × HR
Stroke volume (SV)	The amount of blood ejected by the heart in one contraction.	—
Heart rate (HR)	The number of heartbeats per minute.	—
Systemic vascular resistance (SVR)	The resistance offered by the systemic blood vessels.	—

the force produced when cardiac muscle contracts from a defined length. It can be estimated by the ejection fraction, where ejection fraction = stroke volume/end-diastolic volume. Contractility is decreased in neonates and young children compared with adults because of fewer contractile components and increased connective tissue. Therefore they have reduced ability to adjust SV. Afterload is the resistance the ventricle pumps against when ejecting blood and is influenced by arterial blood pressure and vascular tone. Afterload applies to the pressure from the aorta for the left ventricle to pump against and pulmonary artery for the right ventricle to pump against. Thus high blood pressure increases afterload and decreases SV. Drugs that lead to significantly elevated tachycardia (1) will not permit filling of the ventricles with an adequate end-diastolic volume reducing CO, and (2) reduce left ventricle coronary artery blood flow during diastole and elevate myocardial oxygen demand, which may result in ischemia of cardiac muscle. Medications for patients with heart failure may reduce the heart rate, increase end-diastolic volume, and increase CO.[24,26,27]

Conclusion

The anatomy and physiology of children differ from that of adults. However, as the child matures, the anatomy and physiology become similar to that of adults. It is important for the pediatric dentist to recollect the changes from embryologic to term neonate to childhood as pathology may be correlated to these changes. Providers who choose to sedate children for care or treat children with health conditions outside the norm should be familiar with head, neck, and cardiopulmonary changes during childhood growth and development.

Visit eBooks.Health.Elsevier.com to see full list of references.

PART 2

A Clinical Guide to Treating the Pediatric Patient

8

Infant Oral Health and the Toddler: Ages 0 to 3

KARIN WEBER-GASPARONI

CHAPTER OUTLINE

Introduction

In 1986 the American Academy of Pediatric Dentistry (AAPD) adopted a position on infant oral health, recommending that the first visit occur within 6 months of the eruption of the first primary tooth.[1] This bold recommendation was based on the recognition that many 3-year-old children had already experienced dental caries and, more troubling, that those who had experienced caries remained susceptible to future decay, even with subsequent preventive intervention.[2] Before the adoption of this policy, physicians claimed responsibility for the oral health of the child younger than 36 months of age.[3] The rationale, although somewhat circuitous, assumed that children visited a physician at regular intervals soon after birth but did not see a dentist until later in life. Despite efforts by the medical profession to involve pediatric primary care providers in delivering oral healthcare services to young children, few practitioners in remote areas have taken on this role. To address this gap, it is essential to enhance education on preventive oral healthcare in medical schools and residency programs, expand access to continuing education programs nationwide, advocate for policy changes to ensure reimbursement for pediatric oral healthcare services, and foster stronger collaboration between dentistry and medicine.

Dental caries in pediatric patients continues to be a serious health problem. National data on dental caries among children and adolescents in the United States, collected from 2017 to March 2020 before the COVID-19 pandemic, reveal that 22% of children aged 2 to 5 years have experienced dental caries in their primary teeth. This prevalence increases significantly in older age groups, with 48.1% of children aged 6 to 11 and 56% of adolescents aged 12 to 19 having experienced dental caries in their permanent teeth.[4] Therefore it remains to be seen whether the medical community involvement and interventions can effect a change in that pattern.

Implementing a major shift in health philosophy, such as instituting infant oral health visits to dentists, is not without problems. Some dentists remain reluctant to see these young children because of expectations of negative behavior, complex dental needs, a lack of understanding of preventive opportunities, and concern about reimbursement for procedures.[5]

The purpose of this chapter is to describe the objectives, rationale, and procedures for infant oral health. The goal would be that dentists would gain a better knowledge of these practices and become more comfortable in treating patients in this age group.

Infant Oral Health: Definition, Rationale, and Goals

Infant oral health is defined as the child's first dental visit occurring within 6 months after the eruption of the first primary tooth or no later than 12 months of age.[6] Infant oral health serves as the foundation for interventions designed to prevent common pediatric oral diseases and conditions such as dental caries, oral injuries, and malocclusion. Furthermore, infant oral health fosters the development of a strong relationship among the infant, their family, and the dental team, significantly increasing the likelihood that the child will enjoy a lifetime free from oral disease. Initiating oral healthcare during infancy is ideal for several reasons: dental caries have not had time to develop, detrimental habits have not yet formed, and a full range of preventive dental measures is available.[7] Infant oral health provides a unique opportunity to start fresh, with the overall goal of maintaining good oral health throughout life. Early oral examinations, combined with oral health risk assessments and anticipatory guidance, are effective methods of true primary prevention, as they facilitate the timely identification and management of oral health issues, which not only proves cost-effective but also leads to satisfactory outcomes. Children who receive prevention-focused dental examinations before the age of 2 are more likely to require fewer dental treatments in the future compared with those who have their initial visit after age 2.[8] At no other point in life will the dentist have the same level of parental concern, attention, and compliance. The goals of infant oral health can be summarized by the following six tenets.

Break the Cycle of Early Childhood Caries

Although early childhood caries is relatively inexpensive to prevent, it is a pandemic disease among select populations, including very young children of low-income, racial, and ethnic minority groups. The prevalence of early childhood caries in disadvantaged groups in the United States can be as high as 70%.[9] A global systematic review showed that almost half of preschool children are affected by early childhood caries.[10] Untreated cases of early childhood caries can lead to potentially life-threatening infection, pain, failure to thrive, learning difficulties, hospitalizations, and emergency department visits.[1,11] Early childhood caries progresses rapidly, and by the time treatment is sought, the disease can be extensive enough to warrant the use of sedation or general anesthesia. Consequently, the overall costs to treat early childhood caries are quite high.[12] Of concern is the cyclic nature of early childhood caries, in which children afflicted remain at risk throughout childhood, even when preventive services are available.[2]

Disrupt the Acquisition of Harmful Microflora

Research suggests that children are inoculated with caries-initiating bacteria by vertical transmission from caretakers, primarily mothers. The relationship between maternal salivary levels of mutans streptococci (MS) and the risk of infant infection seems to be relatively strong because mothers with high levels of MS tend to have children with high levels, whereas those with low levels tend to have children with low levels.[13] If a child's caretaker harbors virulent organisms, then transmission via kissing, sharing food and eating utensils, or other contact can occur and initiate the caries process.[14] This process is described in detail in Chapter 12. On the plus side of this acquisition model is the potential to prevent transmission by reducing the caretaker's bacterial inoculum through dental treatment, increased oral health literacy, improved oral health dietary and hygiene habits,[15] and, to a lesser extent, the use of antibacterial chemotherapeutic agents.[16] Recent preventive strategies emphasize the importance of maintaining a child's favorable oral health environment and healthy biofilm by establishing a low-sugar diet, adequate fluoride exposure, and effective oral hygiene practices.[17]

Prenatal counseling coupled with maternal oral health and infant oral health forms the chain for prevention of bacterial acquisition. Hormonal changes during pregnancy can increase expectant mothers' vulnerability to preventable oral health issues, including gingivitis and tooth decay. As a result, perinatal oral healthcare plays a critical role in ensuring that comprehensive and accessible oral health services are available to expectant mothers and their infants. This approach helps enhance oral health outcomes for both mothers and infants while addressing disparities in access to care. It is crucial for oral healthcare to begin as early as possible for all females of childbearing age, allowing for the identification and management of potential risk factors through education, prevention, and early interventions aimed at both mothers and their children.[18]

Manage the Risk/Benefit of Habits

Infancy gives rise to many habits, and those affecting the oral cavity are described later in this chapter in the section "Nonnutritive Sucking Habits." Traditionally, dentists were usually called on only to deal with lingering habits in older children that were causing deleterious dental problems. The opportunity to provide counseling to parents during infant oral health visits allows the dentist to enter the habit continuum and work with the family to mitigate deleterious effects and transition the child out of the habit. The goal would be a gentle waning of the habit, which would negate the need to correct habit-related malocclusions.

Establish a Dental Home

The concept of a dental home is defined by the AAPD as an "ongoing relationship between the dentist and the patient, inclusive of all aspects of oral health care delivered in a safe, culturally-sensitive, individualized, comprehensive, continuous, accessible, coordinated, compassionate, and patient- and family-centered way regardless of race, ethnicity, religion, sexual or gender identity, medical status, family structure, or financial circumstances. The dental home should be established no later than 12 months of age to help children, and their families institute a lifetime of optimal oral health."[19] A dental home offers a comprehensive assessment of oral diseases and conditions, evidence-based oral healthcare that encompasses both acute and preventive services according to AAPD periodicity schedules, and personalized preventive programs tailored to caries and periodontal disease risk assessments, while providing anticipatory guidance, management of acute and chronic oral pain and infections, long-term follow-up for acute dental trauma, prevention, diagnosis, and treatment of oral diseases, as well as referrals to dental specialists when necessary.[20] The dental home concept is derived from the American Academy of Pediatrics (AAP) definition of a medical home.[21] Our physician colleagues understand the benefits of establishing a doctor-family relationship. Care is initiated with nonthreatening preventive services, and if an emergency occurs, parents know where to turn. If questions arise, reliable and trusted information is available, and if treatment is needed, a firm foundation of trust has been built. As with the medical home, the early establishment of a dental home has the potential to provide more effective preventive services and less costly dental care when compared with dental care provided in emergency care facilities or hospitals.[22] In a systematic review, authors reported that establishing a dental home early in life can be particularly crucial for children whose caregivers have low health literacy or face socioeconomic challenges as well as for those generally at high risk for dental issues.[23] Research has shown that early preventive oral healthcare targeted to high-risk populations can lower overall dental costs and yield better oral health outcomes, making the use of a caries risk assessment tool to guide the delivery of preventive interventions to children at the highest dental caries risk both economically attractive and beneficial.[24] Reports of preschool-aged, Medicaid-enrolled children have shown that the earlier a preventive dental visit occurred, the more likely these children were to use subsequent preventive services and experience lower dentally related costs.[25] In addition, the number and cost of dental procedures among high-risk children have been reported to be less for children seen at an earlier age versus later, confirming the fact that the sooner a child is seen by a dentist, the less treatment needs they are likely to have in the future.[26]

Impart Optimal Fluoride Protection

Fluoride remains dentistry's best preventive tool, and optimal fluoride exposure is the foundation of early intervention (see Chapter 14). Community water fluoridation is a beneficial and cost-effective approach that is accessible to entire communities, including those at high risk for cavities, and remains a key strategy in the primary prevention of caries.[27] Systematic reviews support the efficacy of fluoride toothpaste and in-office fluoride varnish applications as effective measures for early childhood caries prevention.[28,29] The daily use of fluoride toothpaste initiated immediately after the eruption of the first tooth is regarded as the best clinical preventive practice for early childhood caries.[28] The AAPD recognizes that drinking fluoridated water and brushing with fluoridated toothpaste are perhaps the *most effective* method in reducing dental caries prevalence in children.[27]

Arming the Parents Through Anticipatory Guidance

Parental involvement is a cornerstone of child healthcare, especially in the realm of infant oral health, which relies heavily on protective factors at home. In this context, parents become co-therapists. Dentists should empower parents not only to implement effective preventive measures at home but also to anticipate the oral health changes that occur as their child grows. This is achieved through anticipatory guidance, a concept detailed later in this chapter.

Normal Findings

The dentist should expect to see a healthy oral cavity in most infants. Table 8.1 shows some common oral conditions of infants and their management. In addition, Chapter 19 addresses some uncommon pathologic conditions of infancy, including dental lamina cysts (Bohn nodules and Epstein pearls), congenital epuli, eruption cysts, and neuroectodermal tumors of infancy. It is important for the dentist to understand the normal head, neck, and oral presentations of an infant so that they are more likely to recognize abnormal presentations. These normal findings are described in Table 8.2, and more detailed information about pediatric physiology and anatomy can be found in Chapter 7.

Preparing for Your Patient

Office Readiness for Infant Oral Health

Infant care deviates from routine office practice in several ways. To increase efficiency, a significant part of the infant oral health visit is handled by auxiliary personnel (e.g., dental assistants, expanded function dental assistants, dental hygienists) under the direct supervision of the dentist, focusing on preventive and educational tasks.[20] Meanwhile, the dentist remains responsible for conducting examinations, diagnosing oral conditions, and creating treatment plans. It does not routinely require the same armamentarium that would be used for an older patient. The examination location can be in the operatory but can just as well be in a well-lit, comfortable conference room or play area. Radiographs are typically not required during most infant visits, except when assessing traumatic dental injuries, carious lesions, and/or abnormal tooth mobility, where they may be necessary for an accurate diagnosis.

A dental record is still required but may be abbreviated. However, the essentials of a medical and dental history, examination record, treatment plan, and progress note remain. Patient education brochures and other instructional material should be available for this particular age group. The dental team can be enlisted in developing the time, place, and protocol for in-office infant oral health visits. This allows the team the opportunity to use their knowledge to provide parental education and to work with small children, which is a joy for most pediatric dental personnel. Finally, in a busy office, the logistics of the infant dental appointment require some thought because it ties up auxiliaries and, if done outside the dental operatory area, necessitates a change in staff flow patterns.

Elements of the Infant Oral Health Visit

Diagnostic Process

The best way to envision the infant oral health visit is to compare it with the traditional medical model used for the diagnosis of disease. The medical model uses a stepwise approach beginning with a chief complaint, history, physical examination, differential diagnosis, and treatment plan. Infant oral health intervention assumes that the child has no oral disease but may be prone to disease due to risk behaviors such as high consumption of sugar-sweetened beverages or lack of fluoride. Conceptually, these risk factors will eventually lead to disease if not addressed. Conversely, if the risk factors are eliminated, the child will be free of disease.

In infant oral health, the chief complaint may be a generic interest in prevention. The infant oral examination is equivalent to the well-baby visit for oral health. The health history is replaced with a focused risk-based history aimed at predisposing factors for dental conditions. The patient examination looks for existing disease in addition to physical factors that predispose the child to oral disease. The differential diagnosis is replaced with a risk profile that is individualized to the child. Instead of a treatment plan, the family receives anticipatory guidance with directives to eliminate risk and impart protective factors. They are given measurable outcomes to determine progress toward wellness. Both of these factors make the parents a part of the therapeutic alliance. The recall interval is designed to give parents time to address risk and for the dentist to reassess progress, institute preventive measures if needed, and ensure that disease has not manifested.

One of the primary goals of infant oral health is to break the cycle of early childhood caries, which is a dental disease highly prevalent among preschool children, often remaining untreated in children under age 3, and significantly affecting their overall well-being.[30] Therefore it is crucial to ensure clinicians can adequately diagnose this dental disease. Early childhood caries is defined as "the presence of one or more decayed (noncavitated or cavitated lesions), missing (due to caries), or filled tooth surfaces in any primary tooth"[31] in a child under the age of six. The definition of severe early childhood caries is "1) any sign of smooth-surface caries in a child younger than three years of age, 2) from ages three through five, one or more cavitated, missing (due to caries), or filled smooth surfaces in primary maxillary anterior teeth, or 3) a decayed, missing, or filled score of greater than or equal to four (age three), greater than or equal to five (age four), or greater than or equal to six (age five)."[31]

TABLE 8.1 Infant Oral Pathology and Unusual Clinical Findings

Condition Description and Illustration	Clinical Findings and Management
Ankyloglossia (tongue-tie) 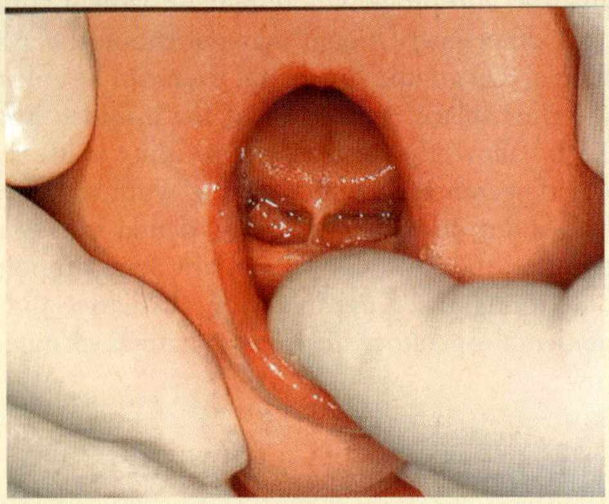	Prevalence reported to range from 2% (using unspecific classifications) to 20% (using Coryllos classification)[85] Coryllos classifications of tongue-tie: type 1, type 2, and type 3 Frenum may be short, thick, muscular or fibrotic May be associated with breastfeeding difficulties, failure to thrive, swallowing, articulation among other complications Frenotomy is a treatment option
Natal and neonatal teeth 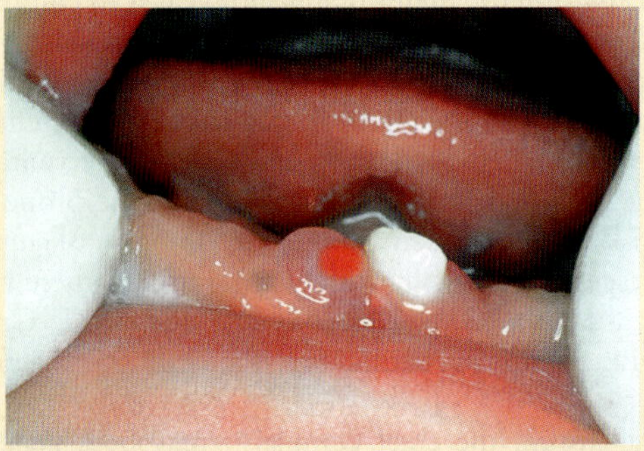	Natal teeth present at birth and neonatal present within 30 days of birth Worldwide prevalence of natal teeth is reported to be 34.55 per 10,000 (1 in 289 newborns), while neonatal 4.52 per 10,000 (1 in 2212 newborns)[86] 90% are primary; 10% supernumerary; 85% mandibular Extract supernumeraries; primary teeth left if not highly mobile Can be aspiration risk; nursing obstacle
Riga-Fede disease 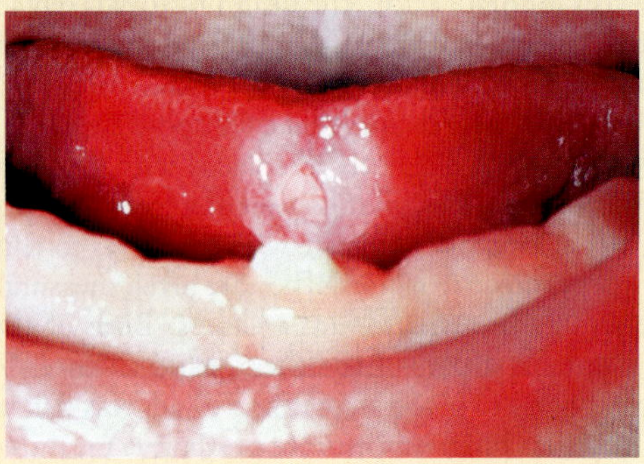	Traumatic ulcer of ventral surface of tongue from rubbing against lower incisors Incidence ranges of natal and neonatal teeth reported from 1:2000 and 1:3500[87] Natal teeth are three times more common than neonatal teeth Greater involvement of the lower incisors May cause active bleeding and discomfort Treatment options are observation, cessation of breastfeeding, or smoothing/removal of the offending tooth

Risk Assessment

The predentate infant presents with a clean slate in terms of acquired dental conditions and diseases, but as the child grows and expands their world, this changes. Considering risks that go beyond infectious disease and encompass trauma and injury, orthodontic problems, and compliance with oral hygiene and dietary practices helps maximize a child's opportunity to achieve good oral health. Risk assessment is defined as identification of factors known or believed to be associated with a condition or disease for purposes of further diagnosis, prevention, monitoring, or treatment. According to the AAPD guidelines, "risk assessment: 1. fosters the treatment of the disease process instead of treating the outcome of the disease. 2. allows an understanding of the disease factors for a specific patient and aids in individualizing preventive discussions. 3. individualizes, selects, and determines frequency of preventive and restorative treatment for a patient. 4. anticipates caries progression or stabilization."[2] An essential part of the infant oral health visit is an individualized review of risk factors, particularly those related to the development of early childhood caries. Caries risk assessment is "the clinical process of establishing the probability of an individual patient to develop caries lesions over a certain period of time or the likelihood that there will be a change in size or activity of lesions already present."[32] Taking into consideration that the etiology of early

TABLE 8.2 Elements of Head and Neck Examination of Infants

Structure	Diagnostic Technique	Normal Characteristics
Head	Visualization	Disproportionately large
Hair	Visualization	Thin and fine
Scalp	Visualization/palpation	Open fontanels
Temporomandibular joint	Palpation/manipulation	Short condyles/flat fossae
Skin	Visualization	Soft, smooth
Neck	Palpation	Weak musculature Soft airway cartilage
Lips	Visualization	Full, cupid's bow
Oral Cavity		
Dental arches	Visualization	Edentulous/tooth bulges
Frenula	Visualization	High placement on alveolus
Palate	Visualization	Prominent median raphe/rugae
Gingivae	Visualization	Pink, hydrated, flaccid around teeth

childhood caries is multifactorial and complex, current caries risk assessment models entail a combination of factors including diet, fluoride exposure, host susceptibility, and microflora analysis, and consideration of how these factors interact with social, cultural, and behavioral factors. More comprehensive models that include social, political, psychological, and environmental determinants of health are also available.[33–35] These multilevel conceptual models recognize the complex interplay of causal factors and describe their influences on oral health behaviors, dental disease rates, and oral health outcomes. Table 8.3 depicts a caries risk assessment form developed by the AAPD, which can be used by dental providers to identify risk factors for dental caries development in children from birth to 5 years of age.[2]

The parent or guardian is the historian for the child, and a thorough general health history is always of utmost importance. The focus of this section is on historical elements related to oral disease risk. eBox 8.1 depicts a risk assessment form for infant oral health.[36] Historical risk elements can be divided into perinatal factors, bacteria transmission, diet and nutrition, fluoride adequacy, oral hygiene, oral habits, injury prevention, and oral development. The clinician should combine the general health history responses with those focused on the risk of oral disease and protective factors for oral health, while balancing them against each other to assess a child's risk of developing early childhood caries. When used in combination, this will form an individualized historical risk profile for the child, which helps in determining preventive and treatment strategies as well as follow-up intervals.

Perinatal factors are important because of the attendant oral effects associated with premature birth. Although experts have concluded that prematurity does not predispose a child to an increased risk of dental caries,[37] some low-birth-weight children receive special diets, have hypoplastic dentitions,[38] and have developmental disabilities that place them at higher risk. The means of *bacteria transmission* from mother/caregiver to the infant and ways to avoid such transmission should be thoroughly discussed. *Diet and nutrition* questions should focus on breastfeeding, bottle and sippy-cup use and the transition to an open cup, frequency of sugar-sweetened beverages and snacks, and special diets. Another component of the infant risk assessment is a determination of *fluoride adequacy* and current oral hygiene practices. Fluoride adequacy refers to a consideration of whether the drinking water (community vs. bottled) provides optimal fluoride. It also addresses the effectiveness of fluoride dentifrice in reducing dental caries and the appropriate amount to decrease the risk of fluorosis. *Oral hygiene practices* are assessed by asking the parents how involved they currently are with cleansing of the oral structures. Such questioning should lead to a discussion of tooth-cleaning implements, timing, frequency, and positioning of the child for oral care and the amount of fluoride toothpaste used. The discussion of *oral habits* establishes a baseline for families and enables the dentist to counsel parents on the risks and benefits of behavioral habits throughout early childhood. Historical information on *injury prevention* moves beyond purely dental trauma to general health issues like play objects, electrical cords, home childproofing, and car seat use. Oral development is covered to assess the presence of teeth, eruptive disorders, and teething problems. Finally, the clinician evaluates the family's *social determinants of health* (e.g., caregiver oral health literacy and educational level, socioeconomic status, food insecurity), and assesses the presence of *clinical factors* (e.g., plaque, white spot lesions, enamel defects) known to place a child at a higher risk for developing early childhood caries.

Oral Examination, Proper Positioning, Toothbrush Prophylaxis, Assessment of Clinical Risk Factors, Fluoride Therapy, Normal Behavior and Development

The oral examination of the infant is a quick process but differs from the typical child examination in several ways:

- Use of a dental chair is unnecessary and the least preferred approach.
- The parent participates as a learner and immobilizer.
- Teaching about the oral cavity occurs during the examination process.
- The child may cry, which should be expected, and may be useful.

Children less than 30 months of age can usually only respond to simple commands such as "sit in the chair" or "open your mouth."[39] At this age they are entirely dependent on parents and have little verbal language. Typical fears of the 2-year-old child are strangers, loud sounds, sudden movement, and falling. Having the parents involved is critical because children in this group are typically very attached to parents. The preferred approach to the infant examination is the knee-to-knee position using gentle active restraint from the dentist and parent in which a parent and a dental provider sit facing each other (Fig. 8.1). Their knees should touch and, ideally, mesh slightly, creating a flat surface on which the child can rest. The infant initially is held facing the parent and then reclined onto the lap of the dentist. The parent has the infant's legs straddling their torso and uses their elbows to hold the child's feet in place. The parent is responsible for holding the child's hands, and the dentist stabilizes the child's head. The examination can occur wherever a suitable light source can be found. The closeness of the parent and provider may concern some parents and should be explained before the procedure begins.

TABLE 8.3 Caries Risk Assessment Form for 0- to 5-Year-Olds

Factors	High Risk	Moderate Risk	Low Risk
Risk factors, social/behavioral/medical			
Mother/primary caregiver has active dental caries	Yes		
Parent/caregiver has lifetime of poverty, low health literacy	Yes		
Child has frequent exposure (>3 times/day) between-meal sugar-containing snacks or beverages per day	Yes		
Child uses bottle or nonspill cup containing natural or added sugar frequently, between meals and/or at bedtime	Yes		
Child is a recent immigrant		Yes	
Child has special healthcare needs[a]		Yes	
Risk factors, clinical			
Child has visible plaque on teeth	Yes		
Child presents with dental enamel defects	Yes		
Protective factors			
Child receives optimally fluoridated drinking water or fluoride supplements			Yes
Child has teeth brushed daily with fluoridated toothpaste			Yes
Child receives topical fluoride from health professional			Yes
Child has dental home/regular dental care			Yes
Disease indicators[b]			
Child has noncavitated (incipient/white spot) caries lesions	Yes		
Child has visible caries lesions	Yes		
Child has recent restorations or missing teeth caused by caries	Yes		

[a]Practitioners may choose a different risk level based on specific medical diagnosis and unique circumstances, especially conditions that affect motor coordination or cooperation.
[b]While these do not cause caries directly or indirectly, they indicate presence of factors that do.
***Instructions**: Circle "Yes" that corresponds with those conditions applying to a specific patient. Use the circled responses to visualize the balance among risk factors, protective factors, and disease indicators. Use this balance or imbalance, together with clinical judgment, to assign a caries risk level of low, moderate, or high based on the preponderance of factors for the individual. Clinical judgment may justify the weighting of one factor (e.g., heavy plaque on the teeth) more than others.*
Overall assessment of the child's dental caries risk: High ❑ Moderate ❑ Low ❑
From American Academy of Pediatric Dentistry. Caries-risk assessment and management for infants, children, and adolescents. In: *The Reference Manual of Pediatric Dentistry.* American Academy of Pediatric Dentistry; 2024:306-312.

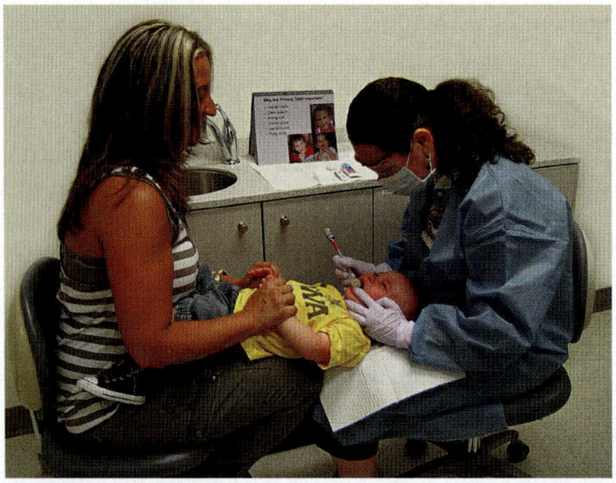

• **Fig. 8.1** Knee-to-Knee Clinical Examination Position for Dentist, Child, and Parent. Parent and dentist face each other with knees touching while parent holds child on lap with child facing parent. Parent carefully lays child in dentist's lap while holding child's hands.

During the examination (Video 8.1), which may take only seconds, the dentist has the opportunity to demonstrate oral hygiene and point out oral structures of importance. A toothbrush coronal polish, which involves using a toothbrush and toothpaste, is a simple procedure used to remove plaque from the surfaces of teeth of young children who cannot tolerate the use of a rotary rubber cup. It also serves as a means to demonstrate proper brushing techniques to caregivers of infants and toddlers.[40] Most infants will cry briefly during the examination, which often results in a wide-open mouth. Alternatively, a toothbrush handle can be used as a mouth prop while counting teeth and assessing soft tissues (e.g., gingival status, soft tissue abnormalities) and hard tissues (e.g., number of teeth present, tooth anomalies, previous dental trauma). Additionally, clinical factors that increase the risk of caries in young children, such as visible plaque, noncavitated/cavitated lesions, presence of restorations, and enamel defects, should be documented. Because of the child's young age, a complete oral cancer screening and occlusion examination are unlikely to be performed.

Applying fluoride varnish in the office is recommended, particularly for children at higher risk of developing early childhood caries. After the fluoride application, caregivers should be advised to avoid brushing the child's teeth or giving them crunchy or sticky foods for the remainder of the day to ensure the fluoride varnish is most effective.

It is important to set appropriate expectations for behavior before any intervention. Parents may need to be assured that crying is a normal response and is to be expected, even for a simple examination at this age. At the completion of the examination, the child is returned to the parent, who can cuddle and console the child as needed. Children of this age are more likely to have seen a physician for regular visits, so delays in cognitive, physical, emotional, and gross motor development are usually known by parents before the first dental visit. However, dentists should be familiar with developmental milestones for children from birth to age 3 years, such as language, social interactions, and gross/fine motor skills (Table 8.4). This knowledge helps in recognizing potential developmental concerns early, advising families on the need for medical evaluations when problems are noted and/or making appropriate referrals to therapeutic services. Additionally, understanding these milestones makes it easier to relate to child behaviors and abilities when providing anticipatory guidance to parents.

Caries Management Protocol for 1- to 2-Year-Olds

The AAPD has developed caries management protocols, with the objective of assisting providers in the decisions regarding individualized treatments. These protocols are based on the patients' caries risk level, age, social, environmental, and economic factors as well as parental compliance with recommended preventive strategies. This aids practitioners in determining the types and frequency of diagnostic, preventive, and restorative care for dental caries management. Such protocols increase the probability of successful and cost-effective treatments. An example of a caries management protocol for children 1 to 2 years of age is shown in Table 8.5.[2]

Anticipatory Guidance

Anticipatory guidance is defined as proactive counseling that addresses the significant physical, emotional, psychological, and developmental changes that will occur in children during the interval between health supervision visits. It presumes that developmental information should cover the period until the next health supervision visit. eBox 8.2 lists anticipatory guidance topics for children under 36 months and the knowledge base needed for each area. Anticipatory guidance is the complement to a risk assessment. It addresses protective factors aimed at preventing oral health problems. An example of anticipatory guidance would be a discussion on ambulation of an infant with a warning about possible tooth trauma that often occurs as the infant learns to stand and walk. Topics to address in this age group include oral development, fluoride adequacy, nonnutritive habits, diet and nutrition, oral hygiene, and injury prevention.[36] These six areas capture the major concerns related to the oral conditions of dental caries, periodontal disease, trauma, and malocclusion. Anticipatory guidance is crucial for improving oral health behaviors and reducing the risk of early childhood caries. It should consider the family's social determinants of health, providing caregivers with practical and realistic strategies to effectively enhance their children's oral health. An example of a basic checklist of anticipatory guidance recommendations for

TABLE 8.4 Selected Developmental Characteristics of the Child Aged 6 Months to 3 Years

6–9 Months	12–13 Months	24 Months+
Intellectual Development		
Opens for a spoon	Copies sounds and actions	3- to 4-word sentences
Imitates actions of adults	Understands simple commands	Puts toys in groups
Turns to locate sounds	Tries to accomplish simple acts	Names five body parts
Gross/Fine Motor Skills		
Rolls over	Stands with hand held	Scribbles; draws shapes
Becomes able to sit independently	Sits without support	Kicks/throws ball
Picks up objects with fingers	Feeds self raisins	Puts on/takes off clothes
Psychological Development		
Laughs and squeals with delight	Shows affection to adults	Changeable feelings
Screams if annoyed	Fear of strangers	Recognizes emotions
Dental implications	Fear of separation	Understands commands
Needs physical support	Sippy cup use	Prone to falls/trauma
Can hold bottle alone		
Physiologic Height (75th percentile)		
Boys = 69.7–74 cm	77.7 cm	89.9 cm
Girls = 67.8–72.4 cm	76.3 cm	88.7 cm
Weight (75th percentile)		
Boys = 8.49–9.88 kg	10.91 kg	13.44 kg
Girls = 7.83–9.24 kg	10.23 kg	12.74 kg
Pulse (90th percentile)		
120 beats/min	120 beats/min	110 beats/min
Respiration (50th percentile)		
30 breaths/min	28 breaths/min	25 breaths/min
Blood Pressure		
105/67 mm Hg	105/69 mm Hg	106/68 mm Hg

infants that can be added to for unique situations is provided in Table 8.6 and discussed as follows.[41]

Oral and dental development

Parents and caregivers should receive anticipatory guidance on what constitutes a normal, healthy oral cavity, which may include discussions on oral facial development, eruption pattern, tooth morphology, spacing, and occlusion. This knowledge enables them to identify any deviations, such as growth delays, tooth abnormalities, traumatic injuries, the presence of cavities, or poor oral hygiene. Chapter 2 discusses the child's oral and dental development in more details.

TABLE 8.5 Example of a Caries Management Pathways for 0- to 5-Year-Olds

Risk Category	Diagnostics	PREVENTIVE INTERVENTIONS: Fluoride	Dietary Counseling	Sealants	Restorative Interventions
Low risk	• Recall every 6 to 12 months • Radiographs every 12 to 24 months	• Drink optimally fluoridated water • Twice daily brushing with fluoridated toothpaste	Yes	Yes	• Surveillance
Moderate risk	• Recall every 6 months • Radiographs every 6 to 12 months	• Drink optimally fluoridated water (alternatively, take fluoride supplements with fluoride-deficient water supplies) • Twice daily brushing with fluoridated toothpaste • Professional topical treatment every 6 months	Yes	Yes	• Active surveillance of noncavitated (white spot) caries lesions • Restore cavitated or enlarging caries lesions
High risk	• Recall every 3 months • Radiographs every 6 months	• Drink optimally fluoridated water (alternatively, take fluoride supplements with fluoride-deficient water supplies) • Twice daily brushing with fluoridated toothpaste • Professional topical treatment every 3 months • Silver diamine fluoride on cavitated lesions	Yes	Yes	• Active surveillance of noncavitated (white spot) caries lesions • Restore cavitated or enlarging caries lesions • Interim therapeutic restorations (ITR) may be used until permanent restorations can be placed

Notes for caries management pathways table:

Twice daily brushing: Parental supervision of a "smear" amount of fluoridated toothpaste for children under age 3, pea-sized amount for children ages 3 through 5.

Surveillance: Periodic monitoring for signs of caries progression; active surveillance: active measures by parents and oral health professionals to reduce cariogenic environment and monitor possible caries progression.

Silver diamine fluoride: Use of 38% silver diamine fluoride to assist in arresting caries lesions; informed consent: particularly highlighting expected staining of treated lesions.

Sealants: The decision to seal primary and permanent molars should account for both the individual-level and tooth-level risks.

From American Academy of Pediatric Dentistry. Caries-risk assessment and management for infants, children, and adolescents. In: *The Reference Manual of Pediatric Dentistry.* American Academy of Pediatric Dentistry; 2024:306-312.

TABLE 8.6 Anticipatory Guidance Knowledge Base for Pre–3-Year-Old Care

Areas of Anticipatory Guidance	Knowledge Base for Area
Oral and Dental Development	
Eruption	Normal range, delay, acceleration and potential etiologies, sequence, occlusion, and exfoliation Eruption problems including malposition, cyst formation, teething, Riga-Fede disease, and bruxism
Teeth	Color, shape, staining causes, role in speech, and chewing
Soft tissue	Mucosal color, ulceration, alveolar anatomy, and congenital abnormalities
Anatomy	Structures, integrity, and color
Fluorides	
Systemic	Water fluoridation procedures, supplementation, fluoride vehicles, timing, storage safety, fluorosis risk, bottled water, breast milk, formula, prenatal fluorides, and halo effect in diet
Topical	Role of dentifrice, storage safety, caries and fluorosis risks, swallowing amounts of dentifrice for age, and supplementation issues (if indicated)
Nonnutritive Habits	
Assessment	Frequency, duration, and intensity Thumbs, fingers, pacifiers, toys, or blankets Perceived emotional benefit to child Effects on oral cavity Interventions currently being used
Management	Interventions to discontinue the habit Techniques, effectiveness, and safety of interventions Life cycle of habits Systemic effects of habits

TABLE 8.6 Anticipatory Guidance Knowledge Base for Pre–3-Year-Old Care—cont'd

Diet and Nutrition	
Feeding	Food in caries paradigm Breastfeeding, weaning, and effect(s) on teeth and jaws Formula feeding, frequency, and content of formulas Development of feeding skills
Snacking	Snacking frequency and contents Food choices Safety and general health benefits
Diet	Infant food choices and evolution of pre–3-year-old diet
Problems and issues	Obesity concerns, picky eating, ethnic variations, and food aspiration
Oral Hygiene	
Science	Role of plaque (caries paradigm) Plaque removal goals Developmental issues
Activity	Type of cleaning currently performed Parental involvement Frequency and duration Devices Dentifrice
Problems and issues	Positioning difficulties Child resistance and behavior Taste of dentifrice, choices Technical skills of parents Role of flossing, injury
Injury Prevention	
General issues	Accidental injury awareness Car safety Choking risks of toys and food Matching skills with activity Childproofing and poisoning safety
Oral health issues	Normal anatomy Trauma assessment and management Dental home access numbers for emergency management Snacking safety Fluoride safety Medication use for oral problems Signs of child abuse Helmet safety

From Casamassimo PS, Nowak AJ. Anticipatory guidance. In: Berg JH, Slayton RL, eds. *Early Childhood Oral Health.* 2nd ed. Wiley-Blackwell; 2016.

During the neonatal period (the first 28 days of life), issues related to natal or neonatal teeth may arise. Parents should be advised that potential interventions, such as monitoring, incisal smoothing, or extractions, should be assessed individually. These assessments should consider possible complications for both the baby (e.g., lingual ulcerations known as Riga-Fede disease, risk of aspiration if the teeth are mobile) and the mother (e.g., sore nipples).[42]

Discussions on the management of ankyloglossia and hyperplastic labial frenulum may be particularly relevant for mothers experiencing breastfeeding difficulties. Interventions should be tailored individually, taking into account other potential contributing factors such as craniofacial anomalies and airway or nasal obstructions, to name a few.[43] More detailed information on this topic is found in Chapter 49.

Teething

Teething is a frequent topic inquired by caregivers during their child's tooth eruption process. Symptoms associated with tooth eruption continue to be controversial. Similar opinions regarding teething symptoms have been consistently reported by parents and health professionals for decades across numerous cultures. However, although some studies have reported fever, drooling, diarrhea, irritability, and sleep disturbances to be related to tooth eruption, others found no association of these symptoms with the eruption of teeth.[44] Gingival irritation, irritability, and drooling were the most frequent signs and symptoms of primary tooth eruption in a meta-analysis published between 1969 and 2012.[45] An analysis of body temperature showed that tooth eruption could lead to a rise in temperature not characterized as fever.[45] In a systematic review and meta-analysis on global prevalence of teething problems in infants, an increase in biting was also reported.[46] The discrepancy observed among studies reflects the possible bias and subjectivity of caregivers' reports of teething symptoms. Moreover, teething might be the culprit for the common childhood diseases (e.g., diarrhea, respiratory and ear infections) during the first 3 years of life. Tooth eruption overlaps with the timing when infants are in the oral stage exploring the environment. By introducing objects and fingers into their mouths, infants are at risk of exposure to viruses and bacteria that can cause illnesses. Health professionals should inform caregivers that teething symptoms are generally mild. Parents should consult a physician if their child exhibits severe or persistent symptoms. They should also be advised against using over-the-counter benzocaine products for teething pain relief. The US Food and Drug Administration (FDA) warns that benzocaine can cause methemoglobinemia, a serious condition that reduces oxygen in the bloodstream and can be fatal in severe cases. Therefore the FDA recommends that benzocaine products not be used for children under 2 years old, except under the guidance of a healthcare professional.[47] Additionally, the FDA has issued warnings about the potential dangers of homeopathic teething tablets and gels, advising consumers to discontinue their use due to a lack of proven benefits and reports of adverse effects such as difficulty breathing, seizures, excessive sleepiness, muscle weakness, and constipation.[48] Parents should also be informed about safe teething toys made of nontoxic materials and the risks of strangulation and choking associated with teething necklaces.[47]

Fluoride adequacy

The daily use of fluoride toothpaste initiated immediately after the eruption of the first tooth is regarded as the best clinical preventive practice for early childhood caries.[29] One concern is that children of this age are at greatest risk of developing fluorosis because of excessive amounts of fluoride being ingested. For this reason, the AAPD recommends the use of no more than a smear or rice-sized amount (0.1 mg F) of fluoridated toothpaste for children 3 years of age and younger.[27] Chapter 14 details the safety and toxicity concerns of fluoride in this age group. Because of the risk of ingestion of mouthrinses, the potential harm to children younger than 6 years of age outweighs its possible benefit[49]; therefore it is contraindicated.

To minimize the risk of fluorosis, the US Department of Health and Human Services recommends optimizing community water fluoridation supplies to 0.7 ppm.[50] This is particularly important when reconstituting infant formulas with fluoridated water. Bottled water often has fluoride concentrations below the accepted standards for optimal fluoridation.[51] Therefore parents should be advised that bottled water might not contain optimal levels of fluoride and that daily exposure to fluoridated tap water is proven effective in preventing caries, is readily accessible, and is low-cost.

Concerns regarding the safety of fluoride have been reported as one of the main reasons parents completely refuse fluoride treatments.[52] Communication is key to educate parents about the benefits of fluoride, the evidence-based information about its safety, and the specific rationale for recommending fluoride to their child.

Nonnutritive sucking

Parents often inquire about their child's habits, particularly thumb and pacifier habits. Such questions are common because oral habits are very prevalent in young children and negative effects of long-term habits on the dentition are well documented. Traditionally, dentists' involvement in nonnutritive sucking habits occurred only after prolonged habits produced clear damage to the dentition and raised parental concern. The dentist was consulted for advice on how to stop the nonnutritive sucking habit. This scenario still occurs with frequency, but early anticipatory guidance aimed at preventing the prolonged engagement of oral habits is a more effective role that dentists can have in nonnutritive sucking habits. However, before such guidance can be given, the dentist must have a thorough understanding of how and why nonnutritive sucking habits develop, how they affect oral structures, and what duration of habitual behavior may cause harm that will be described in detail later in this chapter.

Diet and nutrition

The AAP recommends "exclusive breastfeeding for about 6 months, with complementary food introduction at about 6 months, and as mutually desired by mother and child, supports continued breastfeeding until 2 years or beyond."[53] Because of the developmental, economic, health, nutritional, immunologic, psychological, and social advantages that breastfeeding provides to mothers and their children, clinicians should promote and encourage optimal breastfeeding habits.[53,54] Because of the unique biologic properties of human milk, research shows that breastfeeding can reduce the incidence of various acute and chronic pediatric conditions, including sudden infant death syndrome, acute diarrheal disease, otitis media, lower respiratory illnesses, asthma, inflammatory bowel disease, atopic dermatitis, childhood leukemia, diabetes mellitus, and obesity.[53] Breastfeeding mothers also have a lower risk of developing type 2 diabetes, hypertension, and breast, ovarian, and endometrial cancers.[53] In a systematic review,[55] higher frequency of breastfeeding up to 12 months was associated with reduced caries risk. However, with the introduction of other dietary carbohydrates and inadequate oral hygiene, breastfeeding beyond 12 months of age, especially if frequent or nocturnal, increased a child's risk for developing caries.[31] Although human milk alone cannot cause caries, in vitro studies have found breastfeeding in combination with other carbohydrates to be highly cariogenic.[56] Therefore the best recommendation for caries prevention clinicians can provide to mothers who are willing to breastfeed, including at nighttime, is to establish a diet low in simple carbohydrates and sugars when other foods and beverages are introduced in addition to breastfeeding, brush the child's teeth at least twice a day, especially at bedtime, and consider a smear amount of fluoride toothpaste.

When breastfeeding is not possible, infant formula is the ideal liquid nutrition for the first 12 months of life. In fact, infants only require breast milk or infant formula and do not need any other beverages, such as juice, soda, or cow's or goat's milk.[57] Plain fluoridated water should be introduced at 6 months to support hydration and help the child get accustomed to the taste early on, and is recommended as the preferred drink for children aged 1 to 5 when consumed between meals or snacks.[58] To prevent dental caries and reduce the risk of obesity later on, caregivers should be advised to avoid giving children sugar-sweetened beverages such as fruit drinks, regular soda, sports drinks, energy drinks, and tea and coffee drinks that contain added sugars like fructose, corn syrup, and sucrose.[58] It is crucial to emphasize with caregivers that added sugars, especially in the form of sugar-sweetened beverages, are a major contributor to dental caries.[59] Additionally, it is important to limit beverages that naturally contain sugars, such as 100% fruit juice. The AAP recommends not giving juice to infants under 1 year old and limiting juice intake to 4 ounces per day for children aged 1 to 3.[60] Additionally, the American Heart Association recommends avoiding added sugars in the diets of children under 2 years old. Like juice, added sugars provide no nutritional value, can foster a preference for sweet tastes early on, and increase the likelihood of consuming sugary beverages later in life.[61] Many caregivers might believe that diluting juice with water reduces the risk of dental caries. However, this is a misconception. Diluted juice remains cariogenic and can increase the frequency of sugar-sweetened beverage consumption.

Nighttime bottle feeding predominantly occurs before the age of 6 months, which coincides with the eruption of the first primary teeth in most children. If this habit persists beyond 6 months, caregivers should be advised to offer only water in the nighttime baby's bottle to avoid the risk of caries development. The use of bottles should be discontinued around 12 months of age, as this is an ideal time to introduce a cup. At this age, babies are developmentally ready to drink from a cup.[57] Therefore nonspill cups (i.e., sippy cups) are not a necessary intermediary between bottle/breastfeeding and regular cups. Because of their popularity and practicality in preventing spills, caregivers often prefer nonspill cups. However, caregivers should be advised to place only water in them, both during the day and at night, to prevent dental caries.

Infants are ready to start solid foods when they developmentally are able to "control head and neck, opens the mouth when food is offered, swallow food rather than pushes it back out onto the chin, brings objects to the mouth, try to grasp small objects, such as toys or food, transfers food from the front to the back of the tongue to swallow."[62] Introducing healthy snacks like low-sugar infant cereals, proteins such as meats, fruits, vegetables, grains, yogurts, and cheeses is essential. It's equally important to avoid high-carbohydrate, sugary, and sticky snacks. As babies grow, they should transition to three structured meals and two to three snack times per day. Grazing throughout the day and frequently consuming sugary snacks between meals should be discouraged, as these habits increase the risk of dental caries. Therefore children's meals should be scheduled at planned times, with the child seated and supervised by an adult.[57,58,63]

Oral hygiene

When providing anticipatory guidance on oral hygiene, it is important to discuss tooth cleaning tools, the timing and frequency of brushing, the child's positioning during oral care, and the appropriate amount of fluoride toothpaste. Even before infants have their first teeth, parents should be encouraged to clean their infants' mouths and gums daily with a moist washcloth. This practice helps establish crucial oral hygiene habits and makes the child comfortable with future tooth brushing.

Once the first teeth appear, it is essential to switch to a toothbrush, as a washcloth will not clean teeth effectively. Brushing should be done twice daily using a smear amount of fluoridated toothpaste, after breakfast and before bedtime, with the most critical time being right before bed. Children under 6 years old need adult assistance with brushing because they lack the fine motor skills required for thorough cleaning.[31]

Parents should understand that tooth brushing is a vital part of their children's daily hygiene, like bathing and hair washing. Establishing a consistent routine, such as brushing right after breakfast or just before bedtime, can help ensure success. Parents can be advised to use a procedure called "lift-the-lip"[64] to check their child's oral hygiene by lifting the child's lip to look for plaque on the upper front teeth and inspect the gum tissue for signs of inflammation and bleeding.

Injury prevention

Anticipatory guidance on injury prevention for infants should not only include information on dental trauma, but also general health issues like play objects, electrical cords, home childproofing, choking hazards, and car seat use. Children, especially those who are learning to walk, are known to be at higher risk of sustaining oral injuries from falling while carrying a bottle, nonspill cups, and pacifier.[65] Parents should be informed that certain foods, when served uncooked, whole, or in specific shapes or sizes, can pose choking hazards.[66]

The same caution applies to pacifiers.[67] To prevent ingestion of broken parts, the AAP recommends using pacifiers molded in one solid piece. To ensure pacifiers do not pass through the mouth, parents should purchase those appropriate for their child's age, with a firm shield, vent holes, and at least 3.8 cm across. The use of attachments tied to pacifiers is strongly discouraged because of the risk of serious injuries or even death. Because pacifiers deteriorate over time, parents are encouraged to inspect them regularly. In cases of oral or dental trauma, it is crucial for parents to know how to access emergency care, especially after hours.[68]

Special Considerations

Growth and Development Treatment Planning

In rare instances, there may be an orthodontic or craniofacial component to the infant oral health visit, as would be the case with a child with a cleft lip or palate or a significant craniofacial abnormality. These patients should be referred to a craniofacial team for management and followed routinely by the primary care dentist for basic oral health needs.

Parents often express interest in occlusal development and may press the dentist to discuss future orthodontic needs. Growth is difficult to predict at this age, but the dentist should take the opportunity to discuss eruption, spacing, and occlusion with the parents as a part of anticipatory guidance.

Nonnutritive Sucking Habits

Origins of Nonnutritive Sucking Habits

Sucking behaviors are believed to arise from psychological needs, mainly from the physiologic need for nutrition. Normally developed infants have an inherent biologic drive for sucking. Psychoanalytic theorists and learning theorists differ in their explanation of why human infants possess a sucking drive and why it might persist beyond infancy, but they are in agreement that this drive is a normal developmental characteristic.[69] According to the psychoanalytic theory, nonnutritive sucking behaviors (such as pacifier, thumb, or finger sucking) arise out of erotic pleasure derived from oral stimulation. Persistence of substantial nonnutritive sucking beyond the so-called oral phase (approximately 3 years of age) reflects a psychological disturbance suggestive of an inability to manage stress or anxiety. Conversely, the learning theory suggests that nonnutritive sucking is an adaptive response that is often rewarded and that becomes a learned habit without psychological manifestations. Given the prevalence of nonnutritive sucking behaviors in normally developed children, the learning theory explanation is the most widely accepted. An alternative, yet complementary, theory proposed by Larsson and Dahlin[70] suggests that if an infant sucking need is not satisfied at the breast, the infant's fingers will be used as a substitute.

Prevalence of Nonnutritive Sucking Habits

It has been reported that well over 90% of children engaged in nonnutritive sucking at some time during their first year of life.[71] Prolonged nonnutritive sucking habits may have negative consequences to the orofacial structures; therefore habits that continue beyond the toddler years are more concerning than those that terminate earlier. On average, children cease these habits by 24 to 36 months of age, and those who continue tend to be from better educated or higher income families.[72] Numerous studies document that thumb and finger sucking habits are more likely to persist longer than pacifier habits.[71,73] Pacifier habits rarely persist beyond the preschool years because of peer pressure that occurs when children enter kindergarten. This has led to the suggestion that when a digit habit develops, a pacifier should be encouraged as a substitute for the digit.[74,75]

The length of time of actual engagement (duration) of a habit is perhaps the single most important factor to consider when assessing the risk for habit-induced malocclusions. Other factors that also need to be considered include the amount of time a child engages in a particular habit per day (frequency) and the forcefulness (intensity) associated with the child's sucking pattern. For example, a child who sucks on a pacifier for only a few minutes before falling asleep at night would be expected to be at less risk for developing a malocclusion than a child who has a pacifier in the mouth several hours a day with a sucking intensity that results in audible sounds. Therefore parents should be instructed to limit the time a pacifier is in the infant's mouth and avoid ad lib use throughout the day.[76]

Effects and Mechanisms of Nonnutritive Sucking Habits on the Dentition

Studies of the primary dentition have found sucking habits to be associated with a higher prevalence of malocclusion in the primary dentition, including class II canine and molar relationships, anterior open bite, increased overjet, decreased maxillary arch width, and increased mandibular arch width, resulting in an increased likelihood of posterior crossbite. Digit habits are more commonly associated with excessive overjet and anterior open bite, whereas pacifier habits are associated with posterior crossbites and class II canine relationships.[71,73,74,77–79] Pacifier habits, even if discontinued by 2 years of age, represent an increased risk for malocclusion. Open bites tend to resolve with the cessation of pacifier habits, whereas crossbites are more likely to persist after habits stop. One systematic review reported that orthodontic pacifiers (e.g., those with a thin neck) induce less open bite compared with conventional pacifiers.[80] However, another systematic review concluded that there is not enough evidence to confirm that the occurrence of malocclusion traits differs between children who used orthodontic pacifiers and those who used conventional pacifiers.[81]

The differences in digit and pacifier effects on the orofacial structures are likely caused by the different forces applied. Pacifiers, presumably because they extend farther into the mouth, tend to force the tongue downward, applying lateral outward pressure against the lower arch. At the same time, the sucking action activates the muscles surrounding the mouth, which increases cheek pressure and results in greater medial force applied to the upper arch. Pacifiers tend to widen the mandibular arch and narrow the maxillary arch, resulting in posterior crossbites.[80] Fingers or thumbs, because of the weight of the arm, tend to apply forward and slightly upward pressure on the maxillary incisor region, with accompanying backward and downward pressure on mandibular incisors; the net effect of digit habits is greater overjet and a tendency toward open bite.

The risk of acute otitis media (middle ear infection) may be higher among children using pacifiers. Some studies have linked pacifier use to early cessation of breastfeeding,[77] whereas others have concluded that pacifier use is a marker of breastfeeding difficulties, reduced motivation to breastfeed, and parental choice to bottle-feed rather than a true cause of early weaning.[82,83] Some studies have suggested that pacifier use may be beneficial in reducing sudden infant death syndrome, a benefit that potentially far outweighs the risks associated with acute otitis media or possible breastfeeding cessation.[84]

Recommendations

Studies have demonstrated that habits of longer duration are associated with higher prevalence of malocclusions, with some potential harm if habits continue between 24 and 36 months and greater risk for malocclusions if habits persist past 48 months of age.[78,79] Prolonged pacifier or digit habits past 48 months are associated with detrimental effects on the occlusion in the late deciduous dentition[74] and past 60 months in the mixed dentition.[79] Given the physiologic and psychological need for sucking in the first year of life, it is neither prudent nor realistic to recommend elimination of habits before 12 or 24 months of age.[78] Therefore anticipatory guidance to parents during infant oral health visits should advocate for cessation of nonnutritive habits no later than 36 months of age.[67,78,79] Because digit habits are likely to cause malocclusions of greater severity than those caused by pacifier habits and because digit habits are more difficult to overcome than pacifier habits, substitution of a pacifier habit for a digit habit may be advisable.

Visit eBooks.Health.Elsevier.com to see full list of references.

9

The Preschool Child: Ages 3 to 6

MICHAEL KANELLIS

CHAPTER OUTLINE

Normal Findings

By 3 years of age, children should have a full complement of 20 primary teeth. By age 6, many children will have lost some or all their primary incisors, and both permanent incisors and first permanent molars may be present or erupting. The timing of exfoliation of teeth can vary greatly with some children not losing any primary teeth during this period (Table 9.1).

Ideal findings in the primary dentition include homogenous white enamel free from caries, hypomineralization, or fluorosis. Ideal occlusion includes some anterior spacing (Fig. 9.1) between the incisors and minimal positive overjet and overbite. Crowding or a lack of spacing may be present (Fig. 9.2) at this stage and would portend future crowding. The molar relationship should be either mesial step or flush terminal plane. The ideal canine relationship should be class I. The gingival tissues should be healthy, with the attached gingiva having a stippled appearance and no visible inflammation. The gingiva should not bleed when brushed with a soft toothbrush.

Preparing for Your Patient

Effective preparation for patients ages 3 to 6 in the dental office requires advance planning and a child-centric approach. The office environment should be welcoming, colorful, and equipped with age-appropriate distractions to alleviate anxiety and engage young minds (Fig. 9.3). The dental team should be trained in communication techniques tailored to this age group, emphasizing clear, simple language and positive reinforcement.

Creating a setup that allows for the presence of a parent or caregiver during the initial examination helps establish trust and comfort for the child. Additionally, incorporating simple behavior management strategies, like tell-show-do and desensitization, proves invaluable in navigating the unique challenges posed by treating preschool-aged patients. By thoughtfully preparing both the physical space and the dental team, dentists can create an environment conducive to successful and stress-free dental visits for young children.

TABLE 9.1 Timing of Tooth Eruption and Exfoliation

Tooth	Eruption	Exfoliation
PRIMARY DENTITION		
Central incisors	6–10 months	6–7 years
Lateral incisors	8–12 months	7–8 years
Canines (cuspids)	16–20 months	9–12 years
First molars	11–18 months	9–11 years
Second molars	20–30 months	10–12 years
PERMANENT DENTITION		
Central incisors	6–7 years (mandibular), 7–8 years (maxillary)	
Lateral incisors	7–8 years (mandibular), 8–9 years (maxillary)	
Canines (cuspids)	9–10 years (mandibular), 11–12 years (maxillary)	
First molars	6–7 years	
Second molars	11–13 years	

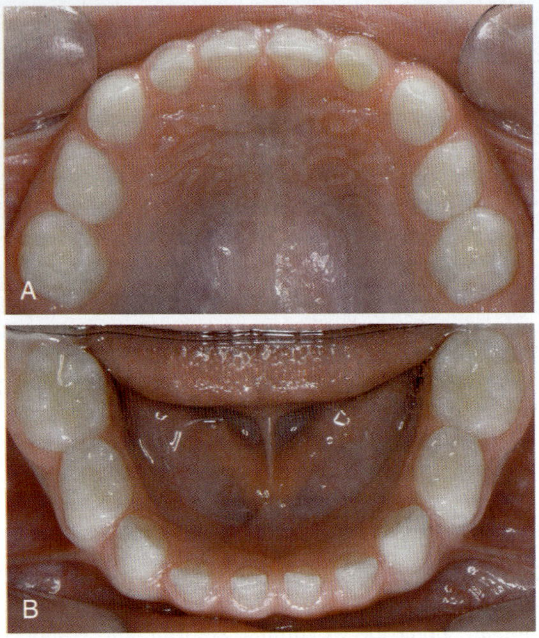

• **Fig. 9.1** Primary maxillary (A) and mandibular (B) arches showing generalized spacing and primate spaces (mesial to the maxillary canines and distal to the mandibular canines).

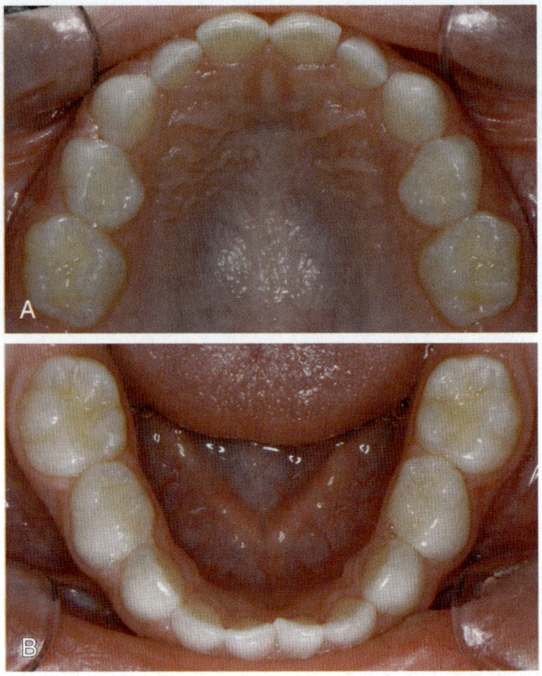

• **Fig. 9.2** These arches, maxillary (A) and mandibular (B), show a lack of primate or developmental spaces and portend future crowding.

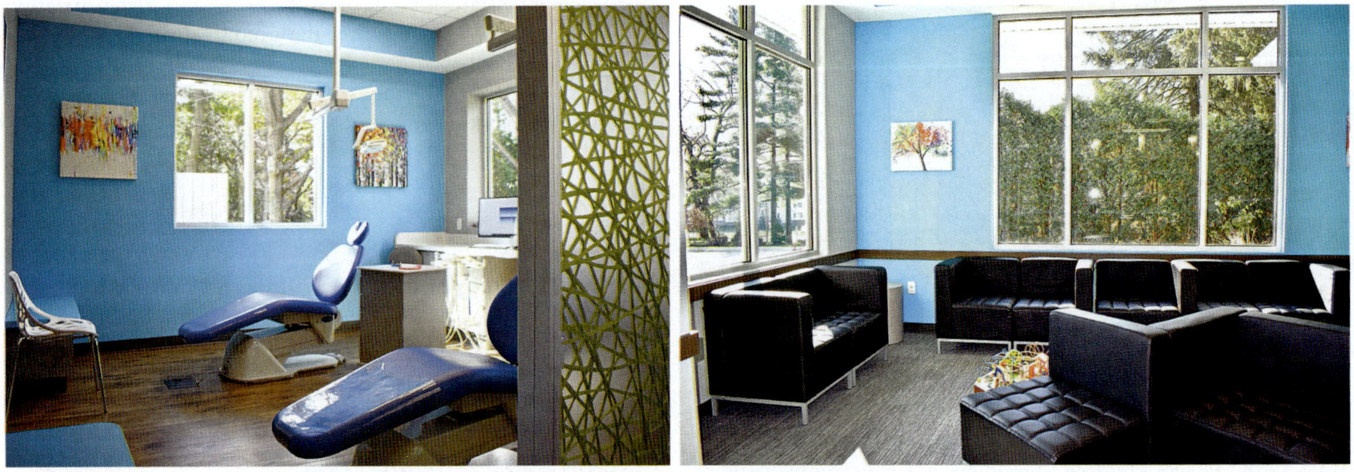

• **Fig. 9.3** This dental office is inviting to young children with distractions built into the décor but also welcoming to older children who may be seen here as well. (Courtesy of Dr. Teresa Geneser.)

Information Gathering

Gathering comprehensive information from young patients is a crucial step in providing tailored and effective pediatric dental care. In this age group, where communication skills are still evolving, obtaining a thorough health history is imperative (Table 9.2). Dental history, encompassing early oral habits, previous dental experiences, and any familial predispositions, aids in assessing potential risks and tailoring preventive measures. Social history plays a pivotal role, shedding light on dietary habits, oral hygiene practices, and environmental factors that may influence oral health.

Behavior Guidance

Language improves dramatically during the ages of 3 to 6, improving the success of basic behavior guidance in dental care. By age 4 years, all children should be competent in the domain of language, unless an abnormality is present in their

TABLE 9.2 Selected Health History Considerations With Common Findings in the 3- to 6-Year-Old Group

Area of Concern	Common Findings
General Health	
Allergies	Probably related to food and other environmental allergens; may have allergy to medications such as antibiotics; rash is common manifestation; false allergies often reported
Asthma	May be reported; triggering factors usually known; medications also well known; impact of dental intervention usually not known
Bleeding	Parent may suggest excessive bruising without real problem
Blood transfusion	May have been performed at birth
Childhood infections	Immunizations will have occurred, or there is a clear history of having had a specific illness such as measles or chickenpox
Development	Poor parental knowledge for normal children; for those with developmental delays, a good history of diagnostic procedures and status
Heart	Functional murmur may exist, or parent may have been told of a murmur
Hypertension	Usually unknown unless child has chronic problem
Illnesses	Probable history of upper respiratory infections
Jaundice	Possible at birth
Medications	Probably has taken acetaminophen (Tylenol) as necessary; may have received amoxicillin or other antibiotic
Seizures	Possibly febrile; may be on seizure medication for only one seizure
Surgical procedures	Possible tonsillectomy or adenoidectomy; possible ear tubes; circumcision seldom noted as procedure
Dental Health	
Bottle use	Probably considered not to contribute to decay
Developmental/eruption	Knowledge may be limited to eruption dates of first teeth unless consistently very early or late
Fluoride	May know water status; possible vitamin with fluoride supplementation
Habits (thumb-sucking)	Will be well known to parent if present
Home care	Usually confined to toothbrushing; may be largely left to child
Previous care	Possibly none; no dentist or care rendered
Reaction to care (behavior)	Possibly none; likely poor or tentative
Trauma to teeth and chin	Possible, but usually left untreated unless serious; commonly upper teeth and chin

This table suggests usual or common responses to questions asked of parents about the average child in this age group, but it does not suggest a norm or most frequent response for all children.

psychological development. At this age, clear communication by the dentist is critical. Table 9.3 shows expected developmental milestones for children in these age groups. These children may need more time and patience than others, but the outcomes can be rewarding. An undemanding, introductory appointment with emphasis on "tell-show-do" (TSD) is especially beneficial. TSD is a universally applied strategy with this age group, along with positive reinforcement, distraction, and desensitization.

TABLE 9.3 Selected Developmental Characteristics of the 3- to 6-Year-Old Group

3-Year-Old	4-Year-Old	6-Year-Old
Intellectual Development		
Gives first and last name	Recognizes colors	Names 4 colors
Counts 3 objects	Counts 4 objects	Counts 10 objects
States own age and sex	Tells a story	Asks about the meaning of words
Gross/Fine Motor Skills		
Puts on shoes	Dresses without supervision	Dresses and undresses
Pedals tricycle	Balances on one foot	Hops on one foot
Copies a circle	Copies cross and square	Draws a triangle
Psychological		
The 3- to 6-year-old is in the *phallic* stage of development. During this period, the child undergoes *oedipal* conflicts, which may lead to opposite-sex parental preference. The child may exhibit some aggression with siblings. By age 6 years, the child may be ready to surrender some dependency on parents		
Dental Implications		
Needs maternal presence, especially during stress	May be difficult and aggressive	Should leave parent for treatment
Fear of separation	Responds to verbal direction	Proud of possessions
Visual fear	Auditory fear	Bodily harm fear
Physiologic Height (75th Percentile)		
Boys = 97.5 cm	Boys = 106 cm	Boys = 113 cm
Girls = 97 cm	Girls = 104.5 cm	Girls = 111.5 cm
(Growth rate for this period is approximately 6–8 cm per year)		
Weight (75th Percentile)		
Boys = 15.5 kg	Boys = 18 kg	Boys = 20 kg
Girls = 15.5 kg	Girls = 17.5 kg	Girls = 19.5 kg
(Growth rate for this period is approximately 2 kg per year)		
Pulse (90th Percentile)		
105 beats/min	100 beats/min	100 beats/min
Respiration (90th Percentile)		
30 breaths/min	28 breaths/min	26 breaths/min
Blood Pressure		
100/60 mm Hg	100/60 mm Hg	100/60 mm Hg

These behavioral guidance techniques, along with others, allow children to become familiarized and desensitized to each step of the dental visit.[1] A more complete discussion of behavior guidance techniques can be found in Chapter 26.

Younger children in this age group may be startled by the chair moving back, so it is advisable to have the chair in a supine position at the beginning of the appointment or to have the dentist present the experience of the chair going back as a "spaceship ride." These young patients will respond best to clear, single-step instructions, followed by positive reinforcement. The key to successful desensitization is to build upon each visit. Even though a toothbrush may adequately remove plaque deposits at this age, use of the rotary prophy cup with child's toothpaste may desensitize the child to the handpiece and give insight into compliance for planned operative treatments. Appointments should be short and efficient to not overwhelm the child's coping abilities.

Clinical Examination

Conducting a thorough clinical examination for patients aged 3 to 6 necessitates a strategic and patient-centered approach. Proper positioning of the child is critical. For the most part, the operatory setup for this age group would be the same as for older children. However, although most children in this age group are capable of reclining in a dental chair, some in the younger range may still benefit from a knee-to-knee examination with a parent present, so the provider should be prepared to modify their approach based on the development level of the child.

There are multiple components (Table 9.4) of a comprehensive clinical examination.[2] Initiating the examination from the periphery and gradually progressing to the oral cavity allows the child to acclimate to the dental setting gradually. Beginning with extraoral observations, assessing facial symmetry, lip competence, and oral habits provides valuable information. Moving inward, an assessment

TABLE 9.4 Elements of the Head and Neck Examination

Structure	Diagnostic Technique	Normal Characteristics	Selected Abnormal Findings/Possible Causes
Head			
Hair	Visualization	Quality	Dryness/malnutrition, ectodermal dysplasia
		Thickness	Baldness/child abuse, self-abuse, chemotherapy
		Color	Infestation/neglect
Scalp	Visualization	Skin color	Scaling/dermatitis
		Dryness	Lesions/abuse, infection, neglect
		Ulceration	
Ears	Visualization	Intact and normally formed external ear and auditory canal	Malformed ears and canals/genetic malformation syndrome (e.g., Treacher Collins)
	Palpation		Conductive and neurologic hearing loss/trauma, developmental disability
	Assessment of hearing	Gross normal hearing	
Eyes	Visualization	Position and orientation intact	Variation in separation and orientation/genetic malformation syndromes
	Assessment of vision	Movement of eyes Vision Reaction to light	Cranial nerve damage/trauma, developmental disability
Nose	Visualization	Normal size, shape, function, and location	Malposition/genetic malformation syndrome (e.g., median facial cleft) Misshapen/ectodermal dysplasia, congenital syphilis, achondroplasia Discharge/URI, asthma, allergy Poor smell, cranial nerve damage
Lip	Visualization	Speech, closure	Poor closure/lip incompetence
	Assessment of function	Integrity	Clefting/genetic clefting syndrome
		Absence of lesions	Asymmetry/Bell palsy or cranial nerve damage
			Ulceration/herpes infection
Temporomandibular joint	Visualization	Symmetry in function	Deviation/trauma
	Palpation	Smooth movement	Crepitus, pain/temporomandibular joint disorder
	Auscultation	Absence of pain	Limitation/arthritis, trauma
		Range of motion (maximum)	

TABLE 9.4 Elements of the Head and Neck Examination—cont'd

Structure	Diagnostic Technique	Normal Characteristics	Selected Abnormal Findings/Possible Causes
Skin	Visualization	Color	Edema cellulitis, renal disorder
		Tone	Redness/allergic response
		Moisture	Dryness/dehydration, ectodermal dysplasia
		Absence of lesions	ulceration/infectious disease, abuse
Chin	Visualization	Absence of scar	Scar indicates previous mandibular trauma
Neck			
Lymph nodes	Palpation	Normal size, mobility	Increased size/infection, neoplasia Fixation/neoplasia
Thyroid	Palpation	Normal size	Increased size/goiter, tumor
Oral Cavity			
Palates	Visualization	Integrity	Cleft/genetic syndrome
	Palpation	Absence of lesion	Ulceration/herpes, mononucleosis, or other infection, abuse
	Assessment of function	Normal function	Petechiae/sexual abuse
			Deviation/cranial nerve damage
Pharynx	Visualization	Normal color Normal size of tonsils	Redness/URI, tonsillitis
Tongue	Visualization	Normal color	Redness/glossitis
	Palpation	Range of motion	Ulceration/herpes, aphthous, or other infection, trauma
	Assessment of function	Absence of lesions	Deviation/cranial nerve damage
			Limited movement/cerebral palsy
Floor of mouth	Visualization	Salivary function	Swelling/mucocele, sialolith
	Palpation	Absence of swelling	Ulceration/aphthous ulceration or other infection, abuse
		Absence of lesions	
Buccal mucosa	Visualization	Absence of lesions	Ulceration/cheek bite, abuse
	Palpation	Absence of swelling	Swelling/salivary gland infection, mumps
		Salivary function	
Teeth	Visualization	Normal development	Absence/delayed eruption/congenital absence, genetic syndromes
	Palpation	Morphologic appearance	
	Percussion	Occlusion	Extra teeth/supernumerary, cleidocranial dysplasia
		Color Integrity Mobility Hygiene	Abnormal morphologic appearance/microdontia, macrodontia, fusion Abnormal color/amelogenesis or dentinogenesis imperfecta, staining, pulpal necrosis, caries Fracture/trauma, abuse, caries Mobility/periapical infection, trauma, bone loss conditions, exfoliation Malposition/malocclusion, trauma Pain/periapical involvement

URI, Upper respiratory tract infection.

of the oral cavity includes examination of the soft tissues, dentition, and occlusion (Figs. 9.4 and 9.5). The focus should be on discerning normal development from common abnormalities, such as early signs of malocclusion, dental caries, or abnormal oral habits. Engaging the child in a nonthreatening manner, incorporating positive reinforcement, and emphasizing a fun, exploratory atmosphere contributes to a successful clinical examination for this age group, promoting both oral health and a positive dental experience.

Radiographic Examination

Obtaining radiographs for patients aged 3 to 6 is a careful and selective process designed to balance diagnostic necessity with the

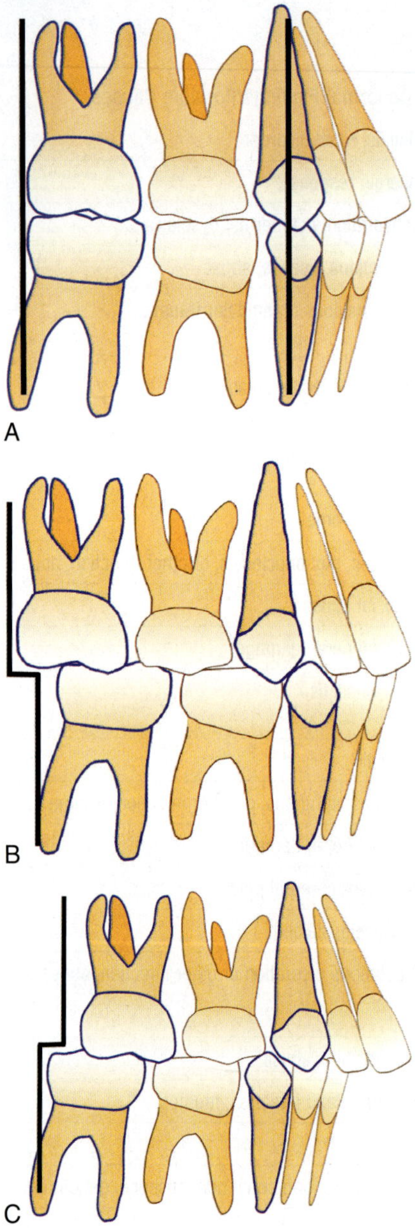

• **Fig. 9.4** In the primary dentition, the occlusion is classified by the relationship of the mandibular second molars and canines to the maxillary second molars and canines. (A) A "flush terminal plane" relationship and an end-to-end canine relationship. (B) A "mesial step terminal plane" relationship where the distal surface of the mandibular molar is mesial to the distal surface of the maxillary molar. The maxillary canine in this example is positioned in the embrasure between the mandibular canine and the first primary molar. This is termed a class I canine relationship. (C) An example where the distal surface of the mandibular molar is distal to the distal surface of the maxillary second molar. This is called a "distal step terminal plane". The maxillary canine in this example is positioned in the embrasure between the mandibular lateral incisor and the mandibular canine. This is termed a class II canine relationship.

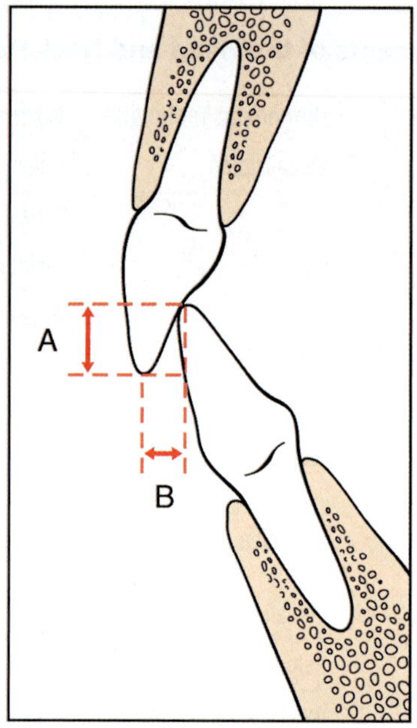

• **Fig. 9.5** Overbite (A) is the vertical overlap of the incisors, while overjet (B) is the horizontal overlap of these same incisors. (Redrawn from Friedman MH, Weisberg J. The temporomandibular joint. In: Gould JA, ed. *Orthopedics and Sports Physical Therapy*. Mosby; 1990.)

child's comfort and ability to cooperate. Dentists should prescribe dental radiographs only when they expect that the diagnostic yield will benefit patient care, enhance patient safety, or substantially improve clinical outcomes.[3]

Common radiographs (Table 9.5) in this age group include bitewing radiographs, typically used for detecting dental caries

TABLE 9.5 Selection Criteria and Guidelines for Pediatric Radiographs in the 3- to 6-Year-Old Group

Projection	Criteria	Frequency
Posterior bitewing	Proximal surfaces of posterior teeth cannot be examined clinically Child is cooperative	At initial examination if contacts closed Semiannually if interproximal surfaces have been restored, until child achieves low-risk status[a] or is caries free; also 6- to 12-month intervals if child is at increased risk[b] Annually to 24-month interval if child is caries free at initial bitewing examination
Posterior periapical	Suspected pathosis Confirmed pathosis Child is cooperative	As needed to diagnose and monitor treatment or patient condition
Anterior occlusal	Suspected pathosis Confirmed pathosis Child is cooperative	Same as above or as a caries-detecting radiograph if closed contacts preclude thorough examination

[a]Consider child cooperation in decision making.
[b]Increased risk for dental caries may be associated with (1) poor oral hygiene, (2) fluoride deficiency, (3) prolonged nursing, (4) high-carbohydrate diet, (5) poor family dental health, (6) developmental enamel defects, (7) developmental disability or acute medical problem, or (8) genetic abnormality.
Modified from American Dental Association, US Department of Health and Human Services. *The Selection of Patients for Dental Radiographic Examination*. 2012.

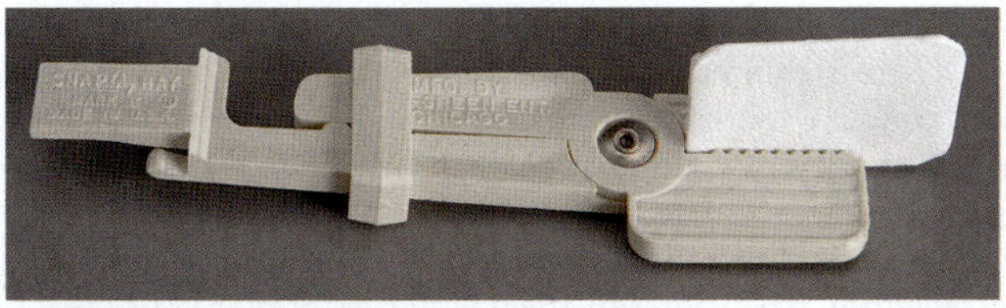

• **Fig. 9.6** Snap-a-Ray Film Holder. (From Boyd LRB. *Dental Instruments: A Pocket Guide*. 4th ed. Saunders; 2012.)

between primary teeth, and occlusal (periapical) radiographs of anterior teeth. Once permanent teeth are erupting, a panoramic radiograph should be considered. Panoramic radiographs offer a comprehensive view of the entire dentition and supporting structures, providing insight into overall dental development and identifying potential issues such as congenitally missing teeth or anomalies.

Modifications to technique, such as the use of film holders (Fig. 9.6), are important to consider, providing comfort and allowing for radiographs to be made of these younger children. Abdominal and thyroid shielding during intraoral and panoramic radiographs is no longer recommended, and the use of these forms of protective shielding can be discontinued as routine practice.[3]

Caries Risk Assessment

The American Academy of Pediatric Dentistry recommends the use of two clinically validated tools to determine which children are at higher risk for dental caries: Caries Management by Risk Assessment (CAMBRA) and Cariogram.[4] Based on an accurate assessment of risk factors and disease indicators, patients can be put into either low-risk, moderate-risk, or high-risk categories. These categories in turn can guide the practitioner in developing targeted preventive strategies that can maintain optimal oral health in their patients.

To accurately assign a risk category to a patient in this age group, practitioners need to carefully evaluate social, behavioral, and medical risk factors. Examples of potential risk factors in these categories include the following: (1) mother or primary caregiver has active dental caries, (2) patient's family is low income or has low health literacy, (3) child has daily frequent exposures to sugar-containing snacks or beverages, (4) child is a recent immigrant, or (5) child has special healthcare needs. Clinical risk factors contributing to a higher risk categorization include (1) visible plaque on teeth and (2) presence of enamel defects.

Some children have protective factors that can put them at less risk for developing caries. These factors include (1) optimally fluoridated drinking water, (2) daily brushing with fluoridated toothpaste, (3) topical fluoride application from health professionals, and (4) a dental home and regular dental care.

One final group of factors automatically puts children in a higher risk group. Disease indicators include (1) incipient or white spot carious lesions, (2) visible carious lesions, and (3) presence of recent restorations or teeth missing because of caries.

Risk assessment should be performed at each regular recare appointment because contributory factors can change over time. An accurate assessment of caries risk can help the practitioner plan effective intervention and education strategies.

TABLE 9.6 Basic Preventive Dental Care Recommendations, Ages 3 to 6

Recommendation	Details
Dental visits	Schedule regular dental checkups every 6 months.
Oral hygiene	Brush teeth twice daily with fluoride toothpaste and floss daily.
Fluoride use	Use fluoride toothpaste and consider fluoride varnish applications.
Dietary counseling	Limit sugary snacks and drinks; encourage a balanced diet.
Sealants	Apply dental sealants to prevent cavities in molars with deep grooves.
Caries risk assessment	Conduct regular assessments to identify and manage risk factors for caries.
Anticipatory guidance	Provide guidance on oral habits, injury prevention, and oral development.
Radiographic assessment	Take dental x-rays when necessary, based on individual risk factors.

Prevention

The American Academy of Pediatric Dentistry (AAPD) has established guidelines for preventive dental care for children of all ages.[5] Establishing effective preventive regimens for children aged 3 to 6 (and communicating these regimens effectively to caregivers) is an essential component of attaining and maintain excellent oral health throughout childhood (Table 9.6).

Preventive services that can be carried out in a professional setting for this age group include oral prophylaxis, topical fluoride application, application of caries-arresting medicaments, placement of dental sealants, oral hygiene instruction, and dietary counseling. Recommendations for which services should be provided, and how often, are spelled out in the AAPD's periodicity schedule of preventive services.[5]

Preventive strategies for home care should include recommendations that parents or guardians assist with the brushing. A common recommendation is to allow children to brush first and then to have an adult brush to make sure the teeth are clean. Children in this age range do not typically have the manual dexterity required to effectively remove plaque from their teeth while brushing. Parental involvement is also recommended for placing toothpaste on the toothbrush.

The importance of a healthy diet cannot be overstated. Frequent exposure to sugary snacks and liquids is one of the primary causes of tooth decay in children.

Toothpaste Recommendations

The AAPD recommends the use of a fluoridated toothpaste for this age group.[6] The fluoride concentration should typically be around 1000 parts per million (ppm). Toothbrushing should be done twice a day and should be supervised by an adult. A pea-sized amount of toothpaste is advised for this age group. Children should be encouraged to spit after brushing. Ingesting too much fluoridated toothpaste in this age group could lead to dental fluorosis in the permanent teeth and the potential for gastrointestinal upset.

Nonfluoride Preventive Adjuncts

In addition to using fluoride toothpaste, nonfluoride preventive adjuncts (see Chapter 14) play a significant role in promoting optimal oral health for children in this age group. The use of pit and fissure sealants can prevent and arrest occlusal carious lesions on both primary and permanent molars.[7] Xylitol-containing products, such as chewing gum or lozenges, have demonstrated potential in reducing caries risk by inhibiting bacterial growth.[7] Silver diamine fluoride (SDF) has proven effective in slowing or arresting caries progression.[7] Oral hygiene aids like soft-bristled brushes, flossers, or interdental brushes, when introduced with parental guidance, contribute to a more comprehensive and effective home care routine. By incorporating these nonfluoride preventive adjuncts into the oral care regimen for young children, dentists can tailor their approach to individual needs, promoting a holistic strategy for preserving the oral health of the primary dentition.

Nutrition Advice

Nutrition advice for children ages 3 to 6 should emphasize a balanced and tooth-friendly diet as essential, encouraging the consumption of nutrient-rich foods such as fruits, vegetables, dairy products, and whole grains. Limiting the intake of sugary snacks, candies, and sugary beverages is crucial in preventing the development of dental caries. AAPD guidelines for healthy beverage consumption recommend no more than 4 to 6 ounces of juice per day.[7] Encouraging regular meals and snacks while minimizing prolonged exposure to sugars aids in maintaining a healthy oral environment. Proper assessment and parent education are key to lowering the child's caries risk. See Chapter 16 for an in-depth discussion of pediatric nutrition.

Restorative Considerations

Selecting appropriate restorative materials for pediatric patients aged 3 to 6 requires careful consideration of their unique dental needs and developmental stage. For primary teeth affected by dental caries, glass ionomer cement (GIC) and resin-modified glass ionomer cement (RMGIC) are often preferred choices because of their fluoride release properties and ability to bond chemically to tooth structure. These materials provide durability and are suitable for smaller cavities or lesions in primary teeth. Additionally, stainless steel crowns (SSCs) are frequently employed for extensive carious lesions in posterior primary teeth, offering strength, longevity, and ease of placement. Aesthetic tooth-colored composite resins may be utilized for anterior or posterior restorations, balancing both functional and cosmetic considerations. The selection of restorative materials for young children involves a tailored approach, considering the specific clinical situation, patient cooperation, and the need for a reliable, long-lasting solution to preserve the integrity of the primary dentition during this critical developmental period.

Minimally Invasive Dentistry

Minimally invasive dentistry (MID) has emerged as an approach to managing caries in young children when more conventional restorative approaches are problematic. MID is defined as a philosophy of dental care concerned with early identification of disease, factors contributing to the disease, intervention to arrest the disease, and, if needed, restorative treatment.[8] The goal of MID is to stabilize the disease process, prevent disease progression, conserve tooth structure, avoid pulp exposure in vital teeth, reduce anxiety in young patients, and facilitate a positive dental experience.[9]

Examples of techniques that can be considered MID include (1) Hall SSCs, (2) interim therapeutic restorations (IRT/ART), (3) SDF, (4) silver modified atraumatic restorative technique (SMART), (5) guided enamel regeneration,[10] (6) resin infiltration, (7) fluoride varnish, (8) povidone-iodine, and (9) sealants.

Selective (incomplete) caries removal has also emerged as an acceptable form of MID in primary teeth. When a decision is made to incompletely excavate caries, it is important that the pretreatment diagnosis was reversible pulpitis and that restorations have sealed margins with a plan in place for reevaluation. Active surveillance of caries lesions, monitoring for pain or signs/symptoms of infection, and more frequent professional recare can also be an important component of MID.[11]

MID can be especially helpful in managing caries in young children who are not yet cooperative in a dental environment. These situations often leave few options outside of conscious sedation or general anesthesia, so MID may serve as an interim treatment approach until patients are able to cooperate for more traditional treatment. It is also possible, depending on the severity of the disease, that MID can be considered definitive treatment, with no need for reentry or retreatment.

Referrals

Although most dental needs in children ages 3 to 6 can be adequately met by a general dentist, there are times when referral to a pediatric dentist is merited. Examples might include (1) severe caries, (2) dental anxiety or uncooperative behavior, (3) dental trauma, (4) complicated medical history, or (5) complicated developmental disability. Orthodontic concerns can be another reason for referring a child patient to a pediatric dentist or an orthodontist. By involving specialists in their patient's care, general dentists can ensure their patients will receive comprehensive care tailored to their specific needs.

Special Considerations

Oral Habits

Before age 3, children often engage in oral habits (Fig. 9.7) such as thumb-sucking, pacifier use, and tongue thrusting. Although

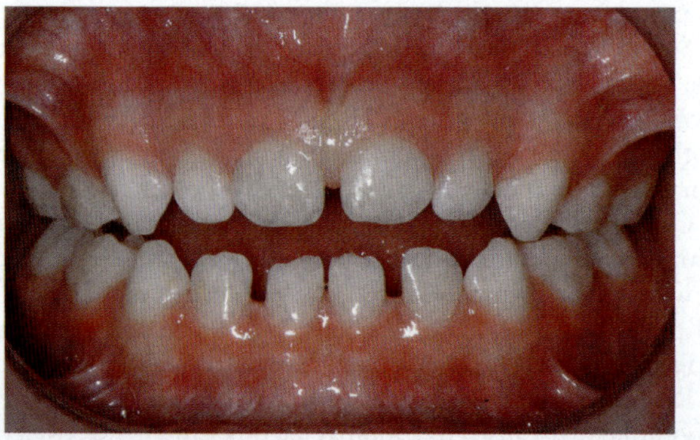

• **Fig. 9.7** This child presents with an anterior open bite, commonly caused by nonnutritive sucking habits such as digit sucking or prolonged pacifier use.

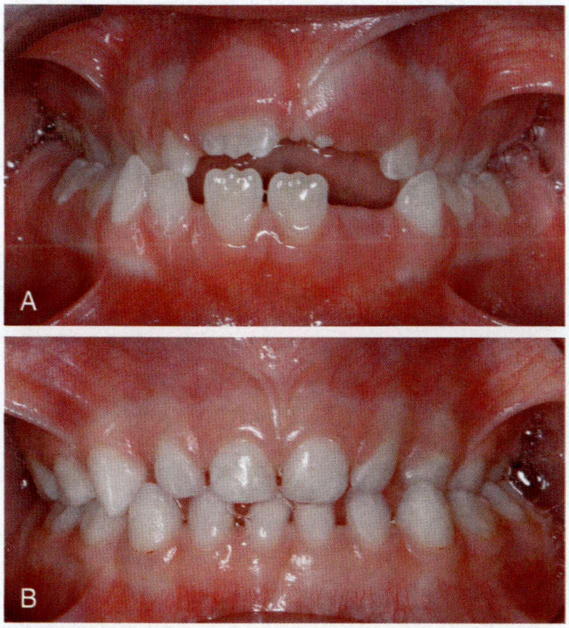

• **Fig. 9.8** Evaluation of this age group may reveal a constriction of the palate and resulting crossbite. Patient A has a bilateral crossbite when the child is in centric relation. Patient B has a unilateral crossbite when the patient is in centric relation. The treatment approaches for these two children will vary because of these relationships. (See Chapter 24 and 25 for a more detailed description of these treatment approaches.)

these behaviors are typically normal and comforting for infants and toddlers, prolonged or intense habits carried over into the 3- to 6-year-old age group can lead to issues such as malocclusion, misalignment of teeth, and changes in the palate (Fig. 9.8). It is crucial for dentists to monitor these habits and provide guidance to parents and caregivers on how to manage and, if necessary, curb them to prevent long-term dental complications. Early intervention and positive reinforcement can help establish healthier oral practices, ensuring better dental outcomes as children grow.

Occlusion

Orthodontic problems and malocclusions in children aged 3 through 6 can significantly affect their dental development and overall well-being. Early identification and treatment of issues such as crossbites, open bites, and severe crowding are crucial in this age group. Malocclusions at this stage may result from prolonged habits like thumb-sucking or pacifier use, genetic factors, or early loss of primary teeth. Addressing these problems early can help guide the proper growth of the jaw and prevent more severe issues as the child ages.

Space Maintenance

Primary teeth act as placeholders for the permanent teeth that will eventually erupt. When a primary tooth is lost prematurely because of decay, trauma, or other factors, the surrounding teeth may shift into the empty space, leading to misalignment and crowding of the future permanent teeth. This can result in complications such as malocclusion, difficulty in chewing, and potential speech issues. Space maintainers help prevent these problems by holding the space open, ensuring that the permanent teeth have adequate room to emerge in their proper positions. By using space maintainers (see Chapter 22 for a thorough discussion of options), dentists can help guide the proper development of the child's dental arch, promoting better oral health and reducing the need for orthodontic treatment in the future.

Visit eBooks.Health.Elsevier.com to see full list of references.

10

The School-aged Child: Ages 6 to 12

HEIDI M. STEINKAMP

CHAPTER OUTLINE

Normal Findings

Dental change is a hallmark feature of children aged 6 to 12. Dentists must recognize that there is a wide continuum of what is considered "normal" within this age range. However, it is key to understand normal eruption and exfoliation sequences to ensure early identification of potential dental anomalies or growth and development problems (Table 10.1).

Although there is wide variability in dental development, by 6 years of age, it is common that many children will have exfoliated some or all primary incisors. Additionally, permanent incisors and first ("six-year") molars may be present or erupting. However, it is important to note that having full primary dentition with no permanent teeth present is not unusual at age 6. By age 12 some children may have exfoliated all primary teeth with second permanent molars present or erupting. However, it is not uncommon for some 12-year-olds to have primary second molars and maxillary canines still present.

Ideal findings include enamel free from hypomineralization, hypoplasia, or fluorosis. It is important to note that primary teeth appear significantly whiter relative to their permanent counterparts,[1] which may be of concern to parents and some pediatric patients who will need reassurance that this is a normal finding (Fig. 10.1). Ideal occlusion includes class I molars (for children with erupted permanent first molars) and class I canines, with approximately 2 mm of overbite and overjet for children with fully erupted permanent incisors.[2] During this time period it is not uncommon to observe minor crowding in the mixed dentition; however, once full permanent dentition has fully erupted, ideally there should be no crowding or spacing present in the dental arches.

The gingiva should be healthy, with attached gingiva exhibiting a stippled appearance with knife-edge papilla (Fig. 10.2). There should be no signs of inflammation, such as bulbous, erythematous gingiva, or bleeding during prophylaxis or dental probing. However, it is important to note that gingivitis occurs in 50% of children aged 4 to 5 and peaks to nearly 100% at puberty.[3]

Preparing for Your Patient

Preparation needed for dental treatment of children aged 6 to 12 is very similar to that of younger age groups, including a welcoming, child-centric office. Age-appropriate distractions to reduce anxiety may include a wide continuum of items from handheld tactile objects (such as fidget spinners and pop-its)[4] to overhead televisions and virtual reality headsets.[5] Dental offices should consider having a website with content that includes child-friendly introductions to team members and operatory setups to help children understand some of the faces and items they may see at their dental visit.[6] And, as with earlier age groups, a dental team trained in communication techniques with children and preteens who recognizes that this age group is quite variable in their development is key in guiding children through their dental visits during these transitional ages.

Equipment needed for children this age includes a dental chair that can accommodate a range of pediatric body sizes; radiography equipment that allows for bitewing, periapical, and panoramic

TABLE 10.1 **Dental Growth and Development**

PRIMARY DENTITION						
			ERUPTION		EXFOLIATION	
	Calcification Begins at	Formation Complete at	Maxillary	Mandibular	Maxillary	Mandibular
Central incisors	4th fetal mo	18–24 mo	6–10 mo	5–8 mo	7–8 y	6–7 y
Lateral incisors	4th fetal mo	18–24 mo	8–12 mo	7–10 mo	8–9 y	7–8 y
Canines	4th fetal mo	30–39 mo	16–20 mo	16–20 mo	11–12 y	9–11 y
First molars	4th fetal mo	24–30 mo	11–18 mo	11–18 mo	9–11 y	10–12 y
Second molars	4th fetal mo	36 mo	20–30 mo	20–30 mo	9–12 y	11–13 y

PERMANENT DENTITION					
			ROOTS	ERUPTION[a]	
	Calcification Begins at	Crown (Enamel) Complete at	Complete at	Maxillary	Mandibular
Central incisors	3–4 mo	4–5 y	9–10 y	7–8 y (3)	6–7 y (2)
Lateral incisors	Maxilla: 10–12 mo Mandible: 3–4 mo	4–5 y 4–5 y	11 y 10 y	8–9 y (5)	7–8 y (4)
Canines	4–5 mo	6–7 y	12–15 y	11–12 y (11)	9–11 y (6)
First premolars	18–24 mo	5–6 y	12–13 y	10–11 y (7)	10–12 y (8)
Second premolars	24–30 mo	6–7 y	12–14 y	10–12 y (9)	11–13 y (10)
First molars	Birth	30–36 mo	9–10 y	5.5–7 y (1)	5.5–7 y (1a)
Second molars	30–36 mo	7–8 y	14–16 y	12–14 y (12)	12–14 y (12a)
Third molars	Maxilla: 7–9 y Mandible: 8–10 y			17–30 y (13)	17–30 y (13a)

[a]Figures in parentheses indicate order of eruption. Many otherwise normal infants do not conform strictly to the stated schedule.

Adapted from Logan WHG, Kronfeld R. Development of the human jaws and surrounding structures from birth to the age of fifteen years. *J Am Dent Assoc* 1933;20(3):379-427.

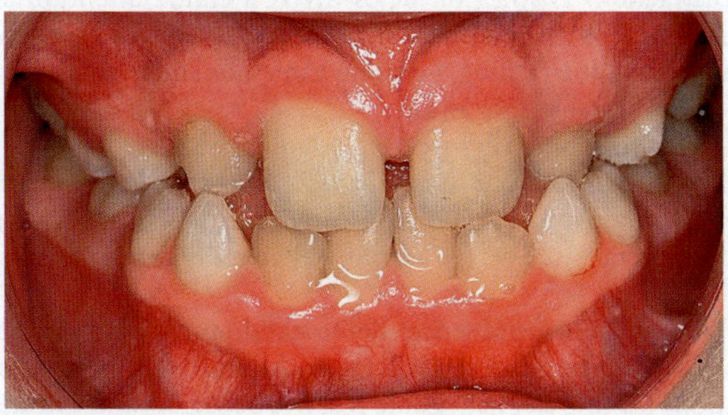

• **Fig. 10.1** The mixed dentition can raise concern for families. Reassurance can be given that crowding is a normal finding and that the color differences between the primary lower canines and the newly erupted permanent incisors is expected due to differences in enamel thickness. (Photo courtesy Dr. Steve Marshall.)

imaging; and supplies needed for nitrous oxide administration. Restorative supplies to have on hand include rubber dam setups and vacuum-based isolations systems, stainless steel crowns (SSCs), and primary and permanent strip crown forms as well as sealant material and restorative supplies.

Information Gathering

Obtaining an accurate health history is key to providing safe dental treatment to pediatric patients. A review of systems approach can be helpful to understand chronic conditions as well as gathering information about allergies, medications, surgical history, previous hospitalizations, and special healthcare needs. For children with complex medical histories and/or special healthcare needs, consultation with their primary care pediatrician or medical specialty team may be necessary to ensure the safest delivery of dental care. It is also important to understand that children who have a history of extensive medical care—such as pediatric cancers or cleft lip and palate—may be more anxious about dental care. Furthermore, children with special healthcare needs may require modifications in behavior guidance and treatment planning (see Chapter 36 for more details).

Obtaining a comprehensive dental history (see Box 10.1) is important in assessing caries risk and understanding how behavior may have impacted past dental visits. Identifying when the last dental visit was and requesting previous records will help better understand individual dental needs and aid in judicious prescribing of radiographs. Inquiring about previous dental trauma is important to ensure proper follow-up and anticipatory guidance

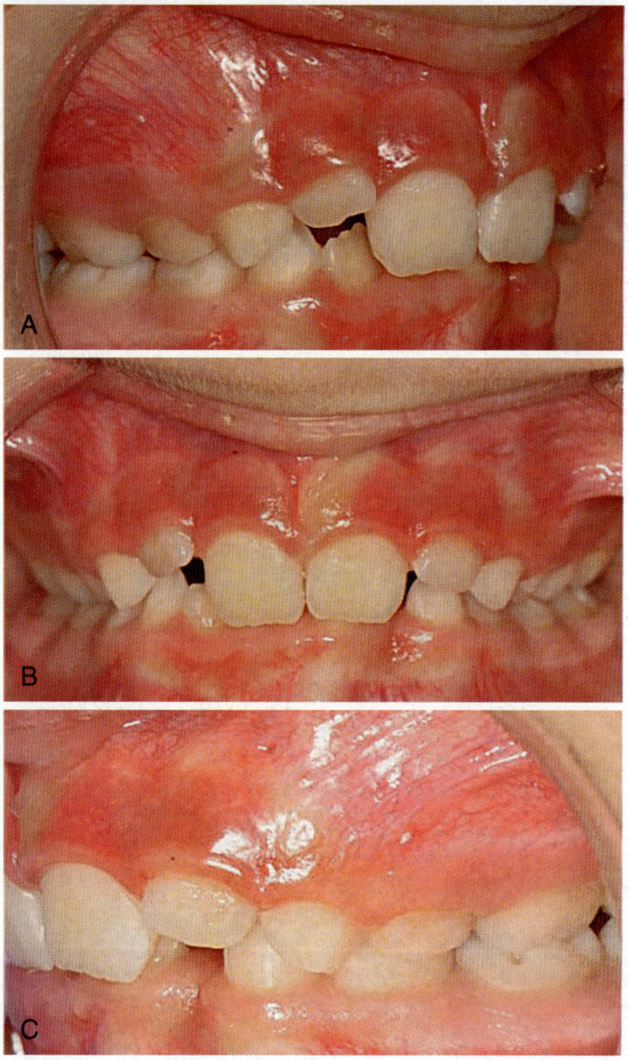

• **Fig. 10.2** Normal gingival appearance in the mixed dentition: (A) right side, (B) anterior, (C) left side. Note areas of localized gingivitis secondary to suboptimal oral hygiene. Healthy, knife-edged papilla can also be seen along with stippling. (Photo courtesy Dr. Matt Geneser.)

for possible trauma sequelae. Inquiring about home oral hygiene, diet, and oral habits is important to facilitate patient education and home care recommendations.

Understanding a child's social history is important for several reasons. From a medicolegal standpoint it is important to know who the child's legal guardian(s) are and who participates in medical/dental decision making. It is also important to understand whether the child spends a significant amount of time in another parent or guardian's household, as oral hygiene and diet practices may be very different in different households.

Behavior Guidance

Appropriate behavior guidance for techniques for children aged 6 to 12 is critical to helping many children through potentially difficult dental visits. It is very important to recognize that there is a great deal of variability within this age range with regard to maturity and coping skills, so having several behavioral guidance strategies available and utilizing an individualized approach with each patient are key. For this age group, school provides children with the experience of separating from parents, responding to instructions from strangers, and cooperating in a structured environment. However, new experiences may be a source of stress for the child, which can manifest in the dental environment.[7] Nash suggests three skills that can be used for effective communication with children: (1) reflective listening, (2) self-disclosing assertiveness (i.e., "I cannot see the teeth when the mouth is closed"), and (3) descriptive praise. In addition, this age group is especially receptive to play and humor.[8] Playing games and telling jokes can be useful to build rapport and make the visit more enjoyable.[9] These techniques are appropriate in all age groups but are especially helpful in this age group of patients because they become more sophisticated in their relationships with adults outside the home.

It is very important to recognize that many outside influences can affect how children behave at dental visits, such as parental perceptions of dental care, the child's temperament and personality, the presence of pain, the presence of special healthcare needs, a history of previous stressful medical or dental visits, and the child's native language.[6] Although those factors are out of your control, you can ensure that you and your staff employ effective behavior guidance strategies.

Some behavior guidance techniques to consider for this age group include[6] (but are not limited to):

- Positive previsit imagery: As mentioned previously, having videos or images on a practice website or having guidebooks in reception areas can help introduce children to the dental team and the dental armamentarium.
- Tell-show-do (TSD): TSD is a universal technique that helps prepare children by initially explaining what is going to happen (tell), demonstrating what will happen in a nonthreatening way (show), and then implementing the dental procedure (do). TSD aids in desensitization and helps set expectations for the child.
- Positive reinforcement: Provide positive feedback to reward a child who is behaving well during treatment. This could include verbal praise (be specific), facial expressions, and prizes.
- Distraction: Distraction helps divert a child's attention away from a potentially unpleasant procedure. This can be accomplished by storytelling, guessing games, or audiovisuals such as television, tablets, or music.
- Desensitization: Very fearful or apprehensive patients can slowly be introduced to new aspects of dental care in a systematic, progressive fashion. This approach is gradual and may take several visits before a child will be ready for a "traditional" dental visit.
- Parental presence/absence: Some children may behave better without a parent present chairside. Alternatively, in some situations parents can help guide positive behaviors and extinguish unwanted behaviors during treatment. However, it is important to note that many parents will expect to be present with their child during their dental visits.
- Nitrous oxide: Nitrous oxide is a safe and proven mechanism to help alleviate anxiety during dental treatment. It is important to titrate to the minimal dose needed to achieve anxiolysis for an individual child. Practitioners must possess the skills and necessary training to safely administer nitrous oxide in compliance with state dental laws and recognize factors that could be contraindications to use.
- Oral sedation: Oral conscious sedation is an advanced behavior guidance technique that may need to be employed for the

• BOX 10.1 Components of a Comprehensive Dental History

Obtaining and understanding a **comprehensive dental history** is essential for every dental practitioner. While the core components apply to patients of all ages, certain areas may become more important depending on the patient's age and developmental stage.

A thorough dental history should include evaluation of the following components:

1. **Chief Complaint**
   - Document in the **patient's own words**
   - Clarify onset, duration, severity, and associated symptoms
2. **Fluoride Use and Exposure**
   - Community water fluoridation
   - Fluoridated toothpaste, supplements, varnishes
   - Any **hesitancy or parental concerns**
3. **Oral Hygiene Practices**
   - Brushing frequency
   - Solo or assisted brushing
   - Use of floss, mouth rinse, or other adjuncts
4. **Previous Dental History**
   - Prior dental experiences (positive or negative)
   - History of radiographs, sealants, restorations, extractions
   - Access to dental care and frequency of previous visits
5. **Dietary Habits**
   - Level of caregiver or personal control over diet
   - Carbohydrate exposure and timing
   - Snacking frequency
   - Use of bottles, sippy cups, or nighttime feeding (for pediatric patients)
6. **Oral Habits**
   - Current or past habits such as:
   - Thumb/finger sucking, pacifier use, bruxism, nail biting, cheek biting
7. **Trauma History**
   - Prior **dental or facial trauma**
   - History of **TMJ dysfunction**, clicking, pain, or limitation of movement
8. **Sports and Activity Level**
   - Participation in contact sports
   - **Mouthguard** usage
   - Helmet use when appropriate (biking, skateboarding, etc.)
9. **Family Dental History**
   - Caries experience
   - Hypomineralization or enamel defects
   - Missing or extra teeth
   - Genetic or hereditary dental conditions
10. **Social Development**
    - Age-appropriate behavior and communication
    - Ability to socialize
    - Willingness to separate from a guardian
    - Understanding and tolerance for dental procedures

most apprehensive patients. Administration of sedative agents to children in this age group requires advanced training and often requires special permitting or licensure. See Chapter 27 for a thorough review of pharmacologic behavior guidance techniques.

Other factors to consider when treating this age group are avoiding terms that could cause fear such as "shot" or "needle" and not showing children needles or other instruments that could cause fear. Furthermore, it is important not to deny or ignore pain because this can undermine the child's trust in you and your dental team. And finally, instructing children to do specific actions versus asking them whether they want to do something can help avoid situations in which a child refuses to do something because they believe they were given a choice. A thorough discussion of nonpharmacologic behavior guidance techniques can be found in Chapter 26.

Clinical Examination

A thorough clinical examination is key to identifying anomalies that may be present intraorally or extraorally. Position patients in the dental chair as you would a teenage or adult patient, with the operator chairside or behind the patient during examination. Begin with an extraoral examination that assesses facial symmetry, lip competence, and the presence, size, and location of any extraoral soft tissue findings such as cicatrices or nevi. The temporomandibular joint should be assessed for tenderness and/or clicks or deviations upon opening and closing, and any palpable or tender head and neck lymph nodes should be noted.

After the extraoral examination a thorough intraoral examination will include a soft tissue evaluation, including examination and assessment of the lips, tongue, hard and soft palates, buccal tissues, sublingual space, and gingiva. Gingival health should be noted, including the presence of healthy gingiva or the presence of gingivitis (including severity), bleeding, pigmentation, and/or recession. For cooperative patients in this age range certain fully erupted teeth can be selected for periodontal probing. Abnormal periodontal probing depths may warrant full mouth probing for patients able to cooperate. Oral hygiene should be documented, including the presence, level, and location of plaque and calculus.

After the soft tissue examination, a hard tissue examination should take place. Begin by noting which teeth are present, bearing in mind that this age group is characterized by dental change and there is a continuum of "normal" dental compositions that may vary by patient. Note the location and presence of clinically evident caries, fractures, or attrition. Document the location and condition of existing restorations. Finally, perform an occlusal analysis, noting canine and molar relationships, overbite, overjet, crossbites, crowding, and/or spacing present.

Radiographic Examination

Radiographs should be prescribed on an individual basis following a thorough intraoral examination, with consideration of clinical findings, caries risk, and patient history. The American Academy of Pediatric Dentistry (AAPD) has recommendations for prescribing dental radiographs that were developed using Americans with Disabilities Act and US Food and Drug Administration guidelines and should be used in conjunction with professional judgment.

Bitewing radiographs are the most prescribed films in this age group. These films allow for the detection of interproximal caries and assessment of crestal bone height. The frequency of bitewing radiographs can be anywhere between 6 and 36 months, taking into consideration caries risk, dentition present, and the presence/absence of existing interproximal caries or incipient lesions.[10]

Select periapical films can be considered in situations in which patients are reporting dental pain or there are deep caries present in close approximation to pulp to assess furcal or periapical bone health. Periapical films may also be indicated if there is a history of dental trauma. Furthermore, periapical or occlusal films may be taken to identify supernumerary anterior teeth or to assess canine eruption paths.

After the eruption of permanent teeth begins, panoramic radiograph imaging should be considered to allow practitioners a comprehensive view of the dentition—including both erupted and unerupted teeth and supporting structures. Panoramic films can also allow for early detection of congenitally missing teeth, ectopic eruption paths, and pathology. Panoramic films are often taken every 3 to 5 years to allow for continued monitoring of growth and development and surveillance of dental pathology.

Prevention

An in-office and home preventive plan should be developed for every child. Development of an individualized prevention approach (versus a "one size fits all") is key to caries prevention and management. The first step in an individualized plan is determining appropriate recalls for in-office dental care. Although 6-month recall intervals are acceptable for many children aged 6 to 12, some high-risk patients may benefit from more frequent visits, such as 3- or 4-month recall intervals. In-office preventive care may include dental prophylaxis, sealant application, application of topical fluorides, application of caries-arresting medicaments, oral hygiene instruction, and dietary counseling.

The importance of a practical and implementable home care preventive plan cannot be overstated. Twice daily brushing for 2 minutes with fluoridated toothpaste should be stressed as well as the introduction of once-a-day flossing if it has not already been implemented into a home care plan. It is important to note that this age group will begin to transition from assisted and/or supervised brushing to autonomous brushing, so home care advice and correct techniques should be directed to both patients and caregivers. Many caregivers will ask what age children can begin to brush independently, but it is important to stress that many factors play into children's ability to brush independently, such as maturity and manual dexterity. One study found that children who play musical instruments independently and wash dishes are more effective at plaque removal.[11]

A thorough caries risk assessment for each child based on individual risk factors is key to guiding both in-office and home care regimens and caries management plans. AAPD has a caries risk assessment form to help providers determine whether a child is at low, moderate, or high caries risk (Table 10.2). By assessing each child's individual risk level based on dental, medical, social, and clinical risk factors, in addition to protective factors, providers can determine appropriate intervals for recall visits, the need for prescription fluoride applications, and the periodicity of dental radiographs.

Fluoride remains the key component of caries-prevention plans, but some non-fluoride preventive adjuncts could be considered for children aged 6 to 12. Xylitol and other sugar alcohols used in the manufacturing of products such as gum, mints, lozenges, and candy can serve as noncariogenic sugar substitutes.[12] Calcium and phosphate-containing dentifrices such as MI paste (Minimal Intervention paste) may be recommended for children with white spot lesions or hypomineralized enamel. Although newer dentifrices containing hydroxyapatite[13] and arginine show promise in reducing dental caries,[14] further research is needed (see Chapter 14).

Dietary counseling with both patients and caregivers should be performed at each dental visit. Recommendations should include eating nutrient-dense lean or low-fat foods from each of the five food groups (fruits, vegetables, proteins, grains, and dairy) and limiting intake of excess sugars and saturated fats.[15] Limiting snacking to discrete times should be emphasized, with recommendations for fresh fruits, vegetables, nuts, and cheeses. In addition, discussing healthy beverage choices is also important, with emphasis given to limiting or eliminating sugar-sweetened beverages.[15] Milk should ideally be consumed at mealtimes only, and fluoridated water should be recommended as the preferred beverage of choice.

Restorative Considerations

When treatment planning restorative care for children aged 6 to 12, many factors must be considered, such as primary versus permanent tooth caries, remaining intraoral time (for primary teeth), lesion size, caries risk, parent preferences, and the ability of the child to cooperate for restorative care (Fig. 10.3). For cooperative children with lesions on permanent teeth, a traditional restorative dental approach can be taken, following ideal preparation and restoration principles. For uncooperative children with lesions on permanent teeth, interim treatment modalities may have to be implemented such as silver diamine fluoride (SDF) application[16] or transitional glass ionomer restorations[17] until the child is able to cooperate for more definitive restorations.

For children with primary tooth caries, remaining intraoral time, lesions size, and caries risk will factor heavily into treatment planning. Class II resin, resin-modified glass ionomer, or amalgam restorations may be appropriate in some situations, particularly for children with few or isolated class II carious lesions. SSCs are the ideal treatment for any posterior tooth with mesial and distal caries that is not approaching natural exfoliation and for posterior teeth with large carious lesions that exhibit marginal ridge breakdown. SSCs are also a reasonable option for young children who are high caries risk with one or two surface lesions present on posterior teeth with longer remaining intraoral times. In addition, SSCs are often better restorative options for posterior primary teeth in children with limited cooperation because they are less technique sensitive. SSCs can also be placed with no preparation, via the Hall technique, which can be done without the need for local anesthetic.[18]

For cooperative children with mesio-occlusal (MO) or disto-occlusal (DO) caries present on posterior primary teeth or with anterior class III or class V lesions, both composite resins and resin-modified glass ionomers are good restorative options. Composite restorations have the benefit of better aesthetics and wear resistance over time, whereas resin-modified glass ionomers may be chosen for their fluoride-releasing properties, and they have the benefit of being less technique sensitive. Zirconia crowns can be considered for cooperative children with mesial and distal caries on posterior teeth or posterior teeth with marginal ridge breakdown or on anterior teeth with extensive caries. However, evidence is limited on their long-term success, and their preparation often requires longer appointment times compared with SSCs. Composite or glass ionomer strip crowns may also present a good restorative option for children with extensive caries on anterior primary teeth with longer remaining intraoral times and for permanent anterior teeth with extensive breakdown caused by caries or dental trauma.[18]

Active surveillance or medical management with SDF may be appropriate for children with caries on primary teeth that are nearing natural exfoliation. SDF can also be considered for incipient lesions that have not crossed the dentino-enamel junction (DEJ) in children of all ages. In addition, SDF or glass ionomer interim restorations could be considered for very uncooperative children with cavitated lesions that do not involve the pulp.[16,17] For children with caries

TABLE 10.2 Caries Risk Assessment Form for Ages 6+

Use of this tool will help the healthcare provider assess the child's risk for developing caries lesions. In addition, reviewing specific factors will help the practitioner and patient/parent understand the variable influences that contribute to or protect from dental caries.

Factors	High Risk	Moderate Risk	Low Risk
Risk factors, social/behavioral/medical			
Patient has lifetime of poverty, low health literacy	Yes		
Patient has frequent exposure (>3 times/day) to between-meal sugar-containing snacks or beverages per day	Yes		
Child is a recent immigrant		Yes	
Patient uses hyposalivatory medication(s)		Yes	
Patient has special healthcare needs[a]		Yes	
Risk factors, clinical			
Patient has low salivary flow	Yes		
Patient has visible plaque on teeth	Yes		
Patient presents with dental enamel defects	Yes		
Patient wears an intraoral appliance		Yes	
Patient has defective restorations		Yes	
Protective factors			
Patient receives optimally fluoridated drinking water			Yes
Patient has teeth brushed daily with fluoridated toothpaste			Yes
Patient receives topical fluoride from health professional			Yes
Patient has dental home/regular dental care			Yes
Disease indicators[b]			
Patient has interproximal caries lesion(s)	Yes		
Patient has new noncavitated (white spot) caries lesions	Yes		
Patient has new cavitated caries lesions or lesions into dentin radiographically	Yes		
Patient has restorations that were placed in the past 3 years (new patient) or in the past 12 months (patient of record)	Yes		

[a]Practitioners may choose a different risk level based on specific medical diagnosis and unique circumstances, especially conditions that affect motor coordination or cooperation.

[b]Although these do not cause caries directly or indirectly, they indicate presence factors that do.

Instructions: *Circle "yes" that corresponds with host conditions that apply to a specific patient. Use the circled responses to visualize the balance among risk factors, protective factors, and disease indicators. Use this balance or imbalance, together with clinical judgment, to assign a caries risk level of low, moderate, or high based on the preponderance of factors for the individual. Clinical judgment may justify the weighting of one factor (e.g., heavy plaque on the teeth) more than others.*

Overall assessment of the dental caries risk: High ❑ Moderate ❑ Low ❑

From American Academy of Pediatric Dentistry. Caries-risk assessment and management for infants, children, and adolescents. *The Reference Manual of Pediatric Dentistry.* Chicago, IL: American Academy of Pediatric Dentistry; 2025:325-31.

Adapted from Featherstone JBD, Domejean-Orliaguet S, Jenson L, et al. Caries risk assessment in practice for age 6 through adult. *J Calif Dent Assoc.* 2007;35(10):703-713.

being managed by interim therapeutics or active surveillance, it is very important to provide thorough informed consent to caregivers.

Referrals

Sometimes specialty referrals are necessary for comprehensive dental care. Some specialty referrals for children aged 6 to 12 could include:

- Orthodontics: Orthodontists can help manage dental malocclusions and dental and skeletal growth issues. The American Academy of Orthodontists recommends an orthodontic consultation for all children by the age of 7.
- Oral and maxillofacial surgery: Referral may be necessary to manage supernumerary or ankylosed tooth extractions, biopsy of pathologic lesions, or management of severe facial traumas.
- Periodontics: Periodontists can help manage aggressive periodontitis or recession.
- Endodontics: Endodontic referrals may be necessary for management of root canal therapies on permanent teeth secondary to caries or dental trauma.
- Prosthodontics: Referral to a prosthodontist may be indicated for children in this age group with anodontia, oligodontia, or congenital dental defects of enamel or dentin such as amelogenesis imperfecta or dentinogenesis imperfecta.

Special Considerations

Management of Hypomineralized Molars

Management of molar hypomineralization (MH) in this age group can be a major challenge (see Chapter 31, online case). MH often occurs with incisor hypomineralization; however, MH tends to be more problematic because masticatory forces can cause rapid wear and breakdown of these teeth. The prevalence of MH in the United States is approximately 10% to 13%. Risk factors for hypomineralization are believed to include infections, persistent fevers, antibiotic use in early childhood, preterm birth, maternal smoking during pregnancy, and traumatic birth/hypoxia at birth. Restorative management can vary depending on the severity, timing, number of teeth affected, parental preferences, and patient

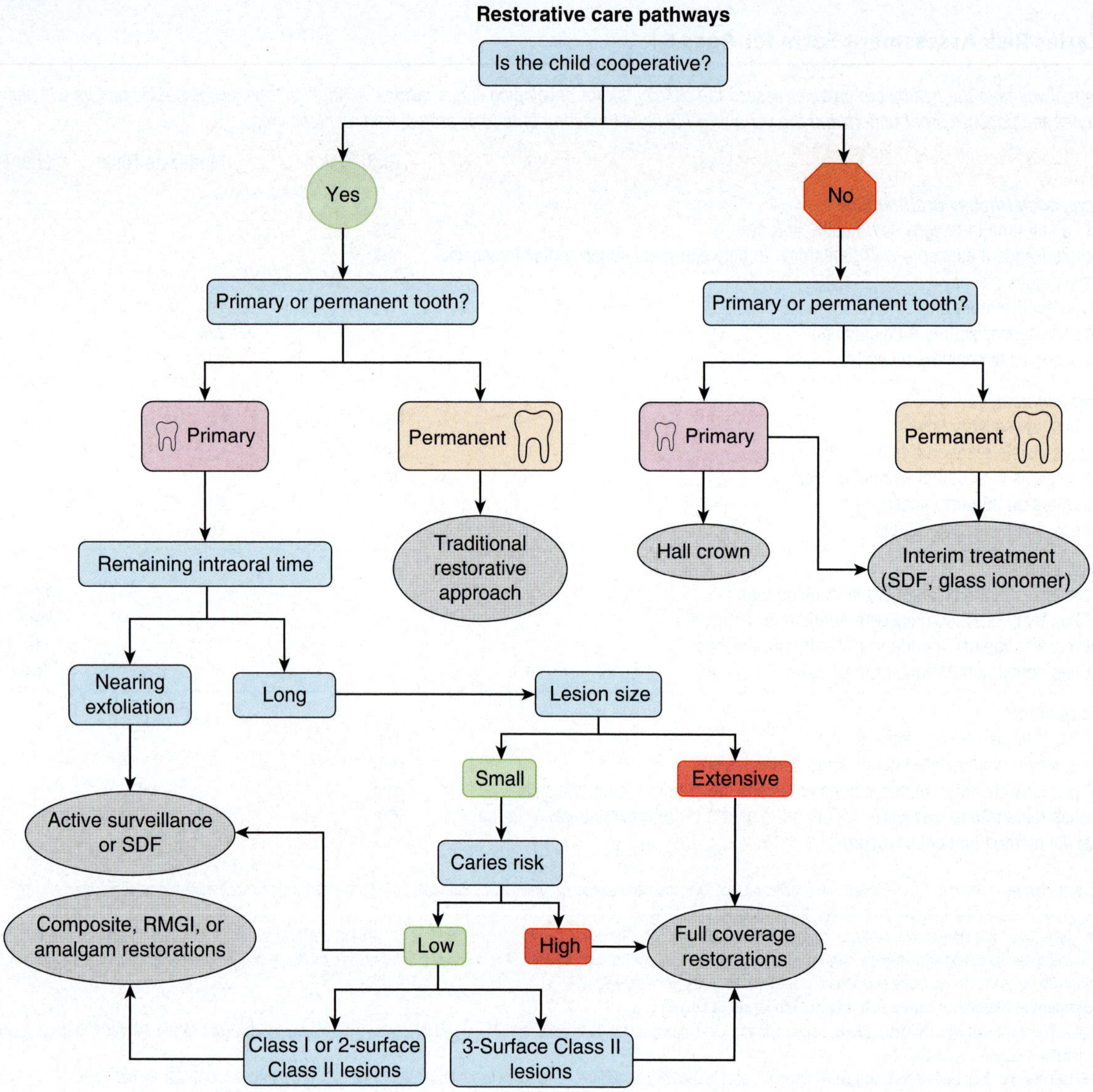

• **Fig. 10.3** Restorative treatment planning decision tree. *RMGI,* Resin-modified glass ionomer; *SDF,* silver diamine fluoride.

cooperation. In some instances, mild cases can be managed with remineralizing agents, SDF, and sealants. However, in more severe cases full coverage restorations such as SSCs or orthodontic bands with glass ionomer occlusal coverage can be considered as well as extraction of hypomineralized teeth. Factors in support of maintaining hypomineralized molars include hypodontia; dental spacing; the need for anchorage in orthodontic therapy; and in situations where only one molar is affected, extraction may cause supraeruption of the opposing dentition. Factors in favor of extraction include severely affected molars (often with pulpal or periapical pathology), dental crowding, acute hypersensitivity, poor patient cooperation, and barriers to dental care.[19]

Pulp Therapy for Primary Teeth

Vital pulp therapy for primary teeth can include liners, indirect pulp treatment, direct pulp caps, and pulpotomies (see Chapter 32). Liners may be placed over dentin in deeper areas of cavity preparations that may be in close approximation to the pulp to help promote pulp tissue healing. Liners can include mineral trioxide aggregate (MTA), trisilicate cements, calcium hydroxide, glass ionomers, or other biocompatible materials. Indirect pulp therapy involves leaving the deepest carious dentin adjacent to the pulp undisturbed to avoid a pulp exposure. This affected dentin should be covered with a biocompatible material such as dentin bonding agents, glass ionomer, MTA, calcium hydroxide, or other biocompatible materials to produce a biologic seal. Direct pulp capping can be performed when a pinpoint exposure less than 1 mm occurs during cavity preparation or because of a traumatic pulp exposure. Biocompatible radiopaque materials such as MTA or calcium hydroxide should be placed over the exposed pulp tissue. Pulpotomies are indicated in primary teeth after a caries removal or trauma causes a pulp exposure in teeth that do not have clinical or radiograph signs or symptoms of irreversible pulpitis or necrosis. Coronal tissue is amputated, and after the remaining radicular tissue is deemed vital with adequate hemostasis, MTA is the material of choice to be applied over the exposed pulp stumps. After any vital pulp therapy, a restoration that seals the tooth from microleakage should be chosen for the best long-term prognosis.[20]

Nonvital pulp therapies for primary teeth with irreversible pulpitis or necrosis include pulpectomies and lesion sterilization/tissue repair (LSTR). In primary tooth pulpectomies root canals are debrided with files and then irrigated with dilute NaOCl (1% to 5%), chlorhexidine, or sterile water or saline. After the canals are dried a resorbable material such as zinc oxide eugenol (ZOE) or iodoform paste is used to seal the canals. In LSTR a triple antibiotic paste composed of clindamycin, metronidazole, and ciprofloxacin is placed in the pulp chamber of the tooth, with no canal instrumentation. LSTR is preferred over pulpectomy when a tooth has limited remaining intraoral time (less than 12 months) or exhibits resorption.[20]

Pulp Therapy for Young Permanent Teeth

Vital pulp therapy for immature permanent teeth can include liners, indirect pulp treatment, direct pulp capping, partial pulpotomies, and complete pulpotomies (see Chapter 33). Protective liners, indirect pulp treatment, and direct pulp capping follow the same principles outlined previously for primary pulp therapy. Partial pulpotomies can be performed following both carious pulp exposures and traumatic pulp exposures (Cvek pulpotomies). In both types of partial pulpotomies the outermost inflamed pulp tissue is removed to a depth of 1 to 3 mm or deeper to reach healthy pulp tissue. Hemostasis should be achieved by application of cotton pellets soaked in NaOCl, chlorhexidine, or sterile water to the pulp tissue. The exposure should then be covered with calcium hydroxide, MTA, or other biocompatible agents such as tricalcium silicate. It is very important to note that MTA can cause gray staining of teeth, so its use as a pulpal medicament in anterior teeth should be avoided if possible. Complete pulpotomy involves the complete removal of coronal pulp tissue, followed by irrigation with cotton pellets soaked in NaOCl, chlorhexidine, or sterile water, and then placement of MTA or tricalcium silicate over the pulp stumps. As with primary teeth, after any vital pulp therapy, a restoration that seals the tooth from microleakage should be chosen for the best long-term prognosis. The goal of vital pulp therapy in immature teeth is apexogenesis—continued apex closure and dentinal wall deposition.[20]

Nonvital pulp therapies for immature permanent teeth include pulpectomy, apexification, and regenerative endodontics. A pulpectomy in young permanent teeth is conventional root canal therapy in teeth with closed apices. Apexification is a method to induce apical closure in teeth with irreversible pulpitis or necrosis with open apices. After extirpation of pulp tissue, calcium hydroxide is placed into the canal system to disinfect the canal space for 2 to 4 weeks. After this, an MTA plug is placed to create a barrier at the open apices, and gutta percha is used to fill the remaining canal space. During regenerative endodontics, bioactive material containing stem cells and growth factors is placed into the disinfected root canal space to promote increased width of root walls and root length.[20] Most nonvital pulp therapies for young permanent teeth are best managed by endodontists because of the complexity of the procedure.

Management and Prevention of Traumatic Dental Injuries

Effective management and prevention of traumatic dental injuries in children aged 6 to 12 is important, as 25% of all school-aged children experience a dental trauma.[21] If a child reports to your office immediately after a dental trauma, it is extremely important to determine whether there was loss of consciousness or if the child is exhibiting an altered state of consciousness. If this is the case, the child should immediately be referred to the nearest emergency department for medical assessment and management of a possible closed head injury.

Traumatic dental injuries include a wide range of clinical presentations, including enamel infraction, uncomplicated crown (enamel-only and enamel-dentin) fractures, complicated crown fractures (enamel-dentin fracture with pulp exposure), uncomplicated crown-root fractures (without pulp exposure), complicated crown-root fractures (with pulp exposure), root fractures, alveolar fractures, concussions, subluxations, extrusive luxations, lateral luxations, intrusive luxations, and avulsions. The AAPD follows the trauma guidelines developed by the International Association of Dental Traumatology for the management of traumatic dental injuries, which outlines clinical findings, radiographic and treatment recommendations, recommended follow-up, favorable outcomes, and unfavorable outcomes.[21,22] In addition to these published guidelines, the online Dental Trauma Guide offers visual and video resources to members[23] to help dental professionals manage traumatic dental injuries. A thorough review of dental trauma can be found in Chapters 40 and 41.

A key aspect to dental injury management is prevention. Identifying patients at risk of dental injuries such as children who participate in contact sports[24] or children with excess overjet[25] is an important aspect of comprehensive dental care. Mouthguard use should be advocated for children participating in contact sports,[24] and an orthodontic consultation may be valuable for children with excess overjet, although evidence is limited as to whether early orthodontic intervention mitigates the incidence of dental trauma.[26] Anticipatory guidance on what to do if a dental injury occurs should be provided to all patients and caregivers in your dental practice.

Orthodontic Management in Mixed Dentition

With appropriate training, many general dentists and pediatric dentists can manage minor orthodontic problems encountered in children with mixed dentition. Orthodontic management could be as simple as space maintenance after dental extractions, serial extractions to help guide permanent tooth eruption, habit appliances in children with nonnutritive sucking habits, or management of single-tooth anterior crossbites with finger spring appliances.[27] Patients needing phase I (interceptive) and/or phase II (comprehensive) orthodontic care will likely be best served by orthodontists or by pediatric dentists working in close collaboration with orthodontic colleagues. See Chapters 24 and 25 for a more detailed review of orthodontic treatment in children.

Visit eBooks.Health.Elsevier.com to see full list of references.

11
Adolescent Oral Health

NATALIE M. STINTON

CHAPTER OUTLINE

Introduction

The World Health Organization defines adolescence as the transition from childhood to adulthood, ranging from ages 10 to 19, although many think of this population as "teenagers." Treating adolescent dental patients is an important part of dentistry that is often shouldered by the pediatric dental provider. It is crucial that all dentists are educated in treating patients within this age group because preventive care is of utmost importance to establish good oral hygiene habits and prevent dental issues such as caries, gum disease, and malocclusion. During this time frame patients are becoming more autonomous, and thus the responsibility for home care is transitioned away from the parents and rests largely, if not solely, on the adolescent.

Orthodontic evaluation and intervention are also key components of dental care in this time frame. Many adolescents will require orthodontic treatment to correct malalignment of teeth. Timely evaluation can allow for early identification of concerns and initiation of treatment at the appropriate time to maximize success and minimize the amount of time required in active orthodontic care. Patients are in active growth during this phase, and thus alignment concerns can develop over time that may not have been evident earlier in development. Esthetic concerns also become more evident during this period as patients start to be more self-aware of their own appearance. Helping guide patients toward well-timed orthodontic interventions is a key component of the pediatric dental care of these patients.

Many patients are also active in organized sports in this phase, and providing education regarding sports-related injuries can help prevent a damaging loss of tooth structure. During this time frame patients are also more likely to start substance abuse; thus guiding them on the detrimental effects this can have on their systemic and oral health can help prevent unnecessary mortality and morbidity over time.

Many of these considerations are unique to the adolescent population and thus must be taken into account by oral healthcare professionals who care for this group of individuals. Historically a group of oral healthcare providers for this population most often includes:

- Restorative dentists (general or pediatric): Pediatric dentists are often used when behavioral concerns are present. General dentists are often used when the restorative needs match closest to an adult patient.
- Dental hygienists: Hygienists often work alongside dentists to provide preventive dental care including cleanings, fluoride treatments, oral hygiene education, and anticipatory guidance. They play a vital role in promoting oral health and preventing dental issues in adolescents.
- Orthodontists: Orthodontists specialize in the diagnosis, prevention, and treatment of dental and facial irregularities including misaligned teeth and jaws.
- Oral and maxillofacial surgeons: Oral and maxillofacial surgeons specialize in surgical procedures involving the mouth, jaws, and face. They may provide surgical treatment for adolescents requiring third molar removal, corrective jaw surgery, or surgical expose and bond procedures for impacted teeth.

Normal Findings

Normal findings in the adolescent age group vary widely based on the age and stage of development. Patients who are in early adolescence often still have primary teeth and have not reached their growth spurt; however, they may have also reached puberty and have full adolescent dentition. By the end of adolescence, primary teeth should have all exfoliated and all permanent teeth (apart from third molars) should have erupted.

From a soft tissue findings perspective, it has been reported that more than 90% of patients during puberty have gingivitis.[1] This may be related to any number of factors including hormonal changes during this time and poor oral hygiene as they transition to more autonomous care.

Careful records should be maintained on patients, including intraoral photos, when possible, to help track changes over time. These can also be especially helpful in the event of a future dental trauma and determining how to restore the patient to prior function and esthetics.

Preparing for Your Patient

The equipment needed to treat adolescent dental patients is very similar to those in the younger population. You will want to make sure that you have a dental chair that can accommodate their larger size and consider purchasing one with a weight limit of at least 350 pounds. You will also want to make sure that you have appropriate radiographic film sizes. Although many smaller children use a size 0 or size 1 film for intraoral images, an adolescent will need a size 2 film in order to view appropriate anatomy. If you do not have a panorex in your own office, you will want to make sure that you have access to obtaining a panoramic image to screen for pathology and appropriate growth and development.

Other equipment considerations include larger sizes for nitrous oxide nasal hoods, rubber dam clamps, and isolation systems. Different types of dental matrix systems can make restoring permanent teeth easier. A practitioner seeing a large number of adolescent patients may also wish to keep in stock permanent tooth preformed crown options and adult strip crown sizes for teeth that require full-coverage restorations.

Many pediatric offices are designed to be very child friendly, but, when possible, it would be ideal to have at least one room that is more neutral or less geared toward the young child so that an adolescent feels comfortable and welcome. The same principle should be applied to what is playing on any media devices including televisions or music played on the speaker. If an adolescent does not feel welcome in a space, they are less likely to be willing participants in their care.

Patient History

No matter the age of the patient, it is of utmost importance to gather information regarding their past medical history, dental history, and social history. This allows the dental practitioner to safely and appropriately treat the patient. A consideration should be made for gathering information such as the social history directly from the patient out of earshot of the parent in order to give them the opportunity to disclose any sensitive information that they would not want their guardian to hear.

A complete health history includes asking questions regarding any chronic medical conditions, allergies, medications, and prior surgical history or hospitalizations. Depending on the age and sex of the patient, it is important to ask if there is a chance of pregnancy as well, as that may affect treatment. Some facilities require or strongly recommend a pregnancy test before any form of sedation including nitrous oxide analgesia.

Pertinent dental history is important to ascertain because this can affect treatment planning recommendations as well. It is important to know if the patient has had previous dental procedures and their level of anxiety with these procedures. Understanding where and when their last dental examination was completed and obtaining previous records can also be helpful, especially to reduce redundant radiograph exposure if recent diagnostic films are available. It is important to know if the patient has any history of dental trauma so that appropriate reevaluation guidelines can be followed. You also want to get an accurate idea of their oral hygiene habits including how often and when they floss, brushing habits, fluoride exposure, and whether they are using any other oral health products regularly such as mouth rinse or whitening products. If the child has had orthodontic care previously, understanding the type of retainer use and frequency of use will also be important in providing appropriate anticipatory guidance.

The social history for your patient is also important to obtain because several factors could put them at an increased risk for future disease. You want to understand your patient's dietary habits including frequency of sugar consumption and intake of acidic or erosive foods and beverages. Caffeine drinks and sports drinks, as well as sugary coffee drinks, are prevalent in this population. You want to know if your patient has any oral habits (e.g., nail biting, teeth grinding, frequent gum chewing) and if they have any oral piercings. It is important to know if the patient is involved in organized sports because that can influence the risk for dental trauma and the need for mouthguards.

As mentioned previously, risky behaviors also start to arise in this age group. Most often, if you do not ask the question specifically, you will not find out if these behaviors exist. Asking about tobacco use, including smoking, vaping, or smokeless tobacco, is important as it puts the child at risk for certain oral pathology including squamous cell carcinoma. The same is true for alcohol consumption, and understanding frequency and quantity, as this can have interactions with medications (particularly if the patient is going to be sedated) and also puts them at a risk for future oropharyngeal cancer. It is also important to find out if they are sexually active—not only for pregnancy risk but also for sexually transmitted infections including the human papillomavirus (HPV). Some adolescents may not feel that it is necessary to disclose this, or they may feel that oral sex does not "count," so being specific may be necessary to obtain an accurate history.

It is also important to assess the adolescent's support system. Do they have involved, reliable parents, or will it be difficult to get to appointments and maintain adequate home care without the necessary supplies? Do they have a supportive group of friends, or are they isolated and bullied? Factors such as these can put the child at risk for suicidal thoughts, which we know now is approximately tied with homicide as the second leading cause of death in teenagers aged 13 to 18.[2] A positive support system can help prevent adolescents from gravitating toward risky social behaviors as well, which will influence their overall health.

Behavior and Coping Skills

The anticipated behavior and coping skills for an adolescent dental patient may vary widely based on factors such as age, previous dental and medical experiences, and individual temperament. Patients who have had a history of positive dental experiences and are not actively in any acute pain are generally thought to be able to cooperate and follow directions with minimal behavior guidance techniques required. Those who have had previous painful dental experiences and are currently in acute pain due to an active infection or injury are much more likely to be fearful and anxious in the dental clinic. This is one reason to have a thorough understanding of a patient's dental history so that the provider can be sensitive to each patient's potential fears.

The patient should be made aware before any treatment is rendered that it is their responsibility to inform the dental professional if they are experiencing discomfort. Sometimes discomfort can occur because of positioning of dental equipment, the presence of ulcers, chapped or cracked lips, or inadequate local anesthesia. If the patient can communicate this discomfort effectively with members of the dental team, adjustments can quickly be made to make it a more positive and enjoyable experience for the patient. Likewise, the dental team should be on the lookout for signs of discomfort including wincing, white knuckles, shallow breathing, and tears. Taking pauses to specifically ask what is bothering the patient can allow you to take swift action to relieve discomfort and help build a trusting relationship.

Sometimes discomfort is unavoidable, and being truthful with the patient to manage their expectations can still help maintain that trusting relationship. If you are dismissive of a patient's fears or their description of what they are experiencing, this will heighten anxiety and lower the pain threshold.

Behavior management techniques for adolescent dental patients should aim to create a positive and supportive environment while addressing any anxiety or fear they may have. These methods range from basic to advanced and may include:

- Positive reinforcement: Offer praise and encouragement to help build rapport and motivate adolescents. This is particularly helpful in maintaining proper home care.
- Distraction: Provide distractions such as music, television, or handheld devices to help adolescents focus their attention away from the dental procedure. Engaging in conversation about topics of interest can also serve as a distraction.
- Relaxation techniques: Teaching techniques such as deep breathing or progressive muscle relaxation can help adolescents manage anxiety and stress during dental procedures. These procedures can be practiced at home between the treatment planning visit and the procedure visit.
- Choice and control: Adolescents often appreciate the opportunity to have a say in their care. Whether this means something such as isolation method (rubber dam vs. isolating suction system), which tooth to fix first, or a flavor of topical or fluoride, the ability to have a say in their care often improves compliance during the visit.
- Nitrous oxide analgesia: Use of nitrous oxide analgesia can help adolescents who have significant anxiety or fear to help induce relaxation and reduce discomfort during dental procedures.
- Oral sedation: For the very fearful patient, advanced behavior guidance techniques such as sedation with medications like diazepam can allow the patient to tolerate more treatment.

Clinical Examination

It is important to have an idea of what to expect when beginning a clinical examination of a patient. Table 11.1 reveals some common clinical findings in the adolescent population. Every clinical examination begins with an extraoral examination. The patient should be evaluated for face and neck asymmetry, swelling, or abnormalities. Palpate the temporomandibular joint (TMJ) for tenderness or clicking. Assess lymph nodes for enlargement or tenderness.

TABLE 11.1 Possible Clinical Findings in Examination of the Adolescent

Structure	Finding	Comment
Extraoral Evaluation		
Skin	Acne	May be painful locally
		Adolescent may take antibiotics
		May appear as radiopacity on some radiographs if calcification occurs
	Cosmetics use	Can complicate evaluation of the skin
		Can cause local allergic response
Neck	Hematoma	From suction; indicates kissing and possible sexual activity
Ears	Healing or scarred punctures	Multiple ear piercings common in both sexes
Hair	Coloring and preparation	Can complicate examination of the scalp
Intraoral Examination		
Mucosa	Generalized erythema	Effect of smoking Sexually transmitted infection
Buccal mucosa	Erythema, hyperkeratosis	Use of smokeless tobacco
Tongue	Coating, odor	Smoking; poor hygiene; fungal overgrowth from medication
Breath	Acetone; alcohol	Excessive dieting, alcohol abuse, metabolic disorders (e.g., diabetes)
Gingiva	Inflammation	Hormonal changes (e.g., puberty gingivitis) Poor oral hygiene
	Pregnancy tumor	Use of oral contraceptives Pregnancy
Teeth	Erosion	Bulimia, gastroesophageal reflux disease
	Wear facets	Temporomandibular joint disorders/bruxism
	Excessive stain	Tobacco use Coffee or tea use
	Discoloration	Existing pulpal pathosis from trauma

Once the extraoral examination is complete, the intraoral examination can begin. Start with soft tissue assessment including evaluating the lips for dryness, lesions, or swelling, Inspect the buccal mucosa for ulcerations and red or white patches. Examine the dorsal and ventral surfaces, sides, and base of the tongue for lesions. Examine how far the tongue can protrude and evaluate frenal attachments. Inspect the hard and soft palate. Evaluate the floor of the mouth for masses, swellings, or ulcerations.

The soft tissues around the dentition can then be inspected. The gingiva should be evaluated for color, contour, and the presence of bleeding or inflammation. Periodontal pocket depths should be measured to evaluate for bone loss or pseudopocketing. Areas of recession should also be noted as well as thin gingival types that will put the patient at higher risk for future recession. During this time, oral hygiene should also be assessed for plaque accumulation and calculus deposits.

Once a thorough evaluation of the soft tissues is complete, the teeth can be examined. First the teeth should be counted to evaluate for extra or missing teeth. Examine for caries, fractures, erosion, or abrasion lesions. Evaluate the integrity and margins of existing restorations. Assess for malocclusion, crossbites, or occlusal interferences. Evaluate crowding, spacing, overbite, and overjet.

All of these findings should be documented thoroughly in the patient's health record in a standard systematic form so that it can be easily accessed for future reference.

Radiographic Examination

Radiographs should be ordered based on individual patient needs. These needs are adjusted for dates of last films, caries risk, and presence of pathology. The American Academy of Pediatric Dentistry created a chart (Table 11.2) with recommendations that include factors such as dentition type and caries risk.[3] Bitewing radiographs are the most common films taken in this age group. When second molars are erupted and the distal surface of the second molar cannot be visualized in the same film as the distal surface of the canine, two bitewings on each side are recommended. These films allow for the evaluation of interproximal caries as well as the crestal bone height. Depending on the dentition present and caries risk, these films are taken anywhere between 6 and 36 month intervals.

Select periapical films may be needed to assess the root apex, periapical tissues, and surrounding bone. These films are necessary when there has been a history of trauma, previous pulp therapy, or large caries extending close to the pulp. They are also necessary when there are signs of pathology such as a fistula or large swelling on clinical examination, or if pain has been noted on the patient history. Periapical films can help assess whether a tooth is likely necrotic or not.

Panoramic radiographs are excellent for providing an overview of the entire dentition, including unerupted teeth, jawbones, the TMJs, and surrounding structures. These films can be used to evaluate dental age, assess the positioning of third molars, and screen for pathology. In the absence of a new significant finding, these films are typically taken every 3 to 5 years.

Other less commonly taken films include cephalometric radiographs and occlusal films. Cephalometric radiographs are often needed before and during treatment to assess growth patterns and the skeletal and dental relationship. Occlusal radiographs may be helpful in determining the presence of supernumerary teeth or the positioning of impacted canines. Mandibular occlusal films may also be helpful in diagnosing the presence of salivary stones. When three-dimensional imaging is necessary, cone beam computed tomography can help diagnose things like vertical tooth fractures or the positioning of a canine in relation to the roots of maxillary incisors.

Whatever radiographic examination is deemed necessary, it is important to adhere to ALARA (as low as reasonably achievable) principles to minimize radiation exposure. These recommendations are summarized in Table 11.3.

Prevention

Preventive care in the adolescent population is extremely important as they begin to be more autonomous with their home hygiene habits. Recommendations can be split into two categories: in-office prevention and home care.

In-office preventive regiments include regular dental examinations and professional cleanings. Sealants may be applied on deep pits and fissures that are at risk for dental decay. Professional fluoride applications such as 5% sodium fluoride varnish may be

TABLE 11.2 Radiographic Periodicity Recommendations

	PATIENT AGE AND DENTAL DEVELOPMENTAL STAGE			
Type of Encounter	Child With Primary Dentition (before eruption of first permanent tooth)	Child With Transitional Dentition (after eruption of first permanent tooth)	Adolescent With Permanent Dentition (before eruption of third molars)	Adult, Dentate, or Partially Edentulous
New Patient[a] being evaluated for oral diseases.	Individualized radiographic exam consisting of elected periapical/occlusal views and/or posterior bitewings if proximal surfaces cannot be visualized or probed. Patients without evidence of disease and with open proximal contacts may not require a radiographic exam at this time.	Individualized radiographic exam consisting of posterior bitewings with panoramic exam or posterior bitewings and selected periapical images.	Individualized radiographic exam consisting of posterior bitewings with panoramic exam or posterior bitewings and selected periapical images. A full mouth intraoral radiographic exam is preferred when the patient has clinical evidence of generalized oral disease or a history of extensive dental treatment.	
Recall Patient[a] with clinical caries or at increased risk for caries.[b]	Posterior bitewing exam at 6- to 12-month intervals if proximal surfaces cannot be examined visually or with a probe.			Posterior bitewing exam at 6- to 18-month intervals.
Recall Patient[a] with no clinical caries and not at increased risk for caries.[b]	Posterior bitewing exam at 12- to 24-month intervals if proximal surfaces cannot be examined visually or with a probe.		Posterior bitewing exam at 18- to 36-month intervals.	Posterior bitewing exam at 24- to 36-month intervals.

Continued

TABLE 11.2 Radiographic Periodicity Recommendations—cont'd

	PATIENT AGE AND DENTAL DEVELOPMENTAL STAGE			
Type of Encounter	**Child With Primary Dentition (before eruption of first permanent tooth)**	**Child With Transitional Dentition (after eruption of first permanent tooth)**	**Adolescent With Permanent Dentition (before eruption of third molars)**	**Adult, Dentate, or Partially Edentulous**
Patient (New and Recall) for monitoring of dentofacial growth and development, and/or assessment of dental/skeletal relationships.	Clinical judgment as to need for and type of radiographic images for evaluation and/or monitoring of dentofacial growth and development or assessment of dental and skeletal relationships.		Clinical judgment as to need for and type of radiographic images for evaluation and/or monitoring of dentofacial growth and development, or assessment of dental and skeletal relationships. Panoramic or periapical exam to assess developing third molars.	Usually not indicated for monitoring of growth and development. Clinical judgment as to the need for and type of radiographic image for evaluation of dental and skeletal relationships.
Patient with other circumstances including, but not limited to, proposed or existing implants, other dental and craniofacial pathoses, restorative/endodontic needs, treated periodontal disease, and caries remineralization.	Clinical judgment as to the need for and type of radiographic images for evaluation and/or monitoring in these conditions.			

[a]Clinical situations for which radiographs may be indicated include, but are not limited to:

A. *Positive Historical Findings*
  1. Previous periodontal or endodontic treatment
  2. History of pain or trauma
  3. Familial history of dental anomalies
  4. Postoperative evaluation of healing
  5. Remineralization monitoring
  6. Presence of implants, previous implant-related pathosis, or evaluation for implant placement

B. *Positive Clinical Signs/Symptoms*
  1. Clinical evidence of periodontal disease
  2. Large or deep restorations
  3. Deep Carious Lesions (C-A-R-I-O-U-S)
  4. Malposed or clinically impacted teeth
  5. Swelling
  6. Evidence of dentofacial trauma
  7. Mobility of tooth
  8. Sinus tract (fistula)
  9. Clinically suspected sinus pathosis
  10. Growth abnormalities
  11. Oral involvement in known or suspected systemic disease
  12. Positive neurologic findings in the head and neck
  13. Evidence of foreign objects
  14. Pain and/or dysfunction of the temporomandibular joint
  15. Facial asymmetry
  16. Abutment teeth for fixed or removable partial prosthesis
  17. Unexplained bleeding
  18. Unexplained sensitivity of teeth
  10. Unusual eruption, spacing, or migration of teeth
  20. Unusual tooth morphology, calcification, or color
  21. Unexplained absence of teeth
  22. Clinical tooth erosion
  23. Peri-implantitis

[b]Factors increasing risk for caries may be assessed using the ADA Caries Risk Assessment forms (0–6 years of age and over 6 years of age).

From AAPD.org.

recommended to help remineralize enamel and inhibit progression of early carious lesions. It can also be very effective to reduce thermal sensitivity.

Home care recommendations may be limited to over-the-counter supplies, or they may include prescription products for those who are at higher caries risk. Encouraging adolescents to brush at least twice a day with fluoride toothpaste, using an effective technique, is of vital importance. Daily flossing is also an important component of a home care regimen. Higher concentration of fluoride toothpaste (5000 ppm) can be recommended

TABLE 11.3 Suggested Imaging for Adolescent Patient

Imaging Type	Description	Frequency	Comments
Full mouth survey	• 3–5 size 1 maxillary anterior periapicals • 3 size 1 mandibular anterior periapicals • 4 size 2 bitewing films (2 per side) • 4–8 size 2 posterior periapicals (1–2 per quad)	If indicated, every 3–5 years	In presence of generalized dental disease only
Bitewing radiographs	• 1 or 2 films per side to open contacts from second molars to distal of canines • Size 2 films	• Dependent on caries risk assessment • Every 18–36 months for low caries risk • Every 12 months for moderate caries risk • Every 6 months to evaluate active incipient lesions (high caries risk)	Recommended interval should be reevaluated at every periodic examination and adjusted for patient's current caries risk (see Table 11.2)
Periapical radiographs	• Size 1 or size 2 films may be needed based on location and anatomy	• Refer to trauma guidelines for recommended intervals • Take as needed for symptomatic teeth	Used most often to evaluate the periodontal ligament (PDL) in areas of possible pulpal pathology caused by caries or trauma
Panoramic films	Evaluates all oral hard tissues in one film	3–5 years or as indicated by clinical examination	Helpful to visualize third molars and positioning of maxillary canines before eruption. Recommend taking first time upon eruption of maxillary lateral incisors.
Cephalometric films	Side view of oral hard tissues	Interval dictated by growth and development and orthodontic intervention	• May be useful in orthodontic treatment planning • May help identify airway concerns by evaluating tonsil and adenoid size
Occlusal films	Size 4 most useful; angle will depend on diagnostic need	Taken as needed	May be useful in evaluation of trauma, or diagnosis of salivary stones
Cone beam computed tomography (CBCT)	CBCT three-dimensional imaging	Taken as needed (often in follow-up to other films)	Helpful to diagnose concerns not visible in two-dimensional imaging: positioning of impacted teeth, vertical root fractures, airway volume, location of pathology

when there are white spot lesions, orthodontic appliances, or interproximal incipient lesions. Mouth rinses may be appropriate as well, particularly for those struggling with gingivitis.

There are also several nonfluoride-based preventive measures that can be taken including xylitol products (like sugar-free chewing gum). These can help clear food debris after meals, stimulate salivary flow, and even prevent more snacking. Although it is debatable whether the amount of xylitol in these products has any therapeutic effect, other benefits can be seen. Calcium and phosphate products such as MI Paste (GC America) may be beneficial for patients with early signs of enamel demineralization or molar incisor hypomineralization. There are newer products out containing hydroxyapatite, though there are minimal studies at the present time that conclude preventive benefits equal to that of fluoride-based dentifrice. See Chapter 14 for more detail.

Prevention also extends to healthy dietary habits. Recommend avoiding sugary or acidic beverages, especially at sports practices, where prolonged exposure via sipping is likely. Water should be the primary beverage of choice, and education regarding the lack of benefit of sports drinks compared with water may be necessary to combat misleading marketing. Limit snacking between meals, and when snacks are necessary, promote fresh vegetables, cheese, or nuts. These snacks are low in sugar and are unlikely to contribute to decay.

Caries Risk Assessment

It is important to assess the risk of a patient acquiring caries to help guide treatment decisions. Patients who are at low risk require less frequent radiographs and standard prevention protocols. Patients at a high risk require more frequent radiographs to evaluate caries progression, a more aggressive treatment planning approach for early lesions, and a more involved recare and home care program.

The American Academy of Pediatric Dentistry has created a table for assessing a patient's risk for caries, shown in Table 11.4.[4]

By evaluating a patient's social, behavioral, and medical history, along with their clinical examination and protective factors, an oral healthcare professional can see if the patient trends toward a high risk overall, has moderate factors combined with protective factors, or truly is at low risk for caries. Further inquiry can be completed by bacterial activity testing and evaluating salivary flow rate and buffering capacity.

Periodontal Risk Assessment

It is important to evaluate the periodontal health of adolescent patients (Fig. 11.1). Bone levels should be evaluated on bitewing radiographs, assessing for the presence of vertical or horizontal

TABLE 11.4 Caries Risk Assessment

Use of this tool will help the healthcare provider assess the child's risk for developing carious lesions. In addition, reviewing specific factors will help the practitioner and patient/parent understand the variable influences that contribute to or protect from dental caries.

Factors	High Risk	Moderate Risk	Low Risk
Risk factors, social/behavioral medical			
Patient has lifetime of poverty, low health literacy	Yes		
Patient has frequent exposure (>3 times/day) to between-meal sugar-containing snacks or beverages per day	Yes		
Child is a recent immigrant		Yes	
Patient uses hyposalivatory medication(s)		Yes	
Patient has special healthcare needs[a]		Yes	
Risk factors, clinical			
Patient has low salivary flow	Yes		
Patient has visible plaque on teeth	Yes		
Patient presents with dental enamel defects	Yes		
Patient wears an intraoral appliance		Yes	
Patient has defective restorations		Yes	
Protective factors			
Patient receives optimally fluoridated drinking water			Yes
Patient has teeth brushed daily with fluoridated toothpaste			Yes
Patient receives topical fluoride from health professional			Yes
Patient has dental home/regular dental care			Yes
Disease indicators[b]			
Patient has interproximal caries lesion(s)	Yes		
Patient has new noncavitated (white spot) caries lesions	Yes		
Patient has new cavitated caries lesions or lesions into dentin radiographically	Yes		
Patient has restorations that were placed in the past 3 years (new patient) or in the past 12 months (patient of record)	Yes		

[a]Practitioners may choose a different risk level based on specific medical diagnosis and unique circumstances, especially conditions that affect motor coordination or cooperation.

[b]Although these do not cause caries directly or indirectly, they indicate presence of factors that do.

Instructions: *Circle "Yes" that corresponds with those conditions that apply so a specific patient. Use the circled responses to visualize the balance among risk factors, protective factors, and disease indicators. Use this balance or imbalance, together with clinical judgment, to assign a caries risk level of low, moderate, or high based on the preponderance of factors for the individual. Clinical judgment may justify the weighting of one factor (e.g., heavy plaque on the teeth) more than others.*

Overall assessment of the dental caries risk: High ☐ Moderate ☐ Low ☐

bone loss. Recession levels, particularly in patients who have thin gingival subtypes and a history of crossbite or orthodontics, should be evaluated. Probing depths should be completed either with the periodontal screening and recording (PSR) system or the basic periodontal examination (BPE) to assess their periodontal status and identify areas of concern.

The PSR system divides the mouth into sextants and uses a specially banded probe (with demarcations at 0.5 mm, 3.5 mm, and 5.5 mm) to check six sites on each tooth as well as bleeding and calculus. These factors combined determines a score of 0 to 4, and only the highest score is charted in each sextant. This is not intended to replace a full-mouth probing and recording but can serve as an efficient and effective screening tool. The methods and criteria of this screening system are very similar to the BPE, with slightly different definitions. When either screening system is used, scores of 3 and 4 are indicative of the need for a more detailed periodontal assessment, with charting recording for six surfaces of every tooth. See Chapter 21 for a complete discussion of periodontal disease in the pediatric population.

Assessing for Third Molars

Late adolescence frequently marks the period for determining the presence and likelihood of eruption of the third molars. These teeth are typically best evaluated on a panorex (Fig. 11.2), though the coronal portion can often be visible on bitewings. The position and angulation of third molars relative to the adjacent teeth and jawbone can help determine the likelihood of erupting. The risk of pathology should also be assessed as far as the bone level on the distal of the second molar, and the size and appearance of the dental follicle. The decision to remove the third molars should be made before the middle of the third decade (age 25) to reduce the risk of complications postoperatively.[5] There is no clear-cut guidance on whether removing disease-free impacted third molars is beneficial or harmful to the patient.

Restorative Considerations

When treatment planning for adolescents, there are several factors that must be taken into account compared with other age groups.

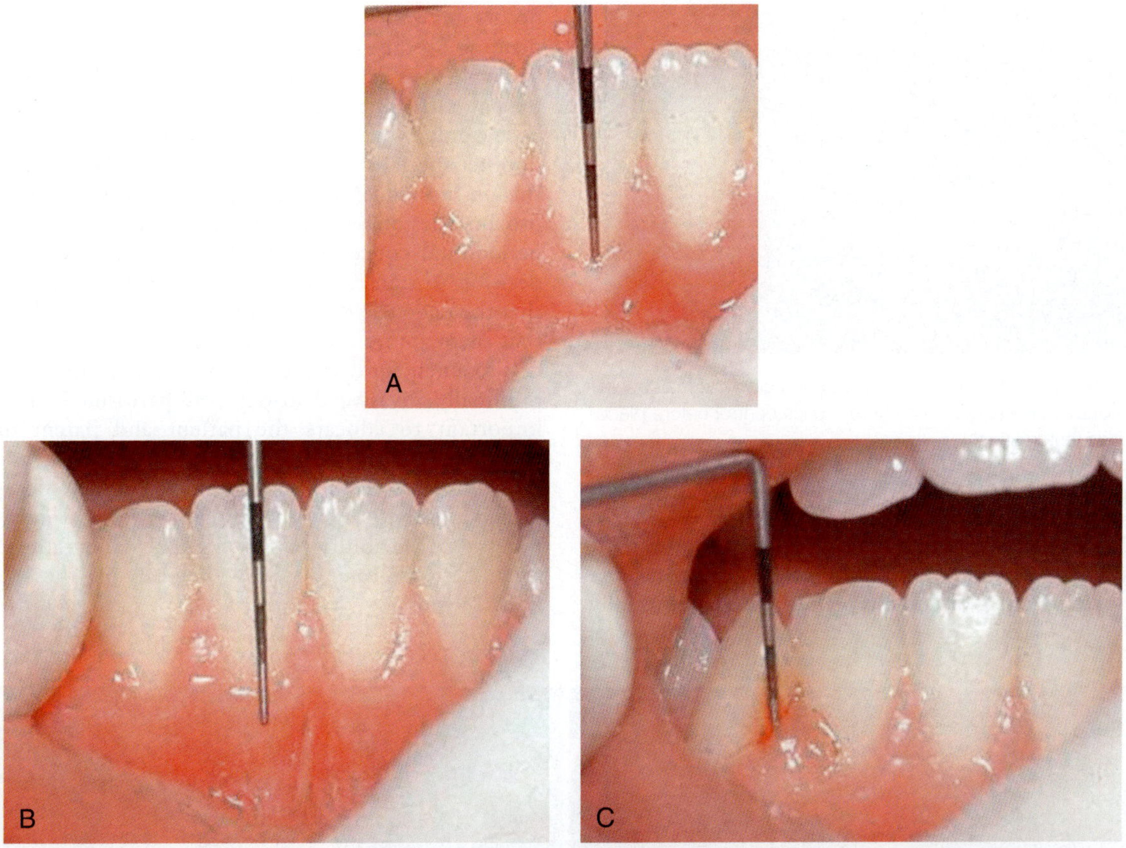

• **Fig. 11.1** The prevalence of periodontal disease begins to increase in the adolescent patient; therefore it is especially necessary to perform a thorough evaluation of the periodontium. A periodontal probe is used to measure pocket depth (A) and the width of the keratinized gingiva (B). Probing is also used to establish a bleeding index (C).

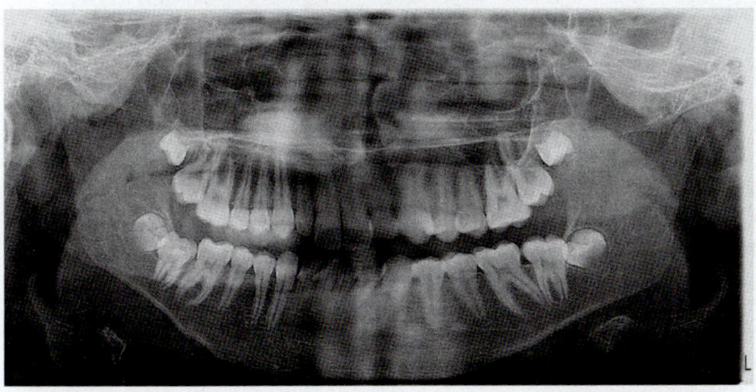

• **Fig. 11.2** Panorex of adolescent used to determine presence and positioning of third molars.

One such factor is how long a tooth is expected to be present. A carious lesion on a primary tooth in adolescence may not be as concerning as a permanent tooth lesion if it is unlikely that the caries will progress to the point of pain or infection before exfoliation. That being said, caries on primary teeth should not be ignored, especially when interproximal lesions are adjacent to a permanent tooth surface. Management of these lesions may involve medical management with agents like silver diamine fluoride, interim therapeutic restorations while waiting for exfoliation or extraction, depending on the severity of decay and the estimated time until exfoliation.

When considering full-coverage restoration, for esthetics or largely compromised teeth, the growth of the patient must be factored into treatment decisions. Particularly in the esthetic zone, the patient will continue to have vertical growth over time and crown margins may become visible as the patient grows. On teeth that have maintained vitality, it is important to consider that the pulp chamber is considerably larger than in an older adult, and therefore care must be taken to not expose or irritate the nerve during preparation. It is also important to consider whether the adjacent contacts have been established for interproximal contouring of the crown. Whenever possible, without compromising the long-term maintenance of the tooth, full-coverage restorations should be deferred until the patient has completed growth.

In patients who have several large carious lesions on permanent teeth and lesions along the gingival margin with significant gingivitis (Fig. 11.3), sometimes doing gross caries removal (or "caries control") is the fastest way to address the abundant needs and prevent further progression. This often involves slow-speed or spoon excavation of carious tooth structure and placing a glass ionomer cement to recontour the tooth. Once gingival health is restored with improved home care, and possibly chlorhexidine if required, more complete esthetic restorations can be placed. Often it is difficult to address more than a couple of permanent teeth at one visit, so this can be an effective management tool to prevent pulp necrosis when patients are unable to be seen for multiple visits in a short time span.

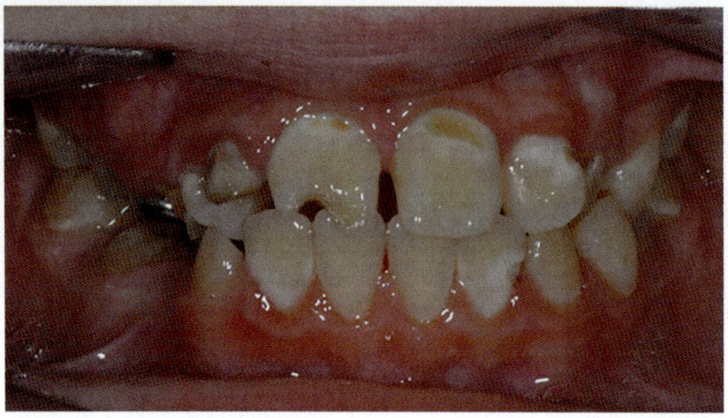

• **Fig. 11.3** Eleven-year-old with rampant decay and gingivitis may benefit from a gross caries removal appointment for caries control before placement of definitive restorations.

Transitioning to the Adult Dental Home

The transition of an adolescent pediatric dental patient to their adult dental home is an important milestone in the dental care journey of a young adult or adolescent. The transition usually occurs anywhere from age 12 to 18 or even college-aged, depending on the resources available within the community, the pediatric dentist's personal preference, and the dental needs of the patient. Some pediatric dentists make this process standard by age only, which may vary on patient population and density of other specialists in the community. Other dentists may base this on individual patient needs, such as when there are interproximal lesions on permanent dentition or when there are periodontal concerns. Whatever the factor that leads to the decision to transfer to a general dentist's care, it is important that the pediatric dentist ensures this is a smooth transition so that there are no gaps in coverage. The patient must have access to emergent dental care until the transition is complete. If minimally invasive dentistry was performed, it is especially important to educate the patient and parent on areas of treatment such as silver diamine fluoride application or resin infiltration, as these areas may look like new decay to a new provider, prompting a more aggressive treatment plan than necessary. The ability to supply serial radiographs monitoring these lesions can be very helpful in these discussions (Fig. 11.4).

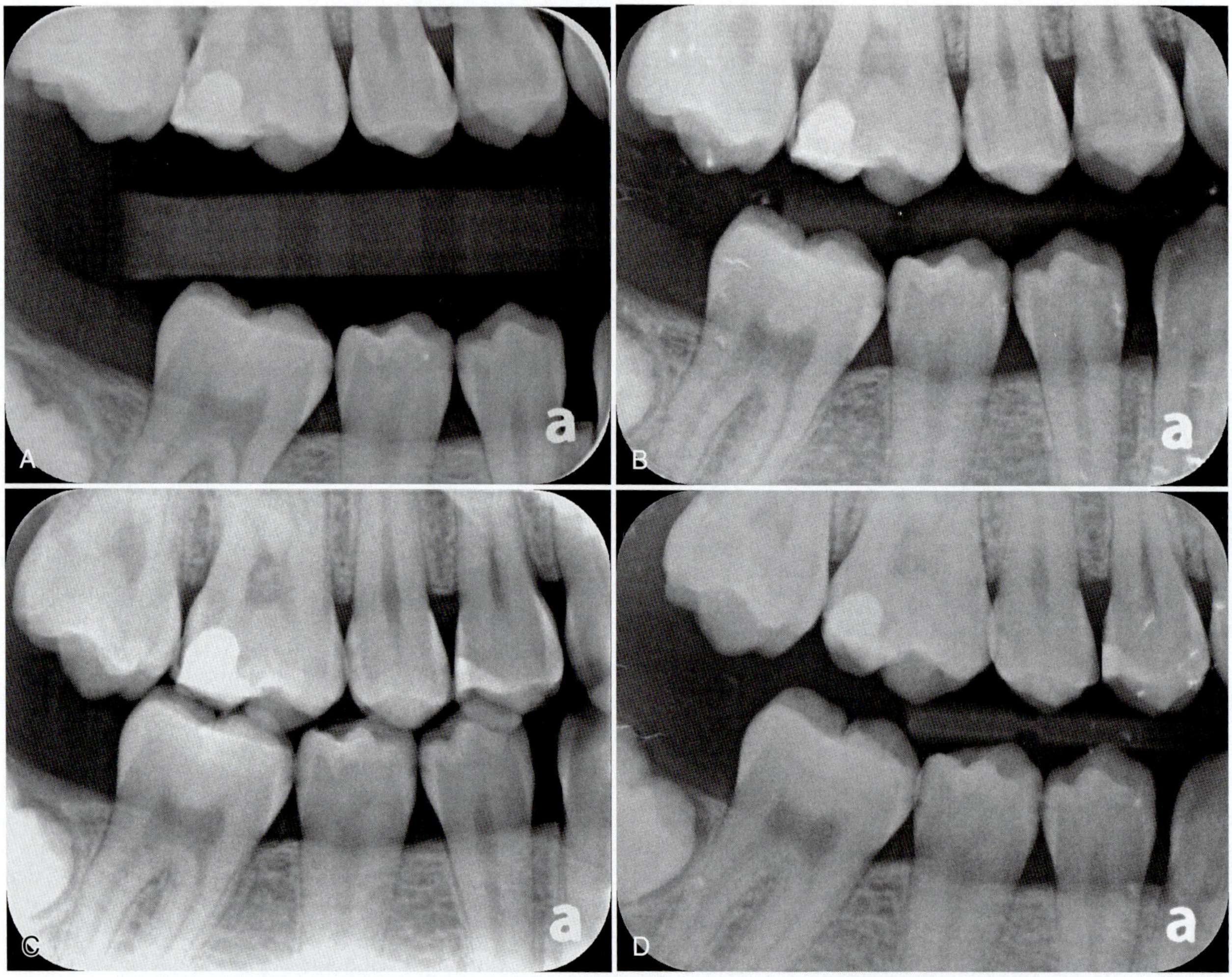

• **Fig. 11.4** Serial radiographs can be important to include in records transfer to a new dental home to show whether they have progressed over time. (A) Initial diagnosis of incipient interproximal lesions and beginning of placement of silver diamine fluoride. (B) Twelve months later show little to no progression. (C) Eighteen months after initial film. (D) Thirty-three months after initial film. Without these films a new dental home may have been more likely to treatment plan interproximal restorations on the lower right.

Special Considerations

There are several special considerations when treating adolescent dental patients, and for each it is important to understand the patient's developmental stage. Adolescents are undergoing physical, emotional, and cognitive development. This can affect their behavior, communication style, and level of understanding. A dentist must tailor their approach to accommodate the developmental stage of each adolescent patient.

Adolescents value their autonomy and independence. Dentists should make sure to involve them in decision making regarding their dental care whenever possible and respect their preferences and opinions. Although often they are not of age to provide consent, providing assent to treatment is an important factor in this age group. There may also be privacy and confidentiality concerns for adolescents, especially regarding sensitive topics such as health history or social behaviors. Dentists should create a safe and confidential environment where adolescents feel comfortable discussing these issues. There are also state-specific laws about the age range that parents can have full access to their child's medical records for these reasons, so the dentist must be familiar with confidentiality laws in their state.

Dental Bleaching

Bleaching, or tooth whitening, in the adolescent population requires careful consideration because of several factors unique to this age group. Adolescents may not have fully erupted dentition, and it can be difficult to get shades to match over time if the entire "social six" front teeth are not being whitened at the same time. The maturing dentitions also have very large pulp chambers in comparison with teeth that have been erupted for a longer period of time. Whitening can lead to sensitivity because of a thinner layer of dentin present to insulate the pulp. Especially with professional whitening regimens, it can be recommended to alternate whitening and desensitizing protocols, such as with a fluoride tray (Fig. 11.5). Lastly, it is crucial that adolescents understand the importance of adhering to at-home bleaching protocols. At times they may not grasp the full understanding of possible complications when protocols are not followed, such as soft tissue damage, enamel erosion, or obtaining the desired outcomes.

Orthodontic Management of Permanent Dentition

As mentioned earlier, the adolescent period is frequently the time when orthodontic concerns such as malocclusion and misalignment are addressed. All patients should be evaluated for crowding,

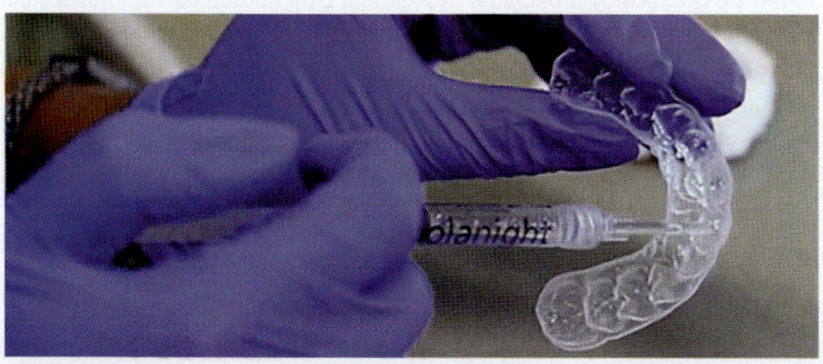

• **Fig. 11.5** A professional whitening tray, which can double as a fluoride tray for patients experiencing sensitivity. (Image from www.electricteeth.co.uk/whitening)

spacing, overbite, overjet, and Angle's classification for canines and molars. Patients should be counseled on whether orthodontics is recommended for the longevity of their function versus whether the benefit would be mostly esthetic in nature.

When a patient is in active orthodontic care, it may be beneficial to see them back for recare appointments more frequently. This is particularly true if they have active white spot lesions or poor oral hygiene while in appliances. Caution must even be exercised with clear aligner therapy, as sugary or acidic liquids can pool in the retainer if they are not removed while drinking. Counseling the patients on proper home care and prescribing adjunctive agents such as fluoride rinses and a high-concentration fluoride dentifrice can help prevent carious lesions.

It is important that the restorative dentist partners with the orthodontic treatment provider to make sure the course of therapy is understood. It may be necessary to coordinate appointments so that appliances are temporarily removed for restorative care. Some orthodontists have hygienists in their practices and are comfortable combining prophylaxis and bitewing visits with appointments when wires are being changed. This can allow for improved visualization of interproximal caries, so they can be detected as early as possible. Chapter 25 discusses orthodontic treatment in the permanent dentition in more detail.

Temporomandibular Joint Disorder

Temporomandibular joint disorder (TMD) often first presents during the adolescent time frame. It is important to evaluate the patient's TMJ at each recall visit for jaw pain, clicking or popping sounds, deviation, or limited opening. It is unlikely that treatment would be recommended for asymptomatic sounds, but anything that causes pain or restricts movement should be evaluated further (see Chapter 45). Usually, conservative management is the first approach including lifestyle modifications, avoiding biting into apples and large sandwiches, limiting gum chewing, and using heat and ice therapy. Sometimes these are combined with nonsteroidal antiinflammatories until the condition is under control, and an occlusal splint may also be recommended.

Many times, the treatment of TMD involves a multidisciplinary approach including physiotherapy, psychology, and the oral healthcare professional. The oral health specialist most often involved in care of these patients is an oral and maxillofacial surgeon, who can also determine whether the condition is severe enough to warrant more invasive treatment such as Botox trigger point injections, arthroscopy, or joint surgery.

Sports Dentistry

Many adolescents are involved in organized sports. Mouthguards are recommended to help prevent dentoalveolar injuries in a number of sports, and there are some sports where the use is required by national regulatory bodies. The National Federation of State High School Associations requires the use of mouthguards for football, lacrosse, field hockey, ice hockey, and wrestling (if the participant has braces). However, a custom-fit mouthguard is recommended in any contact and collision sport. The sport most associated with dental injuries in the 7- to 12-year-old age group is baseball, whereas the highest incidence of injuries in high school boys is basketball. High school girls have the highest rate of dentoalveolar injury in field hockey.[6]

The use of a type I custom-fabricated mouthguard made by vacuum form or heat pressure lamination techniques can help reduce the severity of injury to dentoalveolar structures by spreading out the force of impact. It should be a minimum of 3 mm thick for adequate protection.[6] The dental team plays an important role in educating their patients on the importance of wearing a mouthguard to prevent life-altering trauma to the dentoalveolar structures.

The dentist can also be helpful from a public health perspective in educating coaches and league associations on the use of mouthguards and what to do in case of an injury. By educating those who will be closest to the patient in the event of a sports-related injury, the teeth can be addressed in as short of time frame as possible (such as reimplantation or placing in milk in the case of an avulsion) and dramatically improve the long-term success of the tooth.

Eating Disorders

Adolescence marks a time of heightened awareness of body image and peer influence. This can lend itself to body dysmorphia and eating disorders. The eating disorder that is most associated with oral health changes is bulimia nervosa. This is related to a period of binge eating followed by compensatory behaviors such as self-induced vomiting, excessive exercise, or misuse of laxatives and diuretics. When vomiting is used as a compensatory behavior the repeated exposure of teeth to stomach acid can lead to erosion of tooth enamel, particularly on the lingual surfaces of the maxillary dentition (Fig. 11.6). This is known as perimolysis.

Other forms of eating disorders should also be closely monitored as they can affect electrolyte levels and malnutrition. This can cause issues with normal growth and development, healing, and gingivitis. When oral findings or extraoral examination lend itself to a differential of an eating disorder, it is important to speak to the patient with compassion and in a private setting. Appropriate referrals to psychology and primary care physician involvement are important in getting the patient the help and resources they need. Gaining the trust of the patient in order to disclose this sensitive information is an important part of the relationship of a pediatric dentist with their patient over the long term (Box 11.1).

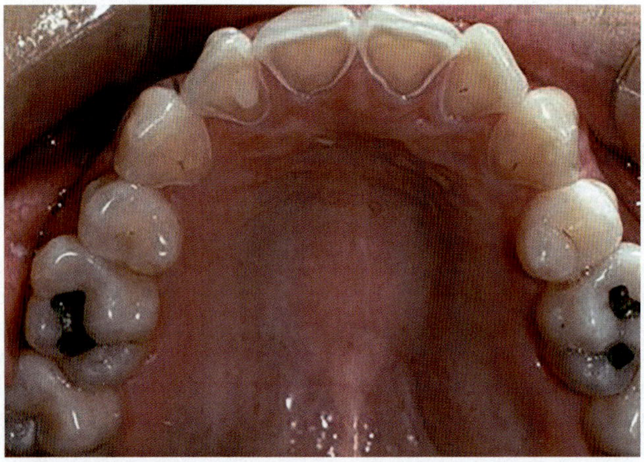

• **Fig. 11.6** Erosion on lingual surfaces for a patient with a history of bulimia. The facial surface of the permanent maxillary central incisors has been covered with veneer restorations. (From Bath-Balogh M, Fehrenbach MK. *Illustrated Dental Embryology, Histology, and Anatomy*. 3rd ed. Saunders; 2011.)

Human Papillomavirus Vaccinations

HPV vaccines are designed to prevent infection with certain strains of HPV known to cause various cancers and genital warts. Multiple formulations of the vaccine exist, but perhaps the most common is the 9-valent option, which helps protect against HPV-6, 11, 16, 18, 31, 33, 45, 52, and 58. These types are associated with cervical cancers, anal cancers, and genital warts. HPV-16 is by far the most related to oropharyngeal cancers.[7]

HPV vaccination is recommended for both male and female adolescents, starting around age 11 or 12. This can provide optimal protection before potential exposure to HPV through sexual activity, including oral intercourse. The recommended vaccination schedule is to have two doses spaced 6 to 12 months apart for patients age 11 to 15. Those who are age 15 to 26 may require three doses for optimal protection. Oral healthcare professionals can play a vital role in promoting HPV vaccination by providing education and guidance to adolescent patients and their caregivers.

Treating the Pregnant Adolescent Patient

Occasionally in a pediatric dental practice there will be the need to treat a patient who is pregnant. There will be a few considerations for the oral healthcare provider when that time comes. Pregnancy hormones such as estrogen and progesterone can affect the oral cavity, leading to an increased risk of gingivitis and pathology such as pyogenic granulomas. Patients may also experience nausea that is exacerbated by activities such as tooth brushing, leading to poor oral hygiene. If there are frequent bouts of emesis this can cause erosion and lead to faster rates of decay. Pregnancy often prompts a change in dietary habits, including cravings for more frequent ingestion of snacks that can put a patient at risk for decay. For all these reasons it is recommended to see a pregnant patient on a more frequent recall interval in order to catch any concerns early, complete a thorough cleaning, and apply fluoride varnish more frequently.

BOX 11.1 Referrals

Sometimes referring patients out for specialist treatment is necessary for their comprehensive care. Such specialists may include:

- Orthodontists: Orthodontists can help treat dental and facial irregularities including malocclusion and facial asymmetry.
- Oral and maxillofacial surgeons: These surgeons may be needed for impacted tooth removal, severe facial trauma involving cortical bone, and the placement of dental implants.
- Restorative dentist: Sometimes general dentists refer adolescents to pediatric dental specialists due to behavioral concerns. Likewise, adolescents may be referred by a pediatric dentist to a general dentist when their needs match those more similar to an adult patient. This may include crowns, large permanent tooth restorations, veneers, or implant restorations.
- Periodontist: Periodontists can help treat aggressive periodontitis, recession, or place implants.
- Endodontists: Endodontists help manage patients with trauma or carious pulp exposures. Endodontists have the tools and training to be able to perform root canal therapy on smaller canals such as the fourth canal on maxillary first permanent molars.
- Prosthodontists: Prosthodontists can be helpful in restoring patients who have had significant bite collapse or replacing multiple teeth in the cases of extensive dental trauma or caries. Prosthodontists specialize in replacement of tooth structure with removable or fixed appliances.

The prescription of doxycycline, tetracycline, alprazolam, and diazepam should be avoided for a pregnant patient. The use of nitrous oxide analgesia should be avoided in the first trimester of pregnancy. To have a complete medical history of the patient and the risk to the developing fetus, oral healthcare providers should consult with the patient's obstetrician if prescriptions are needed.[8]

When a pregnant patient requires treatment, it is beneficial to the fetus to have this treatment completed as quickly as possible. Elective care, such as orthodontics, should be deferred, but anything that could result in inflammation should be mitigated as quickly as possible.[8] Topical and local anesthetics can be safely used, and it is much better to prevent an active infection in a pregnant patient than to defer treatment until after delivery. High rates of inflammation, such as from periodontal disease, are associated with preterm labor and low birth weight.[9] To keep a patient comfortable in the third trimester, it can be beneficial to position them with the right hip elevated so that they are tilted toward their left side. This can help relieve pressure on the inferior vena cava.

Another important factor to consider for a pregnant adolescent is the age of consent. This is considered state specific, but many states have laws regarding confidentiality of care of patients who are pregnant as well as the ability for them to give consent to their own care regardless of their age. The dentist should be aware of their own state's regulations regarding caring for a pregnant patient.

Intraoral and Perioral Piercing

Intraoral jewelry (Fig. 11.7) presents several concerns from a dental perspective. Piercings in the tongue, lips, cheeks, or uvula can lead to soft tissue damage including lacerations, bruising, swelling, and inflammation. Improper placement or poor-quality jewelry can exacerbate these issues. Even in the absence of infection, piercings on the tongue or lip can repeatedly traumatize the gingival tissues, leading to gingival recession, abrasions, and ulcerations. Chronic trauma from oral jewelry may contribute to periodontal disease and tooth mobility. They can also fracture the teeth upon repeated contact, especially during speech, eating, or accidental biting.

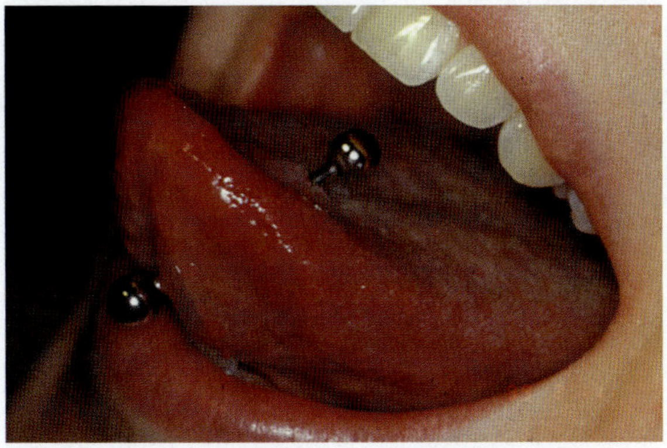

• **Fig. 11.7** Photo of a tongue piercing known as a dumbbell, which is associated with enamel fracture.

Some individuals may have allergic reactions to the metals in oral jewelry such as nickel or cobalt. These can present as inflammation, itching, or dermatitis around the piercing site. Piercings also present difficulty with dental treatment including positioning of equipment and adding artifact to radiographs. It is recommended that, when possible, jewelry is removed for dental visits.

Intraoral Tattoos

Tattoos involve the application of pigmented ink or dyes to the soft tissue, and while not as common as intraoral and perioral piercings, they may be seen in the adolescent population. During the placement of tattoos there is a risk for infection, particularly if proper sterilization techniques are not followed. The pigmentation can make it difficult to detect the presence of oral lesions, mucosal abnormalities, or early signs of pathology. Unlike skin tattoos, mucosal tattoos are challenging to remove due to the delicate nature of the oral mucosa. Laser removal is not recommended because of the risk of tissue damage and complications.

Substance Misuse

Substance misuse among adolescent dental patients poses significant concerns. Counseling regarding prevention or cessation of use from an oral health professional can help change the course of a patient's life. Drugs and alcohol can have detrimental effects on oral health, including a higher risk for dental caries, periodontal disease, xerostomia, mucositis, bruxism, and erosion. These oral health issues can lead to pain, functional problems, and a compromised quality of life for adolescent patients.

The risk of dental trauma is also increased in adolescents who engage in substance misuse. This is related to impaired judgment and coordination. Accidents or injuries resulting from substance-related behaviors such as falls, motor vehicle accidents, or violence can lead to tooth fractures, avulsions, and soft tissue injuries.

Substance misuse can also interfere with dental treatment and compromise treatment outcomes. Adolescents who are misusing stimulants can have hypertensive crises when local anesthesia with epinephrine is used. If they are using depressants their respiratory function may be impaired, particularly in combination with other sedatives that may be used. Long-term use can also impair the healing process when invasive dental treatment is needed.

There are significant systemic health concerns as well. Substance misuse is related to cirrhosis, hepatitis, depression, and acquired immunodeficiency syndrome. It can result in death caused by overdose or accidents such as motor vehicles or drowning. Addiction can happen after just one use of some restricted substances, particularly to those who are predisposed.

Dental professionals play a vital role in promoting preventive measures and providing education on the risks of substance misuse to adolescent patients.

Visit eBooks.Health.Elsevier.com to see full list of references.

PART 3

Fundamentals

12 Cariology

JOEL H. BERG

CHAPTER OUTLINE

Introduction

Brief Overview of Caries

Dental caries, commonly known as tooth decay, is a chronic, multifactorial, infectious disease affecting a significant portion of the global population. It is caused by the demineralization of tooth enamel due to the acidic by-products produced by bacterial fermentation of dietary carbohydrates. Caries primarily affects the hard tissues of the teeth, namely enamel, dentin, and cementum, leading to structural damage and cavities if left untreated.

The development of caries involves a dynamic process of demineralization and remineralization, influenced by various factors such as oral hygiene, diet, fluoride exposure, saliva flow and composition, and the presence of cariogenic microorganisms, particularly *Streptococcus mutans* and *Lactobacillus* species. The disease process can be asymptomatic in its early stages but can lead to pain, infection, and tooth loss as it progresses.

Caries is classified based on its location, such as pit and fissure (Fig. 12.1) or smooth surface (Fig. 12.2), and the extent of the lesion (Fig. 12.3). The management of caries includes preventive measures such as fluoride application, dietary counseling, and oral hygiene education and restorative treatments like fillings, crowns, and, in severe cases, tooth extractions.

Importance of Understanding Cariology in Pediatric Dentistry

Understanding cariology—the study of dental caries and cariogenesis—is crucial in pediatric dentistry for several reasons:

1. **Prevalence in children:** Dental caries is one of the most common chronic diseases in children. Early childhood caries (ECC) can have a significant effect on a child's health, development, and quality of life. It can cause pain, infection, and difficulty in eating, speaking, and learning.
2. **Prevention and early intervention:** Knowledge of cariology enables pediatric dentists to implement effective preventive strategies and early interventions. This includes educating parents and children on proper oral hygiene practices, the importance of a balanced diet, and the use of fluoride and dental sealants to protect teeth from decay.
3. **Risk assessment:** Understanding the risk factors associated with caries allows for the development of individualized caries risk assessment models. These models help in identifying high-risk children who may benefit from more intensive preventive measures and monitoring.

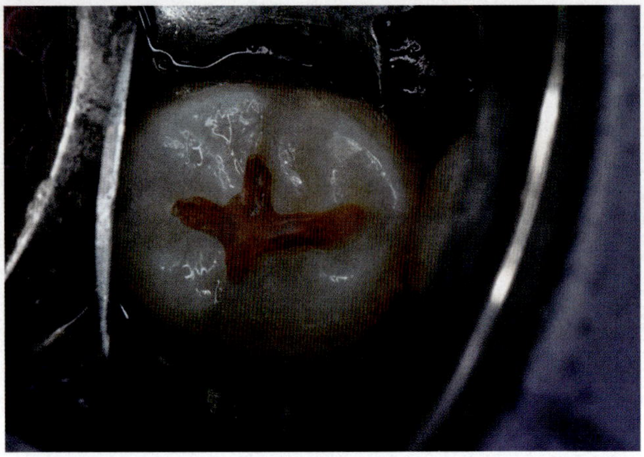

• **Fig. 12.1** Occlusal caries lesion prepared to receive a restoration.

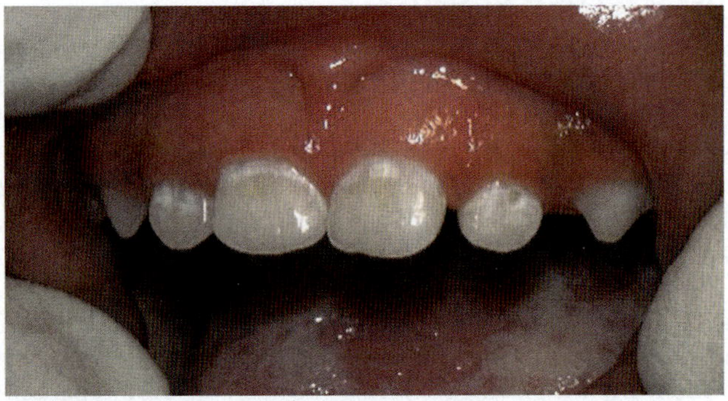

• **Fig. 12.2** Early stages of smooth surface caries lesions manifesting as "white spot lesions".

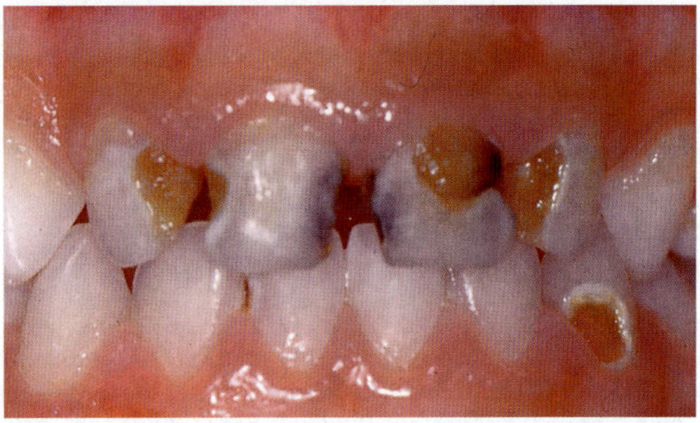

• **Fig. 12.3** Rampant tooth decay seen as multi-surface caries lesions.

4. **Management of caries:** Pediatric dentists must be skilled in managing caries at various stages of development. This includes the ability to detect early lesions, provide minimally invasive treatments, and perform restorative procedures suitable for young patients.
5. **Psychosocial impact:** Caries can have a profound psychosocial impact on children, affecting their self-esteem and social interactions. Pediatric dentists play a vital role in addressing these issues by providing compassionate care and promoting positive dental experiences.
6. **Foundation for lifelong oral health:** Early education and preventive care in childhood lay the foundation for lifelong oral health. By instilling good oral hygiene habits and preventive practices from an early age, pediatric dentists can significantly reduce the burden of dental caries in the population.

Historical Introduction

Timeline of Dentistry With Pivot Points

Dentistry has evolved significantly over the centuries, with several pivotal moments shaping the field as we know it today. The timeline of dentistry includes critical advancements in techniques, materials, and understanding of oral diseases, leading to the modern practice of dental care.

1. Ancient dentistry (7000 BCE–1700s CE):
   - **7000 BCE:** Evidence of dental work, including the use of flint drill bits in ancient Pakistan.
   - **5000 BCE:** Descriptions of tooth decay and its treatment found in Sumerian texts.
   - **1700s CE:** Pierre Fauchard, often called the "father of modern dentistry," published his influential book *Le Chirurgien Dentiste,* laying the foundation for modern dental practices.
2. 19th century:
   - **1839:** Establishment of the first dental school, Baltimore College of Dental Surgery.
   - **1870s:** Introduction of the foot-treadle dental engine, which improved efficiency in dental procedures.
   - **1890:** Willoughby D. Miller's chemo-parasitic theory of dental caries, highlighting the microbial cause of caries.
3. 20th century:
   - **1908:** Publication of *Operative Dentistry* by G.V. Black, which standardized cavity preparations and caries classification.
   - **1940s:** Introduction of fluoride in water supplies, significantly reducing the incidence of dental caries.
   - **1960s:** Development of dental implants by Dr. Per-Ingvar Brånemark.
4. 21st century:
   - **2000s:** Advancements in dental materials, including composite resins and computer-aided design (CAD)/computer-aided manufacturing (CAM) technology for restorations.
   - **2010s:** Implementation of digital dentistry and artificial intelligence (AI) in diagnostics and treatment planning.
   - **2020s:** Ongoing research into regenerative dentistry and the use of stem cells for tooth regeneration and the transition into "chronic disease management" from merely "prevention" (Fig. 12.4).

Historical Findings by Miller, Black, Keyes, and Stephan

The contributions of four key figures—W.D. Miller, G.V. Black, Paul H. Keyes, and Robert M. Stephan—have significantly shaped the field of cariology and modern dentistry.

- **W.D. Miller:** Willoughby D. Miller (1853–1907) is regarded as the father of modern dental microbiology. His pioneering work, including the chemo-parasitic theory of caries proposed in 1890, established that dental caries result from acids produced by oral bacteria fermenting dietary carbohydrates. This

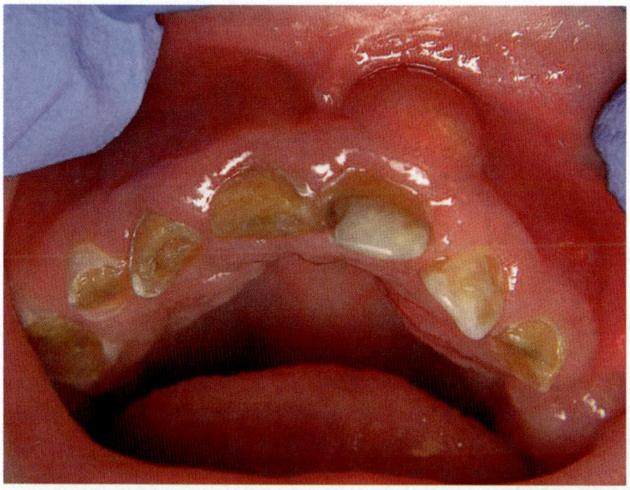

• **Fig. 12.4** Extensive tooth decay along with infection in the soft tissues, both related to lack of disease prevention.

foundational theory highlighted the microbial involvement in caries development and laid the groundwork for understanding the prevention and management of dental caries.

- **G.V. Black:** Known as the "father of modern dentistry," Greene Vardiman Black (1836–1915) made numerous contributions to operative dentistry and cariology. He developed standardized principles for cavity preparation and classification of carious lesions, known as "Black's Classification of Caries Lesions." His extensive research on dental amalgam improved its properties and durability, and his advocacy for preventive dentistry emphasized the importance of regular checkups and proper oral hygiene (Fig. 12.5).
- **Paul H. Keyes:** Dr. Keyes is recognized for his multifactorial caries theory, which identifies three primary factors necessary for caries development: a susceptible tooth surface, fermentable carbohydrates, and acidogenic bacteria, primarily *S. mutans* and *Lactobacillus* species. His research underscored the importance of oral bacteria and diet in caries formation, leading to advancements in preventive dentistry and dental hygiene practices.
- **Robert M. Stephan:** Dr. Stephan's pioneering work on the Stephan curve, which describes changes in plaque pH in response to sugar exposure, provided critical insights into the dynamic relationship between diet, bacterial activity, and the pH of dental plaque. His research showed how dietary sugars cause a rapid drop in pH, leading to demineralization of the tooth enamel and promoting caries development. This understanding has informed strategies for caries prevention through dietary modifications and the use of fluoride to enhance remineralization.

Caries Microbiota and Oral Biofilm

Composition and Role of Oral Microbiota in Caries Development

The oral microbiota, a diverse and complex microbial community, plays a crucial role in maintaining oral health and contributing to the development of dental caries. This microbiota consists of bacteria, fungi, viruses, and protozoa, which exist in a delicate balance within the oral cavity. The oral biofilm, also known as dental plaque, is a structured community of these

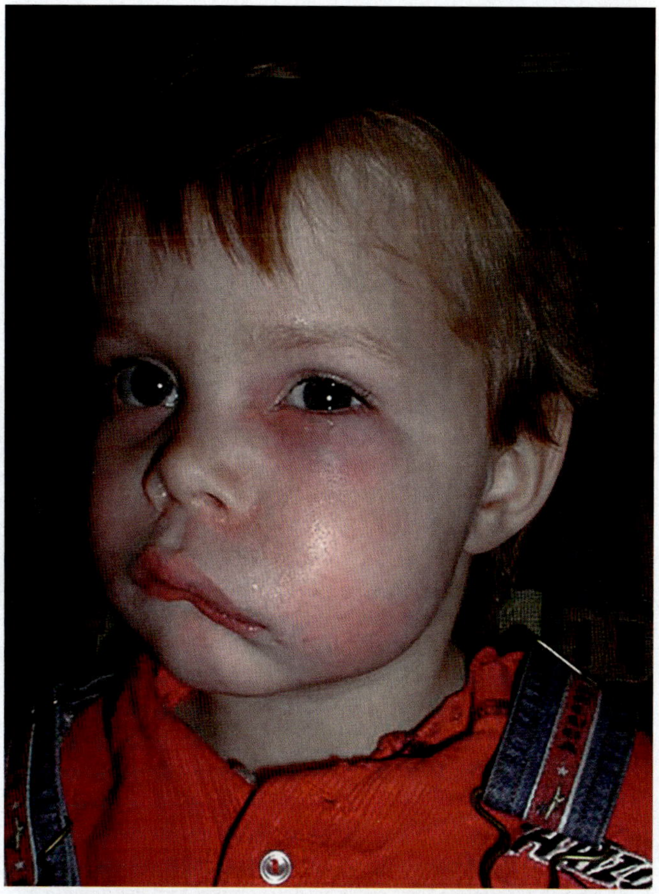

• **Fig. 12.5** Dental caries can manifest in a dangerous form of cellulitis.

microorganisms embedded in a self-produced extracellular matrix composed of polysaccharides, proteins, and nucleic acids.[1]

The oral biofilm's composition and the interactions among its microbial inhabitants are central to the caries process. When the balance of the oral microbiota is disrupted, typically due to dietary sugars and poor oral hygiene, acidogenic (acid-producing) and aciduric (acid-tolerant) bacteria become predominant. These bacteria metabolize fermentable carbohydrates, producing acids that lower the pH in the biofilm. This acidic environment leads to the demineralization of the tooth enamel, initiating the caries process. The protective mechanisms of saliva, such as its buffering capacity and antimicrobial properties, are often overwhelmed, allowing caries to progress (Fig. 12.6).

Key Bacterial Species Involved

Several key bacterial species are implicated in the development of dental caries, with *S. mutans* and *Lactobacillus* species as the most significant.[2]

- ***S. mutans:*** This species is considered the primary pathogen in dental caries.[3] *S. mutans* has a high affinity for tooth surfaces and can rapidly metabolize sucrose to produce lactic acid, contributing to a low pH environment that demineralizes enamel.[4] Additionally, *S. mutans* synthesizes extracellular polysaccharides from sucrose, which enhance bacterial adhesion and biofilm formation.[5]
- ***Lactobacillus:*** Species of *Lactobacillus* are highly acidogenic and aciduric, thriving in the low pH environments created

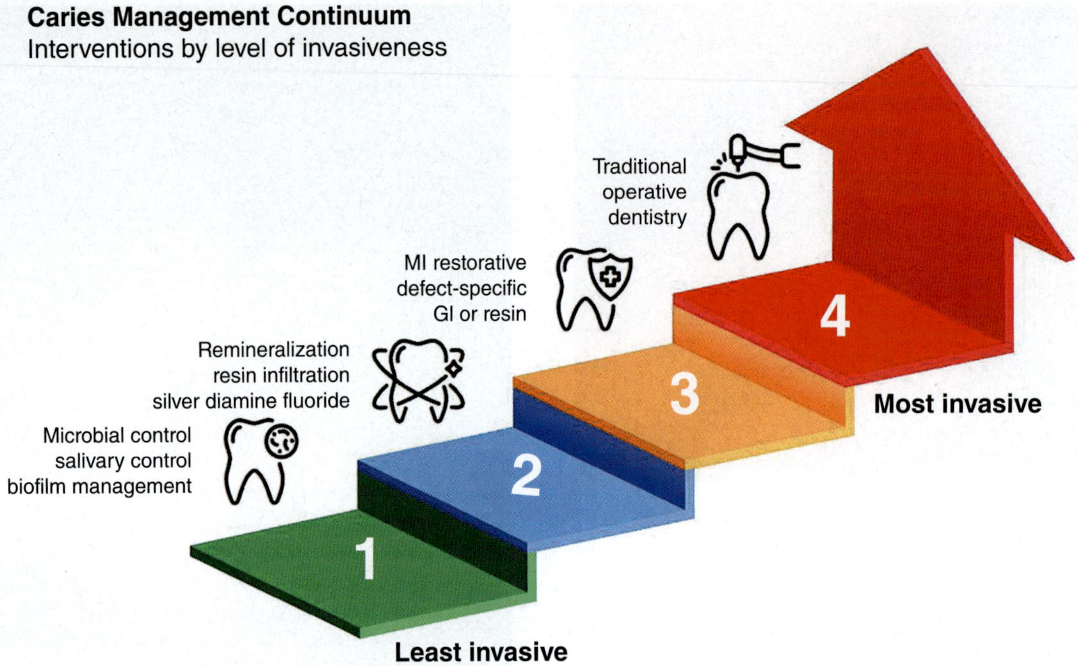

• **Fig. 12.6** Infographic showing the continuum of caries management from etiologic factors to restorative therapy. *GI,* glass Ionomer; *MI,* minimally invasive.

by *S. mutans.* They are often found in deeper carious lesions and play a significant role in the progression of dental caries by maintaining the acidic environment necessary for caries development.

Other bacterial species such as *Actinomyces* and *Veillonella* also contribute to caries by participating in the complex microbial interactions within the biofilm. These bacteria support the metabolic activities of *S. mutans* and *Lactobacillus,* further lowering the pH and enhancing the cariogenic potential of the biofilm.

Research on the Ecologic Shifts and Dysbiosis Leading to Caries

Research into the ecologic shifts and dysbiosis within the oral microbiota has provided significant insights into the mechanisms underlying dental caries. Dysbiosis refers to the imbalance in the microbial community that favors the proliferation of pathogenic bacteria over commensal (beneficial) bacteria.[6]

Studies using advanced molecular techniques, such as next-generation sequencing (NGS) and metagenomics, have revealed that caries is associated with a shift from a healthy, diverse microbial community to a less diverse community dominated by acidogenic and aciduric species. This shift is often driven by frequent consumption of fermentable carbohydrates and inadequate oral hygiene practices.[7]

Ecologic shifts in the biofilm are characterized by an increase in the relative abundance of cariogenic species like *S. mutans* and *Lactobacillus,* and a decrease in beneficial bacteria that contributes to oral health. For instance, *Streptococcus sanguinis* and *Streptococcus gordonii,* which are known to inhibit the growth of *S. mutans,* are often depleted in carious lesions.[8]

Furthermore, the acidification of the biofilm environment not only promotes the growth of acid-tolerant bacteria but also inhibits the growth of acid-sensitive beneficial bacteria.[9,10] This feedback loop exacerbates the dysbiotic state, leading to the progression of dental caries. Research continues to explore the precise interactions and regulatory mechanisms within the oral biofilm to develop targeted strategies for preventing and managing dental caries by restoring a healthy microbial balance.[11]

Role of Saliva

Saliva's Protective Functions Against Caries

Saliva plays a crucial role in protecting the oral cavity against dental caries through several mechanisms. One of its primary functions is to maintain the integrity of tooth enamel by providing a continuous supply of calcium and phosphate ions necessary for remineralization. This process helps repair early carious lesions and prevent the progression of decay.[12–15]

Saliva also has a significant buffering capacity, neutralizing acids produced by cariogenic bacteria in the dental biofilm.[16] This buffering action helps maintain a stable pH in the oral environment, preventing the demineralization of enamel that leads to caries formation. Additionally, saliva's flow helps wash away food particles and bacteria, reducing the substrate available for bacterial fermentation and acid production.[14,15,17–24]

Moreover, saliva contains antimicrobial proteins and enzymes that inhibit the growth of pathogenic microorganisms. These include lysozyme, lactoferrin, and immunoglobulins, which contribute to the control of bacterial populations and the prevention of dental caries.

Components of Saliva and Their Roles

The protective functions of saliva are mediated by its various components, each playing a specific role in maintaining oral health.

- **Enzymes:** Saliva contains several enzymes that contribute to its protective functions. For example, amylase helps in the digestion of dietary starches, reducing the amount of fermentable carbohydrates available for bacterial metabolism. Lysozyme exhibits antibacterial activity by breaking down the cell walls of certain bacteria, while lactoperoxidase produces hypothiocyanite, an antimicrobial agent that inhibits bacterial growth.

- **Buffering capacity:** The bicarbonate, phosphate, and protein systems in saliva are responsible for its buffering capacity. Bicarbonate is the primary buffer that neutralizes acids in the oral cavity, helping maintain a neutral pH and protect against enamel demineralization. Phosphate and protein buffers also contribute to this acid-neutralizing effect.
- **Calcium and phosphate ions:** These ions are essential for the remineralization process. Saliva is supersaturated with calcium and phosphate, which helps maintain the integrity of the enamel and facilitates the repair of early carious lesions. Fluoride, when present in saliva, enhances this remineralization process by forming fluorapatite, a more acid-resistant mineral than hydroxyapatite.
- **Antimicrobial proteins:** Immunoglobulins (primarily IgA), lactoferrin, and histatins are some of the antimicrobial proteins found in saliva. IgA prevents bacterial adhesion to tooth surfaces, lactoferrin binds iron required for bacterial growth, and histatins have antifungal and antibacterial properties, protecting against a wide range of oral pathogens.

Impact of Saliva Flow and Composition on Caries Risk

The flow rate and composition of saliva are critical factors influencing the risk of dental caries. Adequate saliva flow is essential for its protective functions, including buffering capacity, mechanical clearance of food and bacteria, and the delivery of essential ions for remineralization. Reduced saliva flow, a condition known as xerostomia, significantly increases the risk of caries as it impairs these protective mechanisms.[25]

Changes in saliva composition can also affect caries risk. For example, lower levels of calcium, phosphate, and fluoride reduce the saliva's ability to remineralize enamel.[26] Similarly, a decrease in the concentration of antimicrobial proteins can lead to an overgrowth of cariogenic bacteria. Various factors, including medication use, systemic diseases, and radiation therapy, can alter saliva composition and flow, thereby increasing the susceptibility to dental caries (Fig. 12.7).

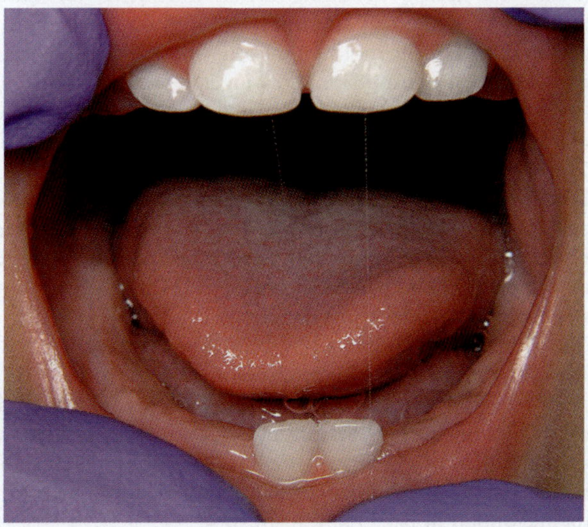

• **Fig. 12.7** Thickened saliva can increase the chance of significant dental caries manifestations.

Saliva plays a multifaceted role in protecting against dental caries. Its components work synergistically to maintain oral health by neutralizing acids, inhibiting bacterial growth, and promoting the remineralization of tooth enamel.[27] Understanding the functions and composition of saliva, as well as the factors affecting its flow, is crucial for developing effective strategies to prevent and manage dental caries.

Remineralization and Regenerative Technology

Remineralization

Importance and Mechanism

Remineralization is a cornerstone of modern, minimally invasive dentistry, particularly valuable in pediatric care where preserving natural tooth structure is paramount. Through remineralization, essential minerals like calcium and phosphate are redeposited into early enamel lesions, reversing demineralization and bolstering enamel resistance to future acid challenges. This process hinges on the diffusion of minerals, often aided by fluoride, which encourages the formation of fluorapatite, an acid-resistant crystalline structure in enamel that acts as a barrier to further decay.[28–31]

Current Remineralization Agents and Techniques

Fluoride remains the most extensively utilized agent in remineralization, available in varnishes, gels, and toothpaste, where it facilitates the uptake of minerals into the enamel surface. In recent years, however, new approaches and materials are enhancing the way remineralization can be achieved.[32–36] Casein phosphopeptide-amorphous calcium phosphate (CPP-ACP) complexes, for example, provide bioavailable calcium and phosphate directly to demineralized enamel, creating a stable reservoir of minerals.[37,38] Similarly, nanohydroxyapatite, which mimics the crystalline structure of natural enamel, has shown significant promise in integrating into weakened enamel surfaces and restoring hardness, making it an effective, nontoxic option for both children and adults.[39,40]

Emerging Research and Biomimetic Innovations

Recent advancements in biomimetic materials are shaping the future of dentistry by closely replicating the natural formation and structure of enamel.[41,42] One of the most promising developments is the creation of protein-based matrices, such as elastin-like recombinamers (ELRs), designed to mimic the structure and function of the enamel matrix present during tooth development.[43–45] When applied to eroded or damaged enamel surfaces, these ELR matrices can guide the organized deposition of hydroxyapatite crystals, aligning along the natural c-axis orientation of enamel and thereby reconstructing its intricate, layered structure. This organized crystal growth is achieved through epitaxial mineralization, a process wherein new crystals[46,47] grow in direct continuity with the natural enamel structure, creating a seamless bond that enhances durability and resistance to acid erosion and mechanical wear.

The ELR-based matrix offers several advantages over traditional approaches. It not only replicates the enamel's natural architecture but also forms a resilient, integrated layer that can withstand daily wear from tooth brushing, mastication, and acidic foods. Studies on this biomimetic matrix have shown that it can form mineralized layers up to 10 μm thick, reconstituting both prismatic and aprismatic enamel regions. The material's durability is tested to resist complex oral environments, making it particularly valuable for pediatric patients who benefit from long-term protection against caries progression.

The Future of Dentistry: Biomimetic and Regenerative Approaches

As research continues to advance, biomimetic remineralization strategies are emerging as the future of preventive and restorative dentistry. Unlike traditional treatments, which merely protect existing enamel, these new approaches aim to regenerate and reinforce the natural tooth structure. This vision of remineralization aligns with a broader shift in dental care toward regenerative practices that not only preserve but also restore lost dental tissues. Biomimetic agents, with their ability to closely replicate natural processes, are setting a new standard for treatment efficacy, durability, and biocompatibility.

In pediatric dentistry, where the longevity of dental treatments is especially critical, the adoption of biomimetic remineralization materials could reshape standard practice. Clinically friendly formulations, like the ELR-based matrix, support minimally invasive approaches that are easy to apply, efficient, and safe for young patients. By educating caregivers and integrating these advanced remineralization options into preventive care routines, dental professionals can offer children a stronger foundation for lifelong oral health.

With ongoing research refining these materials and exploring even more sophisticated biomimetic and regenerative solutions, remineralization is poised to become a central component of dental care. This progress underscores a future where dentistry moves beyond traditional repair, embracing a regenerative paradigm that has the potential to transform how caries and tooth erosion are managed across all patient populations.

Transmission of Caries

Mechanisms of Caries Transmission (Vertical and Horizontal)

Dental caries, a multifactorial infectious disease, primarily involves the transmission of cariogenic bacteria such as *S. mutans* and *Lactobacillus* species. These bacteria are key players in the etiology of caries due to their ability to metabolize sugars into acids that demineralize tooth enamel. The transmission of these bacteria can occur both vertically and horizontally.[48]

- **Vertical transmission:** This refers to the transfer of cariogenic bacteria from parents, particularly mothers, to their children.[49] This transmission typically occurs through direct contact, such as kissing, sharing utensils, or tasting food before feeding the child. The colonization of the child's oral cavity with these bacteria can begin even before the eruption of primary teeth, as the bacteria can inhabit the oral mucosa and other surfaces. Studies have shown that children whose mothers have high levels of *S. mutans* are at a greater risk of early colonization and subsequent caries development.
- **Horizontal transmission:** This involves the spread of cariogenic bacteria between individuals who are in close contact but not necessarily related. This can occur in settings such as day care centers and schools or among siblings.[50] Horizontal transmission is facilitated through the sharing of utensils, toys, or other objects that come into contact with saliva. Research indicates that children in communal living environments are more likely to share similar strains of *S. mutans*,[51] highlighting the significance of horizontal transmission in the spread of dental caries.

Role of Caregivers and Siblings in Transmission

Caregivers, particularly mothers, play a crucial role in the vertical transmission of cariogenic bacteria. The oral health behaviors and hygiene practices of caregivers significantly affect the bacterial load in their oral cavity, which in turn affects the likelihood of transmitting these bacteria to children. For instance, mothers with untreated dental caries or poor oral hygiene are more likely to transmit *S. mutans* to their children. Preventive measures such as improving maternal oral hygiene and treating dental caries can reduce the bacterial load and subsequently lower the risk of transmission.[52,53]

Siblings also play a role in the horizontal transmission of cariogenic bacteria. In families with multiple children, older siblings can be a source of bacterial transmission to younger ones. Shared activities and close contact among siblings facilitate the exchange of saliva and bacteria, contributing to the spread of cariogenic bacteria within the family unit. Ensuring good oral hygiene practices for all family members and educating children about the importance of not sharing utensils or toothbrushes can help mitigate this risk.

Preventive Measures to Reduce Transmission Risk

Effective prevention of caries transmission involves a combination of improving oral hygiene practices, reducing bacterial load in caregivers, and educating families about the risks of bacterial transmission.

- **Improving oral hygiene:** Educating caregivers about proper oral hygiene practices, such as regular tooth brushing with fluoride toothpaste, flossing, and routine dental checkups, is essential. Caregivers should be encouraged to maintain their oral health to minimize the risk of transmitting cariogenic bacteria to their children. Implementing good oral hygiene practices early in a child's life can also help establish lifelong habits that reduce caries risk.[54–56]
- **Maternal oral health:** Interventions aimed at improving maternal oral health, including dental treatments for existing caries and professional cleanings, can significantly reduce the bacterial load in the mother's mouth. This, in turn, lowers the risk of vertical transmission of cariogenic bacteria to the child. Pregnant patients should be educated about the importance of maintaining their oral health and the potential impact on their child's oral health.
- **Dietary modifications:** Reducing the intake of sugary foods and beverages is crucial in preventing caries development. Educating families about the importance of a balanced diet that limits fermentable carbohydrates can help reduce the substrate available for cariogenic bacteria, thereby lowering the risk of caries development.[57–59]
- **Avoiding saliva sharing practices:** Caregivers should be advised to avoid practices that involve the transfer of saliva to their children, such as sharing utensils, cleaning pacifiers with their mouths, or kissing on the lips. Educating parents about these risks and promoting alternative practices can help reduce the likelihood of bacterial transmission.
- **Regular dental visits:** Encouraging regular dental visits for both caregivers and children can help in the early detection

and management of caries. Dental professionals can provide tailored advice on oral hygiene practices, dietary recommendations, and preventive treatments such as fluoride varnishes or dental sealants, which can help protect against caries.[60,61]

Understanding the mechanisms of caries transmission and the roles of caregivers and siblings is essential for developing effective preventive strategies. By improving oral hygiene practices, addressing maternal oral health, making dietary modifications, avoiding saliva-sharing practices, and encouraging regular dental visits, the risk of caries transmission can be significantly reduced, promoting better oral health outcomes for children.

Risk Assessments

Updated Caries Risk Assessment Models

Caries risk assessment models have evolved significantly over the years, integrating new research findings and advanced technologies to improve accuracy and effectiveness. These models aim to identify individuals at high risk for developing dental caries, allowing for targeted preventive and therapeutic interventions.[62]

One of the widely used models is the Caries Management by Risk Assessment (CAMBRA) approach, which considers various factors such as caries history, oral hygiene practices, dietary habits, fluoride exposure, and socioeconomic status. CAMBRA categorizes patients into low, moderate, high, and extreme risk levels and recommends tailored preventive and therapeutic strategies for each risk category.[63]

The Cariogram is another comprehensive model that uses a computer-based program to assess caries risk. It incorporates factors like bacterial load, diet, plaque control, saliva flow, and fluoride usage to generate a visual representation of caries risk, helping clinicians and patients understand the balance between protective and risk factors.

Recent advancements in caries risk assessment also include the use of genetic markers and salivary diagnostics. Genetic testing can identify individuals with genetic predispositions to caries, while salivary diagnostics analyze saliva for biomarkers[64] indicative of caries risk. These innovative approaches enhance the precision of risk assessments and enable more personalized dental care.

Factors Influencing Caries Risk (e.g., Genetic, Environmental, Behavioral)

Caries risk is influenced by a complex interplay of genetic, environmental, and behavioral factors.

- **Genetic factors:** Genetic predisposition plays a significant role in caries susceptibility. Variations in genes related to enamel formation, saliva composition, and immune response can affect an individual's risk of developing caries. For instance, genetic polymorphisms in the genes encoding enamel matrix proteins and salivary proteins have been associated with increased caries risk.
- **Environmental factors:** Environmental factors, such as fluoride exposure, access to dental care, and socioeconomic status, significantly impact caries risk. Fluoride exposure, through drinking water or dental products, enhances enamel resistance to demineralization and promotes remineralization. Limited access to dental care and low socioeconomic status are associated with higher caries prevalence due to inadequate preventive measures and treatments.
- **Behavioral factors:** Behavioral factors, including dietary habits, oral hygiene practices, and health behaviors, are critical determinants of caries risk. Frequent consumption of sugary foods and beverages provides a substrate for cariogenic bacteria, leading to acid production and enamel demineralization. Poor oral hygiene practices, such as infrequent tooth brushing and lack of flossing, result in plaque accumulation and increased bacterial load. Additionally, tobacco use and certain medications that reduce saliva flow can elevate caries risk.

Integration of Risk Assessments Into Clinical Practice

Integrating caries risk assessments into clinical practice involves systematically evaluating risk factors, educating patients, and implementing individualized preventive and therapeutic strategies.

- **Systematic evaluation:** Clinicians should routinely perform comprehensive risk assessments during dental visits. This includes reviewing medical and dental history, conducting clinical examinations, and utilizing risk assessment tools such as CAMBRA or Cariogram. Incorporating genetic testing and salivary diagnostics can further enhance the accuracy of risk assessments.[65–67]
- **Patient education:** Educating patients about their caries risk and the importance of preventive measures is crucial. Dentists should discuss the findings of the risk assessment with patients, highlighting specific risk factors and recommending tailored preventive strategies. This may include dietary counseling, oral hygiene instructions, and the use of fluoride products.
- **Individualized preventive and therapeutic strategies:** Based on the risk assessment, clinicians should develop individualized care plans. For low-risk patients, routine preventive measures such as regular checkups and cleanings may suffice. High-risk patients may require more intensive interventions, including fluoride treatments, sealants, and more frequent dental visits. Monitoring and adjusting the care plan based on changes in risk factors over time are essential for effective caries management.

In conclusion, updated caries risk assessment models, a comprehensive understanding of the factors influencing caries risk, and the integration of these assessments into clinical practice are vital for effective caries prevention and management. By identifying high-risk individuals and providing personalized care, dental professionals can significantly reduce the prevalence and impact of dental caries.

Emerging Diagnostic Methodologies

Early Caries Lesion Detection

Early detection of dental caries lesions is crucial for effective management and prevention of disease progression. Traditional methods such as visual-tactile examination and radiography have been the cornerstone of caries lesion detection, but they have limitations in identifying early lesions (Fig. 12.8). Advances in diagnostic technologies have led to the development of more sensitive and accurate methods for early caries lesion detection.[68–74]

- **Quantitative light-induced fluorescence (QLF) technologies:** QLF technologies utilize blue light to induce fluorescence in teeth, detecting changes in fluorescence intensity that correlate with demineralization. QLF can identify early enamel lesions and quantify the extent of mineral loss, allowing for

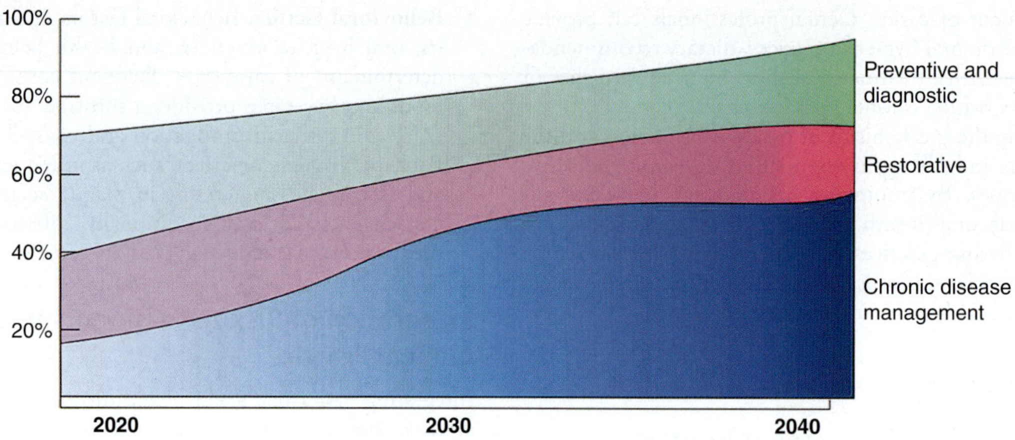

• **Fig. 12.8** Shift from only prevention and restorative to chronic disease management in the decades ahead.

monitoring of lesion progression or remineralization over time. This method is particularly useful for longitudinal studies and patient education.

- **Electrical conductance and impedance spectroscopy technologies:** Techniques like electrical conductance measurement (ECM) and impedance spectroscopy measure the electrical properties of tooth tissues to detect caries. These methods are based on the principle that demineralized tissues have different electrical properties compared with sound enamel. They are useful for detecting early enamel lesions and monitoring changes during remineralization treatments.[75,76]

Salivary Diagnostics

Saliva is a valuable diagnostic fluid due to its ease of collection and the wealth of biologic information it contains. Salivary diagnostics have gained attention for their potential in early caries lesion detection and overall oral health assessment.

- **Biomarkers:** Saliva contains various biomarkers, including proteins, enzymes, and nucleic acids, that can indicate the presence of caries or other oral diseases. For example, elevated levels of matrix metalloproteinases (MMPs) and pro-inflammatory cytokines in saliva have been associated with active caries lesions. Identifying and quantifying these biomarkers can aid in early diagnosis and monitoring of caries progression.[77,78]
- **Microbial analysis:** Salivary diagnostics can also involve analyzing the microbial composition of saliva. Techniques such as polymerase chain reaction (PCR) and NGS can identify and quantify cariogenic bacteria like *S. mutans* and *Lactobacillus* species. This information helps in assessing caries risk and tailoring preventive strategies accordingly.
- **Point-of-care (POC) testing:** The development of POC diagnostic devices enables rapid and chairside analysis of saliva. These devices can measure salivary flow rates, pH, and specific biomarkers, providing immediate feedback to clinicians and patients. POC testing enhances the efficiency of caries risk assessment and facilitates timely interventions.

Biofilm/Microbiota Biomarkers

Oral biofilm, or dental plaque, is a complex microbial community that plays a pivotal role in caries development. Analyzing the composition and activity of the biofilm can provide insights into caries risk and progression.

- **Microbiota profiling:** Advanced molecular techniques such as 16S rRNA sequencing and metagenomics allow for comprehensive profiling of the oral microbiota. These techniques can identify shifts in microbial composition associated with caries development, such as an increase in cariogenic bacteria and a decrease in beneficial species. Monitoring these changes can help in predicting caries risk and evaluating the effectiveness of preventive measures.
- **Metabolomic analysis:** Metabolomics involves the study of metabolites produced by the oral microbiota. Analyzing the metabolic by-products in dental plaque can reveal the biochemical pathways active in caries development. For instance, increased production of lactic acid and other organic acids is indicative of cariogenic activity. Metabolomic analysis provides a deeper understanding of the functional aspects of the biofilm and its role in caries.
- **Plaque pH measurement:** The pH of dental plaque is a critical factor in caries development. Techniques for measuring plaque pH, such as microelectrodes and pH-sensitive dyes, can provide real-time data on the acidity of the biofilm environment. Low plaque pH indicates active acid production by cariogenic bacteria, highlighting areas at risk for demineralization. Regular monitoring of plaque pH can guide preventive and therapeutic interventions.

Evidence-Based Dentistry and Ethical Use of Diagnostic Technology: Role of Artificial Intelligence

- **Evidence-based dentistry (EBD):** EBD integrates clinical expertise, patient values, and the best available scientific evidence to guide decision making. The use of diagnostic technologies in caries lesion detection should be grounded in robust clinical evidence. Systematic reviews and meta-analyses of diagnostic tools ensure that they are validated and effective. EBD promotes the adoption of technologies that improve diagnostic accuracy and patient outcomes.
- **Ethical considerations:** The ethical use of diagnostic technologies involves ensuring patient safety, privacy, and informed consent. Clinicians must be transparent about the benefits and limitations of diagnostic tools and involve patients in decision

making. Additionally, the use of technology should not replace the clinician's judgment but rather augment it to provide comprehensive care.

- **Role of AI:** AI has the potential to revolutionize caries diagnosis and management. Machine learning algorithms can analyze vast amounts of data from diagnostic tools, identifying patterns and predicting caries risk with high accuracy. AI can assist in interpreting imaging data, such as radiographs and QLF images, reducing human error and enhancing diagnostic precision. Moreover, AI-driven decision support systems can provide personalized recommendations for preventive and therapeutic strategies, improving patient care.

Emerging diagnostic methodologies, including early caries lesion detection technologies, salivary diagnostics, biofilm biomarkers, and the integration of AI, hold great promise for advancing caries prevention and management. These innovations, grounded in evidence-based practice and ethical considerations, have the potential to transform dental care and improve oral health outcomes.

Antimicrobials and Vaccines

Use of Antimicrobial Agents in Caries Prevention and Management

Antimicrobial agents play a crucial role in the prevention and management of dental caries by targeting the cariogenic bacteria that contribute to the disease. These agents can be delivered through various forms, including mouth rinses, varnishes, gels, and toothpastes, providing a multifaceted approach to caries control.

- **Chlorhexidine:** Chlorhexidine is a widely used antimicrobial agent effective against a broad spectrum of bacteria. It is available in mouth rinses, gels, and varnishes and is often used in the management of high-risk caries patients.[79] Chlorhexidine works by disrupting bacterial cell membranes and inhibiting bacterial colonization and biofilm formation. Its use has been shown to reduce the levels of *S. mutans* in the oral cavity, thereby decreasing caries incidence. However, long-term use of chlorhexidine can lead to side effects such as tooth staining and altered taste perception.
- **Fluoride:** Fluoride has both antimicrobial properties and the ability to enhance enamel remineralization. Topical fluoride applications, including varnishes, gels, and toothpaste, help reduce cariogenic bacteria and promote the formation of fluorapatite, a more acid-resistant form of enamel. Fluoride's antimicrobial effect is due to its ability to inhibit bacterial enzymes involved in acid production, thus reducing the acidogenic potential of dental plaque.[80–84]
- **Essential oils:** Mouth rinses containing essential oils, such as thymol, eucalyptol, and menthol, have demonstrated antimicrobial activity against cariogenic bacteria. These oils disrupt bacterial cell walls and inhibit enzyme activity, leading to reduced plaque and gingivitis. Essential oil-based mouth rinses are often used as an adjunct to mechanical plaque control methods.
- **Xylitol:** Xylitol, a sugar alcohol used in chewing gums and lozenges, has been shown to reduce the levels of *S. mutans* by disrupting its energy production processes. Regular use of xylitol-containing products can lead to a decrease in caries incidence, making it a valuable adjunct in caries prevention strategies.

Current and Emerging Vaccines Targeting Cariogenic Bacteria

The development of vaccines targeting cariogenic bacteria represents a promising approach to caries prevention. These vaccines aim to induce an immune response against specific bacterial antigens, reducing bacterial colonization and subsequent caries development.

- **Current vaccines:** Research has focused on vaccines targeting *S. mutans,* the primary pathogen associated with dental caries. Various strategies have been explored, including subunit vaccines using recombinant proteins from *S. mutans,* such as glucosyltransferases (GTFs) and adhesins. These proteins are critical for bacterial adherence and biofilm formation. Immunization with these antigens has shown to reduce *S. mutans* colonization and caries incidence in animal models.
- **Emerging vaccines:** Advancements in molecular biology and immunology have led to the development of novel vaccine candidates. DNA vaccines encoding *S. mutans* antigens and peptide vaccines targeting specific bacterial epitopes are currently under investigation. Additionally, mucosal vaccines delivered via nasal or oral routes are being explored to induce local immune responses in the oral cavity. These vaccines aim to provide long-lasting immunity and reduce the reliance on traditional antimicrobial treatments.[85–87]

Future Directions in Cariology Research

Several areas in cariology research hold promise for advancing our understanding and management of dental caries:

- **Microbiome research:** Continued exploration of the oral microbiome and its interactions with host factors will provide deeper insights into the mechanisms underlying caries development and progression.
- **Genetic and epigenetic studies:** Investigating genetic predispositions and epigenetic modifications associated with caries susceptibility will pave the way for personalized caries risk assessments and targeted interventions.
- **Regenerative dentistry:** Advances in regenerative technology, including the use of stem cells and biomimetic materials, offer potential for developing innovative treatments to repair and regenerate damaged dental tissues.[88]
- **Vaccine development:** Ongoing research on caries vaccines aims to develop effective immunizations that provide long-lasting protection against cariogenic bacteria, reducing the burden of dental caries.
- **AI:** The application of AI in diagnostic and treatment planning will continue to evolve, enhancing the accuracy of caries lesion detection and the efficiency of dental care delivery.

Implications for Pediatric Dental Practice

Several areas in cariology research hold promise for advancing our understanding and management of dental caries (Fig. 12.9):

- **Early detection and prevention:** Emphasizing early detection and preventive measures is crucial in pediatric dentistry. Implementing advanced diagnostic tools and caries risk assessments can identify high-risk children and guide preventive strategies.
- **Personalized care:** Integrating personalized care plans based on individual risk assessments and genetic predispositions will improve the effectiveness of caries prevention and management in children.

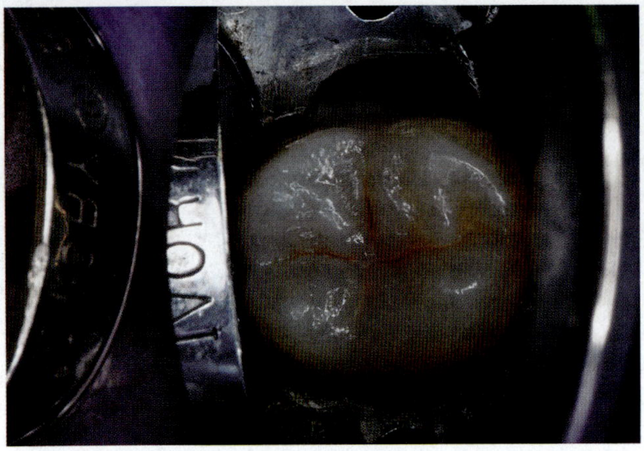

• **Fig. 12.9** Early detection of caries lesions will allow improved non-restorative management of smaller caries lesions.

- **Parental education and involvement:** Educating parents about the importance of oral hygiene, dietary habits, and the prevention of bacterial transmission is essential for reducing caries risk in children.
- **Interdisciplinary collaboration:** Collaborating with other healthcare professionals, including pediatricians and nutritionists, can enhance the overall approach to managing caries and promoting oral health in children.
- **Embracing technology:** Adopting emerging technologies, such as AI and salivary diagnostics, will revolutionize pediatric dental practice, offering more precise and efficient care for young patients.

The comprehensive understanding of cariology and the integration of advanced diagnostic and preventive methodologies are essential for improving oral health outcomes in children. By staying informed about the latest research and embracing innovative technologies, pediatric dentists can effectively combat dental caries and promote lifelong oral health in children.

Visit eBooks.Health.Elsevier.com to see full list of references.

13

Prevention in Pediatric Dentistry in Today's Healthcare

PAUL S. CASAMASSIMO, KERI DISCEPOLO, CHELSEA FOSSE, JESSICA A. MEESKE, AND KIMBERLY J. HAMMERSMITH

CHAPTER OUTLINE

Introduction

In the early 2000s, Fisher-Owens and colleagues published a conceptual model of caries initiation that built upon the half-century-old Keyes model and brought the whole child, family, society, and the system into the caries initiation paradigm.[1] This model recognized that the biology of the mouth was only the beginning of the caries process which was simultaneously influenced by factors from the environment around the mouth (Fig. 13.1). In 2021, the National Institutes of Dental and Craniofacial Research (NIDCR) published the landmark report, *Oral Health in America: Advances and Challenges,* which validated a variety of factors such as social determinants of health (SDOH), health literacy, system limitations, and others that also affect the initiation and continuation of dental caries.[2]

This chapter puts the traditional intraoral caries model into the perspective of the Fisher-Owens orbits of influence and describes those factors, and how to address them, in caries prevention in children and persons with special healthcare needs. Pediatric dentists disproportionately care for children covered by Medicaid, whose caries profile is highly influenced by external caries factors.[3] Pediatric dentists, also by specialty definition and training, treat persons with special healthcare needs,[4] whose oral health is strongly influenced by medical and care-taking factors. Within this chapter, a more global set of considerations provides a framework for more individualized approaches to prevention in the context of a high-volume, diverse, pediatric dentistry private practice system. The role of the traditional optimal fluoride-good oral hygiene-reduced sugar approach, explained in detail in subsequent chapters, will be characterized by the influence of systemic health, social, and systems factors, which if ignored will prevent success, but if managed, will improve the chances for good oral health.

The Whole Patient

To understand why dental care should not have a one-size-fits-all approach, one must broaden awareness and understand the complicated behavioral, medical, social, and other issues touching on caries initiation and prevention. Examining an individual's sugar consumption or fluoride exposure alone does not give the full caries risk picture. Dentists must look at the whole child and take a patient-centered care approach, rather than apply rigid care models that may be wasteful and ineffective for individual patients (Table 13.1).

Children with certain medical conditions (e.g., congenital heart disease, cystic fibrosis, metabolic disorders, HIV, cancer) have increased energy needs or inefficient energy utilization requiring more frequent feedings to increase caloric intake. These special diets increase caries risk. Moreover, much of the caloric supplementation for these children is high in carbohydrates, further increasing caries risk. For all children, calorie restriction is also difficult during growth periods, including much of childhood, as energy needs are higher. Rather than recommending children stop nutrition supplements, families and children can be counseled on increasing caloric intake by using noncarbohydrate sources, such as fat and/or protein and drinking water after any feedings.[5]

Diet in otherwise healthy children is also directly related to caries prevention and management. Culturally driven, highly processed food choices, packaging (lid-tops, snack-size packaging), and access to certain types of food will affect the intake and frequency of a child's diet. Dentists should discourage grazing all day on food, and any portable beverage container should contain only water or sugar-free alternatives.

Obesity, diabetes, and related heart disease are increasing among children. Dentists should gather height and weight during office visits to calculate body mass index (BMI), counsel families, and refer overweight children to physicians or specialists when needed. Although obesity can lead to a myriad of health complications in later life, it may lead to accelerated growth and development sooner. While a strong association between weight and caries in children has not been found,[6] a common culprit in obesity is added dietary sugar. Increased BMI is a relative contraindication for dentists to use sedation as an advanced behavior management technique in anxious children.

Allergies and sensitivities can affect oral intake and caries risk in children. Children must sometimes find food substitutes, and those substitutes may be more processed or have higher sugar content. Children with sensitivity to additives in toothpaste like sodium lauryl sulfate or dyes may choose to forgo the preventive effect of

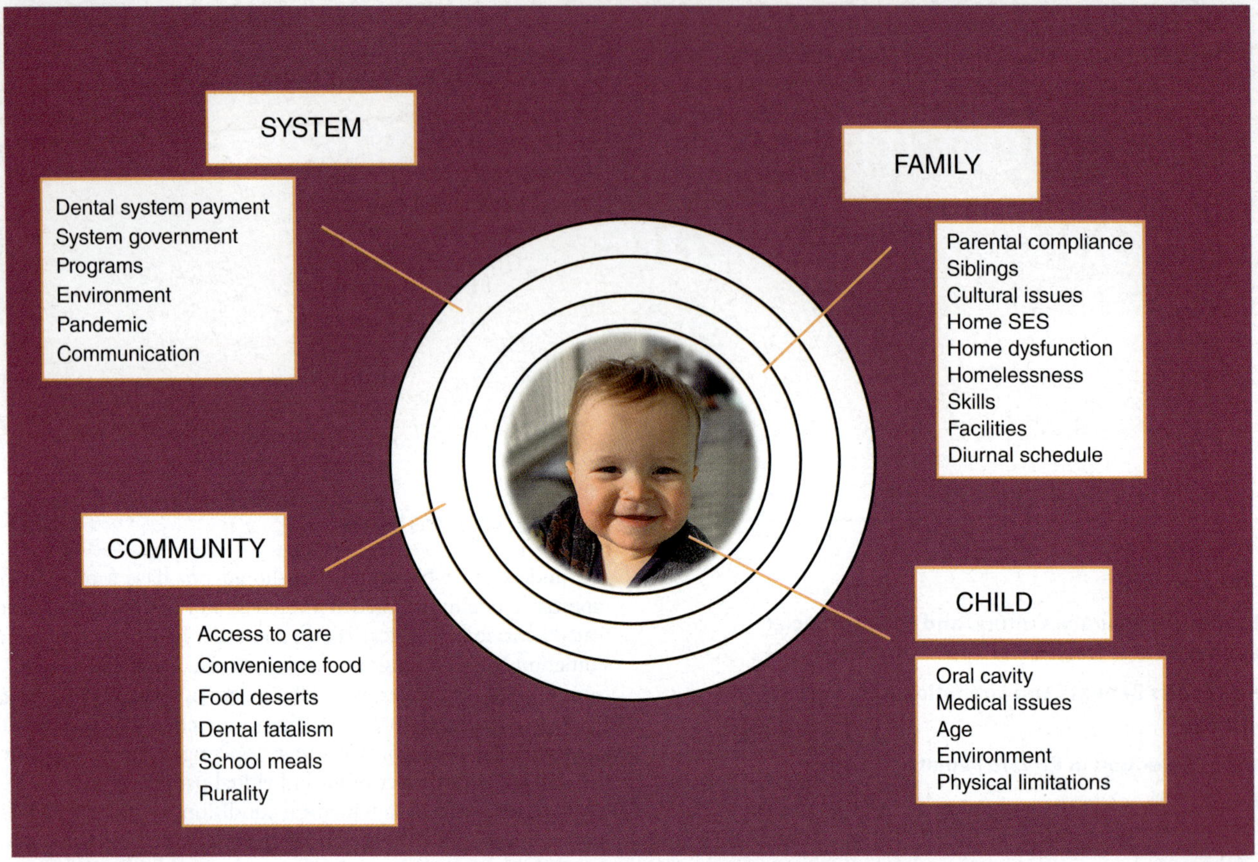

• **Fig. 13.1** Caries initiation model applied to caries prevention. (Adapted from Fisher-Owens SA, Gansky SA, Platt LJ, et al. Influences on children's oral health: a conceptual model. *Pediatrics.* 2007; 120[3]:e510-e520.)

fluoride toothpaste and/or use nonfluoridated substitutes instead. Dentists should provide recommendations for fluoride-containing toothpastes without the additives that the patient wishes to avoid.

Xerostomia results from various types of medications, including those for allergies or asthma, or as a side effect from radiation. Xerostomic children may benefit from use of oral lubricating agents, saliva stimulants including sugarless candies and gum, and prescribed medications. Chewing crunchy foods and sipping on water can help manage the potential detrimental effects of xerostomia.

Children with chronic medical conditions also frequently must take daily medications. Many liquid formulations, even over-the-counter pain relievers, are sweetened with sucrose. Dentists can recommend that these patients take nonliquid or sugar-free forms when possible or take their liquid medications with meals unless this affects the potency of the medication. Additionally, patients can be counseled to rinse with water after medication.

Poor oral hygiene may result from reduced manual dexterity due to a disability, discomfort due to oral mucositis, or lack of parental oversight, all reducing consistent oral hygiene practices. Children need aid from their parents until they can effectively, manually debride their teeth on their own.[7] Toothbrushes should be used when possible, and foam brushes used only for short durations during acute pain. Fixed orthodontic appliances, common in children and adolescents, also make oral hygiene difficult, and children can be counseled on effective means of cleaning around these appliances.

Media and marketing influence the public's perception of athleticism and exercise, the need for nutritional supplements, and the benefits of specific diets and types of hydration, usually other than water. Sports drinks are commonly consumed by young children and adolescents due to the positive effects perceived by their parents; however, they have high sugar content. National beverage consumption guidelines for early and later childhood exist,[8,9] but the plethora of available drink types for purchase and their packaging may make it overwhelmingly difficult for parents to understand and choose correctly. Dentists should guide parents in understanding nutrition labels and encouraging water over these sugar-sweetened sports beverages.

Caries prevention and management is as multifaceted as caries etiology. Overall, children at increased risk for caries due to these factors should be placed on more frequent recall intervals to increase the frequency of professionally applied fluoride as well as reinforcement of home hygiene and diet factors. Antimicrobials such as chlorhexidine, iodine, and xylitol may be used alongside, albeit separately from, fluoride in a preventive regimen. Minimally invasive dental techniques can arrest the progression of caries. Importantly, connecting with families in a way that improves preventive compliance is vital; it may not happen in an isolated dental setting and may require engagement of medical, social, and behavioral specialists.

Integrating oral health into primary care has been shown to be an effective way to promote oral health and involves increasing training of nondental staff, enacting policy changes, and overcoming system-level obstacles.[10] Integrated care can appear as colocation of medical and dental facilities, school-based healthcare, nurses or physicians providing oral health education or fluoride varnish treatment to patients, and telehealth.[11] Dentists can support these as additional means to accomplish oral health goals.

TABLE 13.1 Whole Patient Considerations in Prevention of Dental Caries

Specific Areas of Concern	Queries and Data Collection	Strategies for Prevention
Special, high-calorie diets for children with chronic illnesses	Higher frequency of feedings, caloric supplementation with carbohydrates	• Rinse with or drink water after feedings • Encourage caloric supplementation with fats and proteins • Consider more frequent recalls or limited examinations to monitor or achieve early detection and early intervention
Cultural eating practices and availability of snacks	• Snacking on highly processed foods, and sipping on sugar-containing liquids • Use of food reinforcers • Content of culturally driven diet	• Sip on water outside of mealtime • Discourage grazing • Encourage scheduled snack times • Offer mitigation strategies consistent with child and family abilities • Inform parents how to communicate with grandparents that may be overindulging grandchildren with sugary foods
Obesity, diabetes, and related heart disease	May be related to dietary sugar	• Counsel families of children with high BMI • Refer to specialists
Allergies and sensitivities	Alternatives may have higher sugar content or less fluoride	• Investigate lower-carbohydrate alternatives • Provide recommendations for fluoride-containing toothpastes
Xerostomia	Increases caries risk	• Encourage saliva stimulants • Recommend chewing crunchy foods and/or sipping on water
Daily medications for chronic illnesses	Liquid medicines contain sugar sweeteners	• Encourage nonliquid forms, sugar-free versions when available • Taking medication with meals when possible • Rinse with water afterward
Poor oral hygiene	Increases caries risk	• Encourage parents to help until children can clean mouth effectively
Society and marketing emphasis on athletics and hydration	Sugar-containing beverages increase caries risk	• Educate parents how to read packaging • Encourage water between meals
Caries prevention	High-risk versus low-risk determinants per individual child, characterized in a risk and protective format	• Higher risk necessitates more frequent recalls, fluoride applications, and adjuncts
Primary care: oral health integration	May take many forms and engagement of nondental professionals	Support these efforts to complement preventive strategies in the dental office
Developmental	• Is physical and speech development age appropriate • Ask parent if they have any concerns	• Inform parent that public school district does free speech screenings • Refer to child's primary care physician for physical health evaluation
Behavioral	• Determine whether behavior is age appropriate • Does parent seem unusually stressed	Let parent know that this is common and early intervention from a behavioral health therapist can be life changing for the child and family
Dental anomalies or malocclusion	• Ask about history of missing teeth, extra teeth, or any known conditions that affect child's enamel • Note early malocclusions if they impact child's ability to keep teeth clean	• Counsel parent on future treatment of dental anomalies and risk for dental disease • Let parents know when malocclusion exists, early treatment, such as arch development and alleviation of crowding, can make oral hygiene easier for the child

The Family, Community, Culture, and Society: Social Determinants of Health

The biologic imbalance of dental caries is dynamic and affected by the setting in which individuals live as well as by genetic factors. SDOH are nonmedical factors that affect health and contribute to inequality in achieving optimal health.[12] SDOH are social, economic, and physical conditions which, when negative, create individual disadvantages contributing to greater incidence of chronic diseases and affect preventive success (Table 13.2).

Health equity is defined as all individuals in a group having equal opportunity to achieve the highest level of health.[13] Oral health equity is not easily realized for those individuals experiencing community-related structural factors such as low socioeconomic status (SES), racial/ethnic barriers, reduced access to dental care, and family-level barriers.

SES is described as the economic resources available to an individual relating to overall income level, employment status, and educational level.[14,15] In the United States, children (aged 2 to 19 years) from low-income households experience three times more untreated dental caries than those from higher incomes.[16]

TABLE 13.2 Social Determinants of Health: The Family, Community, Culture, and Society Considerations in Prevention of Dental Caries

Specific Areas of Concern	Queries and Data Collection	Strategies for Prevention
Socioeconomic status (SES)	• Financial stress • Inability to pay for dental care • No dental insurance, limited insurance	• Direct families to state-funded insurances, sliding fee scales, payment plans • Encourage preventive visits with rationale
Adversely affected populations	Marginalized or minority background	• Foster inclusivity • Interpreter services
Accessibility	Work or school hours in conflict with dental office hours	• Value of continuity of care • Support with letter of attendance for working parents and school-aged children • Scheduling multiple services in same day such as adding sealants to recall, avoiding an additional visit
Transportation	• No transportation • Relies on public transportation • Unreliable vehicle • Parent or caregiver without a driver's license	• Medical taxi support • Offer office hours or appointments that work with public transportation schedules
Rural access	• No transportation • No public transportation • Dentist too far from home	• Mobile dental care, vans, school-based clinics, medical taxis when travel to office is needed • Option for teledentistry • Use of public health permit hygienists
Unsafe neighborhoods	No safe neighborhood playground; no safe place to shop for food/oral hygiene supplies	• Strategize on better health of the child, afterschool programs, food shopping • Provide oral hygiene products
ACE	Understanding individual and family allostatic load	• Strategies to help support the stressed family • Alternative or flexible dental appointments • Referral to appropriate mental health provider
Food insecurity	Sugar consumption Processed food consumption	• Coach families on healthy and less costly alternatives such as water over juice • Review resources to support buying food • Determine whether family qualifies for state and federal food programs such as free and reduced lunch at school

ACE, Adverse childhood experience.

SES negatively affects access to care and utilization of dental care, and often, ability to pay for dental care.[17,18] Often, SES is an indication of other SDOH obstacles for the family, such as food insecurity (FI), housing insecurity, and transportation barriers.

Observations regarding global health equity have shown poorer oral health in affected populations, specifically that children's caries prevalence is higher in racial minorities.[17,19] Mexican-American and non-Hispanic Black children aged 2 to 5 experience more caries in their primary teeth compared with non-Hispanic White children. Indigenous children have decay rates five times greater than the US population, with significantly more early childhood caries (ECC) treatments requiring general anesthesia.[20,21] When controlling for SDOH factors, Black children do not experience decay at a higher rate than White children, so by addressing SDOH, greater health equity can be achieved.[16]

Accessibility to and availability of dental care are ongoing problems in the United States, especially for racial and ethnic minorities.[22] When a child's first visit to the dentist is after 12 months of age, the child is more likely to have dental caries.[23] Children with a dental visit within the past year have lower odds of dental caries.[15] Routine dental visits, via establishing a dental home, are associated with less untreated dental decay, and conversely, children who frequently missed dental appointments were found to be 1.7 times more likely to be at high caries risk.[15,24–27]

The ability to obtain and maintain dental insurance is an important modulator of care utilization. For individuals who are underinsured, coverage may be sparse, where only preventive services are covered.[15] With broader Medicaid and Children's Health Insurance Program (CHIP) coverage in the United States, this barrier has been reduced for many.[28] Transportation insecurity relates to other SDOH, such as accessing healthful food, medications, and medical and dental care.[29] One study demonstrated that children insured by Medicaid in Colorado had significantly higher travel distances, and thus travel times, for dental treatment compared with children with private insurance.[30] Inconvenient timing, insufficient time off from work to attend routine dental checkups, and other work-related factors affect access to care.[31] Other factors related to access and travel are missed work or school, dependency on public transportation, and medical taxis.

Family and neighborhood dynamics play a role in experiencing dental caries.[31] Rural children are less likely to have fluoridated drinking water, preventive dental care, and optimal oral health than urban inhabitants.[32,33] Oral health fatalism can be transferred from parent to child, resulting in a pessimistic thought process on whether preventive care will result in better oral health.[34] Households with negative SDOH have been shown to have high sugar consumption, reduced tooth brushing, and lower dental care–seeking behavior.[35,36] Lack of social supports such as family or community groups is associated with poorer oral health.[31] Neighborhoods can be unsafe, exposing children to violence and crime. Parental fears of unsafe environments reduce opportunities for children to play outside, contributing to less physical activity and increased risk for other chronic conditions such as obesity.[37,38] Cumulative adverse childhood experiences (ACEs) (see Chapter 43) are related to both short- and long-term negative health outcomes.[39] ACEs create lifelong adversity due to neurologic changes, which generate higher risk health behaviors, predilection to chronic diseases, and higher mental health disorders due to increased allostatic load,[39] which is the increased "wear and tear" on the body from cortisol produced by chronic stress. The prefrontal cortex, amygdala, and hippocampus are activated possibly resulting in the dysregulation of the hypothalamic-pituitary-adrenal and sympathoadrenal medullary axes.[40] Metabolic, inflammatory, and cardiovascular changes result.[40] This stress is associated with higher rates of periodontal disease and dental caries.[40,41] ACEs are associated with poorer oral health and there is a dose-response relationship with more ACEs attributing to greater disease.[42] When a dental provider recognizes a patient's individual challenges and responds by integrating that information into clinical interventions, they are then delivering what is termed trauma-informed care.[39]

FI is the economic and social condition of limited or uncertain access to adequate food at the household level.[43] FI is defined as hunger and multiple episodes of reduced food intake,[44] and FI negatively affects caries experienced in children and adolescents and is a risk factor for unmet oral health needs.[45–48] Those experiencing the most FI have been shown to consume more sugar than food-secure groups.[49] FI families are likely to be of low SES, have less than a high school education, and be uninsured or underinsured.[49] Non-Hispanic Black or Mexican-American children are more likely to experience FI than their White counterparts.[49] These families struggle to obtain healthful and less processed foods, mostly due to food deserts, often found in low-income neighborhoods, and described by limited proximity to grocery stores selling fresh fruits and vegetables.[2,31] Sugar-sweetened beverage consumption contributes to dental caries experience, but more research is required to understand the SDOH that modulate exposure.[36] Families with multiple children create challenges for diet modification, with research suggesting that changes may need to be incremental or focused on one child at a time, rather than attempting to make wholesale changes to the family's diet. These topics and others are discussed in more detail in Chapter 16.

The System: Its Benefits and Limitations

The dental care financing and delivery system is complex and affects disease prevention. By the time a child engages the dental care system, it too often has already failed to meet the first goal of preventing dental disease. Dentistry relies upon many other healthcare and social service programs and partners in its efforts to prevent disease and comprehensively treat disease when necessary. A multitude of opportunities exist to reach children at the earliest possible stages to prevent dental disease, and to connect those who need it to high-quality dental care. The systems considerations presented here provide a broader context to prevention and are intended to add both immediate and long-term positive preventive outcomes. As previously discussed, SDOH will dictate the ability of a child, or a family on the child's behalf, to access the dental care system. Children's access to dental care at the population level can best be measured by looking at "realized" access or having a dental visit. Race, ethnicity, family income level, and other social factors impact access, but insurance status, a systems issue, presents the starkest disparities in children's access to dental care (Fig. 13.2).[50]

The current dental delivery system remains largely comprised of private practices, mostly small businesses. Gradual consolidation of practices has occurred over time,[51] but dentistry is still decades away from medicine's consolidation. Greater involvement of corporations, dental service organizations (DSOs), and private equity[52] are more apparent now. As powerful business interests influence the field, support for prevention may improve, but it will be even more important that dentists ensure the primary focus of the care process remains achieving optimal oral health for patients.

Zooming out, it is important to note that the United States has made great gains in children's oral health in the past half-century.[53] However, if dentistry aims to "move the needle" on preventing dental disease and connecting more children to dental care, opportunity lies in addressing disparities by insurance status, income, and race and ethnicity. Our current delivery system is not yet optimized to meet the needs of all children, so the following considerations for local action, notably within Medicaid and with other community partners, may be important in individual preventive care.

Medicaid

Medicaid is the public health coverage program that is state and federally funded, operated at the state level, and overseen at the federal level by the Centers for Medicare and Medicaid Services (CMS). As of June 2024, nearly 38 million children in the United States were enrolled in Medicaid or CHIP.[54] Much of the success in children's oral health at the US population level can be attributed to Medicaid. Recently, dental Medicaid programs have benefited from extraordinarily strong oral health leadership in CMS, where oral health has been featured as an agency-wide cross-cutting initiative.[55]

Prevention is directed and controlled by Medicaid provisions in states. The Medicaid program has a provision termed Early and Periodic Screening, Diagnostic and Treatment (EPSDT), which provides parameters that states must adhere to in their Medicaid programs. CMS states, "the goal of EPSDT is to ensure that individual eligible children get the healthcare they need, when they need it, in the most appropriate setting."[56] Consideration of the opportunities and limitations of services can be important in a preventive plan for children covered by Medicaid.

These aspects of Medicaid programs, while variable across states, offer a glimpse into the possibilities of addressing SDOH from a dental vantage point[57] and thus can affect prevention.

Transportation Services

Nonemergency medical transportation is an embedded benefit so enrollees can get to and from healthcare appointments.[58] This is an underutilized service in dentistry, although larger institutions like hospitals and health centers use the service for their patients. There is a significant opportunity to make better use of this in dentistry to improve preventive and care compliance.

Periodicity Schedules

CMS requires states to identify a *dental-specific* periodicity schedule so providers know what services they must be paid to do, and enrollees/families have a sense of what to expect from their dental visits. In preventive planning, monitoring can play an important role and be impacted by this schedule of allowable visits.

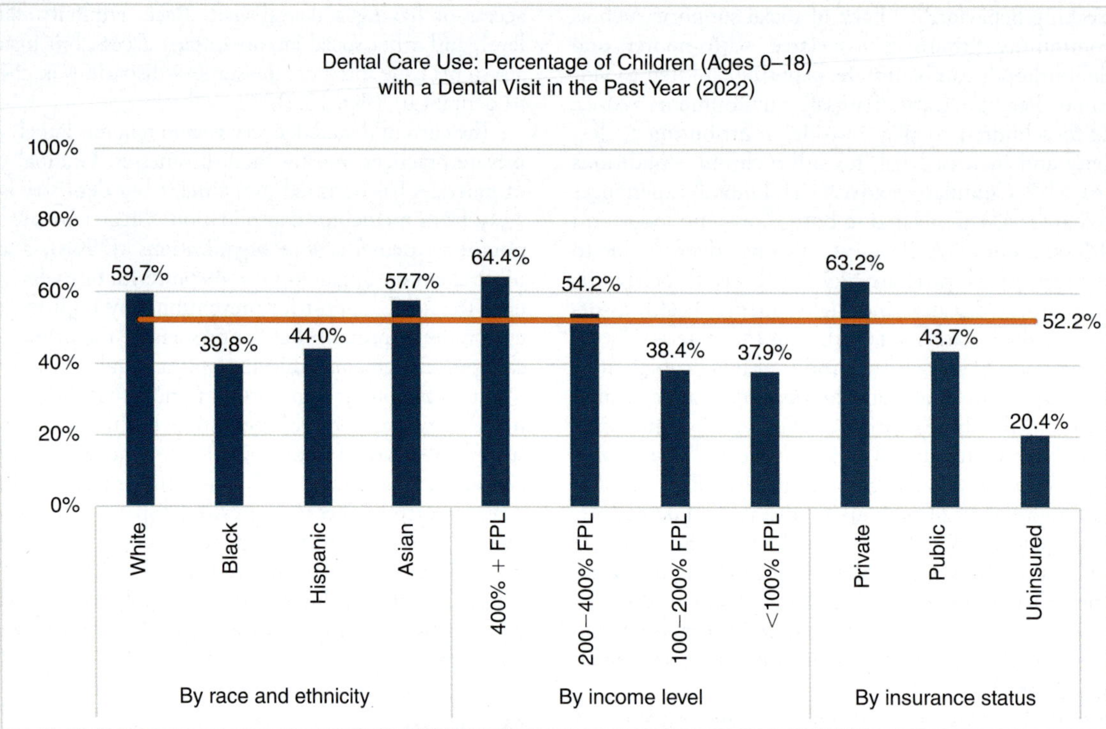

• **Fig. 13.2** Dental care use by race, poverty status, and coverage. *FPL,* Federal poverty level. (From ADA Health Policy Institute, September 2024.)

Teledentistry

Recognizing that populations in need of dental care are often located the furthest from it, many Medicaid agencies have authorized teledentistry in accordance with state practice acts.

Translation and interpretation

Although variable across the United States, some states provide translation and interpretation services to providers and/or enrollees.[59]

Continuous Coverage

As of 2024, states are required to provide at least one full year of coverage for children in their Medicaid programs to reduce the administrative burden for parents/caregivers and providers and minimize chances of delayed care. Some states, such as Oregon, have gone further in supporting this concept, in their implementation of continuous coverage from birth to age 6 years.[60]

Most Medicaid enrollees nationwide are now in managed care. The initial concept was to achieve greater efficiency in these programs, but occasional and numerous concerns that managed care organizations (MCOs) have compromised patient care, eroded patient or provider trust, and/or deteriorated provider networks, thereby reducing access to care. The managed care system's effects on prevention can negate office-based initiatives. As pediatric dentists do their part to provide care to children enrolled in Medicaid, when time and energy allow, dentists are encouraged to get involved with their Medicaid Advisory Committees,[61] offer subject matter expertise in the dental contracting process,[62] and voice concerns directly to state Medicaid agencies.

Community partnerships can offer support in mitigating disease and should be considered a part of a preventive plan, as children and families access other support services, often with greater ease than dental care. Dentists should learn how to collaborate with community partners, adopt the "no wrong door" approach to reach populations not yet benefiting from dental care access. Dietary aspects of prevention illustrate this effect. The Supplemental Nutrition Assistance Program (SNAP) and its Women, Infants, and Children (WIC) program may have more "touchpoints" in communities with more accessible locations and hours, better outreach communications, and perhaps stronger rapport with clients.[63,64] Within the education system, there may be opportunities for partnerships in school-based health programs, to initiate or strengthen an oral health component. Additionally, districts may be able to guide healthcare providers to children and families most in need of care, such as those eligible for the National School Lunch Program.[65] Other potential partners to reach high-need populations include state child welfare agencies (https://www.childwelfare.gov/resources/states-territories-tribes/) and state disabilities agencies (https://www.nasddds.org/state-agencies/). All of these agencies should be assessed when preventive planning for children and families dependent on community services (Table 13.3).

Typically, preventive planning is rooted in the present, but this chapter adds long-term aspects to preventive care. Investing in children's oral health today can have a lasting positive effect at the individual, family, and community levels well into the future. Research indicates that children who have health coverage perform better in school, end up in higher paying jobs, and achieve better overall health as adults. Parent and family coverage matters, too. Children are more likely to access dental care if parents also have insurance and access care.[66] Children of adults who have dental coverage experience lower untreated caries rates compared with children of adults without their own dental coverage.[67] In the last part of this chapter, a practice's readiness for care requires staying abreast of policy determinants of health in that state, such as dental coverage for pregnant and postpartum people and adults generally.[68]

TABLE 13.3 The System of Care and Prevention of Dental Caries

Specific Areas of Concern	Queries and Data Collection	Strategies for Prevention
Insurance coverage	Identify coverage for oral and general health	• Educate parents that it may be challenging to refer older children to a dentist who accepts Medicaid • Make a proactive transfer when indicated • Inform parents of importance of keeping adult children on their medical and dental plans until they age out
Community programs	Family has fiscal difficulty and limitations affecting oral health disease prevention	Review with parents those programs applicable or refer to social services
Diet and food programs	Dietary recommendations are unachievable	• Identify family's unique needs and identify services • Have practice knowledge of available community resources • Establish relationships with social and nutrition services in the community • Be able to provide contact and written information to families
Disability programs	Patient has a disability affecting prevention	• Know community resources • Establish relationships with county boards of IDD, special education in school systems • Liaison with sheltered workshops and group homes

IDD, Intellectual and Developmental Disabilities.

Targeted Prevention in Private Pediatric Dentistry

The preventive challenges in treating very young children, those living in poverty, and children with special needs have been described previously. This section outlines a stepwise prevention readiness plan for a practice (Table 13.4).

A practitioner needs to first establish a practice vision inclusive of these groups. The next step is to build a highly trained team, create a culture of inclusivity, and balance a payer mix that allows comprehensive patient-focused prevention. Implementation of a prevention program in a diverse population requires attention to responsibilities and scheduling. Prevention plans can be presented by the dentist, hygienist, or well-trained dental assistant with an approach that is empathetic and nonjudgmental. Dental hygienists are well trained in the science of caries prevention. Dental assistants trained in motivational interviewing (MI) training or as a community dental health coordinator, a broad skill set now offered at community colleges and online can also be utilized. Staff must embrace the vision and translate it to meet patient and practice goals. For example, parents will ask about straightening teeth, even when caries risk is high. Staff need to be able to explain to parents that their child would benefit from orthodontic treatment, but must have good control of diet, homecare, and behavior before orthodontics.

Scheduling becomes an important factor in successful prevention. It is important that new patient visits are scheduled when the team's full attention can be given to child and parent. The new patient interview is the foundation that knits the story of a child's life thus far, the medical and dental history, with the SDOH the family brings with them. Ideally, the professional delegated to preventive intervention is a skilled interviewer trained in MI, a technique that asks open-ended questions and seeks to help parents recognize areas of concern and pathways for improvement. Once the preventive therapist understands the child's medical, dental, and social history, and has completed a caries risk assessment, the dentist's examination findings are added to craft individualized prevention and treatment plans.

Meeting the child and their family where they are, and not where the dental professional thinks they should be, is crucial to presenting a preventive treatment plan. For example, brushing and flossing may be the norm desired, but this may not be the norm in the patient's home. Taking the time to explain why brushing teeth with fluoride toothpaste, by a parent, if necessary, is important and establishing tooth-cleaning goals that fit into the family's life circumstances are critical to success. Diet and sugar management will often require similar individualized focus based on individual, family, and external influences, like FI. Identifying those factors and how to address them may require incremental steps, such as looking for one to three small changes a family can make and asking them to pick a date for accomplishing those. For example, with infants, it may be a choice among discontinuing a nighttime bottle at age 1 year or recommending only milk or water be placed in a bottle until weaning. Children who have high-risk feeding practices are often placed on a 3-month recall schedule with the focus on stopping the detrimental habit.

A secondary element of scheduling is follow-through and assessment of achievement of goals and expected outcomes. Establishing the interval between dental appointments is based on caries risk assessment, the need to practice good behavior for a period of time (desensitization), any urgent treatment needs, and the patient's insurance benefits, all factors illustrating the links between patient, environment, and system critical to successful prevention.

Another factor for successful prevention is documentation. Today, images taken with a phone, camera, intraoral camera, or intraoral scanner are used for patient and parent education and to supplement the patient record. Intraoral cameras and phones make photographic documentation easy, even with very young children in the knee-to-knee examination position. Documentation of social and systemic factors affecting prevention is also a new but important aspect of recordkeeping. A record may state rationale for the plan, with language needed for prior approval with payers such as "Due to the patient's high risk for ECC as result of nighttime bottle use, more frequent visits are necessary to both prevent caries and detect caries progression in its earliest states to avoid general anesthesia." This terminology may provide

TABLE 13.4 Practice Considerations for Prevention of Dental Caries

Specific Areas of Concern	Strategies and Steps
Establish vision for prevention	• Goals for practice population(s) • Establish patient and practice fiscal convergence • Incorporation of long-term preventive goals, transition to other providers, provision of life span information for child and parents • Evaluation and quality measures
Train preventive dental staff	• Identify key personnel • Train to competence in office and external aspects • Confirm and monitor commitment to vision • Techniques to develop cooperation and compliance (e.g., no charge orientation visits)
Documentation	• Establish individualized plan components • Bring recordkeeping and other records into concert • Identify and record patient-specific resources, needs, and partners • Add intraoral photos to document poor oral hygiene, carious lesions, and other pathology
Community partnerships	• Learn community and system requirements and opportunities • Establish relationships • Share preventive plans and roles • Provide needed information and training • Grandparenting guidelines • WIC, Head Start, Health Departments, school nurse contacts and relationships • Transitional general dentists for emerging adults and special needs patients • Include school nurses and request tooth brushing be added to IEPs if needed
Coverage limitations and practice opportunities	• Establish opportunities and limitations per individual patients for coverage (e.g., Medicaid, school lunch, WIC) • Include public and private individualized parts when applicable (Americans with Disabilities, county IDD boards, food pantries) • Policies to maximize efficiency and fiscal health such as conversion of preventive visits to treatment to fill broken appointments and determining balance of payer mix

IDD, Intellectual and Developmental Disabilities; *IEP*, individualized education program; *WIC*, Women, Infants, and Children.

justification for Medicaid programs to provide payment for limited examinations up to twice per year and fluoride varnish four times per year and customize prevention in a cost-based benefit to both patient and the practice.

Previous sections of this chapter outline system and community factors that can impact prevention. It is also important to determine and document resources and barriers in the home that may make prevention difficult. For example, some families lack running water or water is turned off due to unpaid utility bills. Awareness of social interventions for this type of preventive impasse are critical to success. For children with special needs or with family structures that make oral hygiene difficult at home, a school nurse or director of special education may help in a formal request that tooth brushing by an education aide be added to an individualized education program (IEP) or 504 plan. To achieve the level of practice staff training mentioned earlier in this section, a staff member may travel to a school and demonstrate patient positioning and brushing as well as gain understanding of the capabilities of that facility to partner in prevention. Parents are largely accepting of having a school add tooth brushing to their child's day and schools appreciate reduction in school days lost because of dental-related reasons. Older patients with special healthcare needs may benefit from chlorhexidine rinses, so similar visits and demonstrations to group homes and sheltered work environments serve the same purpose at the community level and should be part of the preventive plan.

A low SES population may miss more scheduled dental appointments. A team should understand a family's unique circumstances, reasons for the missed or canceled appointment, and how to empower them to find solutions to help them attend future appointments, rather than blame them. Policies to accomplish this may include having proactive patient reminders matched to the families' preferred mode of communication and asking open-ended questions about reasons that might keep them from attending dental appointments.

Summary

Current preventive approaches limited to intraoral strategies have likely achieved their therapeutic optimization in children and this chapter proposes a next generation of prevention. The recognition of SDOH and the influence of nonclinical factors on oral health is a start to penetrating that group of children who have not responded to traditional prevention. This last section provides illustrations of what might best be described as patient- and family-centered prevention applied in practice, beginning with identified intraoral needs then expanding interventions to address the factors surrounding the caries process in a child's life. Combining the framework provided in this chapter with the in-depth coverage of elements of the preventive armamentarium in subsequent chapters should provide practitioners with a complete conceptual and scientific approach to dental caries prevention in children.

Visit eBooks.Health.Elsevier.com to see full list of references.

14

Fluoride and Nonfluoride Caries Preventive Agents

JOHN WARREN AND AMY B. MIERS

CHAPTER OUTLINE

Introduction

Untreated dental caries is the most common long-term health condition in the world,[1] and for many, treatment is out of reach. Therefore, from a global perspective, preventing dental caries is of paramount importance. However, preventing dental caries is also vitally important from an individual patient perspective in that dental caries can have a deleterious effect on many aspects of life, particularly for children. Numerous studies have demonstrated that children with untreated dental caries often experience pain,[2] have compromised nutrition,[3] have difficulty concentrating in school[4] (Blumenshine), and may have difficulty in sleeping.[2]

Fortunately, there are many modalities that have been shown to be effective in dental caries prevention, notably the various fluoride agents. In addition, various nonfluoride modalities, including antimicrobial agents, and diet modification have shown promise in reducing caries. This chapter will review fluoride in its many forms and its uses across the age spectrum from birth through adolescence and will also review a variety of nonfluoride preventive therapies.

Fluoride

Fluoride is the cornerstone of dental caries prevention. Fluoride is widely found in nature, including nearly every source of water, and its presence in water led to the discovery of its caries-preventive properties. In the early 1900s, a recent dental graduate of the University of Pennsylvania, Frederick McKay, began practicing in Colorado Springs, Colorado, where he noticed many of his patients had "mottled" enamel, which became known as the "Colorado Brown Stain."[5,6] With careful observation, Dr. McKay noted that patients with mottled enamel rarely suffered from dental caries (very unusual for those times), and he suspected that something in the water supply produced not only the brown stain, but also provided protection from dental caries.[6] With further investigation, he and others were able to pinpoint water sources that produced these effects on the teeth. In the early 1930s, with advances in technology allowing for the detection of trace elements, fluoride was identified as the substance in water responsible for what is now known as dental fluorosis, and for the prevention of dental caries in Dr. McKay's patients.[7]

With the discovery of fluoride's effects on the teeth, a series of studies led by Dr. H. Trendley Dean of the United States Public Health Service found that water fluoride concentrations of around 1.0 parts per million (ppm) were associated with low levels of both dental fluorosis and dental caries in children.[8] As a result of these studies, it was postulated that adding fluoride to community water supplies to a concentration of 1.0 ppm would reduce the prevalence of dental caries; subsequently, Grand Rapids, Michigan, was the first community to add fluoride to its water supply to prevent dental caries.[7] The efforts in Grand Rapids and three other cities proved to be very beneficial, as caries rates among children in these cities declined markedly compared with those in nearby communities with low (<0.3 ppm) levels of fluoride.[7,9]

As the success of community water fluoridation became apparent, efforts began to find other means of delivering fluoride for caries prevention. Initial efforts in the 1950s resulted in dietary fluoride supplements and fluoride dentifrice, and these were followed by the introduction of office- and home-use fluoride gels and mouth rinses in the 1960s and 1970s. During this same time, fluoride varnish and silver diamine fluoride (SDF) were developed in other countries but were not approved for use in the United States until 1994 and 2014, respectively, and in both cases, were approved for treating sensitivity (not caries). Each of these modalities will be discussed separately in later parts of this chapter; however, before doing so, it is important to understand how fluoride works, and the metabolism of fluoride in the human body. These topics are discussed in the next section.

Fluoride Mechanism of Action

Although a systemic mechanism, incorporating fluoride into the developing teeth, may contribute to fluoride's caries preventive effects to some degree, fluoride primarily acts on a topical level.[10] That is, fluoride acts primarily after teeth have erupted. Fluoride, when retained in plaque and saliva, acts to inhibit demineralization of enamel (i.e., loss of calcium, phosphate, and carbonate from healthy enamel) and to enhance remineralization of demineralized enamel. This process occurs when cariogenic bacteria (e.g., the mutans streptococci) metabolize sugars and other carbohydrates, producing acids that dissolve (demineralize) enamel, while the lower pH promotes release of fluoride from plaque and saliva.[9] The released fluoride then is readily taken up by the enamel, forming enamel with enhanced crystal structure, which is more resistant to demineralization. Thus it is necessary that fluoride be retained in plaque and saliva to serve as reservoir for remineralization, which in turn, requires regular exposures of fluoride from diet (water), dentifrice, and other sources.[10] High concentration fluoride products are thought to act by enhancing the fluoride reservoir in plaque and saliva and by creating a long-lasting layer on the enamel surface itself, making more fluoride available for remineralization.[9,10] There is also evidence that higher concentrations of fluoride inhibit acid production of cariogenic bacteria and interferes with their production of adhesive glycans that bind to the teeth.[9,10]

Metabolism

Fluoride, in the form of hydrogen fluoride (HF), is readily absorbed in the stomach due to its low pH environment, which allows HF to cross cell membranes.[11] Because of the rapid absorption in the stomach, and continued absorption in the small intestine, most fluoride (estimated at 80% to 90%) ingested is absorbed in the digestive tract, with most unabsorbed fluoride excreted in urine. With this rapid absorption, plasma fluoride levels increase markedly after ingestion, and the plasma distributes fluoride throughout the body, including saliva.[11] Most of the absorbed fluoride remaining in the body is deposited in the mineralized tissues, such as the bones and developing teeth. Thus chronic high fluoride ingestion during tooth development can result in dental fluorosis, whereas longer-term chronically high intakes can result in skeletal fluorosis.[11] These conditions are discussed later in this chapter.

Fluoride Modalities

Community Water Fluoridation

As described previously, the work of Dr. H. Trendley Dean led to the establishment of the optimal water fluoride concentration of 1.0 ppm to effectively prevent caries and minimize fluorosis risk.[8,12] A modification of that recommendation in the early 1960s, based on climate and water consumption patterns, established a range of 0.7 to 1.2 ppm as the optimal water fluoride concentration, with lower concentrations recommended for those living in warm climates with higher water consumption, and higher concentrations for colder climates with lower water consumption.[13] More recently, with many additional sources of fluoride today, and indications that dental fluorosis prevalence had increased, the recommended water fluoride concentration was reduced to 0.7 ppm for all areas in the United States in 2015.[14]

Initial studies in Grand Rapids and elsewhere found that optimally fluoridated water reduced caries by half (50%) or more.[7] More recently, with the advent of fluoride toothpaste and other products, as well as the distribution of fluoridated water's benefits through the so-called "halo" effect, optimally fluoridated water has been found to reduce caries by approximately 15% to 30%.[15,16] It is important to remember, however, that given water fluoridation is community based, it is not possible to conduct any sort of randomized trials to assess its effectiveness or to completely control for the many factors, including other sources of fluoride, that affect caries incidence.

Because of its effectiveness, low cost, and ability to reach children across all socioeconomic strata, community water fluoridation was named as one of the 10 great public health achievements in the United States during the 20th century.[17] Although it is important to use caution in mixing fluoridated tap water with infant formula concentrates to avoid over ingestion (see Chapter 8), drinking fluoridated water is recommended for children of all ages.

Fluoride Supplements

Fluoride supplements were introduced during the 1950s, primarily for children without access to optimally fluoridated water.[18] The rationale for supplements was that fluoride's anticaries effects were systemic, and thus a means to provide systemic fluoride equivalent to that of optimally fluoridated water was needed. Early studies of supplement effectiveness demonstrated results similar to those for optimally fluoridated water[19]; again, these studies were completed at a time when there were few other fluoride products, such as fluoride toothpaste, available, and caries prevalence was much higher than it is today.

Fluoride supplements require a prescription by a dentist or physician, with dosage based on the child's age and home water fluoride concentration. The fluoride supplement dosage schedule has been revised downward several times since their introduction, to reduce the risk of dental fluorosis. The current schedule remains unchanged from the 1990s but was reaffirmed by the American Dental Association in 2010,[20] and the American Academy of Pediatric Dentistry in 2023.[21] In the current schedule (Table 14.1), no supplements are recommended for children under 6 months of age, or for those with drinking water fluoride levels greater than 0.6 ppm. Thus it is important that clinicians have information on a patient's home water fluoride concentration before prescribing supplements. A good source of information on water fluoridation is the Centers for Disease Control and Prevention's My Water's Fluoride website (https://nccd.cdc.gov/DOH_MWF/Default/Default.aspx; accessed March 1, 2024).

Fluoride supplements for children under 3 years of age are in the form of liquid drops, whereas for those 3 years and older,

TABLE 14.1 Fluoride Supplementation Recommendations

Age Group	<0.3 ppm F	0.3–0.6 ppm F	>0.6 ppm F
Birth to 6 months	0	0	0
6 months to 3 years	0.25 mg	0	0
3–6 years	0.50 mg	0.25 mg	0
6–16 years	1.00 mg	0.50 mg	0

From AAPD.org.

supplements are in the form of chewable tablets. Given that fluoride's primary mechanism in preventing caries is topical, recommendations for liquid fluoride supplement use include placing the drops directly on the teeth and/or spreading the drops on the child's teeth with a finger. Older children should be encouraged to "chew and swish" the chewable tablets so the tablets will dissolve in the mouth before swallowing.[20] Although these recommendations are reasonable, parental compliance with fluoride supplements has been shown to be low overall[22]; thus it is unclear whether these more detailed recommendations are realistic.

Other important considerations in prescribing fluoride supplements include the actual source of patients' drinking water and its fluoride concentration, as many patients rarely drink tap water. This is evidenced by the sales volume of bottled water, which has nearly doubled over the past decade, and follows a long trend of increased bottled water usage (https://www.statista.com/statistics/237832/volume-of-bottled-water-in-the-us/). Moreover, there has been an increase in home water filtration systems in recent years, including reverse osmosis systems that remove fluoride from drinking water. In addition, there continues to be a significant number of people who have private wells or are otherwise not on public water systems. Testing of private water sources for fluoride concentrations is available but is inconvenient and can be costly; thus it is not often done. Together, these factors can make it difficult to discern how much fluoridated water, if any, an individual child is consuming, making appropriate prescriptions for fluoride supplements especially challenging.

As stated previously, early studies showed that fluoride supplements were very effective in preventing caries; however, recent studies in the era of multiple fluoride sources and lower overall caries prevalence are lacking. Thus the evidence for routine use of fluoride supplements is weak, and current recommendations suggest that supplements only be used for patients at high caries risk.[20] Given the many other fluoride regimens that are currently available, and the challenges in prescribing appropriate dosing for them, fluoride supplements are considered second-line caries preventive agents, reserved for use in high caries risk patients where other regimens have been ineffective or inadequate.

Fluoride Dentifrice

With the demonstrated effectiveness of water fluoridation, efforts began to incorporate fluoride into toothpaste. In the 1950s, Procter & Gamble teamed with a group of researchers at Indiana University to develop and test a fluoride-containing toothpaste.[23] This toothpaste, eventually sold under the brand name "Crest," was shown to reduce caries in children by nearly half, which led to the nationwide launch of Crest toothpaste in 1956 (https://crest.com/en-us/oral-care-tips/toothpaste/history-toothpaste). Today, the vast majority of toothpaste sold in the United States contains fluoride, with many products flavored or tailored to children.

Fluoride-containing toothpaste has been shown to be very effective in preventing dental caries, with a recent meta-analysis showing the preventive fraction of 31% for caries in the primary dentition.[24] A Cochrane review found a preventive fraction of 22% for standard (1000 ppm) toothpaste compared with placebo in children and adolescents.[25] Because fluoride toothpaste is effective and readily available, it is also a cornerstone for caries prevention in children. However, due to its fluoride concentration (1000 ppm), some caution is warranted in younger children to minimize the risk of dental fluorosis.

Young children are not capable of spitting out excess toothpaste, thus they swallow most of the toothpaste used when brushing.[26] For this reason, it is important to limit the amount of toothpaste placed on the toothbrush. For very young children, a "smear" amount or "grain of rice" amount of toothpaste is appropriate for caries prevention, while minimizing the risk for dental fluorosis (Fig. 14.1). As children get older during the preschool years, this amount can be increased to a "pea-sized" amount, and slowly increased until a child can reliably spit out the excess, usually age 5 or 6 years.[21,27] For young children, it is important that parents should be involved in placing the appropriate amount of toothpaste on the toothbrush to prevent excess fluoride ingestion. Also, children do not have the manual dexterity to brush their teeth thoroughly and effectively on their own before age 9 or 10; thus parents should also brush the child's teeth (or help them to brush), until well into their elementary school years.[21]

The standard fluoride concentration of over-the-counter toothpastes sold in the United States is 1000 ppm; however, toothpastes with a concentration of 5000 ppm are available by prescription. Such high-fluoride formulations should only be prescribed for older children and adolescents who are no longer at risk for developing dental fluorosis but are at high risk for caries. Studies have demonstrated that higher concentration fluoride toothpastes provide significantly greater caries prevention than standard 1000 ppm formulations.[28,29]

Fluoride Mouth Rinse

Fluoride mouth rinses were developed as a means to provide fluoride exposures to children in communities without water fluoridation. A study published in 1971[30] provided strong evidence that weekly rinsing with a 0.2% sodium fluoride solution could reduce the incidence of dental caries in children. These results led to many additional trials and demonstration projects, which, on average, demonstrated reductions in caries incidence of approximately 30%. During the 1970s and 1980s, school-based fluoride mouth rinse programs, which, like the 1971 study, utilized weekly rinses with 0.2% sodium fluoride, became fairly common in nonfluoridated communities.[31] With the recognition during the 1980s of a decline in dental caries prevalence among children, and

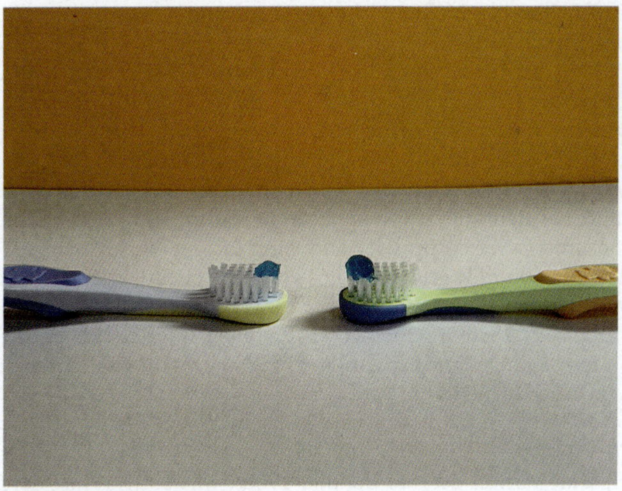

• **Fig. 14.1** Fluoride Dentifrice Amounts. A smear amount *(left)* is recommended for young children once teeth have erupted into the mouth. A pea-sized amount *(right)* is recommended for older children who can reliably spit out the excess.

given the time involved in administering such programs and availability of other fluoride therapies, school-based fluoride mouth rinse programs largely disappeared by the turn of the century.

The decline in school-based fluoride mouth rinse programs due to reduced overall caries prevalence coincided with the rise in efforts to prioritize caries prevention efforts to those at high risk. One such approach for caries prevention for high-risk children that developed during this time was daily over-the-counter fluoride mouth rinses, with sodium fluoride concentrations of 0.05%. These mouth rinses continue to be important options in caries prevention, as they are readily available and relatively inexpensive. They can be used in addition to fluoride toothpastes for those who need additional preventive measures or whose brushing is irregular or inefficient. Because these products are rinses and intended to be spit out, they are recommended only for children aged 6 or over who can expectorate, as ingestion of these rinses could pose risk for acute toxicity (e.g., nausea) and/or development of dental fluorosis in younger children.[9] The original formulation (0.2% sodium fluoride) is available by prescription on a weekly or daily basis, and can be used for those at higher caries risk or when more convenient for the patient.[29]

Similar to early findings of its effectiveness, a recent Cochrane systematic review found that use of fluoride mouth rinses resulted in average caries reductions of 27%. The authors of the review commented that such reductions appeared to be independent of the effects of water fluoridation or use of fluoride toothpaste.[32]

Professionally Applied Fluoride Gels and Foams

Like fluoride mouth rinse, professionally applied fluoride gels and (later) foams were developed to enhance caries prevention beyond the effects of water fluoridation and toothpaste for those at higher risk for caries. Early gel formulations typically contained stannous fluoride (0.4%), which was painted on the teeth during dental visits. Subsequently, gel products containing 1.23% acidulated phosphate fluoride (APF), and later 1.1% sodium fluoride, were developed and often applied using foam trays left in the child's mouth for 1 to 4 minutes, with 4 minutes being the recommended duration.[9,21] Use of these gels, however, often resulted in minor acute toxicity (nausea and vomiting) as a result of swallowing the fluoride gel and were gradually replaced by foam products of the same concentrations.[21,29] These foam products offered similar fluoride exposures, but required much less volume, thus reducing the occurrence of acute toxicity.

Early studies of fluoride gel effectiveness found that they reduced caries incidence by 40% or more[33] (van Rijkom et al.), whereas a later systematic review found average reductions of 21%.[34,35] With the advent of fluoride varnish in the United States during the 1990s, in-office use of fluoride gels and foams declined, as fluoride varnish application was found to be less time-consuming, less expensive, and more acceptable to patients.[36] Although fluoride gels and foams are less frequently used in dental offices today, they are available for home use by older children. Specifically, these products (0.4% stannous fluoride) are brushed on for 1 minute (and expectorated) by children 12 years and older who are at high risk for caries.[9,29]

Fluoride Varnish

Fluoride varnish dates to the mid-1960s, where it was first developed in Europe and was commercially marketed under the name "Duraphat" beginning in 1968. However, fluoride varnish did not become available in the United States until 1994, when the US Food and Drug Administration (FDA) approved it for treating root sensitivity and as a cavity liner.[37] Since that time, fluoride varnish (5% sodium fluoride) has been marketed by numerous companies, and in many flavors. It has become very widely used "off-label" for caries prevention and has been shown by numerous studies to be very effective in caries prevention. For example, two early studies found fluoride varnish to be effective in arresting initial lesions,[38] and that there was a dose-response relationship whereby administering varnish twice per year was more effective than annual applications, and that both were superior to placebo.[39] A Cochrane systematic review reported in 2013 found the preventive fraction for fluoride varnish compared with placebo was 43%.[40]

Despite its high fluoride concentration (22,400 ppm F), the small amount used per application and its slow rate of fluoride release, fluoride varnishes can be safely used with all children, including infants and toddlers. As stated by the American Academy of Pediatric Dentistry's recommendations for fluoride therapy, "unit doses of five percent fluoride varnish are the only professional topical fluoride agents recommended for children younger than age six."[21]

Silver Diamine Fluoride

Like fluoride varnish, SDF was initially developed in the 1960s but was not approved for use in the United States until much later; in the case of SDF, the FDA approved its use for treatment of dentinal sensitivity in 2014.[21] Like fluoride varnish, it is used off-label for caries prevention and arrest. SDF has its origins in silver nitrate compounds, which have been used in dentistry since the mid-1800s to "sanitize" and arrest carious lesions. In addition to silver, SDF contains a high fluoride concentration (approximately 44,800 ppm), and works to block exposed dentinal tubules, reduce bacterial levels, promote remineralization, and inhibit collagen degradation.[41] Due to the presence of silver, SDF stains treated carious lesions black, and can also stain soft tissues, supplies, and equipment if not used with great caution.[21]

Although SDF can act as a primary preventive agent, its primary use is in arresting existing carious lesions, that is, it acts as a secondary preventive agent to prevent progression of such lesions.[21] Several studies have shown that SDF is effective in arresting carious lesions in children. For example, a 30-month study of 308 3- to 5-year-old children in Hong Kong found that annual application of SDF arrested significantly more lesions than did fluoride varnish or placebo.[42] Similarly, a 36-month trial of biannual SDF application conducted in Cuba found that among 373 6-year-olds who were divided into SDF and control groups, those in the SDF group had an average of 0.29 new decayed surfaces in the primary dentition compared with 1.43 in the control group. This study also found that approximately 77% of existing lesions became arrested.[43] More recently, a phase III randomized placebo-controlled clinical trial was conducted in the United States that compared rates of carious lesion arrest among 599 1- to 5-year-old children who were treated with SDF or placebo. Preliminary results after 8 months were that 54% of lesions became arrested in the SDF group compared with 21% in the control group ($P < 0.001$).[44]

Side Effects of Fluoride Exposure

Acute Toxicity

Acute toxicity occurs when a relatively large amount of fluoride is ingested at a single point in time. In all but the rarest events, acute fluoride toxicity produces only mild symptoms, primarily nausea and vomiting. Although not precisely known, acute toxic effects may occur when 5 mg of fluoride are consumed for each kilogram of body weight.[45] For a child weighing 10 kg, ingesting 50 mg of fluoride, approximately 1 to 2 ounces of toothpaste, may cause nausea and vomiting. For a child weighing 20 kg, 100 mg, corresponding to 12 to 16 ounces of fluoride mouth rinse, may produce such symptoms.

More serious complications, including hospitalization and death, can occur when fluoride ingestion as low as 15 mg/kg body weight occurs. For a 10-kg child, this corresponds to 5 ounces of toothpaste; for a 20-kg child, as little as 1 ounce of professionally applied fluoride gel may produce serious complications.[45] Thus given their low body weight, extreme caution is necessary in prescribing high-fluoride products for younger children. Fortunately, serious, or fatal events are extremely rare, with only one known fatality in the United States over the past 50+ years. This fatal case was due to lack of oversight of a 3-year-old child in a dental office where fluoride gel was to be applied, and initial failure to recognize the circumstances and symptoms that resulted in this tragic accident.[46]

Chronic Toxicity

Chronic toxicity is more common and is almost always manifested as dental fluorosis. Dental fluorosis is a dose-dependent discoloration of the enamel that is caused by fluoride ingestion during tooth development. Dental fluorosis can range from very mild, characterized by a few lacy streaks or flecks on the enamel that may not be noticeable unless the teeth are dry, to severe forms characterized by brown staining and pitting of the enamel. Most dental fluorosis in the United States is in the very mild or mild categories,[47] generally posing only slight cosmetic concerns; severe fluorosis is rare (<1% prevalence), but due to the pitting of enamel, may increase risk for caries, in addition to cosmetic concerns (Fig. 14.2). Similarly, dental fluorosis may be limited in scope, affecting only a few teeth, which developed in the same timeframe, or can be seen throughout the mouth. Dental fluorosis can occur in the primary dentition, but generally only affects teeth that form after birth or the second primary molars.[48]

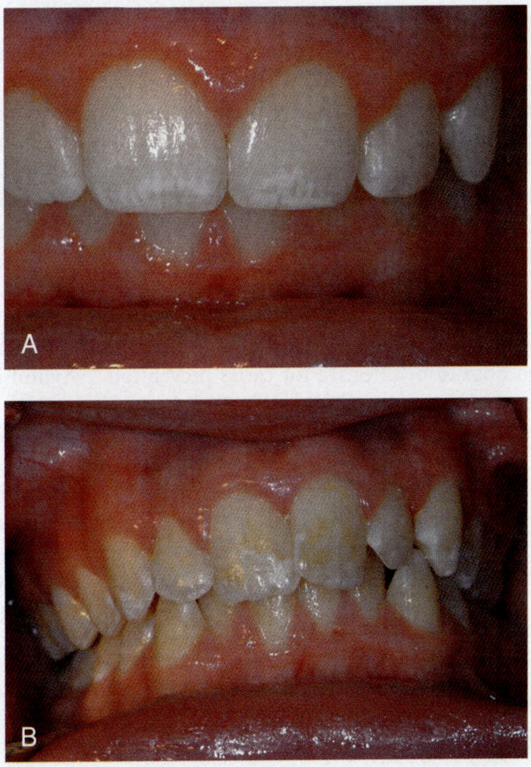

• **Fig. 14.2** Dental Fluorosis. Examples of mild (A) and moderate (B) fluorosis.

Many studies have attempted to identify the critical period for fluoride ingestion that leads to fluorosis of the esthetically important permanent maxillary incisors, but presumably due to variability of tooth development, there is no consensus on a specific window of time that is most critical for development of fluorosis on these teeth. More broadly, fluoride ingestion during the first 4 years of life is associated with fluorosis on the maxillary incisors, whereas risk for fluorosis on posterior teeth may extend to age 10 or older.[49]

The amount of fluoride ingestion necessary to result in dental fluorosis is also largely unknown, but the longitudinal Iowa Fluoride Study found that average fluoride intakes of 0.06 mg fluoride per kilogram of body weight or higher during the first few years of life were associated with substantially higher prevalence of fluorosis, compared with lower intakes.[49]

In addition to dental fluorosis, chronic excessive fluoride ingestion can lead to skeletal fluorosis, a debilitating bone disease. Fortunately, skeletal fluorosis is extremely rare in the United States, with only one documented case over the past 50+ years.[50]

Misinformation About Fluoride

Dental and skeletal fluorosis are the only established risks associated with nonacute fluoride exposures; however, many claims have been made about the safety of fluoride, particularly community water fluoridation. The vast majority of these claims represent misinformation, such as deliberate attempts to mislead the public and create fear. Misinformation about community water fluoridation began shortly after its adoption in number of communities during the 1950s, with claims that fluoride was "poison," caused cancer, led to premature death, or was a communist plot.[51] This latter claim was the basis for the plot of the famous motion picture, *Dr. Strangelove,* a dark comedy about the Cold War, nuclear weapons, and water fluoridation. All these claims were based on very questionable science and were uniformly refuted by government agencies.[51]

More recently, studies purporting to demonstrate links between water fluoridation and various diseases or conditions have become more sophisticated, but from a scientific viewpoint, are deeply flawed. Among the more recent claims was a study suggesting that water fluoridation was linked to thyroid disease, but for this ecologic study without individuals' data, the authors compared two communities in the United Kingdom with differing water fluoride concentrations on their thyroid disease rates, without taking into account data pertinent to thyroid disease (such as iodine intakes or deficiencies).[52] A series of studies conducted in Canada purported to show that drinking fluoridated water during pregnancy resulted in young children with slightly lower IQs; however, these results were widely criticized because the measurement of fluoride intakes and IQ measurements of younger children were not valid.[53] Based on these later studies, the National Toxicology Program (NTP) released a lengthy report suggesting that drinking water with fluoride concentrations greater than 1.5 ppm (1.5 mg/L) were associated with lower IQ in children.[54] In response to the NTP report, the American Dental Association (ADA) issued a statement that pointed out that the threshold concentration cited in the NTP report as being associated with lower IQ (1.5 ppm) was more than twice that recommend for community water fluoridation in the United States (0.7 ppm).[55]

The ADA also criticized the NTP report for using "unorthodox research methods, flawed analyses ... and failed to follow the norms of peer review."[55] The ADA's statement specifically criticized many reviewed studies' use of spot urinary fluoride as not being a valid biomarker for long-term fluoride exposure.

Misinformation about fluoride will likely continue, but it is important to note the extensive research cited in this chapter and elsewhere that confirms not only fluoride's effectiveness, but also its safety when used as recommended. However, because many individuals (including parents) are susceptible to misinformation about fluoride and may be hesitant to accept fluoride for their children,[56] it is important to note that there are other, nonfluoride options available for caries prevention. Nonfluoride caries prevention strategies are discussed in the next section.

NONFLUORIDE PREVENTIVE AGENTS

Although fluoride has been shown to be the most effective agent for caries prevention, other agents can be considered for those who refuse fluorides or as adjunctive therapy for those who still develop caries despite adequate exposure to fluoride.

Chlorhexidine

Chlorhexidine gluconate is commonly utilized in dentistry for plaque control to reduce gingival inflammation.[57] It is available in a variety of forms including varnishes, mouth rinses, and gels. Chlorohexidine has been shown to suppress *Streptococcus mutans* by altering the function of the cell membrane.[58] Because *S. mutans* is associated with dental caries, chlorhexidine has been studied as a caries preventive agent. A 3-year placebo-controlled trial of 1% chlorhexidine gel in 4-year-olds found that approximal caries was reduced by 38% in the chlorhexidine group compared with the control group that received a placebo gel.[59] This trial led to a series of others with mixed results. For example, a randomized clinical trial found that the weekly use of 0.2% chlorhexidine gel in 10-month-old infants with high initial levels of *S. mutans* did not significantly reduce *S. mutans* counts.[60] In children with low initial *S. mutans* counts, there was a significant reduction in *S. mutans* temporarily, but only within the first 3 months after cessation.[60] Another study showed that 40% chlorhexidine varnish was effective in reducing caries (37.3% reduction) in high-risk Chinese preschoolers after 2 years of twice-yearly applications.[61] In contrast, an 18-month study of 211 3-year-olds in Italy found that although there were significantly lower *S. mutans* counts in the chlorhexidine group compared with controls, there were no differences in caries increment.[62] A study looking at preventing the vertical transmission of bacteria from American Indian and Alaskan Native mothers to their children found that 10% chlorhexidine varnish did not change the number of new carious lesions in the children or the proportion of children with caries.[63] A Cochrane review of clinical trials further revealed the inconsistent data regarding the effectiveness of chlorhexidine gels and varnishes in the prevention of dental caries in children and adolescents and in reducing *S. mutans* counts.[64] Although chlorhexidine is readily available in many dental clinic settings, and it has been shown to reduce levels of *S. mutans*, its ability to prevent caries remains questionable.

Povidone Iodine

Povidone iodine is another topical antimicrobial agent that is noted to be effective against *S. mutans*. It is FDA approved for intraoral and extraoral uses and is used in a variety of medical settings. A randomized controlled trial in Micronesia found that the addition of 10% povidone iodine into 5% NaF varnish decreased caries increment in primary teeth by 28% after 2 years compared with NaF varnish alone.[65] A systematic review and meta-analysis comparing the combination of topical fluoride and povidone iodine with topical fluoride alone noted that dental caries incidence was found to be lowered in the combined therapy group, but there was overall a low quality of evidence.[66] Although there are some indications that povidone iodine may provide an additional benefit when combined with topical fluoride, the evidence is very limited regarding the use of povidone iodine in the prevention of caries at this time.

Arginine

Arginine is an amino acid that can be metabolized by certain types of bacteria to form ammonia. Ammonia can raise the pH levels of the mouth preventing demineralization of enamel. Arginine has been mostly studied as an additive to toothpastes with fluoride. A randomized controlled trial in Thailand found that toothpastes containing 1.5% arginine with 1450 ppm fluoride were associated with a reduction in carious teeth after 2 years compared with those only using fluoride toothpastes.[67] However, a systematic review found that there was insufficient evidence to support the added costs of including arginine in toothpastes at this time.[68] Although arginine dental products are not readily available in the United States, the Association of State and Territorial Dental Directors recommended that caregivers consider feeding children a diet high in natural sources of arginine, like spinach, soy, seafood, and nuts, to help prevent early childhood caries.[69]

Xylitol

Xylitol is a sugar alcohol that has been associated with inhibiting *S. mutans.* A systematic review and meta-analysis found that daily use of xylitol was associated with an annual reduction in dfms/DMFS (The number of **D**ecayed, **M**issing and **F**illed tooth **S**urfaces) scores of 1.09.[70] A Cochrane review found that there is some, low-quality evidence that fluoride toothpaste containing xylitol may be more effective than fluoride toothpastes without xylitol in preventing caries (13% over 3 years).[71] However, other xylitol-containing products like lozenges, sucking tablets, and wipes had even less evidence.[71] A benefit of xylitol is that it can be used as a sugar substitute for cariogenic sugars, but a limitation of this approach is that most xylitol products do not contain a high enough dose to be effective for caries prevention.[72] Xylitol is also very expensive compared with other sugar substitutes and it can cause gastrointestinal distress in some patients.[72] Recently a Cleveland Clinic study correlated xylitol-sweetened drink consumption with an increased risk of heart attack and stroke in adults, although further research is ongoing.[73] Overall, xylitol appears to provide minimal caries prevention as the US Preventive Services Task Force concluded that "three trials reported no clear effects of xylitol on caries incidence" and "there is currently not enough evidence to formally recommend its routine use in caries prevention."[74]

Casein Phosphopeptide-Amorphous Calcium Phosphate

Casein phosphopeptide-amorphous calcium phosphate (CPP-ACP) is a product derived from milk that can serve as a reservoir of calcium and phosphate to assist with remineralization. It has been studied extensively in the treatment of white spot or incipient carious lesions. A randomized clinical trial looked at the effect of CPP-ACP pastes on white spot lesions after orthodontic treatment compared with a nonfluoride control toothpaste and found no significant differences.[75] A systematic review and meta-analysis found that fluoride combined with CPP-ACP showed better efficacy on early occlusal lesions than fluoride alone, but they performed the same for smooth surface lesions.[76] The benefits of CPP-ACP might be most pronounced in individuals with reduced saliva,[77] but it is of questionable efficacy in children.

Hydroxyapatite

Hydroxyapatite is the inorganic component of enamel and is made up of calcium and phosphate ions.[78] Hydroxyapatite particles can assist with remineralization by becoming incorporated into demineralized enamel.[79] Toothpastes and varnishes with hydroxyapatite have recently become more readily available, but research on their effectiveness in preventing caries is ongoing. A randomized control trial comparing caries development in Polish children over 1 year using 10% hydroxyapatite toothpaste and 500 ppm fluoride toothpaste found no significant differences, but more research and longer-term studies are needed.[80]

For the prevention of dental caries, fluoride remains the gold standard. The long-term research on its efficacy and safety far surpasses the other caries preventive agents currently available.[81] Although fluoride is very effective in the prevention of caries, there is still a role for other types of preventive agents in high-risk individuals in the prevention and management of early carious lesions. Further research in the identification and development of these products is needed.

Visit eBooks.Health.Elsevier.com to see full list of references.

15

Pit and Fissure Sealants: Scientific and Clinical Rationale

MARTHA H. WELLS AND MARY AUSTIN SMITH

CHAPTER OUTLINE

Dental caries is a chronic disease affecting nearly half of American children ages 2 to 19 years and more than 90% of adults aged 20 to 64.[1,2] Although chronic diseases are among the most common and costly of all health problems, they are also among the most preventable. One of the most powerful prevention tools that the dental health profession has is the dental sealant.

Epidemiology of Pit and Fissure Caries

Despite advances in caries prevention and a decline in overall rates since the early 1970s, dental caries remains the most common chronic disease among children.[3] Data from National Health and Nutrition Examination Surveys show that 17% of children ages 6 to 11 years have had dental caries in their permanent teeth, and by age 19 nearly 57% of adolescents have had caries in their permanent teeth.[3] This trend underscores that caries is a cumulative experience, meaning once the disease is initiated, it progresses over time. The occlusal surfaces of permanent first molars, followed by second molars, remain the sites most frequently attacked by caries[4] with data suggesting that approximately 90% of caries in permanent teeth of children occur in pits and fissures.[5] Like permanent teeth, the pits and fissures of primary teeth are also at risk, as roughly 44% of carious lesions in the primary teeth affect the occlusal surfaces of molars.[5]

The occlusal surface is prone to caries for several reasons. The pit and fissure morphology provides an environment for plaque retention and bacteria proliferation. The enamel is thinner in pits and fissures and may experience accelerated demineralization. In addition, the molars take a relatively long time to fully erupt (1.5 to 2.5 years compared with just several months for premolars).[6] Partly erupted teeth have shown higher plaque accumulation because oral hygiene can be more challenging.[4] Toothbrush bristles have difficulty reaching the occlusal surface when it is out of the plane of occlusion, and the operculum covering the distal portion of the tooth may increase plaque retention. Additionally, occlusal surfaces harbor food particles longer than other surfaces, particularly highly retentive foods like crackers, cookies, sticky candies, or fruit snacks.[7] Accordingly, consistent and supervised daily oral hygiene is essential for the prevention of occlusal caries in children. Dental sealants also serve as an important adjunctive preventive measure.

Sealant Effectiveness

Unquestionably, dental sealants prevent pit and fissure caries in both primary and permanent teeth. The long-term benefit of caries reduction from using sealants on permanent teeth has been well documented, as decades worth of research has shown clear evidence of a reduction in caries and clinical practice guidelines have been developed.[5,8] Wright et al. provide a summary of the evidence of sealant efficacy in caries reduction[8]:

The results of this systematic review suggest that children and adolescents who receive sealants in sound occlusal surfaces or in noncavitated pit-and-fissure carious lesions in their primary or permanent molars (compared with a control without sealants) experience a 76% reduction in the risk of developing new carious lesions after 2 years of follow-up. Even after 7 or more years of follow-up, children and adolescents with sealants had a caries incidence of 29%, whereas those without sealants had a caries incidence of 74%.

The 2016 Clinical Practice Guidelines of the American Dental Association strongly recommend the use of sealants in permanent molars, meaning that the evidence of caries reduction by sealants was of moderate to high quality.[8] In addition, longitudinal data comparing the "life course" of sealed teeth to unsealed teeth show that teeth that receive sealants are less likely to require subsequent restorative treatment compared with unsealed teeth. If restorative treatment is required, the time until the first restorative treatment is greater than that for unsealed molars, and the restoration is likely to be less extensive.[9] The effectiveness of sealants in preventing caries is so well recognized in the literature that a study design with a "sealant-free" control group is no longer considered ethically acceptable.[10]

Current Sealant Utilization

Given the long clinical history and effectiveness of sealants, one would expect that sealants would be widely used by the dental profession. However, sealants are still underused.[3] Approximately 42% of children aged 6–11 years and 48% of adolescents aged 12–19 have at least one dental sealant. However, utilization remains lower among children from low-income households and minority populations.[3,11,12] Only 39% of children in low-income families have sealants compared with 45% in higher-income households.[3,12] Furthermore, the prevalence of sealants is significantly lower among non-Hispanic Black, Hispanic, and Asian children compared with non-Hispanic White children.[12]

Low utilization has been attributed to a lack of confidence in the bonding of sealants to enamel, concern for sealing over caries, difficulty achieving isolation, lack of reimbursement, and concerns for bisphenol A (BPA) exposure.[13] A common misperception of dentists is that sealants should not be placed over initial, early carious lesions.[13–15] This topic will be discussed in detail later in this chapter. Another significant reason cited for limiting sealant usage is the lack of or low reimbursement for sealant placement.[16] However, Medicaid programs have made significant strides in making sealants a covered benefit. All 50 states have included sealants in their Medicaid programs since the mid-1990s, and all reimburse for placement of sealants on permanent first and second molars.[17] However, few provide reimbursement for sealants on primary teeth or permanent premolars, and some reimburse sealant application only once per tooth per lifetime (not covering reapplication as necessary).[17] Clinical practice guidelines recommend sealant application in any teeth at risk for caries (primary and permanent molars and premolars) and reapplication as necessary because sealants prevent caries, are cost-effective, and are worthy of reimbursement.[8]

Types of Sealants

Three types of materials are used as sealants: resin, glass ionomer (conventional and resin-modified), and hybrid.[18] Generally, the most accepted material is the resin-based sealant because it has shown superior retention rates compared with glass ionomer sealants.[19] The resin-based sealant uses the principles of adhesive dentistry as it is retained by micromechanical retention. Resin-based sealants are available with various properties: unfilled, filled, clear, colored, fluoride-releasing, and hydrophilic. For the adhesion of the sealant to enamel, the tooth must be clean (no plaque or food debris) and remain completely dry because the resin is hydrophobic. Tooth enamel is etched with 35% to 37% phosphoric acid, creating surface irregularities in which the sealant material flows and forms resin tags (Fig. 15.1). The resin is polymerized with a curing light and forms a thin, plastic coating over the pits and fissures of the occlusal surface. This physical barrier is essential in preventing the carious process (Fig. 15.2).

Glass ionomer sealants have a different bonding mechanism. They adhere to the enamel through both mechanical retention and chemical bonding, known as chelation. However, the chemical bond alone is weak. Glass ionomers are hydrophilic and can withstand some minimal moisture. For the glass ionomer sealant, the tooth is cleaned, and a tooth conditioner of polyacrylic acid is applied. The tooth is rinsed and dried, and the glass ionomer is placed on the occlusal surface and chemically sets with an acid-base reaction, or if it is resin-modified, it sets with both light and chemical curing.

Hybrid materials include compomer (polyacid-modified composite resin) and giomer (composed of prereacted glass ionomer filler and resin-based monomer matrix). The superiority of sealant material remains inconclusive; thus the dentist should understand the properties of various sealant materials and choose a material for its clinical advantages. Tables 15.1 offer characteristics of various commercially available dental sealant products.

Properties of Sealant Materials

Color of Resin Sealants

Sealants are often available as clear or opaque white. The advantages to an opaque sealant are that it is easy to see during application and easy to monitor its retention at a recall visit. Clear sealant allows a surface to be visualized and monitored over time.[20] However, assessment of a clear sealant requires tactile exploration of the sealed surface. One study examining the visibility of clear and opaque sealants found that the error rate for identifying an opaque sealant was less than 2%, whereas for clear resin it was nearly 23%. The most common error for the examiners was to incorrectly state that a clear resin sealant was present on a tooth that had never been treated.[21] No apparent difference in the clinical efficacy of either type of sealants, has been reported. However, as will be discussed later, for resin-based sealants, retention is critical for the caries preventive effect; hence being able to quickly and correctly assess sealant retention is clinically important.

One additional sealant material is available with color-changing properties. Clinpro (3M ESPE, St. Paul, MN) is a sealant that is pink upon application and turns white when cured. This color

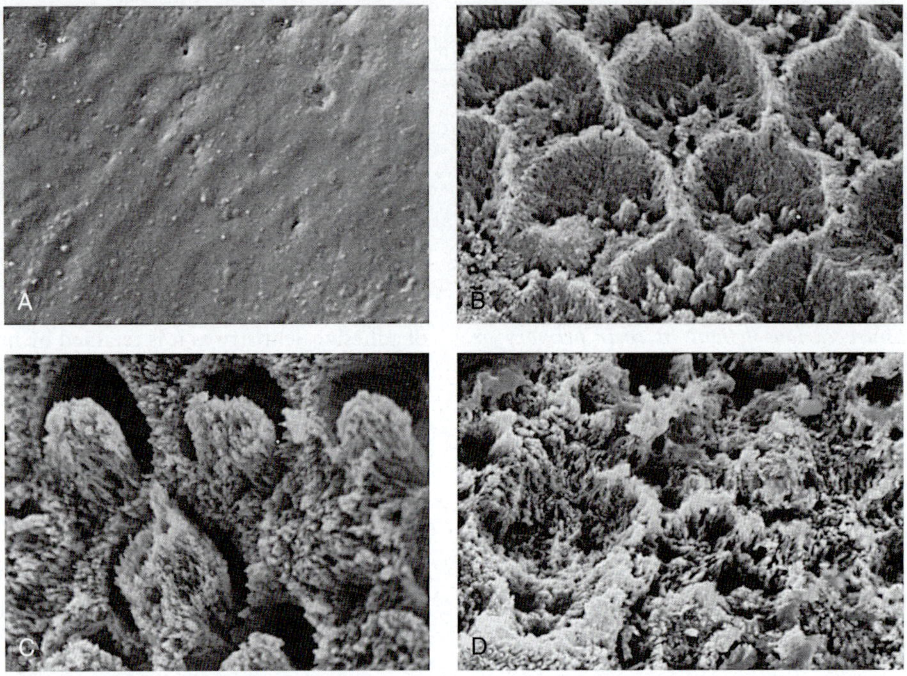

• **Fig. 15.1** Effects of the Acid-Etch Technique on Surface Morphology (Scanning Electron Microscopy). (A) The surface of sound enamel is relatively smooth, with occasional depressions representing terminations of enamel prisms. Several different patterns of etching can occur: (B) the loss of prism cores after etching; (C) the loss of prism peripheries after etching; and (D) surface porosities occur, but without a distinct prism morphologic appearance.

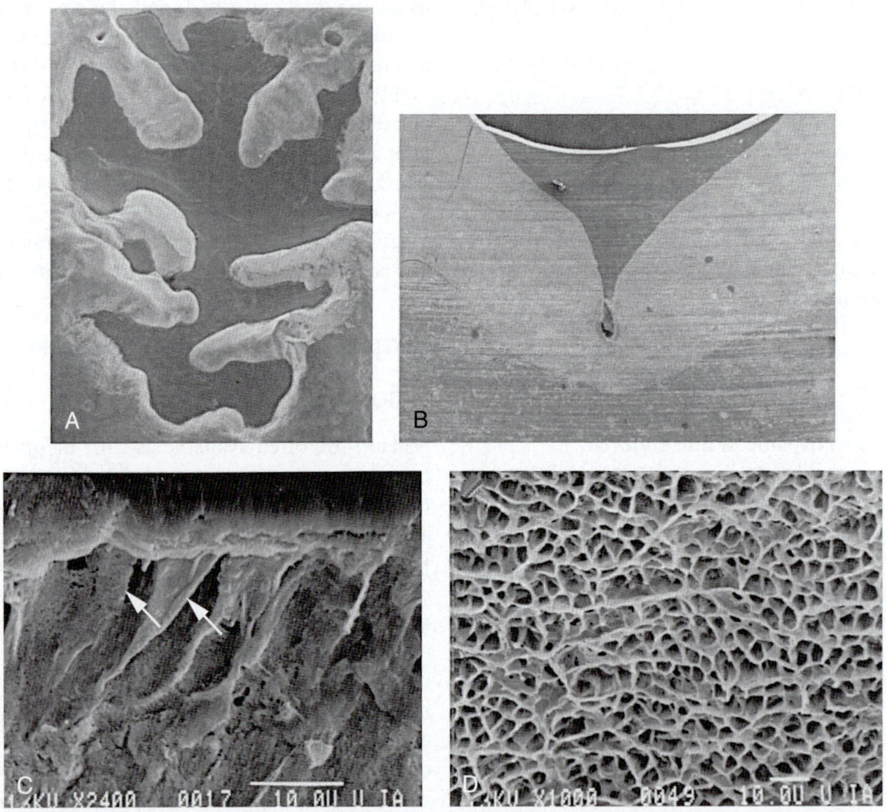

• **Fig. 15.2** The Enamel-Resin Interface (Scanning Electron Microscopy). (A) After sealant placement, the pits and fissures on this occlusal surface are protected from cariogenic challenges by the physical barrier of the sealant. (B) The interface between the enamel forming the fissure and the sealant appears to be an intimate one, with no apparent space between the etched enamel and sealant. (C) After partial demineralization of enamel that has been sealed, resin tags *(arrows)* may be seen in the etched enamel. (D) Complete demineralization of enamel that has been sealed allows one to visualize the appearance of the acid-resistant resin tags.

TABLE 15.1 Characteristics of Commercially Used Resin Dental Sealants

Product Name	Manufacturer	Filler (Percentage if Available)	Contains Fluoride	Color
Clinpro Sealant	3M ESPE	Unfilled	Yes	Pink then white
Conseal F	SDI	Unfilled	Yes	White
Delton Plus	Dentsply	Filled (38%)	Yes	White
Fissurit FX	Voco	Filled (55%)	Yes	White
Grandio Seal	Voco	Nanohybrid Filled, (70%)	Yes	White
Helioseal F	Ivoclar	Filled (40%)	Yes	White
Helioseal F Plus	Ivoclar	Filled	Yes	White
Helioseal Clear		Unfilled	No	Clear
Teethmate F-1	Kuraray	Unfilled	Yes	Natural and opaque (white)
Ultraseal XT Plus	Ultradent	Filled (58%)	Yes	White
Ultraseal XT hydro	Ultradent	Filled (53%) Hydrophilic chemistry	Yes	Natural and opaque (white)
Embrace Wetbond	Pulpdent	Filled (36.6%) and "Low fill" (7.9%) Hydrophilic chemistry	Yes	Natural and white

change is not an indication that the sealant has been adequately cured beyond surface hardness. Thus the color change provides no clinical advantage and has been described as a "perceived marketing benefit."[22] However, this material has similar properties to and is as caries-protective as other resin-based sealants; thus it may be chosen for its other properties (unfilled, fluoride-releasing).[23–25]

Filler Content of Resin Sealants

Sealants are also available with various filler content. For the most part, the filler content dictates the sealant's physical characteristics regarding viscosity, flow ability, and resistance to wear. Unfilled sealants have some advantages: lower rates of microleakage,[26] better penetration into the fissures due to their low viscosity,[27,28] and occlusal adjustment is not necessary. Unfilled sealant will abrade rapidly if left in occlusion, whereas filled sealants require occlusal adjustment because individuals are not able to abrade occlusal interferences to a comfortable level.[29] The necessity to adjust the occlusion may increase the time and cost of the procedure and may prevent delegation of sealant placement to auxiliaries.[22] However, filled materials also have advantages: greater wear resistance, lower shrinkage, and less porosity. For example, several studies have examined flowable composite as a sealant material; its retention is at least equal to conventional resin-based sealant materials.[30,31] The use of a bonding agent with flowable composite improves fissure penetration and decreases microleakage.[32] Using flowable composite may be appropriate when using the material for other applications in the same appointment. Although a resin-based sealant may be chosen for its various properties, no sealant material has been found to be superior for retention or caries prevention.[33]

Fluoride-Releasing Resin Sealants

Based on the benefits of fluoride release from glass ionomer materials, dental manufacturers have also developed fluoride-releasing resin sealants (FRSs).[34] FRSs exhibit variable releasing capabilities with the greatest release of fluoride shortly after placement, which decreases over time.[35] Studies have shown no long-lasting release of fluoride to plaque and saliva.[36,37] One should not consider FRSs as a fluoride reservoir with long-term release of fluoride into the immediately adjacent environment. Clinical studies have not demonstrated significant caries prevention of FRSs over the benefits obtained from conventional sealants.[18,38] Retention rates of FRSs compare with those of conventional sealants.[39,40] Given that the evidence is inconclusive as to the benefit of sealants containing fluoride, dentists should not choose a sealant material based on this property.

Hydrophilic Resin Sealant

There have been significant efforts to develop moisture-tolerant resin sealants. These sealants contain no bisphenol A glycidyl methacrylate (bis-GMA) or BPA, and they use a unique chemistry to achieve a carefully designed hydrophilic-hydrophobic balance.[41] They are thought to overcome the challenge of moisture in the oral environment. Additionally, these sealants have been shown to form longer resin tags than other resin sealants in in vitro studies, presumably because of their thixotropic nature.[42] Longer resin tags may improve their ability to seal the fissure and be retained.

One systematic review and meta-analysis found no difference in sealant retention or caries prevention between hydrophilic sealants and resin-based or glass ionomer sealants.[43] The review identified 13 studies of which only 6 met the inclusion criteria and only 5 were included in the meta-analysis. All 5 studies in the analysis evaluated Embrace™ WetBond™ (Pulpdent, Watertown, MA). The only clinical study to evaluate Ultraseal XT™ hydro (Ultradent, South Jordan, UT) did favor the hydrophilic material but had a very short follow-up time of 3 months. Based on the meta-analysis findings, the authors suggest glass ionomer sealant might be preferred over the use of hydrophilic resin sealants when a dry field is not possible.[43] However, because hydrophilic sealants have similar retention and caries prevention rates to conventional sealants, they may be chosen for their other properties.

Glass Ionomer

Glass ionomer cement sealants were introduced as an alternative to resin-based sealants based on their fluoride-releasing and recharging ability, their higher moisture toleration, and their easy application. In many early clinical studies, long-term retention was the principal evaluation criterion, as it is used as a surrogate measure of effectiveness in preventing caries.[39] When comparing retention, patients who receive glass ionomer sealants have a five times greater chance of experiencing sealant loss at 2 to 3 years.[44] However, a more appropriate measure of the effectiveness of sealants should be to determine a sealant material's ability to prevent caries. Studies have shown that although glass ionomer sealants are not retained as well, the caries preventive effect is similar to resin-based sealants.[44–48] From the most recent meta-analyses comparing different types of sealant material, there is insufficient evidence to judge superior effectiveness of one type of sealant.[48]

The theories for the protective benefit of glass ionomer material (despite its poor retention rates) are that (1) the glass ionomer material remains in the deepest parts of the fissures, still providing a physical barrier, even though it is not clinically visible, or (2) the fluoride release of glass ionomer imparts a long-term benefit to the tooth such that the fissures are more resistant to demineralization. Studies suggest that the residual cariostatic property of glass ionomer sealant is most likely due to a physical barrier of remaining glass ionomer in the fissures rather than a chemical effect on demineralization inhibition (Fig. 15.3).[49–51]

Glass ionomer sealants are widely used as part of the atraumatic restorative treatment (ART) technique, and several studies have shown the caries-preventive effect of ART sealants.[24,52,53] (See Chapter 30 for a discussion of ART.) Different glass ionomer products have been used, but high-viscosity materials are better retained than those of low to medium viscosity.[53]

Glass carbomer sealants are developed from conventional glass ionomer cements and contain nanoparticles of hydroxyapatite and fluorapatite. They are a type of glass ionomer sealant for which laboratory studies have shown improved mechanical properties and command setting with a curing light. They have comparable fluoride release and bond strengths to conventional glass ionomer.[54] Like conventional glass ionomers they show poorer retention rates compared with resin-based sealants but similar effectiveness in preventing caries.[54] However, this material is insufficiently researched and is not regarded as a first-line option.

Although resin-based sealants are widely used and demonstrate proven effectiveness, substantial evidence supports high-viscosity glass ionomer sealants. These materials are more tolerant of minor moisture contamination than resin sealants; however, they still require a controlled clinical environment and are not suitable for placement under completely wet conditions. Their simplified application may reduce chair time and enhance cost-effectiveness.[55,56] Clinical practice guidelines have not been able to provide specific recommendations for the best sealant material to use for caries prevention because the evidence of the head-to-head comparisons is of low quality. Dentists should choose the type of material most appropriate for particular clinical scenarios. For instance, when a child is cooperative and the tooth can be adequately isolated, either material may be selected. However, if isolation is difficult, the operator is working alone, the tooth is not fully erupted, or the child has less than ideal cooperation, a glass ionomer is more appropriate.[8,55]

Hybrid

Hybrid sealants, such as compomers and giomers, integrate the esthetic properties of composite resins with the fluoride-releasing capabilities of glass ionomers. Compomers are hydrophobic, set by a polymerization reaction, lack the ability to bond to tooth structure, and require bonding agents similar to conventional composites.[57] Although they possess fluoride-releasing properties, their fluoride release is significantly lower than that of glass ionomers. As sealant materials, polyacid-modified resin composites demonstrate lower fluoride release compared with glass ionomer cements and inferior retention compared with conventional resin composites.[40,58–60]

Giomer is a tooth-colored material that uses a resin base and prereacted glass ionomer technology and has fluoride-releasing and recharging properties.[61] As sealants, giomer sealants have a self-etching primer that eliminates the need for phosphoric acid etching. Clinical data show poorer retention rates compared with conventional resin sealants.[62]

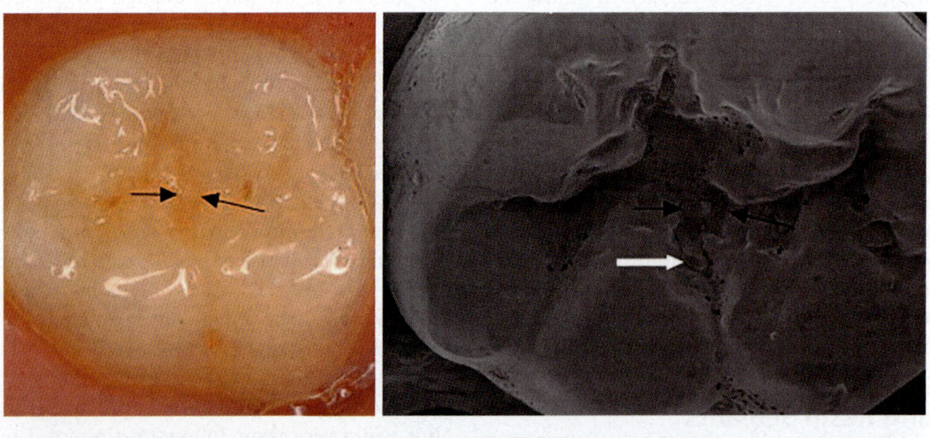

• **Fig. 15.3** Clinically undetected glass ionomer material (Fuji IX) that is visible on scanning electron microscope (SEM) images 13 years after sealant placement. *Left:* the glass ionomer sealant appears to end clinically where the *black arrows* are positioned. The SEM image (12x) shows an extension of glass ionomer *(white arrow).* Copyright JE Frencken. (© JE Frencken.)

The Necessity of Sealants

Caries Risk Assessment

Sealant placement should be based on individual caries risk rather than applied routinely, as low-risk teeth gain minimal benefit, and it is not cost-effective.[63] Both the patient and tooth should be evaluated, with sealants recommended for high-risk cases, including patients with moderate to high caries risk or teeth with deep fissures, occlusal decalcification, or hypomineralization. Research shows sealants provide minimal benefit for sound teeth in low-risk individuals (4.5% reduction in caries) but significantly reduce caries progression (41%) in teeth with incipient lesions (defined by dark staining of the grooves, chalky appearance, or a slight explorer catch; Fig. 15.4; see Fig. 15.16B). Therefore sealants are indicated when a dentist determines a patient or tooth is at risk.[5]

Sealant and Fluoride Varnish

Fluoride varnish reduces caries in permanent teeth.[64] Along with reducing the incidence of smooth surface lesions, varnish has also been shown to reduce pit and fissure caries, perhaps because it adheres to the deeper part of the fissures for a long period of time allowing a high uptake of fluoride ions. Although the 2016 Clinical Practice Guidelines recommended sealants for caries prevention compared to varnish,[8] the most current evidence suggests there may be no difference in efficacy.[65] However, concurrent placement of sealants and varnish is superior to varnish application alone.[65]

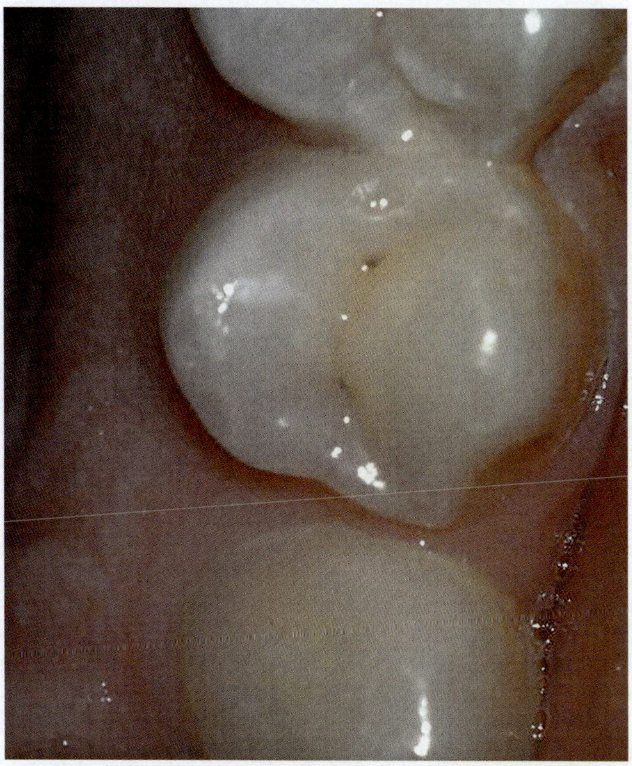

• **Fig. 15.4** Early, noncavitated incipient caries exhibited by distinct, brown early caries in the pits of the premolar. This tooth would benefit from a sealant and would not require mechanical preparation before sealant placement.

Age at Placement

Studies from the 1950s to 1960s showed peak caries incidence shortly after eruption, then tapering, indicating the occlusal surface was most vulnerable early on. Risk dropped significantly after this period. Current evidence highlights thick plaque accumulation and partial eruption as key factors because partially erupted teeth are harder to clean.[4] Although molars face the highest risk soon after eruption, postfluoridation data show new caries develop annually.[66] Fluorides may delay the onset of pit and fissure caries, leading to occlusal surfaces that decay at a later age.[67]

Caries trends (1999 to 2016) show an overall decline in decay among children and adolescents under 19, except for ages 6 to 8 and 12 to 19, where no change is reported. Meanwhile, caries prevalence has slightly increased in adults over age 20.[67] The nature of caries is shifting from a rapidly progressing childhood disease to a slow, lifelong progression.[67]

Evidence-based recommendations support sealants for both children and adults at risk of caries. Sealant placement should be based on the clinical impression of whether a sealant is necessary to prevent caries rather than eruption timing.[5] Fig. 15.5 provides a decision-making tree to guide dentists.

Which Teeth Should Be Sealed?

Traditionally, sealants were used for noncarious first and second permanent molars with deep fissures. However, recommendations now include any at-risk tooth, such as primary teeth, premolars, and permanent molars with incipient, noncavitated lesions.[5] Two recent systematic reviews found insufficient evidence on sealants' effectiveness in preventing or arresting caries in primary molars, calling for further research.[18,68] Gag reflex is noted as a potential issue during placement.[19] Despite this, sealants are recommended for high-risk children who can cooperate.[5]

The indications for sealant placement include (1) deep, retentive pits and fissures (Fig. 15.6); (2) stained pits and fissures with minimal appearance of decalcification or opacification (i.e., incipient caries with no cavitation; see Fig. 15.4); and (3) the possibility of adequate isolation from salivary contamination. Additional considerations are (1) no radiographic or clinical evidence of interproximal caries in need of restoration, though the occlusal surface could still benefit from sealant protection, and (2) other preventive treatment, such as fluoride therapy, to inhibit interproximal caries formation should be initiated because the patient is at higher risk for caries.

Relative contraindications for sealant placement include (1) well-coalesced, self-cleaning pits and fissures; (2) radiographic or clinical evidence of interproximal caries in need of restoration; (3) the presence of many interproximal lesions or restorations with no preventive plan/treatment to inhibit caries formation; (4) limited life expectancy of the primary tooth; and (5) no possibility of adequate isolation from salivary contamination either due to eruption status or patient behavior.

Diagnosing Occlusal Caries

Occlusal caries diagnosis is challenging, with dentists correctly identifying cases only 42% of the time.[69] Experts have challenged the long-held belief that probing an occlusal groove with an explorer is necessary to diagnose a carious lesion.[70] Research disputes the need for explorers, as visual inspection of a clean, dry tooth is equally effective. Forceful probing can damage enamel,

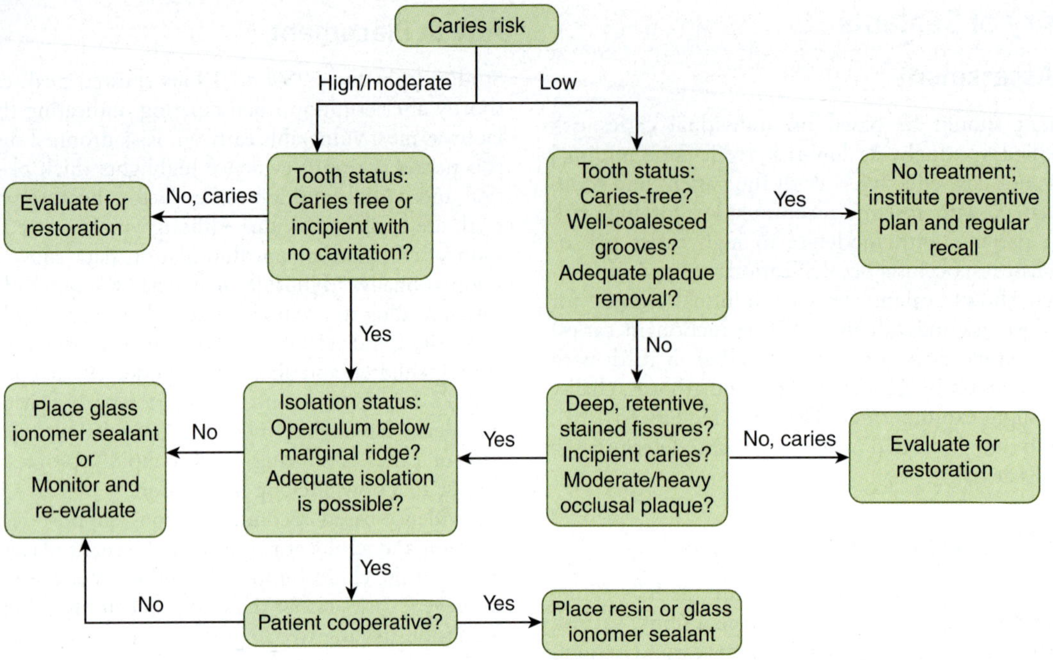

• **Fig. 15.5** Flow chart to aid in making decisions about sealant placement.

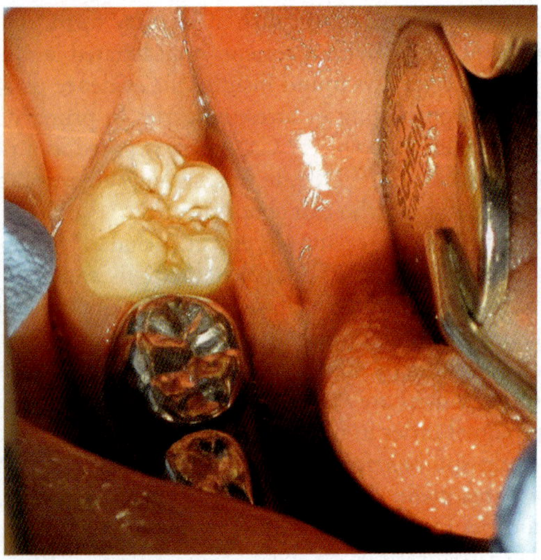

• **Fig. 15.6** Molar with deep, retentive grooves, an ideal candidate for sealant placement—especially because the patient has existing stainless steel crown restorations that indicate a high caries risk assessment.

resulting in possible caries development or progression by causing cavitation of a previously noncavitated lesion.[40,71,72] In one study, a dentist was asked to gently probe a sample of third molars, half of which had initial carious lesions and half of which had sound occlusal surfaces. Using electron microscopy, the study found enamel defects in all probed carious lesions and some sound surfaces.[40] Experts recommend using explorers gently to assess surface roughness rather than forcefully probing fissures.[70] Visual examination remains the primary diagnostic method; the concept of using moderate, firm pressure to find a "catch" in the fissure is no longer the most contemporary approach to caries diagnosis and management.[5,69]

Several noninvasive technologies have shown promise to aid in caries diagnosis and in caries monitoring over time: light-induced and infrared laser fluorescence devices, the electronic caries detector, quantitative laser fluorescence, and transillumination. Although emerging noninvasive technologies show promise, they cannot replace clinical judgment.

Sealing Over Incipient Caries

A paradigm shift in caries management has moved away from complete caries removal. The 2015 International Caries Consensus Collaboration recommends restoring a tooth only if the lesion is cavitated and extends into dentin. Noncavitated enamel or early dentin lesions should be managed through biofilm removal, remineralization, or sealing.[73] What is the science behind this decision? If sealants are applied properly and are monitored periodically, caries arrest beneath a sealant, as demonstrated by numerous studies.[20,74,75] Oong et al. found sealants lowered progression risk by over 70%. Sealants reduce bacteria through acid etching (eliminating 75% of viable microorganisms) and depriving bacteria of nutrients, preventing acid production. Sealing over caries is associated with a 100-fold reduction in mean total viable bacteria counts.[76]

Despite expert recommendations, some US dentists hesitate to seal carious teeth, fearing lesion progression.[14,15] Fontana et al. addressed this concern by sealing noncavitated lesions with clear sealants and monitoring them with visual inspection, radiography, and laser fluorescence. After nearly 4 years, sealants (reapplied yearly when needed) were 98% effective in preventing lesion progression[20] (Fig. 15.7; see Fig. 15.16B).

Some practitioners opt for invasive approaches, mistakenly labeling fissurotomies or enameloplasty as "preventive resin restorations" (PRRs). A true PRR (conservative adhesive restoration) involves restoring a cavitated lesion extending into dentin while sealing intact pits and fissures. (See Chapter 30 for a detailed discussion of conservative adhesive restorations.)

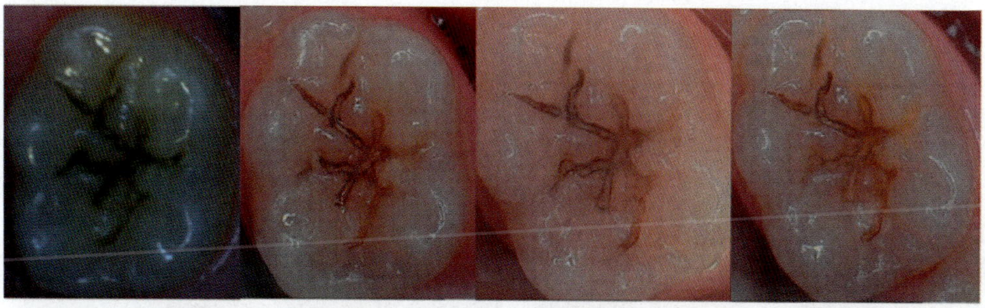

• **Fig. 15.7** Sealed carious permanent molars monitored over 44 months. *ICDAS,* International Caries Detection and Assessment System. (From Fontana M, Platt JA, Eckert GJ, et al. Monitoring of sound and carious surfaces under sealants over 44 months. *J Dent Res*. 2014;93:1070-1075.)

As an example, in a permanent maxillary first molar, if only the distal pit is carious while other fissures remain intact, the caries is removed, and a restorative material is placed without opening unaffected areas. Sealant is applied over the central pit and remaining intact fissures, making this a true PRR. When properly maintained, PRRs are effective, but mechanical preparation of noncavitated lesions is unnecessary. Preparing a tooth with a bur initiates a cycle of repeated restorations, which can ultimately compromise tooth longevity. Fig. 15.8 is a diagram of the continuum of caries and the recommended clinical management.[77] As one can appreciate, surgical intervention is much further down the continuum. Caries management should prioritize sealing rather than surgical intervention unless cavitation extends into dentin.[73]

Preparing the Tooth for a Sealant

Cleaning the Tooth

For a sealant to flow into the fissures of the tooth, the fissures must be free of debris. Debris can be cleaned with pumice slurry and a prophy cup or bristle brush, using an explorer through the fissures and forcefully rinsing with air-water spray,[39] or with a dry bristle toothbrush[78] (Box 15.1). One clinical study showed improved retention with the pumice slurry and rubber cup cleaning method.[78] Complete debridement of the fissures is very difficult, and as a result, complete penetration of the sealant rarely occurs with conventional cleaning methods. The utilization of an air-polishing system such as a Prophy Jet Cavitron Prophy Jet (Dentsply Sirona, Charlotte, NC) is a superior cleaning method as it removes more debris and allows greater sealant penetration into the fissures resulting in an increased number of resin tags for micromechanical retention.[79] However, air polishing never has become the standard for pit and fissure sealant application because of the increased equipment cost and complexity of the procedure.

Mechanical Preparation

For noncavitated surfaces, removal of tooth structure by a bur is unnecessary. Fissurotomy and enameloplasty techniques involve using a small bur to remove any residual debris and/or dubious enamel tissue as well as to widen the fissure. In laboratory studies, enameloplasty allows deeper sealant penetration and better adaptation and increases the surface area for acid etching,[80] but clinical studies are conflicting regarding any clinical benefit from mechanical preparation. Several studies have reported increased retention of sealants after mechanical preparation of the fissures,[81,82] but other studies have not shown a superior retention rate or enhanced performance of the sealant.[83,84] Furthermore, loss of sealants from teeth that have been prepared significantly predisposes those teeth to the development of caries, most likely because of inadequate hygiene and plaque accumulation in the prepared fissures.[81] Additionally, mechanical preparation prevents the delegation of sealant placement to auxiliaries, which decreases cost-effectiveness.[85] The European Academy of Pediatric Dentistry summarizes the evidence well in its guidelines that state the following: "purposeful removal of enamel or enameloplasty just to widen the base of a fissure in a sound tooth is an invasive technique, which disturbs the equilibrium of the fissure system and exposes a child unnecessarily to the use of a handpiece or air abrasion."[86] There is robust evidence that supports high sealant retention without the use of a bur.

A limited number of studies have shown that air abrasion in combination with acid etching results in improved retention of sealants.[87,88] Evidence for other preparation methods such as with a laser is lacking, and neither air abrasion nor preparing the enamel with a laser alone can be a substitute for acid etching.[89,90]

Effect of a Recent Professionally Applied Fluoride Treatment

Dentists may prefer to place or repair sealants during a patient's examination. However, because many patients receive prophylaxis and fluoride before the examination, concerns have arisen about fluoride affecting sealant bond strength. Studies confirm that fluoride gels or foams do not compromise bond strength or retention, allowing sealant application immediately after.[91,92] However, for offices using fluoride varnish, sealants should be placed before varnish application.

Factors Affecting Sealant Success

Etchant

Etchants are available as separate phosphoric acid etchants, self-etching systems, liquids, and gels. Historically the clinical sealant procedure involved an etching time of 60 seconds and a rinsing time of at least 10 seconds. However, multiple studies have shown similar bond strengths for both permanent and primary teeth,

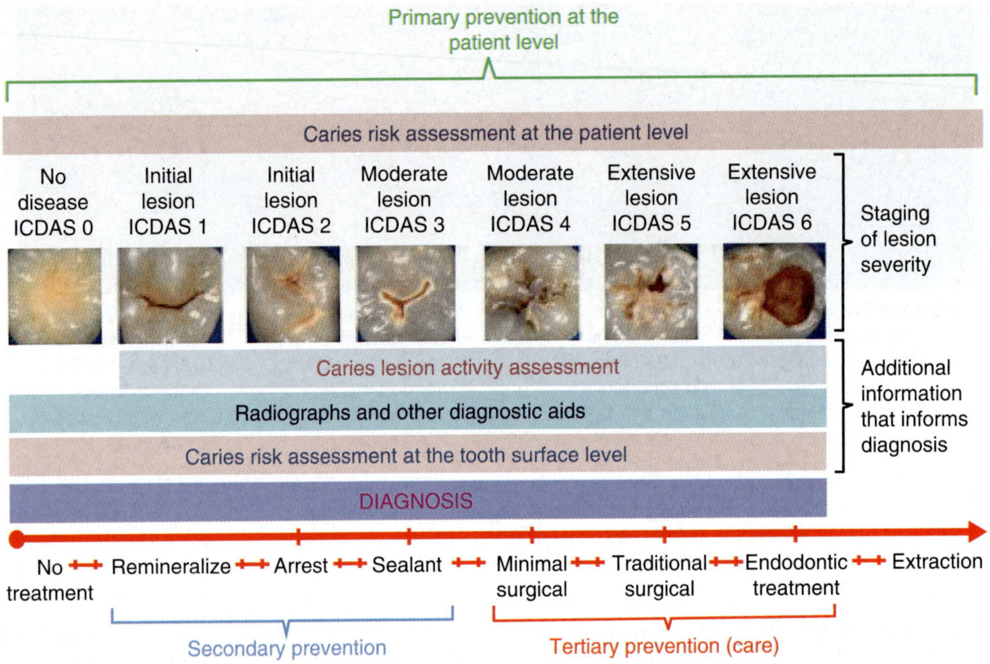

• **Fig. 15.8** Caries diagnosis and management system continuum. *ICDAS,* International Caries Detection and Assessment System. (From Zero DT, Zandona AF, Vail MM, Spolnik KJ. Dental caries and pulpal disease. *Dent Clin North Am.* 2011;55:29-46.)

• BOX 15.1 The Resin-Based Dental Sealant Clinical Procedure

1. Cleaning: Clean the occlusal surface with a toothbrush or bristled rotary brush and pumice slurry.
2. Isolation: Achieve isolation by rubber dam, cotton rolls, or intraoral vacuum suction.
3. Etching: Once isolated, etch the tooth, most commonly with 37% phosphoric acid. The etchant should remain on the surface for 15 to 20 seconds or per the manufacturer's instructions.
4. Rinse and dry: Rinse the tooth utilizing the air-water spray and high-volume suction. The tooth must remain dry and uncontaminated from this point forward.
5. Apply sealant: If a bonding agent is to be used, place it with a microbrush, lightly dry and cure. Apply the sealant to all pits and fissures, and take care to not overfill the sealant. If overfilling occurs remove excess material with a small brush and tease small bubbles out before polymerization.
6. Polymerization: Once the sealant is placed, position the curing light tip as closely as possible to the surface, and cure the sealant for the amount of time recommended by the manufacturer, which is usually 20 seconds.
7. Evaluate: Once cured, visually and tactilely examine the sealant before removing the isolation materials. If bubbles, voids, or areas of deficient material are discovered, add material and cure. Attempt to dislodge the sealant with an explorer. If material de-bonds, see Box 15.3.
8. Limit BPA exposure: Remove the unpolymerized layer by rubbing the surface with pumice on a cotton roll or by rinsing the surface for 30 seconds.
9. Verify occlusion: Make occlusal adjustments if necessary.
10. Periodic evaluation: Evaluate sealants at every recall. Maintain, repair, and replace sealants as needed.
11. Repair: Attempt to dislodge any partially remaining sealants with an explorer. If the partially remaining sealant is retained, do not remove it. Instead, clean the tooth with pumice and rubber cup, and etch both the enamel and remaining sealant before applying additional material.

with lower etching times of 15 to 30 seconds.[93–95] Etching time should be increased for fluorotic teeth. The etchant can be applied liberally (2 to 3 mm beyond the anticipated margin of the sealant) and should flow onto all susceptible pits and fissures, including lingual grooves of maxillary molars and buccal pits of mandibular molars[96] (Fig. 15.9). The different forms of etchant (i.e., gel or liquid) have been shown to perform similarly in regard to penetration, bond strength, and clinical retention.[94,97]

The usual recommendation for rinsing is 20 to 30 seconds. A few studies have shown that a shorter rinse time yields similar enamel bond strengths as a 20-second rinse time.[98,99] The best practice is to follow the manufacturer's instructions for use of the selected etchant.

Different types of etchants do not provide similar results. Self-etching systems yield significantly lower bond strengths than separate etch systems and exhibit much lower retention rates in clinical trials.[100–102] Self-etching systems have decreased bond strengths on uncut enamel; thus utilizing a self-etching bonding system without the use of a separate etch step is not recommended.[5,100]

For glass ionomer sealants, conditioning the enamel with polyacrylic acid increases the chance of a chelation reaction between the calcium of the enamel and polyacrylic acid in the glass ionomer matrix, establishing a more stable bonding surface. After applying the polyacrylic acid, the tooth is rinsed and dried (Box 15.2).

Drying Agents and Time

Given the hydrophobic nature of resins, drying agents such as alcohol or acetone have been explored as possible treatments after the etchant step, before sealant placement. However, a laboratory

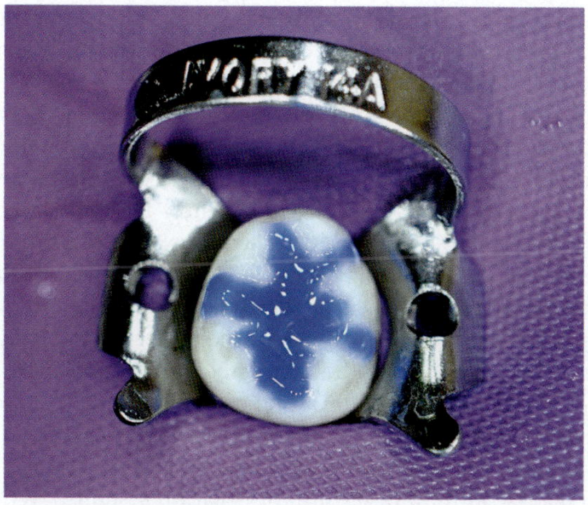

• **Fig. 15.9** Etchant Application to a Mandibular Molar. Note how the etchant extends onto the buccal and lingual grooves.

• BOX 15.2 The Glass Ionomer Dental Sealant Clinical Procedure

1. Cleaning: Clean the occlusal surface with a toothbrush or bristled rotary brush and pumice slurry.
2. Isolation: Maintain a clean, dry field with cotton rolls, a vacuum isolation system, or a rubber dam.
3. Conditioning: Apply 20% polyacrylic acid cavity conditioner with a microbrush for 15 seconds.
4. Rinse and dry: Rinse with water for 10 seconds. Dry the tooth with cotton pellets or gently air dry. Do not desiccate.
5. Sealant application: Apply high-viscosity glass ionomer to occlusal surface. Using a petroleum jelly–coated index finger, press the glass ionomer into the fissures with finger pressure. After 10 to 15 seconds remove the finger sideways with downward pressure. Remove excess material with an instrument or wet cotton tip applicator.
6. End of procedure: Check bite. Apply a layer of petroleum jelly over the sealant. Ask the patient not to eat for at least 1 hour.

From Nicholson JW. Polyacid-modified composite resins ("compomers") and their use in clinical dentistry. *Dent Mater.* 2007;23(5):615-622.

study showed that the use of drying agents did not decrease microleakage or increase sealant penetration.[103] Furthermore, one clinical investigation showed no significant improvements of retention rates with the use of drying agents.[104]

There is no recommended drying time. Rather, a specific result should be obtained. The occlusal surface should have a chalky or frosted appearance (Fig. 15.10). Unlike dentin bonding, in which the collagen fibrils should remain moist to prevent collapsing, the enamel keeps its crystalline structure. This means that the enamel should be thoroughly dried or desiccated to maximize the penetration of the hydrophobic sealant. If the chalky white result is not obtained after thorough drying, the tooth should be re-etched.

For glass ionomers, unlike phosphoric acid etching and rinsing in the resin-based sealant technique, the enamel should not be desiccated. The surface should remain slightly moist as glass ionomer needs some moisture to set, although too much water or contamination is detrimental to the material's properties. Thus lightly drying with air or drying with a cotton pellet is appropriate.

Sealant Application and Polymerization

Sealant should be applied to all pits and fissures including the lingual grooves of maxillary molars and the buccal pits of mandibular molars (Fig. 15.11). Sealant may be applied with a variety of instruments: an explorer tip, a PICH instrument (a calcium hydroxide, or Dycal, placer), or a small brush. Many manufacturers offer their own delivery system. The sealant should not be overfilled to ensure that the sealant material does not extend past the etched area, to limit the amount of occlusal interference created, and to ensure optimal depth of cure. If overfilling occurs, the excess material may be removed with a small brush. If small bubbles form within the sealant material, these should be teased out before polymerization.

Assuming scrupulous isolation can be maintained, a practitioner might be able to improve retention of the sealant by delaying polymerization for several seconds after sealant application. A study by Chosack and Eidelman found that the longer sealants were allowed to remain on the etched surface before polymerization (20 seconds vs. 5 or 10 seconds), the more sealant material penetrated into microporosities, creating longer resin tags, which are critical for micromechanical retention.[105]

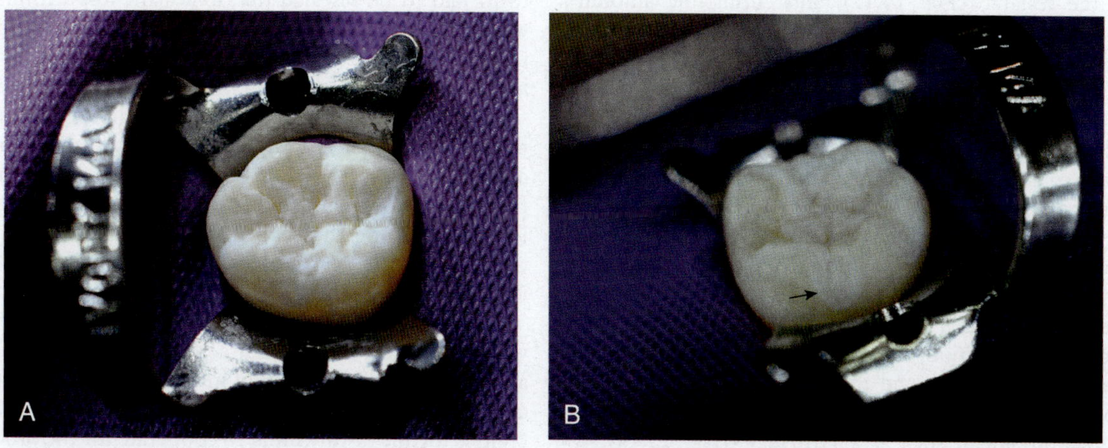

• **Fig. 15.10** (A) Etched enamel displaying frosted appearance. (B) Note the demarcation between the chalky, etched enamel *(arrow)* and the shiny unetched enamel of the buccal surface.

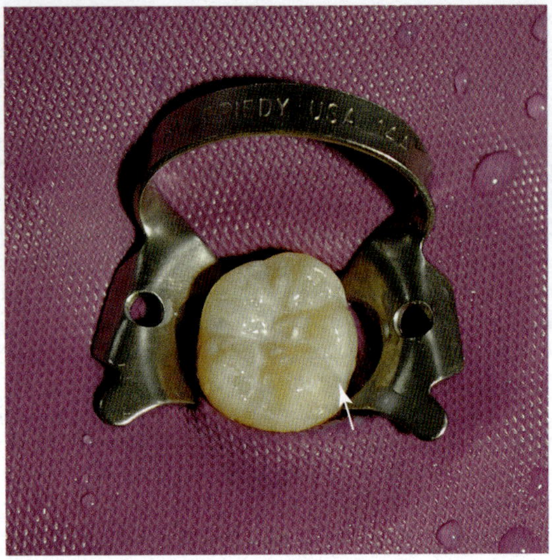

• **Fig. 15.11** Sealed Mandibular Molar. Note how the sealant extends into all susceptible fissures, including the buccal groove *(arrow)*.

A sealant must be adequately cured for it to obtain its physical properties. If the curing time is insufficient, the bonding is poor and decreases in hardness may result, leading to subsequent sealant failure.[106] Several types of curing lights are available (see Chapter 29). Most manufacturers recommend a 20-second exposure time. However, practitioners must consider which kind of curing light is being used because not all perform equally. In vitro studies have examined the depth of cure of dental sealant with LED units that offer high energy and very short curing times, and found these very short curing times (3 to 5 seconds) to be inadequate to optimally cure dental sealant, especially opaque material.[107,108] Short curing times will result in the top or surface of the sealant feeling hard to an explorer, but top hardness is not a valid measure of adequate depth of cure. Several factors affect the level of cure, including shade of the material, the filler content, the thickness of the material, the intensity of the curing light, and the distance of the light source from the material.[109] Additionally, long time exposures and overcuring can be dangerous to the pulp or other oral tissues.[110] When using LED curing lights, clinicians should ensure optimal curing by using a light source with an output of at least 1000 mW/cm^2, placing the light tip as close as possible to the sealant (eFig. 15.12), and curing the amount of time recommended by the sealant material manufacturer (generally 20 seconds).

Isolation

Resin-based sealants are hydrophobic and moisture sensitive. Rubber dam is considered the gold standard for isolation, particularly when using resin materials.[111] However, several studies have shown that cotton roll isolation is comparable to rubber dam isolation for sealant placement,[112–114] though a systematic review and recent clinical trial noted that retention is increased when rubber dam isolation is used[39,115] (Fig. 15.13).

For cotton roll application, the patient is in a supine position with the head extended back and the chin up because this improves visibility and moisture control. For maxillary isolation, a triangular isolation shield, such as a Dri-Angle (Fig. 15.14), is placed against the buccal mucosa and a cotton roll may be placed in the maxillary vestibule to hold the tissue away from the tooth. The mouth mirror is used and should be left in position throughout the procedure until polymerization of the sealant is achieved. Besides providing indirect vision, it also acts as a shield for the tongue. For mandibular isolation, cotton rolls are placed on both the buccal and lingual sides of the teeth. A cotton roll holder may be utilized, or the rolls may be held in place with the fingers. Alternatively, a triangular isolation shield may be used as a tongue shield (Fig. 15.15). Excess moisture can be evacuated from the area with the suction. Utilizing a four-handed delivery method can increase the ease and success of achieving adequate isolation.[116]

Intraoral vacuum systems such as the Isolite (Zyris, Inc., Santa Barbara, CA), DryShield (Solmetex, Northborough, MA, MA), and Mr. Thirsty (Zirc Dental Products, Buffalo, MN) have been shown to produce sealant retention rates comparable to those placed under cotton roll and rubber dam isolation.[112,117,118] (See Chapter 30 for a discussion of isolation systems.) Whenever possible, especially if concurrent operative treatment is provided, rubber dam isolation should be used. However, given the discomfort that can be associated with rubber dam placement on nonanesthetized tissues, rubber dam isolation is not imperative if the operator can maintain a dry field with alternative techniques.

Saliva contamination significantly lowers bond strengths because it prevents the formation of resin tags and results in decreased retention.[119,120] At times, practitioners who are placing sealants will notice that a small amount of saliva seeps onto the tooth from the tongue or the cotton roll, and the practitioner erroneously believes that if the tooth is rinsed and dried well, sealant retention will not be affected. However, even minimal exposure to saliva forms a surface coating that cannot be completely removed by rinsing.[121] The acid-etch step creates microporosities in the enamel, and if saliva touches the tooth, these porosities are occluded so the sealant cannot form resin tags to micromechanically bond to the tooth. Achieving adequate isolation is a critical step to the success of the sealant and is considered a key concept in the clinical procedure[122] (Box 15.3).

Timing of Sealant Placement

Sealants placed on partially erupted teeth require repair or replacement more often than fully erupted teeth.[123] Retention of resin sealant material is critical to its success. One-time placement does not impart long-term protection if the physical barrier over the fissure, the sealant, does not remain intact. Dennison et al. concluded that when the operculum of the gingiva extended over the distal marginal ridge of the tooth, more than 50% of the teeth had to be resealed due to sealant loss within 36 months; when the operculum was at the level of the marginal ridge, retreatment fell to 26%.[124] For partially erupted teeth, which are at high risk for experiencing caries, the best practice is to place a sealant and repair or replace it as necessary as well as to reinforce the importance of adequate hygiene and plaque control. Partial or complete loss of a resin sealant in any groove or pit renders that pit or fissure susceptible to caries attack and equally at risk for caries as one that had never been sealed (Fig. 15.16). For these teeth, the best sealant material is a high-viscosity glass ionomer[5,55] (Fig. 15.17).

Not only should tooth eruption be considered when deciding when to place a sealant, but a child's level of cooperation must also be considered. The child must tolerate the isolation method and the procedure length to place a successful sealant. If the child is unable or unwilling to cooperate for the procedure, placing sealants should be delayed until the level of cooperation is adequate.

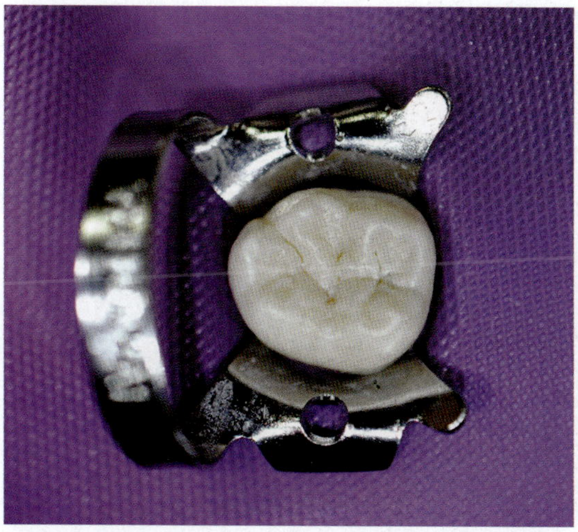

• **Fig. 15.13** Rubber dam isolation can be single tooth or quadrant depending on the needs of the patient and will assist the practitioner in keeping saliva from contaminating any of the fissures once they have been etched.

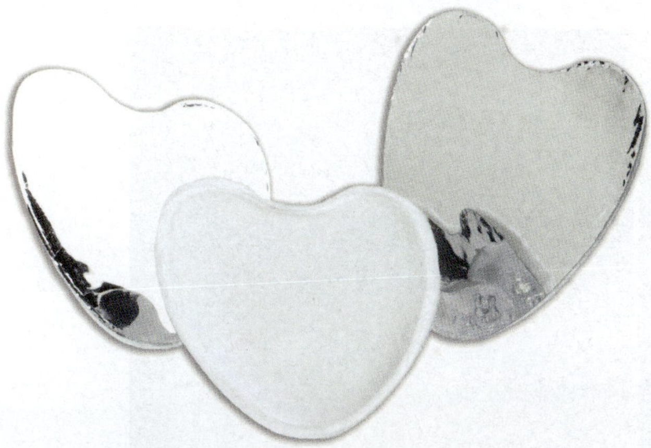

• **Fig. 15.14** Dri-Angle isolation shield. (Courtesy Dental Health Products, Inc., Niagara Falls, NY.)

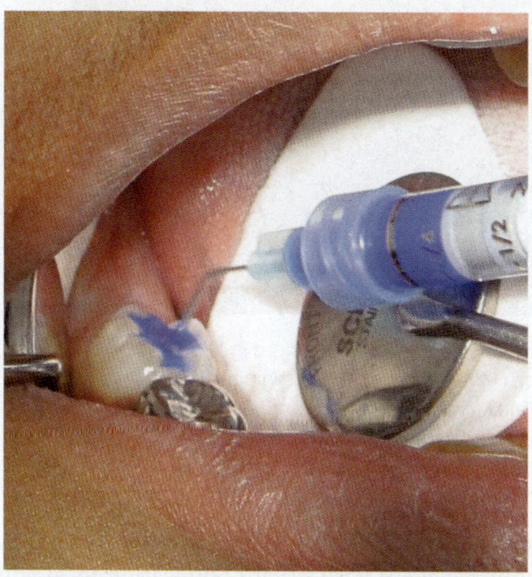

• **Fig. 15.15** Isolation of a Mandibular Molar Using a Cotton Triangle to Shield the Tongue. Note that when sealant is applied with four-handed delivery, the operator has extra help in maintaining adequate isolation (in this case, the operator is able to retract the cheek while the assistant retracts the tongue with mirrors).

• BOX 15.3 Troubleshooting Resin Sealant Placement

Sealant placement is very technique sensitive. If sealant material de-bonds upon immediate evaluation, one of the following three explanations is the most likely cause:

1. Debris remains in the fissure. The tooth must be clean. If plaque remains in the fissure, the resin cannot flow into the fissure to form tags and micromechanically bond to the enamel. Clean the fissures with a toothbrush, re-etch, and complete the application steps again.
2. Saliva contaminated the enamel. If isolation was not meticulously maintained and saliva contacted the occlusal surface, then saliva pooled in the microporosities created by the etchant step. Viscous saliva cannot be removed by rinsing and drying alone. The resin sealant will "float" on the saliva and cannot form resin tags. In this case the tooth should be re-etched, dried, and resealed with no saliva contamination. If perfect isolation is not attainable, a resin sealant should not be used. Glass ionomer may be a more appropriate material.
3. The tooth was not completely dry after the rinsing step. If the tooth does not appear chalky after an adequate etching time, it is most likely not dry. Enamel bonding is different from dentin adhesion. In restorative dentistry, one is advised not to desiccate the dentin; however, enamel must be dry before resin sealant application. Hydrophobic resin will "float" on top of any water in the enamel porosities and will not form resin tags. Again, no micromechanical bonding will occur, and the sealant will de-bond when evaluated with an explorer.

Use of Intermediate Bonding Agent

Resin-based dental sealants are hydrophobic. Because of this property, they cannot tolerate even slight moisture contamination. Dentinal bonding agents have hydrophilic properties so that they can infiltrate wet dentin. Using a layer of bonding agent between the enamel and hydrophobic resin sealant has been studied to determine whether this additional step could enhance retention rates. Numerous laboratory studies have found decreased microleakage and enhanced penetration of sealant material into the fissures with the adjunct of a bonding agent.[125–127] A systematic review and meta-analysis examined five studies that indicated that adhesive systems beneath fissure sealants had a significant positive benefit on retention and thus caries prevention.[33] The authors note that the positive effect was seen in studies that used fifth-generation bonding agents (those that require a separate etch and rinse step but have the "prime" and "bond" together as one step). The use of a bonding agent should be used only with hydrophobic resin-based sealant materials. Glass ionomers chemically bond to the enamel, so using a bonding agent under this material is not logical.

Despite some positive effects for the use of a bonding agent, there are two main disadvantages to this technique. Using a bonding agent increases the cost of the procedure and increases chair time.[128] Several studies have found this step to be unnecessary,[129–131] and they highlight the importance of proper sealant placement technique: fastidious isolation and proper placement negate the need for this additional step. If a clinician is providing resin-operative dentistry in the same appointment and is already using bond for another application, then using a bonding agent under the sealant would be sensible. Additionally, a bonding agent should be used when "in the opinion of the dental professional, the bonding agent would enhance sealant retention in the clinical situation."[5]

Hypomineralized Enamel

Molars affected by enamel hypomineralization (EH; also referred to as molar-incisor hypomineralization) often present a challenge

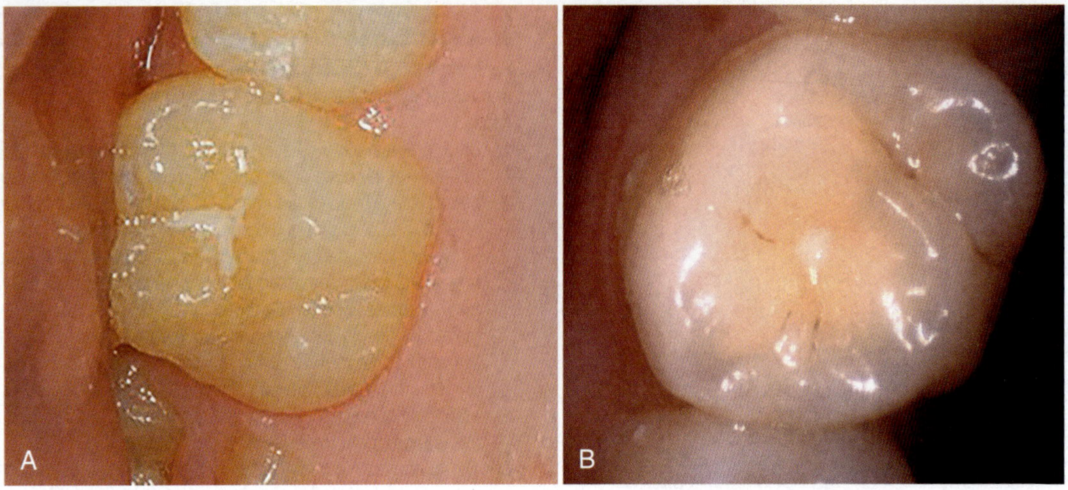

• **Fig. 15.16** (A) Sealant material is missing from the distal pit and lingual groove of this maxillary molar, leaving these areas susceptible to caries. (B) Sealant only remains in the central pit of this maxillary molar. Sealant should be reapplied to radiating fissures, which have acquired stain indicative of incipient caries (no mechanical preparation of this tooth is necessary).

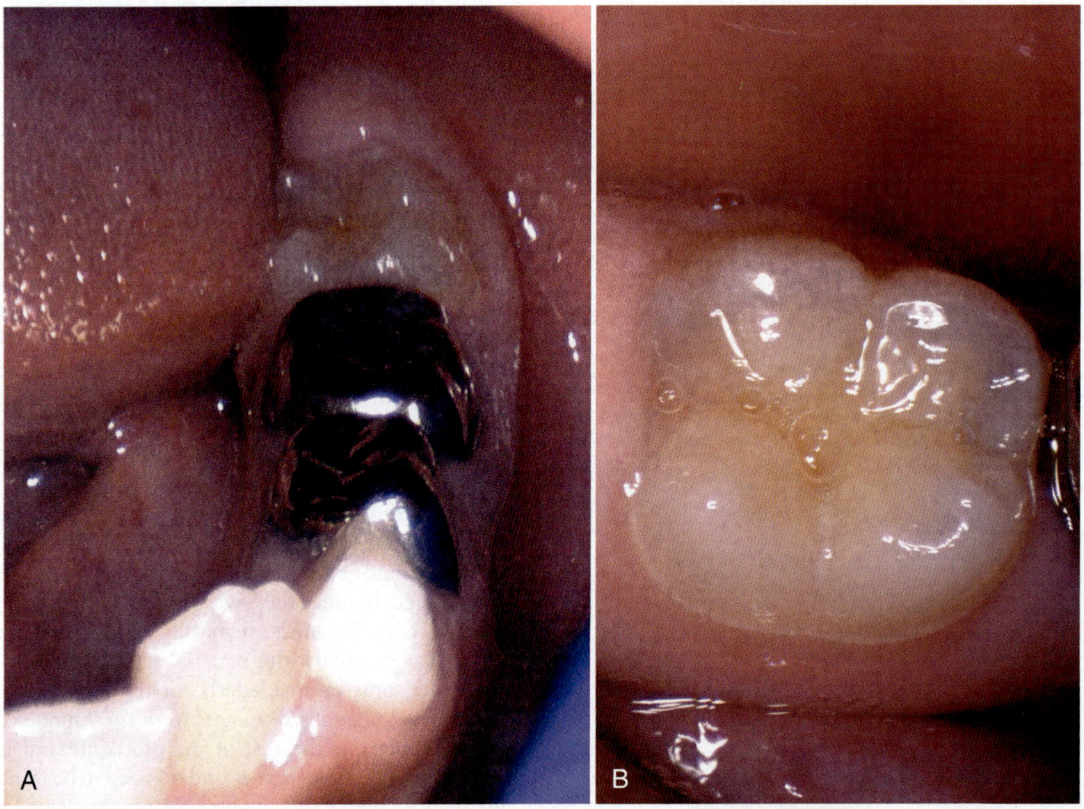

• **Fig. 15.17** (A) The occlusal surface of the permanent molar could benefit from sealant placement in this patient who is at high risk for caries (note the stainless steel crown restorations on the molars). (B) The gingival operculum covers the distal marginal ridge. This tooth will be difficult to isolate for a resin-based sealant. Given the high caries risk of the patient, a sealant should be placed and a glass ionomer sealant is preferred over resin.

for the dentist regarding adhesive dentistry (see Chapter 31). These teeth often have enamel defects and are at higher risk for eventually needing restorative treatment compared with "normal" teeth.[132] Hence these teeth are excellent candidates for preventive efforts. However, research has shown that hypomineralized teeth need to be retreated with resin sealant application after a much shorter time period than teeth in the control group.[133] The addition of a bonding agent with sealant application in hypomineralized teeth can increase fissure sealant retention compared with acid etching alone.[134]

Glass ionomer sealants have been recommended for teeth affected by EH. Glass ionomer sealants have the advantages of moisture tolerance and fluoride release, and they may also decrease hypersensitivity in EH-affected molars, enabling better plaque removal by the patient.[135] In a recent study, glass ionomer sealants significantly decreased the incidence of caries in EH-affected teeth but were not able to prevent posteruptive breakdown (chipping/fracture of weak enamel under masticatory forces),[136] which may require other treatment modalities (see Chapter 31).

Auxiliary Application

Well-trained dental auxiliaries are proficient in applying sealants.[137–139] In studies addressing sealant longevity by operator, researchers found that proper education of personnel and following up on each individual's aptitude in sealant placement are essential, as individual operator, rather than provider type (dentist vs. auxiliary), was correlated to sealant success or failure.[140,141] Both dental assistants and hygienists are as proficient in sealant application as the dentist, and delegating sealant application is cost-effective and results in increased sealant usage.[137]

Four-Handed Delivery

Having an assistant during sealant application may improve the quality and efficiency of sealant placement, improve isolation, shorten placement time, reduce operator fatigue, and enhance patient care. Although no clinical trials have addressed two-handed versus four-handed delivery on the retention of pit and fissure sealants, Griffin et al. found a positive association for four-handed delivery and increased retention rates.[116] When possible, sealants should be applied with the assistance of trained personnel.[5]

School-Based Sealant Programs

School-based sealant programs have been developed to increase sealant usage to reduce caries and to provide prevention services to children less likely to receive dental care, such as those children from minority or low-income backgrounds. School-based sealant programs can (1) help serve low-income children who are at high risk of developing caries and are less likely than their higher-income counterparts to have a dental visit, (2) connect participating students with sources of dental care in the community, and (3) enroll eligible children in public insurance programs.[142] In 2019 approximately 65% of states and the District of Columbia reported having a school-based dental sealant program, which was lower than the 76% reported in 2010.[143] Lack of funding was often cited as a key challenge to expanding school dental sealant programs.

School-based sealant programs save society money and remain cost-effective. According to the Centers for Disease Control and Prevention (CDC), applying sealants in schools to the teeth of nearly 7 million low-income children would prevent more than 3 million cavities and save up to $300 million in dental treatment costs among these children.[11] They are "an important and effective public health approach that complements clinical care systems in promoting the oral health of children and adolescents."[142]

Other Uses for Sealant

Interproximal Dental Sealant

Two techniques can be utilized for sealing interproximal lesions, which have been termed "microinvasive" interventions. The first is to use the same resin sealant material used for occlusal surfaces with phosphoric acid etching, rinsing, applying resin sealant, and light curing. If the lesion is visible, such as the mesial of a permanent first molar when the second primary molar exfoliates, the sealant can be directly applied (Fig. 15.18). Otherwise, orthodontic separators are placed, and the material is applied at a later date when the teeth are separated and the lesion is visible. The second technique is to utilize a resin infiltration system, such as ICON (DMG America, Englewood, NJ). (See Chapter 31 for a more detailed discussion of the technique.) A Cochrane systematic review concluded that microinvasive treatments (i.e., interproximal sealants) arrest noncavitated enamel and early dentinal lesions (limited to the outer third of dentin, Fig. 15.19). These treatments are significantly more effective at arresting lesions compared with other preventive methods like fluoride varnish or recommending flossing.[144] This Cochrane review was completed before the widespread use of silver diamine fluoride (SDF). No head-to-head comparisons exist for which preventive measure (interproximal sealant or SDF application) is more effective at preventing lesion progression.

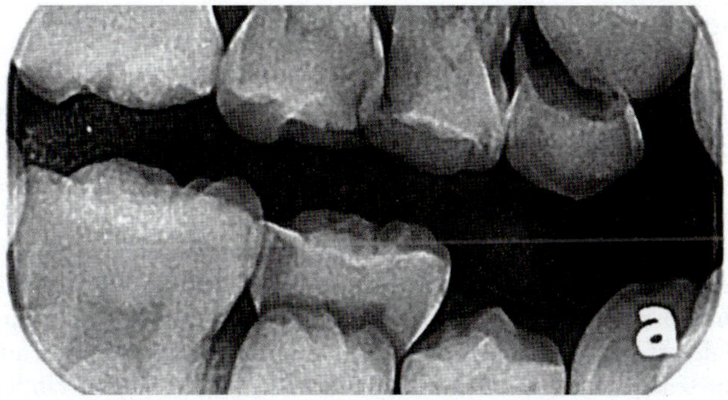

• **Fig. 15.18** This right bitewing shows large caries on the distal of the mandibular primary second molar (tooth K). When this tooth exfoliates, resin-based sealant material could be applied directly to the mesial surface of the permanent first molar (tooth 30).

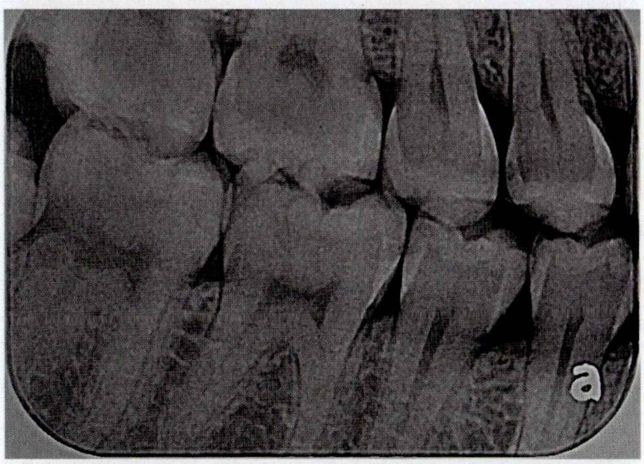

• **Fig. 15.19** Left bitewing of a patient showing interproximal carious lesions confined to enamel on the mesial surface of the mandibular first molar (tooth 30) and distal surface of the second premolar (tooth 29). These teeth would be candidates for resin infiltration compared with the distal lesion on the maxillary first premolar (tooth 4), which is into dentin and requires restoration.

Sealing Restorations

Several studies have shown that restoration longevity can be increased by applying sealant along the margins of both composite and amalgam restorations.[145–147] Mertz-Fairhurst et al. compared conventional amalgams with both sealed amalgam restorations and with sealed composite restorations placed over frank caries without caries removal (only a 1 mm bevel was placed around the lesion in intact enamel). In the 10-year follow-up, they found that the conventional amalgam restorations had the highest occurrence of open margins and the highest rate of recurrent caries, and the sealed amalgams had the best outcomes with only one clinical failure noted in the entire group.[145]

Sealing over restorations significantly reduces microleakage, decreases incidences of recurrent caries, and can increase the longevity of restorations through repair of marginal defects.[148,149] Fig. 15.20 shows a restored mandibular first molar that could have benefited from a sealant placed over the restoration as the patient is experiencing recurrent caries in unfilled fissures and at the margins of the restoration. Several studies have shown success in repairing marginal defects with sealant.[146,149] Serious consideration should be given to repairing marginal defects over replacement of the restoration, because repair is the most conservative treatment option, as it does not result in any further loss of tooth structure and it also lowers the cost of replacement.[149] Practitioners should seal restorations immediately after they are placed[150] and repair margins with a sealant whenever possible.[151] Sealed restorations are superior to unsealed restorations in conserving sound tooth structure, protecting margins, preventing recurrent caries, and prolonging the clinical survival of the restorations.

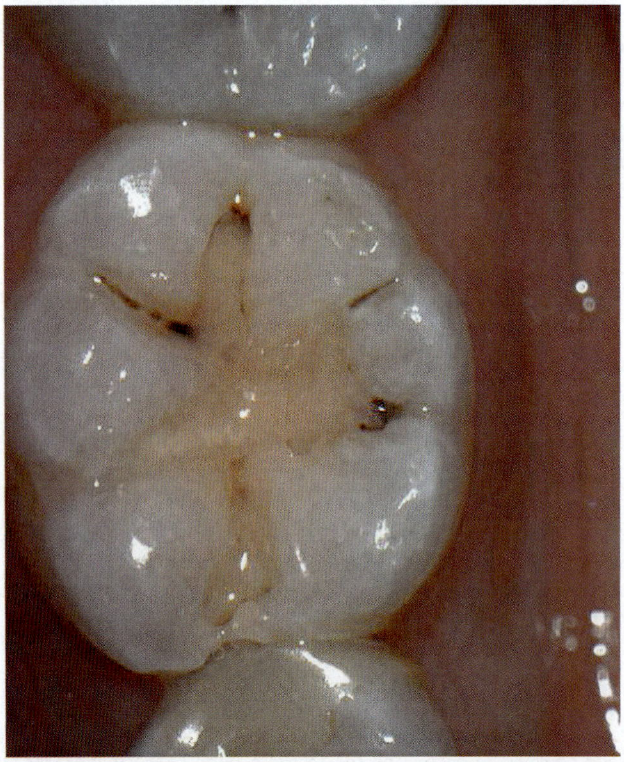

• **Fig. 15.20** Mandibular molar with occlusal composite restoration showing discoloration, staining, and recurrent caries at margins of restoration. Sealing over restorations reduces recurrent caries by reducing microleakage and by sealing susceptible unprepped fissures.

Preventing White Spot Lesions

A complication of poor oral hygiene during orthodontic treatment is the development of demineralized enamel around the orthodontic brackets, commonly called "white spot lesion" (WSL) (see Fig. 15.21). The most recent and comprehensive systematic review evaluating sealants for preventing WSL reviewed 24 studies and showed that use of a sealant significantly decreased the initiation of WSLs compared with its nonuse.[152] No significant difference could be found between fluoride-releasing agents and nonfluoridated agents. Sealants provide a physical barrier that prevents acid diffusion into the enamel and consequently prevents mineral loss.[152] However, the additional time and expense of using sealant to prevent decalcification must be considered. There were many limitations to the studies included such as concerns with subjective scoring or classifying the lesions, short follow-up times, and sealant loss without reapplication. No gold standard prevention strategy of WSLs during orthodontic therapy can be established. However, clinicians could consider using sealants for patients with less than ideal hygiene and those with higher caries risk along with other preventive measures such as oral hygiene instructions and increasing fluoride exposure through fluoride varnish or 5000 parts per million fluoridated toothpaste.

Sealant Safety

In 1996, Olea et al. confirmed the estrogenicity of a bis-GMA–based sealant and detected free BPA in saliva after placement, sparking safety concerns.[153] BPA, a synthetic resin in plastics, is widely present in humans; a CDC study found it in nearly all 2517 tested individuals.[154] Some animal studies link BPA exposure to fetal and infant harm,[155] and the National Toxicology Program has "some concern" about its effects on brain, behavior, and prostate development.

However, BPA exposure from sealants is transient[156] and negligible compared with daily exposure,[157] and poses no known risk.[158] Clinicians can further minimize exposure (see Table 33.2). Given the benefits of resin-based sealants and the fact that BPA exposure from sealants appears transient and can be controlled, concerns about BPA should not discourage their use.[8] Alternatively, glass ionomer could be utilized as has it is similarly effective in preventing caries when compared with resin and contains no plastic components.

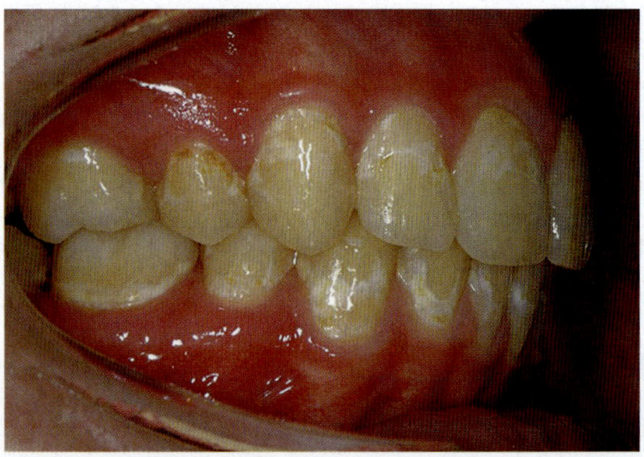

• **Fig. 15.21** Generalized demineralization after orthodontic treatment. (From Cobourne MT, DiBiase AT. *Handbook of Orthodontics*. Mosby; 2010.)

TABLE 15.2 Recommendations to Limit Patient Exposure to Bisphenol A From Resin-Based Dental Sealant

Recommendation	Rationale
Select a product that is BPA-free or one that contains bis-GMA instead of BPA dimethacrylate (bis-DMA)	Saliva can hydrolyze bis-DMA into free BPA
Utilize rubber dam isolation	Ideal isolation will limit exposure
After light curing, rub the surface with pumice on a cotton roll or rinse the sealant for 30 s	The most significant exposure to BPA occurs immediately after sealant placement because residual monomer remains in the unpolymerized, oxygen-inhibited layer

bis-DMA, Bisphenol A diglycidyl ether methacrylate; *bis-GMA*, bisphenol A glycidyl dimethacrylate; *BPA*, bisphenol A.

Future Advances

There is insufficient evidence to establish the best sealant material for caries prevention. Long follow-up time trials are needed to research the effectiveness of different sealant material types. Dental sealants must be applied in a moisture-free environment or they will fail; thus attention can be focused on developing and evaluating the caries-prevention effectiveness of hydrophilic sealants. Additionally, incorporating antibacterial or remineralization properties (such as silver or calcium fluoride nanoparticles) into dental sealant are being studied.[159] New sealant materials should be rigorously evaluated with in vitro and pilot clinical studies before practitioners adopt them into clinical practice. Some practitioners have switched to newer products and been disappointed when, owing to their poor clinical performance, they were removed from the market. Dental professionals should select dental products based on the best available science.

Summary

Extensive research supports sealant efficacy, yet some practitioners report failures. Liebenberg emphasizes the importance of proper technique, material and case selection, and ongoing maintenance to ensure success.[160] However, sealants, when applied correctly, can significantly enhance oral health outcomes.

Visit eBooks.Health.Elsevier.com to see full list of references.

16

Pediatric Diet and Nutrition for Oral Health

TERESA A. MARSHALL

CHAPTER OUTLINE

Normal Nutrition

Normal nutrition refers to the nutritional requirements of the healthy individual, that is the child or adolescent without a metabolic condition or disease affecting their nutrient requirements. Nutrients are substances within foods that provide energy and are necessary to support growth and development. The six major classes of nutrients include carbohydrates, proteins, fats, vitamins, minerals, and water. Foods vary in the type and quantity of nutrients they contain. *Diet* refers to the foods consumed; *dietary pattern* is a term used to describe food intakes characteristic of specific populations.

The Food and Nutrition Board of the National Academy of Sciences regularly evaluates new science to estimate nutrient requirements to prevent nutrient deficiencies, promote health, and prevent diet-related disease.[1] Age- and sex-specific nutrient requirements published as the Daily Reference Intakes (DRIs) include four categories: estimated average requirements (EARs), recommended dietary allowances (RDAs), adequate intakes (AIs), and tolerable upper intake levels (ULs). The Dietary Guidelines for Americans (DGA) are based on the DRIs and provide general guidance on what to eat to promote health, reduce risk of chronic disease, and meet nutrient requirements.[2] The DGA are published by the US Department of Agriculture (USDA) and are used by policymakers to design nutrition-related food programs. MyPlate (Fig. 16.1) is a food guide designed by the USDA to translate the DGA to food recommendations enabling the consumer to select foods containing adequate but not excessive nutrient intakes.[3]

Measures of diet quality have been developed to estimate the extent to which an individual's or population's dietary intake achieves their nutrient requirements while limiting intakes of less desirable food components associated with chronic disease (i.e., added sugars, sodium, saturated fat). Individual foods vary significantly in their proportions of energy and nutrients; the terms *energy-dense* (i.e., foods high in energy) and *nutrient-dense* (i.e., foods high in nutrients) are used to categorize foods based on their nutrient compositions. The Healthy Eating Index (HEI) is a contemporary measure of overall diet quality based on agreement with the DGA.[4] Points are awarded for consuming recommended intakes of desirable foods (i.e., fruits, vegetables) and low intakes of less healthy food components (i.e., added sugars, saturated fat) with higher scores reflecting healthier diets. The overall diet quality of children aged 2 to 17 years in the United States improved between 1999 and 2016[5]; however, the mean HEI score of 50.7 out of 100 suggests that diet quality remained low in 2019 to 2020.[6]

Historically, meal patterns were defined by structured eating events described as meals or snacks. Meals including breakfast,

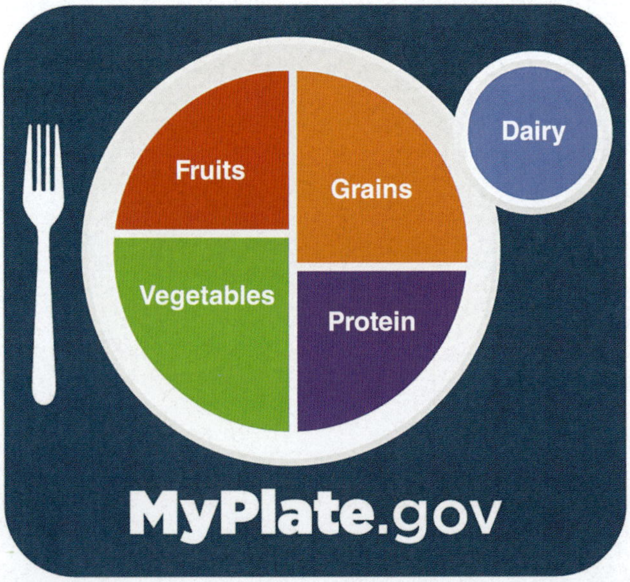

• **Fig. 16.1** MyPlate Food Guide. (Courtesy the USDA [myplate.gov].)

lunch/dinner, and dinner/supper were generally composed of prepared foods representing most food groups, whereas snacks occurring in the morning, afternoon, and evening were simpler selections from one or two food groups. For a variety of reasons, traditional meal patterns have evolved with many individuals consuming fewer meals throughout the day and snacking for extended periods of time. Unstructured meal patterns have been associated with lower overall diet quality and increased intakes of energy-dense foods.[7,8]

Infants, children, and adolescents presenting with metabolic conditions or disease states may require changes to normal nutrition guidance to support their growth and development. Infants having inborn errors of metabolism (e.g., phenylketonuria) are unable to metabolize specific compounds in foods; their food sources are modified to prevent adverse outcomes.[9] Children or adolescents who develop type 1 diabetes must match their carbohydrate intakes to exogenous insulin with consideration for physical activity and illness.[10] Children and adolescents with earlier presentation of chronic systemic disease (i.e., obesity, cardiometabolic disease) might also have specialized dietary patterns.

The DGA and MyPlate provide relatively generalized guidance for choosing a healthy diet. In reality, there are multiple cultural, environmental, and economic factors that influence an individual's food choices. Although the dietary influencers are defined in the nutrition literature, their actual effect on or significance for diet quality is less certain. Common influencers and their nutrition relevance include the following:

1. *Food processing:* Technically, food processing refers to any food preparation (i.e., washing, cooking) that makes foods more edible. Advances in food processing have resulted in the development of energy-dense foods with few, if any, nutrients. The NOVA classification of food processing (Fig. 16.2) has been studied most with respect to diet quality and chronic disease risk.[11] In the NOVA system, unprocessed or minimally processed foods are natural foods with no added sugars, fats, or other compounds.[12] Processed foods are typically combinations of natural foods with some added salt, sugar, and/or fat. Ultraprocessed (UP) foods are composed of substances originating from foods, developed in a laboratory, and/or subject to manufacturing techniques not available to the home cook. As a result, UP foods tend to be higher in added sugars than less processed foods.[13] Examples of UP foods and beverages include sugar-sweetened beverages (SSBs), hot dogs, breakfast cereals, and sweet/savory snack foods. Most dietary guidelines emphasize natural or processed foods and recommend limited UP foods. Although multiple studies have reported associations between UP foods and lower diet quality,[14,15] it is important to remember that some UP foods (e.g., chocolate, ice cream) consumed in limited quantities are appropriate for social and hedonistic purposes.
2. *Organic foods:* The USDA certifies organic foods based on avoidance of synthetic fertilizers and pesticides, antibiotics, or hormones and consideration of growing techniques.[16] Generally, organic farming is more sustainable and has a smaller carbon footprint than conventional farming. The nutritional benefits of organically produced foods is unclear. Furthermore, organic foods generally cost more than conventional foods limiting their accessibility and/or reducing overall fruit and vegetable intakes.
3. *Vegetarian diets:* Vegetarian diets exclude foods containing meat, seafood, and products produced by animals (e.g., milk, eggs) with varying definitions determined by the extent of exclusion. Vegetarian diets consistent with MyPlate recommendations provide adequate energy and nutrient intakes to support growth and development and have been associated with lower risk of systemic disease.[17] The overall quality of a vegetarian diet is determined by food choices; those not consistent with MyPlate and/or composed of UP foods offer few benefits. Children and adolescents following vegetarian diets for weight control purposes are at increased risk of eating disorders.[18]
4. *Food insecurity:* Security is defined by the USDA as "access by all people at all times to enough food for an active, healthy life."[19] Food insecurity is defined as limited or uncertain access to safe and nutritious food to support growth and development and an active and healthy life.[20] Food insecurity is associated with lower-quality diets and increased risk of both oral and systemic disease in children and adolescents.[21–25]

Growth and Development

Physical growth is defined as a gradual increase in weight, length, and head circumference paralleling a standard growth trajectory

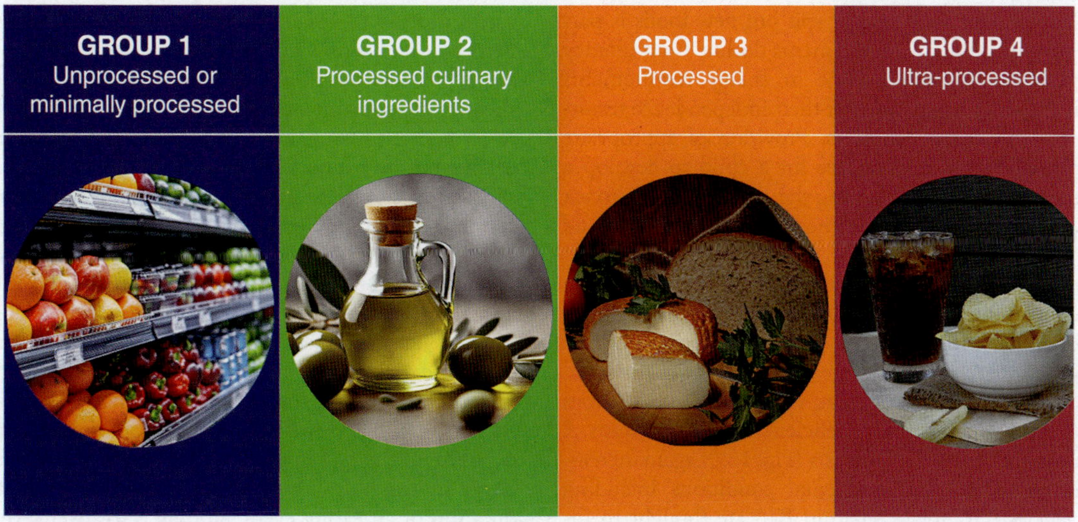
GROUP 1
Unprocessed or minimally processed
GROUP 2
Processed culinary ingredients
GROUP 3
Processed
GROUP 4
Ultra-processed

• **Fig. 16.2** NOVA Classification of Food Processing.

leading to achievement of an adult size consistent with genetic potential. Physical growth is most rapid during infancy with spurts occurring during childhood and adolescence. Development is defined as the progressive physical, emotional, psychological, and cognitive maturation leading to a functional mature state. The balance of healthy versus less healthy food choices throughout infancy, childhood, and adolescence has the potential to enhance or limit physical growth and development. Standardized growth charts are used to monitor growth to ensure that adequate, but not excessive, energy and nutrient intakes are appropriate to achieve expected growth and development.

Nutrient and energy requirements to support physical growth are outlined by the DRIs.[1] The choice of foods and beverages to deliver nutrients is determined by the child's oral motor development.[26,27] Infants are born with rooting and sucking reflexes that require liquid nutrition delivered via a nipple. Although human milk (i.e., breastfeeding) is considered ideal, commercial formulas are designed to meet an infant's nutritional needs. Infants are also born with an extrusion reflex that precludes safe intake of solid foods at birth. As the infant develops, the extrusion reflex relaxes, tongue movements mature, swallowing matures, and head control and sitting skills develop. Achievement of these developmental milestones suggests the infant is ready to transition to solid foods. In addition, intestinal development during this time enables the infant to digest and absorb nutrients from solid foods. Additional development of fine motor skills and lip closure enable the child to finger feed and transition from nipple to cup drinking. Discontinuation of the bottle is appropriate when the toddler can consume adequate liquids by cup. Biting and chewing skills continue to mature throughout early childhood. To prevent risk of choking, large round foods should be cut into small pieces or avoided, and foods should be avoided during active play.

Beyond meeting the nutritional needs for physical growth and development, foods and beverages nurture the infant. Infants bond with their caregivers during the feeding process; regular and adequate nutrition facilitates emotional attachment. Substitution of food for emotional feedback, offering food rewards, and withholding food as punishment can lead to unhealthy relationships with food.[28]

New flavors and textures challenge the toddler's as well as adults' senses; repeated food exposures are often necessary before children are willing to taste and/or eat novel foods.[29] Allowing children to play with the food and/or spit out new foods is part of the learning process. Energy requirements decline from infancy through early childhood; this decline in energy requirements often occurs as the child begins to exert their independence resulting in unpleasant mealtime behaviors. Provision of appropriate foods at appropriate times is necessary for a child to develop a healthy relationship with food; allowing the child to choose to eat or not to eat without parental interference reduces food fights and facilitates the child's independence.[30]

Nutrient and/or energy deficiencies occurring in utero, during infancy, or during childhood can disrupt the development of oral tissues. For example, protein-energy malnutrition might delay tooth eruption, affect tooth size, decrease enamel solubility, and contribute to salivary gland dysfunction, which can increase caries susceptibility.[31] Individual nutrient deficiencies (i.e., vitamins A and D) increase risk of enamel hypoplasia (Fig. 16.3) again increasing caries susceptibility.[31] Environmental conditions including nutrient deficiencies (i.e., folate, vitamin B_{12}) are thought to increase risk of cleft lip and palate disorders in genetically susceptible individuals.[32,33] Thus both prenatal and postnatal nutrition is important for a healthy mouth throughout the entirety of the life cycle.

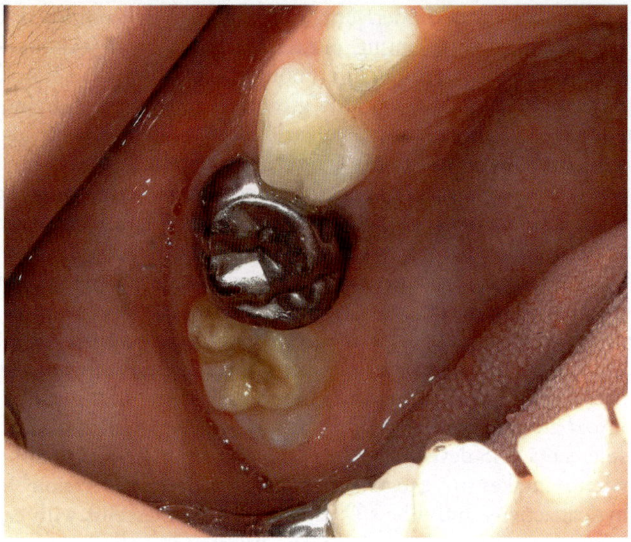

• **Fig. 16.3** Hypomineralized Permanent First Molar in a Child in the Mixed Dentition.

Oral Health and Disease

Oral health is more than the absence of disease; oral health is a component of overall health and well-being. Both the World Dental Federation's and the World Health Organization's definitions emphasize the ability to complete oral functions such as speaking, smiling, and eating with confidence and without pain, discomfort, or embarrassment.[34,35] Oral diseases are abnormalities or conditions that adversely affect oral function, cause oral pain, and impair overall health and well-being. Diet-related oral diseases observed during childhood and adolescence include dental caries, periodontal disease, and tooth wear.

Dental Caries

Fermentable carbohydrates of dietary origin are necessary for the caries process to occur. Fermentable carbohydrates are metabolized by oral bacteria at the tooth surface to produce acid, which then demineralizes the enamel and/or dentin. Although sugars are the primary substrate for oral bacteria, starches are also susceptible to fermentation. Starches that have been altered during food processing for their functional or sensory properties generally contain short glucose chains and are more cariogenic than the original starch. These "modified" starches are a common ingredient in UP foods (i.e., cereals, crackers, snack foods). Baked goods composed of sugars and starches and/or foods that stick to the teeth are retained in the mouth, which can increase their cariogenicity.

Although dietary carbohydrates are essential for the caries process, caries risk is influenced by meal patterns and eating behaviors. Unstructured eating or chronic snacking and eating behaviors, such as holding or swishing beverages in the mouth, will increase exposure of the oral microbiome to the fermentable carbohydrate. Exposure time can be considered a function of the frequency and duration of an eating event; sipping SSBs over several hours prolongs exposure. The prolonged exposure increases the opportunity for carbohydrate fermentation, acid production, and demineralization to occur, thereby increasing caries risk. Toddlers with immature or children with reduced oral motor skills might pocket foods or have reduced oral clearance which can also increase exposure time.

The World Health Organization (WHO) sponsored a systematic review that identified evidence of moderate quality supported a lower caries risk when free sugars intakes were less than 10% of energy consumption, and has recommended that free sugars be restricted to less than 10% of energy intake.[36,37] Similarly, the DGA also recommended that added sugars be restricted to less than 10% total energy to ensure adequate nutrient intake within energy requirements.[2] Between 2001 and 2018, added sugars intakes by children 2 to 8 years of age fell from 15.6% to 12.6% and by adolescents 9 to 18 years from 18.4% to 14.3% of energy requirements, but still exceeded recommendations.[38] Food group recommendations within MyPlate are designed to meet age and sex nutrient requirements; care must be taken to ensure that food selections are primarily composed of few UP foods to limit added sugars intakes.

Early childhood caries (ECC) is defined as the presence of a carious lesion in the primary tooth of a child younger than 5 years of age[39]; the primary risk factor is frequent intake of added sugars including high intakes of SSBs. Although 100% juice does not contain added sugars and most reported research does not support a strong association between 100% juice intakes and ECC,[40,41] 100% juice is an energy-dense, high-sugared beverage containing few nutrients. As such, the American Academy of Pediatrics recommends no 100% juice before 12 months of age, at most 4 oz/day from 12 months through 3 years, and at most 4 to 6 oz from 4 through 6 years.[42] Breastfeeding beyond 12 months of age has also been associated with increased risk of ECC.[43] Unfortunately, the meal patterns and structure of breastfed infants and toddlers have not been thoroughly investigated, and it is unclear as to whether the increased risk is due to the composition of breast milk, nocturnal feedings, frequent exposure, or complementary foods and beverages. Because human milk is considered the gold standard for infant nutrition and easily accessible, recommendations for exclusive breastfeeding through 6 months of age complimented by the introduction of solid foods after 6 months are supported by most public health guidelines.[2,44–46]

Periodontal Disease

Periodontal disease is a chronic disease resulting from the interaction of pathogenic bacteria and the host-inflammatory response. The presence of an inflammatory state at the gingival margin increases risk of both supporting alveolar bone and tooth loss. Although dietary and nutrient factors do not cause periodontal disease, they affect the oral and systemic conditions favoring the disease process. Systemic conditions associated with periodontal disease include obesity and cardiometabolic conditions (e.g., diabetes and cardiovascular disease), which are inflammatory diseases of dietary origin. Thus periodontal disease is a nutrient-related disease. Malnutrition is known to disrupt the oral microbiome, impair tissue health, and compromise the immune system.[47,48] Diets both of low overall diet quality and individual nutrient deficiencies (i.e., vitamins C, D, and B_{12}) have been associated with oral infections and periodontal disease.[47–54] Dietary patterns consistent with MyPlate guidelines meeting energy requirements are appropriate to reduce diet-related risk and/or exacerbation of periodontal disease.

Tooth Wear

Abrasion is a type of mechanical wear associated with repeated contact between teeth and nontooth materials. Abrasion is often observed in individuals with very high intakes of minimally processed whole grains, fruits, and vegetables. Erosion is a chemical process during which internal or external acids dissolve enamel and/or dentin during repeated exposures. Exposure to gastric acid is typically secondary to gastrointestinal reflux, rumination, or repeated vomiting occurring with eating disorders.[55] Ethnic diets high in acidic foods and beverages increase risk of erosion. Similarly, behaviors such as holding or pocketing acid foods or swishing acidic beverages increase exposure and subsequent risk of erosion.

Outcome of Oral Disease

Caries, periodontal disease, and erosion increase risk of tooth loss and oral pain, both of which contribute to oral dysfunction.[56] Oral dysfunction can be defined as impaired biting, oral motility, and swallowing, which negatively influence food choices. An increased reliance on soft foods and beverages that are typically UP and of high energy and low nutrient density compromises overall diet quality. Compromised diet quality (i.e., a diet inconsistent with the DGA or MyPlate recommendations) further exacerbates oral health and compromises systemic health. Diet-related chronic systemic diseases including obesity, cardiometabolic diseases, and cancers share the same dietary risk factors as oral disease. Identification of and addressing diet-related oral risk factors during childhood is necessary to support adult health and well-being. ECC is observed in children with high intakes of added sugars and lower-quality diets, which over time increase risk of diet-related systemic disease. Thus early recognition of ECC presents an opportunity for dietary intervention, disruption of the disease process, and improved overall quality of life throughout adulthood.

Dietary Counseling

The objective of dietary counseling is to improve overall quality of life and well-being by reducing risk of oral and systemic disease. The process involves identification of current food choices and behaviors; medical, social, and environmental factors that influence food choices; and the patient's ability, willingness, and motivation to change current behaviors. All patients should be screened at each appointment to identify dietary habits that increase risk of disease. Patients having dietary behaviors that increase risk or presenting with diet-related oral disease require additional assessment to fully appreciate their overall dietary intake and habits. The assessment provides the foundation for developing dietary recommendations. For children and adolescents, the family food culture should be considered. Caregivers of young children and their children can be interviewed together, whereas adolescents should be interviewed separately from their caregivers to elicit more honest responses.

Pediatric dietary screens focus on factors related to caries risk and diet quality, and include eating frequency and structure, SSB frequency and duration, and compliance with MyPlate. Children who eat more than four to five times per day, lack meal structure, consume SSBs for extended periods of time, and avoid food groups require additional assessment. Additional assessment includes the usual 24-hour daily intake for consideration of meal structure, MyPlate compliance, UP food choices, and beverage choices. For children approximately 6 to 18 months, exploration

TABLE 16.1 Feeding Skills: Birth to 36 Months

Age (mo)	Feeding/Oral Sensorimotor Skills
Birth to 4–6	Nipple feeding, breast or bottle, hand on bottle during feeding (2–4 mo) Maintains semiflexed posture during feeding Promotion of infant-parent interaction
6–9 (transition feeding)	Head and neck control Feeding more in upright position Spoon-feeding thin, pureed foods Both hands to hold bottle Finger feeding of easily dissolvable solids introduced Vertical munching of easily dissolvable solids
9–12	Cup drinking Eats lumpy, mashed food Finger feeding for easily dissolvable solids Chewing includes rotary jaw action
12–18	Self-feeding; grasps spoon with whole hand Holds cup with two hands Drinking with four to five consecutive swallows Holding and tipping bottle
>18–24	Swallowing with lip closure Self-feeding predominates Chewing broad range of food Up-down tongue movements
24–36	Circulatory jaw rotations Chewing with lips closed One-handed cup holding and open cup drinking with no spilling Using fingers to fill spoon Eating wide range of solid food Total self-feeding, using fork

Adapted from Arvedson JC. Swallowing and feeding in infants and young children. *GI Motility Online.* 2006

of feeding skills (Table 16.1), transition to cup drinking, nocturnal feeding (breast or bottle), and mealtime struggles are necessary to facilitate behavioral guidance. For older children and adolescents, exploration of disordered eating, food resources, and the eating environment will facilitate targeted dietary recommendations. Screening household food security status will enable referral for resources enabling patients to comply with recommendations. A two-item screener (Box 16.1) has been validated in the pediatric dental clinic.[57] The screener should only be used if one is prepared to refer to appropriate resources.

After the information gathering stage, relationships between disease risk, food intake, and feeding behaviors should be communicated to the caregiver and their child or adolescent. Consideration of the caregiver's and their child or adolescent's perspective of identified problems is necessary to understand their willingness to consider recommended dietary changes. Healthy dietary behaviors are most successful when supported by caregivers and modeled within the family. When providing recommendations, it is important to acknowledge that changing dietary habits is difficult. Multiple strategies to address dietary behaviors to gradually achieve better habits should be communicated. Prioritization by the pediatric oral healthcare practitioner

• BOX 16.1 Food Security Screener

Questions:

1. "(I/We) worried whether (my/our) food would run out before (I/we) got money to buy more." Was that often true, sometimes true, or never true for (you/your household) in the last 12 months?
   a. Often true
   b. Sometimes true
   c. Never true
   d. Don't know or Refused
2. "The food that (I/we) bought just didn't last, and (I/we) didn't have money to get more." Was that often, sometimes, or never true for (you/your household) in the last 12 months?
   a. Often true
   b. Sometimes true
   c. Never true
   d. Don't know or Refused

Interpretation: Food insecurity is defined by "often true" or "sometimes true" to either question. Food security is defined by "never true" to both questions.

From Radandt NE, Corbridge T, Johnson DB, Kim AS, Scott JM, Coldwell SE. Validation of a 2-item food security screening tool in a dental setting. *J Dent Child (Chic).* 2018;85(3):114-119.

(OHCP), caregiver, and/or child or adolescent of the proposed recommendations is less overwhelming than fixing the entire diet in one swoop. Discussion of barriers and provision of anticipatory guidance will facilitate success. The dietary plan should address factors associated with both oral and systemic disease—they are the same—and include food choices including UP foods, meal patterns, SSB intakes, and use of food rewards. Published oral health-related dietary counseling resources provide more detailed information on added sugars, SSBs, erosion, chairside caries risk, and overall dietary counseling.[27,55,58–62]

The pediatric OHCP is not solely responsible for their patient's dietary choices and should engage with other healthcare and resource providers within their community. The OHCP is responsible for identifying the etiology of the patient's unhealthy dietary choices and/or behaviors, the impact of the unhealthy diet on the patient's health, and the appropriate treatment. The nature and severity of the dietary concern will determine whether the problem is within the OHCP's scope of practice and/or if referral is appropriate. The OHCP's scope of dietary practice includes identifying and addressing diet-related factors associated with oral disease and providing dietary guidance consistent with MyPlate recommendations. Referrals to registered dietitians for in-depth dietary counseling, physicians for undiagnosed medical concerns, counselors for mealtime struggles, eating disorder specialists for suspected eating disorders, and social workers for resources are appropriate to enable change that leads to improved overall quality of life and well-being. Awareness of and referral to government-sponsored food programs (i.e., Special Supplemental Nutrition Program for Women, Infants, and Children [WIC] and Supplemental Nutrition Assistance Program [SNAP]) and local food resources (i.e., food banks, free meal programs) will enable some caregivers to engage with dietary recommendations.

Conclusion

A healthy relationship with food as evidenced by appropriate food choices and dietary behaviors consistent with the DGA and MyPlate is necessary for optimal growth and development.

Food choices high in added sugars and/or of low nutrient density increase risk of both oral and systemic disease and can compromise overall quality of life and well-being. The pediatric OHCP is uniquely suited to identify diet-related oral disease early in the life course, provide dietary counseling, and/or engage with community healthcare professionals to change the disease trajectory and improve their patients' health throughout their life span.

Visit eBooks.Health.Elsevier.com to see full list of references.

17

Radiology for the Pediatric Dental Patient

MIGUEL A. SIMANCAS-PALLARES AND JOHN R. CHRISTENSEN

CHAPTER OUTLINE

Introduction and General Concepts

Imaging constitutes one of the most important diagnostic aids for the dental practitioner. Several imaging modalities are available and usually their recommendations and contraindications are conceived depending on each patient's context, including cooperation in the dental chair, medical history, treatment context (chair vs. general anesthesia [GA]), dental developmental status, presence of malocclusions, severe periodontal disease, dental trauma, clinical evidence of disease, and caries risk. Although understanding the technique for imaging acquisition is of paramount importance for the dental practitioner, often dental assistants and/or radiology technicians will obtain images for the dentist. Detailed concepts and discussions on techniques for image acquisition are beyond the scope of this chapter and can be found in specialized references in the field of oral and maxillofacial radiology. Therefore this chapter will focus on more clinically oriented topics.

As widely known for the pediatric dental patient, several decisions are mediated by the limited cooperation in the chair, which in some scenarios can be linked to a complex medical history. For the safety of the patient, parent/caregiver, dental provider, and their staff, imaging always remains elective, and the comprehensive information gathered from families and supplemented with clinical findings should govern clinical decisions. Patients with limited cooperation in the dental chair and with complex medical history will require dental treatment under GA and in that setting, a full intraoral series of x-rays may be obtained if indicated. Better image quality leads to more ideal dental treatment outcomes.

One of the topics of relevance for the pediatric dental patient has been the dosage of radiation to which the patient is being exposed and its effects on health. Historically, the concern has been tissue reactions and there is growing concern among caretakers regarding this, which has led to many misconceptions, and hesitancy. Furthermore, with the number of radiographs and the dose used to obtain radiographs, there is low to no risk of tissue reactions from dentomaxillofacial radiography.[1] Nevertheless, efforts should be always centered to minimize dose reduction—the historically known ALARA (as low as reasonably achievable) principle that should always guide imaging decisions. Extensively described in the dental radiology literature, dose-reduction efforts typically include adequate selection criteria, collimation (i.e., rectangular), type of image receptors and exposure optimization (i.e., photostimulable phosphor [PSP] x-ray plate or digital sensor), and shielding. Recent recommendations from the American Academy of Oral and Maxillofacial Radiology on patient shielding during dentomaxillofacial radiography suggest discontinuing the routine patient shielding including pediatric patients.[1–10] These recommendations stem from the fact that external scattered radiation is limited by using beam collimation, and lead aprons do not reduce dose from internal scattered radiation. In addition to this, the size and weight of lead aprons (especially in young patients with questionable cooperation in the chair) could lead to motion during imaging introducing artifacts in the obtained x-ray. Although publicly available, these recommendations are rather recent and the rates of adoption in private practice and university-based setting across the United States remains unknown.

A routine question the clinician should ask themselves while in the decision-making process of diagnosis and treatment planning and considering obtaining radiographs is "will this radiograph change my treatment?" Often, the comprehensive information gathering steps and the exercise of asking and answering this question will help in the process of imaging acquisition after safe radiation principles resulting in an increased diagnostic value of the radiograph. It is important to keep in mind that in some clinical scenarios (e.g., traumatic dental injuries [TDIs]) obtaining radiographs at initial and follow-up encounters is strongly recommended as they are part of the guidelines for assessment and management. In the case of an initial encounter, this can facilitate, for instance, the detection of root fractures. Imaging obtained at TDI follow-up visits can facilitate the detection of sequelae such as root resorption or pulp necrosis, therefore changing the patient's prognosis and long-term management options.[11–13]

There are widely known and accepted recommendations for radiograph prescription for the pediatric dental patient. These guidelines have been developed using expert panel consensus via cross-collaboration across several dental organizations and have been endorsed by the American Academy of Pediatric Dentistry (AAPD).[14] In this algorithm (Table 17.1), two main domains are taken into consideration while prescribing dental imaging including:

1. *Patient age and dental developmental stage:* Child with primary dentition, child with mixed dentition, adolescent with permanent dentition, and adult, dentate or partially edentulous
2. *Type of encounter:* New patient examination (NPE), recall patient, and patient with other circumstances such as monitoring for growth and development relevant conditions or periodontal diseases

A logical combination of these factors then formulates several recommendations for different types of dental radiographs (e.g., periapical, bitewing, panoramic), and time intervals at which they should be obtained. The NPE is usually the timepoint where the highest possible amount of information is gathered from the patient and family. In some cases, patients are being referred from other practices where radiographs were previously obtained. In these circumstances, the clinician should make every effort to obtain these images and, whenever possible, use them in the decision-making process of obtaining new images (or deferring them until the next visit). These guidelines should be only conceived as recommendations; final decisions on the number and type of x-rays should be left to the discretion of the clinician after taking into consideration the findings from the clinical examination. It is suggested that radiographs should always follow a clinical examination.

Depending on the positioning of the receptor, dental radiographs can be broadly classified into two main types: (1) intraoral (periapical and bitewing) and (2) extraoral (panoramic and cephalometric). Essentially, intraoral imaging relies on the placement of a receptor inside the oral cavity. Newer imaging technologies with superior diagnostic capabilities (cone beam computed tomography [CBCT]) are more readily available to the dental practitioner and will be reviewed in this chapter.

Intraoral Imaging Modalities

Periapical Radiograph

The periapical radiograph image is one of the most commonly obtained radiographs in dentistry, especially in the presence of positive historical or clinical signs/symptoms[15] (Fig. 17.1). It adds

TABLE 17.1 Initial Imaging Recommendations Based on Type of Encounter

Type of Encounter (New or Recall Visit)	Child With Primary Dentition (Before Eruption of First Permanent Tooth)	Child With Transitional Dentition (After Eruption of First Permanent Tooth)	Adolescent With Permanent Dentition (Before Eruption of Third Molars)	Adult, Dentate or Partially Edentulous
New Patient Evaluation	Individualized radiographic examination with periapical or occlusal views or posterior bitewing radiographs if proximal surfaces cannot be visualized or probed. Patients without evidence of disease and with open proximal contacts may not require a radiographic examination.	Individualized radiographic examination consisting of posterior bite-wing radiographs with panoramic examination or posterior bite-wing radiographs and selected periapical images.	Individualized radiographic examination consisting of posterior bite-wing radiographs with panoramic examination or posterior bite-wing radiographs and selected periapical images. A full-mouth intraoral radiographic examination is preferred when the patient has clinical evidence of generalized oral disease or a history of extensive dental treatment.	Individualized radiographic examination consisting of posterior bite-wing radiographs with panoramic examination or posterior bite-wing radiographs and selected periapical images. A full-mouth intraoral radiographic examination is preferred when the patient has clinical evidence of generalized oral disease or a history of extensive dental treatment.
Recall Visit, Patient With No Clinical Caries and Not at Increased Risk of Developing Caries	Posterior bite-wing examination at 12- to 24-m intervals if proximal surfaces cannot be examined visually or with a probe.	Posterior bite-wing examination at 12- to 24-m intervals if proximal surfaces cannot be examined visually or with a probe.	Posterior bite-wing examination at 18- to 36-mo intervals.	Posterior bite-wing examination at 24- to 36-mo intervals
Recall Visit, Patient With Clinical Caries or at Increased Risk of Developing Caries	Posterior bite-wing examination at 6- to 12-mo intervals if proximal surfaces cannot be examined visually or with a probe.	Posterior bite-wing examination at 6- to 12-mo intervals if proximal surfaces cannot be examined visually or with a probe.	Posterior bite-wing examination at 6- to 12-mo intervals if proximal surfaces cannot be examined visually or with a probe.	Posterior bite-wing examination at 6- to 18-mo intervals.

Continued

TABLE 17.1 Initial Imaging Recommendations Based on Type of Encounter—cont'd

Type of Encounter (New or Recall Visit)	Child With Primary Dentition (Before Eruption of First Permanent Tooth)	Child With Transitional Dentition (After Eruption of First Permanent Tooth)	Adolescent With Permanent Dentition (Before Eruption of Third Molars)	Adult, Dentate or Partially Edentulous
Recall Visit, Patient With Periodontal Disease	Clinical judgment as to the need for and type of radiographic images for evaluation of periodontal disease. Imaging may consist of, but is not limited to, selected bite-wing or periapical images of areas where periodontal disease (other than nonspecific gingivitis) can be found clinically.	Clinical judgment as to the need for and type of radiographic images for evaluation of periodontal disease. Imaging may consist of, but is not limited to, selected bite-wing or periapical images of areas where periodontal disease (other than nonspecific gingivitis) can be found clinically.	Clinical judgment as to the need for and type of radiographic images for evaluation of periodontal disease. Imaging may consist of, but is not limited to, selected bite-wing or periapical images of areas where periodontal disease (other than nonspecific gingivitis) can be found clinically.	Clinical judgment as to the need for and type of radiographic images for evaluation of periodontal disease. Imaging may consist of, but is not limited to, selected bite-wing or periapical images of areas where periodontal disease (other than nonspecific gingivitis) can be found clinically.

From Erika Benavides, DDS, PhD et.al., American Dental Association and American Academy of Oral and Maxillofacial Radiology patient selection for dentalradiography and cone-beam computed tomography Clinical recommendations. JADA 157(1),

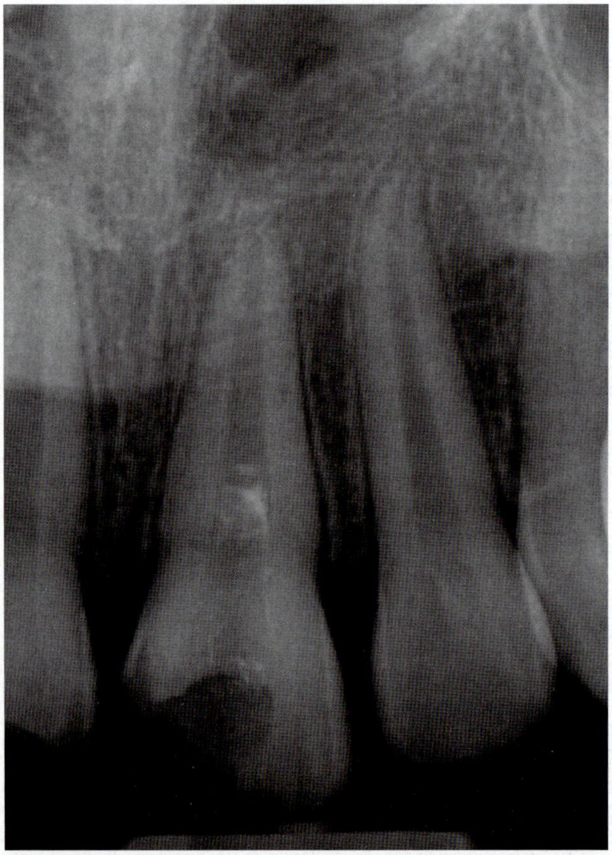

• **Fig. 17.1** Periapical x-ray obtained in a 12-year-old patient with positive history of traumatic dental injury. Teeth #8 through 12 are visible. Bone levels are nonaltered; however, there is discontinuity of lamina dura visible on the mesial aspect of tooth #9. Furthermore, the periodontal ligament space is widened, more so in the distal aspect of the root of tooth #9. A periapical lesion is visible apical to tooth #9. Complicated crown fractures are visible on teeth #8 and 9 and no caries lesions are visible.

diagnostic value in a myriad of clinical scenarios such as TDIs, large cavitated caries lesions in close proximity to the pulp, identification of possible congenitally missing teeth, and treatment (e.g., root canal therapy). For anterior teeth, it is usually obtained in a vertical orientation, whereas for posterior teeth it is usually obtained using a horizontal orientation. Sizing of the receptor should be kept in mind because in very young children the largest size in a vertical orientation can be uncomfortable; however, when oriented horizontally (rotated 90 degrees) for anterior teeth in this same age group it becomes extremely useful and can be regarded as an occlusal radiograph (Fig. 17.2).

Once obtained, it displays a considerable amount of information that is relevant to the dental practitioner. Although a periapical radiograph can be obtained with a particular indication (e.g., to determine the severity of a cavitated caries lesion), all structures that are visible should be interpreted. Typically, the periodontal apparatus, the dentin-pulp complex, and adjacent structures are visible. Basic gross anatomy, dental anatomy, and histology knowledge are necessary for their correct interpretation. As a systematic approach for the interpretation of periapical radiographs, every clinician should account for the following:

1. *Quality of the projection:* The goal is to obtain a quality image that enhances its diagnostic value. The use of positioning devices and the correct time and dose of exposure are of paramount importance. For a periapical radiograph, ideally, the target dental organ that is being exposed should be centered in the image, adjacent anatomical structures should be visible, and there should be a relatively equal distribution of adjacent anatomical structures mesially and distally. No overlaps or foreshortening should be detected, and the dose should be standardized for adequate exposure.
2. *Teeth that are present:* Identify all visible teeth, and a distinction should be made between primary and permanent teeth. A clinical correlation should immediately be made if anomalies in number are detected.
3. *Periodontal apparatus:* Periodontal structures visible in a periapical radiograph include bone, periodontal ligament (PDL)

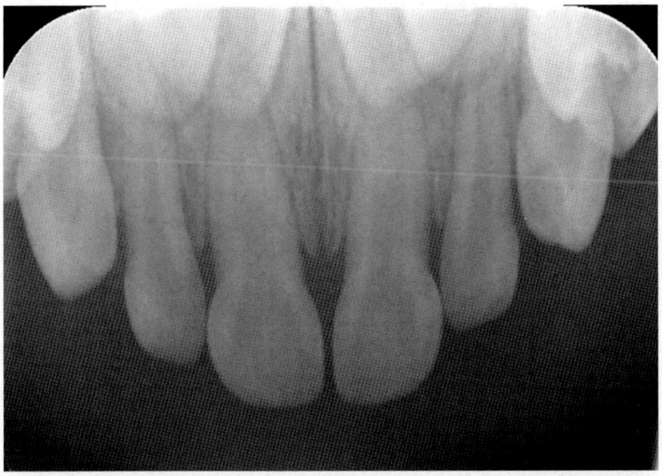

• **Fig. 17.2** Occlusal x-ray from a primary dentition patient (3-year-old) with a positive history of traumatic dental injury. Bone levels are unaltered. There are no visible periodontal findings, and no root fractures are visible. There are no periapical lesions. There are no visible caries lesions.

space (visible as radiolucent because the PDL is all collagen fibers), and lamina dura. On a healthy tooth, there should be no detectable bone loss, and no discontinuity of the lamina dura. On permanent teeth that are fully erupted and in occlusion, the attachment of the periodontal apparatus is already established, therefore a physiologic distance of 0 to 2 mm (between bone crest and cementoenamel junction [CEJ]) is usually visible and this should *not* be considered as bone loss. On partially erupted permanent teeth, this distance often appears to be higher and with the bone crest oriented in an oblique direction rather than a horizontal direction. This finding should not be considered pathologic; a similar situation is often observed for fully erupted primary teeth (Fig. 17.3).

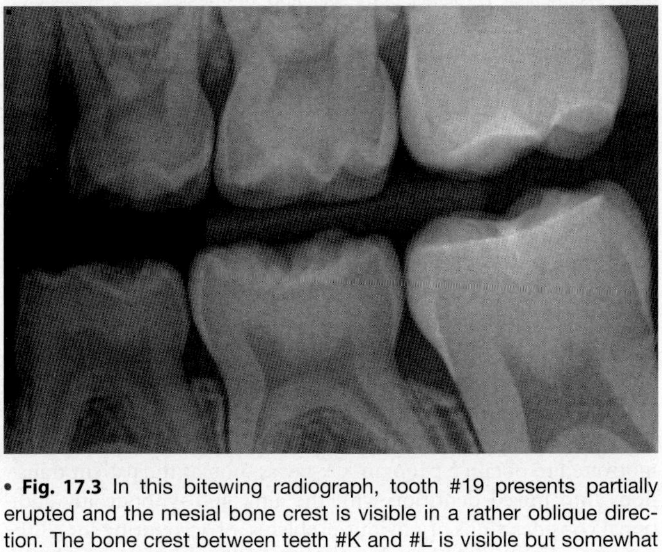

• **Fig. 17.3** In this bitewing radiograph, tooth #19 presents partially erupted and the mesial bone crest is visible in a rather oblique direction. The bone crest between teeth #K and #L is visible but somewhat lower compared with those of fully erupted permanent teeth. None of these findings should be considered compatible with bone loss due to periodontal disease.

4. *Dentin-pulp complex:* The clinician should inspect the appearance of dentin and pulp, especially in the context of deep caries lesions, and teeth with history of TDI wherein pulp canal obliteration (PCO) can be seen. The visible pulp chamber might appear altered in size, which is commonly known as taurodontia (hyper or hypotaurodontism can be visible). Another finding of relevance includes the presence of pulp stones, but this is not necessarily of concern and it is not particularly frequently seen in the pediatric population.
5. *Caries lesions:* Dental radiographs are of high diagnostic value in the detection of caries lesions of proximal surfaces of teeth that have closed contacts. These can be confined to enamel or can extend into dentin as well. A further classification can divide enamel (E) into thirds (1, 2, and 3) and classify lesions accordingly as E1, E2, and E3, wherein E1 is the outermost enamel third and E3 is the innermost (i.e., closer to dentin-enamel junction [DEJ]) enamel third. A similar classification can be applied for those lesions extending into dentin and commonly referred as D1 (outermost dentin third—in contact with enamel DEJ), D2 or D3 (innermost dentin third in contact with the pulp chamber). This coupled with widely known systems for visual caries detection and assessment (International Caries Detection and Assessment System [ICDAS]) can be useful during treatment planning stages.

A special clinical scenario where periapical radiographs gain significant value for diagnosis, treatment planning, and prognosis is during TDIs. In these cases, it is recommended to obtain multiple radiographs.[2] The International Association for Dental Traumatology (IADT) guidelines, and endorsed by the AAPD,[13] recommend the following radiographs:

1. One parallel radiograph aimed through the midline to show the two maxillary central incisors
2. Two parallel radiographs aimed at the lateral incisors (one each and should also show the canine and central incisor)
3. One maxillary occlusal radiograph
4. At least one parallel radiograph of lower incisors

However, the clinician should always evaluate each case and determine the best set of images that can be obtained for the patient. Although three radiographs are not necessarily the recommendation, having multiple images will increase the clinician's ability to detect these additional findings.[11] Along these lines, a set of radiographs that can be obtained during TDIs is as follows:

1. *A long-cone periapical of the injured area:* This radiograph will provide a general visualization of the injured hard tissues and has increased value to quantify the severity of luxation (when present). Horizontal root fractures are usually visible in this projection.
2. *A long-cone periapical with the cone in either a mesial or distal angulation (15 degrees):* This radiograph provides additional value when a root fracture has been suspected. If the findings are consistent in both (long-cone and long-cone with mesial or distal angulation) radiographs, this projection will then confirm (or rule out) the presence of a root fracture. During interpretation steps, the dentist should keep in mind in which direction the cone was positioned.
3. *A soft tissue (lip) radiograph:* It is common for TDIs, especially those that present with crown/alveolar fractures, to result in embedded tooth or bony fragments in the lip. A soft tissue radiograph provides additional diagnostic value. The film (usually size no. 2) is positioned between the lip and the facial surfaces of the injured teeth. The tooth/bone fragments will usually be visible as radiopaque findings.

Bitewing Radiograph

This image has been historically used during new patient or recall examinations *to determine the presence of noncavitated interproximal caries lesions* when contacts are closed; however, this image should not be regarded with that sole purpose as it contains a substantial amount of information that could be useful for the clinician during the examination.[14–17] Typical sizes are available (for PSP plates): 0 (22 × 35 mm); 1 (24 × 40 mm), 2 (31 × 41 mm), 3 (27 × 54 mm), and 4 (57 × 76 mm), where sizes 0 and 1 are the most useful for very young patients. Sensors are of similar size; however, the sensitive area of the receptor is usually smaller compared with PSP. As a rule, if contacts are closed and first permanent molars have not erupted, either a size 0 or 1 should suffice for the needs of bitewing examination. If the contacts are closed, and the first permanent molars have erupted into occlusion, then every effort should be made to obtain bitewing radiographs using a size 2 sensor because it will render information with the highest diagnostic value over the entire buccal segment. If second permanent molars have not erupted, two bitewings (one on each side) generally suffice, and ideally, they capture from the distal surface of the canine to the mesial surface of the first permanent molar (Fig. 17.4). If second permanent molars have erupted and are in occlusion, then four bitewings (two on each side) should be obtained; usually, the mesial bitewing radiograph captures the distal surface of the canine, and the distal bitewing radiograph should capture the distal surface of the second permanent molar. Although premolars are visible on both projections, the difference lies in that usually the mesial image will be rendered without overlaps in contacts in premolars and the distal image will be rendered without overlapping in the molars. The presence of overlap can hinder the clinician's ability to detect noncavitated interproximal caries lesions. Although newer systems such as PSP and sensors work better compared with conventional films, PSP plates have better diagnostic value compared with sensors for assessment of caries lesions (present or not).[18] However, to evaluate lesion severity, sensors might have improved value. Although useful in some circumstances, enhancement features have not been routinely recommended. As there is no overall superiority of one system over the other, the clinician should make every effort to logically use systems and their features as indicated for each patient and each context. In general, the amount of radiation exposure is diminished using PSP or sensors compared with traditional dental films. There is a 50% to 70% reduction in radiation exposure to the patient, a reduction in time between exposure and image generation, elimination of chemical processing of radiographs, and the ability to electronically store patient records. The provider can manipulate the image to provide a clear diagnostic image.[19] Interpretation of a bitewing radiograph should follow the same domains as recommended for periapical radiographs:

1. *Quality of the projection:* The clinician should assess that proportionally the image is displaying the same amount of information for upper and lower teeth. There should be no overlaps or foreshortening.
2. *Teeth that are present:* Examine that for the patient's age and dental developmental status, there are no anomalies in number.
3. *Periodontal anatomy:* Examine lamina dura, bone levels, and furcal space.
4. *Dentin-pulp complex:* Examine presence of pulp stones, PCO, or taurodontism.
5. *Caries lesions:* Examine the presence of interproximal noncavitated caries lesions. If indicated make a distinction for E1, E2 versus E3 lesions and D1, D2, versus D3 lesions.

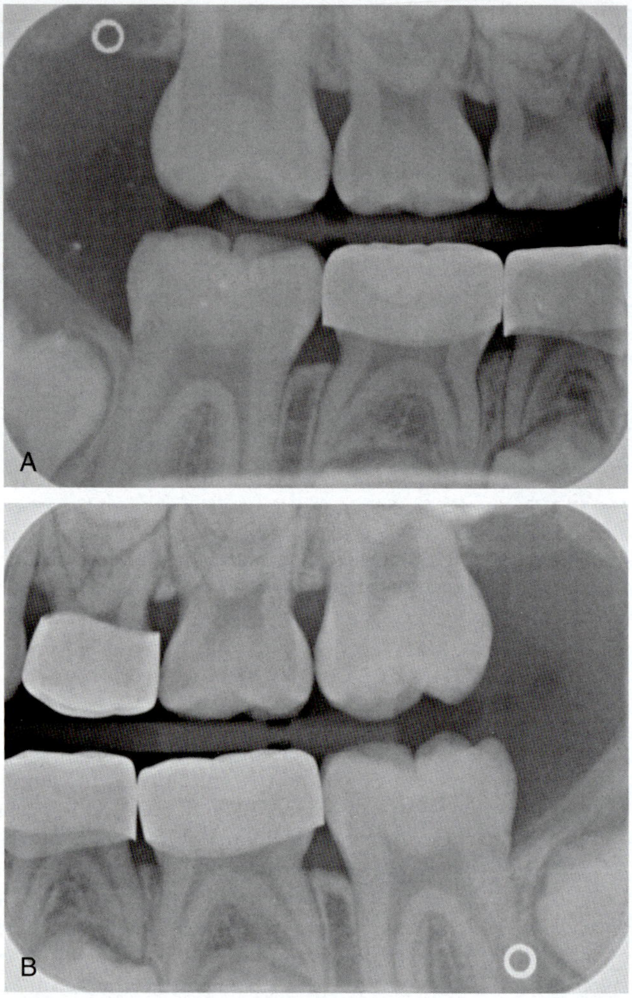

• **Fig. 17.4** (A–B) Two bitewing radiographs obtained in a 7-year-old patient during routine recall examination. Overall, there is good quality of this projection as distal surfaces of upper canines are visible and it also captures the mesial surface of first permanent molars. Overall periodontal structures are without any anomalies and there is no periapical pathology visible. Incipient interproximal caries lesions are visible on teeth #A (mesial), B (distal), J (mesial), and 14 (mesial).

Extraoral Imaging Modalities

Panoramic Radiograph

A panoramic radiograph (Fig. 17.5) is a more comprehensive type of examination given its ability to capture all intraoral structures and some of the extraoral structures.[20] It becomes useful in cases where the clinician is concerned about possible missing teeth, position of third molars, the relationship of teeth with adjacent structures, position of teeth, history of dental trauma where condylar injury (i.e., fracture) is highly suspected, and in cases that would manifest with osseus involvement such as ameloblastoma or florid cemento-osseous dysplasia (FCOD).[20–23] Often, the dentist is motivated to obtain a panoramic x-ray as soon as the patient transitions into mixed dentition with the aim, and without any additional considerations or obvious problems, of accounting for all the permanent teeth.[24] Although current guidelines do endorse obtaining a panoramic radiograph when first permanent molars erupt, a *person-centered* plan is encouraged. Given the low prevalence of

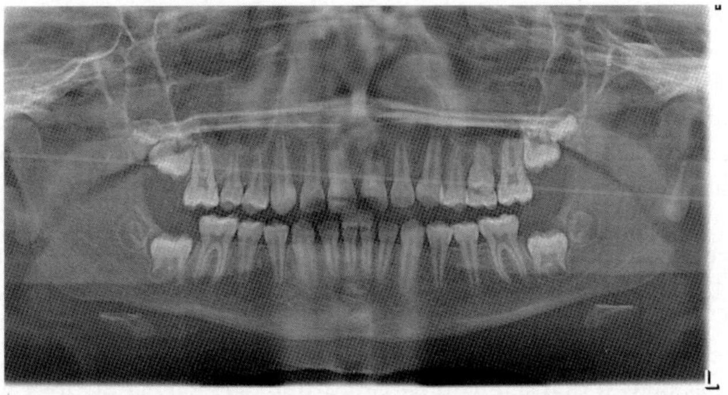

• **Fig. 17.5** Panoramic radiograph obtained in a 10-year-old patient with positive history of traumatic dental injury. Condyles appear unaltered, sinuses appear to be free of pathoses, and the septum is not deviated. Right below the mandible, the hyoid bone is visible. Bone levels appear to be unaltered. All permanent teeth (including third molars) are present and tooth #J is still present and visible. Crown fractures of teeth #8 and #9 are visible. Findings of permanent teeth in development are consistent with the patient's dental developmental status.

abnormalities in (tooth) number, and very little intervention strategies would be indicated at that age, a strong justification for obtaining a panoramic x-ray in this age group should be presented. Although it is understood that at the dosing dentomaxillofacial radiographs are obtained they represent negligible adverse health outcomes, it is strongly discouraged that the dentist would obtain a panoramic radiograph without proper indication or for routine purposes (ALARA principle). Routinely obtained bitewings and/or periapical radiographs should be the first step in the algorithm for deciding when to obtain a panoramic x-ray; if abnormal findings are seen on routine intraoral imaging, then a panoramic radiograph may be considered. In some cases, and upon clinically observed abnormalities, a panoramic x-ray should suffice all radiographic examination for a patient. One example is the adolescent patient where routine bitewing examination is indicated but understanding of the position of third molars is also indicated.[25] If this is the case and given the geometry of the projection due to the position of the teeth, it should be noted that although a panoramic x-ray is not the most ideal imaging to determine the presence of interproximal caries lesions because of overlap, it can be useful when no clinical evidence of caries lesions are visible and with the aim to decrease the dose of radiation. In patients that are candidates for orthodontic treatment, undergoing growth evaluations, and/or in active orthodontic treatment, several panoramic x-rays (in conjunction with other extraoral imaging) are periodically obtained with the aim to diagnose and treatment plan or to monitor for outcomes of the indicated orthodontic therapy. A consideration should be kept for young patients where a panoramic radiograph is indicated because it requires the patient to be able to remain still without moving. Artifacts can be introduced thus hampering the diagnostic value of this radiograph. Another consideration is patients with special healthcare needs (SHCN)—given the technical considerations at acquisition, modifications to the setup including parental presence or larger facilities to accommodate a wheelchair should be considered.

The interpretation of a panoramic radiograph should follow a systematic and comprehensive approach. The "outside-in" approach is often recommended. This system calls for interpretation of structures starting at the outermost structures such as condyles (shape and any evidence of fracture), sigmoidal notch (shape), coronoid process (shape), ramus and body of the mandible, and bone levels. In the maxilla, the status of the maxillary sinuses and nasal septum should be interpreted. Radiologic manifestations that suggest pathologic processes of the sinuses can be visible. The innermost structures to be interpreted include teeth that are present (a systematic approach asks the dentist to count every tooth visible and make distinction between primary and permanent teeth), their position, and any shape anomalies. Findings such as hypertaurodontism or hypercementosis can be visible. The dentist should be able to offer the patient a basic interpretation of the image. If findings indicate the possible presence of pathology that would require intervention, a consultation with an oral and maxillofacial radiologist should be obtained.

Cephalometric Radiograph

A cephalometric radiograph is essentially a projection of the craniofacial structures (cranial vault). Depending on its projection, it can be anteroposterior (AP) or lateral (Fig. 17.6). With the advent of specialized imaging such as CBCT, which renders a three-dimensional (3D) reconstruction of the maxillofacial structures, a cephalometric image is not always indicated because these devices can render a cephalometric radiograph as well. If indicated, the AP cephalometric radiograph, with its subsequent quantitative analysis, yields diagnostic value in patients with marked transverse asymmetry. The most used projection is the lateral (tip of the nose to occipital bone visible) image and it has high diagnostic and prognostic value for orthodontic reasons. The patient should remain standing in the so-called *natural head position* and a visualization of the head, maxilla, mandible, and some cervical vertebrae are displayed. Often, young patients move their head and technical adjustments must be considered at the time of quantitative analysis.

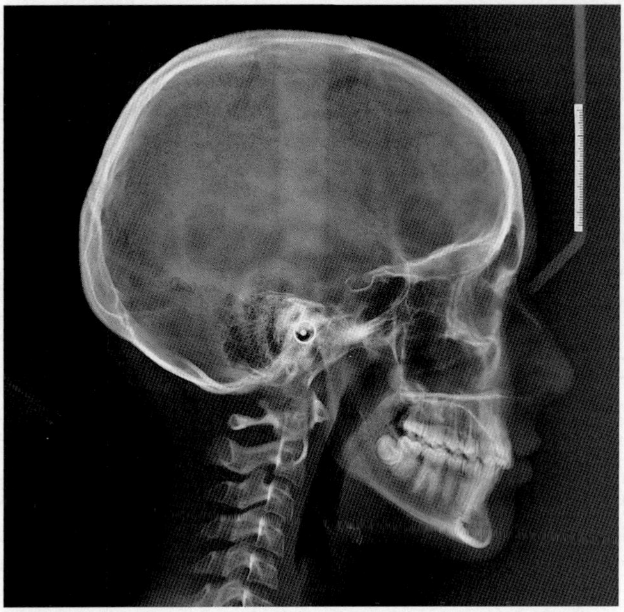

• **Fig. 17.6** Lateral cephalometric radiograph. In the upper right section, the reader can appreciate a ruler. This is intentional as this image is often processed using imaging software for cephalometric analyses. These devices serve in the process of calibration during import of the image (first technical step). The radiograph displays cranial vault, maxilla, mandible, hyoid bone, and vertebrae C1 through C4. A slightly radiopaque projection of the patient's soft tissues is also visible. Using the cervical vertebrae maturation method, this patient can be classified as stage 3.

Although not entirely indicated for these purposes, adjacent soft tissues to these structures can be visible as well. The most common indication of this image is for growth and development reasons; it is useful for patients that are candidates for orthodontic treatment (interceptive or comprehensive), who are in active orthodontic treatment, or who are candidates for orthognathic surgery. There are two main purposes for a cephalometric radiograph: the first is to understand the relationships of the maxilla and mandible with respect to the cranial base, and the second is to quantify growth and treatment changes. Given its projection (lateral), this image is not indicated to understand anomalies in tooth number or in shape or size, or bone levels and any other pathology. Orthodontic records is a term used to document the baseline or progression of patients during treatment and usually encompasses a panoramic and a cephalometric radiograph. Individualized considerations may include a CBCT, which will be discussed in the subsequent section.

The dentist should be able to offer an overall interpretation of the findings of a cephalometric (lateral) radiograph to classify the patient's skeletal relationships as class I, class II, or class III. Cephalometric lateral radiographs require a comprehensive and systematic interpretation from an orthodontist. With the advances of specialized software (Dolphin Imaging, Dolphin Orthodontic Imaging & Management Software, Chatsworth, CA) an interpretation can be offered. The first step is to determine whether the image meets all technical standards such as no artifacts and correct head position. The software allows digitization of an image calibrated to use accurate units of measurement and selected anatomical points of reference. The software also allows the selection of the patient's race and ethnicity considerations as there are variations in the normative values among population groups. The dentist is also able to select the template for cephalometric analysis (preferred method of analysis). A careful analysis of the numerical outputs is performed, although these numerical values should not dominate the interpretation and treatment decisions for the patient. An integrative look of all diagnostic records should be put in place to guide diagnosis and treatment planning. As mentioned earlier, it is often recommended that growing patients (candidates or in active orthodontic care) undergo periodic (on average every year) cephalometric lateral radiographs to better understand growth and treatment changes. For the growing patient, there is value to analyze the stages of cervical vertebral maturation to determine where in the growth stage the patient stands (cervical vertebrae maturation method).[26]

Cone Beam Computed Tomography (CBCT)

Thus far, all imaging modalities that have been discussed in this chapter render a bidimensional image of 3D structures and this imposes numerous limitations for diagnosis and treatment planning. Tomographies are not new. They have been available in medicine for decades. However, the fields of view for medical tomographies did not necessarily apply to dentomaxillofacial structures as it imposed greater doses. CBCT is the type of imaging that overcomes these limitations with minimal radiation dosing. A 3D reconstruction of the desired dentomaxillofacial structure is rendered with adequate accuracy.

CBCT has become an important imaging tool in contemporary dentistry.[27–30] The use of CBCT imaging in the pediatric dental patient is usually limited until patients begin to transition into permanent dentition. This type of imaging becomes more useful in this age group and in adolescence. There has been extensive debate on how often this image should be used. The debate has not been about the information gained but about the amount of radiation needed (dose) to image the patient. Different machines expose the patient to varying amounts of radiation.[2] There is a uniform agreement that newer machines reduce the amount of radiation needed by limiting the size of the field of view.

CBCT imaging is used to assess the health and position of teeth, supporting structures, and temporomandibular joints (TMJs) after dental trauma (Fig. 17.7). The image can establish if a tooth and bone are injured or if fractures are present. It can determine the location and morphology of the fracture. Guidelines suggest that standard periapical and occlusal radiographs are sufficient for most cases, but as radiation exposure decreases from this technique, CBCT may become the standard in practice in the future. Images obtained shortly after trauma are used to assess the extent of the trauma and help determine the treatment plan and prognosis of injured tissues. After the traumatic incident, CBCT imaging provides a tool to measure the effectiveness of the initial treatment and the current state of healing and potential treatment options.

CBCT is also used to assess the volume of the airway in children with obstructive sleep apnea (OSA) and other airway issues. Currently, there is significant interest in this area to see if CBCT is a reliable screening, diagnostic, and treatment assessment tool. There have been studies to identify what anatomical areas of the airway are most useful to assess the airway during OSA in adults; currently, there is no sufficient evidence that evaluates the diagnostic capabilities of CBCT (i.e., precision and validity) to provide a conclusive answer in adults or in children.[31–34]

CBCT is useful to locate impacted teeth with more precision and accuracy. For example, if a maxillary canine is impacted, traditional panoramic and cephalometric films yield information in two dimensions. The clinician has historically gathered additional information from other radiographs, yet there is still uncertainty of where the canine is positioned.[35] The cone beam scan can give the clinician precise information on the position of the impacted tooth, its angulation, its proximity to other teeth, resorption of teeth, and the amount of bone surrounding the tooth.[36] This allows the orthodontist and the surgeon to make a more detailed plan regarding the status of the impacted or ectopic tooth and the adjacent structures (Fig. 17.8).

In the past, the surgeon would determine the orientation of the tooth and its position of an impacted tooth in relation to adjacent teeth using panoramic radiographs before surgical exposure. The CBCT has allowed the dentist and the surgeon to visualize the orientation of the tooth, its location, and its effect on other teeth before any surgical interventions. In cases of impacted teeth that need exposure and ligation, the orthodontist can direct the surgeon to bond the tooth in a certain position to enhance its movement and provide the most efficient force vector (Fig. 17.9).

CBCT images are also being used to plan orthognathic surgical procedures.[37,38] The images provide a much more accurate picture of the malocclusion and the type of skeletal movement necessary to correct the malocclusion. In addition, new software allows surgeons to complete virtual surgery before the actual surgery and have preformed bone plates and surgical splints that fit with increased accuracy. More recent technologic advances with applications for dental implants and autotransplantation cases allow the surgeon to generate (print) a reconstruction of the entire skull (including transplanted teeth) and obtain accurate surgical guides before the surgical procedure.[30] Further applications of CBCT include software reconstruction to evaluate outcomes of

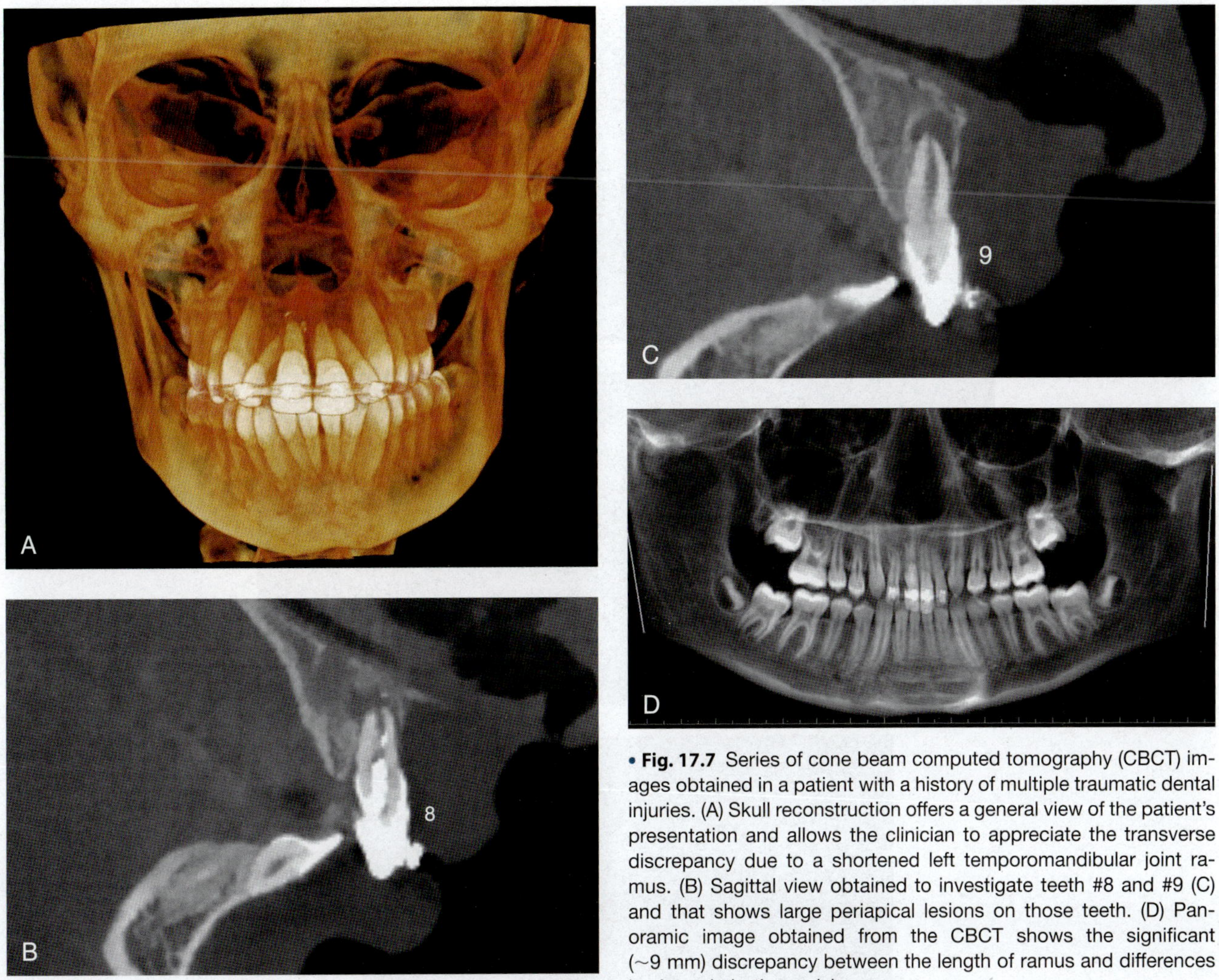

• **Fig. 17.7** Series of cone beam computed tomography (CBCT) images obtained in a patient with a history of multiple traumatic dental injuries. (A) Skull reconstruction offers a general view of the patient's presentation and allows the clinician to appreciate the transverse discrepancy due to a shortened left temporomandibular joint ramus. (B) Sagittal view obtained to investigate teeth #8 and #9 (C) and that shows large periapical lesions on those teeth. (D) Panoramic image obtained from the CBCT shows the significant (~9 mm) discrepancy between the length of ramus and differences in shape in both condyles.

orthodontic treatment (Fig. 17.10) that could be processed using machine learning (ML) algorithms for the prediction of treatment outcomes in similar cases and surgical approaches.[39–42] There is no doubt that as cone beam technology becomes more sophisticated with smaller field size and decreased radiation exposure, the use of traditional two-dimensional (2D) films (PSP and sensors) will decrease.

Considerations Across Pediatric Age Groups

Six months to age 3: It is rare that a pediatric patient in this age group would meet the indications for radiographs. Some instances in which a radiograph would be indicated include patients with TDIs, if the child exhibits a minimal degree of cooperation for this. Usually, this will be by means of an occlusal radiograph (a size no. 2 film positioned horizontally), and a knee-to-knee examination. At this age, the patient generally presents with open contacts and some, but not all primary molars erupted. All surfaces can be readily visualized so radiographs are not indicated to detect interproximal caries lesions. If all the primary molars have erupted with closed contacts and caries lesions at this stage (i.e., closer to 3 years of age) posterior bitewings can be considered if there is cooperation.

Primary dentition years (3 to 6 years): In this age group, the dentist does rely on radiographs to make a comprehensive assessment, diagnosis, and prioritized problem list. Children in this age range may find it difficult to cooperate with radiographic procedures, in which case the radiographic examination should be deferred until cooperation improves or can be managed while preserving the child's well-being and emotional status. Introduction of the child to intraoral radiography can be managed as suggested in Box 17.1.

Radiographs are not indicated when all proximal surfaces can be visualized and examined clinically. This includes both anterior and posterior teeth. Only when proximal surfaces cannot be visualized and clinically examined are bitewing radiographs indicated to determine the presence and severity of interproximal caries (Fig. 17.11).

Other supplemental projections are indicated in the following circumstances: history of pain, deep caries lesions, missing teeth, swelling, dental trauma, mobility of teeth, unexplained bleeding, or a disrupted eruption pattern.[14] These views include the maxillary (Fig. 17.12A) and mandibular (Fig. 17.12B) periapical views and the maxillary (Fig. 17.12C) and mandibular (Fig. 17.12D) occlusal views. A full mouth survey (Fig. 17.12E) is rarely obtained as part of the routine dental care. Technical considerations on the technique for these supplemental views is

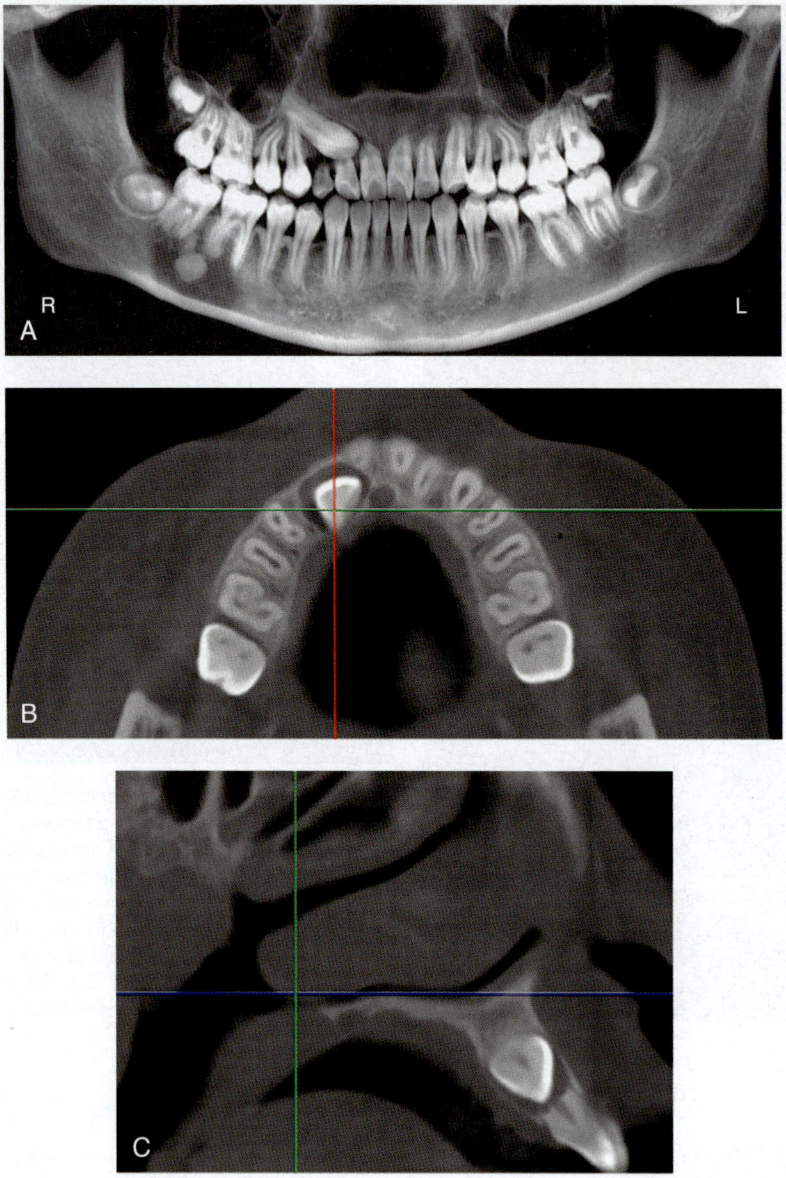

• **Fig. 17.8** (A) Conventional panoramic reconstruction showing the ectopic eruption of the maxillary right canine. The root morphology of the maxillary right lateral and central incisors also looks suspicious. (B) Three-dimensional reconstruction of the patient from a small field of view cone beam computed tomography revealing that the canine is superior to the lateral and central incisors. (C) This view demonstrates the degree of resorption of the central incisor.

presented in Box 17.2. While treating patients in the operating room under GA, typically a set of four, six, or eight x-rays (two occlusal [maxillary and mandibular], two bitewing [left and right], and four periapical [upper right, upper left, lower right, and lower left]) radiographs are obtained. If no deep caries lesions with possible pulpal/furcal/periapical involvement are suspected, this set of eight radiographs can be tailored to each patient's needs and clinical findings (ALARA principle).

Pediatric (size 0) films can be used most often in this age group with the exception of the pediatric occlusal films, which are no. 2 size, turned 90 degrees. If first permanent molars are erupted and in occlusion, then no. 2 size should be used. The Snap-a-Ray (Rinn Corporation, Elgin, IL) (Fig. 17.13) device has been used for film positioning in this age group with great success because of its small size and light weight. Other positioning instruments can be used, but some thought should be given to the size and weight of the instrument that must be placed intraorally.

Typically, a 16-inch or longer cone, which reduces skin exposure and rectangular collimation, should be used, but movement by children of this age may result in less than ideal radiographs with an extremely truncated beam. Before exposure of the radiographs, the ability of the child to cooperate with this procedure must be comprehensively assessed to prevent poor quality radiographs (and unnecessary exposure). When parents assist, they must adequately demonstrate the ability to stabilize the film and patient before exposure. Pregnancy (in the parent) is not a contraindication to obtaining radiographs as recent recommendations concluded the absence of radiation-induced heritable defects in

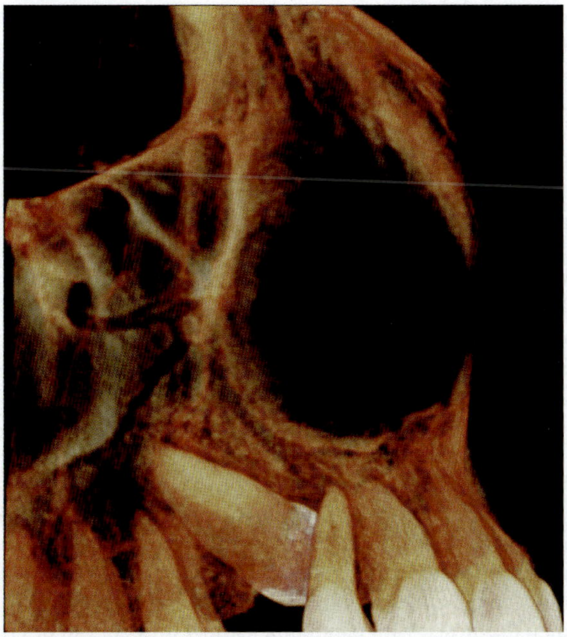

• **Fig. 17.9** A truncated maxillary view (smaller field of view) is a good way to better visualize the position of impacted teeth and to reduce radiation for the patient. This type of information gives the clinician a very precise idea of the position of the tooth.

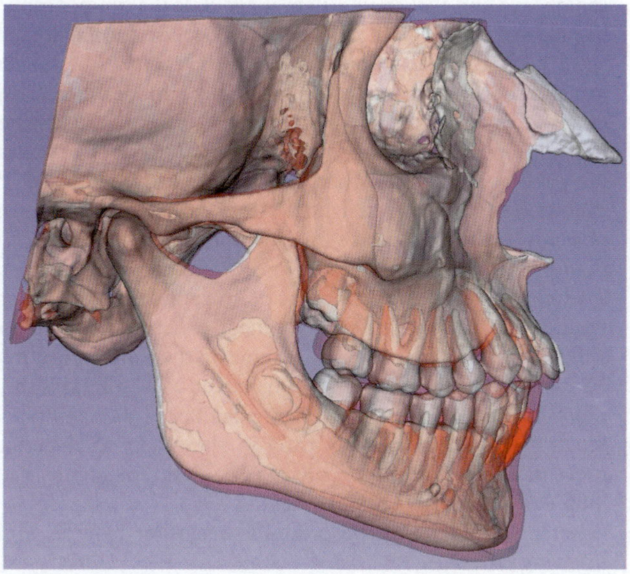

• **Fig. 17.10** Cone beam computed tomography superimposition (of images: pretreatment and posttreatment) featured to evaluate outcomes of orthodontic treatment in the growing patient. This image was rendered via specialized software processing. The image in *white* represents the patient's status before treatment and the image in *red* represents the patient's status after treatment. (Image courtesy Dr. Tung Nguyen, Department of Orthodontics, Adams School of Dentistry, The University of North Carolina at Chapel Hill.)

humans and the negligible dose to the gonads and fetus from dentomaxillofacial radiographs. Therefore thyroid and gonadal shielding are no longer recommended in this population group.[1,8]

A concerned parent may ask about the frequency of taking films. The AAPD[14] advises the use of radiographic exposure at a rate necessary to maximize detection of abnormalities while also minimizing unnecessary exposure (see Fig. 17.1). Table 17.2 lists the selection criteria for pediatric radiographs in the 3- to 6-year-old child. All radiographs should be obtained only after a clinical examination and history has been completed.

The advent of digital intraoral radiography has been both a benefit and a challenge for the pediatric dental patient, particularly for those in the 3- to 6-year-old range. Two different systems predominate. The wired sensor is a solid-state x-ray detector that requires a rather bulky nonflexible intraoral receptor because of the electronics. Sensors are available in typical dental film sizes and are wired to a computer using software to capture and display images. The phosphor plate system uses a flexible receptor much like a traditional dental film and is not attached to any device. The phosphor plate must be processed through a scanning or reading device to convert the image to digital format. Both systems have the following advantages and disadvantages:

1. The PSP plates have some flexibility and are thinner, which is helpful in children and some adults for proper placement and patient comfort compared with the wired sensors.

• BOX 17.1 Introducing a Child to Intraoral Radiography

1 Use tell-show-do, distraction, positive reinforcement, and other conventional communicative behavior guidance techniques to familiarize the patient with the devices—a camera analogy (for the tube) and a cookie (for the receptor) where they have to guess the flavor can be used. It helps to do a dry run, showing an unexposed radiograph to explain the process using analogies including a jacket, putting on a heavy blanket, or guessing the flavor of the cookie. By positioning the film and the x-ray machine, the dentist can also determine whether a child will cooperate for an exposure, preventing unproductive irradiation. Similarly, having the child bite on the Snap-a-Ray (Rinn Corporation, Elgin, IL) without a film provides a good precursor to obtaining necessary images. It is not helpful to ask the patient for permission to do a dry run (i.e., do you want to try this strawberry cookie?) as often they will say no. Rather, use tell-show-do followed by deep praise for all the positive from that step while coaching for the areas that should be improved.

2 Consider the "preoperational" developmental stage of children at this age, or their ability to have one object to represent another.[a] For example, have the x-ray head represent their favorite character that lives inside the x-ray head. You can say: *"Say hello to Elmo who will touch your cheek."*

3 Match film size to comfort. Many children have difficulties with the film impinging on the lingual soft tissue of the mandible. In some cases, bending the anterior corners or using foam covers minimizes the degree of discomfort, but this practice (especially bending), may compromise the diagnostic quality of the radiograph because it can introduce artifacts. Another technique is to place the film vertically to minimize anteroposterior size. However, in this position it can reach the floor of the mouth easily and therefore increase gag reflexes. It is not uncommon that the dentist would downsize the film to adapt to the child's comfort and promote good cooperation.

4 Obtain the least difficult radiograph first to acquaint the child with the procedures. Anterior occlusal films are usually easiest for very young children if indicated (e.g., visible disease or history of dental trauma).

5 Prepare all machine settings and ensure that the device is properly positioned before positioning the film (or sensor). Some children can hold the receptor for only a short period of time because of gag reflexes, discomfort, or a short attention span.

[a]Adapted from Asokan S, Surendran S, Asokan S, et al. Relevance of Piaget's cognitive principles among 4-7 years old children: a descriptive cross-sectional study. *J Indian Soc Pedod Prev Dent.* 2014;32(4):292-296.

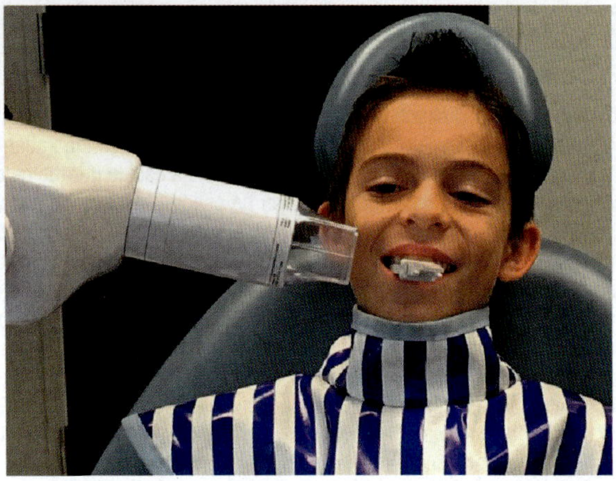

• **Fig. 17.11** The proper technique for obtaining posterior bitewing radiograph (no. 0 or no. 2 film) is critical because it is often used. The tube head should have a vertical angulation of +10 degrees and a horizontal angulation such that the face of the cone is parallel to the receptor; the beam is directed to the open embrasures. The receptor should be placed lingual to the teeth with the child biting on the tab, and anteriorly to obtain a view of the distal surfaces of the canines. Asking the child to smile to show the teeth often helps orient the beam and prevents overlap.

2. Both systems require attention to infection control procedures because the receptors are intended to be reusable. Commercially available transparent plastic sleeves that are inexpensive and disposable can be used to protect the patient.
3. The PSP plates eventually succumb to the wear and tear of use in children, and image deterioration is common. Biting films, common in young children and those unfamiliar with intraoral radiographic techniques, can reduce the quality of images from phosphor plates and hamper the diagnostic value of these images. Bending and light exposure can also affect image quality as well.
4. Wired sensors are expensive and require diligence in handling. Proprietary systems offer replacement warranties at less than the cost of a new sensor.
5. Both systems rely on software, so computer malfunction can render a dental office unable to obtain radiographs.
6. Because of their bulkiness, wired sensors require the operator to develop new placement techniques and they often require purchase of product-specific alternative stabilizing devices that are different from those used with film.
7. The phosphor system requires a processing step, like wet film technology, so it does not offer much in the way of savings, especially in this age group and in patients treated under GA where images should be readily available to decrease exposure time to anesthetic agents. Some processing systems for phosphor plates are cumbersome to use and require space. Wired sensors require storage that places minimal stress on sensors, wire, and attachments.

The Transitional Years: 6 to 12 years

Transition into mixed dentition requires substantial modification of the basic pediatric radiographic examination. Some considerations for radiographs of children in this age group include the following:

1. Identification of missing teeth, supernumerary teeth, and the developmental status of permanent anterior teeth and premolars require greater periapical coverage on films. Furthermore, it must be emphasized that obtaining radiographs with the only concern being the developmental status of teeth is strongly discouraged. In the presence of anomalies of shape and/or number (which is often clinically detectable), additional imaging should be considered. The maxillary lateral incisors should be evident early in this stage of life. The permanent second premolars are usually evident on radiographs at age 4, but they may not be apparent until age 8.
2. Absence of erupted maxillary incisors that are of normal shape and size should be apparent early. If not, they should be confirmed with a panoramic radiograph. The reason for this approach is that the missing or peg-shaped lateral incisors are also associated with missing second premolars, distally erupting mandibular canines, palatally erupting maxillary canines, and transposition of the canines and adjacent teeth.
3. Potential eruption problems may be diagnosed from the radiographs by study of the unerupted teeth. Ectopic eruption of permanent first molars has been discussed and is diagnosed from routine bitewings. Ectopic eruption of incisors and canine impaction, which are other maxillary eruption problems, are often diagnosed with panoramic radiographs but can be erroneously evaluated in this manner if only a panoramic radiograph is used (Fig. 17.14). Often, a maxillary occlusal radiograph followed by a CBCT gains substantial value in these cases.

   A routinely recommended practice part of the intraoral examination is the palpation of soft tissues surrounding the canine area and that should start at age 8. If the canines cannot be palpated on the facial aspect of the alveolus at approximately age 10, labial or palatal positioning of the canine is best determined using a panoramic radiograph to determine whether any of the other associated conditions are also present. The first step in determining the position of the canines is to closely examine the panoramic film and compare the size of the right and left canines. Like using a flashlight to create a shadow, the closer the object is to the light source (or radiation source), the larger the shadow cast. As the object moves away from the light source, the shadow is smaller. The panoramic beam comes from behind the head, so a palatally positioned canine is closer to the beam and will appear larger than the other canine on the panoramic film.[35] Because of the rendering of a 3D object on a 2D film, this technique can still leave questions as to positions of the canines.
4. Small palate size, especially early in the school-aged period, prevents or complicates maxillary periapical radiography via a long-cone film-stabilizing device.
5. Greater AP length in the posterior occlusion requires more bitewing coverage.

In the early mixed dentition period, all tooth-bearing areas should be surveyed (if posterior contacts are closed). Supernumerary, missing, and impacted teeth are the most common issues revealed in the radiographic examination. The AAPD[14] recommends posterior bitewing films and a panoramic radiograph or posterior bitewing films and selected periapical radiographs. If significant findings are seen on a bitewing radiograph, then periapical radiographs can be obtained. The panoramic radiograph offers the advantage of showing the TMJ. Definitive TMJ films are indicated when there are clinical signs of dysfunction, history of TMJ abnormalities, or history of trauma with suspected TMJ involvement. If a more traditional intraoral film survey is considered, it should include appropriate anterior occlusal views, at least one periapical view in each posterior quadrant, and posterior bitewings (Fig. 17.15). An appropriate radiographic examination in this age group consists of anterior

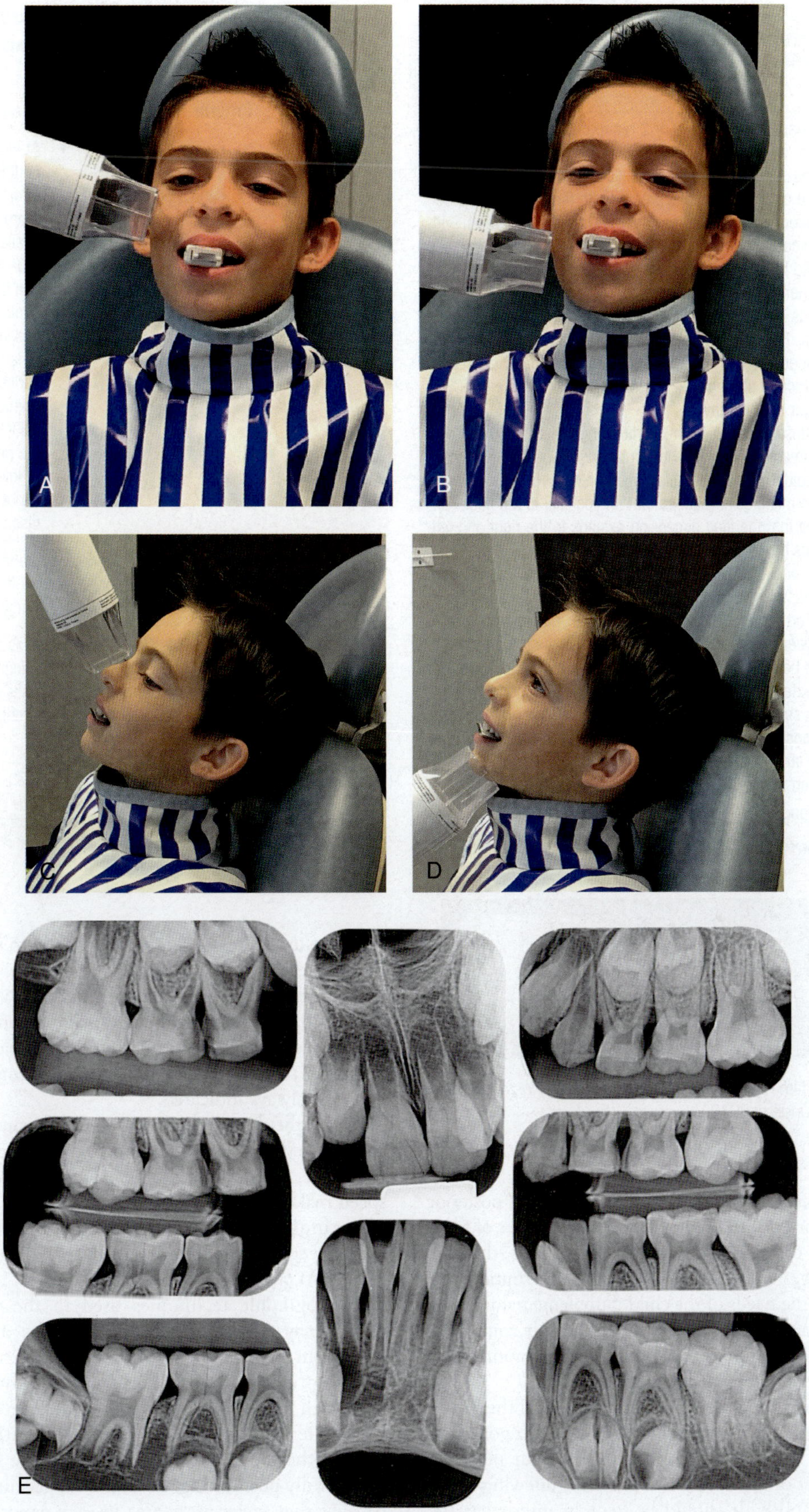

• **Fig. 17.12** The following techniques are commonly used to obtain supplemental views. (A–B) Maxillary periapical view. (C) Maxillary occlusal view. (D) Mandibular occlusal view. (E) Full mouth series.

• BOX 17.2 Techniques Used to Obtain Supplemental Views

Fig. 17.12	Technique
A	Maxillary periapical view (no. 0 or 2 receptor). Vertical angulation: the beam is at a right angle to the film; starting angle is +30 degrees. Horizontal angulation: face to cone is parallel to facial surface of teeth. Film placement: with film in jaw of holder, holder is placed between the maxillary and mandibular teeth with the sensitive component of a receptor against the lingual surfaces of teeth. Child bites on larger sides of jaws.
B	Mandibular periapical view (no. 0 or 2 receptor). Vertical angulation: beam is at a right angle to the film; starting angle is ~5 degrees. Film placement: with film in jaws of holder, and holder is placed between the maxillary and mandibular teeth with dimpled surface of film against the lingual surfaces of teeth. Child bites on larger sides of jaws.
C	Maxillary occlusal view (no. 2 film). Vertical angulation: + 60 degrees, with beam directed downward. Horizontal angulation: beam directed along midsagittal plane. Film placement: film is placed between maxillary and mandibular teeth so that it is parallel to the floor. Film is oriented so that the long dimension extends to the right and left. The child bites gently on the film while seated upright.
D	Mandibular occlusal view (no. 2 film). Vertical angulation: ~15 degrees, with beam directed upward. Horizontal angulation: beam directed along midsagittal plane. Film placement: film is placed between the maxillary and mandibular teeth, and child is instructed to bite gently on the film. The patient is reclining so that the chin is extended. Bisecting angle technique is used.
E	A full mouth series comprising all of the above films. To minimize a child's exposure to radiation, dentists often reduce the number of films in a survey if tooth and supporting tissues can be viewed adequately on fewer films.

(Courtesy Dr. Stephanie Furlong).

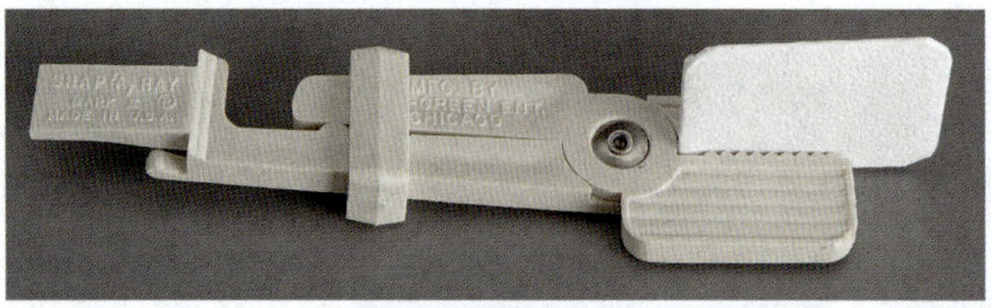

• Fig. 17.13 Snap-a-Ray film holder. (From Boyd LRB. *Dental Instruments: A Pocket Guide.* 4th ed. Saunders; 2012.)

occlusal radiographs, at least one periapical film in each posterior quadrant, and posterior bitewing radiographs. The number of films should be dictated by the size of the tooth-bearing areas, the adequacy of tissue coverage by the size of the films, the eruption and exfoliation status, and the needs of the child. Supplemental imaging at this age such as panoramic radiographs should be only considered in the presence of clinical findings that would suggest anomalies in shape, size, or number and not just for routine purposes.

The number of films should be dictated by the size of the tooth-bearing areas, the adequacy of tissue coverage by the size of films, and the needs of the child. An eight-film survey (four posterior periapical, two anterior occlusal, and two posterior bitewing films) should suffice for an NPE. It should be kept in mind that the mixed dentition stage is characterized by exfoliation of primary and eruption of permanent teeth. Often, individualization of these rules (with the aim of decreasing unnecessary radiation) is considered because there are mobile teeth close to exfoliation or partially erupted teeth that are not in close contact with adjacent teeth. The radiographs can be deferred until the next visits. Therefore in this age group, two bitewing radiographs (one on each side) will suffice for the radiographic examination for the patient. In patients that are being treated under GA in the operating room, an eight-film survey is always indicated.

TABLE 17.2 Selection Criteria and Frequency for Obtaining Intraoral Pediatric Radiographs in the 3-to-6-Year-Old Child

Projection	Criteria	Frequency
Posterior bitewing	a. Proximal surfaces of posterior teeth cannot be examined clinically b. Child is cooperative[a]	• At initial examination if contacts closed (make every effort to obtain x-rays from a previous practitioner if available) • A 6- to 12-month interval can be considered if contacts are closed, the child has visible caries lesions, or is at increased risk for caries[b] • Annually to 24-month interval if contacts are closed; the child does not have any visible caries lesions and is not at increased risk for disease.
Posterior periapical	a. Suspected pathosis b. Confirmed pathosis c. Child is cooperative	As needed to diagnose and monitor treatment or patient condition
Anterior occlusal	a. Suspected pathosis b. Confirmed pathosis c. Child is cooperative	Same as above or as a radiograph to aid during caries examination and if child is considered high caries risk

[a]Consider child cooperation in the decision-making process.
[b]Factors increasing caries risk may be assessed using the ADA Caries Risk Assessment form for patients 0–6 years of age and over 6 years of age. Last updated July, 2023.
Modified from American Dental Association caries risk assessment system (2023), and the, US Department of Health and Human services. *The Selection of Patients for Dental Radiographic Examination (revised 2012).*

It is difficult to determine whether a complete film survey or a panoramic/bitewing combination yields a greater effective radiation dose. The variables of machine type, collimation, and film speed make determination difficult. There is ample discussion currently in the dental imaging literature on whether to switch from the concept of ALARA to "as low as diagnostically acceptable" (ALADA).[29]

Radiographic techniques used in the youngest in this age group may include modifications. The anterior area requires placement of the film positioner deeper in the palate to obtain proper orientation. If indicated, a film-holding device can be used with a bisecting-angle technique (Fig. 17.16). The bitewing technique used in this age group is essentially the same as that used in the preschooler. It may take more skill to open contacts by carefully positioning the beam. Larger films may be preferrable because they cover more area in each exposure.

Selection criteria also apply to this age group. Justification of a full-mouth survey of some type is based on the need to identify dental developmental problems and pathologic processes. The

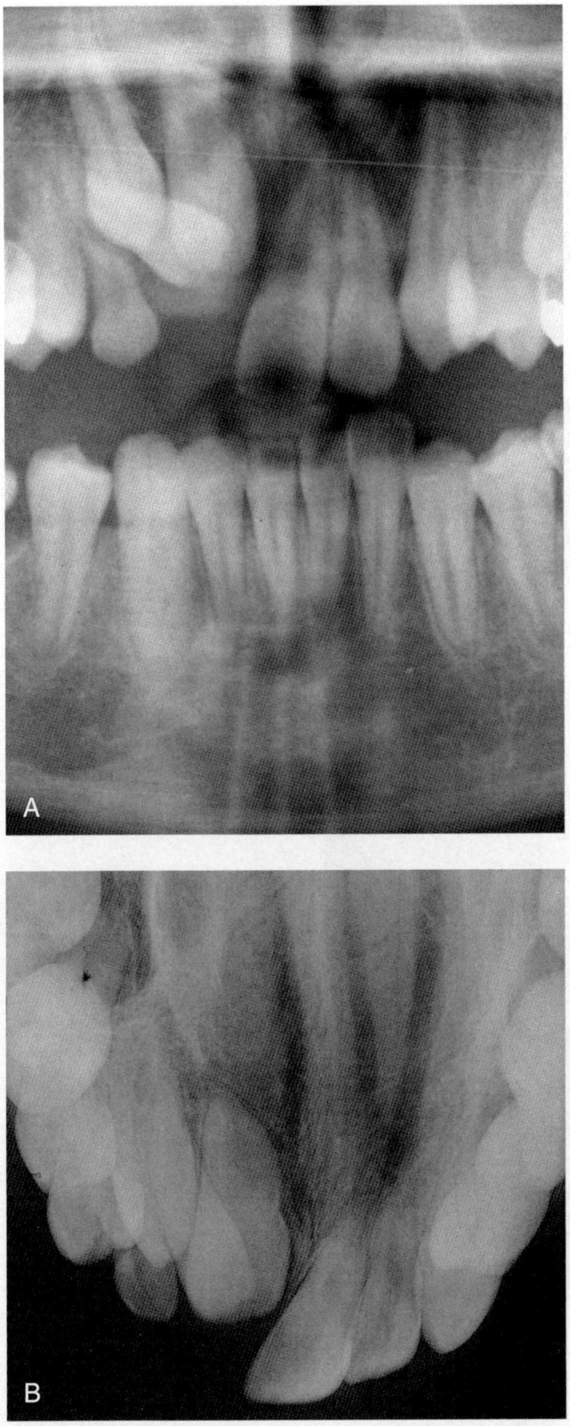

• **Fig. 17.14** Often images of unerupted canines and lateral incisors are distorted on panoramic radiographs and can be better visualized on occlusal radiographs. (A) Panoramic radiograph shows little overlap of the maxillary left canine and lateral incisor. (B) Occlusal radiograph shows considerable overlap of the same canine and lateral incisor.

number of films obtained should reflect the adequacy of composite exposure provided by individual views, using the smallest number possible that still reveal all necessary areas. In the age range of 6 to 12 years, several film combinations are possible. No single set of projections is considered best.

Adolescence

The adolescent radiographic examination ranges from a transitional to an adult multifilm survey including panoramic x-rays and CBCT, depending on the child's dentition, cooperation, and medical history. The types of film to be used should be determined by the number of teeth present, the assessment of closed contacts that are not clinically visible, and the reason for radiographic examination. For the new adolescent patient with no apparent major dental needs, low caries risk and low to no history of previous dental treatment, an individualized examination of posterior bitewings (typically four, no. 2 size) with a panoramic radiograph (to better visualize position of third molars) or selected periapical radiographs should suffice. For the adolescent patient with major dental care needs, high caries risk, and/or extensive history of dental treatment, a full mouth intraoral examination is preferred (see Table 17.1).

The radiographic examination in this age group should also address growth and development concerning findings: the eruption status of unerupted (delayed eruption) premolars and canines. Later in adolescence, the final issue is third molar development. The development of these teeth can be evaluated by using periapical radiographs or a panoramic radiograph. Adolescents should be able to tolerate no. 2 size intraoral films. However, for the child with a small oral cavity, techniques to aid in positioning are described in the mixed dentition stage of dentition. Multiple or serial periapical radiographs are often required for the diagnosis of pathosis or for management of conditions that require significant follow up, such as endodontic therapy for incisors with history of TDIs.

Bitewing radiographs during early adolescence is affected by the developing occlusion and lack of contacts. A thorough clinical examination should determine whether posterior surfaces can be adequately visualized until the premolars have fully erupted. The benefit of exposing bitewing films to examine two or four interproximal surfaces should be weighed against the risk of radiation exposure. In these cases, the caries risk assessment and a current comprehensive clinical examination will help determine whether films are necessary.

The panoramic film has a role in adolescent dentistry as a full-mouth radiographic survey for a new patient who does not have major treatment needs. The panoramic radiograph reveals bone pathosis and orients the examiner to the presence and position of third molars. The panoramic radiograph also grossly displays sinuses and the TMJ, which may be less well displayed on a multifilm intraoral survey. Table 17.3 summarizes the issues that apply to radiography of the adolescent patient.

Visit eBooks.Health.Elsevier.com to see full list of references.

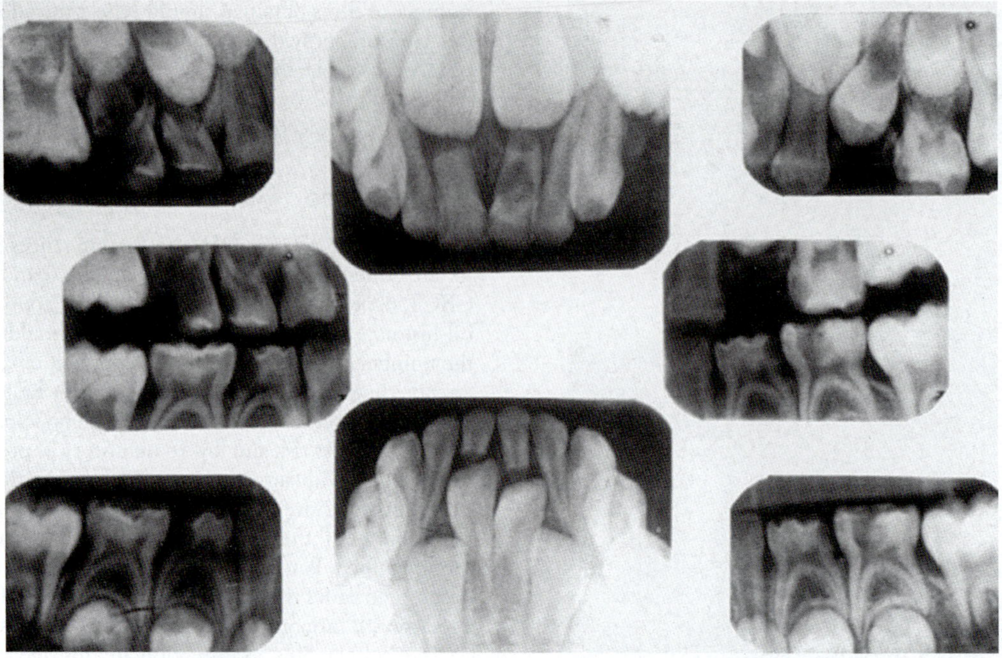

• **Fig. 17.15** Radiographic examination series in the transitional years.

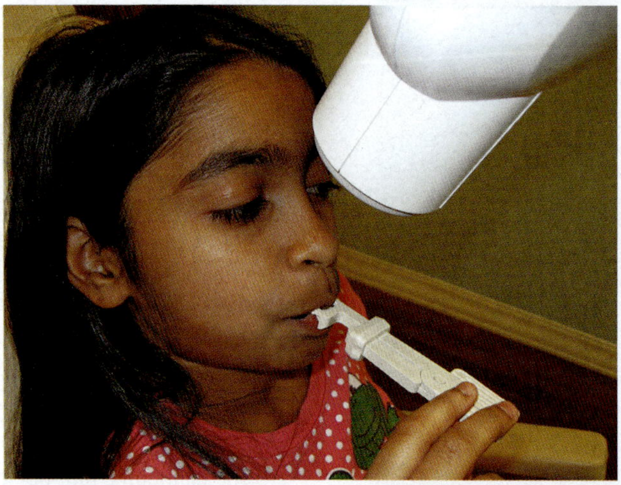

• **Fig. 17.16** A film-holding device similar to the device shown here (Snap-a-Ray film holder).

TABLE 17.3 Current Radiographic Considerations for the Adolescent Patient

Type of Radiograph	Frequency	Number and Size
Full mouth survey	• No suggested frequency or interval • Determined by patient age, dental development, history of dental treatment, and caries risk assessment • Preferred when clinical evidence of generalized dental disease	• Number of films included to be based on tissue coverage needed *Early adolescence (12–15 years):* • Maxillary and mandibular periapical (no. 2 size) • Canine periapical (no. 1 or 2 size) • Bitewing (two films, no. 2 size) • Four posterior quadrant periapical (no. 2 size) to include premolars and erupted molars *Late adolescence (16–21 years):* • Complete set (21-film survey)
Bitewing	• No suggested frequency or interval • Determined by patient age, dental development, and caries risk assessment • Should be taken if caries lesions are visible or high caries risk • Should be taken if multiple interproximal restorations are present and are being followed • Should be taken if incipient caries lesions were noted on previous films and are being monitored • Interval for these situations should be individualized and reevaluated at each periodic examination	• Size determined by oral access, but usually no. 2 is used • One film sufficient until eruption of second permanent molars • Position varies with the location and number of posterior contacts
Periapical	• No suggested frequency or interval • Pathosis or treatment needs should dictate frequency • To evaluate dental trauma • To determine developmental status of third molars	• Size no. 2 is usually used • Size no. 4 is usually used as an occlusal radiograph
Panoramic	• Possible component of a full-mouth survey for a disease-free new patient • Evaluate the mesiodistal position of maxillary canines • To determine position and developmental status of third molars	• Should only be used in the presence of positive signs or findings such as nonerupted canines, premolars or in late adolescence, to evaluate third molars

18

Pediatric Pharmacology

AMY R. GREENWOOD

CHAPTER OUTLINE

The necessity for antimicrobial drug use in pediatric dentistry arises from a variety of circumstances, including odontogenic infections, oral wounds, periodontal disease, candidiasis, and primary herpetic gingivostomatitis. Successful management of infections relies on the practitioner's knowledge of the microbiology of odontogenic and intraoral infections and the spectrum of activity, pharmacology, and adverse effects of the antimicrobial agents being prescribed. In addition, patient-specific factors such as overall health, concomitant medications, and the ability to afford or comply with the prescribed drug regimen must be considered. In the case of pediatric patients, compliance with unpalatable liquid medications can be especially problematic.

Antimicrobial Classification and Use

Microbiology

Antibiotics are defined as substances naturally produced by microorganisms (yeast or fungi) and used to inhibit bacteria and sometimes protozoa. Semisynthetic agents such as sulfonamides and fluoroquinolones also fall into this category.

Maximally effective antimicrobial therapy occurs after a definitive identification of the pathogen is made via culture or serologic testing, which is followed by susceptibility testing to determine which therapeutic agent is most effective against the pathogen. In outpatient dentistry the recognition of common causative pathogens, along with the most efficacious antimicrobial agents against those pathogens, is well established and microbiologic testing is rarely used.[2] However, culture and sensitivity testing can be useful in the treatment of recalcitrant infections, recurrent infections, postoperative infections, or suspected osteomyelitis or when the patient is significantly immunocompromised.[3]

The susceptibility of a microorganism to an antibiotic is based on the minimum inhibitory concentration (MIC), which is the lowest concentration of the drug that prevents growth of the microorganism. The organisms may still be viable, but they are no longer actively dividing.

The process of culture and sensitivity testing may take hours or days to complete. A rapid, preliminary identification of bacteria can often be obtained through a Gram stain (crystal violet) and microscopical evaluation. Bacteria that remain stained from crystal violet have a thick outer layer of peptidoglycan and are called gram-positive bacteria. Gram-negative bacteria have an outermost lipopolysaccharide membrane that does not retain the stain. Microscopical evaluation reveals morphology. Medically significant gram-positive pathogens are frequently cocci (spheres) rather than bacilli (rods).[1] Streptococci tend to appear in pairs or chains, whereas staphylococci form clusters.

Other common microbiologic tests include the following:

- Rapid catalase test: Differentiates between staphylococci and streptococci.
- Blood agar plates (BAPs): Patterns of hemolysis (clearing around colonies) are used to differentiate streptococci. β-Hemolytic activity reveals lysis and complete digestion of red blood cell (RBC) contents. α-Hemolysis *(Streptococcus viridans)* causes partial lysis of RBCs and results in a green/brown appearance on the plate. γ-Hemolysis refers to no hemolytic activity and the plate remains the original red color.
- Coagulase test: Differentiates *Staphylococcus aureus,* a virulent coagulase positive microorganism, from *Staphylococcus epidermidis* (coagulase negative), which is a common blood culture contaminant.[1]

Chemotherapeutic Spectrum of Activity

An antibiotic's *spectrum of activity* refers to the species of microorganisms affected by the drug. Narrow-spectrum antibiotics are active against a single or limited group of microorganisms (e.g., some gram-positive organisms). Extended-spectrum antibiotics are effective against gram-positive organisms and a significant number of gram-negative organisms.

Broad-spectrum antibiotics act against a wide variety of species. These agents are often initially prescribed to neutropenic or critically ill patients while awaiting the results of culture and sensitivity testing. Administering broad-spectrum agents can significantly alter the normal microbial flora by killing of both beneficial and commensal organisms, creating an environment where opportunistic pathogens such as *Candida albicans* can grow, leading to superinfections.[1] Practitioners should choose the narrowest spectrum antibiotic that will target the identified pathogen(s).

Bacteriostatic versus Bactericidal Agents

Antimicrobial agents are classified as either bacteriostatic or bactericidal (Box 18.1). Bacteriostatic drugs limit the spread of the infection by halting bacterial growth and replication. This allows the body's immune system to attack, immobilize, and kill the pathogens. To eradicate the infection, the patient's host defense mechanisms must be intact. Host defense mechanisms can be compromised by a variety of conditions, including alcoholism, diabetes, malnutrition, advanced age, infection with human immunodeficiency virus, and immunosuppressant drugs. The effects of bacteriostatic antibiotics on microorganisms are reversible. If patient compliance is poor or the drug is discontinued before the organisms have been scavenged, a second cycle of the infection may occur because remaining viable bacteria will be able to grow and replicate.

Bactericidal drugs act independently of host immune defenses to cause cell death. These effects are irreversible; the microorganism will ultimately die after adequate drug exposure. Bactericidal drugs are preferred for most infections, including intraoral infections, because they act largely independent of host factors, which is an important consideration for rapidly progressing infections or when the patient is immunocompromised. It should be noted that some antibiotics may be "-cidal" to certain microorganisms and have a static effect on others or the effect may be concentration dependent.[4]

• BOX 18.1 Bactericidal and Bacteriostatic Antibiotics

Bactericidal

Aminoglycosides
Carbapenems
Cephalosporins
Fluoroquinolones
Metronidazole
Penicillins
Vancomycin

Bacteriostatic

Clindamycin[a]
Macrolides[a]
Sulfonamides
Trimethoprim
Tetracyclines

[a]May be bactericidal against some organisms or at higher concentrations.

Data from Flynn TR. Principles of management of odontogenic infections. In: Miloro M, Ghali GE, Larsen PE, Waite PD, eds. *Peterson's Principles of Oral and Maxillofacial Surgery.* 2nd ed. Hamilton, BC Decker, Inc.; 2004. Used with permission of PMPH USA, Ltd., Raleigh, North Carolina.

Many bactericidal drugs, including β-lactam antibiotics and vancomycin, act when the cell is actively growing or dividing. Concomitant administration of a bacteriostatic drug with a β-lactam antibiotic or similarly acting drug can interfere with the effectiveness of the bactericidal antibiotic.[4]

Categories of Antibiotic Use

The clinical use of antibiotics falls into one of three categories: prophylactic, empiric, or definitive. Prophylaxis is the use of antimicrobial chemotherapy to prevent an infection. Prophylactic therapy is intended for patients at high risk for developing an infection. Common reasons include disease states (previous bacterial endocarditis, uncontrolled diabetes), immunosuppressive drug therapy, and high-risk surgery.[1] Due to emerging resistance patterns and risk of superinfection, prophylactic administration of antibiotics should occur only when the benefit outweighs the risk. The duration of the prophylaxis regimen is dictated by the duration of risk.[1]

In medical and dental practice, most antibiotics are prescribed empirically. This approach works particularly well in dentistry, due to the extensive information available on both the causative organisms seen in dental infections and the best agents to eradicate them. Unless the infection is severe or rapidly spreading, a penicillin is generally the drug of choice assuming the patient does not have an allergy. If the infection fails to improve or worsens, then a broader-spectrum drug with good anaerobic activity is chosen.

Definitive antimicrobial therapy occurs after culture and susceptibility tests. Empiric therapy in medical practice often initially uses a broad-spectrum antibiotic, especially if the patient is seriously ill. After the organism is identified, the clinician should then choose an agent that is narrower in spectrum to target the specific pathogen. The failure to transition to definitive therapy and the widespread use of empiric antibiotics in medicine are major factors contributing to the global burden of drug resistance.[1]

Antimicrobial Mechanisms of Action

Antimicrobial agents exert their effects on microorganisms through various mechanisms including the inhibition of cell wall synthesis, inhibition of ribosomal protein synthesis, suppression of deoxyribonucleic acid (DNA) synthesis, disruption of cell membrane integrity, and alteration of cell membrane permeability.[5] Selected antimicrobial agents, and their mechanisms of action are listed in Box 18.2.

In general, antimicrobials that suppress DNA synthesis or affect the cell wall or cell membrane tend to be bactericidal, whereas those that inhibit protein or folic acid synthesis result in a bacteriostatic effect. Understanding the mechanisms of action of antibiotics frequently used in dental practice is an important component of rational prescribing.

Inhibition of Cell Wall Synthesis

The β-lactam antibiotics classified according to their ring structure include penicillins (penams), cephalosporins (cephams), carbapenems, and monobactam, among others. These groups share the four-sided β-lactam ring structure, which imparts similar features of chemistry, mechanism of action, pharmacology, and immunologic characteristics.[6] Most β-lactams are fused to five- or six-membered rings; the exception is monobactam, which contains only the β-lactam ring. These agents selectively act on bacteria because they have cell walls versus mammalian cells that are encased by outer membranes.

β-Lactam antibiotics exert their bactericidal effects by disrupting bacterial cell wall synthesis. Bacterial cell walls consist of peptidoglycan, a cross-linked polymer of polysaccharides and polypeptides. Cross-linkage of peptides is necessary for the formation of a rigid cell wall that can withstand the osmotic pressure of the cytopasm.[6] Penicillin is a structural analog of D-alanine and acts by competitively inhibiting the final transpeptidation reaction (removal of a terminal D-alanine) necessary to complete cross-linkage. Inhibiting transpeptidase (also known as penicillin-binding protein) halts peptidoglycan synthesis and ultimately results in cell death.

In some organisms the presence of β-lactam antibiotics causes the derepression of an endogenous autolysin. Autolysins are enzymes that selectively break down the rigid peptidoglycan matrix to allow for cell growth and division. Excessive amounts of autolysin will weaken the peptidoglycan and result in cell lysis.[6]

Vancomycin is a tricyclic glycopeptide antibiotic that disrupts cell wall synthesis by binding to the terminal D-alanine–D-alanine chains on the peptidoglycan cell wall, preventing elongation of the peptidoglycan chains (one step ahead of β-lactams).[1,6] Vancomycin requires active cell growth to exert bactericidal effects.[6] The large molecular size of the vancomycin molecule prevents the drug from entering gram-negative bacteria, limiting its spectrum of activity to aerobic and anaerobic gram-positive bacteria.[7] Vancomycin is effective against multiple drug-resistant organisms, including methicillin-resistant staphylococci and most enterococci and *Clostridioide difficile.*[1]

Both β-lactam antibiotics and vancomycin exhibit time-dependent bactericidal effects. This means that the bactericidal activity continues as long as the serum concentrations are greater than the minimum bactericidal concentration (MBC) of the antimicrobial agent against the pathogens.

Inhibition of Protein Synthesis

Antimicrobials that inhibit protein synthesis target the bacterial ribosome, which is structurally different from the human ribosome (70S vs. 80S in mammals).[5] The bacterial ribosome functions to translate messenger RNA, adding the correct amino acid to make the protein. The bacterial ribosome is composed of a 50S and 30S subunit. Macrolides and clindamycin both bind irreversibly to the same site on the 50S subunit, inhibiting translocation steps of protein synthesis.[7] Tetracycline antibiotics bind to the 30S subunit, blocking amino acyl-tRNA from adding amino acids to the protein, thus halting protein growth.[5,8]

Aminoglycosides (gentamycin, tobramycin, amikacin) irreversibly bind to the separated 30S ribosomal subunit and interfere with the microbial genetic code, producing a bactericidal effect.[7,9] Susceptible organisms have an oxygen-dependent transport system that allows the drug to enter the cell wall; therefore the agents are effective only against aerobic organisms.[9] A high degree of toxicity (nephrotoxicity and ototoxicity) limits their use. Aminoglycosides (usually gentamycin) are combined with β-lactam antibiotics to produce a synergistic effect. Cell wall inhibition by β-lactams enhances the entry of the aminoglycoside into the cell.[8]

Many agents that inhibit protein or DNA synthesis (aminoglycosides, quinolones) exhibit concentration-dependent killing of bacteria where the rate and extent of killing increases as the peak drug concentration increases.[9] These drugs also exhibit a "post antibiotic effect" where the inhibition of bacterial growth persists, even after a short exposure to the drug. Proposed mechanisms for this effect include slow recovery of bacteria after nonlethal drug exposure, the need to synthesize new proteins, and antibiotic occupation of the binding site.[4] The clinical advantage of drugs with long post antibiotic effects (aminoglycosides, azithromycin, fluoroquinolones) is longer dosing intervals. Fewer doses per day result in increased compliance, which is particularly important when dealing with pediatric patients.

• BOX 18.2 Antimicrobial Mechanisms of Action

Inhibition of Cell Wall Synthesis

β-Lactam antibiotics
- Penicillins (penams)
- Cephalosporins (cephems)
- Monobactams
- Carbapenems

Vancomycin

Inhibition of Protein Synthesis

Bind 50S ribosome
- Clindamycin
- Macrolides

Bind 30S ribosome
- Aminoglycosides
- Tetracyclines

Suppression of DNA Synthesis

Fluoroquinolones

Alteration of Cell Membrane Permeability

Polyene antifungals
Azole antifungals

Data from Carroll KC, Morse A, Mietzner T, Miller S, et al., eds. Antimicrobial chemotherapy. In: *Jawetz, Melnick, & Adelberg's Medical Microbiology.* 27th ed. McGraw-Hill; 2016:363-396.

antimicrobial drugs and dosages for pediatric patients can be found in Table 18.3.

Numerous studies have shown that parents often measure liquid medications incorrectly. When administering liquid medications to children, adults tend to use dosing cups, teaspoons, and droppers.[37] These devices are not as accurate as using an oral syringe, which is the recommended measuring device for pediatric liquids by The Joint Commision.[36] However, oral syringes are used in a minority (perhaps less than 20%) of households.[37] Parents may have the belief that oral syringes are only for babies, and older children may resist taking a medication via oral syringe for the same reason.

Medicine cups are the most frequently reported device used by parents to measure liquid medications. Parents usually dispense an excessive dose when using marked plastic medicine cups to measure a liquid medication.[38] Parents should be educated on the importance of accurate dosing of liquid medications to children. The dose should always be measured via oral syringe to ensure accuracy.[36] Once measured, the liquid can then be placed in a medicine cup for administration if the patient objects to an oral syringe.

Unpalatable Medications

Many children resist taking liquid antimicrobials due to their disagreeable taste or smell or because of previous experiences with other medications. Refusal to take medications can result

TABLE 18.3 Key Antimicrobial Drugs and Dosages for Pediatric Patients

KEY ANTIMICROBIAL DRUGS AND DOSAGES FOR PEDIATRIC PATIENTS	
Antimicrobial Drug	**Indication and Dosing**
Acyclovir *(Zovirax)*	*Preferred antiviral for children <12 years old.* **Usual oral dosing** 15 mg/kg five times a day for 5–7 days *Maximum single dose: 200 mg*
Amoxicillin	**Usual oral dosing** >3 months of age and <40 kg: 20–40 mg/kg/day in divided doses every 8 hours. *Maximum single dose: 500 mg* >3 months of age and <40 kg: 25–45 mg/kg/day in divided doses every 12 hours. *Maximum single dose: 875 mg* **Periodontal disease treatment for select cases (in combination with metronidazole)** 25–35 mg/kg/day in divided doses every 8 hours for 7 days. *Maximum single dose: 500 mg* **Infective Endocarditis** 50 mg/kg *Maximum dose: 2000 mg*
Amoxicillin/clavulanate *(Augmentin)*	*Use the lowest dose of clavulanate combined with amoxicillin to decrease gastrointestinal side effects.* **Usual oral dosing** <40 kg: 25–45 mg/kg/day in divided doses every 12 hours. >40 kg: 500–875 mg every 12 hours. *Maximum single dose: 875 mg of amoxicillin*
Ampicillin	**Infective Endocarditis** 50 mg/kg IM or IV *Maximum dose: 2000 mg*
Azithromycin *(Zithromax)*	**Usual oral dosing** 10–12 mg/kg on day 1 (maximum of 500 mg), followed by 5–6 mg/kg (maximum of 250 mg) once daily on days 2–5. **Periodontal disease treatment for select cases if allergic to penicillin** 10–12 mg/kg once daily for three days *Maximum: 500 mg* **Infective Endocarditis if allergic to penicillin** 15 mg/kg *Maximum dose: 500 mg*
Cephalexin *(Keflex)*	*Should not be used if an individual has a history of anaphylaxis, angioedema, or urticaria with penicillin* **Mild to moderate infections** 20–50 mg/kg/day divided every 6–12 hours *Maximum daily dose: 2000 mg* **Severe infections** 75–100 mg/kg/day divided every 6–8 hours *Maximum daily dose of 4000 mg* **Infective Endocarditis if allergic to penicillin** 50 mg/kg *Maximum: 2000 mg*

Continued

TABLE 18.3 Key Antimicrobial Drugs and Dosages for Pediatric Patients—cont'd

KEY ANTIMICROBIAL DRUGS AND DOSAGES FOR PEDIATRIC PATIENTS	
Antimicrobial Drug	**Indication and Dosing**
Clindamycin *(Cleocin)*	*Clostridioide difficile is a serious adverse reaction with this antibiotic.* *This antibiotic in no longer recommended for endocarditis prophylaxis before dental procedures.* **Usual oral dosing** 20–30 mg/kg/day in divided doses every 8 hours. *Maximum single dose: 450 mg* **Methicillin resistant staphylococcus aureus (MRSA) infections** 30–40 mg/kg/day every 8 hours *Maximum dosing: 300–450 mg every 6–8 hours.*
Doxycycline *(Avidoxy, Doryx)*	*Typically, not recommended for pregnant people and children <8 years old due to potential for permanent tooth discoloration, enamel hypoplasia in developing teeth, and soft tissue hyperpigmentation. Short-term use of drug (<21 days) may be considered due to lack of clinical evidence of tooth discoloration in developing teeth when used for <21 days.* **Usual oral dosing** >8 years old: 2.2 mg/kg every 12 hours. *Maximum single dose: 100 mg* **Infective Endocarditis if allergic to penicillin** <45 kg: 2.2 mg/kg >45 kg: 100 mg *Maximum dose: 100 mg*
Metronidazole *(Flagyl)*	15–50 mg/kg/day in divided doses every 8 hours *Maximum daily dose: 2250 mg* **Periodontal disease treatment for select cases, including necrotizing gingivitis** 10 mg/kg/dose every 8 hours for 7 days *Maximum single dose: 250 mg*
Fluconazole *(Diflucan)*	**Usual oral dosing** >12 months old: 6 mg/kg as one dose on day 1 *(maximum dose of 200 mg),* followed by 3 mg/kg once daily for 7–14 days *(maximum dose of 100 mg).*
Valacyclovir *(Valtrex)*	**Herpes labialis** >12 years old: 2 g at the onset of prodrome, repeat dose in 12 hours *Maximum 4 g/day for 1-day regimens*

IM, Intramuscular.

in battles of will between parents and children that escalate during the course of therapy. This often leads to nonadherence with the dosage regimen and early discontinuation of the medication.

Clindamycin pediatric solution has the deserved reputation of being the worst tasting antibiotic liquid. Thankfully, there are ways to overcome a child's reluctance to take liquid medications, even clindamycin solution. Administering bad-tasting medications with an oral syringe will limit the surface area that comes into contact with the medication. It also masks the medication odor better than a medicine cup. Liquids that do not taste good often have an objectionable smell, and this is especially true with some antimicrobial agents. A common mistake is to not give the parent an action plan regarding drug administration if the child has a history of medication refusal or if the product is known to be problematic. Many liquid medications have flavoring added to increase patient palatability. If the medication does not have a flavor already added, the dispensing pharmacy may be able to add flavoring to the product, but care must be taken when flavoring medications to avoid problems with drug stability or dosing.

Leaving a bad-tasting medication on a child's palate will lead to increased reluctance as the duration of therapy continues. A successful countermeasure for bad-tasting medications is to have a small cup of cold grape soda ready as a "chaser" as soon as the child swallows the medication. Grape is one of the best flavors available to mask foul-tasting and bitter medications. Grape soda is much better than grape juice because the carbonation helps to lift the taste off the palate.

Another method that can be used in difficult situations is a sugar syringe. This is useful if the correct dose of medication is available in capsule form or a tablet that can be split to achieve the desired dose. Parents should be instructed to remove the plunger from an oral syringe and then cap it. Fill the syringe to the 2-mL mark with sugar, then add the finely crushed tablet or capsule contents to the top of the sugar. Layer another 2-mL of sugar on top of the medication. Slowly drip water into the syringe until the sugar at the bottom becomes a slurry. Then add the plunger and immediately administer the contents of the syringe. The bad-tasting medication is surrounded by sugar and often goes down without being noticed by the child.

Clinical Use of Antimicrobials in Pediatric Dentistry

Bacterial Infections

Necrotizing Ulcerative Gingivitis, Necrotizing Ulcerative Periodontitis, Necrotizing Ulcerative Stomatitis

Necrotizing ulcerative gingivitis (NUG), necrotizing ulcerative periodontitis (NUP), and necrotizing ulcerative stomatitis (NUS) are a group of diseases that can affect specific intraoral structures such as gingiva, periodontal tissues, and mucosa. Various microorganisms have been isolated from affected tissues and include *Fusobacterium nucleatum, Borrelia vincentii, Prevotella intermedia, Porphyromonas gingivalis, Selenomonas sputigena,* and other anaerobic organisms.[39] Additional theories for etiology include a role for viruses, such the human herpesviruses (HHVs). Several factors have been identified as potential triggers for these conditions including stress, altered immune status, trauma, illness, smoking, malnutrition, and lack of sleep.[40,41] NUG presents as necrotic, crater-like ulcerations that initially affect the interdental papilla with progression to free gingival margins and extension to adjacent tissues (NUP, NUS). Spontaneous hemorrhage, halitosis, as well as fever, lymphadenopathy, and malaise have also been reported. Management of these conditions includes the debridement of local factors, topical antiseptics, and oral hygiene instructions, as well as antibiotics such as penicillin and metronidazole, which may be indicated in patients with fever and/or lymphadenopathy.

Periapical Abscess

This acute inflammatory condition is associated with pulpal necrosis resulting in purulence within the alveolus at the apex of a nonvital tooth. Both aerobic and anaerobic bacteria have been isolated from these lesions. Periapical abscesses can present with pain to percussion, extrusion of the tooth within the socket, and soft tissue swelling in the periradicular region. If the infection spreads into intraosseous medullary spaces, osteomyelitis can develop.[42] Extension through the cortical plate into adjacent soft tissues can result in sinus tract formation. This condition can be accompanied by fever and lymphadenopathy. Management may include incision and drainage, appropriate therapy for the nonvital tooth (root canal therapy or extraction), and pain control with analgesics. A localized lesion with appropriate drainage does not require antibiotic therapy. Antibiotic therapy using amoxicillin or clindamycin would be indicated for the patient who is immunocompromised or who develops cellulitis.

Periodontal Abscess

A periodontal abscess is an acute infection that presents with purulence in a periodontal pocket. Both aerobic and anaerobic bacteria have been isolated from these lesions. Frequently, foreign material implantation is identified. This condition presents as a localized swelling with redness of the gingiva. There may be pain, tooth mobility, and tenderness to percussion, but the associated tooth responds to vitality testing. If a sinus tract develops, purulent exudate may be noted. The amount of bone loss and attachment loss can be variable. Management includes drainage through the periodontal pocket to avoid fenestration as well as debridement and curettage. Systemic antibiotics may be indicated if fever and/or lymphadenopathy is identified.

Pericoronitis

Pericoronitis is an acute or subacute gingival inflammatory reaction around a partially erupted, impacted, or erupting tooth. When food, debris, and/or microorganisms accumulate underneath the overlying soft tissue, an inflammatory reaction can develop.[39] Pericoronitis has a predilection for mandibular first and second molars in adolescents and mandibular third molars in young adults. Patients may present with severe, painful inflammation of gingiva, soft tissue edema, taste alterations, foul taste or odor, trismus, and abscess formation. Fever, lymphadenopathy, and malaise may also be present. Management includes irrigation below the soft tissue flap, antiseptic rinses, and alleviation of the condition through surgical removal of the overlying soft tissue or tooth extraction. Systemic antibiotics may be indicated if fever and/or lymphadenopathy is identified.

Cervicofacial Cellulitis/Facial Space Infections

Cervicofacial cellulitis develops when an abscess cannot develop a path of drainage. There is extension of acute edema and infection via the spread of the exudate into the adjacent facial soft tissues.[42] Various microorganisms such as *S. aureus,* alpha-hemolytic streptococci, and gram-negative and anaerobic bacteria have been isolated from these lesions. In addition, *Haemophilus influenzae* type B has been identified in cases of buccal cellulitis in infants. These patients present with diffuse swelling of buccal and/or submandibular facial areas. The swelling is firm, ill-defined, red, and warm to the touch. Pain, fever, lymphadenopathy, and malaise have been reported. Depending on the areas of involvement, patients may also present with trismus or dysphagia. The condition is usually diagnosed using blood cultures, fine-needle aspiration, or biopsy. Management includes hospitalization, maintaining a secure airway, and bacterial culture and sensitivity testing. Incision and drainage and systemic antibiotics are indicated.

Acute Suppurative Sialadenitis

Acute suppurative sialadenitis develops when ductal obstruction causes backflow of saliva and retrograde infection of salivary ducts and/or glands. The condition can affect the major or minor salivary glands and can present as unilateral or bilateral involvement. *S. aureus, Streptococcus pyogenes, Streptococcus pneumococci,* and other microorganisms have been identified with this condition.[43] There will be painful, indurated swelling of the affected gland. The area may feel warm to palpation, the ductal orifice may appear inflamed, and purulent drainage may be identified. A sialolith may or may not be present. Malaise, fever, and tender lymphadenopathy can be present, and trismus may be noted. The condition is diagnosed through cultures, magnetic resonance imaging (MRI), or computed tomography (CT) imaging and/or a sialogram. Management includes bacterial culture and antibiotic sensitivity testing with appropriate antibiotic therapy. If present, the sialolith should be removed.

Viral Infections

Primary Herpetic Gingivostomatitis

Primary herpetic gingivostomatitis is the most common acute viral infection affecting the oral mucosa. The condition is caused by infection with HHV-1 or HHV-2, and transmission occurs through direct contact. The condition peaks between 2 and 4 years of age, and lesions are widely distributed on keratinizing and nonkeratinizing tissues. The most frequent sites of involvement include gingiva, tongue, palate, labial mucosa, buccal mucosa, tonsils, and posterior pharynx.[43] The condition presents as an abrupt onset of fever and malaise. Typically, there will be intraoral discomfort and red, swollen mucosa with small vesicles. These vesicles rupture within 24 hours, resulting in shallow, painful, small ulcerations with a pseudomembrane and red halo. The ulcers can progressively coalesce. Lesions continue to develop for 3 to 5 days, and the condition heals within 7 to 10 days without scarring. Bilateral tender lymphadenopathy, fever, malaise, and perioral lesions may be present. Diagnosis can be made using culture, cytology, serology for antibody titers, and/or biopsy. Management includes palliative care and may include systemic antiviral therapy when indicated. Systemic antivirals must be initiated within 72 hours of symptom onset to be effective.[44] Although eating is often painful, fluid intake should be encouraged with the young child to prevent dehydration. Parents should be advised not to use products that contain benzocaine in infants or young children with primary herpetic gingivostomatitis due to reports of benzocaine gel–related cases of methemoglobinemia.

Secondary Herpetic Infections

Secondary herpetic infections occur through reactivation in a patient previously infected with HHV-1 or HHV-2. After the primary infection the virus remains latent in neural ganglion until reactivated. Predisposing factors that have been identified include illness, trauma, stress, UV light, and immunosuppression. The most common sites of involvement include the lips (herpes labialis) and intraoral keratinized tissues such as hard palate, dorsal tongue, and attached gingiva. This condition may present with a prodrome described as burning, tingling, itching, or paresthesia. There will be discrete small vesicles arranged in clusters that rupture within 2 to 3 days, leaving 1- to 3-mm areas of ulceration that heal within 6 to 10 days.[43] Lesions of herpes labialis can also be secondarily infected by skin flora. Recurrent herpes in an immunocompromised patient can present on any mucosal site. Diagnosis can be made using culture, cytology, serology for antibody titers, and/or biopsy. Management includes palliative care and appropriate systemic antiviral therapy ideally given at the time of prodrome.[44]

Varicella

VZV/HHV-3 causes the primary infection of chickenpox and presents as a recurrent infection in the form of herpes zoster (shingles). Patients most at risk for the recurrent infection include elderly, medically complex, and immunocompromised patients. Recurrent infection usually presents in a unilateral distribution along a trigeminal nerve and extends to the midline. Chickenpox presents as a cutaneous rash that initially appears on the face and trunk with extension to other sites. It starts as erythematous skin lesions that progress to vesicles and pustules that rupture into a hardened crust. The vesicles are surrounded by a rim of erythema. The condition can present in successive crops of lesions every 2 to 3 days that remain contagious before the exanthema until all lesions crust. Oral involvement can precede skin involvement and frequent oral sites of involvement include the palate, vermilion border, and buccal mucosa, as well as the gingiva. The intraoral vesicles will rupture and form small round shallow erosions with a red halo. Chickenpox is often accompanied by tender lymphadenopathy, fever, and malaise. Diagnosis is made through cytology, serology, biopsy, or polymerase chain reaction (PCR) testing of vesicular fluid. Management includes palliative care with antiviral medications reserved for individuals at risk for severe disease. Systemic antivirals are also considered for secondary household members.

Fungal Infections

Candidiasis

Candidiasis is the most common intraoral superficial mycosis. It most often involves *C. albicans,* but *C. tropicalis, C. krusei,* and *C. glabrata* have also been identified. Predisposing factors for infection include xerostomia, anemia, uncontrolled diabetes mellitus, malignancies, immunodeficiency, and medications such as antibiotics. The infant with cleft lip and/or palate is particularly susceptible to *Candida* infections because of the pooling of breast milk or formula in the areas of clefting, which serve as a reservoir for the organism. Parents and caregivers should be encouraged to cleanse the oral cavity of the cleft lip/palate infant with a clean, moist washcloth after each feeding.

The most frequent sites of involvement for *Candida* infections include the soft palate, buccal mucosa, and tongue. Pseudomembranous candidiasis (thrush) presents as white removable papules or plaques with erythematous underlying tissue.[45] Patients with thrush may report a burning sensation or pain. Angular cheilitis presents as red, fissuring, and crusting in the commissure region, whereas erythematous candidiasis (which includes denture stomatitis) presents as red patches accompanied by a burning sensation primarily affecting the dorsal tongue and palate. Diagnosis can be made using cytologic smears, culture, and histopathologic examination. Management of most forms of candidiasis includes topical or systemic antifungals, whereas angular cheilitis may have concomitant *S. aureus* infection requiring both antifungal and antibacterial medications.[46]

Antimicrobial Prophylaxis

Antibiotic prophylaxis is recommended for certain dental procedures to lessen the risk of bacteremia-induced infections. The American Heart Association has published guidelines[47] that are focused on prophylaxis 30 to 60 minutes before high-risk procedures that involve manipulation of the gingival tissues or the periapical region of the teeth.

Patients who should be considered for antibiotic prophylaxis include individuals with artificial heart valves, a history of infective endocarditis, heart transplant patients with a history of valvular problems, and some patients with congenital cardiac conditions. Congenital conditions needing prophylaxis may include unrepaired cyanotic congenital heart disease, palliative shunts and conduits, defects repaired with prosthetic material or a device during the first 6 months after repair, and repaired defects with a residual defect remaining at the site or adjacent to the site of the prosthetic patch or prosthetic device.

A major change to the antibiotic prophylaxis guidelines (Table 18.4) is that clindamycin is no longer to be used for this purpose due to significant adverse drug reactions and CDIs.[48] The decision to provide antibiotic prophylaxis is made on an individual basis and the guidelines are updated periodically. If uncertainty exists in terms of the necessity for antibiotic prophylaxis, consultation with the child's cardiologist and medical care team is always recommended before invasive dental treatment.

Visit eBooks.Health.Elsevier.com to see full list of references.

TABLE 18.4 Antibiotic Prophylaxis for a Dental Procedure (Taken 30–60 Minutes Before Procedure)

Situation	Agent	Adults	Children
Oral	Amoxicillin	2 g	50 mg/kg
Unable to take oral medication	Ampicillin OR	2 g IM or IV	50 mg/kg IM or IV
	Cefazolin or ceftriaxone	1 g IM or IV	50 mg/kg IM or IV
Allergic to penicillin or ampicillin—oral	Cephalexin[a,b] OR	2 g	50 mg/kg
	Azithromycin or clarithromycin OR	500 mg	15 mg/kg
	Doxycycline	100 mg	<45 kg, 2.2 mg/kg >45 kg, 100 mg
Allergic to penicillin or ampicillin and unable to take oral medication	Cefazolin or ceftriaxone[b]	1 g IM or IV	50 mg/kg IM or IV

Clindamycin is no longer recommended for antibiotic prophylaxis for a dental procedure.
[a]Or other first- or second-generation oral cephalosporin in equivalent adult or pediatric dosing.
[b]Cephalosporins should not be used in an individual with a history of anaphylaxis, angioedema, or urticarial with penicillin or ampicillin.
IM, Intramuscular.

19

Differential Diagnosis of Oral Lesions and Developmental Anomalies

CATHERINE M. FLAITZ AND CHRISTEL M. HABERLAND

A wide variety of oral lesions and soft tissue anomalies are detected in children, but the low frequency at which many of these entities occur makes them challenging to clinically diagnose. The purpose of this chapter is to highlight selected oral lesions that are most commonly found in children and pathologic entities that primarily develop in this age group. In addition, oral lesions associated with several genetic disorders and specific malignancies, which may mimic benign or inflammatory conditions, are included to broaden the disease scope. The material is outlined in tables to make this comprehensive subject more succinct and easier to review. The brief description for each entity summarizes the most important clinical information that is relevant to the child patient. Representative examples of these conditions are included to illustrate the characteristic clinical or radiographic features.

Each oral lesion is described according to key points: (1) the most common pediatric age group affected and the sex predilection, (2) the characteristic clinical and radiographic findings of the lesion, (3) the most frequent location for the lesion, (4) the pediatric significance of the lesion, (5) the treatment and prognosis for the lesion, and (6) the differential diagnosis that is pertinent to this age group.

Except for the first table on selected developmental anomalies, the other tables are arranged to capture the primary clinical or radiographic characteristics for the purpose of comparison. The sequential headings for each of the tables include the following disease categories:

Developmental anomalies (Table 19.1, Fig. 19.1)
White soft tissue lesions (Table 19.2, Fig. 19.2)
- White surface thickening lesions
- White surface material lesions
- White subsurface lesions

Dark soft tissue lesions (Table 19.3, Fig. 19.3)
- Red or purple-blue lesions
- Brown-black lesions

Ulcerative lesions (Table 19.4, Fig. 19.4)
Soft tissue enlargements (Table 19.5, Fig. 19.5)
- Papillary lesions
- Acute inflammatory lesions
- Tumor and tumor-like lesions

Radiolucent lesions of bone (Table 19.6, Fig. 19.6)
Mixed radiolucent and radiopaque lesions of bone (Table 19.7, Fig. 19.7)
Radiopaque lesions of bone (Table 19.8, Fig. 19.8)

Visit eBooks.Health.Elsevier.com to see full list of references.

TABLE 19.1 Developmental Anomalies (see Fig. 19.1)

Condition	Pediatric Age and Sex	Clinical Findings	Location	Pediatric Significance	Treatment and Prognosis	Differential Diagnosis
Fissured tongue (scrotal tongue)	First and second decades No sex predilection	Deep central groove; multiple, short furrows; tender, if irritated; may occur with *erythema migrans*	Dorsal and lateral tongue	Polygenic or autosomal dominant trait; occurs in *Down syndrome*, dry mouths, diabetes; detected in 1% of children; source of halitosis	Brush tongue; becomes more prominent with age	Erythema migrans Macroglossia with crenations Hemihyperplasia of tongue Orofacial granulomatosis
Ankyloglossia (tongue-tie)	Present at birth Male predilection	Short, thick lingual frenum or attachment to tip of tongue; may cause slight cleft at tip	Ventral tongue and floor of mouth	Occurs in 2%–11% of infants; infrequently causes speech, feeding, swallowing, or periodontal problems; multiple frenula associated with *oral-facial-digital syndrome*	Infrequently frenectomy is indicated; many self-correct with age	Bifid tongue Microglossia Palatoglossal adhesion (ankyloglossia superior) Tongue scar
Lingual thyroid	Second decade Female predilection	Nodular mass with pink or red, smooth surface; may cause dysphagia, dysphonia, or dyspnea	Midline base of tongue; *thyroglossal duct cyst* is variant that occurs in midline neck	Symptoms develop during puberty or pregnancy; normal thyroid absent in 70%; important cause of infantile hypothyroidism	Thyroid hormone therapy, excision, or radioactive iodine ablation; carcinomas arise in <1%	Lymphoid hyperplasia Hemangioma Lymphatic malformation High-rising epiglottis
Commissural lip pits	Second decade Male predilection	Unilateral or bilateral depressions or fistulas; fluid may be expressed	Corners of mouth	Occurs in <1% of children; an association with preauricular pits	None required	Paramedian lip pits Angular cheilitis
Paramedian lip pits (congenital lip pits)	Present at birth No sex predilection	Bilateral and symmetrical depressions or swellings; fluid may be expressed	Adjacent to the midline of the lower lip vermilion	Autosomal dominant trait; associated with cleft lip and palate; *van der Woude* and other syndromes	None required; surgery, if cosmetic problem	Mucocele Soft tissue abscess Median lip fissure Double lip Lip piercing
Retrocuspid papilla	First and second decades Female predilection	Asymptomatic, pink, sessile papule or nodule; usually bilateral	Lingual attached gingiva, adjacent to mandibular canines	Very common in children and regresses with age	None required; normal anatomical variation	Irritation fibroma Giant cell fibroma Soft tissue abscess
Bifid uvula	Present at birth No sex predilection	Midline groove or splitting of uvula; may have speech impairment	Midline, posterior soft palate	Minimal expression of cleft palate; marker for submucous palatal cleft; associated with *Loeys-Dietz syndrome* and others	None required; genetic counseling may be indicated	Traumatic defect

Continued

TABLE 19.1 **Developmental Anomalies (see Fig. 19.1)—cont'd**

Condition	Pediatric Age and Sex	Clinical Findings	Location	Pediatric Significance	Treatment and Prognosis	Differential Diagnosis
Hyperplastic labial frenum	Present at birth No sex predilection	Thick triangular band of pink soft tissue; may be associated with gingival recession or diastema	Midline labial mucosa and gingiva; both maxillary and mandibular lip	Bleeds freely when lacerated; multiple frenula associated with *oral-facial-digital syndrome;* infrequent breastfeeding problems	None required; frenectomy for some large diastemas, gingival recession, or lip mobility problems	Traumatic scar Frenal tag
Torus palatinus (palatal torus)	Second decade Female predilection	Bony hard mass that varies in size and shape; asymptomatic, unless traumatized; may be seen as radiopacity on radiographs	Midline hard palate	Most tori in this age group are slightly elevated with a smooth surface; autosomal dominant inheritance or multifactorial influence	None required; will continue to grow during adulthood	Prominent median palatal raphe Reactive exostosis Median palatal cyst Palatal hamartoma/ choristoma
Torus mandibularis (mandibular torus)	Second decade Male predilection	Bony hard mass that varies in size and shape; asymptomatic, unless traumatized; radiopacity may be superimposed over roots of teeth	Bilateral, lingual mandible	Less common than torus palatinus; genetic and environmental influence	None required; will continue to grow during adulthood	Exostosis Peripheral osteoma Proliferative periostitis Fibrous dysplasia
Exostosis	Second decade No sex predilection	Single or multiple bony hard nodules; asymptomatic, unless traumatized; radiopacity may be superimposed over roots of teeth	Maxillary and mandibular alveolar ridge on the facial aspect; usually bilateral; may occur on the palate	Exostoses that are traumatized mimic odontogenic infection because of the location; may be tender to palpation in children	None required; will continue to grow during adulthood	Peripheral osteoma Proliferative periostitis Ectopic tooth eruption

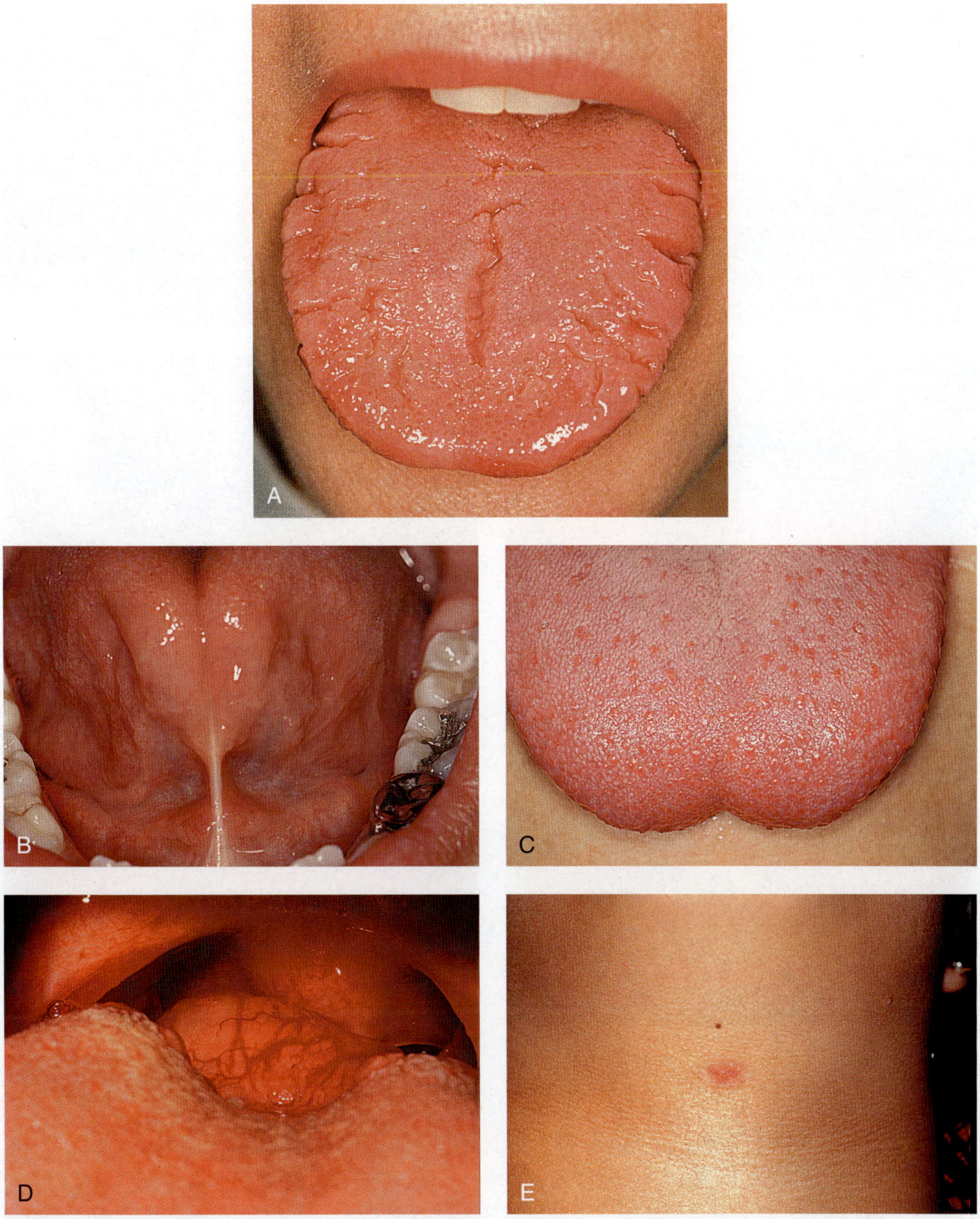

• **Fig. 19.1** Developmental Anomalies. (A) Fissured tongue. (B–C) Partial ankyloglossia with lingual frenum attachment at the tip of the tongue (B). Note the restricted mobility of the tongue with extension (C). (D) Lingual thyroid of the midline base of the tongue. (E) Thyroglossal duct cyst with sinus tract, midline neck.

Continued

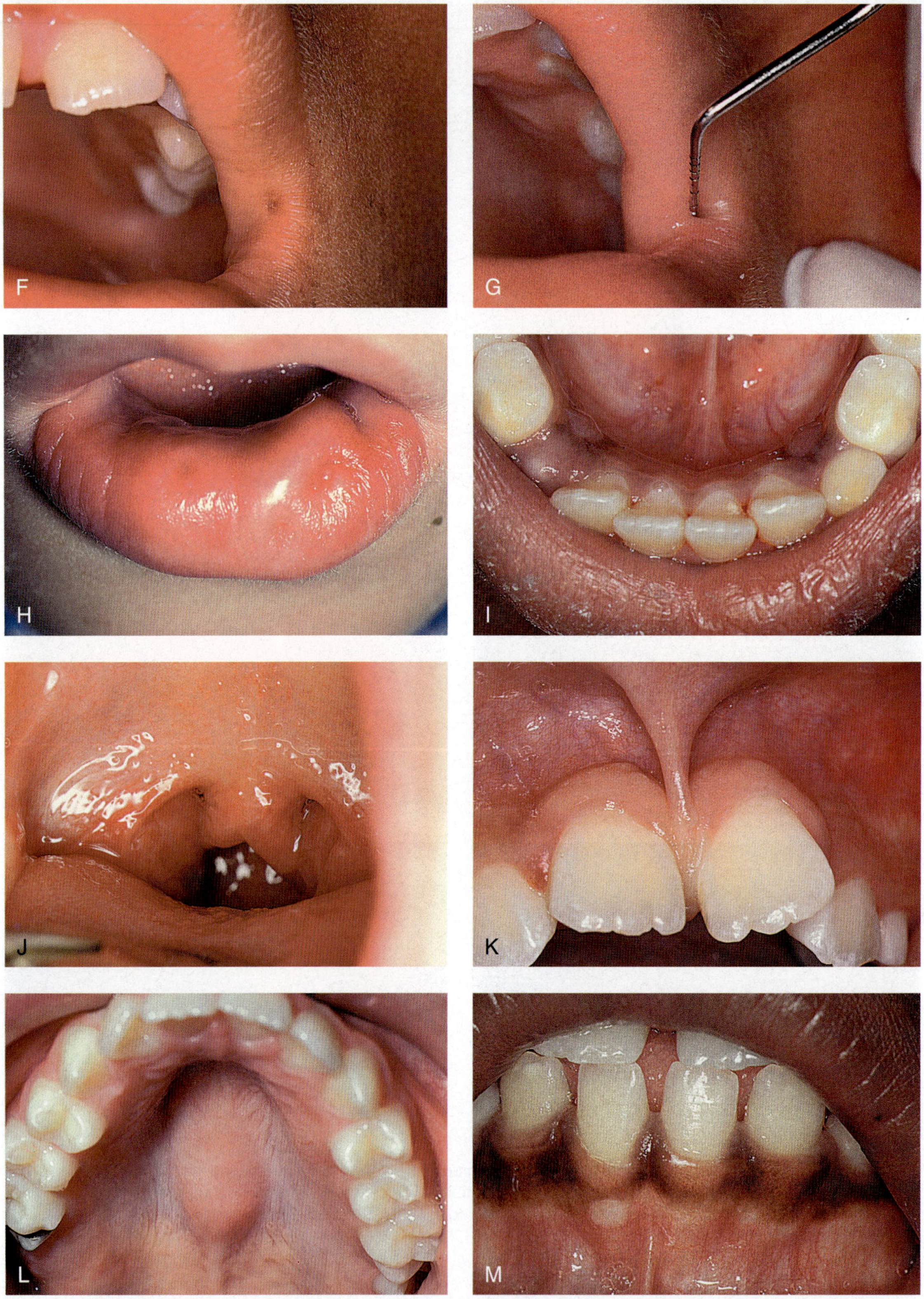

• **Fig. 19.1, cont'd** (F–G) Commissural lip pit (F) with depth illustrated by periodontal probe (G). (H) Paramedian lip pits. (I) Retrocuspid papilla of the lingual mandibular gingiva. (J) Bifid uvula. (K) Hyperplastic maxillary labial frenum. (L) Torus palatinus of the midline hard palate. (M) Small exostosis of the anterior mandibular alveolus, facial aspect. ([D] Courtesy Dr. G.E. Lilly, University of Iowa College of Dentistry.)

TABLE 19.2 White Soft Tissue Lesions (see Fig.19.2)

Lesion	Pediatric Age and Sex	Clinical Findings	Location	Pediatric Significance	Treatment and Prognosis	Differential Diagnosis
White Surface Thickening Lesions						
Frictional keratosis and Morsicatio mucosae oris	First and second decades No sex predilection	Localized to diffuse, white, rough or shredded patches; adherent; asymptomatic	Mucosa adjacent to occlusal plane, including buccal, labial mucosa, lateral tongue; attached gingiva	Caused by chronic nibbling habits *(morsicatio)*, irritation from orthodontic appliances, fractured teeth, and improper tooth brushing	Elimination of cause; lesion regresses; acrylic splint therapy for severe cases of *morsicatio*	Leukoedema Linea alba Smokeless tobacco keratosis Cinnamon contact stomatitis Hyperplastic candidiasis
Smokeless tobacco keratosis (tobacco pouch keratosis)	Second decade Male predilection	Diffuse, white, wrinkled patch; adherent; asymptomatic; gingival recession; tooth staining; caused by snuff or chewing tobacco	Vestibular, labial, and buccal mucosa; usually mandibular site	Addictive habit; develop after 1–5 years of use; increased risk for periodontal disease, dental caries, tooth sensitivity, and halitosis	Discontinuation of habit results in lesion reversal; biopsy of persistent lesions; low risk for malignant transformation	Nicotine pouch keratosis Leukoedema Frictional keratosis Cinnamon contact stomatitis Chronic hyperplastic candidiasis
Leukoedema	First and second decades No sex predilection	Widespread, filmy white, wrinkled mucosa; adherent; disappears when stretched	Bilateral buccal, labial mucosa and soft palate	Most prominent on pigmented mucosa; condition increases with age; more pronounced with cigarette smoking/ vaping	None required; common variant of normal mucosa	Frictional keratosis Irritant contact-related keratosis White sponge nevus
Cinnamon contact stomatitis	Second decade No sex predilection	Oblong to broadly linear, white plaques with a shaggy, thickened surface; diffuse erythema; tender	Gingiva, mucosa adjacent to occlusal plane, including buccal mucosa and lateral tongue	Cinnamon flavoring in candy, chewing gum, toothpaste, mouth rinses	Identify and discontinue use of offending product; lesions resolve within 1 week	Morsicatio mucosae oris Hyperplastic candidiasis Smokeless tobacco keratosis Hairy leukoplakia
Linea alba	Any age after the eruption of teeth; female predilec-tion	Smooth or shaggy white line; may be scalloped; asymptomatic	Bilateral buccal mucosa, along occlusal plane	Associated with biting irritation or sucking habit	None required; may spontaneously regress	Cinnamon contact stomatitis Scar formation Morsicatio mucosae oris
Hairy tongue	Second decade No sex predilection	Cream to brown discoloration; diffuse elongation of filiform papillae	Dorsal tongue	Contributes to halitosis; associated with cigarette smoking, poor oral hygiene, antibiotics, dry mouth, overuse of mouth rinses	Eliminate cause; brush tongue	Coated tongue Hyperplastic candidiasis Chronic lingual papulosis
White sponge nevus	First decade, may be present at birth No sex predilection	Diffuse, symmetrical, corrugated, or velvety white plaques: adherent; asymptomatic; persistent	Bilateral buccal mucosa is most common; also found on labial mucosa, ventral tongue, floor of mouth, and soft palate	Autosomal dominant skin disorder; defect in *keratin 4* and *keratin 13;* extraoral sites may be involved; reaches full expression during adolescence	None required; condition stabilizes in young adulthood; no malignant transformation	Leukoedema Hereditary benign intraepithelial dyskeratosis Frictional keratosis Hyperplastic candidiasis Syndrome-related leukoplakia

Continued

TABLE 19.2 White Soft Tissue Lesions (see Fig.19.2)—cont'd

Lesion	Pediatric Age and Sex	Clinical Findings	Location	Pediatric Significance	Treatment and Prognosis	Differential Diagnosis
White Surface Material Lesions						
Pseudomembranous candidiasis (thrush)	Any age, especially infancy No sex predilection	Widespread, white plaques that wipe off leaving a normal or red, raw base; mild burning	Any mucosal site but common on buccal mucosa, tongue, and palate	Caused by *Candida albicans* and other species; contributing factors are antibiotics, steroids, immune suppression; infants may have diaper rash; pacifiers, orthodontic appliances, and toothbrushes may harbor fungus	Antifungal medication and proper oral hygiene; may recur if cause is not eliminated	Dental plaque biofilm Chemical burn Coated tongue Oral mucosal sloughing Morsicatio mucosae oris Koplik spots of rubeola
Chemical burn	First and second decades No sex predilection	Localized or widespread, white nonadherent plaques, erosions, or ulcers; tender to painful; sudden onset	Any site but common on lips, tongue, buccal mucosa, and gingiva	Multiple chemicals and drugs may cause this reaction, including those used in dentistry—mouth rinses, topical anesthetics, phosphoric acid, whitening agents	Identify and remove cause; ask about homeopathic remedies; symptomatic relief management	Thermal burn Pseudomembranous candidiasis Coated tongue Oral mucosal sloughing Mucous patch of syphilis
Coated tongue (furred tongue)	First and second decades No sex predilection	White or yellow nonadherent coating on tongue; asymptomatic; may be source of halitosis	Dorsal tongue	Common; associated with mouth breathing, febrile illnesses, dehydration, poor oral hygiene, reflux disease	Brushing tongue and adequate hydration; tends to recur	Pseudomembranous candidiasis Hairy tongue White strawberry tongue
Oral mucosal sloughing	Second decade No sex predilection	Translucent to white strips of mucosa that peel off; stringy and slimy in texture; may burn	Buccal and labial mucosa, tongue	Associated with detergents and other ingredients in toothpastes and mouth rinses	Identify and discontinue the oral hygiene product; resolves spontaneously	Dental plaque biofilm Pseudomembranous candidiasis Allergic contact stomatitis Thermal/chemical burn
White Subsurface Lesions						
Scar formation (cicatrix)	First and second decades No sex predilection	White or pale pink line or irregular patch with smooth surface; cross-hatch or starburst pattern; asymptomatic	Any site but common on labial mucosa, lip vermilion, tongue	History of oral trauma or surgery; may represent child abuse or self-mutilation	None required; scar revision if cosmetic concern or if restricts function	Linea alba Mucosal graft Lichen planus
Fordyce granules	Second decade Male predilection	Small, yellow-white, multifocal papules; discrete or clustered; asymptomatic	Bilateral buccal mucosa, retromolar pad, and upper lip vermilion	Oral sebaceous glands occur in 20%–30% of children; puberty stimulates development	No treatment is necessary; may increase in size; laser treatment for cosmetics	Frictional keratosis Scar formation

Oral lymphoepithelial cyst	Second decade No sex predilection	Solitary, soft, pinkish white nodule with superficial fine vascular pattern; usually nontender	Posterior lateral tongue, floor of mouth, soft palate	Mimics an abscess because it may fluctuate in size and discharge contents	Excisional biopsy; does not recur	Soft tissue abscess Lipoma Sialolith Tonsillar concretions Hyperplastic lymphoid aggregate
Sialolithiasis	Second decade No sex predilection	Solitary or multiple, hard, yellowish white globular mass; episodic pain and swelling when eating; obstructive disease of the duct	Usually floor of mouth within Wharton duct, submandibular gland	Occlusal or panoramic radiograph may assist with diagnosis; circular calcified mass	Massage of gland, surgical removal of stone and sometimes the gland; lithotripsy; stone may recur	Soft tissue abscess Oral lymphoepithelial cyst Epidermoid cyst Calcified lymph nodes
Palatal cysts of the newborn	Neonates No sex predilection	Solitary or multiple, discrete or clustered papules with a smooth pearly white surface; usually 1–3 mm in size, asymptomatic	*Epstein pearls:* median palatal raphe *Bohn nodules:* lateral hard and soft palate and junction	Cysts occur in up to 85% of neonates	None required; keratin-filled cysts that spontaneously rupture within first month	Soft tissue abscess Oral lymphoepithelial cyst
Gingival cysts of the newborn (dental lamina cysts)	Neonates No sex predilection	Solitary or multiple, discrete or clustered papules with a smooth translucent to pearly white surface; usually 1–3 mm in size, asymptomatic	Alveolar mucosa, especially maxillary mucosa	Cysts occur in up to 50% of neonates	None required; spontaneously rupture within first 3 months	Natal/neonatal teeth Soft tissue abscess Neonatal alveolar lymphangioma Mucosal calcified nodule

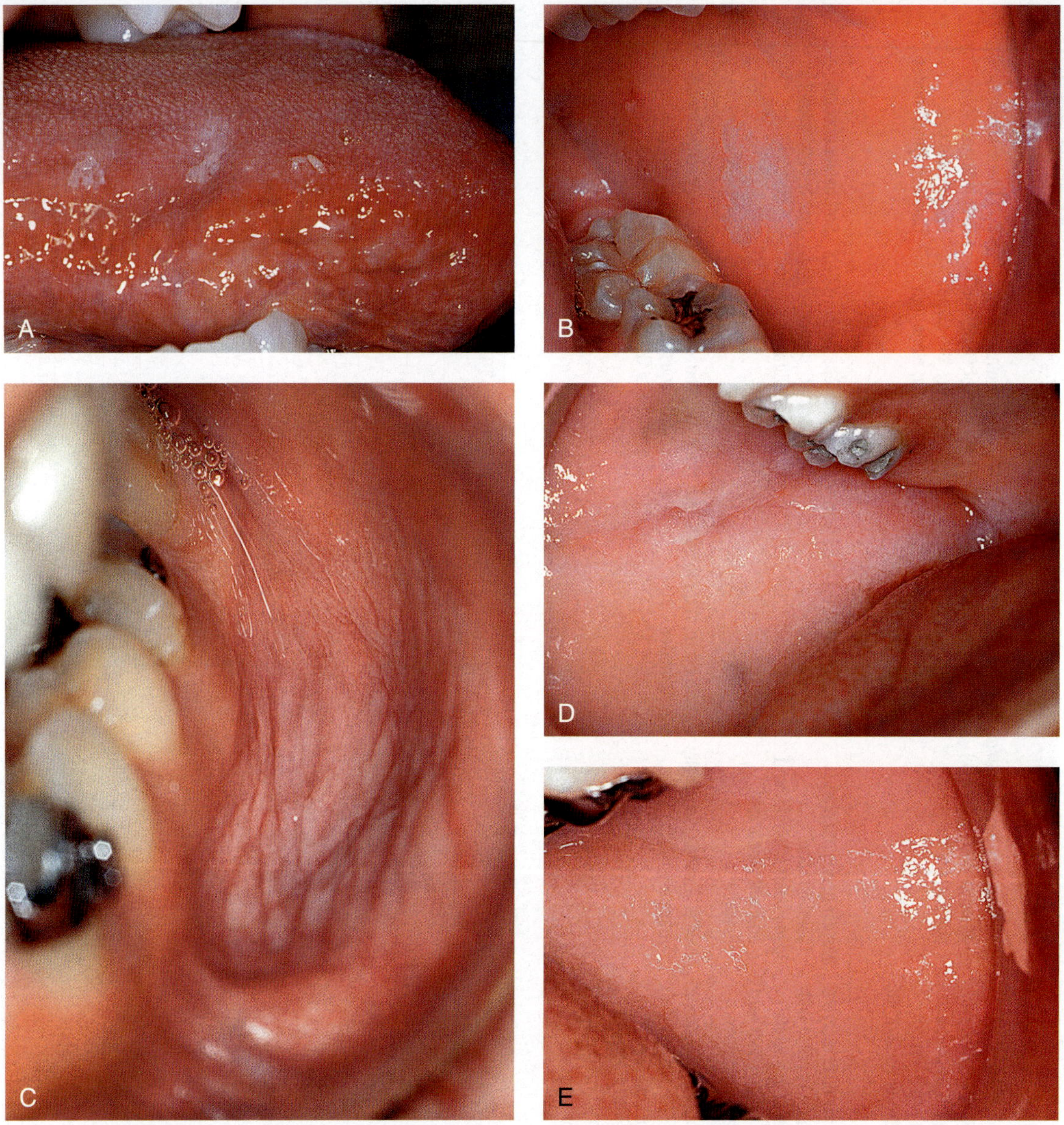

• **Fig. 19.2** White Soft Tissue Lesions. (A–B) Frictional keratosis of the lateral tongue (A) and buccal mucosa (B) from chronic biting of the tissues. (C) Smokeless tobacco keratosis of the posterior mandibular vestibule. (D–E) Leukoedema of the buccal mucosa, bilaterally.

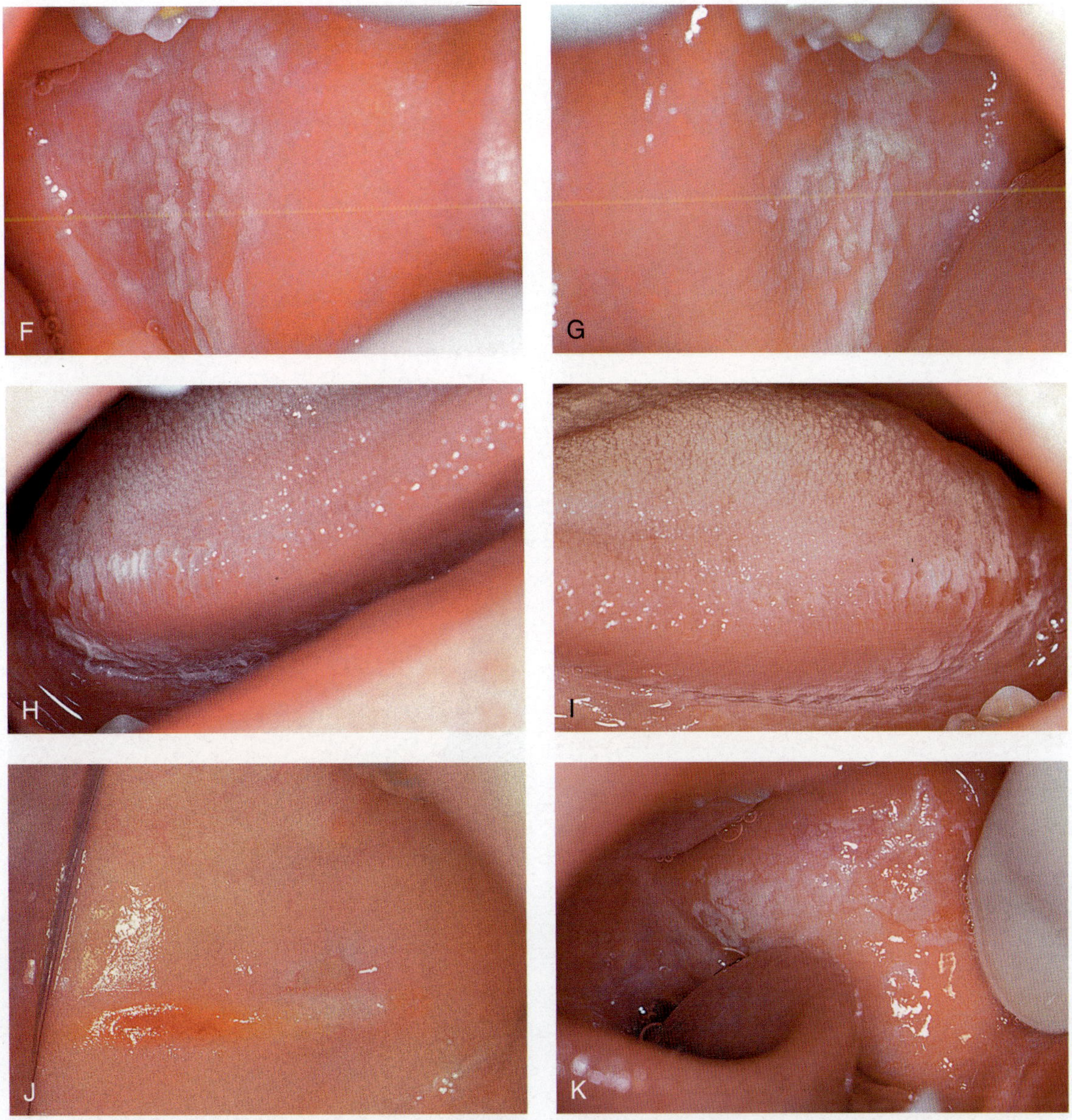

• **Fig. 19.2, cont'd** (F–I) White sponge nevus of the buccal mucosa (F–G) and lateral tongue (H–I). (J) Ulcerated linea alba from aggressive sucking habit. (K) Pseudomembranous candidiasis of the buccal mucosa.

Continued

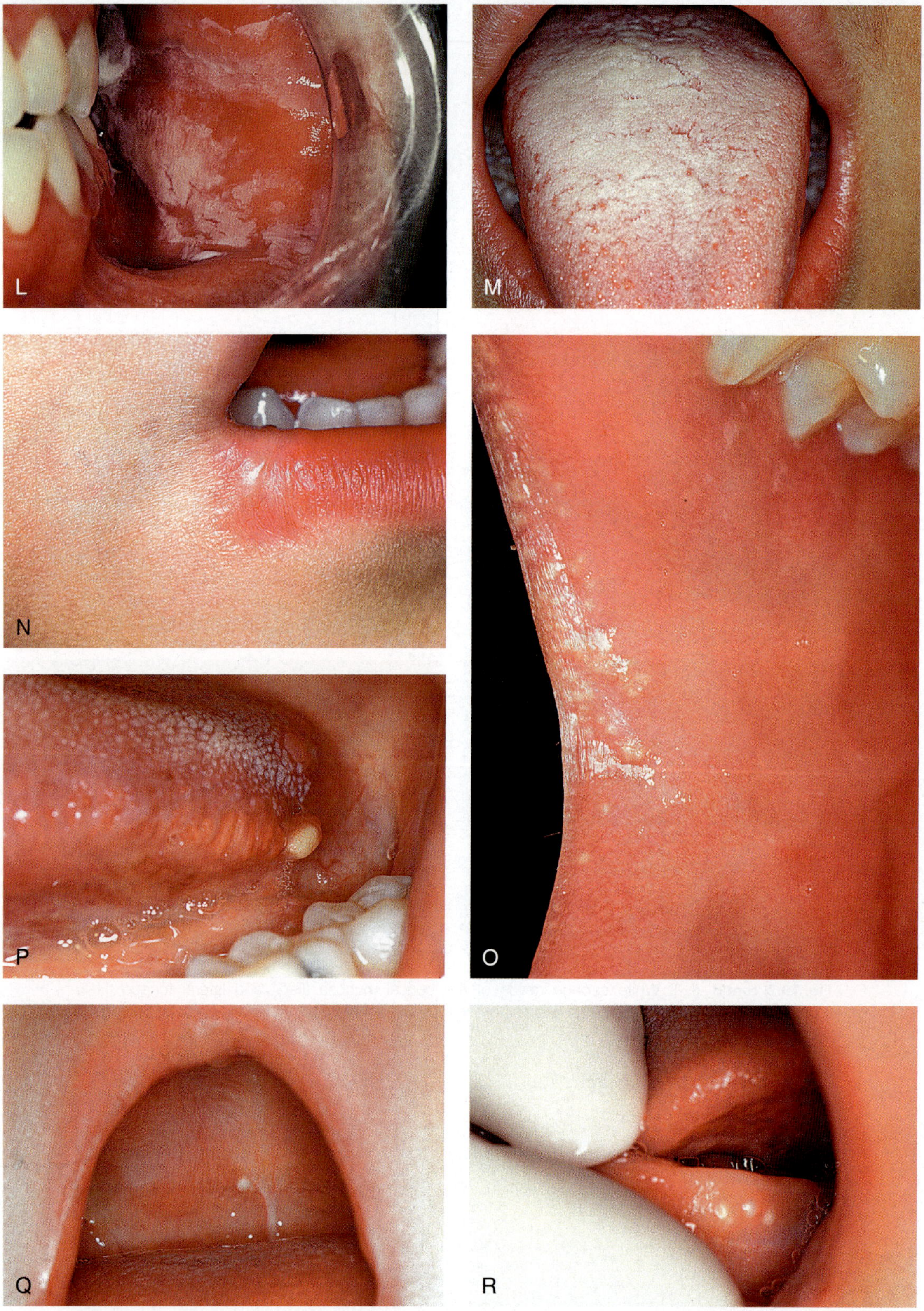

• Fig. 19.2, cont'd (L) Chemical burn from overuse of a topical anesthetic. (M) Coated tongue in a child who is mouth breathing. (N) Fan-shaped scar at the corners of the mouth caused by an electrical burn. (O) Cluster of Fordyce granules of the anterior buccal mucosa. (P) Oral lymphoepithelial cyst of the posterior lateral tongue. (Q) Single palatal cyst of the newborn on the midline hard palate. (R) Cluster of gingival cysts of the newborn on the mandibular alveolar mucosa.

TABLE 19.3 Dark Soft Tissue Lesions (see Fig. 19.3)

Lesion	Pediatric Age and Sex	Clinical Findings	Location	Pediatric Significance	Treatment and Prognosis	Differential Diagnosis
Red or Purple-Blue Lesions						
Port-wine stain (capillary vascular malformation)	Infancy No sex predilection	Localized to diffuse, red to purple macular lesions; variable blanching; bleeds freely; gingival and bony enlargement; grows with child	Face, along distribution of trigeminal nerve, is most common site; may have lip and oral mucosal involvement	Occurs in approximately 1% of newborns; may be sign of *Sturge-Weber syndrome;* bleeding is complication; possible neurologic disease; gingival lesion mimics *pyogenic granuloma*	Laser treatment; persistent lesion that may become darker in color and nodular with age	Nevus simplex Hemangioma Venous and arteriovenous malformation Hereditary hemorrhagic telangiectasia
Submucosal hemorrhage, including petechiae, ecchymosis, and hematoma	First and second decades No sex predilection	Localized to diffuse, pinpoint spots, patches, or swellings with smooth surface; early lesions are red; late lesions are blue-black; may be tender	Buccal mucosa, lips, lateral tongue, and soft palate; may develop concurrently on skin	If multiple lesions, need to exclude child abuse, factitial injury, infectious diseases, such as infectious mononucleosis, and blood disorders including leukemia, thrombocytopenia, anemia, and hemophilia	Identify the cause; no treatment for lesions; spontaneously resolve	Amalgam/graphite tattoo Blue nevus Hemangioma Vascular malformation Erythematous candidiasis Blood dyscrasia
Erythematous candidiasis	First and second decades No sex predilection	Multiple red macules to diffuse red patches; depapillation of tongue; burning sensation; may have *angular cheilitis*	Palate, buccal mucosa, dorsal tongue	Caused by *Candida albicans* and other species; contributing factors are antibiotics, immunosuppression, xerostomia, pacifier, and palatal coverage appliances	Antifungal medication and proper oral hygiene; may recur if cause is not eliminated or managed	Contact allergy Traumatic erythema Erythema migrans Mucosal burn Palatal petechiae Strawberry tongue
Median rhomboid glossitis	First and second decades No sex predilection	Localized red, depapillated patch; oval to rhomboid in shape with smooth or lobulated surface; asymptomatic	Midline posterior dorsal tongue	Caused by candidal infection; localized palatal erythema or "kissing lesion" may be present	Antifungal medication and proper oral hygiene	Erythema migrans Traumatic erosion Contact allergy Hemangioma Vascular malformation Lingual thyroid
Erythema migrans (benign migratory glossitis)	First and second decades Female predilection	Multiple oval or circular red patches with white scalloped borders; loss of filiform papillae; pattern changes; may burn	Dorsal and ventrolateral tongue; rarely at other mucosal sites	More common in children than adults; increased risk in atopic children; may occur with *fissured tongue* and *transient lingual papillitis*	None required; avoidance of hot, spicy, or acidic foods; topical coating agents or steroids in symptomatic cases	Median rhomboid glossitis Contact allergy Erythematous candidiasis Transient lingual papillitis Lichen planus
Eruption hematoma and cyst	First and second decades No sex predilection	Localized patch or swelling; amber, red, or blue in color; overlying an erupting tooth; usually nontender	Alveolar mucosa	Eruption cyst is soft tissue counterpart of *dentigerous cyst;* infrequently delays tooth eruption; minimal bleeding may occur at this site	No treatment is usually necessary; resolves with tooth eruption; uncover tooth if symptomatic	Hemangioma Neonatal alveolar lymphangioma Pyogenic granuloma Herniated dental follicle

Continued

TABLE 19.3 Dark Soft Tissue Lesions (see Fig. 19.3)—cont'd

Lesion	Pediatric Age and Sex	Clinical Findings	Location	Pediatric Significance	Treatment and Prognosis	Differential Diagnosis
Brown-Black Lesions						
Physiologic (racial) pigmentation	First and second decades No sex predilection	Gray, brown, or black patches with smooth surface; patchy to generalized distribution	Any location but attached gingiva is most common	Pigmentation increases with age of child; common in dark-complexioned skin types	None required; common variant of normal mucosa	Postinflammatory hyperpigmentation Drug-induced pigmentation Smoker's melanosis Gingival lead line Oral melanoacanthoma
Amalgam tattoo	Second decade No sex predilection	Gray-blue, black macule with smooth surface and well-defined to irregular margins; radiographs may show opaque fragments	Gingiva, alveolar mucosa, buccal mucosa	Graphite tattoo is found on palate from self-inflicted wound; intentional tattooing on lower labial mucosa	None required unless melanocytic neoplasm cannot be excluded; permanent discoloration	Melanotic macule Graphite tattoo Melanocytic nevus Varix Late ecchymosis Charcoal dentifrice staining
Oral melanotic macule (focal melanosis)	First and second decades Female predilection	Brown, gray, or black oval macule with smooth surface, well-defined margins; single or multiple	Lower lip vermilion, buccal mucosa, gingiva	Most common oral pigmentation of fair-complexioned children; multiple oral and perioral macules in *Peutz-Jeghers syndrome*	None required unless a melanocytic neoplasm cannot be excluded; no malignant transformation	Amalgam tattoo Graphite tattoo Melanocytic nevus Smoker's melanosis Late ecchymosis Drug-induced pigmentation
Melanocytic nevus	Second decade Female predilection	Brown, blue, or black well-defined nodule or macule with smooth surface	Lip vermilion, palate, gingiva	Oral lesions are uncommon but head and neck skin is frequently involved	Excisional biopsy; low risk of malignant transformation	Amalgam tattoo Graphite tattoo Oral melanotic macule Oral melanoacanthoma Melanoma

TABLE 19.4 Ulcerative Lesions (see Fig. 19.4)

Lesion	Pediatric Age and Sex	Clinical Findings	Location	Pediatric Significance	Treatment and Prognosis	Differential Diagnosis
Aphthous ulcer	First and second decades Female predilection	Recurrent, painful ulcers *Minor variant:* 1–5 superficial oval ulcers <1 cm; resolves in 7–10 days *Major variant:* multiple, deep ulcers >1 cm; resolves in 2–6 weeks *Herpetiform variant:* showers of multiple small ulcers	Buccal, labial mucosa, and ventral tongue are most common; primarily occurs on nonkeratinized mucosa	Occurs in 20%–30% of children; T cell–medicated immune reaction; trauma and orthodontic appliances are important factors in children; genetic predisposition; associated with several systemic diseases, food sensitivities, nutritional deficiencies	Topical anesthetics and coating agents for symptomatic relief; topical and systemic steroids, chlorhexidine oral rinse, laser treatment, nutritional supplements Major variant heals with scarring; evaluate for systemic disease with frequent recurrences	Traumatic ulcer Secondary herpetic ulcer Transient lingual papillitis Crohn disease Behçet disease Celiac disease Neutropenic ulcer PFAPA syndrome Gastroesophageal reflux disease
Secondary herpetic ulcer	First and second decades No sex predilection	Multiple, recurrent, small ulcers; painful; preceded by vesicles; clustered pattern; prodromal burning sensation; heals in 7–14 days	Herpes labialis on lip vermilion and perioral skin; intraoral herpetic ulcers on hard palate, attached gingiva; herpetic whitlow on fingers, especially with digit sucking habit	Reactivation of HSV; occurs in one-third of children; ultraviolet light, systemic diseases, trauma, stress, menses are triggering factors	Sunscreen for prevention; topical anesthetics for symptomatic relief; topical antiviral agents, systemic acyclovir, valacyclovir; immunocompromised children should be treated	Traumatic erosion Aphthous ulcer Angular cheilitis Impetigo Contact allergy Transient lingual papillitis Herpes zoster
Angular cheilitis	First and second decades No sex predilection	Red fissures that bleed and may ulcerate; scaling and crusted surface; burning sensation; may be recurrent	Commissures of mouth; may be associated with concurrent oral candidal infection	Caused by *Candida* species and staphylococci; lip incompetence, licking of lips, and drooling are aggravating factors	Lubrication of lips, antifungal, antifungal/steroid ointments; recurring lesions may require oral antifungal treatment	Secondary herpetic ulcer Impetigo Exfoliative cheilitis Traumatic erosions Contact allergy Anemia Vitamin B deficiency
Traumatic ulcer	First and second decades No sex predilection	Usually single ulcer; variable shape with irregular margins; shallow or deep; painful; typically heals in 1–3 weeks	Lateral tongue, buccal mucosa, lips, and gingiva; *Riga-Fede disease* occurs in infants on ventral tongue from rubbing against lower incisors	Most common oral ulcer; may indicate child abuse, neurologic impairment, or factitial injuries when persistent and recurrent	Symptomatic relief; eliminate cause; factitial ulcers are diagnostic problem; may heal with scarring	Aphthous ulcer Mucosal burn Secondary herpetic ulcer Contact allergy

Continued

TABLE 19.4 Ulcerative Lesions (see Fig. 19.4)—cont'd

Lesion	Pediatric Age and Sex	Clinical Findings	Location	Pediatric Significance	Treatment and Prognosis	Differential Diagnosis
Contact allergy	First and second decades No sex predilection	Focal or widespread erythema, vesicles, and ulcers; swelling, burning sensation and pain; if chronic, then white plaques may develop	Any mucosal site that comes in contact with allergen, especially lips, buccal mucosa, and gingiva	Wide variety of allergens including foods, dental materials, oral hygiene products, topical medications, cosmetic products	Identify and eliminate allergen; patch testing helpful in older children; topical steroids to reduce symptoms; lesions recur with reexposure to allergen	Mucosal burn Secondary herpetic ulcer Aphthous ulcer Angular cheilitis Erythema multiforme Angioedema
Erythema multiforme	Second decade Male predilection	Widespread, painful, red macules, vesicles, bullae, and ulcers; blood-crusted lesions on lips; target lesions on skin; acute onset; fever, malaise	Oral lesions on lips, tongue, buccal mucosa, and soft palate Skin lesions on extremities and head and neck region	Common precipitating factors include HSV and medications; minor and major forms of the disease	Withdrawal of medication; lubrication of lips, symptomatic relief; hospitalization if severe; recurrences are common if triggered by HSV	Primary herpetic gingivostomatitis Necrotizing ulcerative gingivitis Hand, foot, and mouth disease Chemical burn Reactive infectious mucocutaneous eruptions
Primary herpetic gingivostomatitis	Usually first decade No sex predilection	Fever, irritability, pain, lymphadenopathy, drooling, multiple vesicles, and ulcers; diffuse erythema; sudden onset; resolves in 7–10 days	Widespread oral and perioral involvement; gingival lesions are usually chief complaint; pharyngeal involvement in adolescents	Caused by HSV; high fever and dehydration are serious complications in children; digital and ocular lesions may occur	Supportive care includes antipyretics, analgesics, palliative oral rinses, hydration; systemic antivirals may be indicated in immunocompromised children	Necrotizing ulcerative gingivitis Erythema multiforme Herpangina Hand, foot, and mouth disease Reactive infectious mucocutaneous eruptions; Scorbutic gingivitis

HSV, Herpes simplex virus; *PFAPA,* periodic fever, aphthous-stomatitis, pharyngitis, adenitis syndrome.

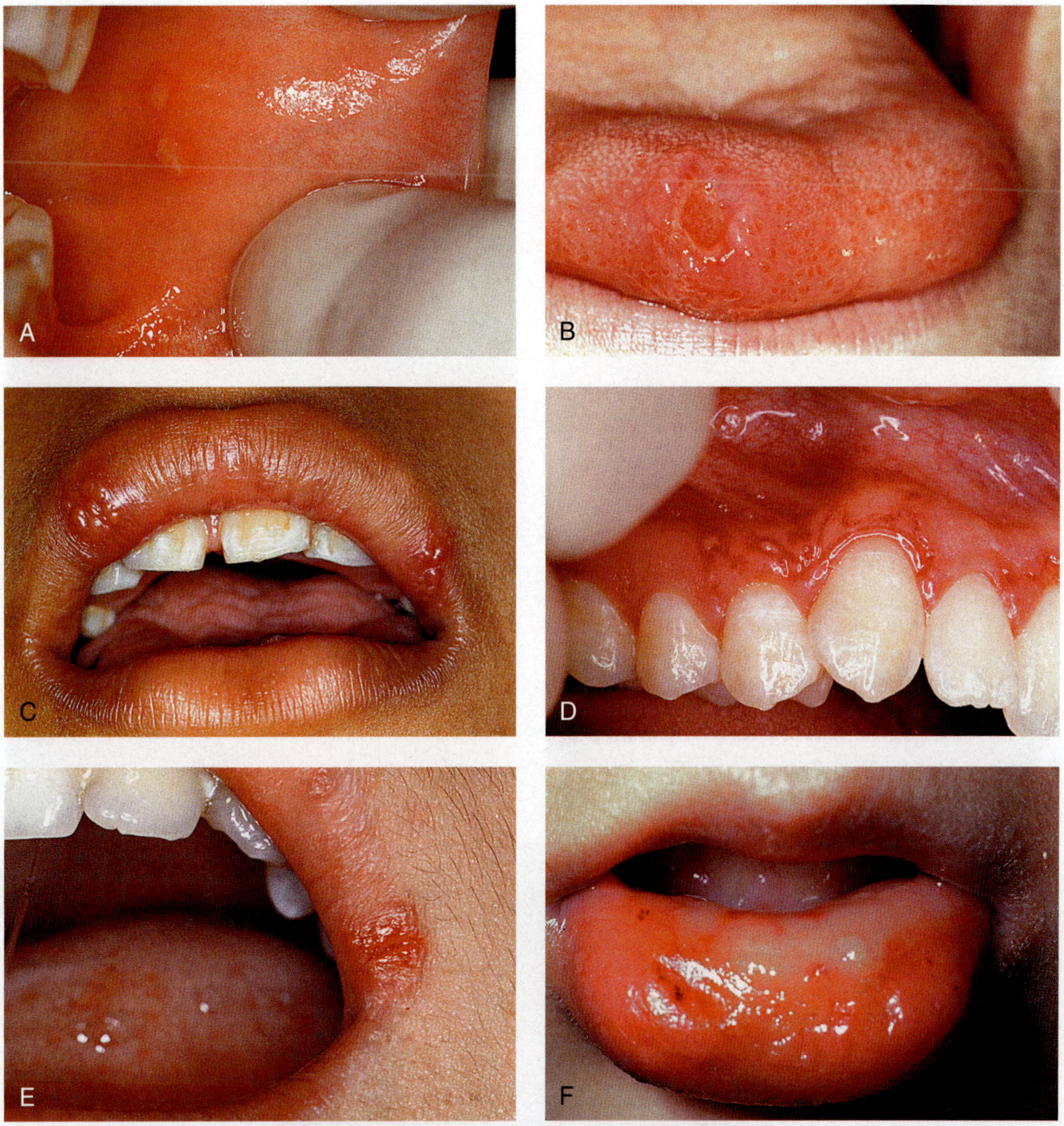

• **Fig. 19.4** Ulcerative Lesions. (A) Aphthous minor ulcer of the posterior buccal mucosa. (B) Aphthous major ulcer of the anterior dorsal tongue. (C) Herpes labialis of the vermilion of the maxillary lip. (D) Secondary herpetic ulcers of the maxillary attached gingiva. (E) Angular cheilitis. (F) Diffuse traumatic ulcer from biting the lip after local anesthesia for restorative treatment.

Continued

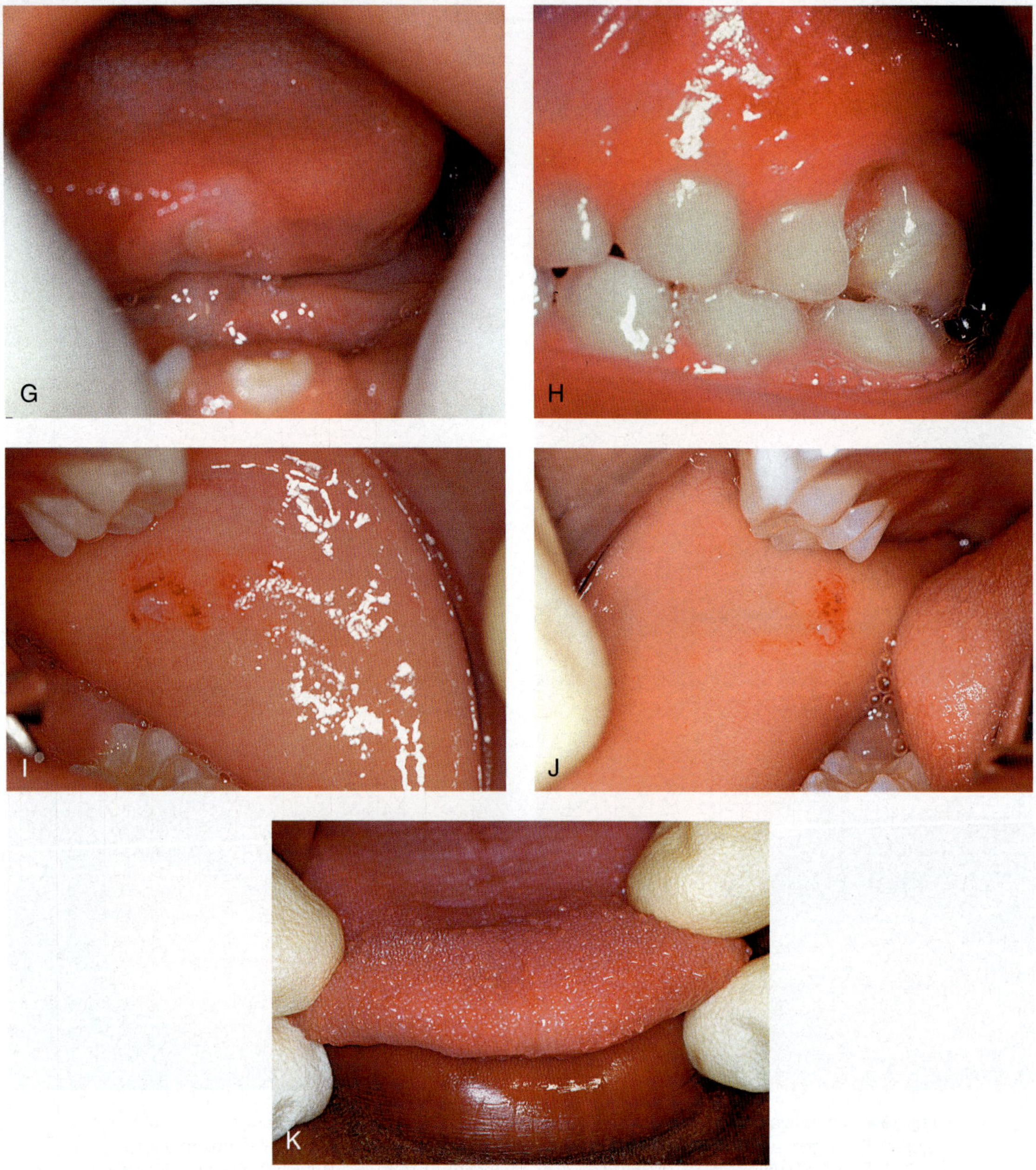

• **Fig. 19.4, cont'd** (G) Riga-Fede disease of the ventral tongue in a child with neonatal teeth. (H) Erythema and recession of the attached gingiva between the primary first and second maxillary molars from picking the tissues with the fingernails. (I–K) Bilateral erosions of the buccal mucosa (I–J) and tenderness of the fungiform papillae at the tip of the tongue (K) from a toothpaste hypersensitivity.

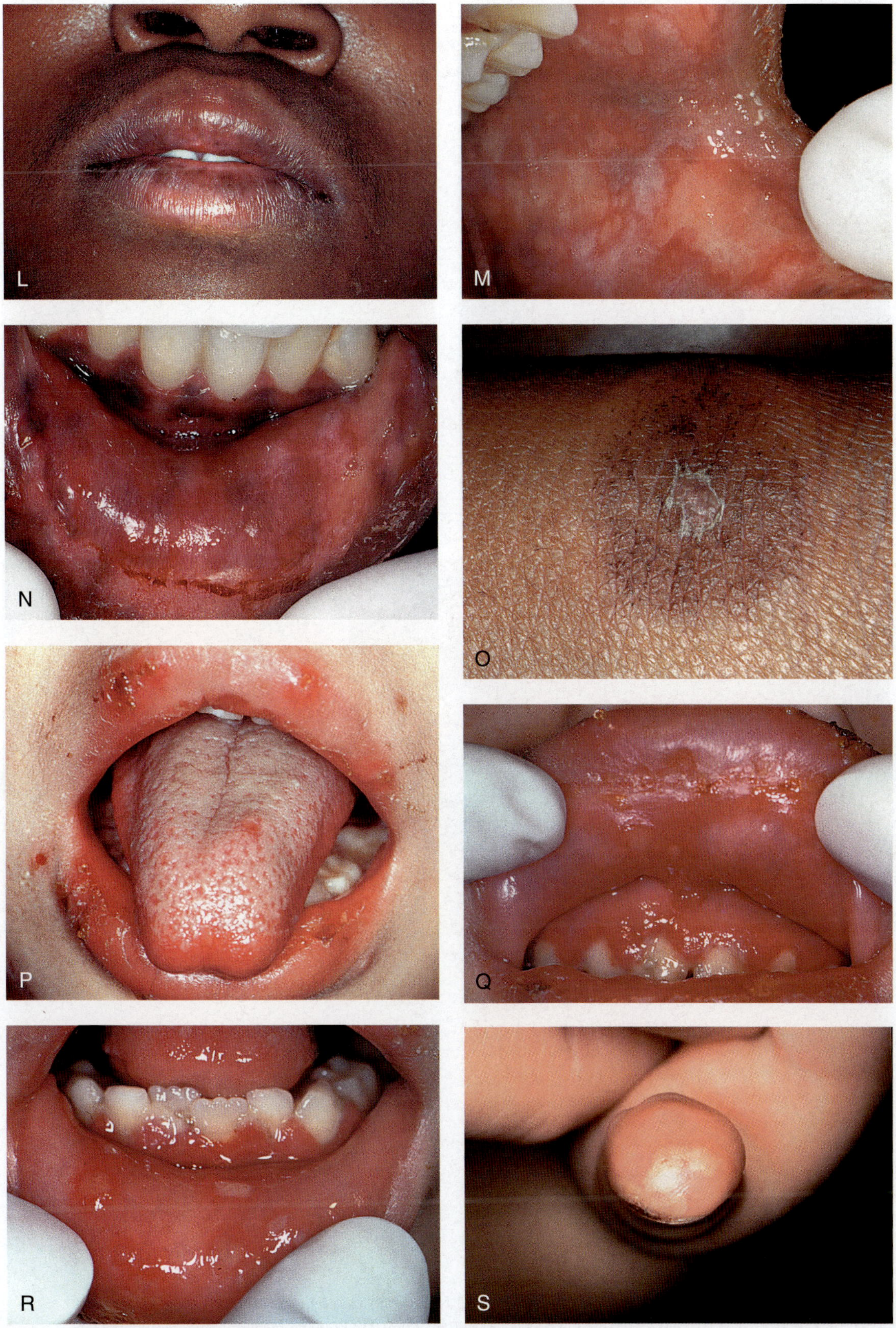

• **Fig. 19.4, cont'd** (L–O) Drug-induced erythema multiforme with swelling of the lips (L), erythema and ulcerations of the buccal mucosa (M) and labial mucosa (N), and target lesions on the skin (O). (P–S) Primary herpetic gingivostomatitis of the tongue and lips (P), maxillary gingiva and labial mucosa (Q) and mandibular gingiva and labial mucosa (R), and vesicles on the thumb (S).

Continued

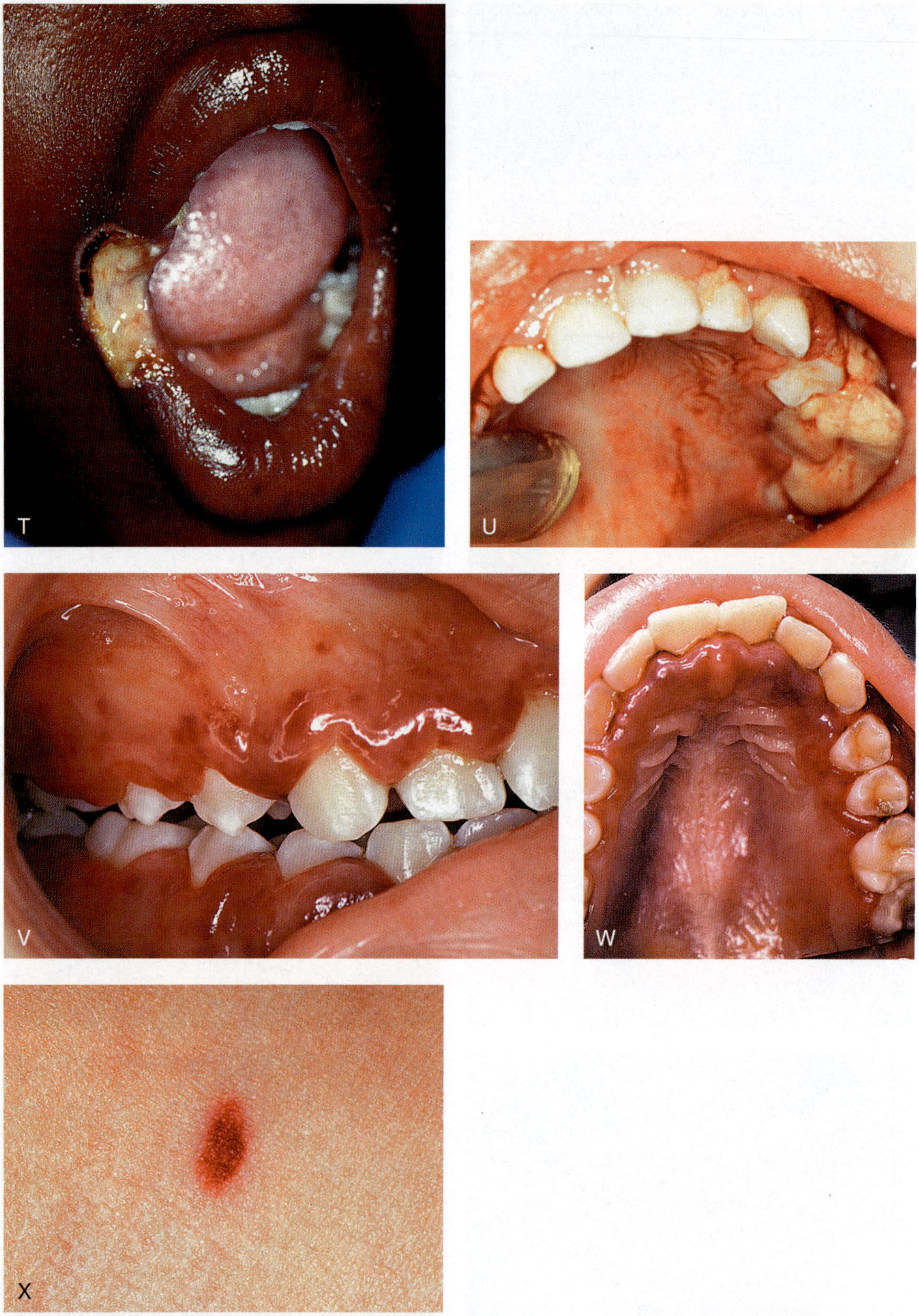

• Fig. 19.4, cont'd (T) Electrical burn of the lip. (U) Necrotizing gingival ulcer with a thick pseudomembrane in a child with acute lymphoblastic leukemia. (V–X) Red-purple enlargements of the buccal gingiva (V), palatal mucosa (W), and skin (X) that represent leukemic infiltrates in a child with acute myeloid leukemia.

TABLE 19.5 Soft Tissue Enlargements (see Fig. 19.5)

Lesion	Pediatric Age and Sex	Clinical Findings	Location	Pediatric Significance	Treatment and Prognosis	Differential Diagnosis
Papillary Lesions						
Squamous papilloma	Second decade No sex predilection	Single, pedunculated nodule with finger-like projections; pink to white; soft and nontender	Any oral site but predilection for the tongue, lips, and soft palate	Caused by HPV, especially types 6, 11; low virulence and infectivity rate	Excisional biopsy; recurrence is rare; no evidence of malignant transformation	Verruca vulgaris Condyloma acuminatum Giant cell fibroma Localized spongiotic gingival hyperplasia
Verruca vulgaris (common wart)	First and second decades No sex predilection	Multiple sessile or pedunculated papules and nodules with rough, pebbly, or papillary surface; white; nontender	Common on skin of hands and face; infrequently found on the lip vermilion, labial mucosa, and anterior tongue	Caused by HPV, especially types 2, 4; spread by autoinoculation to oral site by sucking on fingers or nail biting	Excisional biopsy of oral warts; low risk for recurrence for oral lesions; spontaneous resolution may occur; no risk for malignant transformation	Squamous papilloma Verruca plana Condyloma acuminatum Giant cell fibroma Molluscum contagiosum Frictional keratosis Gingival micropapillomatosis
Condyloma acuminatum (venereal wart)	Second decade No sex predilection	Multiple, discrete, sessile nodules with blunted papillary surface; pink; nontender	Usually anogenital lesions; oral sites include labial mucosa, soft palate, and ventral tongue	Oral lesions caused by HPV 6, 11, 16, 18; oncogenic HPV types 16, 18; autoinoculation, vertical or sexual transmission; may indicate child abuse; HPV vaccine for prevention	Excisional biopsy, laser ablation of oral warts; highly contagious; frequently recur; oral HPV 16, 18 associated with oropharyngeal carcinoma; HPV vaccine available	Squamous papilloma Multifocal epithelial hyperplasia Inflammatory papillary hyperplasia Giant cell fibroma Superficial lymphatic malformation Linear epidermal nevus Condyloma lata
Giant cell fibroma	Second decade Female predilection	Solitary, sessile, or pedunculated nodule with a pebbly surface; pink; nontender	Attached gingiva, dorsal tongue, and hard palate	Fibrous lesion of unknown cause that has a predilection for children; may displace teeth	Excisional biopsy; recurrence is rare	Squamous papilloma Retrocuspid papilla Irritation fibroma Gingival micropapillomatosis
Multifocal epithelial hyperplasia (Heck disease)	First and second decades No sex predilection	Multifocal, sessile papules and nodules with pink grainy to stippled surface; lesions coalesce, display cobblestone appearance; nontender	Usually located on labial and buccal mucosa and tongue	Caused by HPV 13, 32; familial tendency, genetic susceptibility Other risk factors include poor oral hygiene, crowded living conditions, nutritional deficiencies	Excisional biopsy; laser ablation; recurrence is common; spontaneous regression may occur; no malignant transformation potential	Verruca vulgaris Condyloma acuminata Multiple hamartoma syndrome Multiple endocrine neoplasia syndrome 2B

Continued

TABLE 19.5 Soft Tissue Enlargements (see Fig. 19.5)—cont'd

Lesion	Pediatric Age and Sex	Clinical Findings	Location	Pediatric Significance	Treatment and Prognosis	Differential Diagnosis
Localized juvenile spongiotic gingival hyperplasia	Second decade Female predilection	Isolated red, velvety to papillary patch or nodule; bleeds freely; persistent; does not respond to oral hygiene measures	Anterior facial gingiva, usually maxillary gingiva; represents transplanted crevicular or junctional epithelium	Contributing factors appear to be mouth breathing, anterior crowding, orthodontic appliances	Topical steroids; excisional biopsy; may spontaneously resolve; recurs up to 16%	Pyogenic granuloma Inflamed squamous papilloma Giant cell fibroma Gingival lymphatic malformation
Inflammatory papillary hyperplasia	Second decade No sex predilection	Multiple, clustered papules and nodules with pink to red granular surface; cobblestone appearance; nontender	Hard palatal mucosa and adjacent alveolar mucosa	Caused by continuous wear of palatal coverage appliance; other factors include mouth breathing and high palatal vault; candidal infection may be present	Remove and clean appliance; reline appliance if needed; antifungal therapy; excisional biopsy of persistent lesions	Condyloma acuminata Multifocal epithelial hyperplasia Erythematous candidiasis Early nicotine stomatitis
Acute Inflammatory Lesions						
Soft tissue abscess (parulis)	First and second decades No sex predilection	Solitary pinkish white or deep red nodule; purulence; fluctuates in size; tender to painful; may progress to cellulitis	Gingiva and alveolar mucosa are most common sites	Usually caused by odontogenic infection or entrapped foreign body; *pericoronitis* is a gingival abscess associated with erupting molars	Manage source of infection; local debridement; usually antibiotics are not indicated; recurs if infection is not eliminated	Pyogenic granuloma Herniated dental follicle Oral lymphoepithelial cyst Sialolithiasis Tonsillar concretions Gingival cysts of newborn
Cellulitis	First and second decades No sex predilection	Diffuse erythematous swelling of sudden onset; soft to boardlike; warm and painful tissues; fever, headache, airway obstruction, and leukocytosis may be present	Upper or lower face and neck	Caused by odontogenic infection, facial or oral lacerations, insect bites, peritonsillar abscesses, jaw fractures, sialadenitis, sinusitis, and bacteremia	Manage source of infection; antibiotic therapy; incision and drainage in severe cases *Ludwig angina* and *cavernous sinus thrombosis* may be life threatening	Facial hematoma Plunging ranula Emphysema Obstructive sialadenitis Angioedema Acute sinusitis Acute lymphadenitis
Angioedema	First and second decades No sex predilection	Diffuse swelling of sudden onset; soft and nontender; may be associated with urticaria, respiratory and gastrointestinal problems	Lips, tongue, soft palate, and face, and other cutaneous sites	Acquired form is caused by allergic reaction to foods, plants, drugs, insect bites, cold, heat, latex, pressure, stress, and infections; most hereditary forms are caused by C1-INH deficiency	Allergic forms are treated by antihistamines, steroids, or epinephrine; other drugs are used for the hereditary forms; may be life threatening	Cellulitis Emphysema Traumatic edema Contact allergy Orofacial granulomatosis

Mucocele	First and second decades No sex predilection	Fluid-filled nodule with a smooth, translucent, red, or blue surface; sudden onset; fluctuates in size; tender if traumatized; periodically drains	Lower labial mucosa, buccal mucosa, and anterior ventral tongue	Most common lip swelling in children; may be associated with trauma and orthodontic appliances; rare cases are congenital	Excisional biopsy with removal of underlying minor salivary glands; may recur with incomplete removal or repeated trauma	Lymphatic malformation Hemangioma Hematoma Soft fibroma Soft tissue abscess Salivary duct cyst
Ranula	First and second decades No sex predilection	Fluid-filled swelling with smooth, translucent to blue surface of recent onset; fluctuates in size; mildly tender; periodically drains; may elevate tongue	Floor of mouth, lateral to midline; plunging variant results in diffuse swelling of the submandibular region and neck	Usually associated with sublingual gland; rare cases are congenital and caused by aplasia of submandibular excretory duct	Excisional biopsy of sublingual gland or marsupialization; recurrences are common with marsupialization	Lymphatic malformation Hemangioma Mucoepidermoid carcinoma Obstructive sialadenitis Salivary duct cyst Dermoid cyst Heterotopic gastrointestinal cyst
Tumor and Tumor-like Lesions						
Irritation fibroma	First and second decades No sex predilection	Nodule with pink smooth surface; firm and nontender; limited growth potential	Buccal and labial mucosa, tongue, and attached gingiva	Common reactive hyperplastic lesion caused by chronic trauma and mimics a tumor	Conservative excisional biopsy; may recur if irritation continues	Fibrosing mucocele Giant cell fibroma Fibrosing pyogenic granuloma Peripheral ossifying fibroma Benign submucosal neoplasm
Peripheral ossifying fibroma	Second decade Female predilection	Nodule with pink to red surface; frequently ulcerated; firm and nontender; may resorb alveolar bone; limited growth potential	Emanates from interdental papilla of attached gingiva; most common site is anterior region	Reactive hyperplastic lesion with mineralized product from cells of periosteum or periodontal ligament; may displace teeth	Excisional biopsy down to periosteum and removal of local irritation; 16% recurrence rate	Irritation fibroma Peripheral giant cell granuloma Giant cell fibroma Pyogenic granuloma Peripheral odontogenic fibroma
Peripheral giant cell granuloma	Second decade Female predilection	Nodule with red or purple-blue surface; may be ulcerated; firm and nontender; resorb alveolar bone; limited growth potential	Attached gingiva or alveolar mucosa	Reactive hyperplastic lesion caused by irritation; may displace teeth; rare cases associated with hyperparathyroidism	Excisional biopsy to periosteum and remove local irritation; 10%–18% recurrence rate	Pyogenic granuloma Ulcerated irritation fibroma Peripheral ossifying fibroma Hemangioma Foreign body granuloma

Continued

TABLE 19.5 Soft Tissue Enlargements (see Fig. 19.5)—cont'd

Lesion	Pediatric Age and Sex	Clinical Findings	Location	Pediatric Significance	Treatment and Prognosis	Differential Diagnosis
Pyogenic granuloma	First and second decades Female predilection	Nodule with smooth to irregular, red surface; usually ulcerated; bleeds freely; soft and friable; nontender; limited growth potential	Most occur on attached gingiva; other sites include lip, tongue, and buccal mucosa; also occurs on skin	Reactive hyperplastic lesion caused by irritation and poor oral hygiene; may be associated with pregnancy *(pregnancy tumor)* or may develop at extraction site because of bony sequestra *(epulis granulomatosa)*	Excisional biopsy and remove local irritation; recurrence rate is 3%–15%	Ulcerated irritation fibroma Peripheral ossifying fibroma Peripheral giant cell granuloma Soft tissue abscess Hemangioma Localized, spongiotic gingival hyperplasia
Gingival fibromatosis	First and second decades No sex predilection	Localized or generalized gingival enlargements; pink, smooth to stippled surfaces; firm and nontender; affects both dentitions	Attached gingiva and maxillary tuberosity	May be familial or idiopathic; associated with several syndromes; interferes with eruption of teeth; displacement of teeth	Gingivectomy and good oral hygiene; high recurrence rate	Drug-induced gingival overgrowth Mouth breathing gingivitis Chronic hyperplastic gingivitis Leukemic gingival infiltrates Scorbutic gingivitis
Hemangioma	Infancy Female predilection	Localized to diffuse, red, blue, or purple lesion, flat or nodular, soft and compressible; may blanch; bleeds freely; 20% are multiple	60% occur in head and neck region; lips, tongue, and buccal mucosa are most common sites; rarely occurs in jaws	Hemorrhage is potential complication; may cause malocclusion; scarring is common with involution	Involution of lesion within first decade; surgery for select cases and scar revision, laser ablation, corticosteroids, propranolol; does not recur	Vascular malformation Pyogenic granuloma Lymphatic malformation Eruption cyst/hematoma Mucocele
Lymphatic malformation (lymphangioma)	Infancy; most detected by 2 years No sex predilection	Localized to diffuse, translucent to red or purple swelling; smooth or vesicular to pebbly surface; soft and compressible; crepitus may be palpated	Up to 75% occur in head and neck; common oral sites include the tongue, lip, and buccal mucosa	May cause malocclusion, dysphagia, and respiratory problems; *neonatal alveolar lymphangioma* is uncommon variant	Surgical excision; recurrences are common; airway obstruction and death may occur with large neck or tongue lesions	Vascular malformation Squamous papilloma Lingual papillitis Mucocele Plunging ranula Parotitis Branchial cleft cyst
Lipoma	Second decade No sex predilection	Solitary, slowly growing nodule with a yellowish-pink hue; smooth surface with fine capillaries; soft to palpation and nontender	Buccal mucosa and vestibule, tongue, and labial mucosa	In children, it may represent a herniated buccal fat pad. Congenital lipomatous choristomas of the tongue are a feature of *oral-facial-digital syndrome*	Surgical excision; recurrences are rare	Irritation fibroma Oral lymphoepithelial cyst Fibrosing mucocele Schwannoma Eruption cyst

Congenital epulis	Infancy Female predilection	Pedunculated or sessile nodule; pink to red smooth surface; may be ulcerated; 10% are multiple	Anterior alveolar ridge; usually maxilla	May cause feeding problems; usually reaches maximum size at birth	Surgical excision; occasional spontaneous regression; no recurrence; normal tooth development	Hemangioma Pyogenic granuloma Neonatal alveolar lymphangioma Neuroectodermal tumor of infancy
Neurofibroma	Second decade No sex predilection	Single or multiple nodules with smooth surface; discrete or diffuse; soft to firm on palpation; nontender	Tongue, buccal mucosa, and palate; rarely within mandible; syndromic lesions occur at any site, especially skin	*Neurofibromatosis, type 1* is autosomal dominant condition with neurofibromas, café-au-lait macules, axillary freckling, Lisch nodules on iris, enlargement of mandibular canal	Surgical excision if solitary lesion; selective excision of syndrome type; 5% malignant transformation of syndrome type	Schwannoma Mucosal neuroma Irritation fibroma Traumatic neuroma Benign submucosal neoplasm Salivary gland neoplasm
Mucosal neuromas (multiple endocrine neoplasia syndrome, type 2B)	First decade No sex predilection	Multiple, pink papules and nodules; soft and nontender; marfanoid body type; narrow face with full lips	Labial and buccal mucosa, anterior tongue, gingiva; also on conjunctiva and eyelid	Autosomal dominant syndrome; other stigmata include pheochromocytoma and medullary carcinoma of thyroid gland	Surgical excision of neuromas for cosmetics; aggressive thyroid cancer develops in second decade	*Neurofibromatosis, type 1* Multifocal epithelial hyperplasia *Multiple hamartoma syndrome*
Pleomorphic adenoma (benign mixed tumor)	Second decade Slight female predilection	Pink, dome-shaped enlargement with smooth surface; slowly growing; firm and nontender	Parotid gland is most common site; palate is most common oral site	Most common benign salivary gland neoplasm; *mucoepidermoid carcinoma* is most common malignant salivary gland tumor in this age group	Surgical excision with adequate margins; recurrence is low; malignant transformation rate of <4%	Neurofibroma Schwannoma Mucoepidermoid carcinoma Irritation fibroma
Juvenile fibromatosis	First and second decades No sex predilection	Rapidly growing, pink, firm mass with an irregular surface; may be ulcerated; painless; large in size; facial disfigurement; destruction of adjacent bone	Head and neck region; maxillary sinus and paramandibular soft tissues are common intraoral sites	Rare, locally aggressive, and destructive lesion that mimics a malignancy; associated with *familial adenomatous polyposis, Gardner syndrome*	Surgical excision with wide margins; adjunctive chemotherapy and radiotherapy may be indicated; high recurrence rate	Large pyogenic granuloma Myofibroma Fibrosarcoma Rhabdomyosarcoma Metastatic disease
Rhabdomyosarcoma	First and second decades Male predilection	Rapidly growing, infiltrative, and destructive mass; painless	Head and neck region is the most common site; face, orbit, nasal cavity, maxillary sinus, palate	Skeletal muscle malignancy; one of the most common sarcomas in children; extensive long-term orofacial complications with head and neck involvement	Surgical excision, multiagent chemotherapy with or without radiation therapy Pediatric prognosis for intermediate risk is 50%–70% 5-year survival rate	Aggressive Fibromatosis Lymphoma Neuroblastoma Malignant salivary gland tumor Retinoblastoma Juvenile nasopharyngeal angiofibroma

C1-INH, C1-esterase inhibitor; *HPV*, human papillomavirus.

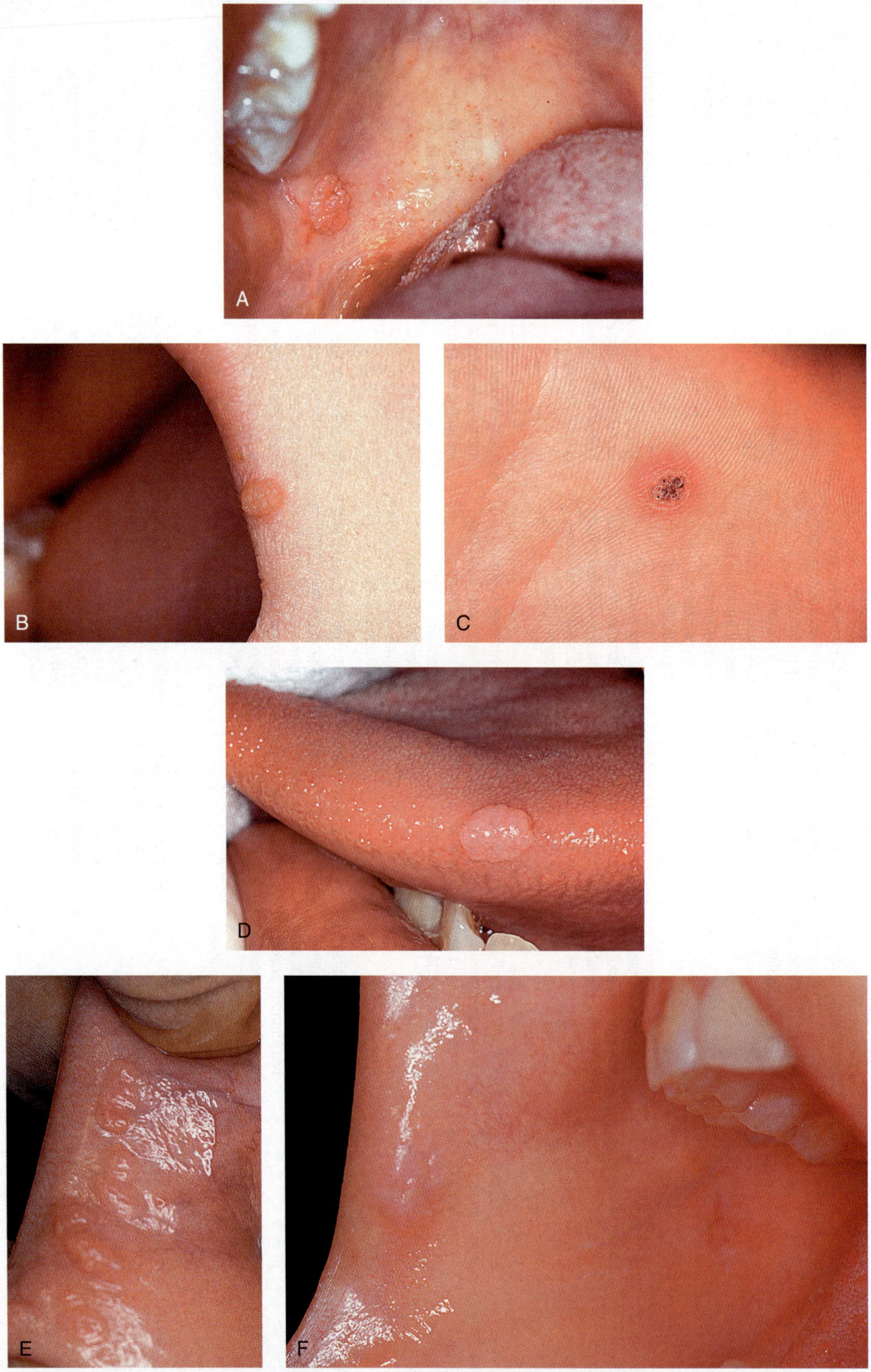

• **Fig. 19.5** Soft Tissue Enlargements. (A) Squamous papilloma of the soft palate. (B–C) Verruca vulgaris of the lip vermilion (B) and hand (C). (D) Giant cell fibroma of the lateral tongue. (E–F) Focal epithelial hyperplasia of the buccal mucosa displaying a cobblestone appearance (E) or a small clustered pattern (F).

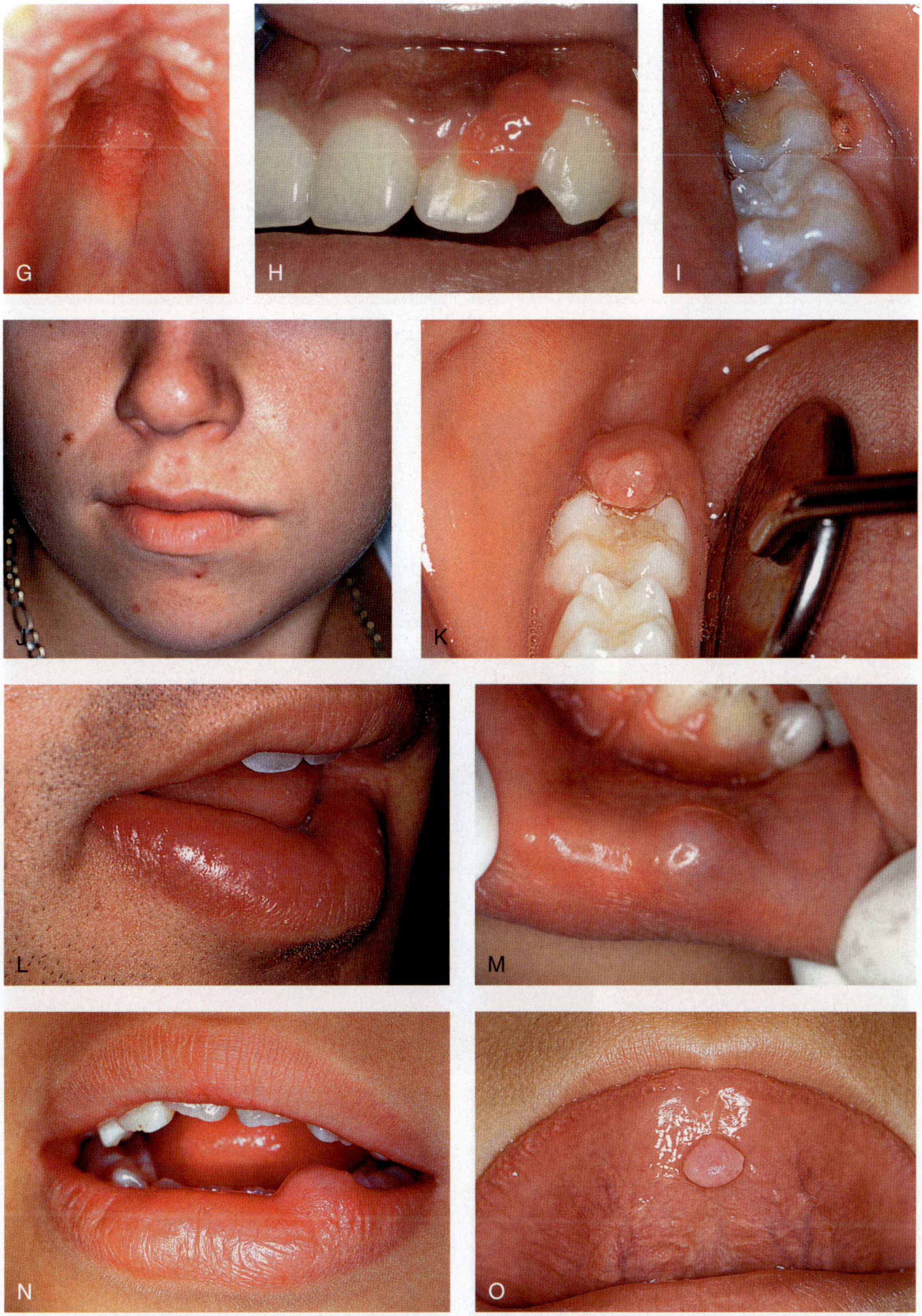

• Fig. 19.5, cont'd (G) Inflammatory papillary hyperplasia of the hard palatal mucosa. (H) Localized juvenile spongiotic gingival hyperplasia. (I–J) Pericoronitis associated with an erupting mandibular molar (I) and a lower face cellulitis (J). (K) Inflamed operculum associated with an erupting mandibular molar. (L) Angioedema of the lips caused by a latex allergy. (M–N) Mucocele of the mandibular labial mucosa (M). The lesion was obvious when the child's lips were at rest (N). (O) Mucocele at the anterior midline ventral tongue.

Continued

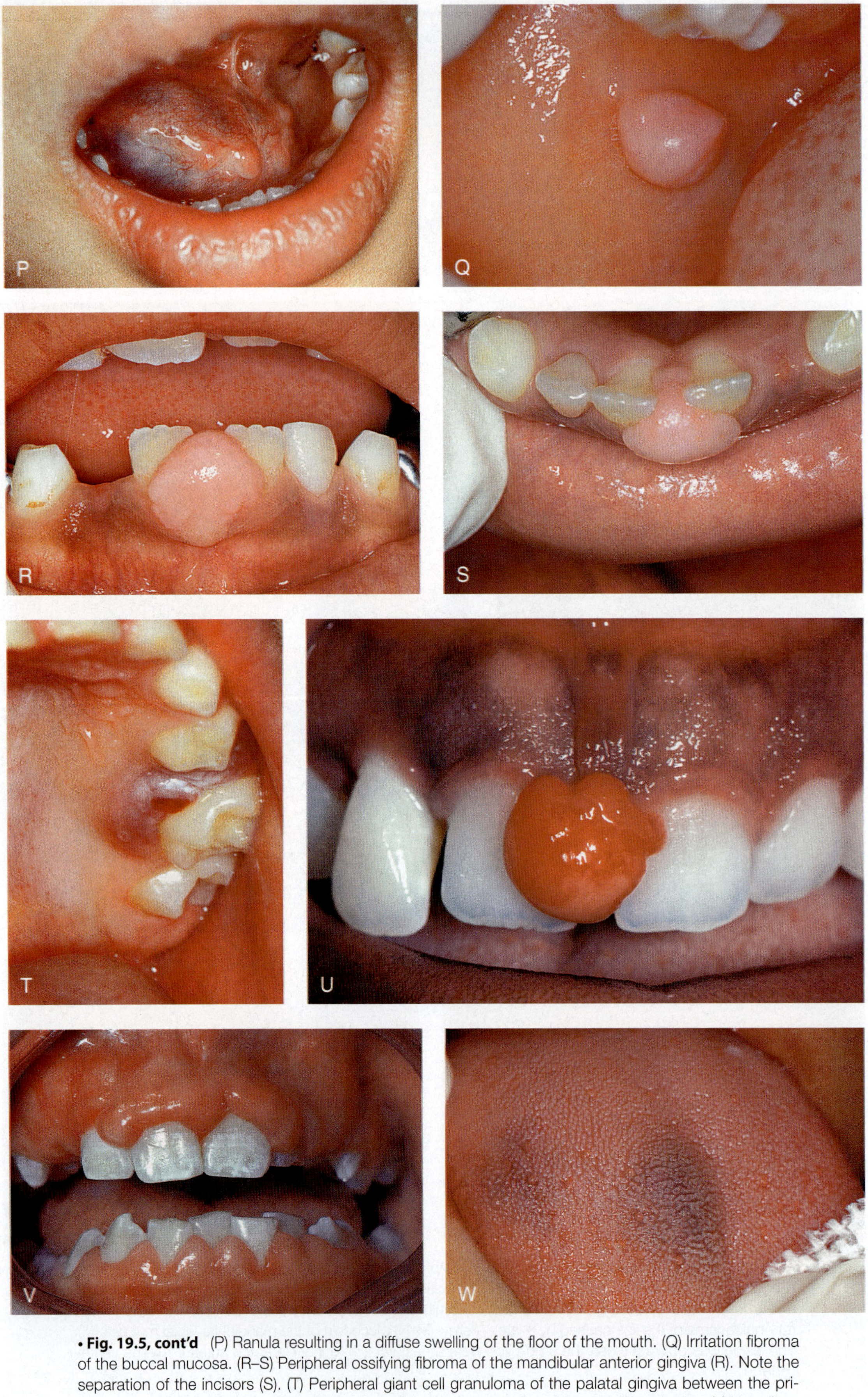

• Fig. 19.5, cont'd (P) Ranula resulting in a diffuse swelling of the floor of the mouth. (Q) Irritation fibroma of the buccal mucosa. (R–S) Peripheral ossifying fibroma of the mandibular anterior gingiva (R). Note the separation of the incisors (S). (T) Peripheral giant cell granuloma of the palatal gingiva between the primary molars. (U) Pyogenic granuloma and physiologic pigmentation of the maxillary gingiva. (V) Hereditary gingival fibromatosis. (W) Hemangioma of the dorsal tongue.

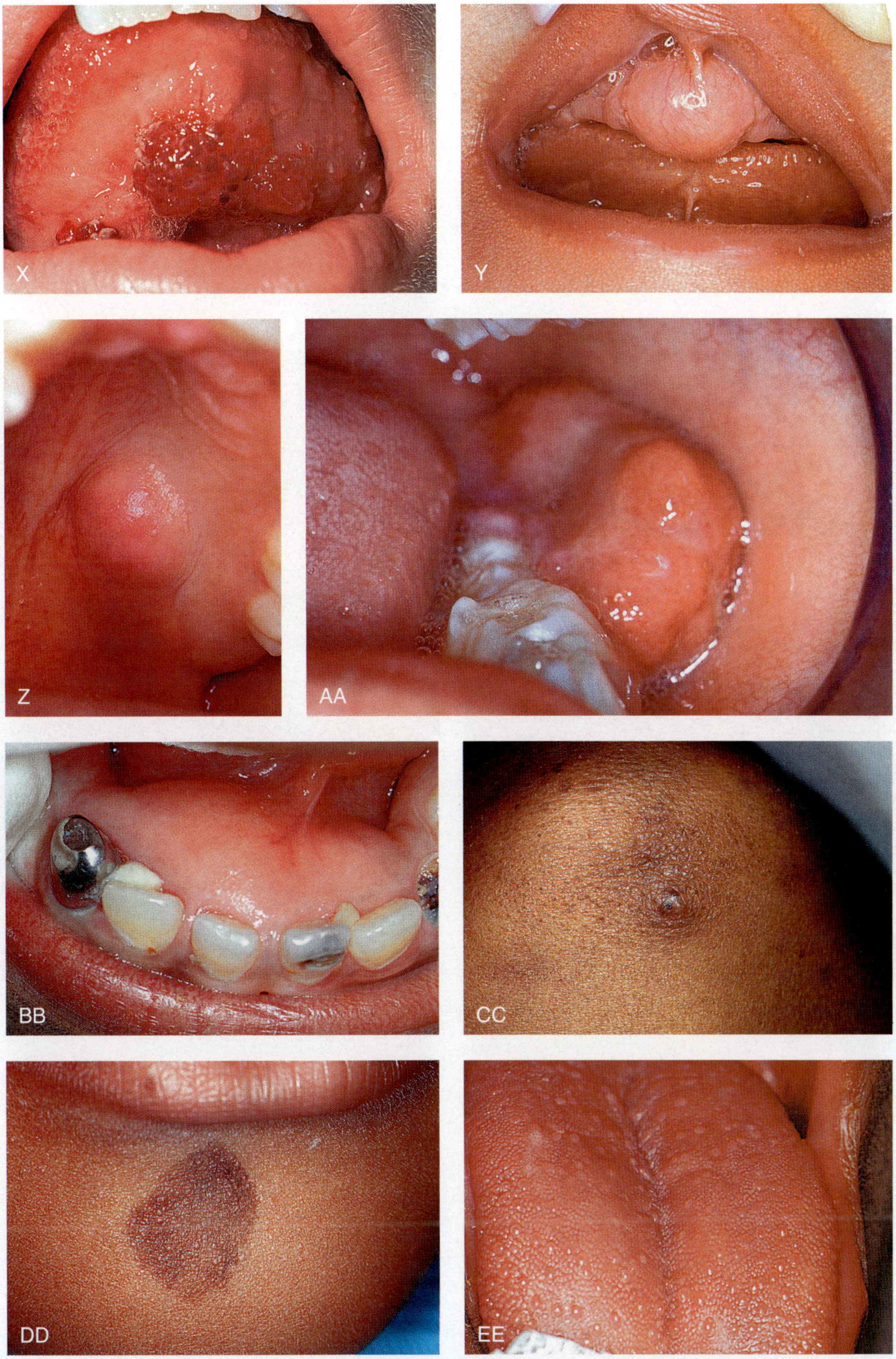

• Fig. 19.5, cont'd (X) Lymphangioma of the ventral tongue. (Y) Congenital epulis of the anterior maxillary alveolar mucosa. (Z) Pleomorphic adenoma of the posterior hard palate. (AA) Juvenile fibromatosis of the posterior mandibular vestibule and gingiva. (BB–EE) Child with neurofibromatosis including neurofibroma of the floor of the mouth (BB), skin of the neck (CC), café-au-lait macule on the chin (DD), and enlarged fungiform papillae (EE).

Continued

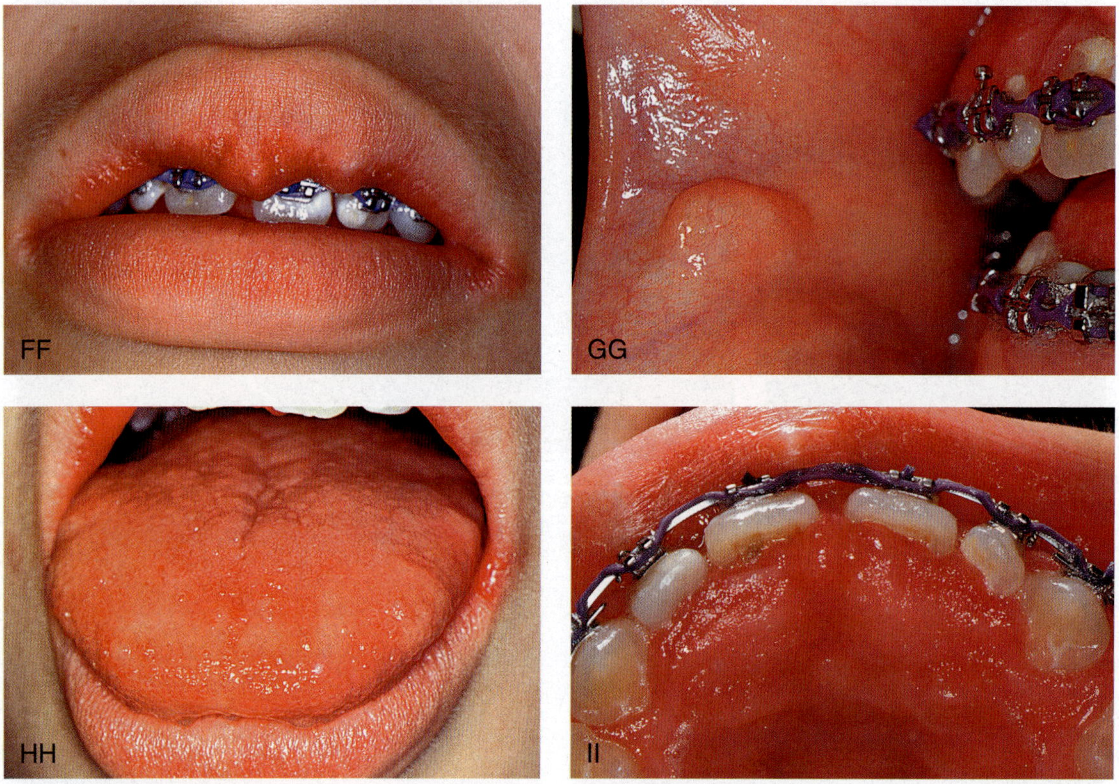

• Fig. 19.5, cont'd (FF–II) Child with multiple endocrine neoplasia syndrome, type 2B, including mucosal neuromas of the lips (FF), buccal mucosa (GG), tongue (HH), and palatal gingiva (II).

TABLE 19.6 Radiolucent Lesions of Bone (see Fig. 19.6)

Lesion	Pediatric Age and Sex	Clinical and Radiographic Findings	Location	Pediatric Significance	Treatment and Prognosis	Differential Diagnosis
Dentigerous cyst	Second decade Slight male predilection	Well-defined, unilocular, radiolucency around crown of unerupted tooth; may displace teeth, cause cortical expansion and root resorption; asymptomatic unless infected	Mandibular and maxillary third molar and canine regions	Common odontogenic cyst in children; growth may be rapid; may involve primary or supernumerary teeth; *eruption cyst* is soft tissue analog	Enucleation; marsupialization if extensive; orthodontic treatment to assist tooth eruption; seldom recur; ameloblastoma and carcinoma are rare complications	Hyperplastic dental follicle Periapical cyst Ameloblastic fibroma Unicystic ameloblastoma Odontogenic keratocyst Adenomatoid odontogenic tumor Buccal bifurcation cyst Primordial odontogenic tumor
Odontogenic keratocyst (keratocystic odontogenic tumor)	Second decade Slight male predilection	Well-defined, unilocular or multilocular radiolucency with thin corticated margins; expansile; 25%–40% associated with unerupted tooth; may resorb and displace teeth; may be painful	Posterior body and ramus of mandible; maxillary third molar and canine regions	Multiple cysts are consistent with *nevoid basal cell carcinoma syndrome* and includes jaw cysts, basal cell carcinomas, palmar-plantar pits, bifid ribs, epidermal cysts, and calcified falx cerebri	Surgical excision; may include peripheral ostectomy or chemical cautery; may treat large cysts by decompression; recurrence rate of 30%	Dentigerous cyst Unicystic ameloblastoma Ameloblastic fibroma Odontogenic myxoma Central vascular malformation Central giant cell granuloma
Ameloblastic fibroma	First and second decades Slight male predilection	Well-defined unilocular or multilocular lesion with sclerotic margins; expansile; 75% associated with unerupted tooth	Posterior mandible (70%)	Rare malignant counterpart, *ameloblastic fibrosarcoma* arises de novo or from preexisting or recurrent tumor	Surgical excision; recurrences are common (18%); long-term follow-up is recommended	Dentigerous cyst Odontogenic keratocyst Central vascular malformation Central giant cell granuloma Ameloblastoma
Ameloblastoma	Second decade No sex predilection	Well-defined, unilocular or multilocular radiolucency; cortical perforation; expansile; slow growing; root displacement and resorption; usually asymptomatic	Mandibular molar and ramus areas	*Unicystic ameloblastoma* is most common variant in children; associated with unerupted molar; treatment varies from enucleation to resection; less aggressive than conventional tumor	Aggressive odontogenic tumor requires marginal or en bloc resection; 50%–90% recurs with curettage; rarely undergoes malignant transformation	Dentigerous cyst Odontogenic keratocyst Odontogenic myxoma Central giant cell granuloma Ameloblastic fibroma
Melanotic neuroectodermal tumor of infancy	Infancy, may be present at birth Slight male predilection	Rapidly expanding bony lesion; may exhibit blue-black pigmented surface; ill-defined, unilocular radiolucency; displacement of tooth buds; "floating tooth" appearance	Anterior maxilla	Lesion mimics malignancy with destructive, rapid growth rate; dental abnormalities due to surgery; high urinary levels of vanillylmandelic acid	Surgical excision or curettage; 20% recurrence rate; reported cases of metastasis	Metastatic sarcoma Central vascular malformation Large eruption cyst Large congenital epulis

Continued

TABLE 19.6 Radiolucent Lesions of Bone (see Fig. 19.6)—cont'd

Lesion	Pediatric Age and Sex	Clinical and Radiographic Findings	Location	Pediatric Significance	Treatment and Prognosis	Differential Diagnosis
Central giant cell granuloma	First and second decades Female predilection	Well-defined, unilocular or multilocular radiolucency with scalloped border; expansile; may displace teeth and cause root resorption; pain and paresthesia may be noted	Most frequently in mandible; anterior to first molar; may cross midline	Aggressive form exists; need to rule out *hyperparathyroidism, cherubism,* and other syndromes, especially with multiple lesions	Thorough curettage; alternative treatments include intralesional corticosteroids, calcitonin, interferon, bisphosphonates; recurrence rate of 20%	Periapical cyst Odontogenic keratocyst Simple bone cyst Odontogenic myxoma Central vascular malformation Aneurysmal bone cyst Ameloblastic fibroma
Cherubism	First decade; usually by 5 years Male predilection	Chubby face appearance; bilateral, symmetrical, painless enlargement of jaws; extensive, multiple, well-defined, multilocular radiolucencies	Maxilla and mandible; in particular, angles of mandible; all four quadrants frequently involved	Autosomal dominant condition; causes premature exfoliation of primary teeth; displacement of tooth buds, severe malocclusion, and malformed teeth	Treatment is controversial; spontaneous regression with onset of puberty; surgery may improve function and cosmetics	Nevoid basal cell carcinoma syndrome Hyperparathyroidism Noonan-like syndrome Ramon syndrome Neurofibromatosis, type 1
Simple bone cyst (traumatic bone cyst)	Second decade No sex predilection for jaw lesions	Well to poorly delineated, unilocular radiolucency with thin, sclerotic border; scalloping between roots of teeth; 20% are expansile; teeth are vital	Posterior and anterior body of mandible and ramus; bilateral lesions are uncommon	Cause is uncertain but may be associated with trauma; extensive, expansile lesions may occur; may be seen with fibro-osseous lesions	Surgical exploration and curettage; low recurrence rate of 1%–2%	Central giant cell granuloma Periapical cyst Odontogenic keratocyst Developing tooth bud
Aneurysmal bone cyst	First and second decades No sex predilection	Painful swelling with rapid growth; unilocular or multilocular radiolucency with ballooning distention of buccal cortex; may be painful; tooth displacement	Posterior mandibular region	Blood-filled pseudocyst; 20% associated with preexisting lesion, including *central giant cell granuloma, fibrous dysplasia, ossifying fibroma*	Curettage or enucleation; hemorrhage control; 2-year recurrence rate is approximately 13%; incomplete removal is common	Ameloblastic fibroma Ameloblastoma Central giant cell granuloma Central vascular malformation Odontogenic keratocyst Odontogenic myxoma
Periapical abscess	First and second decades No sex predilection	Nonvital, mobile tooth; soft tissue swelling with purulence; sinus tract may be present; painful; widening of periodontal ligament space or poorly defined radiolucency	Alveolus; primary dentition is most frequently affected in children	May progress to cellulitis; may result in aborted development or enamel hypoplasia of succedaneous tooth	Endodontic treatment or tooth extraction; antibiotics and analgesics may be needed; serious complications include *cavernous sinus thrombosis* and *Ludwig angina*	Incomplete apexification of erupted tooth Periodontal abscess Periapical granuloma or cyst Buccal bifurcation cyst Langerhans cell histiocytosis

Periapical granuloma and cyst	First and second decades No sex predilection	Nonvital tooth; usually asymptomatic unless acute exacerbation of the lesion; well or poorly defined radiolucency at the root apex; loss of lamina dura; root resorption	Alveolar bone adjacent to root apex and bifurcation	May displace succedaneous teeth and cause dental abnormalities; large lesions in primary dentition resemble a *dentigerous cyst* when a succedaneous tooth is present	Endodontic treatment or tooth extraction and gentle curettage to avoid disturbing permanent tooth bud, if present	Dentigerous cyst Developing tooth bud Solitary bone cyst Central giant cell granuloma Langerhans cell histiocytosis
Acute osteomyelitis	First and second decades Male predilection	Diffuse radiolucency with poorly defined margins; sequestra; fever, swelling, pain, lymphadenopathy, leukocytosis, and draining sinus tracts	Posterior mandible in children; anterior maxilla in infants	Most cases are caused by odontogenic infections or jaw fractures; occasionally caused by bacteremia	Incision and drainage with culture and sensitivity testing; antibiotic coverage; may develop into *chronic osteomyelitis*	Jaw fracture Ewing sarcoma Burkitt lymphoma Langerhans cell histiocytosis Osteosarcoma
Langerhans cell histiocytosis (histiocytosis X)	*Disseminated form:* first decade *Localized form:* second decade Male predilection	Lymphadenopathy, rash, oral pain, gingivitis, ulcers, mobile teeth, multiple punched-out radiolucencies with "floating tooth" appearance without corticated rim; premature tooth loss	Skull, mandible, ribs and vertebrae are most often involved; jaws affected in 20% of cases	Neoplastic disease of myeloid cells; chronic disseminated form includes lytic bone lesions, exophthalmos, diabetes insipidus; all forms mimic periodontal disease or multifocal odontogenic infection	Multiagent chemotherapy, low-dose radiotherapy, surgical curettage, and stem cell transplantation are used, depending on form of disease and location; children younger than 2 years have worst prognosis	Cyclic neutropenia Burkitt lymphoma Leukemia Aggressive periodontitis Periapical abscess or granuloma Acute osteomyelitis
Burkitt lymphoma	First and second decades Male predilection	Lymphadenopathy, facial swelling, tenderness, tooth mobility, extrusion, and premature loss; patchy loss of lamina dura, irregular radiolucencies, "floating tooth" appearance	Posterior mandible is most common site; may involve all four quadrants; African (endemic) form affects the jaws in 50%–70% of cases	Most jaw lesions are misdiagnosed as odontogenic infection; associated with Epstein-Barr virus and chromosomal translocation	Treatment includes multiagent chemotherapy; aggressive malignancy with 5-year survival rate of 75%–95%, depending on disease stage	Acute osteomyelitis Langerhans cell histiocytosis Periapical abscess or granuloma Acute leukemia Aggressive periodontitis

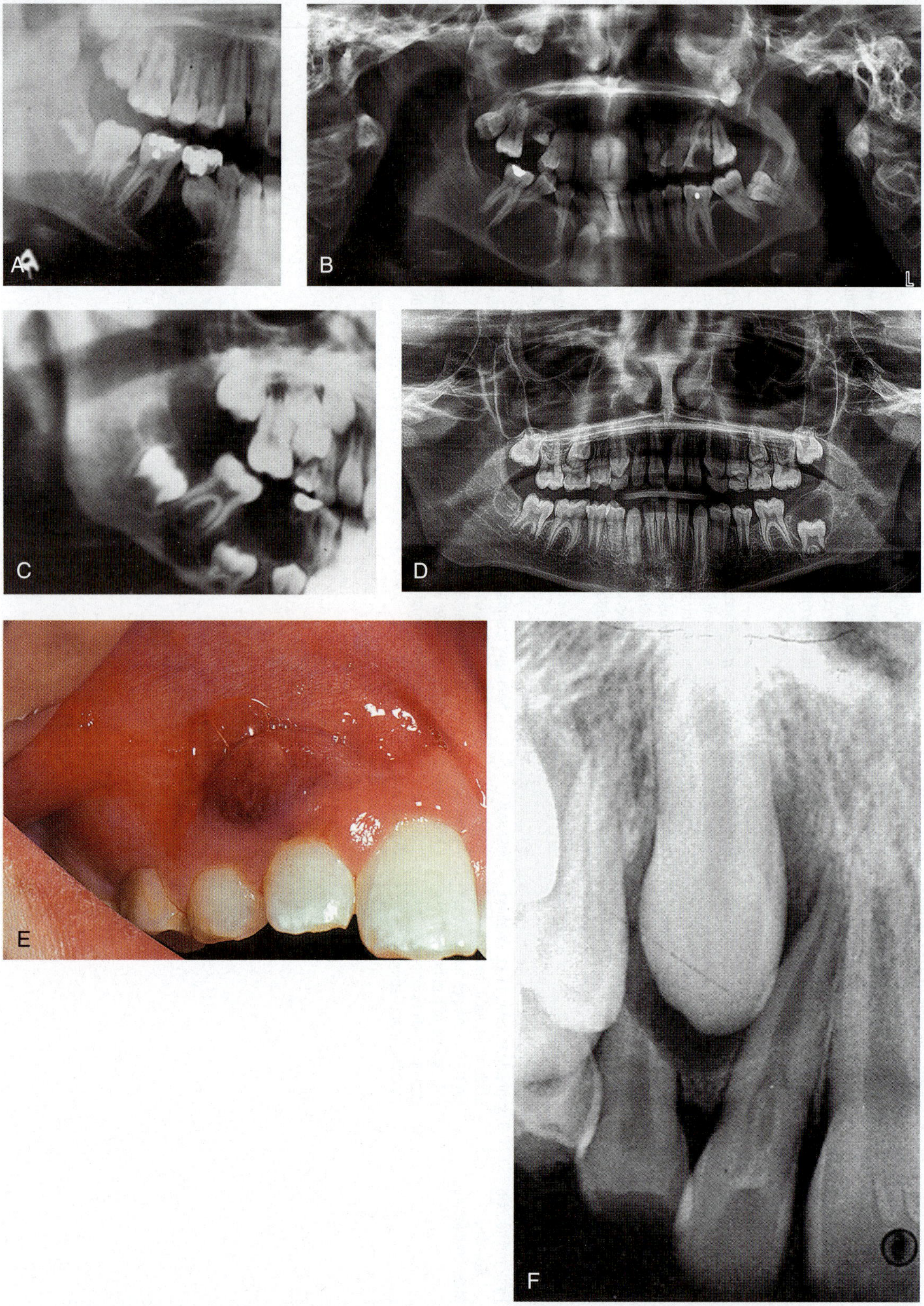

• **Fig. 19.6** Radiolucent Lesions of Bone. (A) Dentigerous cyst of the posterior mandible. (B) Multiple odontogenic keratocysts of the maxilla and mandible associated with nevoid basal cell carcinoma syndrome. (C) Ameloblastic fibroma of the posterior mandible. (D) Ameloblastoma of the posterior mandible associated with impacted second molar. (E–F) Periapical abscess of the maxillary lateral incisor caused by dens invaginatus, parulis (E), and radiographic findings (F). Note the hyperplastic dental follicle surrounding the crown of the permanent canine.

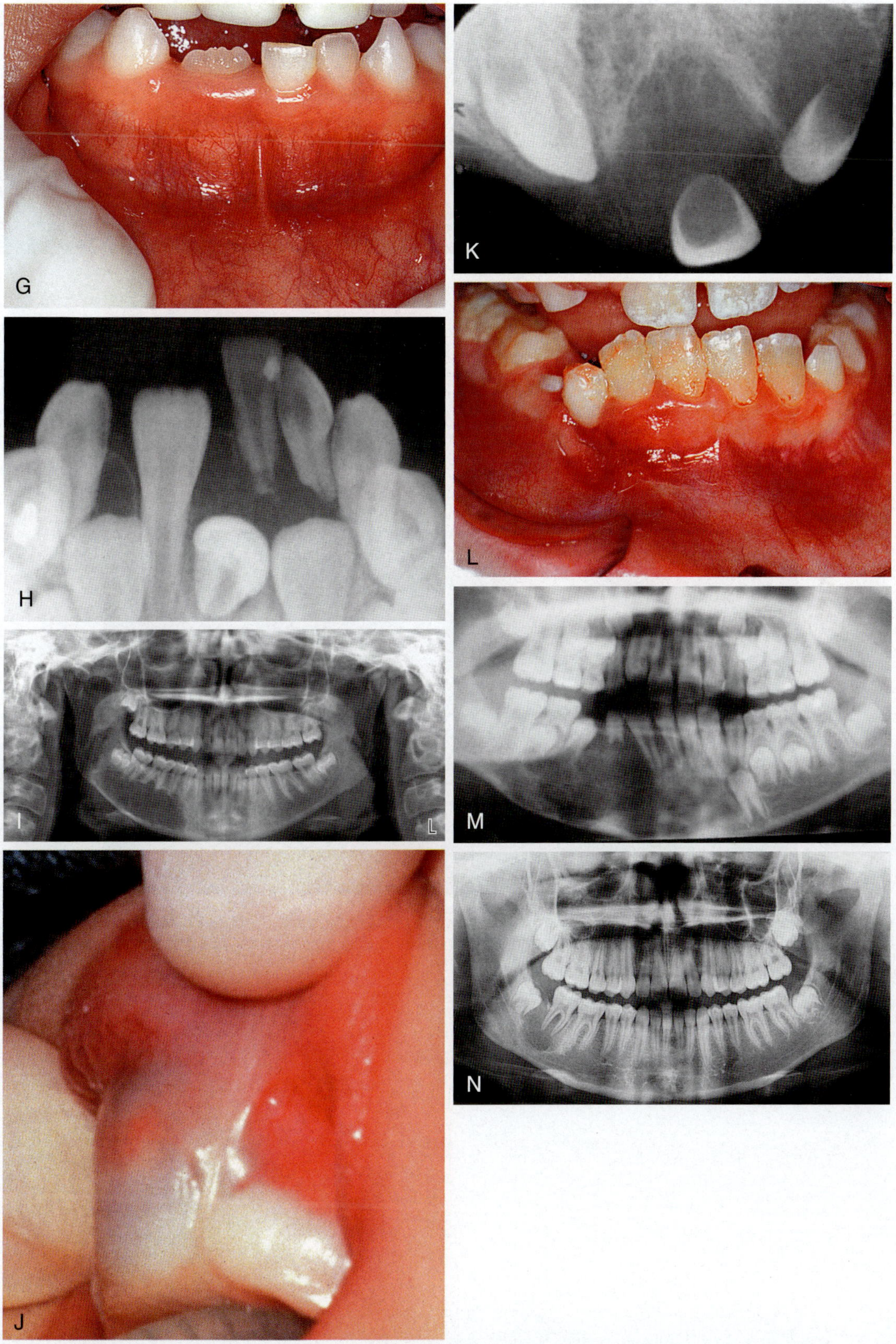

• Fig. 19.6, cont'd (G–H) Periapical cyst with no significant bony expansion, intraoral view (G) and radiographic view (H). (I) Simple bone cyst of the right posterior mandible. (J–K) Melanotic neuroectodermal tumor of infancy of the anterior maxilla, clinical view (J) and radiographic view (K). (L–M) Central giant cell granuloma of the mandible, clinical view (L) and radiographic view (M). (N) Buccal bifurcation cyst, panoramic radiographic view.

Continued

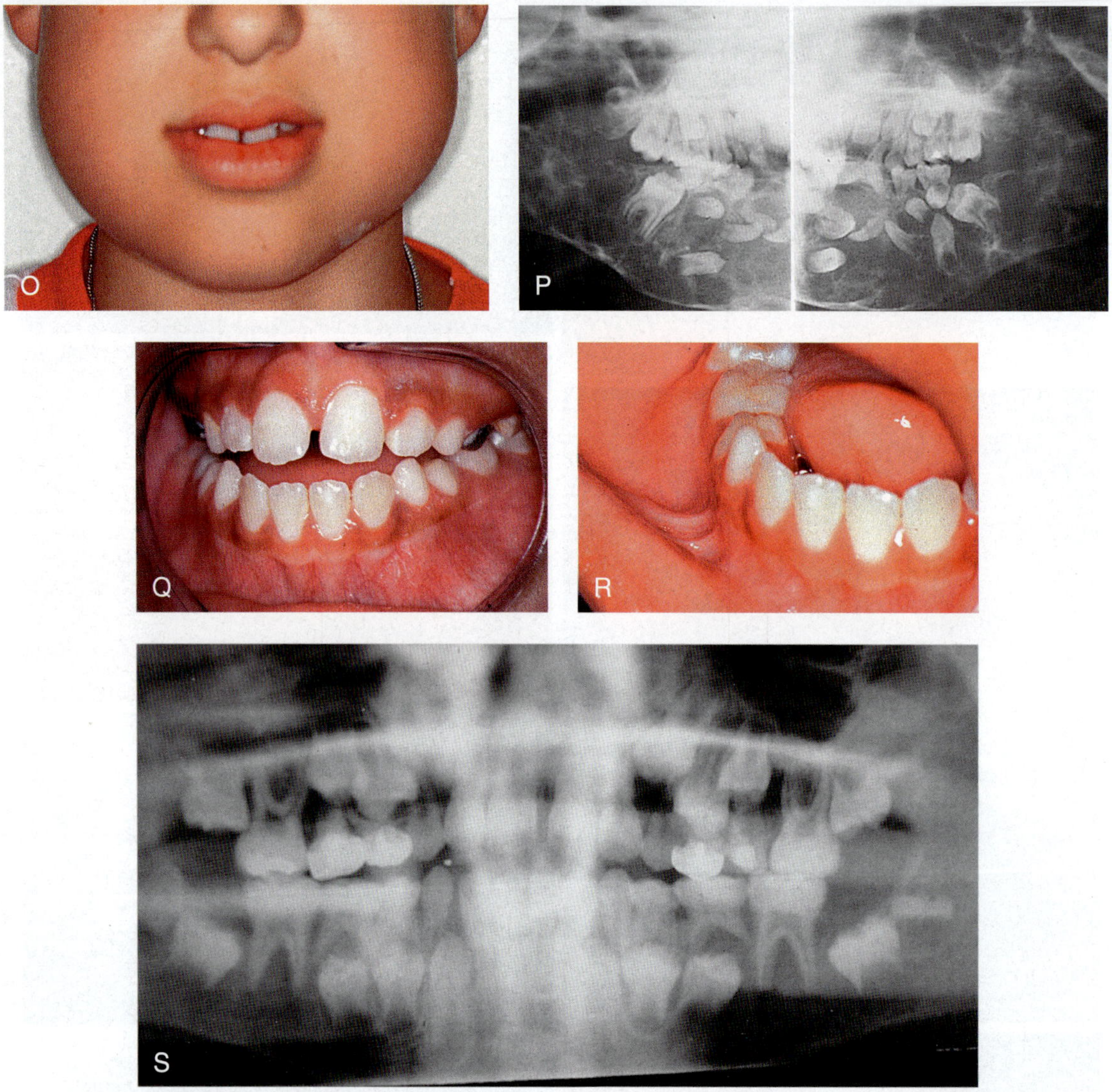

• Fig. 19.6, cont'd (O and P) Cherubism, clinical view (O), radiographic view (P). (Q–S) Burkitt lymphoma, open bite due to extrusion of posterior teeth (Q), mandibular buccal expansion (R), and panoramic radiographic view (S).

TABLE 19.7 Mixed Radiolucent and Radiopaque Lesions of Bone (see Fig. 19.7)

Lesion	Pediatric Age and Sex	Clinical and Radiographic Findings	Location	Pediatric Significance	Treatment and Prognosis	Differential Diagnosis
Calcifying odontogenic cyst (Gorlin cyst)	Second decade No sex predilection	Well-defined, unilocular radiolucency with irregular calcifications or toothlike structures; expansile; 33% associated with unerupted teeth; asymptomatic	Most develop in incisor-canine region of maxilla and mandible; may occur as gingival lesion	In this age group, this odontogenic cyst is often associated with *odontoma*	Enucleation; minimal risk of recurrence; rarely manifests aggressive or malignant behavior	Odontoma Adenomatoid odontogenic tumor Ameloblastic fibro-odontoma Calcifying epithelial odontogenic tumor Central ossifying fibroma
Adenomatoid odontogenic tumor	Second decade Female predilection	Well-defined, unilocular radiolucency with fine snowflake calcifications; most associated with unerupted tooth (canine); root divergence; asymptomatic expansion	Anterior maxilla is most common site, followed by the anterior mandible	Most lesions occur between 10 and 20 years of age; rarely occurs as gingival lesion	Enucleation; does not recur	Dentigerous cyst Calcifying odontogenic cyst Developing odontoma Odontogenic keratocyst
Ameloblastic fibro-odontoma	First and second decades No sex predilection	Well-defined unilocular radiolucency with calcified material and toothlike structures; expansile; often associated with unerupted tooth	Mandibular molar and premolar regions	Odontogenic tumor is frequently diagnosed because tooth fails to erupt; this entity is classified as a developing odontoma and not a unique odontogenic tumor	Conservative curettage; rarely recurs	Developing odontoma Calcifying odontogenic cyst Calcifying epithelial odontogenic tumor Cemento-ossifying fibroma
Cemento-ossifying fibroma	Second decade Female predilection	Painless swelling; circular growth pattern; well-defined, unilocular lesion with sclerotic borders; downward bowing of inferior cortex of mandible; may be radiolucent, mixed, or radiopaque	Premolar and molar region; usually occurs in mandible	Multiple lesions in children are a feature of *hyperparathyroidism-jaw tumor syndrome*	Enucleation or resection; rarely recurs	Fibrous dysplasia Idiopathic osteosclerosis Focal cemento-osseous dysplasia Osteoblastoma Cementoblastoma
Osteomyelitis with proliferative periostitis (Garré osteomyelitis)	First and second decades No sex predilection	Diffuse, poorly defined, mixed radiolucent and opaque lesion; expansile; cortical bone duplication with laminated or onion skin pattern; mild tenderness	Posterior mandible; usually involves first permanent molar	Usually carious molar is noted; occlusal radiograph is helpful for demonstrating cortical laminations	Endodontic treatment or tooth extraction; if necessary, antibiotic therapy; expanded bone usually remodels without surgical recontouring	Fibrous dysplasia Fracture callus Buccal bifurcation cyst Ewing sarcoma Infantile cortical hyperostosis Osteosarcoma

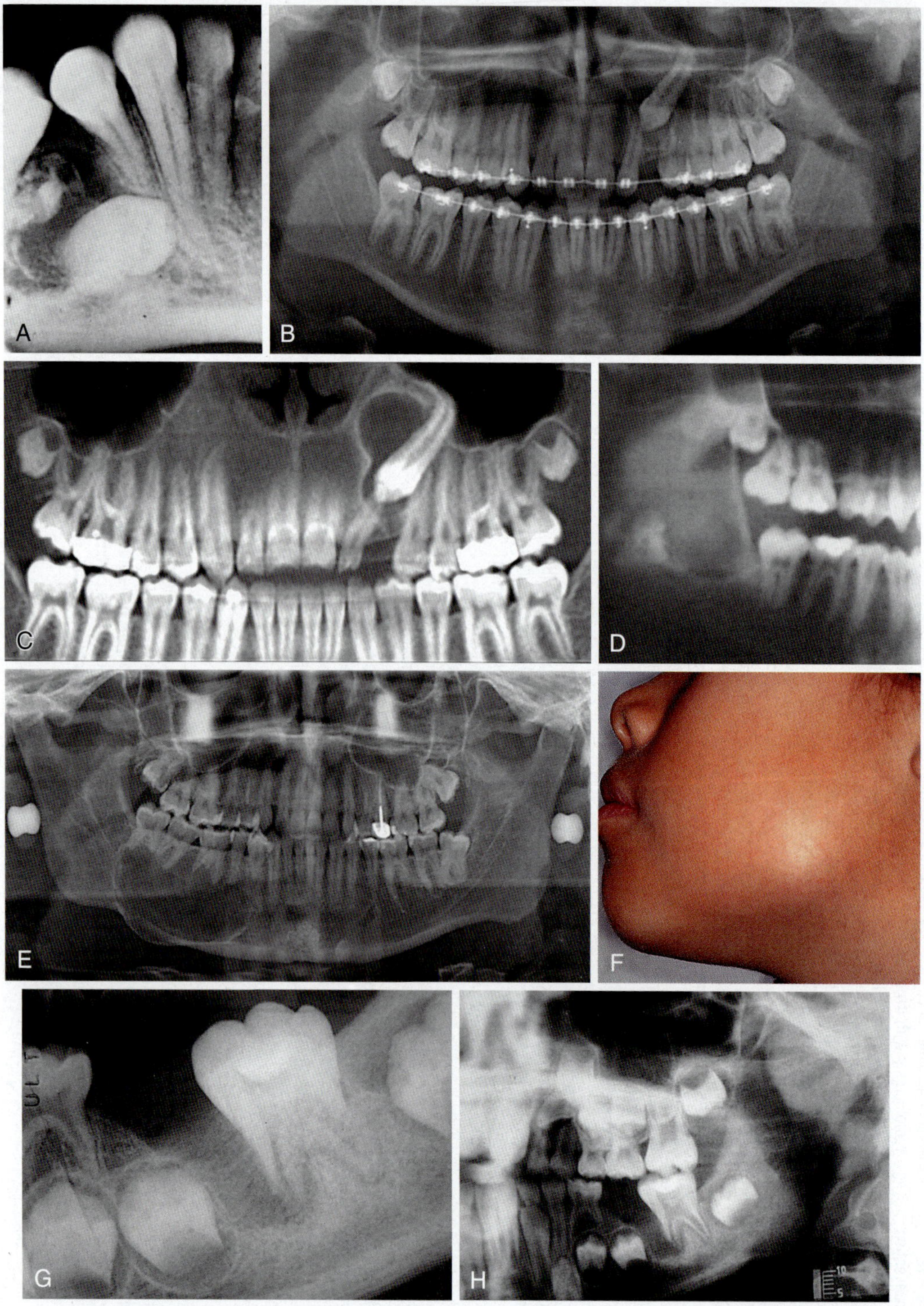

• **Fig. 19.7** Mixed Radiolucent and Radiopaque Lesions of Bone. (A) Calcifying odontogenic cyst of the mandible with displacement of the unerupted premolar. (B–C) Adenomatoid odontogenic tumor of the maxilla associated with impacted maxillary canine, panoramic radiograph (B) and cone-bean computed tomography reconstructed panoramic image (C). (D) Ameloblastic fibro-odontoma of the posterior mandible and ramus. (E) Ossifying fibroma of the right posterior mandible. (F–H) Osteomyelitis with proliferative periostitis, clinical view (F), periapical radiographic view (G), and cropped panoramic view (H).

TABLE 19.8 Radiopaque Lesions of Bone (see Fig. 19.8)

Lesion	Pediatric Age and Sex	Clinical and Radiographic Findings	Location	Pediatric Significance	Treatment and Prognosis	Differential Diagnosis
Odontoma, compound and complex	First and second decades No sex predilection	Well-defined radiopacity surrounded by narrow radiolucent rim; develop in pericoronal or radicular areas *Compound type* resembles miniature teeth; *complex type* is amorphous opaque mass	*Compound type:* anterior maxilla *Complex type:* posterior mandible Rarely occurs in gingiva	Represents a hamartoma; most common odontogenic tumor-like lesion; frequent cause of isolated delayed tooth eruption	Local excision; recurrence is rare	Eruption sequestrum Ameloblastic fibro-odontoma Cementoblastoma Calcifying odontogenic cyst Calcifying epithelial odontogenic tumor
Osteoma	Second decade No sex predilection	Usually solitary, well-defined, spherical radiopacity; slow growing, may be expansile and result in facial deformity	Body of mandible and condyle are most common sites; endosteal or periosteal location	*Gardner syndrome,* autosomal dominant: characterized by osteomas, intestinal polyposis, supernumerary teeth, odontomas, and skin lesions; malignant polyps	Surgical excision; periodically evaluate small lesions; no recurrence	Torus/exostosis Complex odontoma Fibrous dysplasia Condensing osteitis Familial gigantiform cementoma Idiopathic osteosclerosis
Fibrous dysplasia	Second decade No sex predilection	Unilateral, fusiform enlargement; ground-glass radiopacity with ill-defined borders; may displace teeth and delay eruption; slow growing and asymptomatic; facial asymmetry	Maxilla is more frequently affected than mandible; buccal and lingual cortical expansion	*McCune-Albright syndrome* includes polyostotic fibrous dysplasia, café-au-lait macules, and endocrine abnormalities	Osseous recontouring for cosmetic and functional problems; stabilizes after completion of skeletal development; rare malignant transformation	Chronic sclerosing osteomyelitis Cemento-ossifying fibroma Osteoma Segmental odontomaxillary dysplasia
Condensing osteitis (focal sclerosing osteomyelitis)	First and second decades No sex predilection	Localized radiopacity at root apices of pulpally involved tooth; margins blend into surrounding bone; usually asymptomatic	Most cases are in mandibular premolar and molar region	Most common periapical radiopacity; sclerotic bone may impede eruption of succedaneous tooth	No treatment of bony lesion; manage odontogenic infection; may regress after treatment or cause a bone scar	Cementoblastoma Idiopathic osteosclerosis Complex odontoma Exostosis/torus Osteoma
Cementoblastoma	First and second decades No sex predilection	Radiopaque mass surrounded by thin radiolucent rim; may be mixed radiolucent-radiopaque; fused to root of vital tooth; pain and swelling are common	Posterior mandible in molar and premolar region	Rarely involves primary teeth	Surgical extraction of tooth with attached tumor or endodontic treatment with root amputation	Condensing osteitis Osteoblastoma Complex odontoma Hypercementosis
Idiopathic osteosclerosis (bone scar)	First and second decades No sex predilection	Asymptomatic, nonexpansile, uniformly radiopaque lesion that blends into surrounding bone; round or elliptical in shape; adjacent teeth are vital	Molar-premolar mandible; usually by root apices	Rare cases reach >2 cm in size and may interfere with tooth eruption	No treatment is necessary; tend to stabilize in size in young adulthood	Condensing osteitis Residual root tip Exostosis Osteoma Bone graft

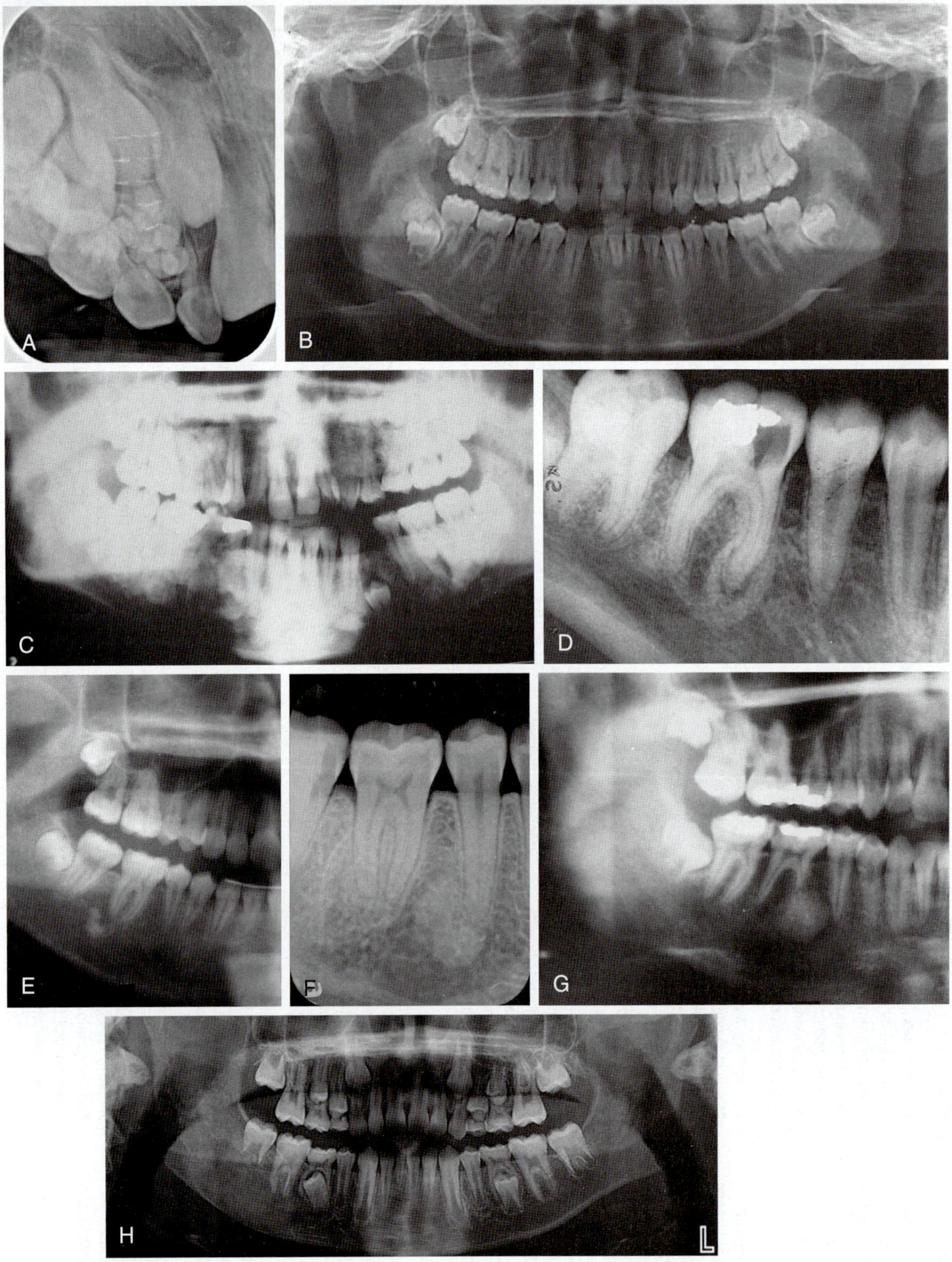

• **Fig. 19.8** Radiopaque Lesions of Bone. (A) Compound odontoma of the right maxilla. (B) Complex odontoma of the right mandible. (C) Multiple osteomas associated with Gardner syndrome. (D) Condensing osteitis associated with carious mandibular molar. (E–F) Idiopathic osteosclerosis of the posterior mandible, cropped panoramic radiographic view (E), periapical example that mimics condensing osteitis (F). (G) Cementoblastoma associated with the mandibular molar. (H) Fibrous dysplasia of the right mandible.

20

Anomalies of the Developing Dentition

J. TIMOTHY WRIGHT AND BEAU D. MEYER

CHAPTER OUTLINE

Developmental Controls and Environmental Interactions

Developmental defects of teeth are clinically heterogeneous in their phenotypes, and as a result they present diverse challenges in their clinical management. Tooth formation involves a complex series of tightly orchestrated events that are highly regulated at the molecular level, with thousands of genes involved.[1,2] Many of these genes are now known to be associated with developmental defects of teeth.[3] The cellular events and processes are sensitive to environmental stressors that can alter cell and tissue function and result in developmental dental defects. The clinician is faced with diagnosing these defects, identifying their underlying etiology (genetic, environmental, combined), understanding how the dental tissues are affected, and then managing these conditions. This chapter's goal is to review some of the more common conditions likely to present to clinicians who provide oral healthcare for the pediatric population.

Making an accurate diagnosis for many hereditary conditions can now be confirmed with molecular testing. The dentist should establish if the patient's presenting condition is likely to have a hereditary basis through evaluation of family history of the trait and, when indicated, referral to the child's pediatrician or a geneticist for further evaluation and any indicated laboratory or genetic tests (such as the family history tutorial found at https://www.genome.gov/genetics-glossary/Family-History). This is becoming increasingly important because new therapies are now available that can effectively treat a variety of conditions (e.g., hypophosphatasia).[4] Being able to optimally treat individuals is predicated on obtaining an accurate and timely diagnosis so that available therapeutics and treatments can be provided. Clinicians should become accustomed to searching databases that provide current information on known hereditary conditions, clinical phenotypes or clinical manifestations, and the molecular basis that causes the condition, such as the Online Mendelian Inheritance in Man (OMIM) website (http://www.omim.org) that provides an electronic catalog of hereditary conditions and their causes. In this chapter we include the OMIM number to designate specific conditions to facilitate the reader who wants to further investigate specific hereditary dental traits.

Anomalies of Tooth Number

Developmental dental defects involving tooth number can be classified in a variety of ways, but for simplicity we will use hypodontia to denote any number of missing teeth and hyperdontia as any number of extra teeth. Other commonly used terms include *oligodontia,* which is defined as missing more than six teeth excluding third molars, and *anodontia,* the complete absence of teeth. Developmental anomalies of tooth number are common, with missing teeth being more prevalent than having extra or supernumerary teeth. Alterations in tooth number often result from abnormalities in the genetic and molecular regulation of tooth development, but any number of environmental stressors can also arrest tooth bud development at later developmental stages.[5]

Environmental stressors such as infection, radiation, and trauma can be associated with changes in tooth number, size, and shape. The effects will depend on the magnitude, duration, and timing of the stressor in relation to tooth development. Radiation and chemotherapy can be associated with hypodontia, small teeth, or teeth with only rudimentary root formation, depending on the dose and timing of treatment and the concomitant stage of dental development. Two of the most implicated chemotherapeutic agents are vincristine and the alkylating agent cyclophosphamide.[6,7] If these agents are administered during tooth formation, the pediatric patient is at risk for developing dental anomalies, including hypodontia.[8] Radiation doses of 30 Gray (Gy) and

10 Gy can arrest tooth development and amelogenesis, respectively (see Chapter 39).[8,9]

Hyperdontia

The presence of supernumerary teeth can be an isolated trait or be associated with a syndrome (Table 20.1, see Chapter 37). The most commonly occurring supernumerary teeth are called *mesiodens,* with a prevalence of approximately 1% in the population (reports vary from 0.15% to 4%).[10] Mesiodens develop in the anterior midline of the maxillary arch. Ninety percent to 98% of supernumerary teeth occur in the maxilla, with the permanent dentition being more frequently affected than the primary dentition. The extra tooth or teeth are often diagnosed during routine radiographic examination or due to asymmetrical tooth eruption of a central incisor whose eruption is being impeded by the supernumerary tooth (Fig. 20.1). There may be one or two extra teeth present; they frequently have a conical or abnormal morphology, can be oriented to either erupt normally or be inverted, and are most often positioned palatal to the permanent incisors.

TABLE 20.1 Syndromes Demonstrating Hyperdontia

Condition	Mode of Inheritance	Phenotype	OMIM #	Gene
Apert syndrome	Autosomal dominant	Scaphocephaly, craniosynostosis, bilateral syndactyly, midface hypoplasia	101200	*FGFR2*
Cleidocranial dysplasia	Autosomal dominant	Aplastic clavicles, frontal bossing, hypoplastic midface	119600	*RUNX2*
Gardner syndrome	Autosomal dominant	Osteomas, epidermoid cysts, odontomas, intestinal polyps	175100	*APC*
Down syndrome	Trisomy 21	Brachycephaly, intellectual disability, epicanthal folds	190685	Many
Crouzon syndrome	Autosomal dominant	Craniosynostosis, exophthalmos, hypoplastic midface	123500	*FGFR2*
Sturge-Weber syndrome	(In progress)	Angiomatosis and calcification of leptomeninges, seizures, port-wine nevi of face	185300	*GNAQ*
Oral-facial-digital syndrome	X-linked dominant (in progress)	Hypoplastic alar cartilage, cleft tongue, clinodactyly	311200	*OFD1*
Oculodentodigital dysplasia	Autosomal recessive (in progress)	Maxillary hypoplasia, micrognathia, enamel hypoplasia	257850	*GJA1*

OMIM, Online Mendelian Inheritance in Man.

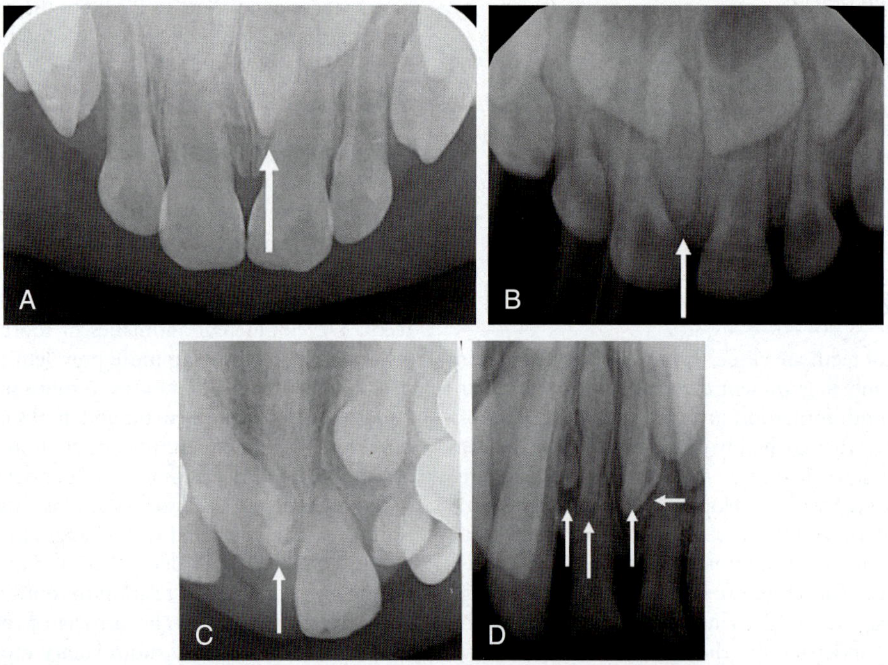

• **Fig. 20.1** Supernumerary teeth can take a variety of presentations in number, shape, and orientation, particularly in the anterior maxilla. These radiographs illustrate (A) a single conically shaped, normally oriented mesiodens *(arrow)*, (B) a single conically shaped, inverted mesiodens *(arrow)*, (C) a single, nebulous-shaped radiopacity *(arrow)*, or (D) multiple conically shaped supernumerary teeth with different orientations. Subsequent three-dimensional imaging is sometimes needed to confirm orientation, fusion, or proximity to erupting teeth.

Mesiodens are thought to be an isolated developmental anomaly and are not known to be associated with syndromes or to be hereditary with an increased familial occurrence.

Supernumerary teeth can be classified as supplemental or rudimentary. Supplemental supernumerary teeth duplicate the typical anatomy of posterior and anterior teeth. Rudimentary supernumerary teeth are dysmorphic and can assume conical forms, tuberculate forms, or shapes that duplicate molar anatomy. From a clinical standpoint, the tuberculate, or barrel-shaped, supernumeraries generate the most severe complications with respect to difficulty of removal and adverse effects on adjacent teeth, such as impaction or ectopic eruption. Additional complications associated with supernumeraries include dentigerous cyst formation, diastema, and crown resorption.[11] The presence of supernumerary teeth has a similar radiographic and clinical presentation as an odontoma, given the similar morphologic characteristics of a compound odontoma.[12]

Supernumerary teeth can occur in nonsyndromic and syndromic cleft lip with or without cleft palate, further complicating management of these patients. Patients with cleft lip and palate have been reported to have an increased incidence of hyperdontia, with reports indicating an incidence of up to 5%.[13] Careful evaluation by the craniofacial team to determine which teeth are best kept and which will require extraction, and the timing of treatment, is essential (see Chapter 38).

There are multiple syndromes associated with supernumerary teeth that are caused by a variety of genetic mutations involving diverse development pathways (see Table 20.1).[14] Gardner syndrome, also known as familial adenomatous polyposis (OMIM #175100), is caused by mutations in the *APC* gene that is involved in the beta catenin pathway (as is the *AXIN2* gene that is associated with congenitally missing teeth).[15] Individuals with this condition are at increased risk for developing intestinal cancer (adenopolyposis carcinoma), making it critical to evaluate the family history for this associated clinical feature (see Chapter 19).

Cleidocranial dysplasia (OMIM #119600) is a syndrome caused by mutations in the *RUNX2* gene, which is important in the development of bone and teeth.[16] Individuals having this condition are typically short in stature and can exhibit the following: frontal bossing and delayed suture closure, multiple supernumerary teeth, and failure of the succedaneous teeth to erupt (Fig. 20.2). Although cleidocranial dysplasia is inherited as an autosomal dominant trait, there often is no family history because the affected individual's condition is caused by a de novo mutation in the *RUNX2* gene. Managing the dental manifestations of this condition can be quite challenging, often requiring a team approach.[17]

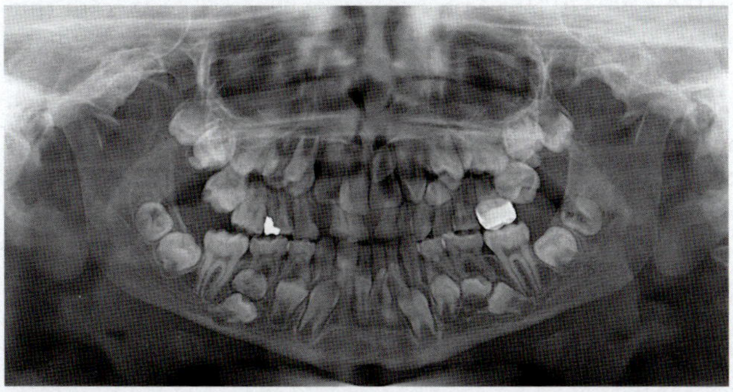

• **Fig. 20.2** This 10-year-old with cleidocranial dysplasia demonstrates failed eruption of the succedaneous teeth and multiple supernumerary visible in this panoramic radiograph.

Hypodontia

Approximately 6% of the White population is missing a tooth other than third permanent molars, and there is racial variance regarding the prevalence of missing teeth. The most frequently occurring congenitally absent permanent tooth, excluding the third molars, tends to be the mandibular second bicuspid (3.4%), followed by the maxillary lateral incisor (2.2%).[18] Missing primary teeth is much less common compared with permanent teeth, with a prevalence of approximately 1%. However, there is a high correlation between having a missing primary tooth and absence of its permanent tooth successor. The greater the number of teeth a person is missing, the more likely they are to have a syndrome such as ectodermal dysplasia. Isolated hypodontia can occur in the absence of syndromic features. Family history will often reveal that the missing tooth trait is present in multiple generations of family members and often demonstrates an autosomal dominant mode of inheritance.

Like hyperdontia, mentioned previously, hypodontia is also seen in nonsyndromic and syndromic cleft lip with or without cleft palate. Patients with cleft lip and palate have been reported to have an increased incidence of hypodontia, with reports indicating an incidence of up to 47% in patients with a cleft diagnosis.[19] In cases of hypodontia associated with cleft lip and palate, there is a 30% incidence of hypodontia outside the cleft site. Multiple genes have been identified as being causative of congenitally missing teeth in the absence of a syndrome including *MSX1, PAX9, WNT10A, AXIN2,* and *EDA* (Table 20.2). Mutations in the

TABLE 20.2 Hereditary Traits Associated With Hypodontia

Condition	Inheritance	OMIM #	Gene
Hypodontia			
Hypodontia: premolar, third molar	Autosomal dominant	106600	*MSX1*
Oligodontia: incisor, molar	Autosomal dominant	604625	*PAX9*
Oligodontia	Autosomal dominant	150400	*WNT10A*
Syndrome/Hypodontia			
Hypohidrotic ectodermal dysplasia	X-linked recessive	305100	*EDA*
Hypohidrotic ectodermal dysplasia	Autosomal dominant–recessive	129490–224900	*DL*
Incontinentia pigmenti	X-linked dominant	308300	*NEMO*
Witkop/tooth and nail syndrome	Autosomal dominant	189500	*MSX1*
Reiger syndrome type I	Autosomal dominant	180500	*RIEG1*
Ellis–van Creveld syndrome	Autosomal recessive	225500	*EVG*
Ectodermal dysplasia, cleft, syndactyly	Autosomal recessive	225000	*PVRL1*

OMIM, Online Mendelian Inheritance in Man.

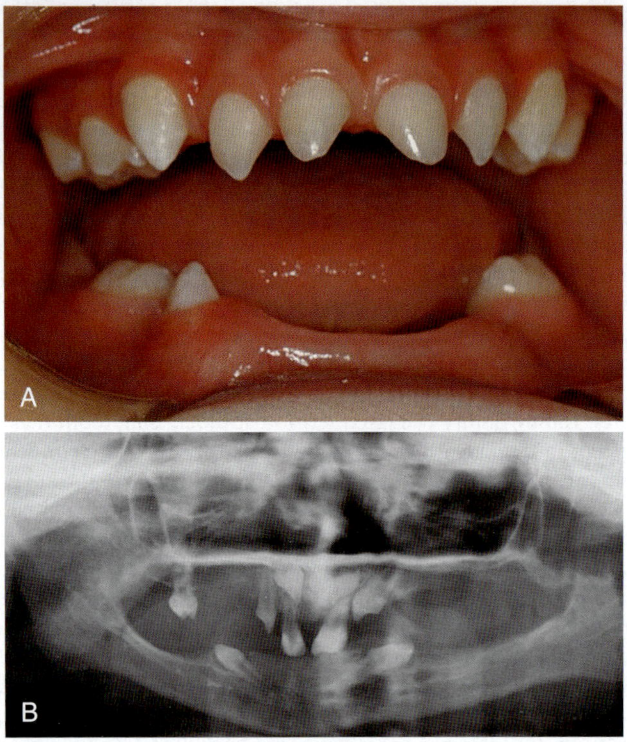

• **Fig. 20.3** (A–B) Conical-shaped incisors and missing teeth are common clinical features of X-linked hypohidrotic ectodermal dysplasia, as seen in these two affected male patients.

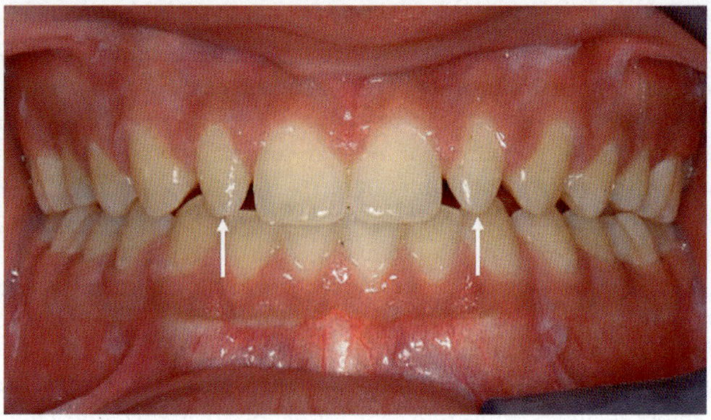

• **Fig. 20.4** This patient has isolated (nonsyndromic), bilateral microdontia in the form of peg-shaped maxillary lateral incisors.

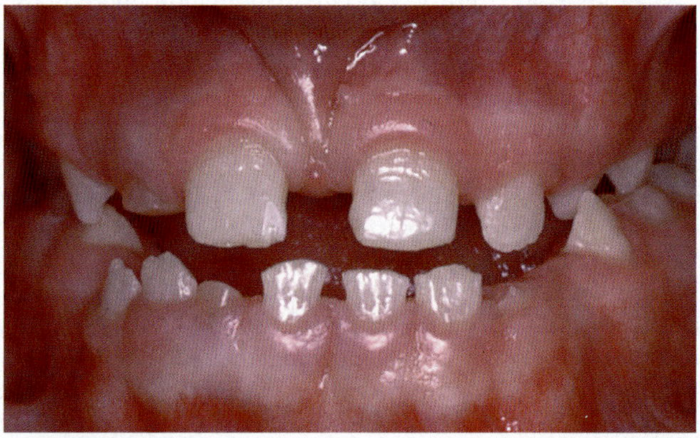

• **Fig. 20.5** Generalized microdontia is seen in the late transitional dentition (permanent incisors) of this child affected with the tricho-dento-osseous syndrome.

WNT10A gene appear to be the most prevalent cause of nonsyndromic hypodontia.[20]

In addition to nonsyndromic hypodontia, there are many syndromes that have missing teeth as a common feature. Ectodermal dysplasia is a term used to describe conditions with two or more tissues of ectodermal derivation (e.g., teeth, hair, sweat glands, mammary glands, salivary glands, fingernails) that demonstrate abnormal development because of genetic causes. In the dentition, this often manifests as conical shaped and missing teeth (Fig. 20.3). There are nearly 100 conditions that can be considered as ectodermal dysplasias, with the X-linked hypohidrotic ectodermal dysplasia (OMIM #305100) being the most common type.[21–23] Numerous other conditions display hypodontia as part of their phenotype. For example, Down syndrome is frequently (20% to 40%) associated with conical-shaped incisors and missing teeth.[24]

Anomalies of Size

Abnormalities in tooth size can be localized, affecting one or several teeth, or generalized, affecting all the teeth. A reduction in tooth size is called *microdontia* and is more common than an increase in tooth size termed *macrodontia*. The peg-shaped maxillary lateral incisor (Fig. 20.4) is an example of localized microdontia and has been linked to mutations in the *WNT10A* gene (OMIM #150400). It is often transmitted as an autosomal dominant trait with variable expressivity and incomplete penetrance. In some cases, patients develop one maxillary lateral incisor that is peg shaped and one that fails to form and is missing.

Not surprisingly, reduced tooth size and conical-shaped teeth are features of many of the ectodermal dysplasias (e.g., OMIM #305100, 604292, 224900, 129490), oculodentodigital dysplasia (OMIM #164200), and many other syndromes, including Down syndrome (OMIM #190685). Furthermore, environmental stressors such as chemotherapy and radiation as part of cancer treatment can interfere with the normal development of tooth size, with many cases resulting in microdontia.[8,25]

Microdontia

Diminished tooth size can result from a change in the overall tooth size or can occur secondary to reduction in the enamel thickness or both. Conditions demonstrating microdontia include many of the ectodermal dysplasias and the tricho-dento-osseous syndrome (OMIM #190320) that can have generally small teeth with thin enamel (Fig. 20.5). A decrease in dental crown size occurs due to generalized thin enamel (e.g., generalized thin hypoplastic amelogenesis imperfecta [AI]) despite the dentin morphology and dimension being normal. The overall tooth size in individuals affected with dentinogenesis imperfecta (DGI) is typically reduced as well.

Macrodontia

Macrodontia can occur as a localized trait and most commonly occurs as gemination (Fig. 20.6). Gemination is the incomplete twinning of primary or permanent teeth and is not known to have any genetic predilection or heritable etiology. This developmental disturbance can result in teeth that are almost twice the width of the normal nontwinned tooth (Fig. 20.7). Fusion of developing teeth also can result in an enlarged tooth, but there will be one less individual tooth in the affected area, whereas gemination manifests with the normal number of teeth present. Gemination and fusion are both rare, with a prevalence of approximately 0.5%.[26] Fusion is more common in the primary dentition compared with the permanent dentition.

Hereditary conditions with macrodontia include otodental syndrome (OMIM #166750) and the rare but quite remarkable Ekman-Westborg and Julin trait.[27] Otodental syndrome/otodental dysplasia (OMIM #166750) is an autosomal dominant condition caused by microdeletion at the *FGF3* gene on chromosome 11q13. It is characterized by grossly enlarged canines and molars and is frequently associated with sensorineural hearing loss and ocular coloboma.

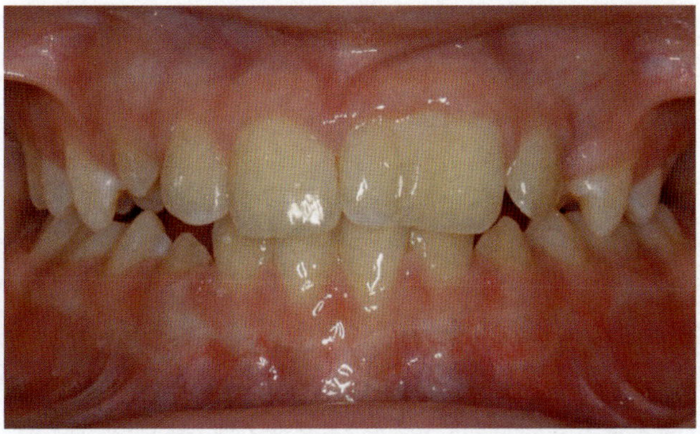

• **Fig. 20.6** Gemination is the incomplete twinning of teeth and presents as macrodontia in a dentition with the normal number of teeth.

Anomalies of Tooth Morphology

Developmental abnormalities in crown and/or root morphology or shape are collectively relatively common and are diverse in both their clinical presentation and apparent etiology. These developmental variances can involve one or more teeth and can affect any portion or component of the tooth (e.g., crown, root, pulp).

Environmental stressors can have a profound influence on tooth shape as well. Infectious conditions such as congenital syphilis, which is caused by the spirochete *Treponema pallidum,* produce classic patterns of hypoplastic and dysmorphic permanent teeth. The tapered and notched incisal edges of anterior teeth with screwdriver shapes are called *Hutchinson incisors,* and the irregular and accentuated occlusal patterns of posterior teeth known as mulberry molars are classic clinical findings for prenatal syphilis infection.[28]

Regional odontodysplasia affects enamel, dentin, and cementum, and typically is localized to one or more teeth in a specific area or developmental field. The affected teeth show marked dysplasia of the crown, root, and pulp morphology and are most often not compatible with a functioning tooth. The prognosis and management for each of these conditions also can be quite variable and should be investigated by further research when clinicians are managing patients with one of these developmental variances.[29]

Crown Size and Morphology

Tooth crown size and morphology are highly regulated at the genetic level, producing quite predictable dental morphologies for each specific primary and permanent tooth. Despite this regulation, a variety of developmental defects present as abnormal crown development, including variable cuspal patterns (talon, dens evaginatus, dens invaginatus, cusp of Carabelli), or more globally, crown shape, such as the marked cervical constriction seen in teeth (especially the posterior teeth) of individuals with DGI.

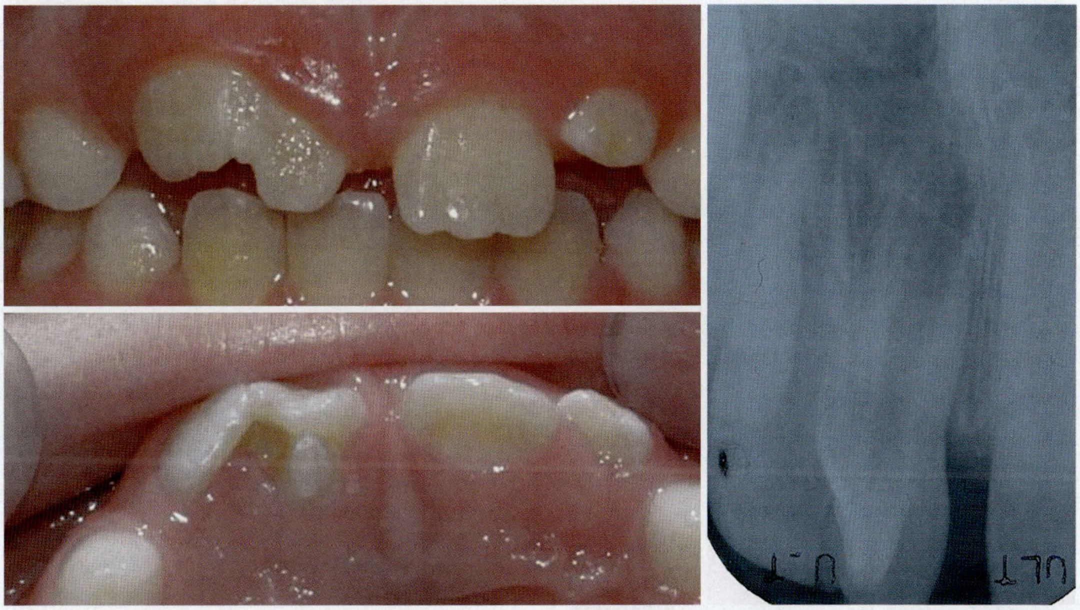

• **Fig. 20.7** As seen in this patient, gemination can produce localized macrodontia (A) and other developmental abnormalities such as a talon cusp in the lingual-cingulum area (B). Discerning whether there is communication between the different dental segments can be difficult using traditional radiography as illustrated in this periapical radiograph (C). Cone beam computed tomography can help determine pulp and root communication status.

Dens Evaginatus/Invaginatus

Dens evaginatus (OMIM #125280) describes an outfolding of the enamel organ that results in an extra cusp, usually in the central groove or ridge of posterior teeth and in the cingulum area of the anterior teeth, sometimes called a talon cusp (see Fig. 20.7). It occurs with a frequency of 1% to 4% and results from the evagination of inner enamel epithelium cells, which are the precursors of ameloblasts. The extra cusp contains enamel, dentin, and pulp tissue; therefore pulp exposure is possible by radically equilibrating the occlusion. Management of this anomaly includes careful enameloplasty or preventive resin restorations.[30]

Dens invaginatus, or dens in dente (OMIM #125300), is a condition resulting from invagination of the inner enamel epithelium producing the appearance of a tooth within a tooth (Fig. 20.8). The prevalence ranges from 0.25% to 3%, with the maxillary lateral incisors being most frequently affected.[31] The clinical significance of this anomaly is the high likelihood of carious and/or pulpal involvement through the communication of the invaginated portion of the lingual surface of the tooth with the outside environment. Therefore prompt diagnosis and preventive care (e.g., sealant, restoration) are crucial in cases of dens in dente.

Root Size and Morphology

Root morphology can be affected by environmental stressors (e.g., trauma to a developing tooth bud resulting in root dilacerations), can be caused by genetic factors that affect only root development, or can be associated with a syndrome. Severe infections such as that which occur in Stevens-Johnson syndrome or meningococcemia can lead to abnormal root formation.[32] Chemotherapy and radiation can lead to V-shaped or stunted roots if administered while tooth roots are developing (Fig. 20.9).[8,25]

Genetic causes of abnormal root formation include truncated root formation caused by mutations in the *IFIH1* gene that is associated with the Singleton-Merten syndrome 1 (OMIM #182250).[33] Individuals with tumoral calcinosis (OMIM #211900) can have short bulbous roots, and the condition is caused by mutations in the *GALNT3* gene.[34] Short dental roots are also seen with spondyloepimetaphyseal dysplasia (OMIM #271510) and Bardet-Biedl syndrome 1 (OMIM #209900).[35,36]

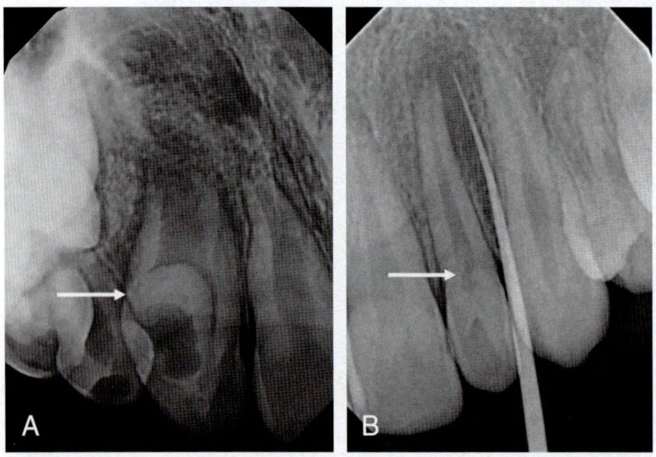

• **Fig. 20.8** These maxillary incisors have undergone pulpal necrosis as a result of dens in dente and presumably communication between the dental pulp and the oral environment. The presentation can be marked (A) or more subtle (B).

Molar Incisor Root Malformation

A novel dental phenotype has recently been described that is characterized by diminished and dysplastic root formation of the first permanent molars and a narrow abnormal pulp chamber (Fig. 20.10).[37] This molar dysmorphology is the cardinal or primary feature of this trait. The second primary molars and other primary and permanent teeth are affected in some cases with developmental changes that appear like those seen in the affected first permanent molars. The permanent anterior teeth can be involved and exhibit cervical crown constrictions and changes in the pulp chamber morphology. These phenotypic features have led to this condition being referred to as molar incisor root malformation (MIRM).[38] The etiology remains unclear; however, many affected individuals have a history of systemic illness or neonatal conditions, such as meningomyelocele or sacral dimple, meningitis, preterm birth, or chronic renal disease to name a few. Clinicians identifying cases of MIRM

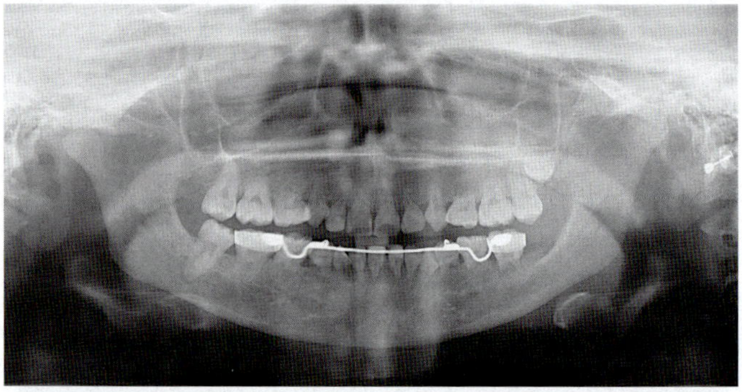

• **Fig. 20.9** This panoramic radiograph of this 18-year-old cancer survivor's dentition displays numerous developmentally missing permanent teeth and marked disruption of the normal root development secondary to aggressive chemotherapy between age 1 and 2 years.

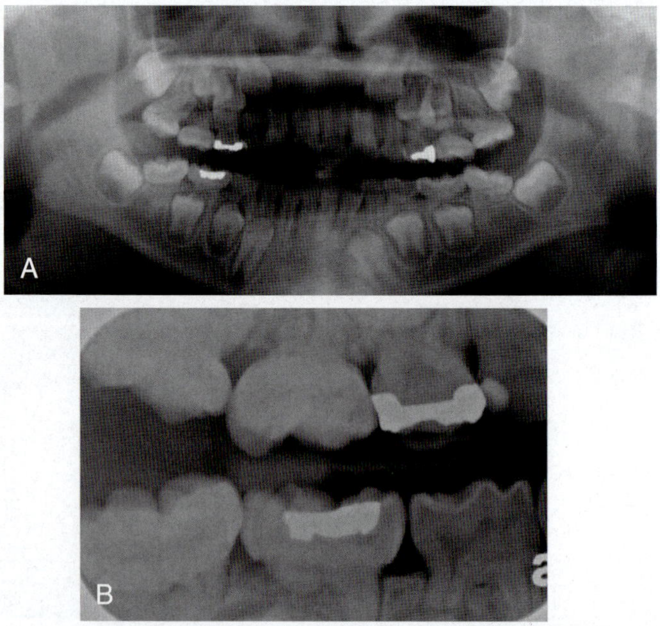

• **Fig. 20.10** Molar incisor root malformation affects the first permanent molars' root and pulp morphology, as seen in the panoramic radiograph, as well as incisors (A). (B) The periapical radiograph of this same child shows the second primary molar, and, to less extent, the first primary molar are also affected.

should carefully evaluate them because of the increased potential of ectopic eruption, pulp necrosis, and permanent incisor malformations.[38]

Short Root Anomaly

First described in the 1970s, short root anomaly is still a poorly understood phenomenon. Central incisors and premolars are the most commonly affected teeth, frequently presenting with shortened, wide, and round roots. Although few epidemiologic studies exist, it is estimated that short root anomaly has a prevalence of 1.3%.[39] The etiology remains unclear, but it is suspected to be of genetic origin and transmitted as an autosomal dominant trait.[40] In syndromic cases of short root anomaly, such as Rothmund-Thomson syndrome (OMIM #268400), specific genes have been associated with the dental anomaly.[41] Many clinicians often misdiagnose this condition as a pathologic resorption, when the two conditions are distinctly different. Correctly diagnosing this condition has major implications for treatment planning decisions because treatment options for an abnormal variant differ from options for a pathologic condition with root resorption. In contrast to short root anomaly, there have been reports of elongated roots in oculofaciocardiodental syndrome (OMIM #300166) caused by mutations in the *BCOR* gene that lead to increased periodontal ligament (PDL) cell proliferation and uncontrolled root growth, particularly of the permanent canines.[42,43]

Hypercementosis

Hypercementosis is the increase in cementum deposition on a root surface resulting in an abnormal root shape, frequently a bulbous tip at the root apex. The prevalence of hypercementosis is estimated to be 1.3%.[44] The etiology can include a reactive response to periapical inflammation, dental trauma to the PDL, or an abnormal developmental process. Several systemic conditions have been related to hypercementosis including atherosclerosis, acromegaly, and Paget disease.

Taurodontism

Taurodontism affects multirooted teeth and is characterized by an elongated pulp chamber due to apical displacement of the pulpal floor. Thus the root furcation moves apically leaving the individual roots variably shortened even though the overall root length may be normal. The prevalence in the general population ranges from 0.5% to 5%, with the permanent molar most often affected. The condition can be classified according to the extent of the pulp chamber elongation.[45] Because root furcation results from invagination of Hertwig's epithelial root sheath, many of the ectodermal dysplasias exhibit taurodontism. Individuals with tricho-dento-osseous syndrome (OMIM #190320) often have quite pronounced taurodontism (Fig. 20.11).[46] Taurodontism has also been associated with a variety of syndromes and has an increased prevalence in individuals with sex chromosome aneuploidy (Table 20.3).

Dental Tissue Composition and Structural Defects

The composition and structure of the dental tissues are unique and highly specialized, giving each tissue the requisite properties related to wear, flexure, fracture resistance, and attachment (tissue to tissue and tooth to bone) to have a viable dentition that can withstand the rigors of oral function. The etiologies of defects involving the composition and/or structure of the dental tissues can be either environmental or hereditary. However, in certain teeth the etiology is not well understood. For example, preeruptive dentinal radiolucencies can be seen on radiographs (Fig. 20.12), and, although no prevalence studies exist for this condition, case reports and case series do document its presence. The etiology is unclear, but the most likely explanation seems to be a combination of developmental anomaly, internal resorption, and/or external resorption.[47] Some have posited that the developmental anomaly is a type of hypoplasia or the inclusion of a noncalcified enamel matrix in dentin.[47,48] The processes involved in development of the dental tissues are highly specialized, so it is not surprising that there are

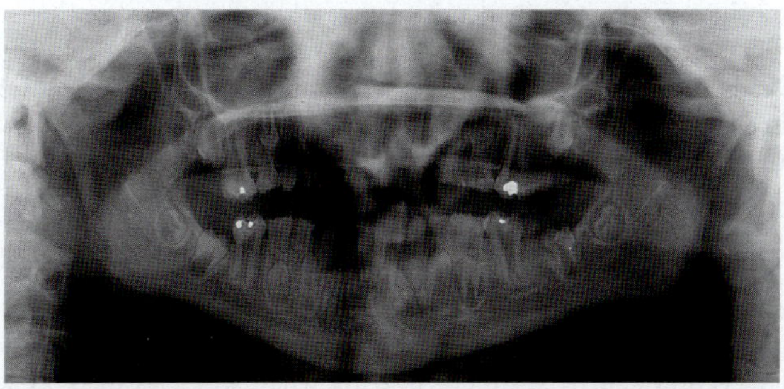

• **Fig. 20.11** This patient with tricho-dento-osseous syndrome demonstrates marked taurodontism of both the first permanent and second primary molars, as seen in this panoramic radiograph of their mixed dentition.

TABLE 20.3 Conditions Demonstrating Taurodontism

Condition	Characteristics	OMIM #	Gene	Mode of Inheritance
Klinefelter syndrome	Aspermatogenesis, mental retardation	400045	46,XX	—
Tricho-dento-osseous syndrome	Sclerotic bones, coarse gnarled hair, enamel defects	190320	*DLX3*	Autosomal dominant
Oral-facial-digital syndrome type 2	Dystrophic nails, hyperplastic frenum, lobed tongue	252100	*OFD2*	Autosomal recessive
Ectodermal dysplasia (hypohidrotic)	Hypotrichosis, aplasia of sweat/sebaceous glands	305100	*EDA*	X-linked recessive
Amelogenesis imperfecta type 4	Enamel hypoplasia and hypomaturation, mottled yellow teeth	104510	*DLX3*	Autosomal dominant
Down syndrome	Brachycephaly, mental retardation, epicanthal fold	190685	Many	Trisomy 21

OMIM, Online Mendelian Inheritance in Man.

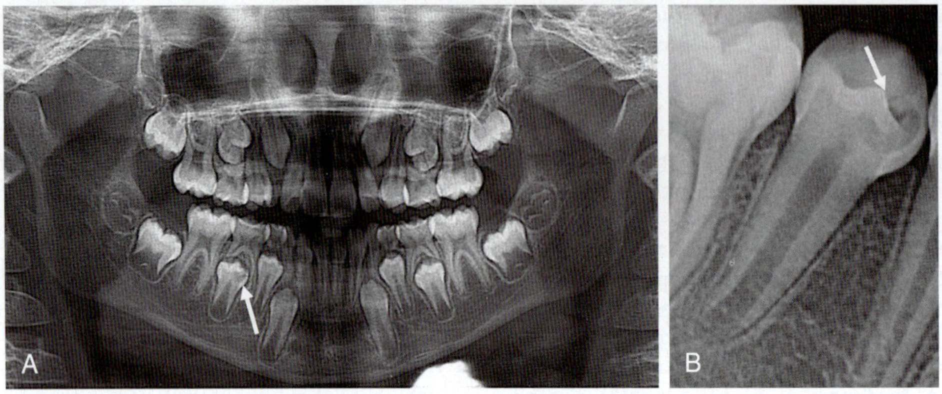

• **Fig. 20.12** This child had showed an approximately 0.5-cm radiolucency just below the dentin enamel junction on this panoramic radiograph *(arrow)* (A). This well-circumscribed lesion *(arrow)* that does not extend through the proximal enamel can be appreciated after the tooth erupted in this periapical radiograph (B).

so many different etiologies and clinical presentations of dental defects involving composition and structure.

Environmental Defects Altering Tooth Color

Enamel development, or amelogenesis, is an exquisitely regulated process at the molecular level but can be disrupted by many environmental factors, such as fever, infection, trauma, changes in oxygen saturation, antibiotics, and many other influences (Table 20.4). In general, the resulting enamel defects can be classified as defects in the amount of enamel (hypoplasia) or deficiencies in the mineral content (hypomineralization). Changes in enamel mineralization result in altered enamel translucency and color. Because enamel is translucent, changes in dentin can result in tooth color changes even when the enamel is unchanged (e.g., tetracycline staining). Enamel hypoplasia or hypomineralization can be generalized throughout the dentition or it can be localized. Environmental stressors of short duration often cause localized defects (e.g., fever), whereas chronic stressors are more likely to be associated with generalized defects (e.g., fluorosis).

Enamel defects are common in the general population, with reports suggesting that between 20% and 80% of people will have an enamel defect.[49,50] The broad range of reported enamel defect prevalence is largely due to what was classified as an enamel defect (actual hypoplasia versus color change indicating hypomineralization). Not all teeth are affected equally, with anterior teeth being more affected than premolars in the permanent dentition. Children who have more frequent and serious illnesses are more likely to have enamel defects. Common causes of intrinsic stains include blood-borne pigments, drug administration, and stressors influencing enamel mineralization such as fluorosis or fever (see Table 20.4). Congenital porphyria, bile duct defects, anemias, and transfusion-reaction hemolysis are examples of conditions with characteristic blood-borne pigments. For example, biliary atresia and the resultant hyperbilirubinemia often cause green teeth (Fig. 20.13).

A classic example of drug-induced intrinsic staining occurs from the tetracycline group of antibiotics. Both dentitions can have severe discoloration from this antibiotic when given over as brief a period as 3 days. Tetracycline hydrochloride has the greatest potential for staining among the cycline antibiotics. The agent forms an orthocalcium phosphate complex with dentin and enamel, which is then oxidized by ultraviolet light. The oxidation process results in pigments that stain the hard tissues. The critical

TABLE 20.4 Environmental Influences on Enamel and/or Tooth Color

Condition	Phenotype
Fever	Hypomineralization to marked enamel hypoplasia
Starvation	Enamel hypoplasia
Excess fluoride exposure	Enamel hypomineralization
Trauma	Hypomineralization to marked enamel hypoplasia, blue-gray to yellow-brown color
Hypoxia (e.g., severe cardiac defect)	Hypomineralization to marked enamel hypoplasia
Infection (e.g., congenital syphilis, cytomegalovirus, congenital rubella)	Hypomineralization to marked enamel hypoplasia
Tetracycline	Blue-gray color, dentin staining possible enamel hypoplasia
Low birth weight	Enamel hypoplasia
Hyperbilirubinemia	Green discoloration

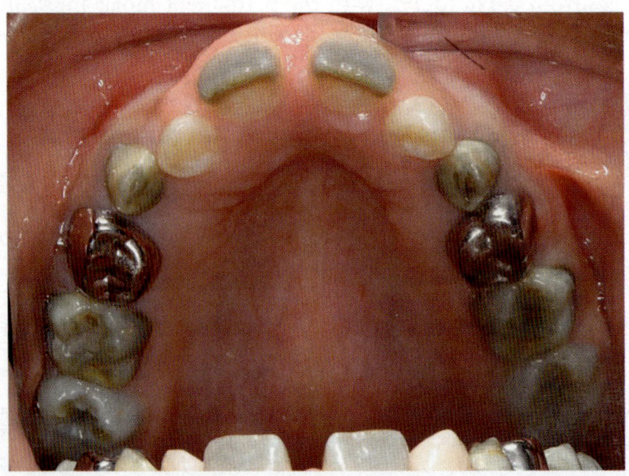

• **Fig. 20.13** This child suffered from hyperbilirubinemia during early development of the primary and permanent dentitions. Note the staining in both primary and some permanent teeth.

period for initiation of primary and permanent tooth staining is that of intrauterine development through 8 years of age. Tetracycline administration must be especially avoided during this time. The International Association of Dental Traumatology (IADT) antibiotics use for avulsion injuries has changed, and due to limited evidence supporting their use, IADT recommends clinician decision based on the case. Caution should be used in considering antibiotics such as tetracycline or doxycycline, as administration may result in discoloration.[51]

Fluorosis

Dental fluorosis is a pathologic condition characterized by hypomineralization of the enamel caused by excessive exposure to fluoride during enamel mineralization. The level of hypomineralization and clinical appearance of the fluorotic enamel varies from mild to severe (Fig. 20.14) and is partially determined by the amount of fluoride in the individual's serum during amelogenesis. Individuals have differing risk and resistance to developing dental fluorosis based on their genetic makeup and health. Studies suggest several genes are important in defining the population's variance for dental fluorosis risk.[52] Fluoride has a variety of actions that contribute to the development of dental fluorosis, including direct effects on the ameloblasts, the developing matrix, and processing of the matrix.[53]

Molar Hypomineralization

Molar hypomineralization, also known as molar incisor hypomineralization, is a developmental defect of the human dentition that primarily affects the enamel of the first permanent molars. Because the cardinal feature of this condition is hypomineralization of the first permanent molars with only 40% of cases involving incisors, the term molar hypomineralization is the more appropriate name. Typically, the second permanent molars and premolars are not involved. This condition has been recognized since approximately 1970 and has been described using a variety of terms (e.g., cheese molars, idiopathic hypomineralization of enamel). The term molar incisor hypomineralization was adopted by leaders in the field that convened at the European Academy of Pediatric Dentistry Annual Meeting in 2000.[54] The clinical characteristics vary from case to case and between teeth in the same individual. The more severely affected the first permanent molars, the more likely it is that there will be incisor involvement. The defects vary from small, well-demarcated areas of color change to extensive hypomineralization that includes the entire dental crown (Fig. 20.15). Affected teeth form with a normal thickness of enamel with the abnormal areas of enamel having a decreased mineral content and increased protein and water content. Thus the defects are not hypoplastic in that the full thickness of enamel develops. Once the tooth begins to erupt and comes into function, rapid enamel loss can make the crown appear hypoplastic, but this is typically the result of enamel fracturing, wear, and dental caries.[55]

Hereditary Enamel Defects

There are thousands of genes expressed by ameloblasts, and there are more than 100 different hereditary conditions associated with

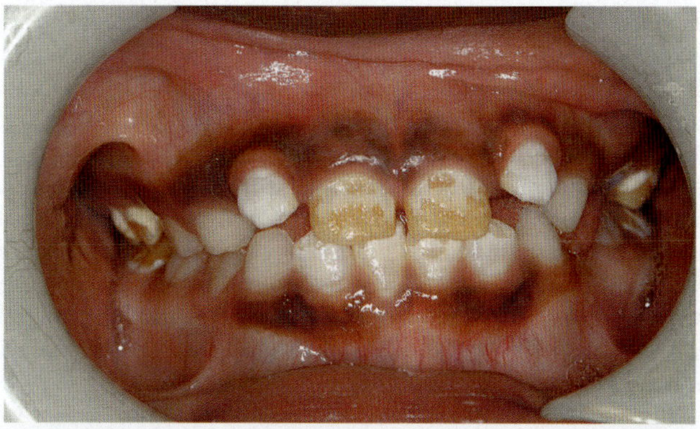

• **Fig. 20.14** This child demonstrates severe fluorosis of the permanent incisors and molars, but the primary dentition appears unaffected as a consequence of reduced fetal fluoride exposure resulting from fluid dynamics and fluoride uptake differentials in the mother and infant.

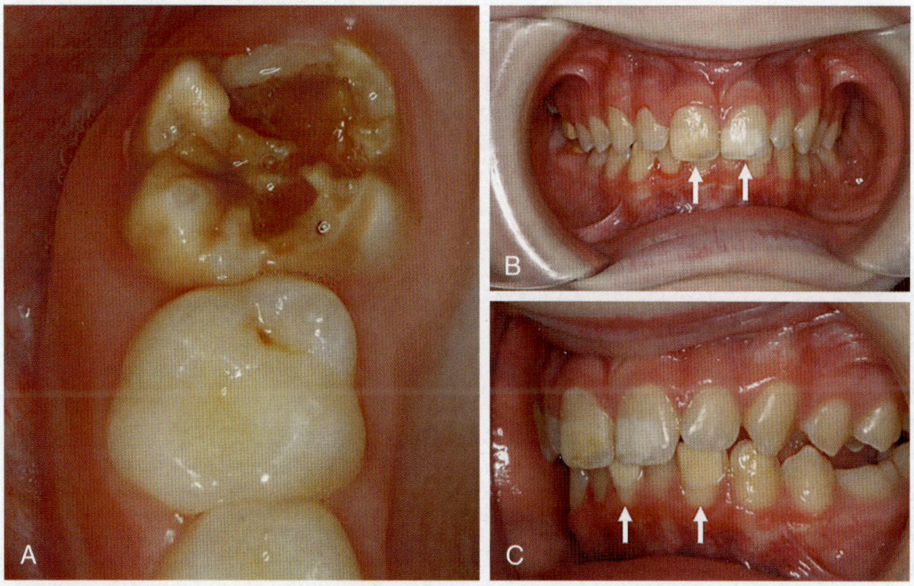

• **Fig. 20.15** Molar incisor hypomineralization is highly variable in its presentation and in severe cases (A) can be associated with early enamel loss and dental sensitivity. Involvement of other teeth is variable as well but often involves the incisors *(arrows)* as seen in this adolescent patient (B–C).

an enamel phenotype.[56] Most hereditary conditions affecting enamel formation are syndromes and have clinical manifestations and phenotypes that extend beyond the dental enamel. Genes with known ameloblastic function cause many of these conditions. The most common resulting enamel phenotype is hypoplasia. For example, junctional epidermolysis bullosa (OMIM #226700) is caused by mutations in genes that are expressed by ameloblasts and are important in cell-to-cell adhesion. The abnormal proteins produced from these genes (e.g., *COL17A1, LAM3, IGbeta6*) result in fragility of the skin that blisters. Abnormal function of these proteins results in ameloblasts that do not adhere to each other, or the stratum intermedium cells, resulting in cell separation and enamel hypoplasia.

Hereditary conditions affecting primarily the enamel have been referred to as amelogenesis imperfecta (AI) (eTable 20.5).[57,58] The prevalence of AI varies around world and is thought to occur in approximately 1 out of 8000 people, although there has only been one epidemiologic study ever conducted in the United States.[57] These disorders have been classified based on their clinical phenotype and mode of inheritance. The AI types were also classified based on the perceived mechanism leading to the enamel defect (i.e., deficient matrix formation leading to hypoplasia, deficient crystal growth and mineralization during the maturation stage of enamel development causing hypomaturation, and abnormal initiation of the enamel crystallites with subsequent abnormal mineralization or hypocalcification). Both hypomaturation and hypocalcification are characterized by deficient enamel mineral or hypomineralization (Fig. 20.16). Hypomineralized AI enamel has greater amounts of protein present compared with normal enamel and will thus have an altered translucency and can be markedly weakened depending on the decrease in mineral content.

Hereditary Dentin Defects

The process of dentin development, or dentinogenesis, is thought to be relatively resistant to environmental insults or systemic conditions compared with tooth enamel formation. It is the mesenchymally derived dentin that is the most abundant tissue in teeth and the tissue that determines much of the crown and root morphology. Normal dentin development and mineralization requires adequate levels of vitamin D (the active form is 1–25 dihydroxy vitamin D or calcitriol). Inadequate vitamin D levels during tooth development can result in decreased dentin production, resulting in large pulp chambers and a decreased dentin mineral content.

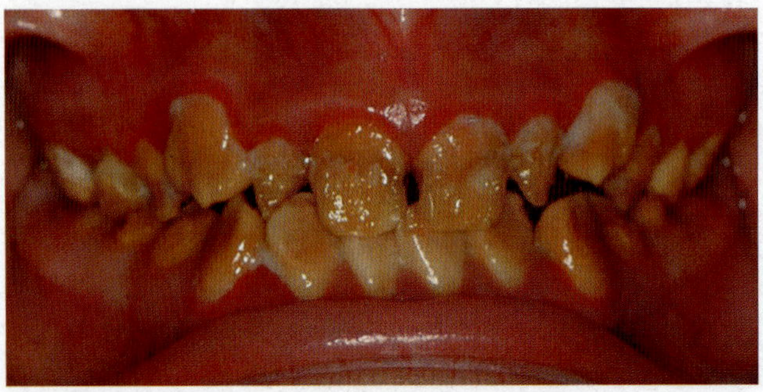

• **Fig. 20.16** This individual with autosomal recessive hypomaturation amelogenesis imperfecta has marked discoloration of her teeth caused by the lack of mineral and therefore limited insulating capacity of the enamel.

Genetic mutations in several genes related to vitamin D can cause similar developmental disturbances such as the X-linked conditions vitamin D–resistant (OMIM #307800) and autosomal dominant vitamin D–dependent rickets (OMIM #193100).

Dentinogenesis Imperfecta

Hereditary dentin defects have been classified as dentinogenesis imperfectas (DGIs) and dentin dysplasias (DDs) (Table 20.6).[59] These hereditary conditions are associated with abnormal dentin mineralization and varying degrees of changes in tooth morphology. DGI type I (OMIM #166200) is associated with osteogenesis imperfecta, whereas the clinically similar DGI type II (OMIM #125490) is not associated with a syndrome and is caused by mutations in the gene encoding dentin sialophosphoprotein *(DSPP)*.[59] Osteogenesis imperfecta or brittle bone disease is caused by mutations in the genes coding for type I collagen or proteins involved in fibrillogenesis. The DGI tooth phenotype is highly variable and is characterized by an opalescent blue-gray to yellow-brown coloration caused by the discolored dentin shining through the normal and translucent enamel (enamel is affected in some cases; Fig. 20.17). The teeth can have a pronounced cervical constriction at the cementoenamel junction area that demarcates the junction of the clinical crown and the tooth root. Individuals with DGI often have dental root structures that are diminished in size and can appear sharp and "tent peg-like." The dentin in DGI teeth or in DD type II is poorly organized structurally and is less mineralized than normal dentin. This abnormal structure and lack of mineral result in the dentin inadequately supporting the enamel that often fractures away from the tooth, leaving it susceptible to undergoing rapid attrition due to the poor wear resistance of the hypomineralized DGI dentin. Enamel loss and subsequent

TABLE 20.6 Hereditary Dentin Anomalies: Shields Classification

Condition	Dental Phenotype	OMIM #	Gene
DI type I	Yellow-brown to blue-gray color, enamel fracturing, diminished tooth size, cervical constriction, enamel fracturing pulp chamber obliteration, typically more severe in primary dentition, short roots	166200	*COL1A1*
			COL1A2
DI type II	Essentially the same as above	125490	*DSPP*
	Primary and permanent frequently affected similarly		
	Risk of periapical abscess		
DI type III	Generally the same as DI type II except initially have large pulp chambers that obliterate with age	125500	*DSPP*
DD type I	Normal clinical crown morphology, and color, short or no roots, pulp chamber obliteration	125400	Unknown

DD, Dentin dysplasia; *DI*, dentinogenesis imperfecta; *OMIM*, Online Mendelian Inheritance in Man.

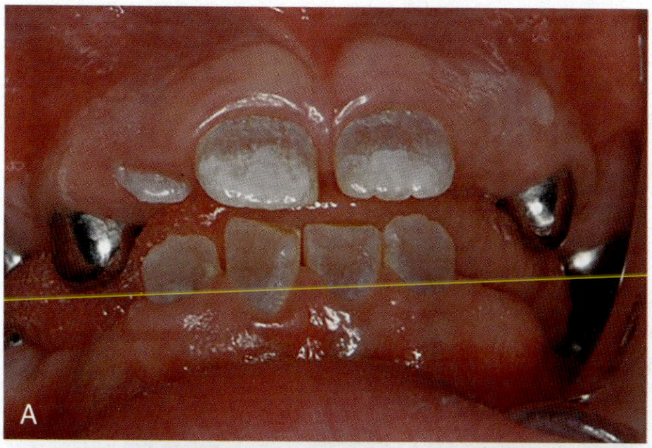

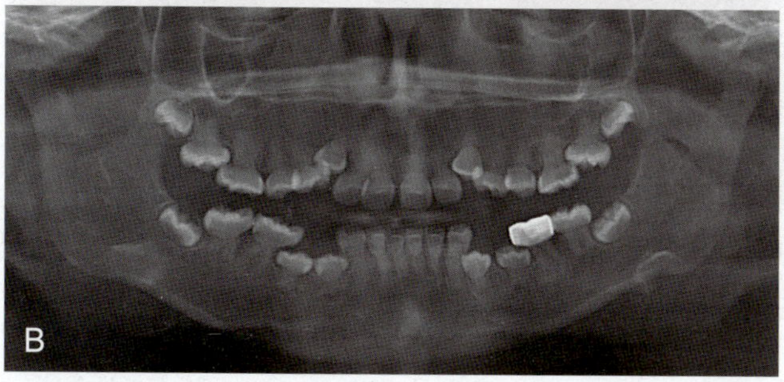

• **Fig. 20.17** Dentinogenesis imperfecta is characterized clinically by variable yellow-brown to blue-gray coloration of the dentition (A). Radiographically the teeth often display pulp obliteration, cervical constriction at the cementoenamel junction, and diminished root formation (B). Ectopic eruption due to the marked cervical coronal constriction also can be a feature of dentinogenesis imperfecta as seen in this panoramic radiograph (B).

rapid attrition is a common but variable feature of DGI. In those cases, in which enamel is lost, the teeth tend to wear very rapidly. Full coverage crowns are typically the treatment of choice once this process begins.

Dentin Dysplasias

DD type II, or the coronal DD type (OMIM #125420), is an allelic disorder of DGI type II caused by *DSPP* mutations. DD type II is characterized by a DGI phenotype in the primary dentition and slight or no discernable clinical phenotype in permanent dentition (e.g., there may be slight discoloration of the dental crown).[60] Radiographically, DD type II permanent teeth often have an abnormal pulp morphology that can present as a thistle tube in the anterior teeth and sometimes a bowtie morphology in the molar teeth. Both DGI type II and DD type II are inherited as autosomal dominant traits and are highly penetrant. Interestingly, individuals with DD type II may not remember having affected primary teeth. This can make the determination of a family history challenging.

The phenotype in DD type I, or radicular DD type (OMIM #125400), is characterized by clinically normal-appearing tooth crowns and markedly altered dentin formation that has a pathognomonic cascading waterfall histologic appearance, pulp chamber obliteration, and abnormal to nearly missing root development. The etiology of this classic DD type I with normal crowns and unique histologic appearance is not known yet.[61]

Hereditary Cementum Defects

Cementum is deposited on the tooth surface by cementoblasts in a process known as cementogenesis. Of the dental hard tissues, cementum is the least mineralized and most cellular with many cementoblasts becoming encased in the developing tooth layer. This cellular cementum is seen more in the apical half of the root, whereas acellular cementum dominates the coronal half.

Hypophosphatasia (OMIM #146300, 241500, 241510) results from mutations in the tissue-nonspecific alkaline phosphatase gene. Alkaline phosphatase is essential for normal mineralization and development of tissues including bone, dentin, and cementum. Osteoporosis, bone fragility, and premature loss of primary incisors are classic clinical features (Fig. 20.18). Abnormal development of cementum results in early loss of primary teeth that occurs without root resorption. Children presenting with early tooth loss, especially without evidence of root resorption or systemic illness, should be evaluated for hypophosphatasia (see Chapter 37). This condition is now treatable with a fusion protein that replaces the lost alkaline phosphatase protein function.

Anomalies of Tooth Eruption

The process of tooth eruption (particularly of permanent teeth) has been described in several stages, namely preemergent and postemergent eruption. Once root formation begins during the preemergent stage, eruption is thought to begin. This process requires resorption of alveolar bone and primary tooth roots and a propulsive movement in an occlusal direction. Some suggest that hard tissue proliferation at the root apex is the primary mechanism for eruption. However, some teeth, for example intruded or luxated teeth, will show eruption/reeruption without apical proliferation. The mechanisms controlling tooth eruption are complex and involve a variety of dental components including the dental follicle and PDL.[62]

The clearance of an eruption path is the primary control for preemergent eruption. In general, so long as a path is cleared, a tooth will erupt into that path and begin its postemergent eruption. However, a blocked eruptive path can lead to eruption anomalies. Inadequate space is thus a common cause of failed tooth eruption. One of the more common eruption anomalies is ectopic eruption, which has a prevalence of approximately 3%, and the most commonly involved teeth are the permanent first molars, lateral incisors, and canines.[63] Aside from ectopic eruption, primary teeth can experience delayed exfoliation, and permanent teeth can experience delayed eruption. Table 20.7 lists a few common syndromes associated with eruption anomalies, including cleidocranial dysplasia, cherubism, and enamel-renal syndrome.

Primary Failure of Eruption

Primary failure of eruption (PFE, OMIM #125350), a nonsyndromic condition affecting tooth eruption, is caused in many cases by mutations in the *PTH1R* gene that is a regulator of bone homeostasis. PFE is characterized by having at least one affected first permanent molar; the teeth distal to the affected first permanent molar also show failed eruption usually with a progressive open bite. The involved teeth tend to have a supracrestal position, meaning they have a completely cleared eruption pathway with no alveolar bone occlusal to the affected tooth.[64] Orthodontic extrusion of affected teeth is unsuccessful and leads to ankylosis.

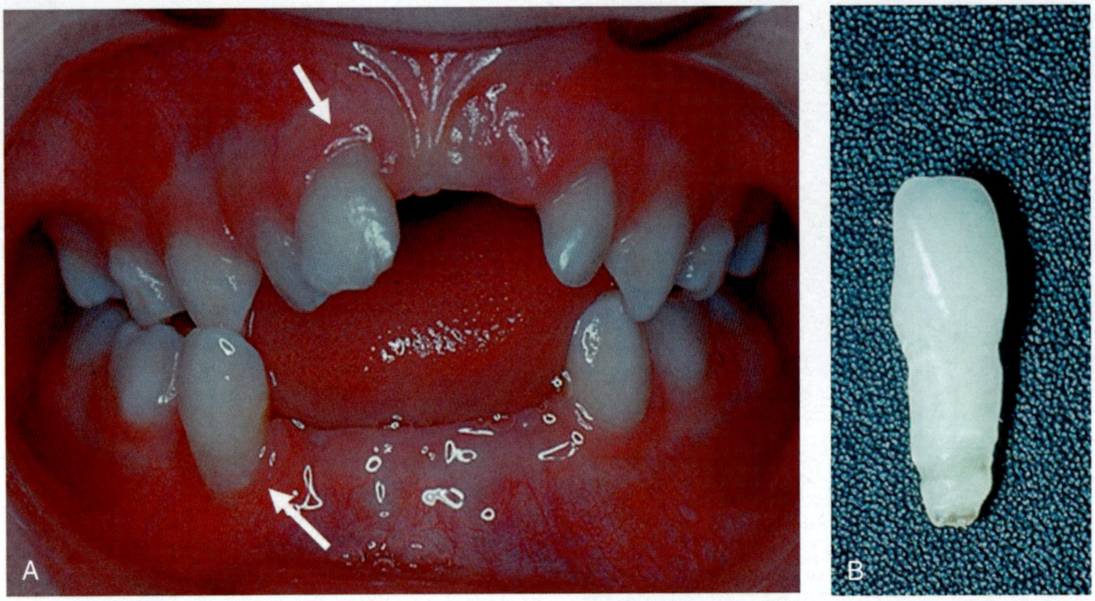

• **Fig. 20.18** (A) Premature tooth loss is a hallmark feature of hypophosphatasia, and as seen in this affected child the teeth exfoliate with minimal inflammation despite gingival recession around the maxillary primary incisor and mandibular canine *(arrows).* Children with teeth exfoliating prematurely without root resorption (B) and soft tissue inflammation should be evaluated for hypophosphatasia.

TABLE 20.7 Conditions With Abnormal Tooth Eruption Phenotype

Condition	Phenotype	OMIM #	Gene	Mode of Inheritance
Cleidocranial dysplasia	Failure of succedaneous tooth to erupt, supernumerary teeth, retention cysts	119600	*RUNX2*	Autosomal dominant
Primary failure of eruption	Failure of posterior teeth to erupt and not orthodontically movable	125350	*PTH1R*	Autosomal dominant
Osteopetrosis	Failure of eruption due to abnormal osteoclast function	259700	*TCIRG1*	Autosomal recessive
Cherubism	Multilocular cystic changes in the jaws that interfere with tooth eruption and facial growth	11840	*SH3BP2*	Autosomal dominant
Mucopolysaccharidosis	Defective enzyme results in accumulation of material around dental follicles	309900	*IDS*	X-linked recessive
Oculodentodigital dysplasia	Small teeth with abnormal eruption	164200	*GJA1*	Autosomal dominant
		257850		Autosomal recessive
Autosomal recessive AI and gingival fibromatosis syndrome (enamel renal syndrome)	Hypoplastic enamel, pulp calcifications, eruption abnormalities	614253	*FAM20A*	Autosomal recessive

AI, Amelogenesis imperfecta; *OMIM,* Online Mendelian Inheritance in Man.

21

Periodontal Problems in Children and Adolescents

ANN L. GRIFFEN, KYULIM LEE, SHAUN ROTENBERG

CHAPTER OUTLINE

Children and adolescents are affected by a variety of periodontal diseases and conditions. Gingivitis is the most common, especially around puberty. Significant loss of periodontal attachment or alveolar bone is more unusual in young patients and can result from systemic disease or occur as isolated dental disease. In addition, gingival anatomical problems, such as lack of attached gingiva, can arise during development and may necessitate early management.

Gingivitis

Gingivitis is characterized by inflammation of the gingival tissues with no loss of attachment or bone. It occurs in response to the microbes that live in biofilms at the gingival margin and in the sulcus.[1] The clinical signs of gingivitis include erythema, bleeding on probing, and edema. In the early primary dentition, gingivitis is uncommon. Younger children have less plaque than adults and appear to be less reactive to the same amount of plaque. This can be explained both by differences in bacterial composition of plaque and by developmental changes in the inflammatory response. Gingivitis occurs in half the population by the age of 4 or 5 years, and the incidence continues to increase with age. Gingivitis is exacerbated by high levels of steroid hormones, and hormone-influenced plaque-induced gingivitis is common around the time of puberty (Fig. 21.1), when the prevalence of gingivitis peaks at close to 100%. After puberty, gingivitis declines slightly and stays constant into adulthood.[2] The peak prevalence of hormone-influenced plaque-induced gingivitis during puberty is at age 10 years in girls and age 13 years in boys. Extensive gingivitis in 12-year-olds, as indicated by bleeding upon probing in more than 15% of sites, has been shown to negatively affect children in how they perceive their oral health as well as their daily lives.[3] Hormone-influenced plaque-induced gingivitis can also occur with the use of oral contraceptive medications or during pregnancy.[4] In these conditions the gingiva may be enlarged and granulomatous changes observed.

Certain local factors may be important contributors to gingivitis in children. Crowded teeth and orthodontic appliances may make oral hygiene more difficult and predispose to gingivitis. Mouth breathing may cause chronically dehydrated gingiva in the maxillary labial area and lead to a characteristic localized gingivitis as shown in Fig. 21.2. Inflammation, especially erythema, often occurs around erupting primary and permanent teeth in the presence of plaque.

Gingivitis is reversible and can be managed with improved plaque control. Appropriately sized toothbrushes and toothpaste flavored to appeal to children may enhance compliance. Young children, especially those younger than 6 years of age, will require parental assistance with their oral hygiene care. Older children and even some adolescents can benefit from some degree of parental supervision.

Localized Juvenile Spongiotic Gingival Hyperplasia

Localized juvenile spongiotic gingival hyperplasia (LJSGH), initially called *juvenile spongiotic gingivitis,* is a unique gingival presentation characterized by a hyperplastic tissue that is bright red, often presenting with a velvet-like texture (Fig. 21.3).[5] LJSGH is

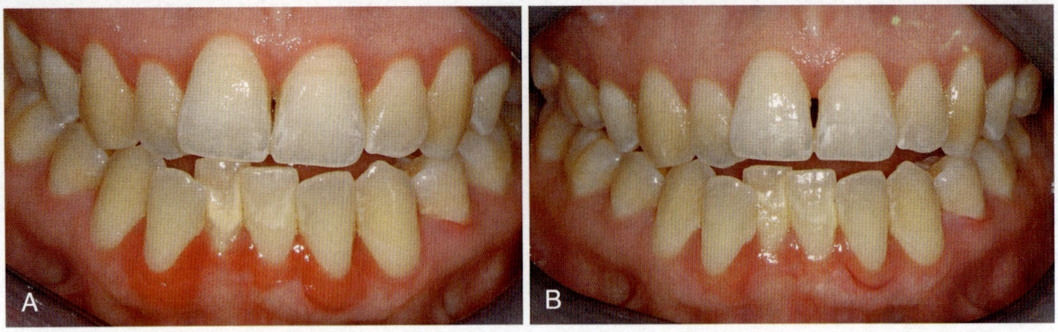

• **Fig. 21.1** (A) Hormone-influenced plaque-induced gingivitis in a 16-year-old female patient. (B) Some resolution seen after 1-month of plaque control.

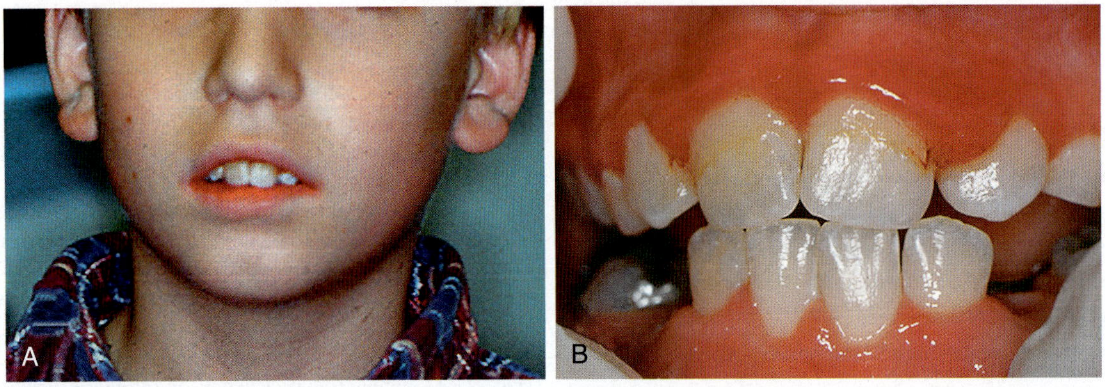

• **Fig. 21.2** (A) The typical oral posture of mouth breathing. (B) The resultant gingivitis of the maxillary facial gingiva.

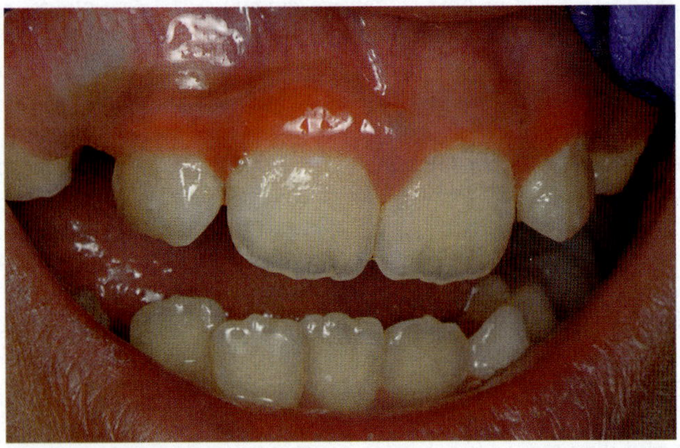

• **Fig. 21.3** Localized juvenile spongiotic gingival hyperplasia. Note erythematous hyperplastic tissue along the gingival margin of maxillary anterior teeth.

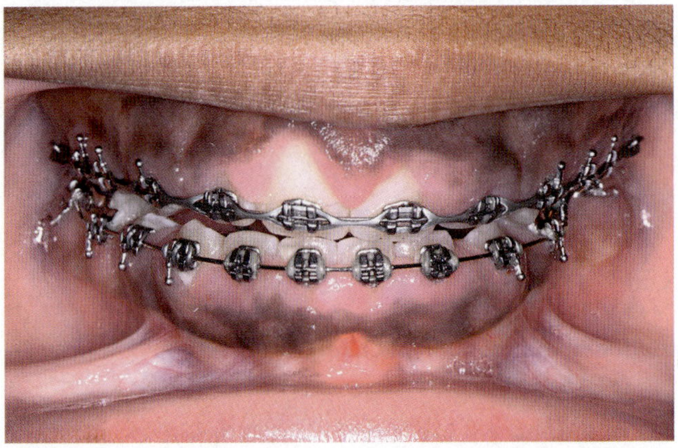

• **Fig. 21.4** Gingival enlargement in response to long-standing plaque accumulation secondary to orthodontic appliances. Note uneven gingival margin on maxillary central incisors and generalized fibrotic surfaces.

most common in the maxillary anterior region of young patients, although it is sometimes seen in adults. It involves the marginal and sometimes the adjacent attached gingiva. LJSGH is not associated with plaque or calculus and does not respond to oral hygiene measures. Although these lesions are often asymptomatic and may resolve spontaneously, LJSGH can pose esthetic concerns. Surgical excision should be recommended with caution given the recurrence rate and risk of gingival recession. The effectiveness of other treatment options, such as cryotherapy, laser ablation, topical steroids, and more, remains inconclusive.[5]

Gingival Enlargement

Chronic Inflammatory Gingival Enlargement

Long-standing gingivitis in young patients sometimes results in chronic inflammatory gingival enlargement, which may be localized or generalized. It commonly occurs when plaque is allowed to accumulate around orthodontic appliances, as shown in Fig. 21.4, or in areas chronically dried by mouth breathing. The interdental papillae and the marginal gingiva become enlarged, and the tissue is usually erythematous and bleeds easily. It may be soft and friable with a smooth, shiny surface, or dense and fibrotic with a matte surface. Inflammatory gingival enlargement often slowly resolves when adequate plaque control is instituted, unless the tissues are fibrotic; in such cases, gingivectomy is often required.

Plaque-Induced, Drug-Influenced Gingival Enlargement

Long-term therapy with certain systemic medications can produce an overgrowth of gingival tissue (Fig. 21.5A–B).[6] It can occur after therapy with anticonvulsants (i.e., phenytoin), immunosuppressants (i.e., cyclosporine), or calcium channel blockers (i.e., nifedipine). The overgrowth is painless and differs from chronic inflammatory enlargement in that it is fibrous, firm, and pale pink, often with little tendency to bleed. The enlargement occurs first in the interdental region and may appear lobular. It gradually spreads to the gingival margin. The condition can become extreme, sometimes covering the crowns of the teeth and interfering with eruption or occlusion (see Fig. 21.5B).

Plaque-induced, drug-influenced gingival enlargement occurs slowly and may resolve to some degree when medication is discontinued. There appears to be a genetic component to susceptibility to gingival enlargement. The severity of the enlargement is also affected by both the adequacy of oral hygiene and the gingival concentration of the medication. If medication cannot be discontinued or changed, the enlargement can be surgically removed, but it will recur. Surgery is indicated when the appearance of the gingiva is unacceptable to the patient, when the enlargement interferes with comfortable functioning, or when enlargement produces periodontal pockets that cannot be maintained in a healthy state. An internal beveled incision approach is recommended for gingivectomy to create a more natural gingival contour and reduce risk of recurrence (see Fig. 21.5C–D). Postoperative discomfort after gingivectomy can be considerable and should be carefully weighed against potential benefits for special needs patients who may not be able to give fully informed consent.

Anatomical Problems

Development and Defects of the Attached Gingiva

When teeth erupt, they pierce through an existing band of keratinized gingiva, and the width of this band and its relationship to the teeth change very little during subsequent growth and development. Deflections in the path of eruption, such as those due to crowding or overretention of primary teeth, may result in a narrowed band of attached gingiva[7] and uneven exposure of the crowns of adjacent teeth. This is particularly common when mandibular incisors erupt labial to the alveolar ridge, as shown in Fig. 21.6A. This usually occurs without loss of attachment and can easily be misdiagnosed as recession on the longer tooth. Careful examination is needed to determine the position of the cementoenamel junction (CEJ). If the band of attached gingiva is very narrow, even a small subsequent loss of attachment can result in a mucogingival defect (which occurs when the pocket depth exceeds the width of keratinized gingiva), and recession may occur, as shown in Fig. 21.6B. Other factors that may contribute to recession in children and adolescents are habit-related self-inflicted injury, oral piercings, and the use of smokeless tobacco.

In situations with a significant loss of attachment, autogenous soft tissue augmentation in the form of a free gingival graft of subepithelial connective tissue may be indicated to stabilize and repair the gingiva. Surgical repair of lingual recession due to oral piercings can be performed but requires more complex treatment than typical labial grafts.[8] Orthodontic movement of a labially malpositioned tooth in the direction of the alveolar ridge may

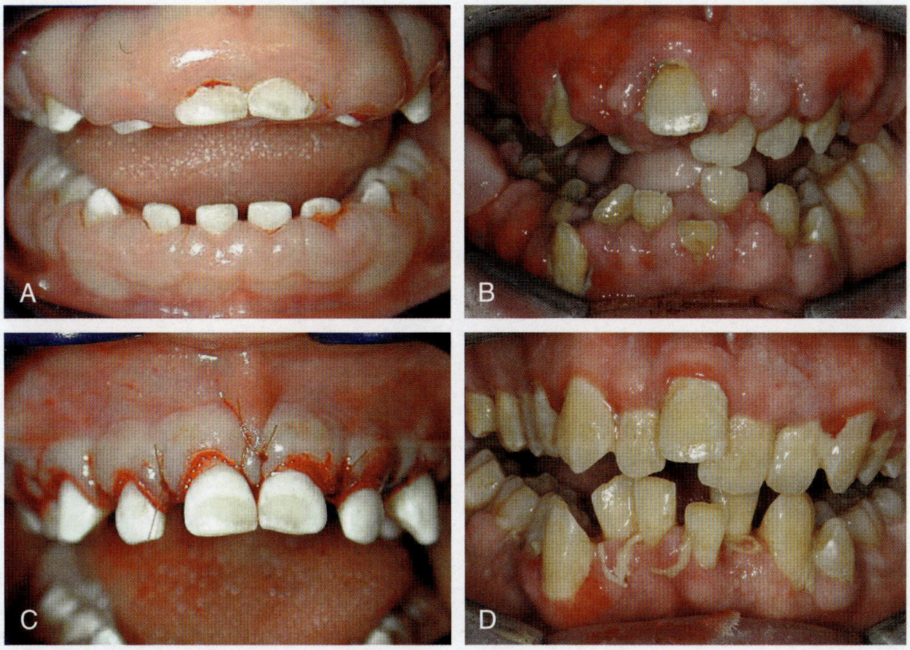

• **Fig. 21.5** Severe gingival enlargement secondary to phenytoin therapy in a (A) 6-year-old or (B) 17-year-old. (C) Gingivectomy using the internal beveled incision approach for patient featured in (A). (D) Postoperative healing two weeks postgingivectomy in patient shown in (B).

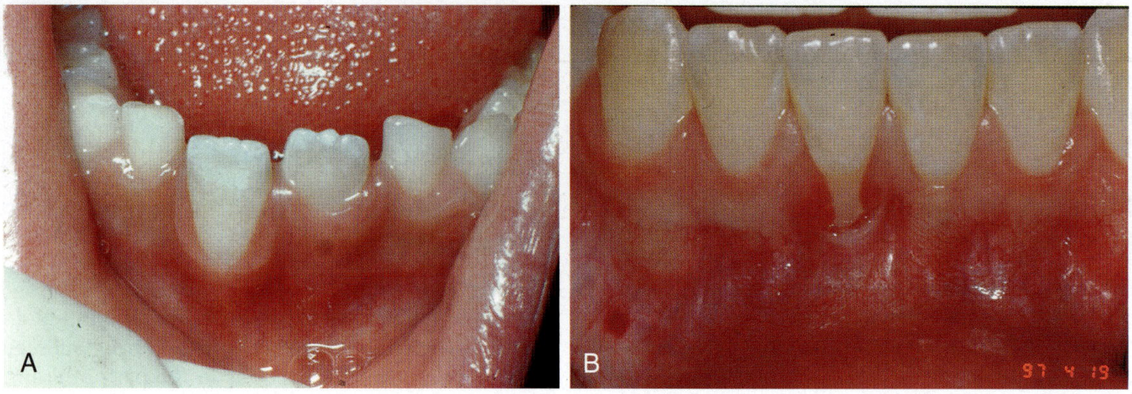

• **Fig. 21.6** (A) A reduction in the width of gingiva resulting from labial eruption of the mandibular right central incisor. In the absence of root exposure, this pseudorecession does not require periodontal intervention. (B) Localized recession occurring on the mandibular right central incisor as a result of inadequate attached gingiva.

produce a small increase in attached gingiva and place the tooth in a periodontally more stable position. Consequently, surgical treatment is often postponed until after orthodontic treatment.

Frena

Periodontal examination of the pediatric patient should include evaluation of the frena. These are mucosal folds with enclosed fibrous connective tissue containing elastic and muscle fibers that serve as attachments for the lips and tongue to the immobile tissue of the mandible and premaxilla. The three primary frena are the maxillary labial, mandibular labial, and lingual frena. Aberrant frena can be related to various problems at different stages of growth and development. Several craniofacial anomalies can also be associated with abnormal frenal attachments. Tethered oral tissues, their effect on oral motor function and management, and special considerations for craniofacial conditions are covered elsewhere in this textbook (see Chapter 48).

Maxillary Frenum

A prominent maxillary frenum, often extending to the incisive papilla and accompanied by a large midline diastema, is a common finding in children (Fig. 21.7). After closure of the diastema a frenum that penetrates the papilla may result in a gingival gap or "black triangle." Prominent frena are often a cause for concern by parents and healthcare providers. In general, surgical treatment of this condition should be delayed until the maxillary canines have fully erupted because they will often cause spontaneous closure of the diastema. If orthodontic therapy is necessary, consideration for surgery can usually be delayed until the completion of active treatment and is only necessary if the diastema presents an esthetic or functional problem at that time. Treatment has traditionally consisted of a Z-plasty procedure that allows removal of fibrous tissue in the bony cleft, but lasers are increasingly used to provide this treatment.

A restrictive maxillary frenum has also been implicated in difficulties with breastfeeding and bottle-feeding in nursing infants,[9] although this relationship remains unclear. As suboptimal breastfeeding/latching is a multifaceted complex issue, a team-based approach is recommended for management, including consultation with other healthcare professionals.[10] See Chapter 48 for an in-depth review of this topic.

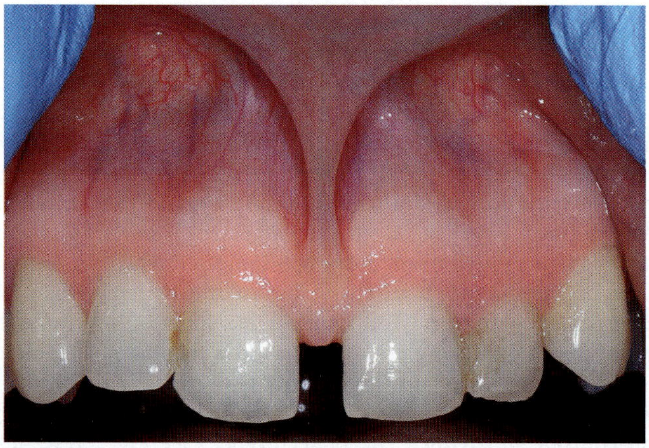

• **Fig. 21.7** Prominent maxillary labial frenum extending to the interdental papilla accompanied by a midline diastema.

Mandibular Labial Frenum

The mandibular labial frenum should normally attach between the mandibular central incisors and apical to the attached gingiva. A frenum with an aberrant attachment near the free gingival margin may be associated with gingival recession. In these cases, treatment is directed at the reconstruction of the attached gingiva and not at the frenum per se. Treatment options consist of periodontal plastic surgery, such as a free gingival graft with vestibular extension or a connective tissue graft. The frenum is relocated to a more apical position as a consequence of the grafting procedure. This is very effective at providing root coverage and gingival stability, in addition to preventing reattachment of the frenum to the free gingival margin.

Lingual Frenum

A restrictive lingual frenum ("tongue tie") is often seen in children (Fig. 21.8). In approximately 3% of children, the attachment may limit normal tongue mobility (ankyloglossia), which can lead to discomfort or difficulties while nursing and can also affect the development of speech. Although some studies have shown marked improvement in speech and language assessment in children who were treated for ankyloglossia and had preexisting speech difficulties,[11] there are insufficient data that correlate

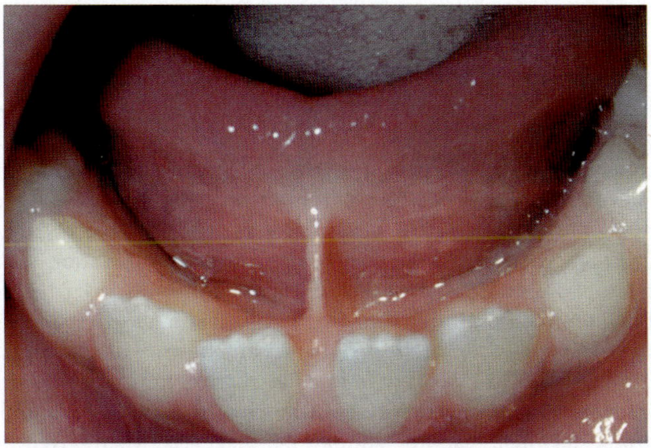

• **Fig. 21.8** Restrictive lingual frenum in a child. Note the relationship of the frenum to the tip of the tongue and the lingual gingiva of the central incisors.

ankyloglossia and speech disorders. Consultation with a speech pathologist is recommended if problems are suspected. Occasionally, the restrictive lingual frenum may affect the lingual gingiva. Treatment generally consists of a simple frenotomy, which can be performed with scissors or with lasers. See Chapter 48 for more information on this topic.

Periodontitis

Most individuals eventually experience loss of periodontal attachment, with both the number and severity of affected sites increasing with age. It usually accumulates so slowly that measurable attachment loss is not present before adulthood. However, approximately 20% of 14- to 17-year-olds in the United States were found to have attachment loss of at least 2 mm at one or more sites,[12,13] demonstrating that for some individuals periodontitis begins in adolescence. This early-stage, low-grade periodontitis responds well to oral hygiene measures and can be arrested when attachment loss is minimal and deep pockets have not developed.

Smoking is a major risk factor for periodontitis. The use of e-cigarettes is increasing faster in younger age groups than use of traditional cigarettes, and e-cigarettes are currently the most used tobacco product among middle- and high-school students.[14] The misconception that e-cigarettes are a harmless alternative to smoking is common, but studies have demonstrated a causal link to periodontal destruction.[15] With the recent legalization of marijuana in many states, the availability to children and adolescents has increased. The frequent use of cannabis is associated with deeper periodontal probing depths, more clinical attachment loss, and increased risk of developing severe periodontitis.[16,17] Smoking crack cocaine and other illicit drugs is also linked to periodontal destruction.[18]

Current and past smoking status should be determined as part of a periodontal assessment for young patients, including detailed questioning about nontraditional smoking and other tobacco use. Appropriate anticipatory guidance and cessation counseling and/or referrals should be provided.

Grade C Periodontitis

Rare, rapidly progressing, high-grade forms of periodontitis also affect children and adolescents who are otherwise healthy. Now categorized as grade C periodontitis,[1] this form of aggressive periodontitis has localized and generalized forms and can occur in the permanent or the primary dentition.

Generalized Grade C Periodontitis

Grade C generalized pattern periodontitis sometimes occurs in adolescents and teenagers. In young adults the same disease was formerly called *rapidly progressive periodontitis.*[19] This generalized pattern may affect the entire dentition and is not self-limiting. Heavy accumulations of plaque and calculus are found in generalized pattern periodontitis, and inflammation may be severe. Unlike molar-incisor pattern periodontitis, discussed later, generalized pattern periodontitis is not associated with high levels of *Aggregatibacter actinomycetemcomitans;* instead it has a microbiologic profile closer to that of adult disease. It should be managed aggressively with local therapy and systemic antibiotics.

Molar-Incisor Pattern Periodontitis in the Permanent Dentition

Molar-incisor pattern periodontitis, formerly called *localized aggressive periodontitis,* is characterized by the loss of attachment and bone around the permanent incisors and first permanent molars. The radiographic appearance is distinctive (Fig. 21.9). The attachment

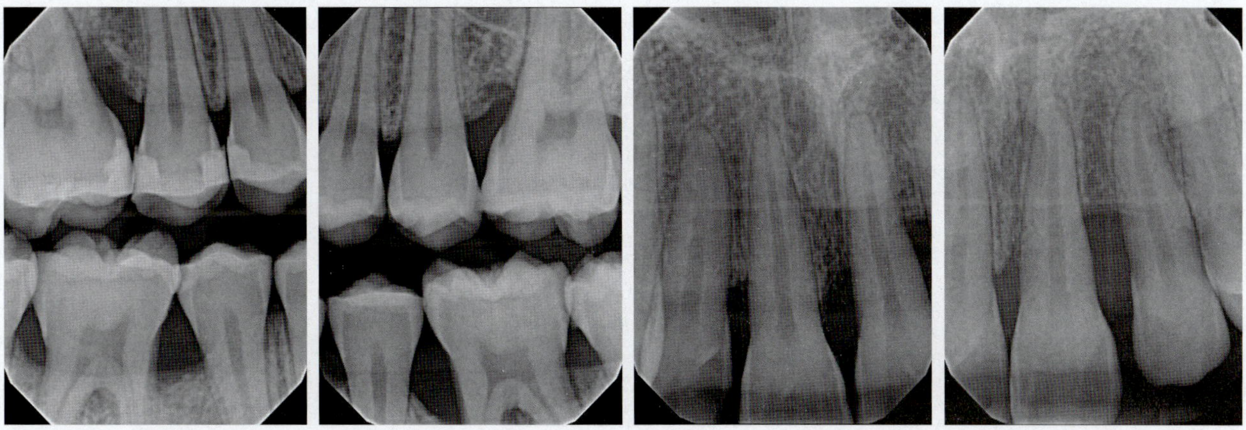

• **Fig. 21.9** Radiographic appearance of molar-incisor pattern periodontitis in the permanent dentition showing the typical bone loss pattern around first molars and central incisors.

loss is rapid, occurring at three times the rate of chronic disease. Inflammation in molar-incisor pattern periodontitis is not as extreme as that occurring in periodontitis associated with systemic disease such as neutropenia, but both inflammation and plaque accumulation are often greater than those found in the typical teenager. The disease is usually detected in early adolescence but may begin in the primary dentition (discussed later). The prevalence of molar-incisor pattern periodontitis is estimated to be approximately 1%, and in the United States it most commonly occurs in the African American population.

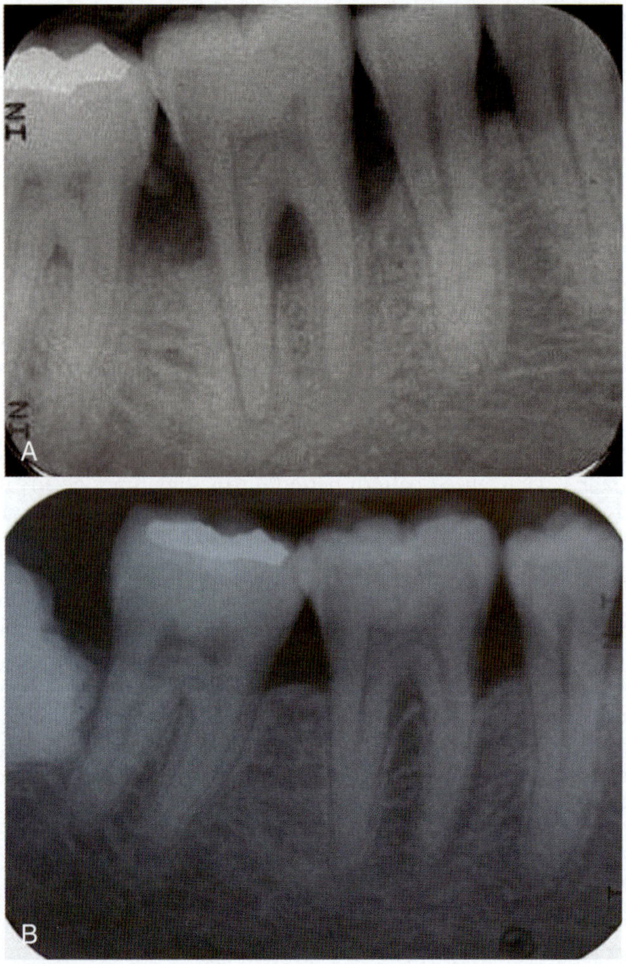

• **Fig. 21.10** (A) Radiographic calculus and localized bone loss around first molar in patient with molar-incisor pattern periodontitis. (B) One year follow-up. Radiographic evidence of spontaneous regeneration around the first molar after disease control phase.

Possible host genetic factors have been linked to molar-incisor pattern periodontitis. It is most clearly linked to the presence of high numbers of *A. actinomycetemcomitans,* and successful treatment outcomes correlate well with eradication of the bacteria. Treatment consists of local debridement in combination with systemic antibiotic therapy and clinical monitoring. Metronidazole alone or in combination with amoxicillin or azithromycin have been shown to be effective in arresting disease progression.[20] Although azithromycin is a safe alternative for patients with penicillin allergy and it may even be preferred due to its simple dosing regimen, caution should be practiced when given to patients with cardiac risk factors. After disease control phase, spontaneous regeneration may occur (Fig. 21.10), but localized surgical intervention may be necessary in some cases to manage any residual defects.

Primary Molar Pattern Periodontitis

Primary molar pattern periodontitis, formerly known as *localized prepubertal periodontitis,* is characterized by localized loss of attachment in the primary dentition. It occurs in children without evidence of systemic disease. The disease most commonly manifests in the molar area, where localized, usually bilaterally symmetrical loss of attachment occurs, with distance from the CEJ to crestal bone greater than 2 mm and frequent furcal involvement (Fig. 21.11). If bone loss without inflammation occurs in the primary incisors, hypophosphatasia should be suspected (see Chapters 20 and 37 for more information). In the United States primary molar pattern periodontitis occurs most commonly in the African American population. It is usually accompanied by mild to moderate inflammation, and heavier than average plaque deposits may be visible. It is commonly first diagnosed during the late primary dentition or early transitional dentition. Primary molar pattern periodontitis may progress to molar-incisor pattern periodontitis in the permanent dentition and may be an age-specific manifestation of the same disease.

Primary molar pattern periodontitis is less well studied than the molar-incisor pattern, but is associated with known periodontal pathogens, usually *A. actinomycetemcomitans,* and possibly with specific, minor host immunologic deficits. The same regimen used for management of molar-incisor pattern periodontitis, antibiotic

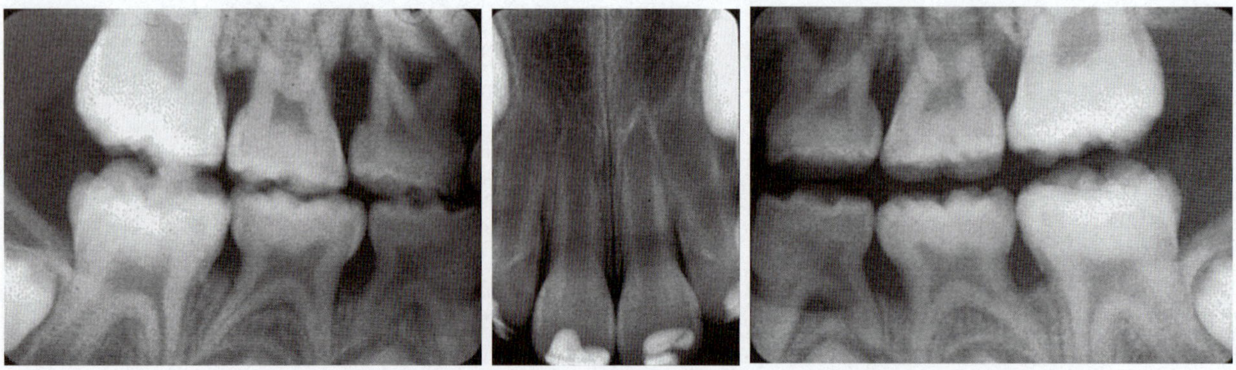

• **Fig. 21.11** Radiographic appearance of primary molar pattern periodontitis showing the characteristic loss of bone around the primary molars. Note adequate bone levels around the maxillary incisors.

therapy combined with local debridement, is recommended and appears to be effective. Tetracyclines are contraindicated due to the potential for staining permanent teeth.

Necrotizing Ulcerative Gingivitis/Periodontitis

Necrotizing ulcerative gingivitis/periodontitis is characterized by the rapid onset of painful gingivitis with interproximal and marginal necrosis and ulceration. The incidence peaks in the late teens and early twenties in North America and Europe, but in less developed countries it is common in young children. Malnutrition, viral infections (especially primary herpetic gingivostomatitis), stress, lack of sleep, and smoking have been reported as predisposing factors. Necrotizing ulcerative gingivitis/periodontitis is associated with high levels of spirochetes and *Prevotella intermedia.* Local debridement usually produces rapid resolution of the disease, but antibiotic therapy with penicillin or metronidazole may be indicated in patients with elevated body temperature and/or lymphadenopathy.

Systemic Diseases and Conditions With Associated Periodontal Problems

Early loss of periodontal attachment in children is often a sign of systemic disease. Periodontitis may occur in the presence of defects in the immune system that result in susceptibility to infection such as leukocyte adhesion deficiency (LAD) or neutropenia, secondary to metabolic disorders such as diabetes, or from the invasion of neoplastic cells as in leukemia.

Diabetes

An increased risk and earlier onset of periodontitis occur in both insulin-dependent and non–insulin-dependent diabetes mellitus.[21] As many as 10% to 15% of teenagers with insulin-dependent diabetes mellitus have significant periodontal disease. Poor metabolic control increases the risk of periodontitis, and untreated periodontitis in turn worsens metabolic control of diabetes. Effective preventive regimens and early diagnosis and treatment of periodontitis are important for the overall health of patients with diabetes.

Down Syndrome

Down syndrome is accompanied by an increased susceptibility to periodontitis. Most Down syndrome patients develop periodontitis by 30 years of age, and it may first occur in the primary dentition.[22] Plaque levels are high in these patients, but the severity of periodontal destruction exceeds that attributable to local factors alone. Minor immune deficits in patients with Down syndrome may be responsible for the increased susceptibility to periodontitis. Severe recession in the mandibular anterior region associated with a coronally positioned labial frenum attachment is also common in Down syndrome.

Leukocyte Adhesion Deficiency

LAD, also called generalized prepubertal periodontitis,[23] is a rare, autosomal recessive immunodeficiency disorder characterized by neutrophil migration defects to infection sites, resulting in increased susceptibility to bacterial infections including periodontitis. Because of the high incidence of skin abscesses, recurrent otitis media, pneumonitis, and other bacterial infections of soft tissues, a diagnosis is usually made before any oral manifestations. Dental symptoms such as generalized rapid bone loss, marked inflammation, tooth mobility, and premature tooth loss are manifested early in the primary dentition. Scrupulous oral hygiene measures are necessary to control the periodontitis associated with LAD.

Neutropenia

Neutropenia is a hematologic disorder characterized by reduced numbers of neutrophils from the blood and bone marrow. There are various types of neutropenia, including acquired (secondary to chemotherapy) or congenital (immune disorders) forms. In addition to increased susceptibility to recurrent infections such as otitis media or respiratory and skin infections, patients with neutropenia generally suffer from severe gingivitis and pronounced alveolar bone loss. Periodontal therapy consists of rigorous local measures to control plaque, but patients are seldom able to maintain the level of oral hygiene necessary to prevent the development and progression of periodontal disease.

Papillon-Lefèvre Syndrome

Papillon-Lefèvre syndrome (PLS) is an autosomal recessive disorder that is caused by loss-of-function mutations in the cathepsin C gene that result in impaired neutrophil function. PLS is characterized by rapidly progressing periodontal manifestations in the primary or transitional dentition, leading to premature tooth loss (Fig. 21.12). Loss of primary teeth usually occurs by 3 to 5 years of age and loss of permanent teeth is seen a few years after eruption. Gingival tissue health typically returns after tooth loss. Hyperkeratosis of the palms and soles will be evident upon clinical examination. Both neutrophil defects and microbiologic factors appear to play a role in the severity of PLS. Therapy consists of aggressive local measures to control plaque formation including frequent scaling and root planing. Successful treatment outcomes in children have been reported with antibiotic therapy.[24,25]

Histiocytosis

Langerhans cell histiocytosis (LCH), previously known as histiocytosis X, is a rare disorder of childhood that presents with histiocytic infiltration of bones, skin, liver, and other organs. In 20% to 30% of cases, the initial infiltrates occur in the oral cavity, usually in the mandible.[26] Typical findings include gingival enlargement; ulcerations; mobility of teeth with alveolar expansion; and discrete, destructive lesions of bone with the appearance of "floating teeth," which can be observed on radiographs and may be confused with periodontitis. LCH may be diagnosed by biopsy. Therapy consists of local measures such as radiation and surgery to remove lesions and systemic chemotherapy or gene inhibitor therapy for disseminated disease. The lesions of LCH and the local therapy used to treat them may result in loss of teeth or arrested development of teeth. Survival rates are generally high with treatment.

Leukemia

Leukemias are the most common form of childhood cancer. Acute lymphoblastic leukemia (ALL) is the most common and has the best prognosis. Acute myeloid leukemia (AML) accounts for

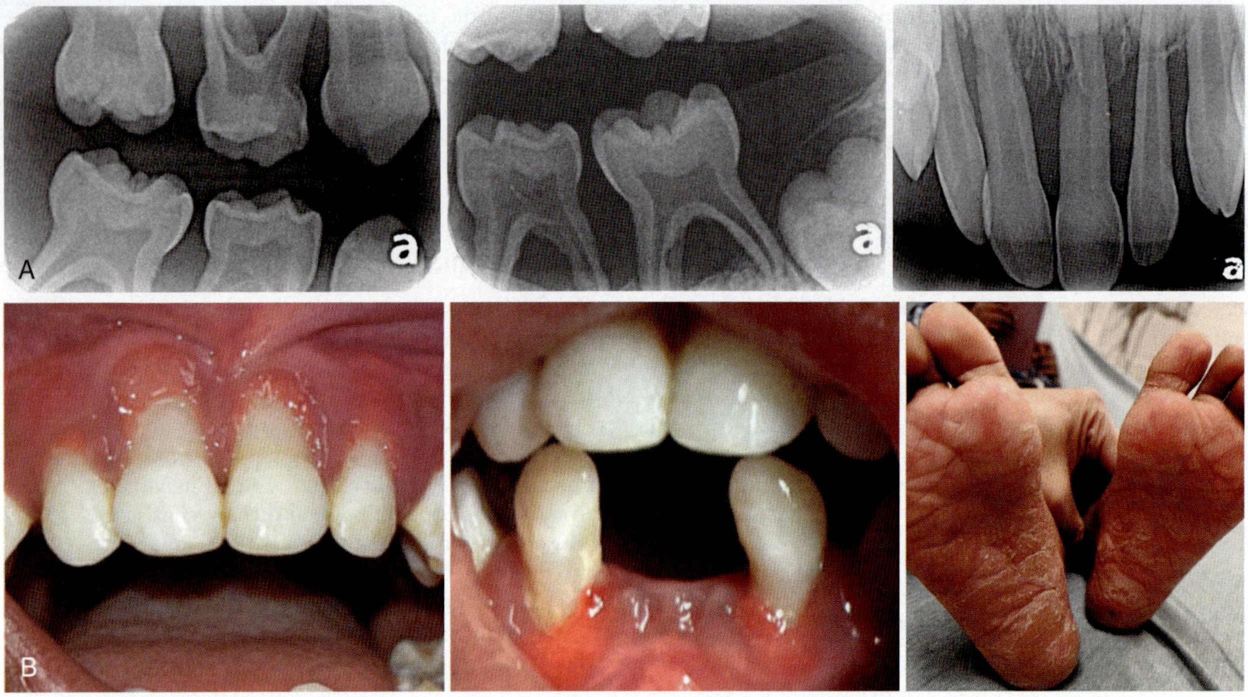

• **Fig. 21.12** (A) Radiographic appearance of grade C generalized pattern periodontitis in a 3-year-old patient with Papillon-Lefèvre syndrome (PLS). (B) Corresponding clinical presentation. Note marked gingival inflammation and recession around the anterior teeth with early loss of mandibular central incisors due to PLS. Hyperkeratosis of the soles is also seen.

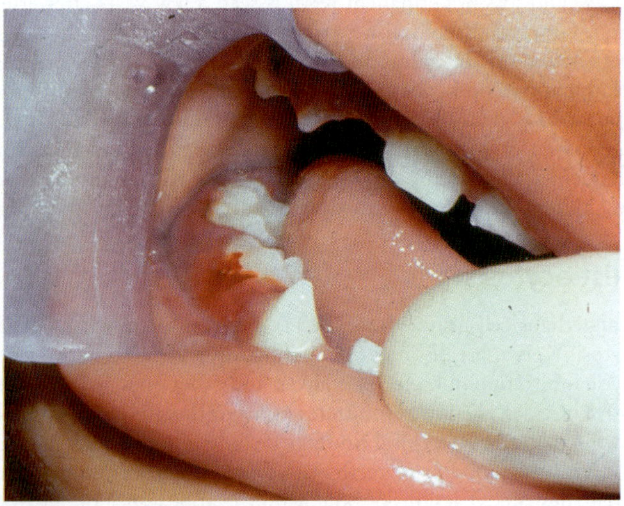

• **Fig. 21.13** Gingival leukemic infiltration in a child with acute myeloid leukemia.

approximately 20% of childhood leukemias and has a poorer long-term survival rate. AML may present with erythematous gingival enlargements caused by infiltrates of leukemic cells (Fig. 21.13) that may sometimes invade bone. This presentation usually does not occur with ALL. In addition to the gingival lesions, the patient may have fever, malaise, gingival or other bleeding, and bone or joint pain. AML may be diagnosed by a complete blood cell count. Anemia, abnormal leukocyte and differential counts, and thrombocytopenia are usually observed (see Chapter 39).

Periodontal Examination of Children

The periodontal health of children and adolescents should be assessed at each examination. The gingival tissues should be examined for redness, edema, bleeding, or enlargement. Oral hygiene may be assessed via a plaque index. Use of a disclosant provides an excellent oral hygiene instruction tool, and a plaque index provides a method for monitoring and documenting oral hygiene practices. Calculus is not as common in young patients as it is in adults, but it is found in approximately 10% of children and one-third of teenagers. Patients of all ages should always be checked for calculus during periodic examinations, and deposits, when noted, should be removed.

Particularly after the eruption of permanent teeth, attachment levels should be determined by periodontal probing. Probing of the permanent incisors and first permanent molars provides a diagnostic screening for molar-incisor pattern periodontitis. Because erupting teeth can be probed all the way to the CEJ, transient deep pockets are a normal finding in the transitional dentition and must be distinguished from true attachment loss by locating the CEJ.

When radiographs are available, bone levels should be examined. Normal crestal height should be within 1 to 2 mm of the CEJ.[27] After permanent teeth have erupted, the patient should also be examined for deficiencies in the width of attached gingiva and areas of recession should be noted.

Visit eBooks.Health.Elsevier.com to see full list of references.

22

Space Maintenance in the Primary and Mixed Dentition

CLARICE LAW EYRE

CHAPTER OUTLINE

General Considerations

The "Best Practices" recommendations of the American Academy of Pediatric Dentistry state that "management of developing dentition and occlusion is an essential part of comprehensive oral health care and that early diagnosis and treatment of abnormalities can aid patients in achieving the goal of a stable, functional, and esthetic occlusion."[1] Premature loss of primary teeth can occur for a variety of reasons, including dental caries, congenital disorders, ectopic eruption of adjacent permanent teeth, and trauma.[2] Premature loss can result in a reduction in the overall space available for the permanent teeth, with malocclusion and orthodontic treatment need as a potential outcome.[2] Thus it is important for the oral health provider to understand the consequences of premature tooth loss for each tooth type, along with the options for managing space in the primary and mixed dentition. Appropriate space management can reduce any harmful effects to the development of the dentition and occlusion during the transition from primary to the permanent dentition.

Reasons for premature tooth loss can be distinguished between those that occur with anterior teeth (incisors and canines) and those with posterior teeth (molars). Anterior tooth loss most frequently occurs as a result of trauma and tooth decay. Toddlers and young children are still developing gross motor skills, so injuries to the primary incisors are common. And despite efforts at promoting preventive care, approximately 23% of US children ages 2 to 5 still suffer from early childhood caries.[3,4] When dental caries results in tooth loss, it can affect multiple teeth, both anterior and posterior, unlike traumatic dental injuries, which may be isolated to the incisors. Premature loss of the primary molars is most frequently caused by dental caries; rarely are primary molars lost to trauma. Ectopic eruption of adjacent teeth is another reason for premature tooth loss. Primary canines often exfoliate prematurely when a crowded incisor segment results in resorption of the canine root by the eruption of the lateral incisor. Primary second molars may be lost due to ectopic eruption of permanent molars.

The key clinical decision in management of premature loss is whether to perform active surveillance, space maintenance, or space regaining. Active surveillance might be appropriate if the permanent successor is expected to erupt before space loss would likely occur or if minimal to no space loss is anticipated to occur. Space maintenance is appropriate if a delay is expected before eruption of the permanent successor and if no space loss has occurred. If space loss has occurred, a comprehensive evaluation should be performed to determine whether space regaining or limited orthodontic treatment is indicated. Overall, the provider must distinguish from localized space loss, which might affect the eruption path or alignment of the successor tooth and adjacent teeth, and loss of arch perimeter, with downstream effects on molar relationship and crowding. Diagnosis and treatment planning of crowding and space loss are addressed in the discussions on orthodontic treatment in the primary and permanent dentition (see Chapters 24 and 25).

Loss of Primary Incisors

There are four basic considerations after premature loss of primary incisors: space maintenance, function, speech, and psychosocial. In terms of the need for space maintenance, most studies address the outcomes of premature loss of maxillary incisors caused by trauma or dental caries.[5] When mandibular incisors are lost, it is most frequently a central incisor, extracted as underdeveloped natal teeth or lost due to trauma, and less frequently studied when lost because of caries.[5] The literature lacks a sufficient number of studies to support a meta-analysis determining the effect of premature loss of maxillary incisors on the dental arch. There is low-quality evidence that early removal of a primary incisor will not result in space loss in most situations.

Dental arch perimeter generally does not show significant decrease after extraction of primary incisors.[6,7] However, in cases where one or more incisors are lost before eruption of primary canines or in cases with minimal interdental spacing, there may be loss of anterior space.[5] A general consensus is that there may be some redistribution of space between the remaining incisors, but there is usually no net loss of space, especially when developmental spacing is present in the primary dentition. Thus the decision to place a space maintainer based on potential space loss in the incisor region is controversial.

Aside from space maintenance, when primary incisors are lost early, the developmental effects on the permanent successors must be considered. Whether lost due to trauma or infection, there is the possibility of developmental defects to the crown of the successor.[6] When a primary incisor is lost at an early age, eruption time of the permanent successor may be affected—usually delayed, sometimes accelerated. It may also erupt out of alignment.[6,8] There is anecdotal evidence that early loss of maxillary primary incisors may result in overeruption of mandibular incisors. With the palatal to buccal eruption path of maxillary incisors, there is the possibility that maxillary incisors will erupt into anterior crossbite. A space-maintaining appliance may reduce the risk of anterior crossbite in these situations. Thus developmental considerations can influence the decision to place a space maintainer to replace prematurely lost maxillary primary incisors, but these must be taken on a case-by-case basis.

Masticatory function is generally not a consideration in premature loss of primary incisors. Incisive function may be affected, particularly if all four maxillary incisors have been extracted, but children have shown excellent adaptive abilities with their eating abilities.[8]

Premature loss of maxillary primary incisors can sometimes increase the risk of speech distortion.[5,8] Sounds made against the incisors ("v," "f," "th," "z," and "s") may be affected, particularly if the child has not yet developed the ability to produce these sounds. Children who have already developed the ability to produce these sounds are usually able to adapt their speech production after tooth loss. Any decision to fabricate a space-maintaining appliance to improve speech should be made in conjunction with a speech pathologist after giving the child an opportunity to adapt.

A commonly overlooked consequence of premature loss of primary incisors is the potential development of an oral habit.[8] An atypical swallow or active tongue thrust has been observed in children with extraction of multiple incisors. Loss of dental arch integrity requires an adaptation in tongue position to achieve a seal for swallow. This is thought to be a transient change, likely to resolve when the permanent incisors erupt. However, there are no studies justifying placement of a space-maintaining appliance to address atypical swallow under these circumstances.

A final consideration in premature loss of primary incisors addresses esthetic concerns. Studies of oral health–related quality of life yield inconsistent findings regarding the psychosocial effect of premature incisor loss.[8,9] Even young children are aware of esthetics, but it is unclear how much influence parents have on a child's motivation to seek replacement of incisors. The decision to pursue placement of an appliance might be justified based on family preferences if the child's behavior allows the provider to construct and place the appliance. If parents do not indicate a desire to replace missing anterior teeth, no treatment is certainly appropriate.

Loss of Primary Canines

Isolated loss of a primary canine as a result of dental caries is rare. Dental disease severe enough to require extraction of primary canines usually results in multiple extractions, in which case the decision on space maintenance will be based on the pattern of primary molar loss, discussed later in this chapter. When unilateral or bilateral loss of primary canines occurs, it is most typically due to ectopic eruption of lateral incisors.[8] A crowded arch can redirect the eruption path of lateral incisors so that resorption of the adjacent primary canine roots and premature exfoliation occurs. Decrease in overall arch perimeter can sometimes occur, from the mesial of the permanent first molar around to the opposite molar.[10] If the loss is bilateral, a decrease in arch perimeter is more likely to occur, from lingual tipping of the incisors.[2,11] If loss of the primary canine is unilateral, there may be a shift of the midline toward the side with loss.[12] In summary, the decision to place a space maintainer in situations with premature canine loss along with multiple other teeth is influenced by pattern of primary molar loss. Otherwise, space maintenance for premature loss of one or more primary canines might be considered as management of crowding.

Loss of Primary Molars

In contrast with premature loss of primary incisors, function, speech, and psychosocial considerations are generally not an issue with loss of primary molars. Reducing the risk of malocclusion is the key priority. Systematic review on the effects of premature loss of primary molars on malocclusion demonstrates a strong justification to strategize for space management. The frequency of malocclusion increases from 80% without premature loss of molars to 90% with the loss of any primary molar. There is an increase in the percentage of permanent first molars in a class III relationship, from mesial drift in the mandible. And mesial drift of maxillary molars could certainly result in a class II molar relationship. Most significantly, there is an increased frequency of crowding.[2]

Premature loss of primary second molars consistently demonstrates an unfavorable effect on malocclusion.[13] The natural mesial drift that occurs with all teeth is unhindered by the absence of the primary second molar, resulting in mesial tipping and bodily movement of both the maxillary and mandibular permanent molars. The outcomes are worse if a primary second molar is extracted before the eruption of the permanent molar. Without a distal root surface to serve as a guide, permanent molars can erupt in a mesial position. Teeth that have translated forward like this are more difficult to move with orthodontic forces than teeth that have erupted according to typical developmental processes and then tipped mesially because of loss of a mesial contact tooth. A space maintainer is almost always indicated when a primary second molar is lost prematurely.[13] The only time one would not consider a space maintainer after loss of a primary second molar is if there is clear evidence of a missing permanent second premolar.

Outcomes of premature loss of primary first molars are somewhat more controversial. Conclusions vary depending on how the outcomes are measured in research studies. Most studies agree that there usually is space loss, from distal drift of canine[13,14] and mesial tipping of the primary second molar. Thus loss of space can occur from both directions (Fig. 22.1). This may result in misaligned incisors and a compromised eruption path for permanent

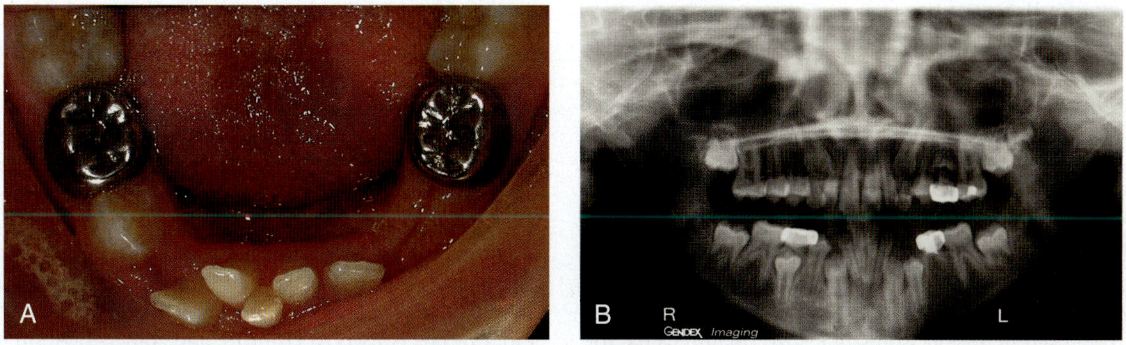

• **Fig. 22.1** Premature loss of the primary first molar can result in loss of space from both directions. (A) Arch perimeter has been lost mesial and distal to the primary first molars. (B) Panoramic radiograph shows the canine and two premolars attempting to erupt into the limited space on the patient's right. The left mandibular second premolar is missing.

canines. However, long-term follow-up suggests no loss in overall arch perimeter.[13,15] A consideration that is not clearly addressed by recent systematic reviews is the eruption status of the permanent first molars when the primary first molar is lost. Classic literature and textbooks suggest that as long as the permanent first molar is well interdigitated with the opposing molar, the risk of overall space loss is reduced.[16] It is proposed that the occlusion keeps the primary second molars and permanent molars from tipping or moving mesially. The one published long-term study of space loss suggests that space maintenance is not needed for premature loss of a maxillary primary molar.

Additional Considerations

The timing of space management is an important consideration in managing premature tooth loss. Most studies of space loss suggest that the greatest amount of space loss occurs within the first 4 months.[13] As a general principle to minimize space loss, a space maintainer should be placed within those first four months. However, developmental status plays into timing also. If a child has interdental spacing and is in the primary dentition before the start of the early mesial shift that occurs before the eruption of the permanent molars (around age 4), the dental arches might be stable enough to defer placement of a space maintainer for a period of time. But from the time of the early mesial shift until the permanent first molar erupts into occlusion, there is a higher probability of space loss from the mesial eruption path of both maxillary and mandibular molars. Space maintenance is very important during this time, particularly with loss of primary second molars and in the mandibular arch. The period after eruption of the permanent molars into occlusion is considered a more stable period, when active surveillance might be an appropriate alternative to placement of a space maintainer.

Developmental effects of tooth loss must also be considered. Teeth lost during the primary dentition years can cause later-than-normal eruption of the succedaneous teeth. This means that the appliances should be monitored, adjusted, and possibly replaced over a longer period of time. Abutment teeth for appliances may exfoliate or interfere with adjacent erupting teeth. Abutment teeth are also at greater risk of decay and decalcification because of plaque retention around the appliance. These aspects of care should be considered during treatment planning.

Overall, effective space management begins with good management of dental caries and restorative dentistry. The dentist should strive for ideal restoration of all interproximal contours because space loss can occur without even losing a primary tooth once an interproximal contact is compromised by cavitation.[17] Early restoration of interproximal caries ensures that no space loss occurs. However, in some instances, large carious lesions may make ideal restoration of the tooth impossible, and space loss is inevitable. Even if the pulpal tissues have been compromised, pulp therapy should be initiated and the tooth maintained, if at all possible, because the natural tooth is still superior to the best space maintainer available; it is functional, it is the correct size, and it exfoliates appropriately. Space loss can also occur when teeth adjacent to an ankylosed tooth continue to erupt and tip over the ankylosed molar because of the loss of a contact point. There are several options in these cases. The tooth can be maintained as is or restored into occlusion until space loss occurs, or it can be extracted and the space maintained.

Space-Maintaining Appliances

The *Code on Dental Procedures and Nomenclature (CDT) 2024* lists four categories for space maintenance appliances[18]: fixed unilateral, fixed bilateral, removable unilateral, and removable bilateral. There is no specificity for the stage of dentition during which these are used. Unilateral appliances are typically used to maintain space for a single missing tooth. Fixed unilateral appliances include the band and loop, crown and loop, and the distal shoe. Interestingly, the distal shoe has a code in the *CDT* distinct from the other fixed unilateral appliances, which all use the same code. Removable unilateral appliances are rarely mentioned in the literature and, if so, with cautions against use because of their small size. Bilateral appliances maintain space for two adjacent teeth or in cases where one or more teeth are missing in different quadrants within the same arch. The Nance appliance, transpalatal arch (TPA), and passive lingual arch or lower lingual holding arch are included as examples of fixed bilateral space maintainers. Removable bilateral appliances are more commonly used than unilateral designs, particularly in cases where multiple teeth have been lost prematurely. These generally consist of variations on the Hawley type retainer.

Fixed Unilateral Appliances

One of the most common appliances used for space maintenance is the band and loop. In the primary dentition, it is frequently used to maintain space for unilateral loss of the primary first molar before or after eruption of the permanent first molar (Fig. 22.2). It is also used for bilateral loss of primary molars before the eruption of the permanent incisors (Fig. 22.3). More discussion on this will take place in the subsequent section on fixed bilateral appliances. The band and loop appliance typically consists of a band that is cemented to the primary second molar with the loop contacting the distal surface of the primary canine. The appliance provides resistance to the pressure of the early mesial shift that occurs as the permanent first molar begins its eruption, as well as the distal drift of the adjacent canine. The band and loop can also be used in the mixed dentition to provide space maintenance for premature loss of a primary second molar but requires the permanent first molar be erupted sufficiently to fully seat a band. In some cases, a variation called the reverse band and loop can be used to hold the space of the missing primary second molar. The band is seated on the intact primary first molar with the loop extending distally to contact the mesial surface of the permanent molar. One caveat for the reverse band and loop is that the occlusal convergence of the crown of the primary first molar makes proper band fit difficult and can increase band fragility. In some cases, a primary first molar stainless steel crown can be cut into a band to make the fit easier and increase the strength of the band.

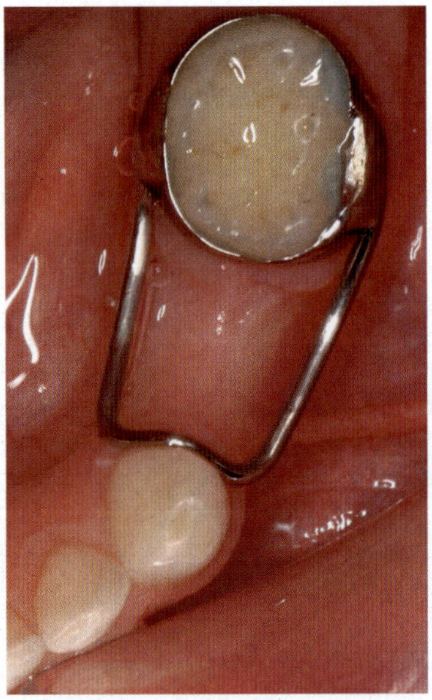

• **Fig. 22.2** The band and loop appliance is used to maintain the space after the premature loss of a single tooth. The traditional band and loop appliance is most frequently used with unilateral loss of a primary first molar before or after the eruption of the permanent first molar. The loop is constructed of .028″–.036″ round wire and is soldered to the band.

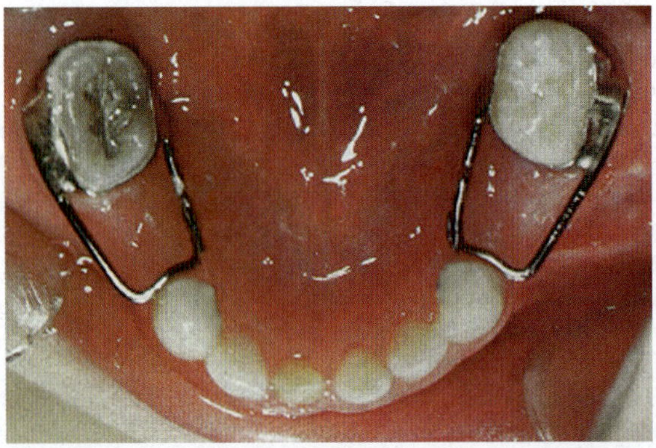

• **Fig. 22.3** If both primary first molars are lost prematurely in the mandibular arch and the permanent incisors have not erupted, bilateral band and loop appliances may be used to maintain space. A lingual arch is not indicated in this situation because it may interfere with the subsequent eruption of the permanent mandibular incisors.

The classic band and loop is a laboratory-fabricated appliance. The typical process involves the fitting of a band on the tooth that will serve as the abutment. An impression or digital scan is made, and a model is used to fabricate and solder the loop to the band. Disadvantages include the chair time to fit a band and the need to make an impression. An additional appointment to deliver the appliance is also necessary. Several years ago, companies began making prefabricated band and loop appliances of a wire and tube design. The most significant advantage is the possibility of same-day delivery. A disadvantage is that chairside placement might not yield as accurate a loop placement as a laboratory-fabricated version. Recent comparisons suggest no difference in longevity between conventional laboratory-fabricated band and loop and prefabricated tube and loop space maintainers.[19,20] More recently, there have been publications regarding three-dimensional printed band and loop appliances. This protocol improves accuracy and fit, and it also reduces chair time and visits.[21,22] Survivability is similar to a laboratory-fabricated band and loop.[23]

Another variation on the band and loop appliance is the crown and loop appliance. This design includes a loop directly attached to a crown and is used when the abutment tooth requires full coverage restoration. Before the development of prefabricated crown and loop kits, the laboratory-fabricated design was not recommended. The disadvantages of having a laboratory take the time to fabricate the appliance outweighed the advantages of having the loop securely fastened to the crown without an additional band around the crown. Care and maintenance of the crown and loop can be more difficult than for the band and loop if there is damage or if modifications are required. If the loop fails or requires adjustment, it is more difficult to adjust the appliance intraorally, as opposed to the band and loop, which can be removed.

The cantilever design of a band and loop indicates that the appliance should only replace a single tooth. Any span greater than a single tooth could result in interference or orthodontic tooth movement for the abutment tooth. Overall, the band and loop appliance is inexpensive and easy to fabricate. However, its use requires continuous supervision and care, and it does not restore the occlusal function of the missing tooth.

Another variation on the fixed unilateral appliance that must be mentioned is the distal shoe appliance. This is specifically used to maintain the space of a primary second molar that has been lost before the eruption of the permanent first molar (Fig. 22.4). An unerupted permanent first molar can drift mesially within the alveolar bone if the primary second molar is lost prematurely. The result of the mesial drift is loss of arch length and possible impaction of the second premolar. The distal shoe appliance has traditionally been controversial in use. Histologic examination shows that complete epithelialization does not occur after placement of the appliance.[24] Because the epithelium is not intact, the distal shoe appliance is contraindicated in immunocompromised patients and patients at risk for infective endocarditis.

The distal shoe can have modifications. It can be fabricated with the crown and distal shoe modification. Although feasible, like the crown and loop, it is difficult to modify and repair.

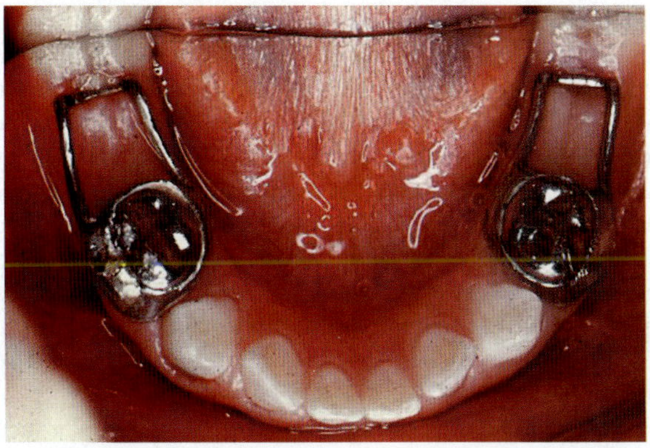

• **Fig. 22.4** The distal shoe appliance is used to maintain the space of a primary second molar that has been lost prematurely before the eruption of the permanent first molar. A stainless steel extension is soldered to the distal end of the band and loop; this extension is positioned 1 mm below the mesial marginal ridge of the unerupted permanent first molar. The extension serves to guide the eruption of the permanent first molar.

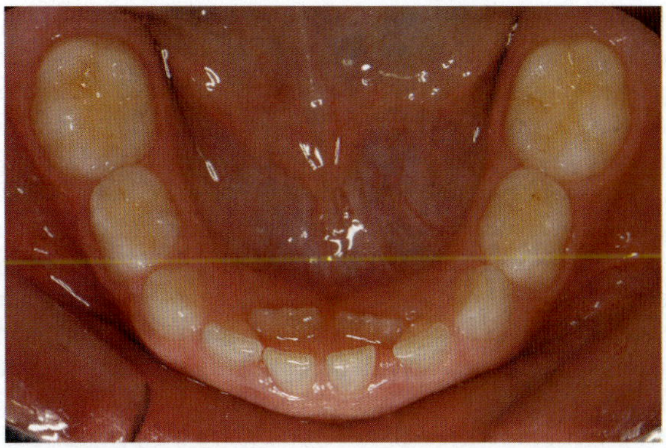

• **Fig. 22.5** The eruption path of the permanent mandibular incisors typically proceeds from lingual to labial. A mandibular lingual arch is not recommended as a space maintainer in the primary dentition because it may interfere with the eruption of these incisors. Bilateral band and loop appliances are recommended when both primary mandibular first molars are lost prematurely.

The reverse band and loop described previously can be used as a substitute for the distal shoe, with the appliance designed so that the wire of the loop rests on the soft tissue (sometimes with mild pressure) approximately where the distal surface of the lost primary second molar was located. And the reverse band and loop configuration can be fabricated with additional supragingival loop to serve as a "distal guide."[25] To date, there are several case reports but no clinical trials to support these modifications. Overall, the goal of any variation of the distal shoe is to minimize mesial movement of the unerupted permanent first molar.

A final appliance that should be mentioned for premature loss of a single primary molar is the fiber-reinforced composite space maintainer. This consists of a ribbon or strip of silanated glass fibers bonded in position between two abutment teeth with composite resin. This particular appliance has been discussed in the European dental journals for many years but has not seemed to gain wide acceptance in the United States. Advantages include chairside placement, a less bulky size, and higher esthetic values. Because this appliance is small and depends on an adhesive bond with enamel, there have been concerns about bond failure and ingestion or aspiration. Studies of longevity suggest that the fiber-reinforced composite space maintainer has fewer failures than band and loop at 6 months, but more failures at 12 months.[26] This type of space maintainer may be considered if there is only a short-term expected need for space maintenance.

Fixed Bilateral Appliances

The second category of appliances used to maintain posterior space in the primary and mixed dentition consists of fixed bilateral appliances. These appliances are indicated when teeth are lost in both quadrants of the same arch or multiple teeth have been lost within a quadrant.

The lower lingual holding arch is commonly used in the mandibular arch during the mixed dentition period. Because the permanent incisor tooth buds develop and erupt lingual to their primary precursors in the lower arch, a mandibular lingual arch is not recommended in the primary dentition; the wire resting adjacent to the primary incisors might interfere with the eruption of the permanent incisors (Fig. 22.5). Instead, two band and loop appliances are recommended when there is bilateral tooth loss in the mandibular arch. When the permanent molars and incisors erupt, a lower lingual holding arch can be considered as a replacement for the band and loop appliances.

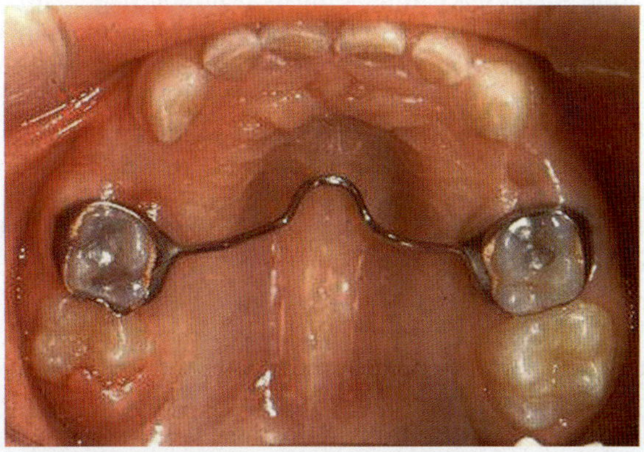

• **Fig. 22.6** The transpalatal arch (TPA) is a fixed lingual arch appliance used to maintain space after bilateral loss of maxillary teeth. The TPA is more hygienic than the Nance appliance because it consists of only the .036″ palatal wire, but it can allow the abutment teeth to tip mesially in some cases, resulting in space loss.

The two most common maxillary fixed bilateral appliance designs are the Nance arch and TPA. These appliances use a large wire (0.036 inches) to connect banded molars on both sides of the arch distal to the extraction site. Bands are more commonly placed on permanent molars, because the arch perimeter loss from mesial movement of these teeth have more direct long-term consequences on crowding of the permanent dentition than mesial movement of primary second molars. Fixed bilateral appliances may be placed on primary second molars, but replacement appliances often need to be considered once the permanent molars erupt. The difference between the two appliances is where the wire is placed in the palate. The Nance arch incorporates an acrylic button that rests directly behind the palatal rugae. The TPA is made from a wire that traverses the palate directly without touching it (Fig. 22.6). In distinguishing between the two appliances, the TPA is a cleaner appliance and is easier to construct. It has the advantage of being able to generate minor orthodontic tooth movement. The acrylic button of the Nance tends to trap food and plaque and may irritate the palatal tissue. However, comparative studies suggest that the TPA allows more mesial molar movement, resulting in space loss.[27] The Nance is considered to be more effective at maintaining space.

Fixed bilateral appliances can also be options for children who have had incisors extracted (Fig. 22.7). Prosthetic primary teeth can be affixed to a lingual arch extending from banded molars to serve as replacements for the missing incisors. These appliances, often called Groper fixed anterior bridges or pediatric partials, generally address esthetics but can serve functional purposes if posterior teeth have been extracted. Because the permanent incisors erupt much sooner than canines and premolars, appliances serving dual functions as esthetic incisor replacements and posterior space maintainers will require alternate options in the mixed dentition.

Removable Appliances

Removable appliances make up the third category of appliances used to maintain space in the primary dentition (Fig. 22.8). Like fixed bilateral appliances, removable appliances are typically used when more than one tooth has been lost in a quadrant. The removable appliance is often the only alternative because there are no suitable abutment teeth and because the cantilever design of the distal shoe or the band and loop appliance is too weak to withstand occlusal forces over a two-tooth span. Removable appliances can also be an alternative to fixed bilateral appliances for the replacement of missing incisors. Not only can the partial denture replace more than one tooth, but it also replaces occlusal function.

Two drawbacks of removal appliances are retention and compliance. Retention is a problem because primary canines do not have large undercuts for clasp engagement. If multiple tooth loss is unilateral, retention problems can be overcome by placing sturdy retention clasps on the opposite side of the arch. However, if multiple teeth are lost bilaterally, retention problems are almost inevitable.

The problem of compliance is closely related to that of retention. Children aged 3 to 6 years will not tolerate an ill-fitting appliance and may not use it. In fact, some children will not tolerate a removable appliance at all. The dentist is then resigned to waiting until the permanent teeth (molars) erupt so that they can be used as abutments for a conventional lingual arch appliance. Partial dentures occasionally require clasp adjustment and acrylic modification to maintain good retention and allow eruption of the underlying or adjacent permanent teeth. Some children are compliant in wearing an appliance but not in cleaning the appliance and the underlying tissue. This can result in decay, tissue irritation, and hyperplasia.

A recent study compared short-term effectiveness of a vacuum-formed space maintainer for a group of children in the mixed dentition.[28] There was no difference in effectiveness between the thermoplastic appliance and a fixed space maintainer at six months. These are promising results that may indicate potential success. With the recognition of clear aligners as an increasingly popular alternative to fixed orthodontic appliances for early orthodontic treatment, the vacuum-formed space maintainer might be a viable solution.

Fabrication and Laboratory Considerations

The classic method of constructing a fixed appliance is a two- or three-visit process. If there is tight interproximal contact of the molars, the first visit is to place separators. If there is interdental spacing or a light contact, a visit to place a separator may be skipped. The initial step in constructing a fixed appliance is to select and fit a band on the abutment tooth or teeth (Fig. 22.9). The next step is to obtain an impression or scan of the banded tooth and edentulous area. Alginate impression material is most commonly used. A quarter-arch tray may be used for the unilateral appliances. The next step varies, depending on the office or laboratory preference. The band(s) is removed from the tooth with a band remover and stabilized in the impression. The impression is poured in stone with the band(s) in place. An alternative approach is to pour the dental casts without the band(s) in place and send the appropriately sized band(s) to the laboratory to be seated by the technician during appliance fabrication. Other offices obtain only impressions and ask the laboratory to fit bands

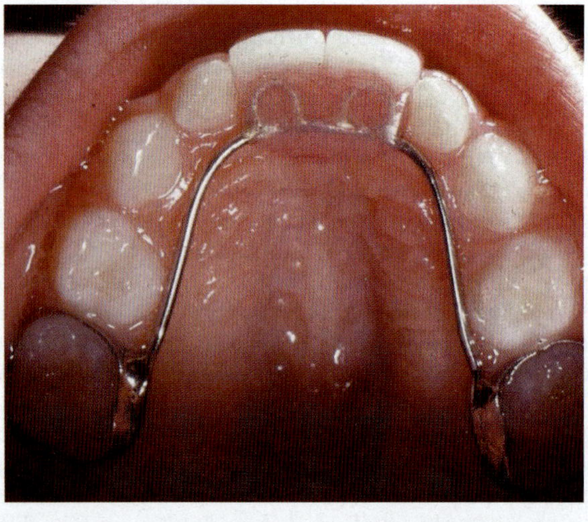

• **Fig. 22.7** A fixed (as shown here) or removable appliance can be used to replace missing anterior teeth in the primary dentition. In most cases the appliance is placed for esthetic reasons rather than to prevent space loss in the anterior dental arch.

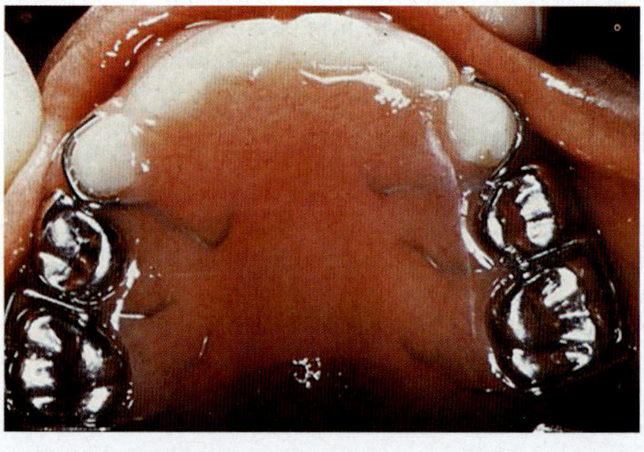

• **Fig. 22.8** A removable partial denture is used to maintain space in the primary dentition when more than one tooth in a quadrant is lost. This appliance is an alternative to the lingual arch with teeth attached. In the patient portrayed here, only anterior teeth have been replaced.

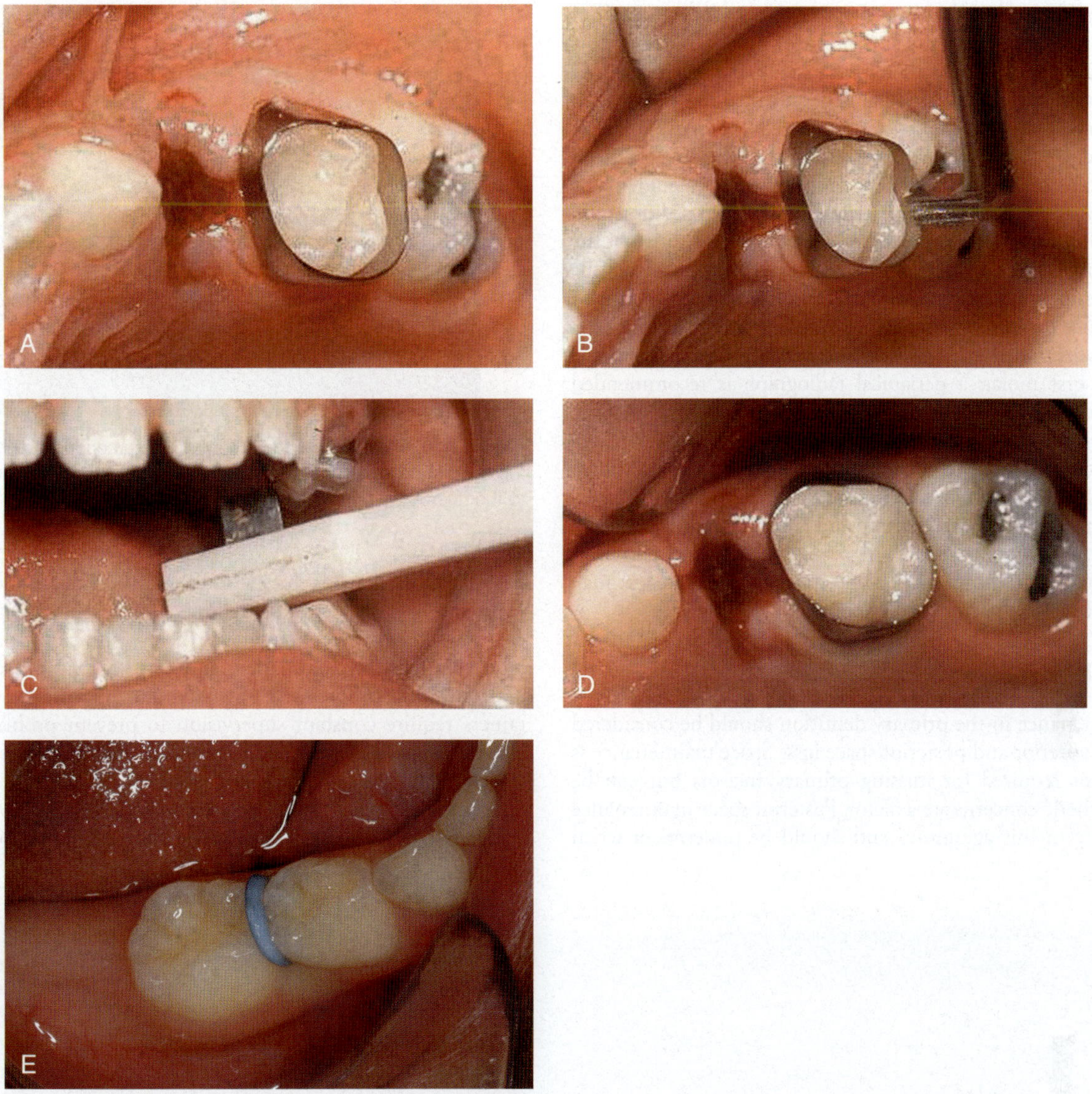

• **Fig. 22.9** (A) The initial step in making a laboratory-fabricated band and loop device is to fit a band on the abutment tooth. Band selection is a trial-and-error procedure and continues until a band can be nearly seated on the tooth with finger pressure. (B) A band pusher may be used to seat the band to a nearly ideal position. The dentist should maintain a good finger rest because soft and hard tissue injury can occur if the pusher slips without proper support. (C) Final occlusogingival position is achieved with a bite stick. In the maxillary arch the bite stick should be placed on the distolingual portion of the band for final positioning. In the mandibular arch the band biter should be placed on the distofacial portion of the band. (D) A properly fitted band is seated approximately 1 mm below the mesial and distal marginal ridges. (E) If a tight interproximal contact prevents the band from seating properly, orthodontic separators are placed to create space for the band material. The separators are removed within 7 to 10 days, and the band is fitted.

and fabricate the appliance on the dental cast. Intraoral scanning may also be used. A digital scan provides information to print a three-dimensional model on which the appliance is constructed. The dentist, an in-office technician, or a commercial dental laboratory will bend a 0.036-inch wire into the appropriate appliance.

The appliance is commonly delivered in a separate visit. First, it is tried in and adjusted to fit. The interior of the band is cleaned thoroughly, and the cement is loaded along the gingival margin. If the cement is loaded on the occlusal side, there is a risk there will be a void in the cement. Next, the band is placed on the clean, dry abutment tooth (teeth), and the excess cement is cleaned. There are several types of cement from which to choose, but glass ionomer cement is recommended. This type of cement releases fluoride over time to protect the tooth from demineralization. The appliance should be checked every 6 months to ensure it still fits properly, cement has not washed out, and the abutment teeth are nonmobile. Eruption of the permanent tooth is an easily recognized indication for removal.

The laboratory-fabricated distal shoe has some variation in the process. The appliance can be constructed from an impression taken after removal of the primary second molar or from an impression taken before the tooth is extracted. In the former situation the gingiva must be incised when the appliance is placed if the extraction site has healed. In the latter situation the construction cast must be modified to simulate loss of the primary second molar, but placement in the extraction site at the time of surgery is straightforward. The appliance is constructed very much like the band and loop. The primary first molar is banded, and the loop is extended to the former distal contact of the primary second molar. A piece of stainless steel is soldered to the distal end of the loop and placed in the extraction site. The stainless steel extension acts as a guide plane for the permanent first molar to erupt into proper position and should be positioned 1 mm below the mesial marginal ridge of the unerupted first permanent molar in the alveolar bone. After the molar has erupted, the extension can be cut off or a new band and loop appliance can be constructed. To ensure that the stainless steel extension is in the proper position and in close proximity to the permanent first molar, a periapical radiograph is recommended before the appliance is cemented (Fig. 22.10).

An alternative to the two-step process is the prefabricated appliance, which comes in band and loop and distal shoe variations. These are fabricated intraorally and save chairside time and laboratory expense. Extra chairside time and equipment are needed to fit and place the appliances. These are a practical and common alternative to the traditional unilateral space maintainers but may lack durability.

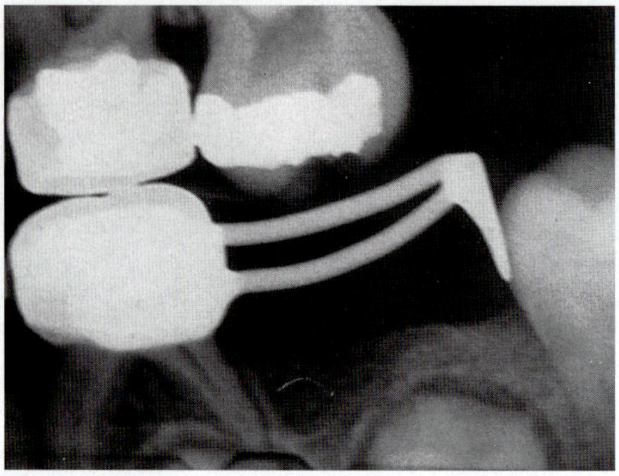

• **Fig. 22.10** A periapical radiograph is recommended before cementing the distal shoe appliance to ensure that it is properly positioned in relation to the unerupted permanent first molar.

Summary

Space maintenance in the primary dentition should be considered in terms of anterior and posterior space loss. Space maintenance is generally not required for missing primary incisors but can be placed if esthetic concerns are a factor. Posterior space maintenance is a necessity in this age group and should be undertaken when primary molars are lost prematurely and the space is adequate. The band and loop appliance is used most frequently; other appliances can be used as different situations dictate. Judicious space maintenance benefits the child patient and may prevent future alignment and crowding problems. Both fixed and removable space maintainers require constant supervision to prevent problems, so the clinician should be prepared to see these children on regular intervals until the space maintainer is no longer required.

Visit eBooks.Health.Elsevier.com to see full list of references.

23

Oral Habits

CLARICE LAW EYRE

CHAPTER OUTLINE

Oral habits are repetitive behaviors that can cause problems in the structure of teeth or the orofacial complex. The urge to suck, which is the origin of an oral habit, is a physiologic necessity in newborns. The ability to suck and swallow develops in utero and is a necessary skill for a newborn to feed effectively from the breast or bottle. Newborns also derive comfort from sucking behaviors. Along with swaddling, rocking, music, and maternal touch, sucking has a soothing effect on a newborn and can even be used to alleviate pain in the postnatal period. As with most repetitive behaviors, problems come with the nature of the habit. Nutritive sucking—breastfeeding and bottle feeding—can evolve from a skill to support nutritional intake to a habit that promotes or facilitates the development of dental caries. Nonnutritive sucking can evolve from a skill to cope with environmental stressors to a habit that promotes malocclusion. In this chapter, the nonnutritive behaviors that are related to somatic and craniofacial growth and development will be discussed.

Nonnutritive Sucking Habits

Thumb/finger and pacifier sucking are very common topics considered by parents. A simple Internet search yields an abundance of resources discussing causes, benefits, side effects, and tips for cessation. Classic literature considers digit and pacifier habits separately, with most conclusions drawn from descriptive research studies. The more recent evidence base of systematic reviews combines the activities together under the heading of nonnutritive sucking habits to provide a higher quality of evidence.

The prevalence of thumb and finger sucking varies substantially worldwide, affecting children representing a variety of socioeconomic and cultural backgrounds.[1] Frequency of any nonnutritive sucking in the first 6 to 12 months can be as high as 85% to 90% of all infants and 70% to 75% of children between 2 and 5 years. Most children generally cease digit and pacifier sucking spontaneously between 3 and 4 years.[1,2] Children who continue with a habit past the age of 4 tend to be digit suckers.[3] Peer pressure is thought to play a role in pacifier cessation at this stage, along with the fact that parents can have more control over use of a pacifier than with a digit. By 6 to 7 years of age, most children begin the transition into the permanent dentition, making habit cessation more important. At this point, approximately 12% of children continue, mostly with digit habits. By the adolescent period, very few nonnutritive habits persist, with a prevalence of 1.9% in 12-year-old children.[1]

Dentists are often questioned about the kinds of problems these habits may cause if they are prolonged. The malocclusions caused by nonnutritive sucking may be more of an individualized response than a highly specific cause-and-effect response. The types of dental changes that a digit habit may cause vary with the amount of force applied to the teeth (force magnitude), the manner in which the digit is positioned in the mouth (force direction), how much time the child engages in the habit (frequency in hours per day), and how long the habit persists (duration in months or years). Clinical experience suggests that 4 to 6 hours of force per day is probably the minimum necessary to cause tooth movement. However, it is the duration of time sucking (in months and years) that probably plays the most critical role in tooth movement caused by a digit habit.[2,4]

The most frequently reported dental outcomes of an active pacifier (Fig. 23.1) or digit (Fig. 23.2) habit are the following[2,3,5,6]:

1. Anterior open bite
2. Increased overjet and/or incisor spacing
3. Posterior crossbite

Anterior open bite, or the lack of vertical overlap of the upper and lower incisors when the posterior teeth are in occlusion, is a common finding in prolonged nonnutritive sucking habits.[2,3,5,6] The open bite develops because the pacifier or digit rests between the maxillary and mandibular incisors (Fig. 23.3). This prevents complete or continued eruption of the incisors, but the posterior teeth are free to erupt. Anterior open bite may also be caused by intrusion of the incisors, which would require force of greater magnitude, frequency, and/or duration. Anterior open bite has been observed in children who continue use of a pacifier and/or digit habits beyond 2 to 4 years of age.[3,6] There is controversy

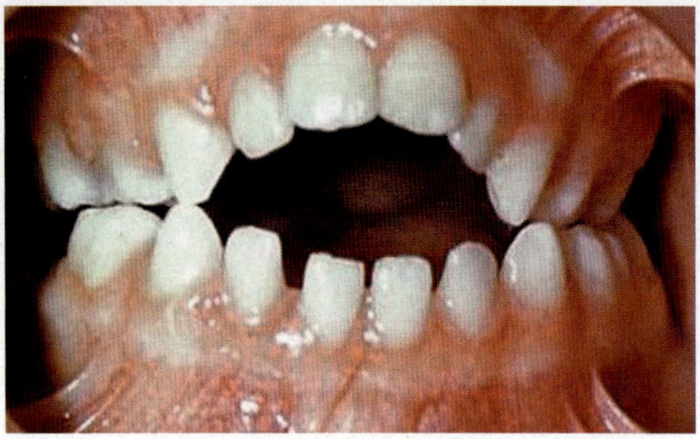

• **Fig. 23.1** A pacifier can result in anterior open bite, increased overjet and/or incisor spacing, and posterior crossbite.

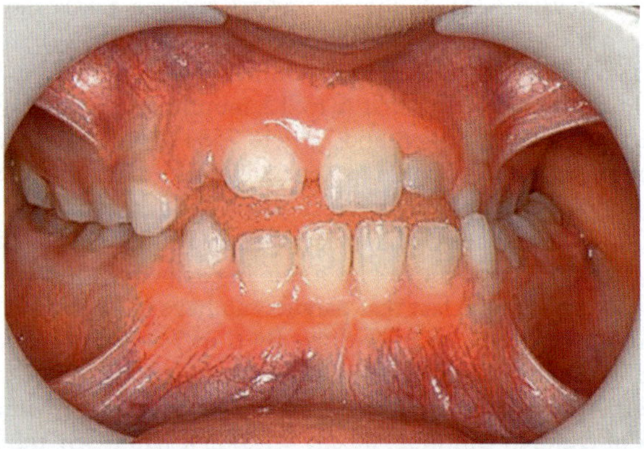

• **Fig. 23.2** A digit habit can result in effects similar to a pacifier. Digit habits tend to persist in older children more frequently than pacifier habits do.

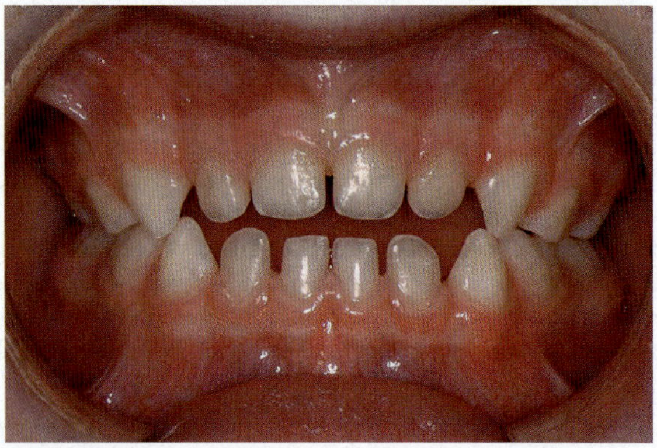

• **Fig. 23.3** This patient's anterior open bite is a direct result of an active thumb-sucking habit. An open bite results when the thumb impedes eruption of the anterior teeth, moves them facially, and allows the posterior teeth to erupt passively. Actual intrusion of the anterior teeth is possible but unlikely.

whether an orthodontic pacifier may reduce effects on malocclusion, with some reports of reduction in anterior open bite with a thinner neck pacifier,[6] and still others that report no difference in any type of malocclusion with an orthodontic pacifier.[7] Fortunately, anterior open bite from pacifier or digit habit has been observed to self-correct without orthodontic intervention. If nonnutritive sucking habits cease by 5 to 6 years of age, 85% to 95% of children can have spontaneous correction of anterior

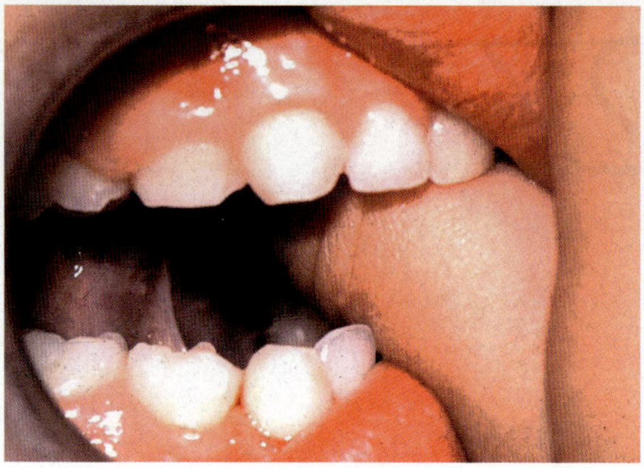

• **Fig. 23.4** With most thumb-sucking habits, the thumb exerts pressure on the lingual surface of the maxillary incisors and on the facial surface of the mandibular incisors. This causes the maxillary incisors to tip facially and the mandibular incisors to tip lingually, resulting in increased overjet.

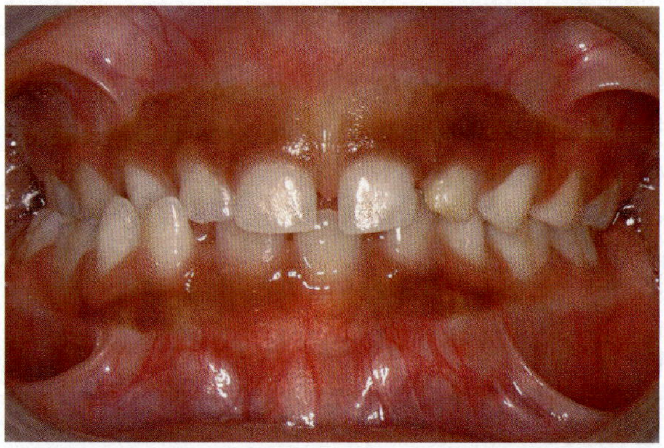

• **Fig. 23.5** This patient exhibits a right maxillary posterior crossbite. A posterior crossbite is often the side effect of a thumb or pacifier habit because the tongue is displaced inferiorly and the orbicularis oris and buccinator muscles exert a force on the upper teeth, constricting the arch.

open bite.[8] It has not been clearly demonstrated whether children who continue habits into the mixed and permanent dentition can still have spontaneous correction of anterior open bite. However, many studies suggest that if incisors have completed active eruption, with full root development, correction is less likely to occur.

Faciolingual movement of the incisors depends on how the pacifier or digit is placed in the mouth. Usually, the thumb is placed so that it exerts pressure on the lingual surfaces of the maxillary incisors and on the labial surfaces of the mandibular incisors (Fig. 23.4). A child who actively sucks can create enough force to tip the upper incisors facially and the lower incisors lingually. The result is an increased overjet and, often, maxillary spacing.

The maxillary arch constriction associated with a posterior crossbite is thought to be caused by the change in equilibrium balance between the oral musculature and the tongue. When the pacifier or digit is placed in the mouth, the tongue is forced down and away from the palate. The orbicularis oris and buccinator muscles continue to exert a force on the buccal surfaces of the maxillary dentition, especially when these muscles are contracted during sucking. Because the tongue no longer exerts a counterbalancing force from the lingual surface, the posterior maxillary arch can collapse into crossbite (Fig. 23.5). Posterior crossbites are at risk of developing when digit or pacifier habits extend beyond 12 to 24 months.[3,6,7,9] Systematic reviews and longitudinal studies indicate that posterior crossbite can develop at a younger age in pacifier users than in digit suckers. The issue of the orthodontic pacifier has been considered with posterior crossbite, with some reports of reduction in posterior crossbite with a wider orthodontic pacifier rather than the symmetrical round nipple pacifier.[9] Overall, it is clear that persistence of any pacifier or digit habit beyond approximately 3 to 4 years of age leaves a child at risk of developing posterior crossbite. Posterior crossbites tend not to resolve spontaneously on habit cessation, as anterior open bites do, so habit cessation before this outcome is preferred to avoid the need for early orthodontic intervention.

Three different approaches to treatment have been advocated, depending on the willingness of the child to stop the habit. It is important to select the approach that is age appropriate and acceptable to parents to increase the odds of successful treatment.

Behavior Modification Techniques

The simplest approach for both digit and pacifier habits is counseling with the patient. This involves discussion between the dentist and the patient of the problems created by nonnutritive sucking. These frank discussions focus on the changes that have occurred because of the sucking and their impact on esthetics. Usually, an appeal is made to the children based on their maturity and responsibility. Clearly, this approach is best aimed at older children who can conceptually grasp the issue and who may be feeling social pressure to stop the habit. Some children are captured by this approach and successfully eliminate their habit.

A reward system is often used in conjunction with counseling. The child, parent(s), and dentist come to an agreement of a specified time period during which the child will work toward discontinuing the habit. The child will receive a reward, which does not need to be extravagant, but special enough to motivate the child. Praise from the parent(s) and dentist has a large role. The more involvement the child has, the more likely it is that the goal will be reached. Involvement may include placing stickers on a homemade calendar for each day the child has successfully avoided the habit. At the end of the specified time, the reward is presented with verbal praise for meeting the conditions of the agreement (Fig. 23.6). The reward system is less successful if the child uses the habit to fall asleep.

In some cultures, rite of passage ceremonies focus on habit cessation. A Scandinavian pacifier company describes one ritual, in which children give up their pacifiers by hanging them on a community tree when they turn 3 years of age.[10] The establishment of a cultural norm probably helps with the child's mindset about the habit.

Because of the subjective nature of the counseling conversation, any related reward system, or cultural tradition, it is difficult to provide any evidence regarding a standardized protocol. Dentists must therefore apply creativity and adapt with increasing clinical experience to develop habit cessation protocols that work within the related developmental factors described in the literature.

Reminder Therapy

The second approach is more applicable for digit habits and is appropriate for those who desire to stop the habit but need external motivators. Reminders involve use of barriers or chemical substances to alert children when they engage in the habit. An adhesive bandage on the offending digit is a common reminder not to place the finger in the mouth (Fig. 23.7). Some clinicians advocate using a mitten or a sock to cover the entire hand. This is especially useful during sleeping hours. Other commercial products such as a plastic thumb guard are available. Another approach is to paint a commercially available bitter substance on the digits that are sucked. The purpose of the intervention should be thoroughly explained to the child. To reduce the likelihood that a child perceives the reminder to be punitive, the child should be included in discussion of the options to be used. Whichever option the child selects should be used routinely during the habit cessation target period.

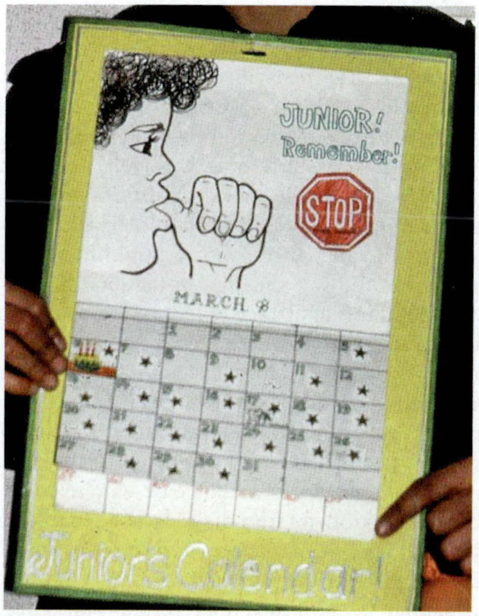

• **Fig. 23.6** A personalized calendar can be used to motivate a child to stop a thumb-sucking habit. Stick-on stars are applied to the calendar on days when the child has successfully avoided the habit. At the end of a month or a specified period of time, a reward and verbal praise can be provided for discontinuing the habit.

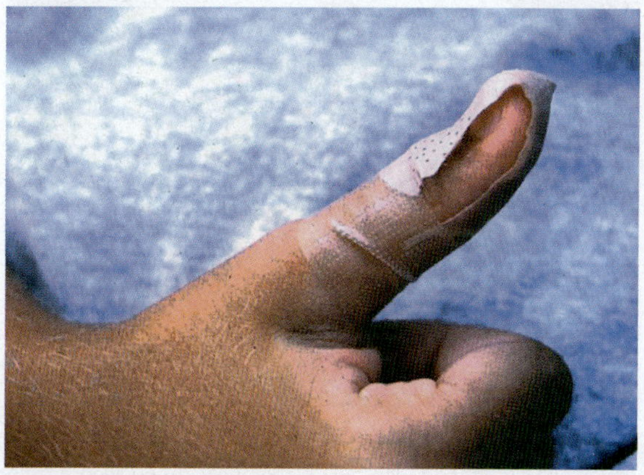

• **Fig. 23.7** One or two adhesive bandages can be secured to a child's digit to serve as a reminder not to place the finger in the mouth. The bandage is worn until the child stops sucking the digit.

Appliance Therapy

If the habit persists after behavior modification and reward therapy and the child continues to be motivated to eliminate the habit, appliances can be placed to physically interrupt the habit. Appliances are almost exclusively used for digit habits and more commonly delayed until the mixed dentition period.[11] As with the chemical reminders, the dentist should explain to the patient and parent that the appliance is not a punishment but rather a fixed reminder not to place the digit in the mouth.

The most common appliance described in systematic reviews to discourage a digit habit is the palatal crib, or tongue crib. The palatal crib is designed to interfere with finger placement and sucking satisfaction. Bands are fitted on the permanent first molars or primary second molars. A heavy lingual arch wire is bent to fit passively in the palate and is soldered to the molar bands. Additional wire is soldered onto this base wire to form a crib or mechanical obstruction for the digit. It is advisable to make a lower cast at the time the appliance is constructed so that the occlusion can be checked for interferences (Fig. 23.8). The parent and child should be informed that certain side effects appear temporarily after the palatal crib is cemented. Eating, speaking, and sleeping patterns may be altered during the first few days after appliance delivery. These difficulties usually subside within a few days. It is not unusual for an imprint of the appliance to appear on the tongue as an indentation. The major problem with the palatal crib is the difficulty of maintaining good oral hygiene. Improvements in overbite and incisor inclination can occur after placement.[12]

An alternative to the palatal crib is the quad helix. This is a fixed appliance commonly used to expand a constricted maxillary arch—a common finding accompanied by posterior crossbite in patients who practice nonnutritive sucking (Fig. 23.9). The anterior extension of the appliance can be designed to cross the palate where the child places the digit and serves as a reminder to the child not to place the digit there. A crib can be added to the appliance for additional effect. The quad helix is a versatile appliance because it can correct a posterior crossbite and discourage a finger habit at the same time.

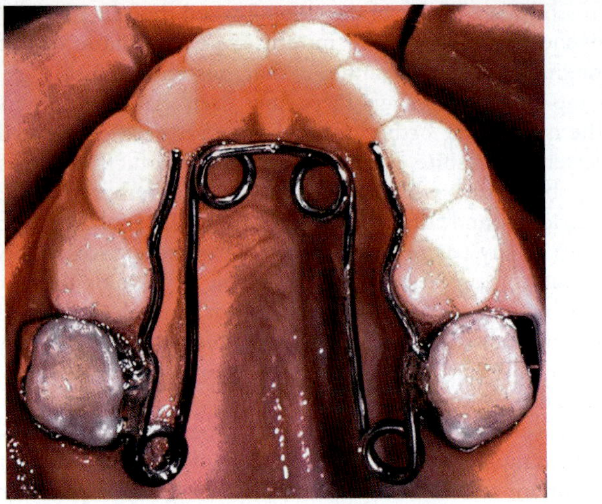

• **Fig. 23.9** The quad helix is a fixed appliance used to expand a constricted maxillary arch. The anterior helices also discourage a sucking habit by reminding the child not to place a finger in the mouth. This appliance is often used in children in whom there is an active sucking habit and a posterior crossbite.

Other appliances have been suggested to accomplish results similar to the palatal crib and the quad helix. The Bluegrass appliance places a Teflon roller in an anterior area of the palate and in the same general area as a Nance arch. The appliance is easier to clean and is less disruptive to eating and speech than the crib. The patient is encouraged to use the tongue to turn the roller, with the idea that the act engaging the tongue will act as a competing habit and decrease the need to suck a thumb or finger for oral gratification. A longitudinal study demonstrated that 40% of children were able to achieve habit cessation within 4 weeks, with a total treatment time of 24 to 30 weeks for up to 80% of the subjects.[13] The Bluegrass appliance can also be combined with a W arch to correct a transverse constriction if it is present (Fig. 23.10).

Appliances should be left in the mouth for 6 to 12 months to allow adequate time for habit cessation and spontaneous correction

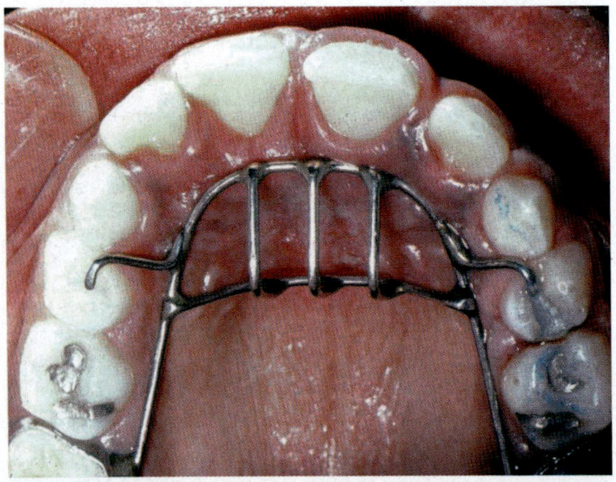

• **Fig. 23.8** A tongue crib is a fixed appliance designed to stop a digit habit by mechanically interfering with digit placement and sucking satisfaction. The parent of the child should expect temporary disturbances in eating, speaking, and sleeping patterns during the first few days after use of the appliance.

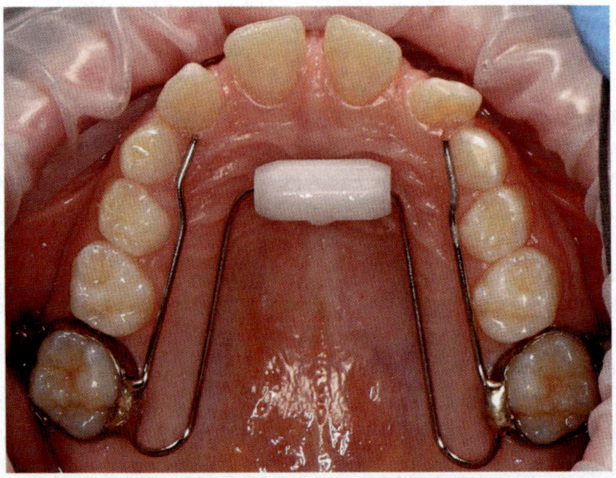

• **Fig. 23.10** This Bluegrass appliance has been combined with a W arch to create an appliance that will help stop a digit habit and at the same time correct the posterior constriction that has resulted from the habit. The Teflon roller is placed in the anterior portion of the palate to disrupt the habit and allow the tongue to turn the roller.

of open bite. The clinician should have the patient return at 1- or 2-month intervals to monitor how the child is doing with the habit and to encourage the patient if indicated. The palatal crib usually stops the child from sucking immediately but often requires another 6 months of wear to extinguish the habit completely. The quad helix also requires a minimum of 6 months of treatment. Three months is typical to correct the crossbite, and 3 months is required to stabilize the movement.

Treatment Interventions

The timing of any intervention for a nonnutritive sucking habit must be strategic. If parents or the child are not ready to engage in treatment, it should not be attempted. Recommendations specific to pacifiers suggest cessation by 2 years, with most children spontaneously stopping by age 4 to 5 years.[5] Digit habits can show changes to the dentition by 3 to 4 years, so treatment is recommended to take place between the ages of 4 and 6 years. The child should first be given an opportunity to stop the habit independently, but certainly before irreversible changes occur or the permanent teeth begin to erupt. Delay until the early school-aged years allows for spontaneous discontinuation of the habit by many children, often through peer pressure at school. If the habit is eliminated before full eruption of the permanent incisors, the eruption process will spontaneously reduce the overjet and open bite as the permanent teeth occupy new positions. It is generally agreed that interception of a digit-sucking habit does no harm to the child's emotional development, nor does it result in habit substitution. However, the dentist should evaluate the child for psychological overtones before embarking on habit elimination. Interventions might be postponed for children who have recently undergone stressful changes in their lives, such as a new sibling, separation or divorce of parents, moving to a new community, or changing schools. Overall, whether a habit appliance is placed, psychological interventions are used, or a combination of the two, some type of intervention is better than nothing in the cessation of a nonnutritive sucking habit.[11] Because there is no high-quality evidence in support of any specific intervention, there is room for creativity and clinical innovation in method of habit cessation.

Atypical Swallowing

Classic literature categorizes "tongue thrust" as an oral habit. The term "tongue thrust" was used in different ways, with some using it to describe a passive anterior posture of the tongue and others describing an active thrust of the tongue forward on swallowing. This latter definition is now described as atypical swallowing,[14] which can be further categorized as primary, with psychological origins for its presence, or secondary, *caused* by oral habits.[15]

The atypical swallow pattern is considered to be normal during the early period of development. The tongue thrust characteristic of the infantile swallow decreases between 12 and 15 months as primary teeth erupt.[15–17] Between ages 3 and 5, prevalence can decrease from 55% to 35%, with prevalence between 5% and 15% reported for older children and adults.[14] Atypical swallow is often associated with prolonged breastfeeding, short frenulum, hypertrophic adenoids and tonsils, oral breathing, allergic rhinitis, and abnormal head, lower jaw, and tongue posture.[14,15] Nonnutritive sucking habits beyond the age of 5 have also been associated with atypical swallowing patterns for 6- to 9-year-old children.[15]

In terms of malocclusion, atypical swallowing has historically been assumed to be correlated with anterior open bite. There is no evidence suggesting that the atypical swallow causes malocclusion, with the frequency, duration, and force magnitude of the thrust insufficient to result in tooth movement. Furthermore, epidemiologic data fail to demonstrate a clear causative relationship for open bite from atypical swallow.[14,17] The passive anterior resting posture of the tongue is thought to have a greater influence on malocclusion than the atypical swallow, with the anterior open bite commonly observed.[18] Thus atypical swallow is often thought of as an "opportunistic behavior" that adapts to the malocclusion rather than being a causative factor. Interestingly, systematic review indicates a significant relationship between atypical swallow and posterior crossbite in children ages 3 to 11, with open bite and excess overjet also observed as comorbidities.[17]

Treatment of tongue thrust varies depending on the origin of the associated problems. If there is a concurrent nonnutritive sucking habit or history of mouth breathing, these issues should be managed first. Limited orthodontics should be considered if the patient exhibits malocclusion. Myofunctional therapy is often suggested, but the body of evidence has not yet clearly demonstrated the effectiveness of the exercises.

Mouth Breathing

Mouth breathing was also once considered a habit. Although it was considered normal for a 3- to 6-year-old to be slightly lip incompetent (Fig. 23.11), persistence beyond that period was considered a habit, related to behaviors or preferences. Mouth breathing is now generally divided into obstructive and functional factors. Obstructive factors include airway obstructions like adenotonsillar hypertrophy, deviated nasal septum, and nasal polyps.[19] Adenoid hypertrophy occurs in approximately 35% of children[20] and is considered the most common cause of mouth breathing in children.[21] Functional factors include persistent oral habits, musculoskeletal issues, or allergic rhinitis/nasal congestion.[19] Asthma also

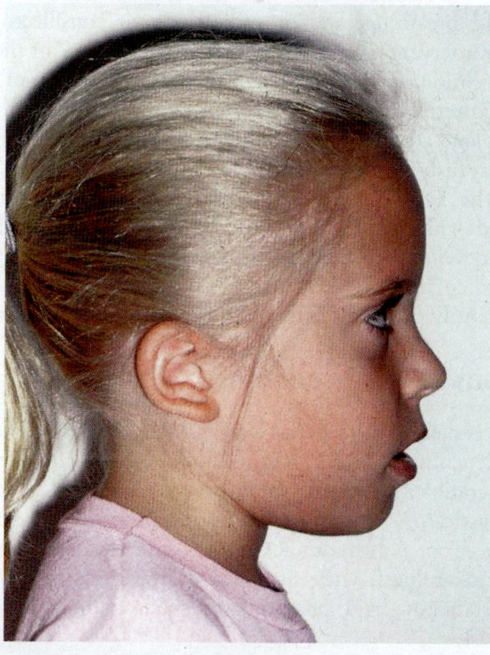

• **Fig. 23.11** The normal relaxed lip posture in the 3- to 6-year-old child is for the lips to be slightly apart or incompetent. These children are often labeled mouth breathers because of this posture, but they may, in fact, be completely nasal breathers.

shows an association with mouth breathing.[22] In sum, the presence of mouth breathing is an indicator that airway issues should be explored in conjunction with the child's physician, as opposed to a behavioral habit that can be retrained.

In terms of the effect of mouth breathing on oral health, the constant airflow through the mouth dries the teeth and mucosa. An association with gingival inflammation has been well established.[23] A higher plaque index is common, along with increased risk of dental caries. Overall, the oral microbiota and salivary environment are affected, making mouth breathers more susceptible to oral diseases.[24]

Beyond oral disease, the role of mouth breathing on malocclusion is also well established. There is stereotypic pattern of "adenoid facies" associated with children with mouth breathing, including small nose and nostrils, short upper lip, prominent display of maxillary incisors, and the unfortunate description of a "vacant facial expression."[25] Facial skeletal development is affected, with systematic reviews indicating downward and backward rotation of the mandible and maxilla, a steep occlusal and/or mandibular plane,[26] and a higher prevalence of class II malocclusion.[27] Other studies indicate a higher frequency of narrow, V-shaped maxilla and posterior crossbite in mouth breathers.[26] There is even an effect on posture, with a higher frequency of children who project their heads forward to improve airflow.[28]

For the dental professional, the most important thing to consider when encountering a child with a tendency toward mouth breathing is whether the child may be at risk for obstructive sleep apnea (OSA) or sleep-disordered breathing. Children with obstructive sleep-disordered breathing are at risk for behavioral problems, with more frequent diagnoses of attention-deficit/hyperactivity disorder (ADHD), and cognitive effects impacting academic performance.[29] There are also long-term health consequences to OSA, including cardiovascular diseases, so appropriate referral and medical management are imperative.

Treatment of mouth breathing is beyond the scope of the dentist if the root cause is airway obstruction. In the case of sleep-disordered breathing, adenotonsillectomy or tonsillectomy are common interventions.[29] As an oral health outcome of the medical intervention, some studies have shown a redirection of vertical growth patterns toward normal after surgery, particularly mandibular plane and anterior face height.[30] However, this does not imply that turbinectomy or adenoidectomy is required to solely to change the facial growth pattern. Considering the stereotype associated with mouth breathing, beyond the oral health and occlusal development benefits of early interventions, the psychosocial and cognitive benefits make it very important for the dentist to identify problems early for appropriate and timely referral.

Bruxism

Bruxism is defined as "repetitive jaw muscle activity characterized by the clenching or grinding of teeth and/or bracing or thrusting of the mandible."[31] Two variations have been defined. Sleep bruxism is masticatory muscle activity during sleep that can be rhythmic (phasic) or nonrhythmic (tonic).[31,32] Awake bruxism occurs during wakefulness, with sustained or repetitive tooth contact and/or static or rigid posturing of the mandible during the day.[31,32]

In general, bruxism is thought to have a physiologic component, maintaining bone homeostasis, promoting alveolar growth, and managing stress.[33] Traditional explanations centered on local, systemic, and psychological factors for excessive bruxism.[34] The local theory suggested that bruxism could be a reaction to an occlusal interference, high restoration, or some irritating dental condition. Systemic factors implicated in bruxism historically included intestinal parasites, subclinical nutritional deficiencies, and endocrine disorders. The psychological theory submits that bruxism is the manifestation of a personality disorder or increased stress, with neuroticism considered to be an influence. Children with ADHD have a higher prevalence of bruxism, sleep or awake.[35] The psychological attributions have mainly been demonstrated in children older than 6 years. Finally, there is an association between sleep bruxism and poor sleep. Children who engage in sleep bruxism have an increased frequency of snoring, mouth breathing, restless sleep, drooling, sleeping on stomach, and sleep deficiencies.[36] It has also been associated with secondhand smoke and environmental factors affecting sleep.[37,38] Most importantly, sleep bruxism can be considered a warning sign of airway obstruction and, consequently, sleep-related breathing disorders to be explored in conjunction with the child's pediatrician.[33,39]

Most children start showing signs of bruxism with the eruption of the first primary teeth. This might be considered local or physiologic bruxism. Prevalence peaks between 9 to 10 and 10 to 14 years of age, decreasing in most cases during adolescence.[31,33] Overall prevalence is highly variable in the literature. However, sleep bruxism appears to be more prevalent in children than adults (between 6% and 50%).[40] Awake bruxism, on the other hand, has a prevalence of approximately 16% to 32%[32] in children, but increases in adulthood, suggestive of psychological origins.

Clinical signs of bruxism that can be identified by the dentist include primary canine wear and dental wear.[41] Rarely does the wear endanger the pulp by proceeding faster than secondary dentin is produced (Fig. 23.12). Children may also report of headache.[41] Masticatory muscle soreness and temporomandibular myofascial pain have also been attributed to bruxism. Long-term activity could increase the risk of temporomandibular disorder in the future.[32]

A grading system has been established to document cases of bruxism.[31,33] Self-reported behaviors are considered "possible" bruxism. Identification of clinical signs of dental wear by the dentist, with or without positive self-report, is considered "probable." And positive signs on instrumental assessment (electromyography or polysomnography), with or without self-report and/or clinical signs, is "definite."

Treatment differs depending on whether the bruxism is an isolated activity or whether it is related to an airway disorder.[33] Isolated cases may be treated with an occlusal splint.[31,33] This has

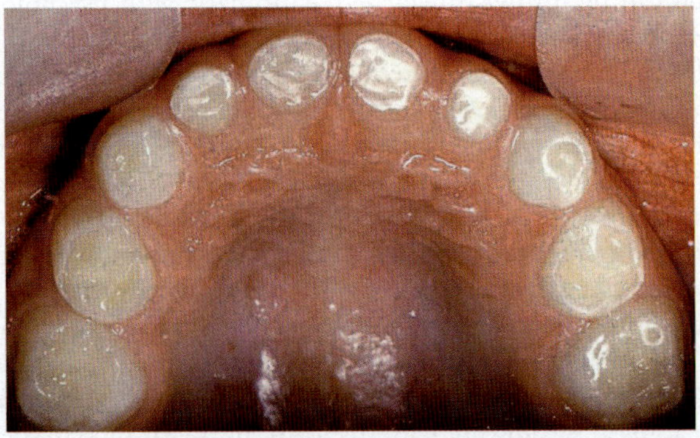

• **Fig. 23.12** This patient's primary maxillary incisors and canines were worn more rapidly due to bruxism.

inconsistent results in eliminating bruxism, but protects the teeth from further damage and reduces reports of headache. Any device covering the occlusal surfaces has to take growth and development into consideration, as exfoliation and continued skeletal growth must be accommodated in the fit of the appliance.[31] The "boil and bite" mouthguards have been proposed. These are inexpensive to purchase and remoldable as the dentition rapidly changes during the mixed dentition years. If the habit is thought to be caused by psychological factors, referral to a child development expert could be considered. Pharmacologic treatment is another option, with the assumption that bruxism is caused by anxiety and stress. Hydroxyzine, an antihistamine, seems to have the best results at decreasing anxiety and improving sleep.[33,42] Benzodiazepines and antidepressants can also be used, but long-term effects of use must be considered.[31] Some homeopathic therapies have been proposed, but these generally do not show effectiveness.[33] Physical therapy can also be effective.[31] Overall, other than the occlusal splint, most treatment options for isolated bruxism should be conducted in conjunction with the patient's pediatrician.

Bruxism associated with airway disorders has different options. The child could be treated with palatal expansion in cases with maxillary constriction, which has shown reductions in bruxism.[31,33] Adenoidectomy is another treatment option that appears to show improvements in bruxism.[33] Again, the root causes of the airway disorder should be directly addressed, with bruxism potentially used as an indicator of the systemic problem.

Children with musculoskeletal disorders (cerebral palsy) and children who are severely developmentally disabled tend to be more susceptible to bruxism. These patients' bruxism is the result of their underlying physical and mental condition and is difficult to manage dentally. On occasion, occlusal wear is so extensive that stainless steel crowns or other restorative options are needed to prevent pulpal exposure or eliminate tooth sensitivity.

Lip Habits

Habits that involve manipulation of the lips and perioral structures are called lip habits. Those that might come to the attention of the dental professional are lip licking, lip biting, and lip sucking. The influence of each on the oral structures is varied, with effects on either soft tissues or malocclusion.

Lip licking is a relatively benign habit as far as dental effects are concerned. Red, inflamed, and chapped lips and perioral tissues are the most apparent signs associated with lip licking (Fig. 23.13). The condition increases in frequency during the dry winter season and is known as lip licking dermatitis. Little can be done to stop this habit effectively. Treatment is usually palliative and limited to moisturizing the lips, although some clinicians have used appliances to interrupt the habits.

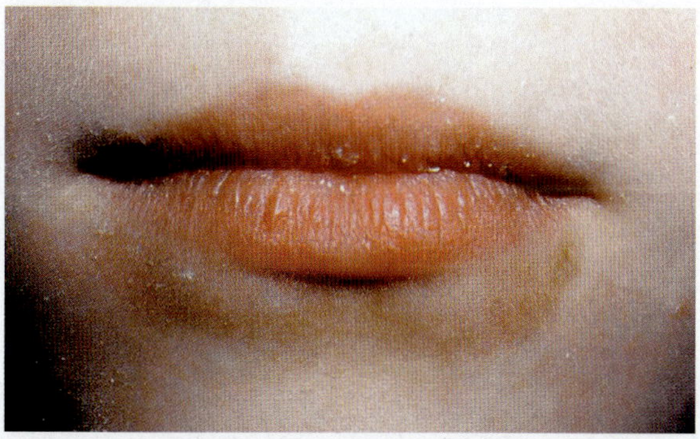

• **Fig. 23.13** Red, inflamed, chapped lips and perioral tissues are often indicative of a lip-sucking or lip-licking habit. These problems are more common and severe during the winter months.

Lip or cheek biting is included in the group of habits known as body-focused repetitive behaviors.[43] These habits have unknown causes, with possible genetic or neurobiologic origins. A recent large-scale study in adults indicated that 75% of adults admitted to engaging in lip/cheek biting at some point in their lives.[43] The most common outcome of lip biting, and the related behavior of cheek biting, is hyperkeratosis or ulcerations and sores, which can become infected. Treatment in the dental setting is palliative, with referral for cognitive behavioral therapy as an appropriate intervention for more severe cases.

Milder forms of lip biting and the related habit of lip sucking generally do not cause dental problems but can maintain an existing malocclusion if the child engages in the habits with adequate intensity, frequency, and duration. Whether these habits can create a malocclusion is a question that is not easily answered. The most common presentation of lip sucking is the lower lip tucked behind the maxillary incisors (Fig. 23.14). This places a lingually directed force on the mandibular teeth and a facial force on the maxillary teeth. The result is a proclination of the maxillary incisors, a retroclination of the mandibular incisors, and increased overjet. This problem is most common in the mixed and permanent dentitions. Treatment depends on the skeletal relationship of the child and on the presence or absence of space in the arch. If the child has a class I skeletal relationship and an increased overjet that is solely the result of tipped teeth, the clinician can tip the teeth to their original or a more normal position with either a fixed or a removable appliance. If a class II skeletal relationship exists, a more involved growth modification procedure is needed to manage the malocclusion.

Nail Biting

Nail biting (onychophagia), like lip biting, is also included among the body-focused repetitive behaviors, with 71% of adults in a

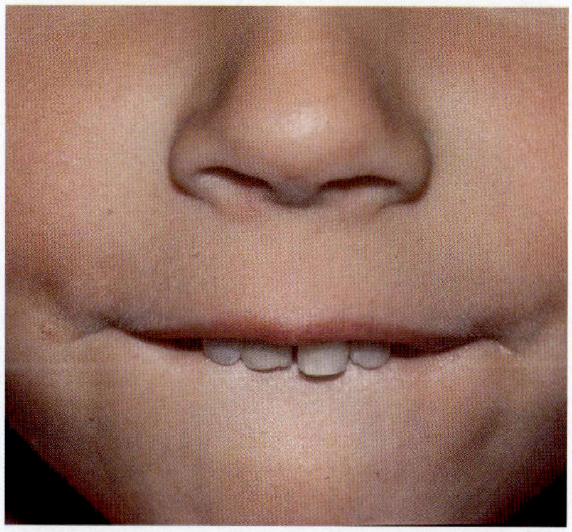

• **Fig. 23.14** The most common habit involving the lips is tucking the lower lip behind the maxillary incisors. The lower lip forces the maxillary teeth facially and the mandibular teeth lingually, resulting in an increased overjet. In addition, the lower lip and other perioral tissues can become chapped and inflamed as a result of constant wetting.

large-scale prevalence study indicating nail biting at some point,[43] and approximately 20% to 30% prevalence overall.[44] It has been suggested that the habit is a manifestation of increased stress. Management may include habit counseling or even referral for behavior therapy. It is a rare habit in persons younger than 4 years. The incidence increases from childhood through adolescence, peaking in young adulthood. There have been suggestions that nail biting may be related to incisor malocclusion, but trauma to the nail bed, warts and vesicular lesions, bacterial infections, and minor enamel fractures are more commonly associated.[44] Other than habit cessation counseling, there is no recommended protocol for the dental professional to address nail biting because dental complications are so mild and appropriate management might be with the mental health professional.

Summary

The oral habits discussed in this chapter were once considered separate behaviors, possibly engaged in by the child as preferences. Current literature is suggesting some connections between groups of habits, with the possibility of systemic rather than just psychological origins for some.

Nonnutritive sucking habits begin as normal infant survival skills, which may have psychological reasons for duration prolonged beyond the typical. The malocclusion that results from a prolonged habit may increase the risk of atypical swallow, which can maintain the changes to the orofacial complex. Habit cessation efforts are within the scope of practice for a dentist and should be initiated before eruption of permanent incisors.

Mouth breathing and bruxism may both be signs of airway obstruction, with systemic and oral health implications for the future. Management of the airway obstruction, if identified, should be conducted by the medical professional. However, the effects on oral disease and malocclusion should be addressed by the dentist.

Lip habits and nail biting most likely have psychological origins and should be addressed by a mental health provider. However, dental effects should also be managed by the dentist.

Overall, a goal should be to address dental and skeletal effects that do not spontaneously resolve and address the habits before irreversible changes occur. Key findings are maxillary constriction, related to both nonnutritive sucking habits and mouth breathing, and dental wear.

Visit eBooks.Health.Elsevier.com to see full list of references.

24

Orthodontic Treatment in the Primary Dentition

POOJAN SHRESTHA AND JOHN R. CHRISTENSEN

CHAPTER OUTLINE

Orthodontic treatment can be considered in each of the developmental stages of the growing patient: primary dentition, mixed dentition, and the permanent dentition. The difficulty is determining what problems should be treated and when they should be treated. If provided too early, the patient may have to go through multiple orthodontic treatments to achieve a functional occlusion. Conversely, if started too late, certain orthodontic treatments are time related and cannot be used if started in a more mature patient. This chapter will provide guidance on treatment for each developmental stage.

Diagnosis is a critical part of providing orthodontic care. Without a baseline of information, the clinician is unable to develop a problem list. It is difficult to develop an appropriate treatment plan without identifying particular problems within the malocclusion.

A clinical examination is necessary for each patient. The clinician reviews the information and develops a prioritized problem list, positive attributes, and treatment goals. The goals should address functional and aesthetic concerns of the patient and the clinician.[1]

After the examination, a problem list is generated, and each problem is ranked in order of severity and possible solutions to each problem listed. The solution list should be comprehensive; that is, all reasonable solutions should be considered for each specific problem without regard for the other problems. After the solution list has been developed, the clinician looks for similar solutions listed for more than one problem. In some cases, the best solution for one problem is the best solution for all problems, and the treatment plan is easily derived. Unfortunately, in most cases a solution to one problem is not the solution for the others and, worse, may magnify the second problem. At this point, interactions, compromises, and cost/benefit decisions should lead to a treatment plan. The treatment plan is presented to the parent and patient and any required adjustments negotiated as needed. The final plan is established and mutually agreed to along with an informed consent presentation. The informed consent process should be directed toward patient understanding and not just a signed form. Treatment planning is not entirely scientific and clinical wisdom and experience are needed to determine a plan in these cases.

If the clinician and the patient are not comfortable with the treatment plan, it is advisable not to proceed with treatment. No one is compelled to provide treatment that does not match their values and professional standards. A recommendation for a second opinion is a useful option in these situations. Motivation for treatment can be reflected in compliance. If the child patient desires to have treatment, cooperation will usually be good during treatment and little parental support will be necessary. This is called internal motivation. External motivation, motivation supplied by the parent for treatment, will require continuous parental support to successfully complete treatment.

Facial Examination

A systematic facial examination is one portion of a complete orthodontic evaluation that describes skeletal and dental relationships in three spatial planes: anteroposterior, vertical, and transverse. The steps include a description of the overall facial pattern, the positions of the maxilla and mandible, and the vertical facial relationships. Next, the position of the lips is determined. Finally, facial symmetry is assessed, and the maxillary dental midline is located relative to the facial midline.

Overall Facial Pattern

The facial profile is evaluated in the anteroposterior plane. An assumption is made that the soft tissue profile reflects the underlying skeletal relationship. To begin the examination, the child should be seated upright, looking at a distant point. Three points on the face are identified: the bridge of the nose, the base of the upper lip, and the chin.

Line segments connecting these points form an angle that describes the profile as convex, straight, or concave (Fig. 24.1). A well-balanced profile in this age group is slightly convex. A well-balanced profile in the anteroposterior dimension has an underlying skeletal relationship that is labeled class I (see Fig. 24.1A). This terminology is used because most class I skeletal relationships also have flush terminal plane or mesial step second primary molar relationships or Angle class I or end-to-end permanent first molar dental relationships if those teeth have erupted. Furthermore, the canine relationships usually will be class I, and there will be overjet of 2 to 5 mm. The Angle dental classification is described in a later section.

An assessment of the overall profile gives a general feeling for skeletal relationships, but this evaluation does not diagnose the reason for the relationships. Some children in this age group have extremely convex profiles (see Fig. 24.1B). This is consistent with a class II skeletal relationship, and these patients usually have distal step second primary molar relationships or class II permanent first molar relationships, class II canine relationships, and increased overjet. Other children have straight or concave profiles (see Fig. 24.1C). These are usually found with mesial step second primary molar relationships or class III permanent first molar relationships, class III canine relationships, and negative overjet.

Positions of the Maxilla and Mandible

If the profile is excessively convex or concave, the clinician can try to determine which skeletal component is contributing to the problem. This is a necessary step if orthodontic treatment is considered. When the problem is known, the appropriate treatment can be tailored to the specific problem.

A vertical reference line is extended from the bridge of the nose (the anterior aspect of the cranial base), and the position of other soft tissue points is noted relative to the reference line (Fig. 24.2). If the maxilla is properly oriented relative to other skeletal structures, the base of the upper lip will be on or near the vertical line. The soft tissue chin will be slightly behind the reference line if the mandible is of proper size and in the correct position. If the maxilla is positioned significantly in front of the vertical reference line, the patient is said to exhibit maxillary protrusion. If the maxilla is substantially behind the line, the patient exhibits maxillary retrusion. The position of the mandible is described in the same way.

So, if the overall skeletal pattern is significantly convex (class II), the maxilla is positioned in front of the line (maxillary protrusion), the mandible is positioned behind the line (mandibular retrusion), or both. Class II skeletal relationships are sometimes caused by one jaw alone but are often the result of some combination of maxillary protrusion and mandibular retrusion.

Conversely, a facial pattern that is straight or extremely concave (class III) results when the maxilla is positioned behind the line (maxillary retrusion), the mandible is positioned in front of the line (mandibular protrusion), or both. Again, both jaws usually contribute to the skeletal dysplasia.

Some caution must be exercised because soft tissue profile relationships do not always accurately reflect the underlying skeletal relationships. Research has shown that the 3- to 6-year-old age group is especially difficult to classify accurately from a profile analysis.[2] In addition, vertical facial relationships influence

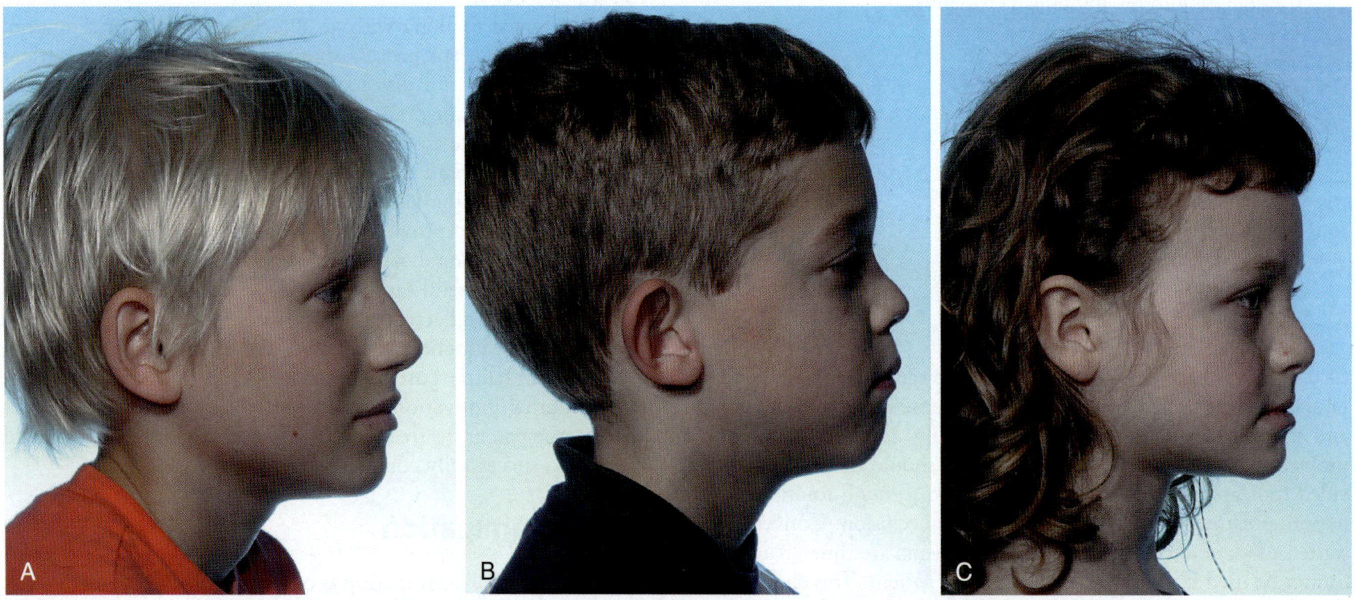

• **Fig. 24.1** (A) A class I skeletal relationship is characterized by a well-balanced profile in the anteroposterior dimension. These relationships can be judged by mentally connecting the points of the bridge of the nose, the base of the upper lip (maxilla), and the soft tissue chin (mandible). This line should be slightly convex. (B) A class II skeletal relationship is characterized by a truly convex profile. (C) A class III skeletal relationship is characterized by a straight or concave profile.

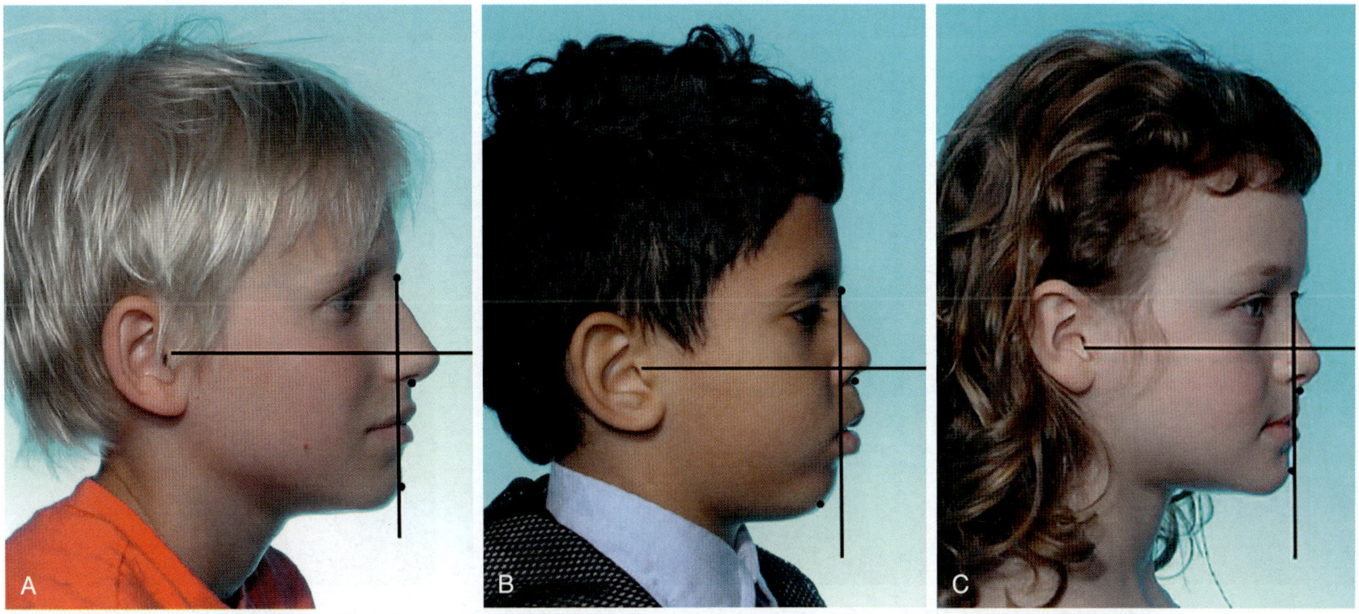

• **Fig. 24.2** The contributions to the skeletal malocclusion can be estimated extraorally by determining the positions of the maxilla and mandible. A perpendicular reference line is established beginning at the soft tissue bridge of the nose. The positions of the maxilla and mandible are related to this line. If the base of the upper lip and nose are anterior to this line, the maxilla is protrusive. If these points are posterior to this line, the maxilla is retrusive. Similarly, the soft tissue chin is determined to be anterior (protrusive) or posterior (retrusive) to this line. (A) This patient has normal relationships for one younger than 6 years. (B) This patient has a significantly convex facial profile (class II), which results from a protrusive maxilla that is ahead of the line and a retrusive mandible that is posterior to the line. (C) This patient has a normal maxilla and a protrusive mandible.

anteroposterior relationships. This interaction between the horizontal and vertical planes of space and its effect on the profile is discussed later.

Vertical Facial Relationships

The third portion of the facial examination is an evaluation of the facial vertical relationships. Proportionality is judged by dividing the face into thirds. The upper third extends from approximately the hairline to the bridge of the nose, the middle third from the bridge of the nose to the base of the upper lip, and the lower third from the base of the upper lip to the bottom of the chin (Fig. 24.3). These thirds are approximately equal, or the lower third is slightly larger in well-proportioned faces.

Vertical problems tend to be manifested below the palate in the lower third of the face.[2] The short-faced person tends to have a lower facial third that is smaller than the other thirds (see Fig. 24.3C). The long-faced patient has a lower facial third that is larger than the other thirds (see Fig. 24.3B).

Lip Position

Next, an evaluation of the anteroposterior lip position gives an estimation of the anteroposterior incisor position. Incisor position is grossly reflected in lip contour and posture. Lip posture is assessed by drawing an imaginary line from the tip of the nose to the most anterior point on the soft tissue chin. The lips normally lie slightly behind this line; however, in the 3- to 6-year-old child, the lower lip is generally 1 mm anterior to the line (Fig. 24.4). Two facts must be kept in mind. First, lip protrusion is characteristic of different ethnic groups, and lips that are considered protrusive in one group may not be considered protrusive in another. For example, African Americans and Asians tend to have more lip protrusion than do people of northern European descent. Second, the lips are evaluated in the context of the nose and chin. A large nose and chin can accommodate more protrusive lips, whereas a small nose and chin require less protrusive lips to be proportional.

Facial Symmetry

Transverse facial dimensions are examined to rule out true facial asymmetry. Facial symmetry is best evaluated with the patient reclined in the dental chair and the dentist seated at the 12 o'clock position. Hair is pulled away from the face, and a piece of dental floss can be stretched down the middle of the upper face to aid in judging lower face symmetry. The mandible should be either at rest or in centric relation position. Maximal intercuspation or centric occlusion positions can be affected by dental interferences during closing.

All faces show a minor degree of asymmetry, but marked asymmetry is not normal (Fig. 24.5). Deviations or asymmetrical positioning of the eyes, ears, or nose may be symptoms of cranial synostosis, an undiagnosed syndrome, or severe trauma. A child with these findings should be referred to appropriate professionals for a complete evaluation.

Asymmetry usually manifests in the lower facial third, whereas upper facial asymmetry is extremely rare. A deviation of the midpoint of the mandible to one side or another may be due to true asymmetry, but it is most often indicative of a posterior crossbite and mandibular shift due to a dental interference.

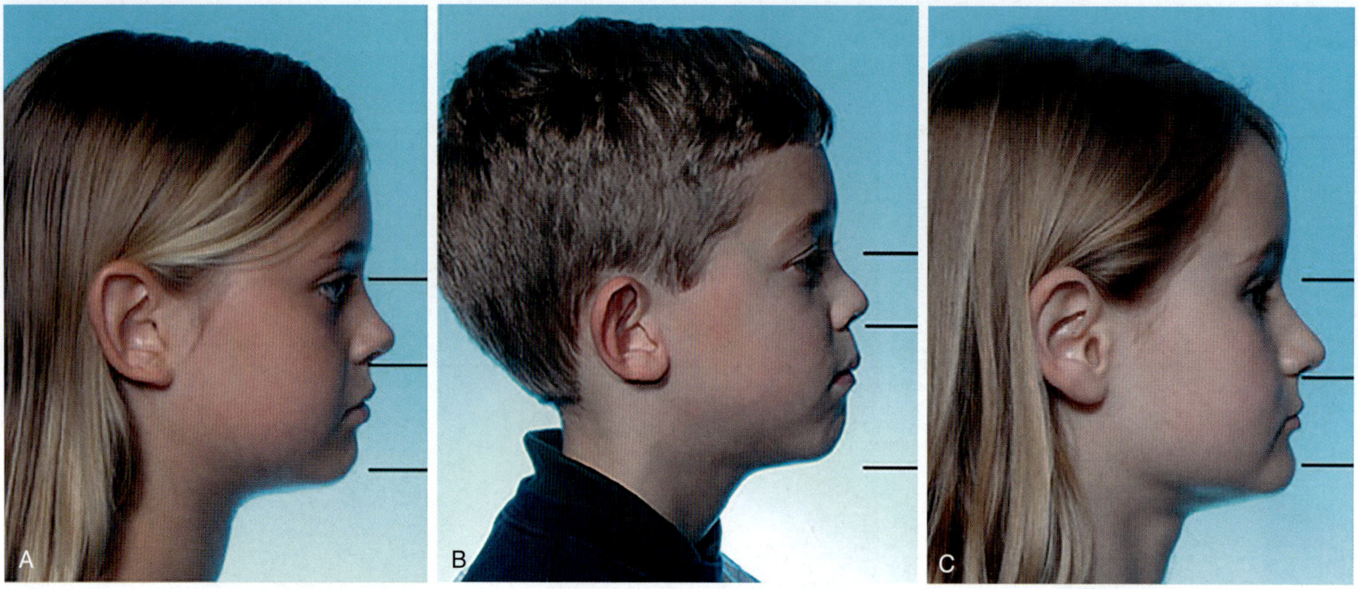

• **Fig. 24.3** Vertical facial proportions can be evaluated by dividing the face into thirds and then comparing the middle third to the lower third. (A) In a well-proportioned face, the facial thirds are equal or the lower third is slightly larger. (B) A child with long lower facial third. (C) A child with short vertical facial dimensions has a proportionately smaller lower facial third.

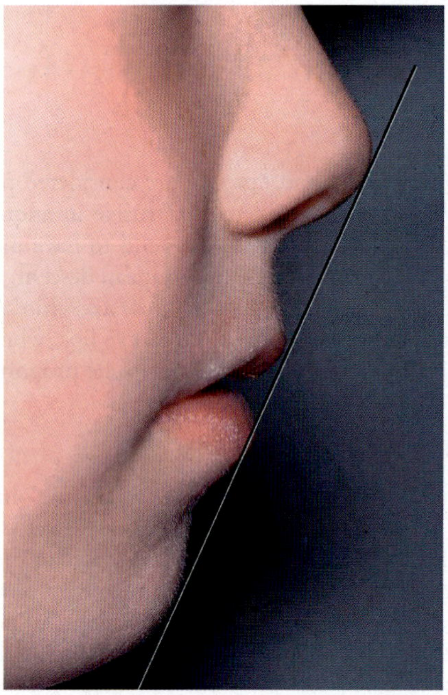

• **Fig. 24.4** The anteroposterior position of the lips is determined by drawing a line from the tip of the nose to the most anterior point on the soft tissue chin. The upper lip normally should lie slightly behind the line, whereas the lower lip should lie slightly in front of this line in the 3- to 6-year-old child.

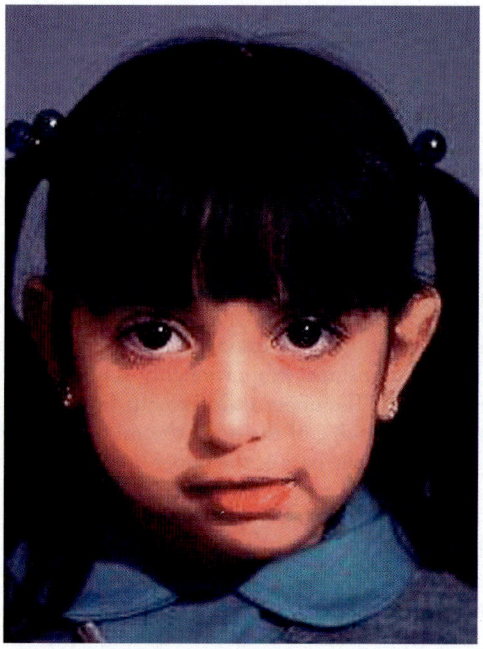

• **Fig. 24.5** This patient exhibits marked asymmetry that is the result of a congenital fusion of the left condyle and coronoid process to the temporal bone.

The maxillary dental midline should be compared with the upper facial midline. This helps determine where the midline of the mandibular teeth is relative to the face when it is compared with the upper dental midline.

During adolescence the face is beginning to assume adult-like features, and treatment decisions can be based more on current rather than projected facial appearance. This does not mean that growth is complete—only that it has slowed considerably from its previous pace during the early adolescent growth spurt. The adult profile tends to be straighter than the adolescent because of continued mandibular skeletal growth. In addition, the soft tissue of the chin increases slightly in thickness. The nose continues to grow in horizontal and vertical directions. Most of this growth is horizontal but the nasal tip tends to drop a small amount. The lips are less protrusive in adults because of these nasal and chin changes combined with a slight thinning of the soft tissue thickness of the lips.

Intraoral Examination

The intraoral examination begins with a review of the oral cavity, noting its general architecture and function. Soft tissue abnormalities of the cheeks, lips, tongue, palate, and floor of the mouth are identified.

Assessing clinical needs and patient oral hygiene skills is part of the examination process. This information should be used to formulate an individual hygiene strategy. If orthodontic treatment is considered, oral hygiene instructions should be given before orthodontic treatment is started and should be consistently reinforced during the treatment. In some cases, it is prudent to delay orthodontic treatment until oral hygiene can be maintained at an acceptable level.

An important portion of the intraoral examination is directed to the teeth. Each tooth should be explored and inspected visually. Selective periodontal probing may be performed, but the yield is likely to be minimal because of the infrequency of irreversible attachment loss in the primary dentition. Periodontal evaluation is more important in the mixed and permanent dentitions when periodontal problems begin to manifest.

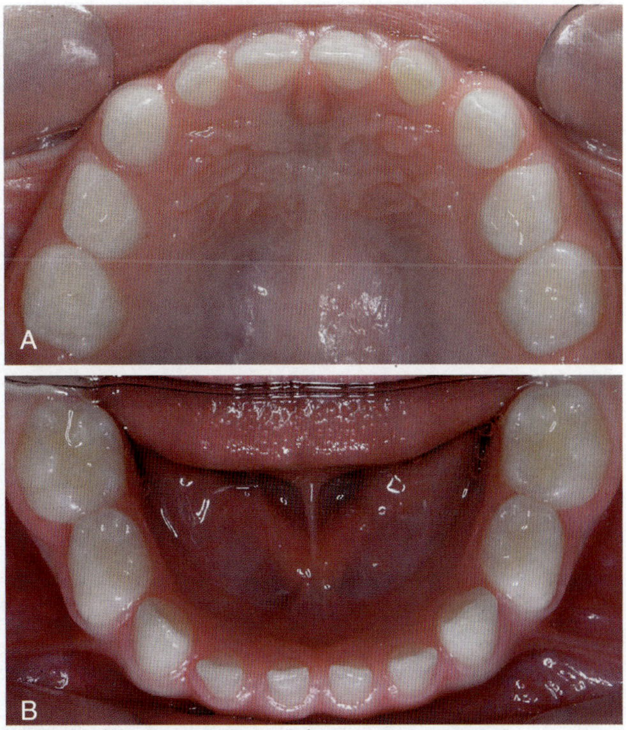

• **Fig. 24.6** These maxillary (A) and mandibular (B) arches show primate spaces (mesial to the maxillary canines and distal to the mandibular canines) and developmental spacing (space between the remaining teeth).

Occlusal Evaluation

The occlusion should be analyzed in three spatial planes. Each dental arch is examined individually to describe arch form and symmetry, spacing and crowding, and the presence or absence of teeth.

Alignment

Dental arches can be categorized as either U-shaped or V-shaped. The mandibular arch is normally U-shaped, whereas the maxillary arch can be either shape. The dental arch should be symmetrical in the anteroposterior and transverse dimensions. Individual teeth are compared with their antimeres to determine whether there is anteroposterior or transverse symmetry.

The ideal arch in the primary dentition has spacing between the teeth. Two types of spaces are identified. The first type, primate space, is located mesial to the maxillary canine and distal to the mandibular canine. Developmental space is the space between the remaining teeth (Fig. 24.6). Anterior spacing is desirable in the primary dentition because the permanent incisors are larger than their primary precursors. Although the presence of primate and developmental spacing does not ensure that the permanent dentition will erupt without crowding, these spaces usually alleviate some crowding during the transition from the primary to the mixed dentition. Crowding or overlapping teeth in the primary dentition may occur, although it is rare. True crowding in the primary dentition is not regarded as encouraging (Fig. 24.7).

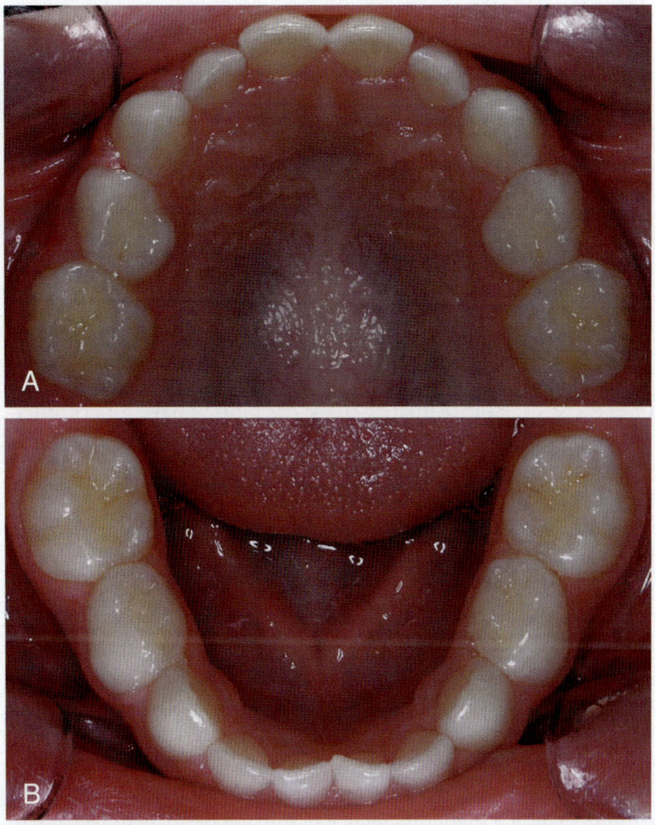

• **Fig. 24.7** These maxillary (A) and mandibular (B) arches show a lack of primate and developmental spaces.

Although it seems elementary, the clinician should carefully count the number of teeth in the mouth. Children in the 3- to 6-year-old age group should have all their primary teeth present. Those with delayed dental eruption may have either a very slow but normal eruption sequence or some isolated eruption problem. To distinguish the two, the eruption sequence of the child

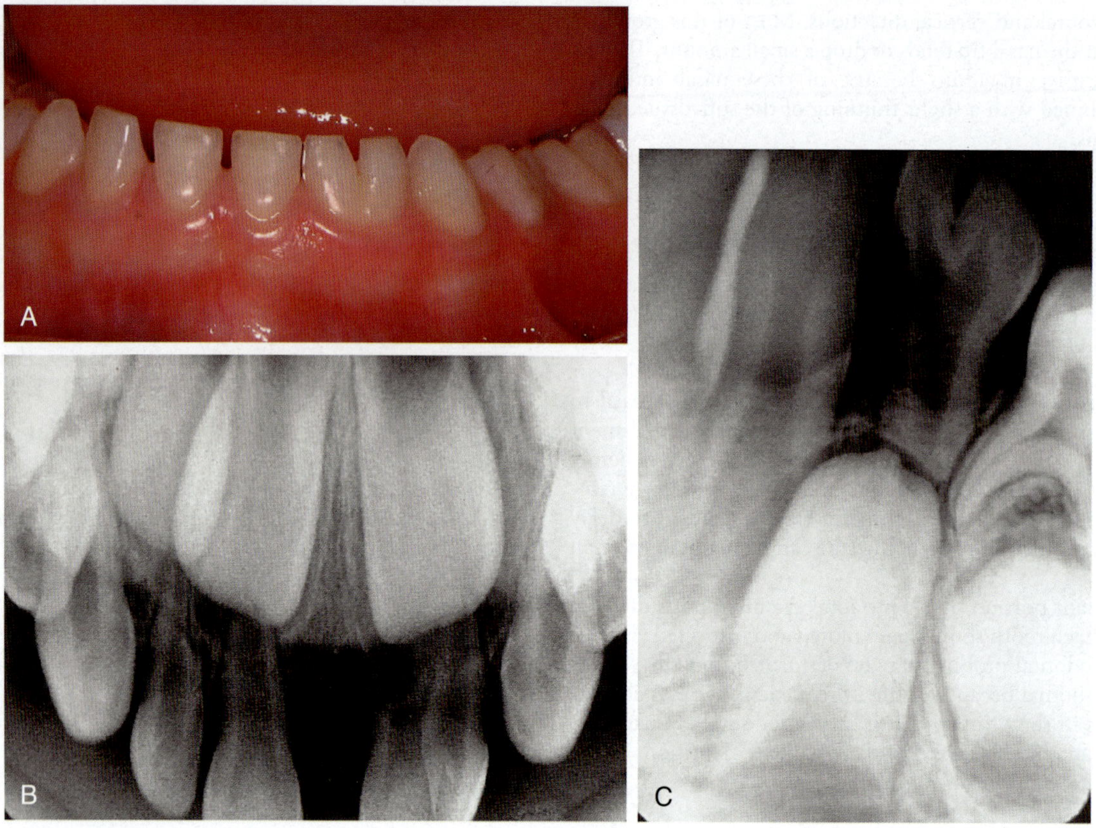

• **Fig. 24.8** (A) This patient shows what appears to be a geminated lower left lateral incisor. Supporting radiographs are often necessary to distinguish fusion from gemination. (B) These fused primary teeth are joined only at the dentin and have independent pulp chambers and canals. (C) This geminated primary tooth has a large crown and a common pulp canal. (Radiographs courtesy Dr. W. F. Vann.)

is compared with the normal sequence of eruption, and the eruption pattern on the right side is compared with that on the left. If the sequence seems to be appropriate, dental development is probably slow. If, however, the patient's eruption pattern deviates from the normal sequence and there are differences between the contralateral sides of the mouth, further investigation is warranted to determine whether teeth are missing or are impeded from erupting. The maxillary lateral incisor is the most common missing tooth in the primary dentition.[3]

Counting the teeth also reveals the presence of supernumerary or extra teeth. Approximately 0.3% of children have supernumerary teeth in the primary dentition. The prevalence of fused and geminated teeth is approximately 0.1% to 0.5%[3] (Fig. 24.8; see Chapter 20).

Disturbances in the initiation and proliferation stage of tooth development may lead to an abnormal number of teeth. Teeth that do not form are referred to as congenitally missing (Fig. 24.9). The most common missing teeth in the permanent dentition, apart from the maxillary and mandibular third molars, are the mandibular second premolar, maxillary lateral incisor, and maxillary second premolar in that order.[4] In general, the most distal tooth in a class of teeth is most liable to be congenitally missing. Some have looked at whether there is a genetic component to missing and impacted teeth. It is reported that patients with palatally impacted canines exhibit a higher incidence of missing permanent teeth than the general population and that several generations in the family will exhibit the same palatal impaction[5] (Fig. 24.10). Recent evidence suggests there are specific genes that cause specific tooth loss when there is a mutation.[6] It is apparent that future genetic study may identify more genes that affect tooth development. The practical implication of a missing anterior tooth is to look elsewhere in the mouth for more eruption or tooth development issues (additional missing teeth, impaction or transpositions).

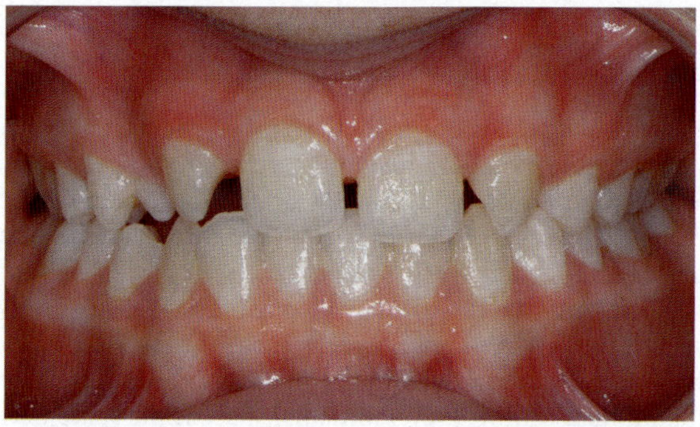

• **Fig. 24.9** This patient is congenitally missing both permanent maxillary lateral incisors, and the permanent maxillary canines have spontaneously substituted in their places. The most common missing teeth in the permanent dentition, besides the third molars, are the maxillary lateral incisor and the mandibular second premolar.

Another cause of missing or malformed teeth is radiation therapy or chemotherapy. This can affect the formation and

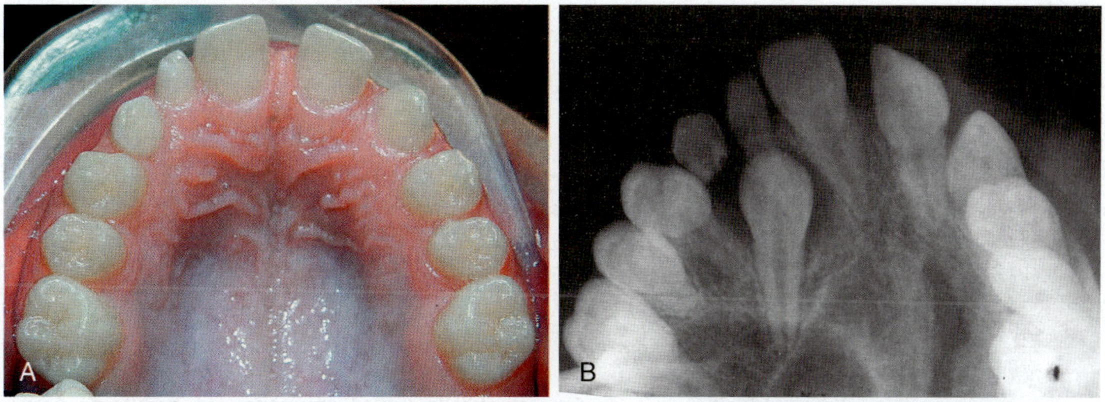

• **Fig. 24.10** (A) The occurrence of multiple anomalies of tooth position, number, and shape linked by genetics is demonstrated in this patient who has an erupted peg-shaped permanent maxillary right lateral incisor, and a retained primary maxillary right canine. (B) The occlusal radiograph shows the peg lateral, the missing permanent maxillary left lateral incisor, and the ectopically erupting permanent maxillary right canine.

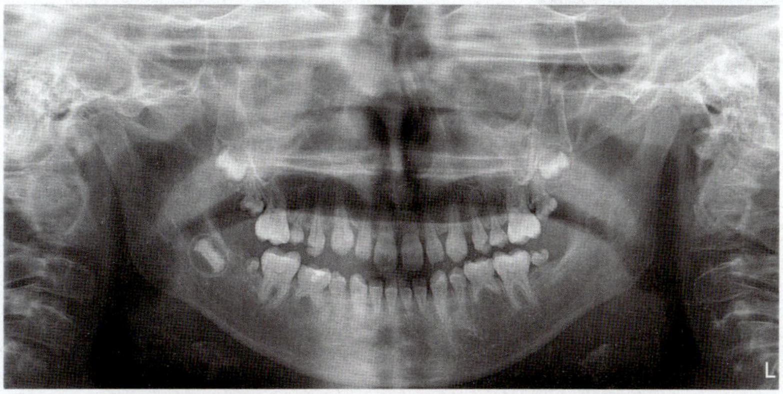

• **Fig. 24.11** This patient was diagnosed with a primitive neuroectodermal tumor and was treated with radiation and chemotherapy from the ages of 2 to 4 years. The teeth developing during that time period are stunted, missing, or have arrested root development. Of interest, the third molars are developing normally because their development started after the end of the therapy.

eruption of the teeth developing at the time or those in the field of the therapeutic beam. Generally, patients treated with radiation before age 5 years will have more anomalies of dental development, but patients receiving chemotherapy and older patients who still have developing teeth are likely affected (Fig. 24.11).[7]

Supernumerary teeth are teeth added to the normal complement of teeth. These teeth are found in about 2% of the population and are most often found in the maxillary midline region.[8] Midline supernumerary teeth are also called mesiodens (Fig. 24.12). Supernumerary teeth are also found distal to the maxillary molars and in the mandibular premolar regions.

Although not a tooth in the strictest sense, the odontoma is discussed in this section on tooth number. The odontoma is a benign mixed tumor of enamel and dentin that is diagnosed radiographically. Two types of odontomas are identified. Odontomas that resemble teeth are called compound odontomas; those that are irregularly shaped are labeled complex odontomas. Both types may interfere with normal tooth eruption and are usually treated by surgical removal before eruption problems arise but late enough to avoid surgical trauma to adjacent developing teeth (Fig. 24.13).

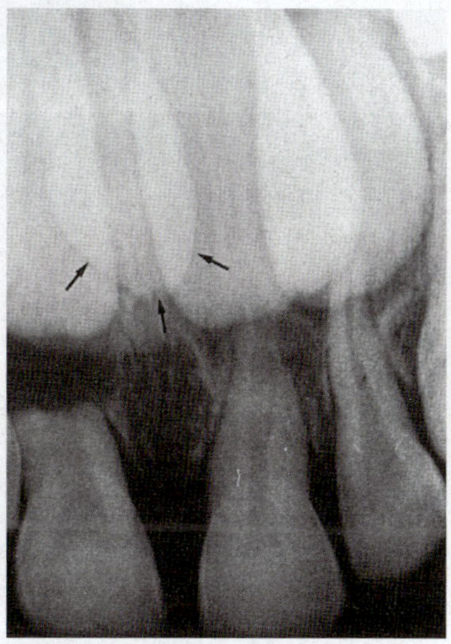

• **Fig. 24.12** A midline supernumerary tooth, or mesiodens, is situated between the unerupted maxillary central incisors. *Arrows* indicate the position of the mesiodens, which can cause disturbances in eruption and adjacent tooth formation.

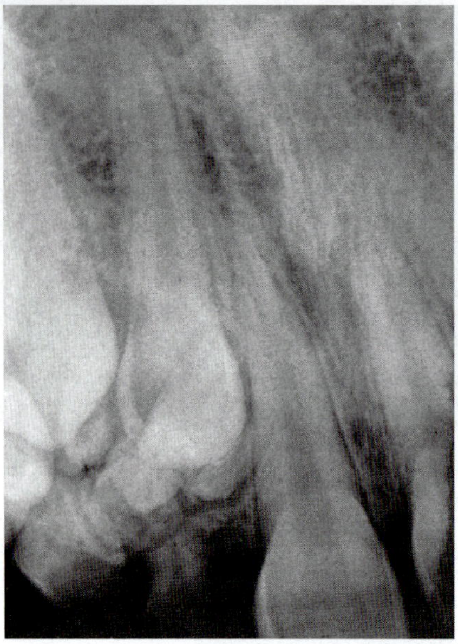

• **Fig. 24.13** An odontoma is impeding the eruption of the maxillary right lateral incisor and canine. The odontoma should be surgically removed before eruption problems arise but late enough to avoid surgical trauma to the adjacent developing teeth. (Courtesy Dr. Phillip R. Parker.)

Tooth Structure

Disturbances in the morphodifferentiation and histodifferentiation stages of tooth development result in alterations of tooth size and shape. Each arch should be examined for generalized large (macrodontia) or small (microdontia) teeth and for localized tooth size discrepancies. Generalized large or small teeth usually can be aligned so that there is a compatible occlusal relationship if the teeth in both arches are equally affected. However, localized tooth size problems make it difficult to establish good dental relationships. Again, the most distal tooth in the dental class is the one most often affected. Undersized maxillary lateral incisors and mandibular second premolars are the most common isolated problems in tooth size (see Fig. 24.10A). These also appear to be genetically linked anomalies, so evaluating patients with peg laterals should include evaluation for palatally displaced canines, additional missing teeth, and transpositions. Sometimes complex orthodontic and restorative treatment is necessary to achieve a harmonious occlusal relationship and satisfy aesthetic requirements when local tooth size problems exist. This type of treatment usually means distributing space between the teeth so that when the teeth are restored to normal size and contour, they fit in a good occlusal relationship with good anterior esthetics (Fig. 24.14). Other times, treatment may mean reducing the mesiodistal dimension of oversized crowns through interproximal reduction (Fig. 24.15).

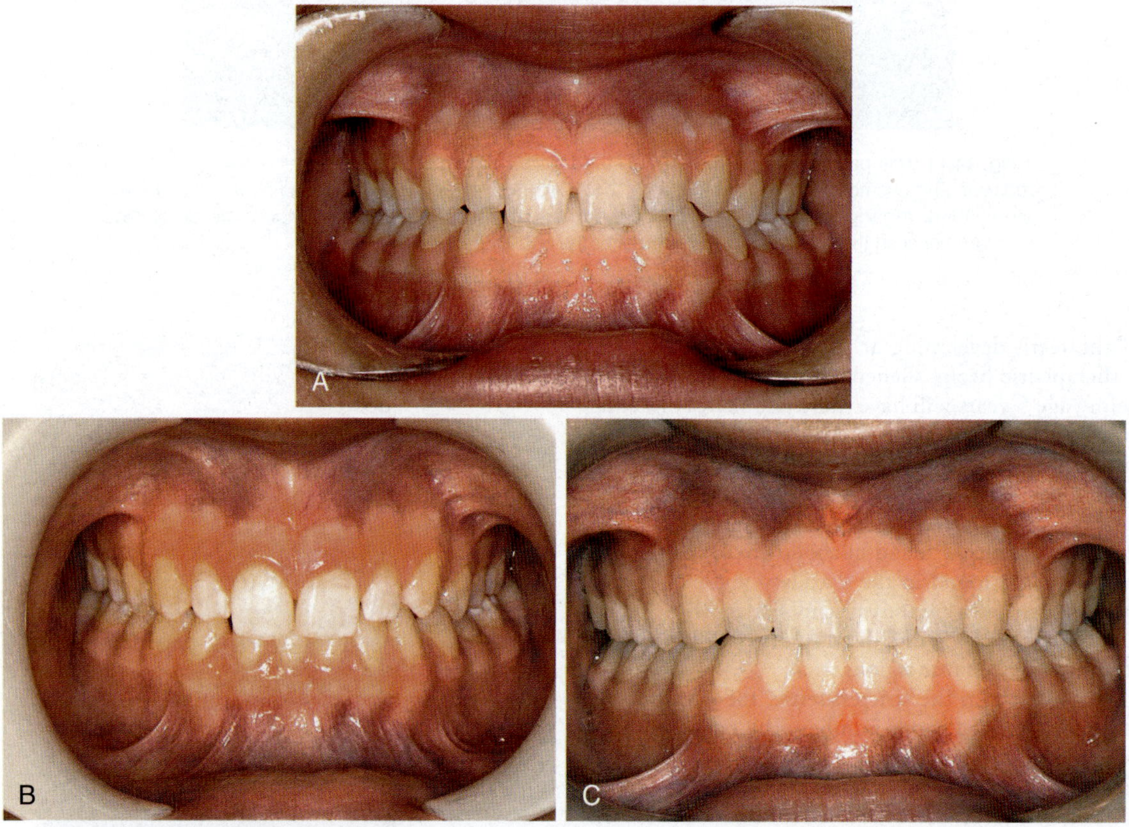

• **Fig. 24.14** (A) In this case, a maxillary tooth size deficiency contributed to the diastema. If the space was closed with orthodontics, the resulting occlusion would not be correct. In addition, the tapered crown form of the central incisor would result in less than ideal aesthetics. (B) Composite resin was added to the mesial surface of both central incisors before orthodontic treatment to correct the tooth size deficiency and give the teeth normal contour. (C) The orthodontic result shows excellent occlusion and aesthetics.

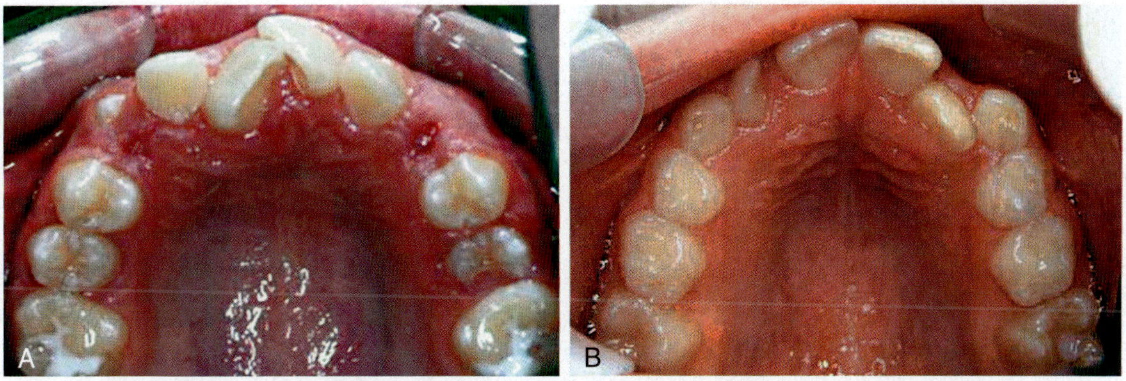

• **Fig. 24.15** (A) The permanent maxillary right central incisor is substantially larger than the contralateral left central incisor. (B) The permanent maxillary left lateral incisor shown here in a lingual position is at least 2 mm larger than normal and the contralateral tooth. Isolated teeth such as these often require mesiodistal interproximal reduction to fit harmoniously in a final occlusion.

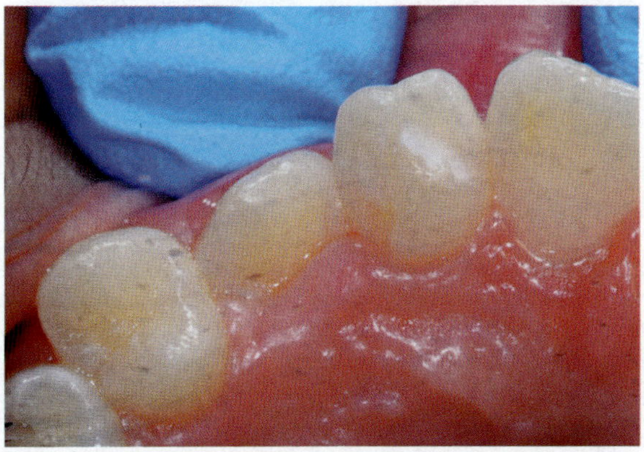

• **Fig. 24.16** This patient has a talon cusp on the maxillary right lateral incisor. The enamel protuberance may have a pulp horn in it and cannot just simply be reduced by abrasion with a bur. These anomalies can cause interference in the occlusion and prohibit normal overbite and overjet. Usually, periodic gradual reduction with a bur will allow the pulp horn to recede, preserve tooth vitality, and improve the morphology toward a normal occlusion.

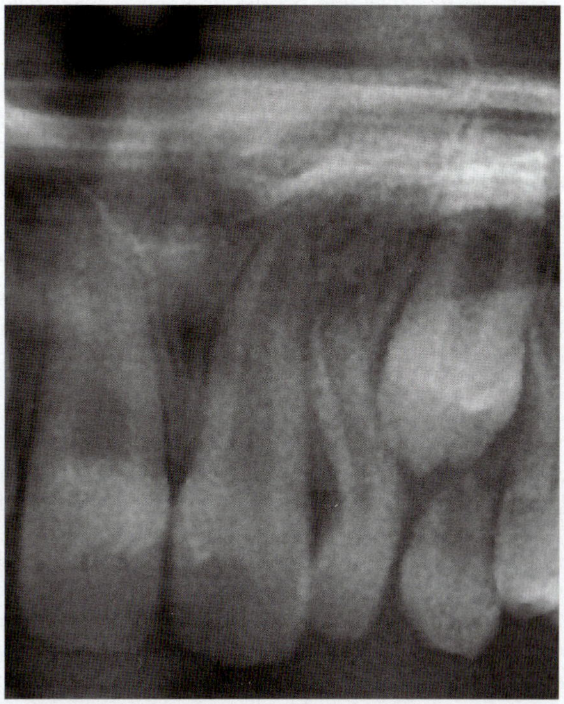

• **Fig. 24.17** Root structure abnormalities, such as this dilacerated maxillary left lateral incisor, make orthodontic movement of teeth very difficult. A dilaceration of this magnitude makes the root more susceptible to apical resorption and complicates the final positioning of the crown and root.

Teeth with abnormal crown and root morphologic characteristics may create occlusal problems. Careful clinical and radiographic examination is necessary to diagnose these problems. If the abnormality involves the crown (maxillary peg lateral or talon cusp), either the crown should be recontoured by addition of restorative material to increase its size or the talon cusp should be reduced in size by selective equilibration to eliminate occlusal interference (Fig. 24.16). Both conditions usually require tooth movement before definitive restorative care to obtain an aesthetically pleasing and functional result. Root structure abnormalities such as significant dilaceration may make orthodontic movement of teeth difficult (Fig. 24.17). Often the portion of the root apical to the irregularity is resorbed or remodeled during tooth movement. If a tooth with root abnormalities is scheduled for extraction, it may be prudent to refer the patient to a specialist because the abnormality will certainly complicate the extraction. Finally, fused or geminated teeth can pose difficulties due to their size. The clinician should consult with other dental specialists because the treatment will often involve a combination of endodontics, surgery, orthodontics, and restorative care.[9,10]

In the early mixed dentition, four upper and lower incisors should be evident early on. When they are not, concern and follow-up are warranted. The clinician should recognize that it is highly unusual for a child of 9 not to have all the upper and lower incisors (Fig. 24.18). If not present, the clinician should investigate why they are not and develop an appropriate treatment plan to address it. Likewise, maxillary permanent canines should be positively palpated, or their existence confirmed radiographically by age 10 years. It appears that cone beam computed tomography (CBCT) images are superior to 2D images for determining the status of canines and the adjacent teeth.[11] A sensible method, then, is to obtain a panoramic radiograph, which

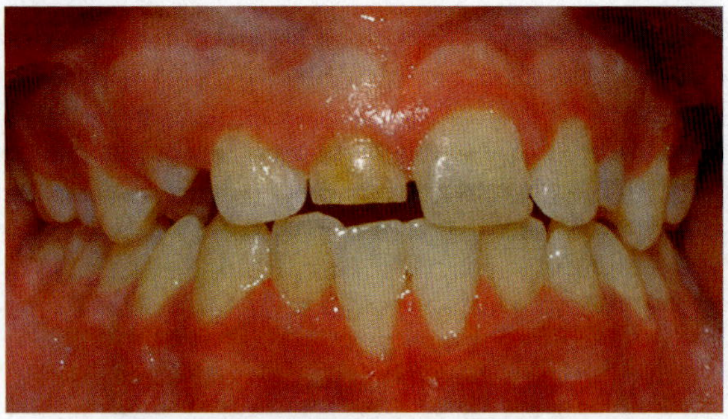

• **Fig. 24.18** All permanent incisors should have erupted by 9 years of age. This patient has a retained primary maxillary central incisor and obvious eruption problems. This clinical sign should not be overlooked and has impact on the developing dentition and the child's self-esteem.

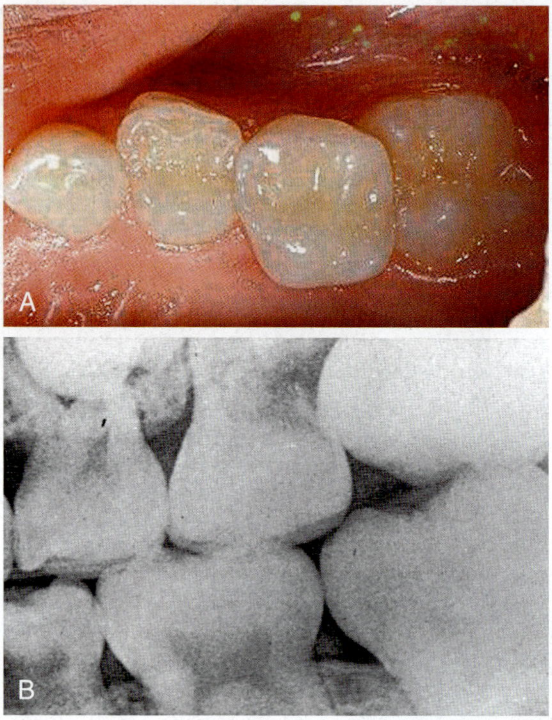

• **Fig. 24.19** In ectopic eruption, the permanent first molar resorbs a portion of the distal root of the primary second molar. (A) In this case, the permanent first molar has lodged under the primary second molar crown. In other cases, the permanent molar spontaneously "jumps" or moves distally and erupts into the normal position. (B) The distal resorption of the primary molar root is evident on this radiograph.

can reveal other related anomalies when missing anterior teeth (lateral incisors or canines) or peg-shaped lateral incisors are encountered. Then, depending on the findings, a small field-of-view CBCT may be indicated. These views can be supplemented with a traditional cephalometric digital image if required for limited or comprehensive orthodontic care. This exposes the patient to less radiation than would be delivered if a full-field CBCT was initially obtained. The details of these examinations are noted in Chapter 17.

Tooth Position

The position of erupted and unerupted permanent teeth in the mixed dentition should be noted and compared with the normal sequence and time of eruption. Minor asymmetry in dental eruption is normal, and there is little cause for concern if less than 6 months difference in eruption exists between contralateral sides of the mouth. Five tooth positioning problems are associated with the mixed dentition: ectopic eruption, transposition, impaction, primary failure of eruption, and the midline diastema. Interestingly, there appears to be a genetic component to some of these tooth position problems. Several studies have shown a genetic link between missing teeth, tooth anomalies, and altered eruption paths.[5,12–14] There seems to be clustering of these problems. If one of these conditions is identified, the clinician should examine the patient for these other related problems as mentioned earlier.

Ectopic eruption describes a path of eruption that causes root resorption of a portion or all the adjacent primary tooth. Ectopic eruption is most often associated with the permanent maxillary first molar, mandibular lateral incisor, and maxillary canine.[15–17] In ectopic eruption of the permanent first molar, a portion of the erupting first molar resorbs the distal root of the primary second molar and is inhibited from erupting by the distal portion of the primary molar (Fig. 24.19). In many cases, the permanent molar spontaneously "jumps" or moves distally and erupts into the correct position. In other cases, the permanent molar lodges under the primary molar crown and no longer erupts. Usually, no pain or discomfort is associated with ectopic eruption unless communication develops between the oral cavity and the pulpal tissue of the primary molar, causing an abscess. Permanent molar ectopic eruption is often detected during clinical examinations and confirmed with routine bitewing radiographs.

The prevalence of permanent first molar ectopic eruption is reported to be 3% to 4%.[18] Several possible causes of ectopic molar eruption have been proposed: (1) the maxillary teeth are larger than normal, (2) the maxilla is smaller than normal, (3) the maxilla is positioned further posteriorly than normal in relation to the cranial base, or (4) the angulation of the erupting maxillary permanent first molar is abnormal.[19,20] Although ectopic molar eruption may occur in the mandibular arch, it is more common in the maxilla.

Ectopic eruption of the permanent lateral incisor is most common in the mandibular arch. The erupting incisor resorbs all or a portion of the primary canine root because the path of eruption is abnormal, there is transitional crowding from the primary to the permanent dentition, or there is a true arch length deficiency. The diagnosis is generally signaled by premature primary canine exfoliation, often accompanied by a midline shift to the side of the ectopic eruption or impeded eruption of the lateral incisor, or it is discovered on an occlusal radiograph (Fig. 24.20).

The third common type of ectopic eruption occurs with maxillary permanent canine eruption and associated resorption of the permanent lateral incisor (Fig. 24.21). Studies have shown that if canines erupt from a more medial position in the dental arch and with a slightly more mesial horizontal path of eruption (an average of 10 degrees), there is a greater risk of lateral incisor resorption. It is recommended to remove the primary canine to promote more ideal canine eruption if the canine cusp on images is positioned medially to the midline of the lateral incisor.[15,21] Some investigations suggest additional treatment to improve canine position, such as primary canine removal in conjunction with maxillary expansion.[22]

A related phenomenon is the lingual eruption of the permanent incisors, predominantly the mandibular incisors (Fig. 24.22). The prevalence of lingually erupting mandibular incisors is about

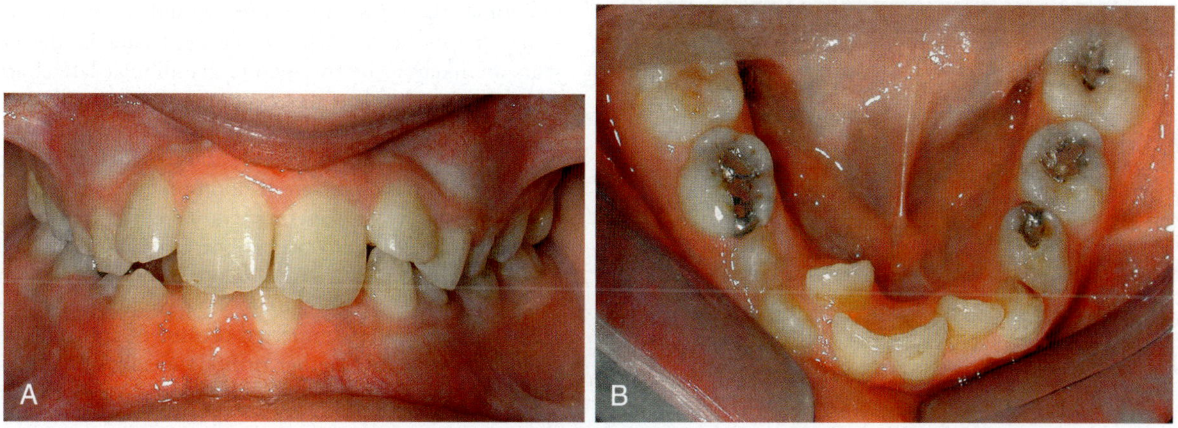

• **Fig. 24.20** When a primary canine is lost because of ectopic eruption of a permanent lateral incisor, the midline often shifts to the side of the lost primary canine. (A) It is apparent from this view that the mandibular midline has shifted to the patient's right. (B) The permanent right lateral incisor is now blocked to the lingual as a consequence of the mandibular midline shift.

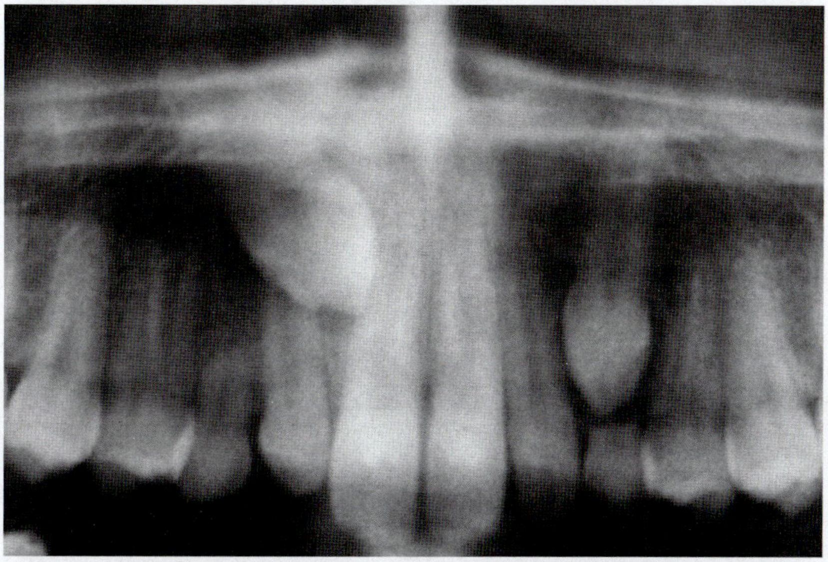

• **Fig. 24.21** The maxillary right canine has erupted into the lateral incisor space and resorbed a portion of the root. This type of resorption is more common than believed, but often not to this extent.

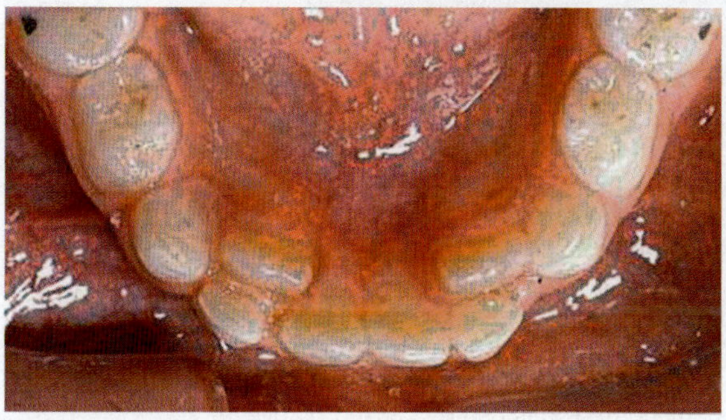

• **Fig. 24.22** Ectopic eruption of the permanent lateral incisors is most common in the mandibular arch. In this example, the mandibular lateral incisors erupted lingual to their ideal position and the primary laterals are still present. In some cases, the lateral incisors erupt into a more normal position but cause premature exfoliation of the primary canine.

10%.[23] The cause of ectopic and lingually erupting incisors is not well established. One explanation suggests that ectopic and lingual eruption of the incisors results from an abnormal pattern of resorption. Alternatively, it has been suggested that lingual eruption is a variation of the normal eruption pattern because the lower incisor tooth buds form lingual to the primary incisors and may not migrate facially.

Transposition occurs when there is "a positional interchange of two adjacent teeth, especially their roots or the development or eruption of a tooth in a position occupied normally by a nonadjacent tooth."[14] Usually transpositions are observed later in the transitional dentition years. The early-stage transposition is uncommon but is the type of transposition observed in the early mixed-dentition years (Fig. 24.23). This usually is a transposition of the mandibular lateral incisor and canine.[13] The lateral incisor will show distal tipping, resorption of the primary canine (and

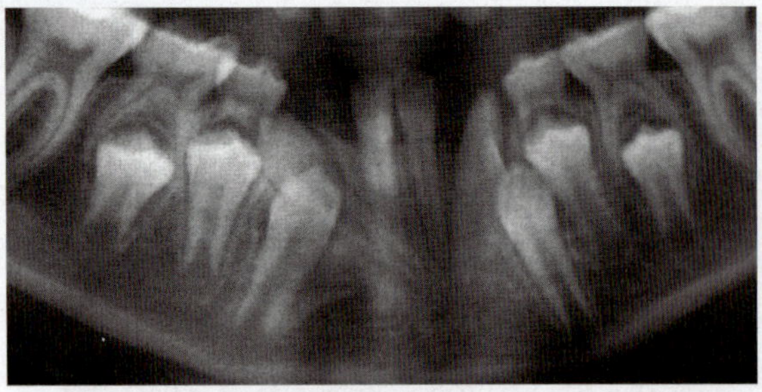

• **Fig. 24.23** Early-stage transposition of the mandibular lateral incisors and the canines. Note that the permanent mandibular right lateral incisor has resorbed the primary canine and the primary first molar is about to be lost. If intercepted early, true transposition will not occur.

sometimes the primary first molar), and rotation as it migrates. Other transpositions that are observed later in the transitional years are likely to be the mature mandibular lateral and canine, and the more prevalent transpositions of the maxillary canine and first premolar and maxillary canine and lateral incisor.[14]

Tooth impaction, as noted earlier, is diagnosed during the clinical examination or from appropriate radiographs. Overretained primary teeth, supernumerary teeth, severe crowding, or a failure in the eruption mechanism can cause impaction of the anterior teeth (Fig. 24.24A). Often the permanent tooth erupts if the overretained primary tooth or supernumerary tooth is removed. If the tooth is impacted because of crowding, it is necessary to provide space either orthodontically or by extraction to allow eruption. Generally, the last tooth to erupt in an arch or

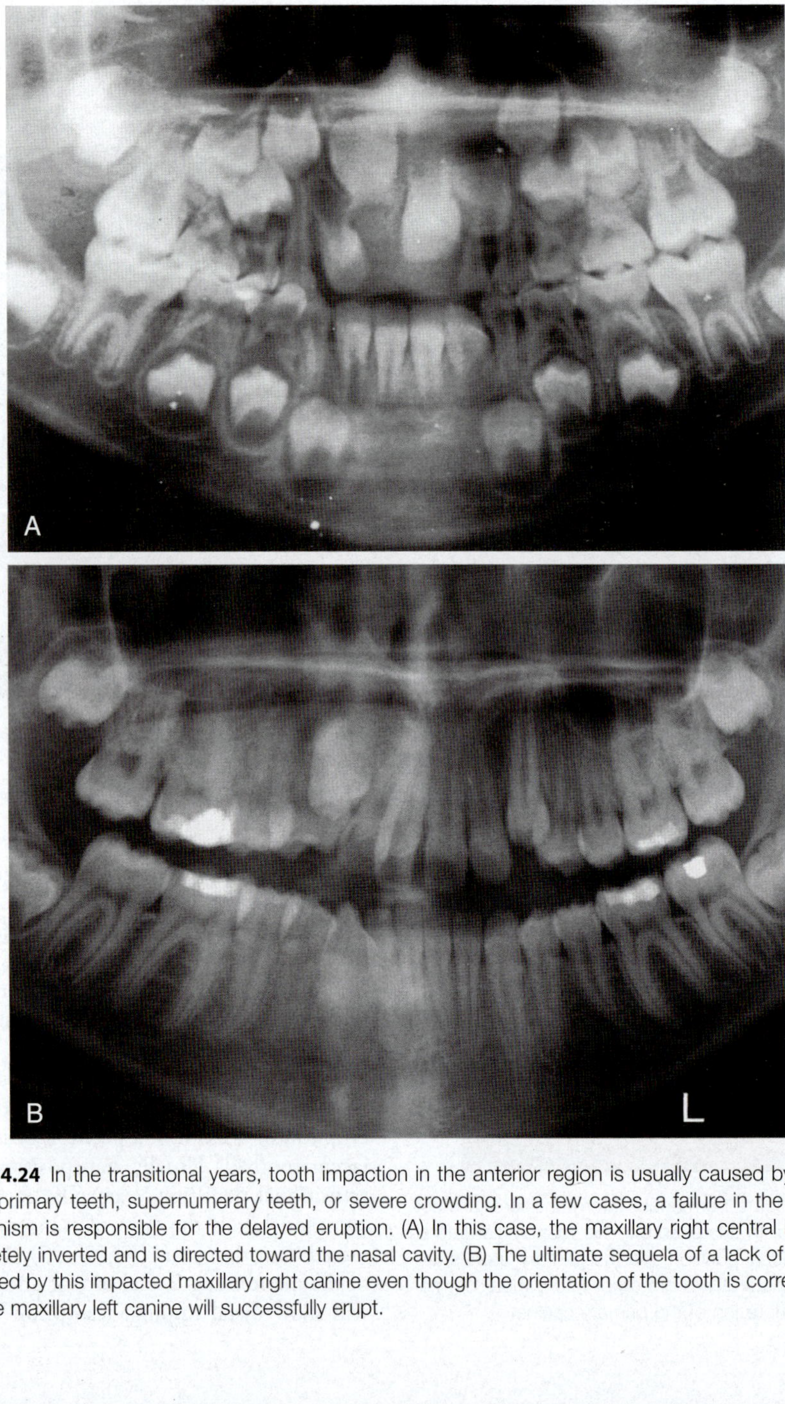

• **Fig. 24.24** In the transitional years, tooth impaction in the anterior region is usually caused by overretained primary teeth, supernumerary teeth, or severe crowding. In a few cases, a failure in the eruption mechanism is responsible for the delayed eruption. (A) In this case, the maxillary right central incisor is completely inverted and is directed toward the nasal cavity. (B) The ultimate sequela of a lack of space is illustrated by this impacted maxillary right canine even though the orientation of the tooth is correct. Note that the maxillary left canine will successfully erupt.

quadrant is impacted because all the space is previously spoken for. This mechanism or the aberrant eruption direction usually is the cause of impaction of the maxillary canine. The maxillary canine is most often the last tooth to erupt into the arch. It also erupts or travels the longest distance to take its place in the arch. These two factors combine to make the maxillary canine the most impacted tooth in the maxillary arch and indeed the mouth (see Fig. 24.24B). Posterior tooth impaction is normally the result of inadequate arch length. Inadequate arch length is caused by a tooth–jaw size discrepancy or space loss because of premature primary tooth loss. If the arch length problem is generalized, either permanent teeth should be removed, or the arch should be expanded to allow eruption of all the permanent teeth. Limited, localized crowding due to space loss can be treated by orthodontically regaining the lost space.

At times the permanent first molar fails to erupt or erupts partially. The dilemma for the clinician is to diagnose the problem. There seem to be three diagnoses for an unerupted permanent molar. The first is primary failure of eruption. Primary failure of eruption is an unusual eruption problem that affects the posterior teeth (Fig. 24.25). It is diagnosed when a tooth fails to erupt despite the presence of adequate space and the absence of overlying hard tissue that prevents eruption. Furthermore, all teeth distal to the affected tooth also fail to erupt. The cause of primary failure of eruption is unknown but appears to have a genetic component.[24–26] The second cause of an unerupted permanent molar is mechanical failure of eruption. Two characteristics distinguish mechanical failure of eruption from primary failure of eruption. The first is that some type of mechanical obstruction can explain the lack of eruption. The path of eruption is not clear like primary failure eruption. Obstruction can be from lack of space, a developmental problem with the tooth, or placement of the tongue. Removal of the obstruction will generally allow tooth movement. The other characteristic distinguishing primary from mechanical failure of eruption is that teeth distal to the affected tooth will erupt. This is difficult to determine early in treatment. Ankylosis of the tooth is the third diagnosis for an unerupted tooth. A tooth with ankylosis will not erupt even if there is space and the teeth distal are not affected.[27]

A small, maxillary midline diastema in the early mixed dentition is normal (Fig. 24.26). Typically, it is caused by the position of the unerupted lateral incisors or canines (Fig. 24.27A). The unerupted teeth are positioned superior and distal to the roots of the central incisors, and they direct the central incisor roots toward the midline and the crowns toward the distal (see Fig. 24.27B). As the lateral incisors or canines erupt, the incisors upright themselves slowly and the midline space begins to close. Treatment to close a diastema is usually delayed until the permanent canines are fully erupted unless the space available for eruption of the lateral incisors or canines is severely limited or the aesthetics are a compelling concern. If the diastema is larger than 2 mm, the cause may be a mesiodens (see Fig. 24.12), a localized tooth size problem, or abnormal incisor positioning. A mesiodens is usually discovered on radiographic examination, and its removal normally allows the diastema to close. A size mismatch between the upper and lower teeth may result in a diastema. In this situation, the maxillary incisor crowns are small or excessively tapered, although the mandibular teeth may be too large in relation to the maxillary teeth. If large spaces are present, a combination of tooth movement and anterior restorations is required to correct the size discrepancy. Abnormal incisor positioning and protrusion also may result in a midline diastema. The abnormal positioning may be due to past or present finger habits or to abnormal eruption. The best treatment is to first eliminate the habit and then to retract the incisors orthodontically and consolidate space.

Anteroposterior Dimension

After the maxillary and mandibular arches have been examined for symmetry, spacing, and number of teeth, the relationship of the two arches to each other is examined. In the anteroposterior dimension, primary molar and canine relationships are determined and compared with the skeletal classification. In the primary dentition, molars are called flush terminal plane, mesial step, or distal step (Fig. 24.28). Primary canines are classified as class I, class II, class III, or end-to-end. These dental classifications generally reflect the skeletal classification.

Primary molar relationships, as described by the distal surfaces of the primary second molar, are worthy of attention not only because they describe the relationship of the primary mandibular teeth to the primary maxillary teeth but also because these surfaces guide the permanent molars into occlusion and determine the permanent molar relationships. Documenting primary molar relationships also allows one to follow the effects of growth or treatment.

In the mixed and permanent dentitions, permanent molar and canine relationships should be noted and compared with the anteroposterior skeletal relationships that were determined during the extraoral examination. Permanent molar and canine

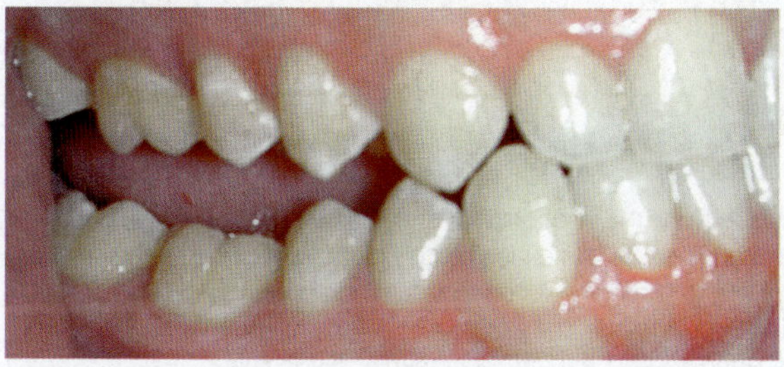

• **Fig. 24.25** Primary failure of eruption usually presents as a posterior segment of open bite. It appears to cause eruption problems with all teeth posterior to the most anterior affected tooth in that quadrant. In this case, given the occlusal plane, it appears that the lower teeth are involved. Treatment can be challenging and the open bite must be closed surgically or prosthetically after growth has ceased.

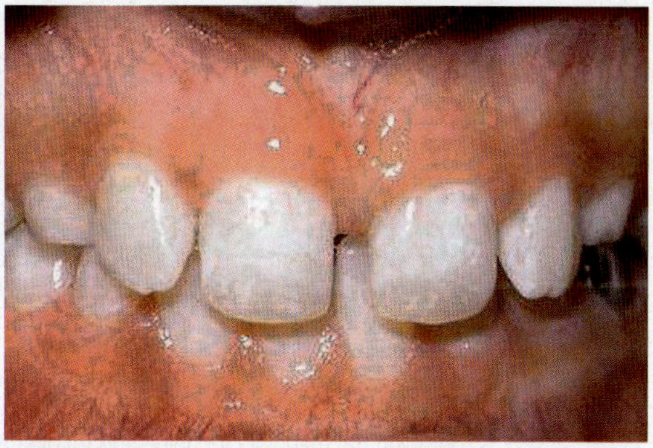

• **Fig. 24.26** A small maxillary midline diastema is normal in the mixed dentition. The diastema tends to close with the eruption of the permanent maxillary lateral incisors and canines.

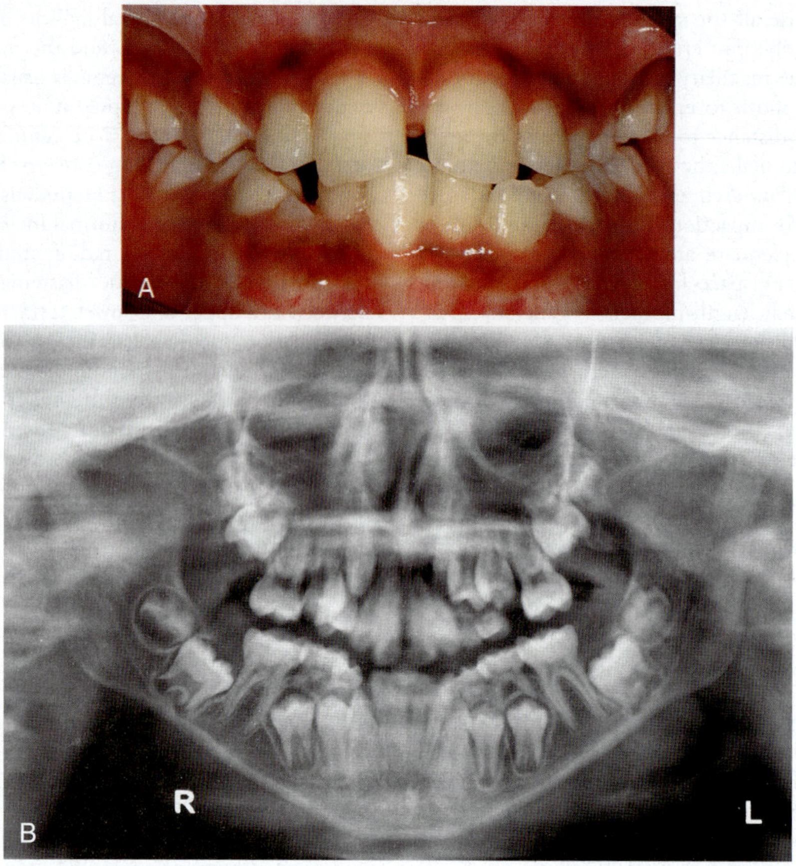

• **Fig. 24.27** (A) The "ugly duckling" stage is evident when the crowns of the lateral incisors tip distally and open diastema between the anterior teeth. (B) The permanent canines are pushing against the roots of the permanent lateral incisors. Some of the anterior space will close with the eruption of the canines.

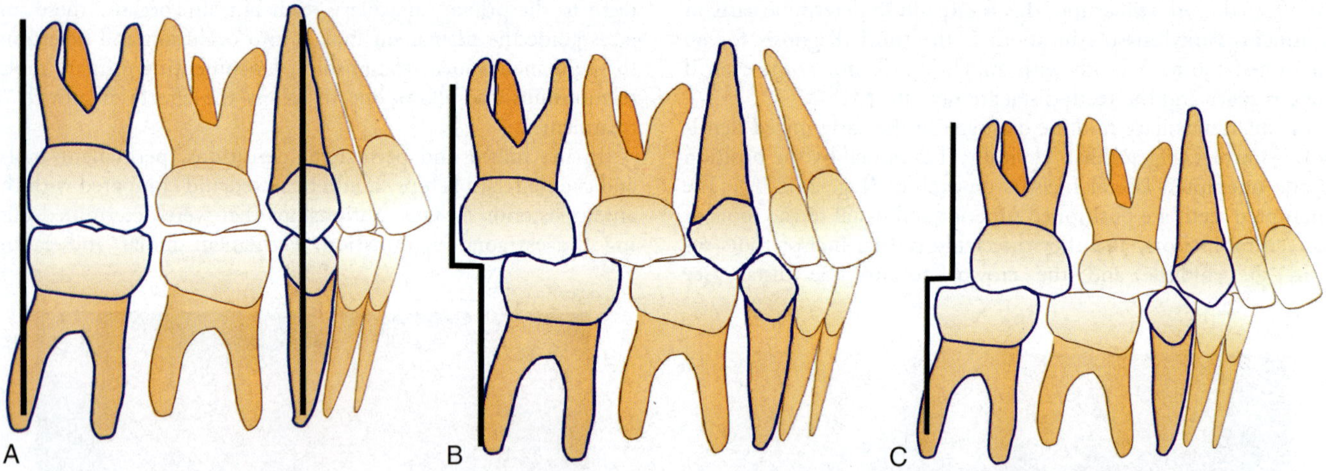

• **Fig. 24.28** (A) In the primary dentition, an occlusion is classified per the relationship of the mandibular second molars and canines to the maxillary second molars and canines. In this example, the distal surface of the mandibular second molar is flush with the distal surface of the maxillary second molar. This primary molar relationship is called flush terminal plane. The long axis of the mandibular canine is coincident with the long axis of the maxillary canine. This is described as an end-to-end canine relationship. (B) In this example, the distal surface of the mandibular molar is mesial to the distal surface of the maxillary molar. This primary molar relationship is termed mesial step. The maxillary canine is positioned in the embrasure between the mandibular canine and the first molar. This is described as a class I canine relationship. (C) In this example, the distal surface of the mandibular molar is distal to the distal surface of the maxillary molar. This primary molar relationship is called distal step. The maxillary canine is positioned in the embrasure between the mandibular canine and the lateral incisor. This is described as a class II canine relationship.

relationships are illustrated in Fig. 24.29. Dental relationships generally reflect the underlying skeletal relationships, including asymmetry, although it is feasible to have different dental and skeletal relationships if teeth are missing or have drifted. For example, a person with a class I skeletal relationship may have a class II molar relationship if there has been posterior space loss and the permanent maxillary first molar drifted forward into the space (Fig. 24.30).

Overjet, the horizontal overlap of the maxillary and mandibular incisors, is measured in millimeters (Fig. 24.31). It may be more helpful to describe overjet as ideal, excessive, or deficient rather than provide its measurement in millimeters.

If the permanent teeth are properly aligned in the alveolar bone at a normal angulation, overjet is a direct measurement of the relationship between the dental arches. Normal overjet is approximately 2 mm; therefore the discrepancy between the arches can be calculated by subtracting 2 mm from the measured overjet. Incisor position is not always ideal, however, and estimates of dental arch discrepancies must be adjusted if both upper and lower anterior teeth are either protrusive or retrusive.

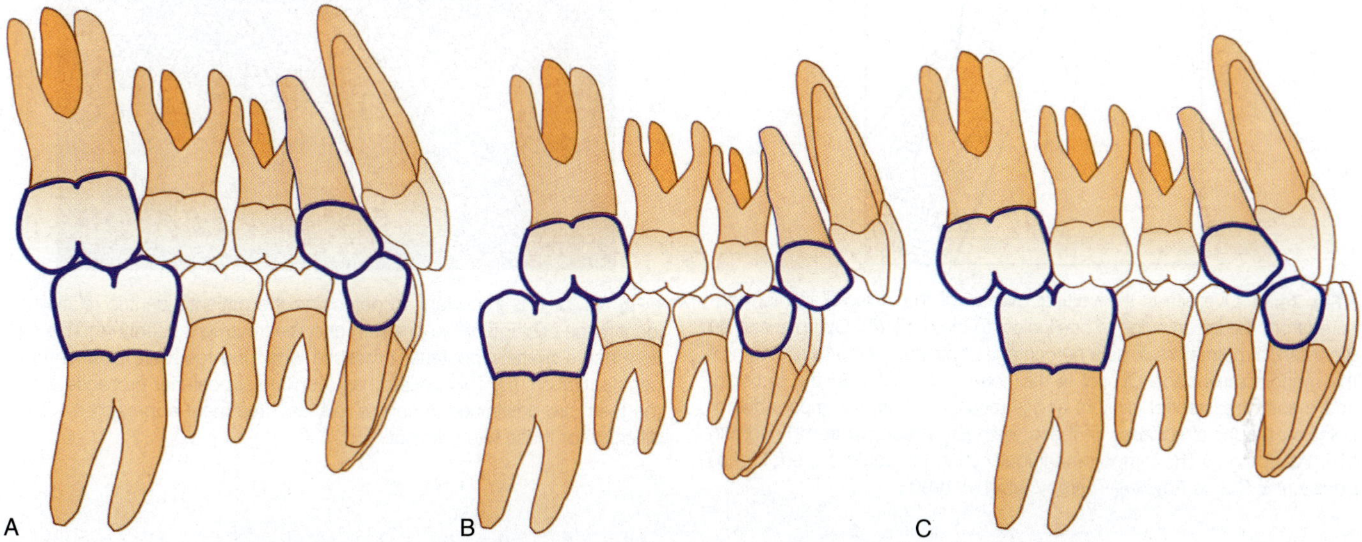

• **Fig. 24.29** (A) In the permanent dentition, permanent molar and canine relationships are determined and compared with the anteroposterior skeletal relationships. To determine molar relationships, the position of the mesiobuccal cusp of the permanent maxillary first molar is related to the position of the facial groove of the permanent mandibular first molar. If the mesiobuccal cusp occludes in the facial groove, the molar relationship is called class I. The canine relationship is determined by the relationship of the maxillary canine to the embrasure between the mandibular canine and the first premolar (or primary first molar). If the maxillary canine occludes in the embrasure, the canine relationship is also called class I. (B) If the mesiobuccal cusp of the permanent maxillary first molar occludes mesial to the mandibular facial groove, the molar relationship is called class II. The canine relationship is called class II if the maxillary canine occludes mesial to the mandibular canine–first premolar embrasure. (C) If the mesiobuccal cusp of the permanent maxillary first molar occludes distal to the mandibular facial groove, the molar relationship is called class III. The canine relationship is class III if the maxillary canine occludes distal to the mandibular canine–first premolar embrasure.

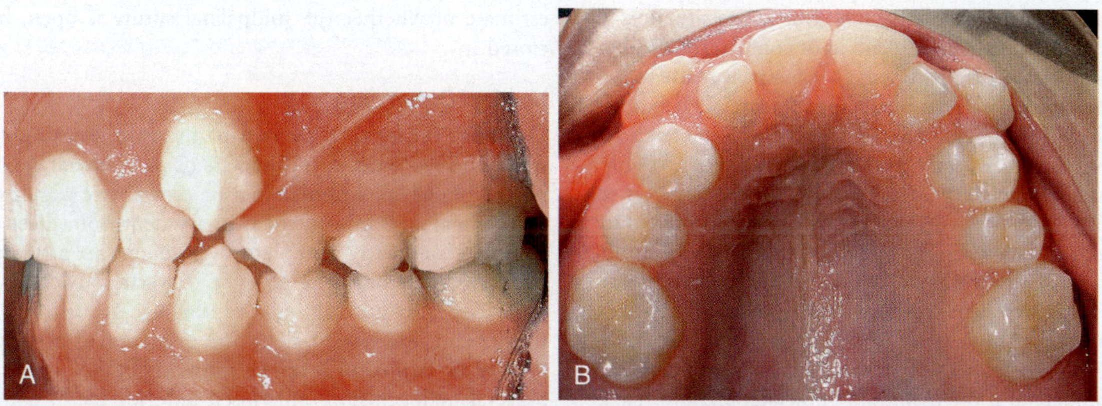

• **Fig. 24.30** Space loss can cause dental relationships to not reflect skeletal relationships. (A) This patient had maxillary posterior space loss with mesial drift so that the molars are class II and not reflective of the skeletal class I relationships. (B) The space loss caused the permanent canines to be blocked to the facial.

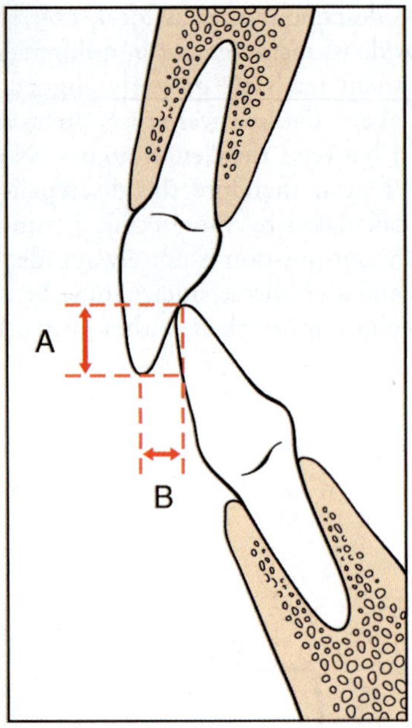

• **Fig. 24.31** Overbite is the vertical overlap of the incisors and is measured from the incisal edge of one incisor to the other *(A)*. Overbite can be recorded in millimeters or as a percentage of overlap of the total length of the mandibular incisor. Overjet is the horizontal overlap of the maxillary and mandibular central incisors and is measured from the most anterior point on the facial surfaces of these teeth *(B)*. (Redrawn from Friedman MH, Weisberg J. The temporomandibular joint. In: Gould JA, ed. *Orthopedics and Sports Physical Therapy.* Mosby; 1990.)

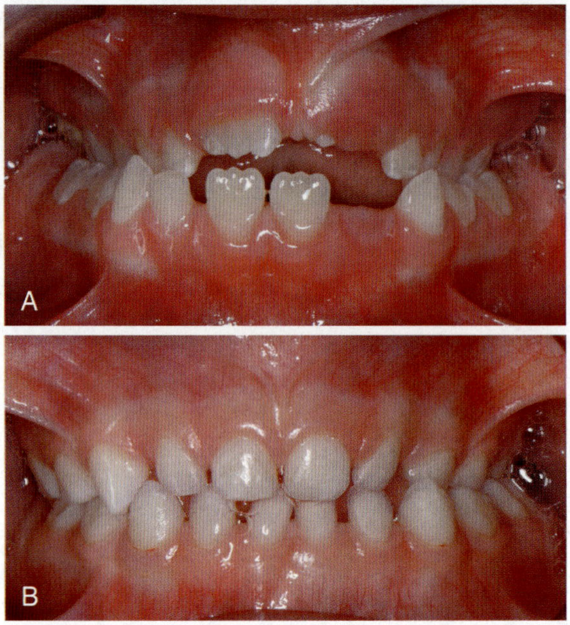

• **Fig. 24.32** It is important to determine the patient's centric relation to identify the etiology of the problem and the treatment needs. (A) This patient has a bilateral posterior crossbite when the teeth are positioned in centric relation. (B) This patient has a unilateral posterior crossbite when the teeth are positioned in centric relation. Treatment approaches will be different for these two patients.

Transverse Relationship

The transverse relationship is examined for midline discrepancies and posterior crossbites. The midline of each arch is compared with the other and with the midsagittal plane. Remember that the upper midline was evaluated to the facial midline during the facial evaluation.

A large midline discrepancy is unusual in the early primary dentition, and clinicians should be suspicious of a mandibular shift. The presence of a mandibular shift is often indicative of a posterior crossbite with a centric relation to centric occlusion shift.

If a posterior crossbite is encountered, the clinician should try to determine the cause. The majority of posterior crossbites are due to constriction of the maxillary arch. This is one situation in which diagnostic casts are helpful to aid in or confirm the diagnosis. After the arch at fault is identified, an attempt is made to determine whether the crossbite is bilateral or unilateral. If models are available, they can be measured to determine whether teeth are equidistant from the midpalatal raphe. If models are not available, the determination must be made clinically. The first step is to guide the mandible into centric relation. If teeth are in crossbite on both sides of the arch when the mandible is in centric relation, the child has a bilateral crossbite. If the teeth are in crossbite on only one side of the arch when the mandible is in centric relation, the crossbite is unilateral (Fig. 24.32). It is important to check that the mandible is in centric relation because a bilateral crossbite appears to be unilateral if the mandible shifts laterally into maximal intercuspation. The child shifts the jaw because the teeth do not fit well together, and the bite is uncomfortable because of dental interferences. A true unilateral crossbite that is due to a unilateral maxillary constriction in the primary dentition is rare but can occur.

In the mixed and permanent dentitions, dental midline deviations are either the result of moderate to severe crowding or ectopic eruption and tooth loss with a shift of the midline as teeth realign in the newly available space (see Fig. 24.20). Functional deviations of the mandible are identified by noting discrepancies between centric relation and centric occlusion. In the early mixed-dentition years, treatments for both skeletal and dental crossbites are essentially the same. As the child becomes older, it becomes more critical to identify whether a crossbite is due to skeletal or dental causes because the midpalatal suture becomes more interdigitated over time. The management of posterior crossbite in the complete permanent dentition varies according to whether the crossbite is skeletal or dental in origin and the estimate of whether the midpalatal suture is open, bridged, or closed.

Vertical Dimension

Overbite, the vertical overlap of the primary incisors, is measured and recorded in millimeters or as a percentage of the total height of the mandibular incisor crown (see Fig. 24.31). It is approximately 2 mm in the primary dentition. Deep bite is the complete or nearly complete overlap of the primary incisors. Anterior open bite, the absence of vertical overlap, is usually indicative of a sucking habit in this age group (Fig. 24.33). If the patient and parent deny the existence of a sucking habit, further investigation into the cause of the open bite is needed. Skeletal malocclusion, ankylosed anterior teeth, condylar fracture or the sequelae of trauma, and degenerative diseases such as juvenile rheumatoid arthritis may account for the open bite and should be investigated.

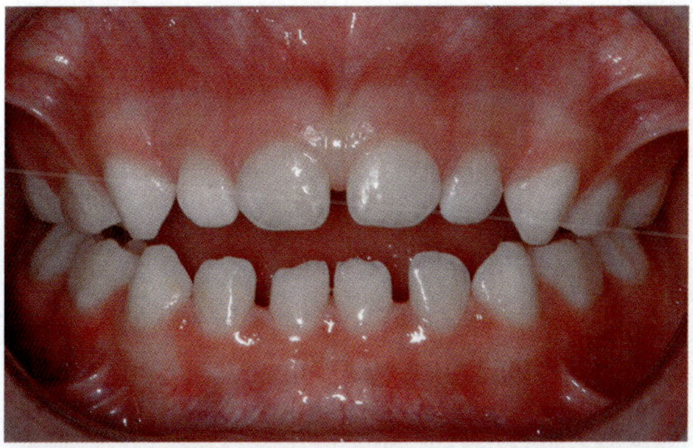

• **Fig. 24.33** This patient exhibits an anterior open bite (the absence of vertical overlap). Anterior open bite, especially an asymmetrical anterior open bite, is most commonly caused by a sucking habit in this age group.

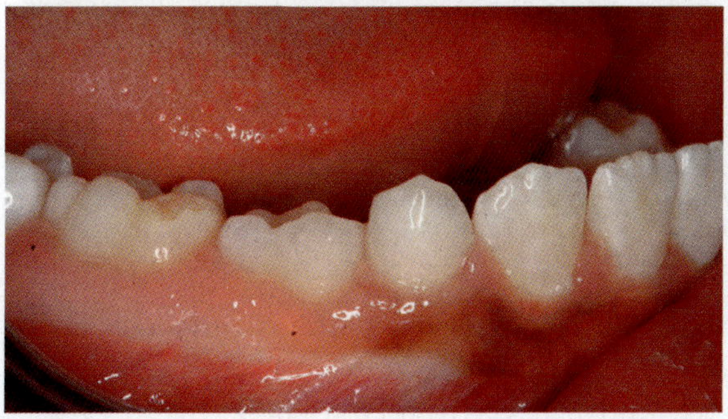

• **Fig. 24.34** Ankylosis, the fusion of tooth to bone, is common in the primary dentition. This patient has an ankylosed primary mandibular first molar that is below the plane of occlusion.

Ankylosis, the fusion of tooth to bone, is common in the primary dentition (Fig. 24.34). Although an ankylosed tooth cannot erupt further, the unaffected adjacent teeth will continue to erupt. This creates the illusion that the ankylosed tooth is submerged in the bone. The prevalence of ankylosed teeth is between 7% and 14% in the primary dentition.[28,29] In addition, 50% of patients with an ankylosed tooth have more than one ankylosis. The following is a list of the most ankylosed teeth in the primary dentition[30]:

1. Mandibular primary first molar
2. Mandibular primary second molar
3. Maxillary primary first molar
4. Maxillary primary second molar

A number of eruption and exfoliation problems have been blamed on ankylosed teeth. However, longitudinal studies indicate that ankylosed primary teeth exfoliate normally and allow normal eruption of succedaneous teeth.[29–31] An ankylosed tooth discovered during this developmental stage should not be removed routinely unless a large marginal ridge discrepancy develops between it and the unaffected adjacent teeth. If a marginal ridge discrepancy develops, the adjacent teeth may tip into the space occupied by the ankylosed tooth and cause space loss. A systematic review of ankylosed primary molars with permanent successors suggested removal of the ankylosed tooth in three situations. The first is if there is an altered eruption path of the permanent successor. The second situation is when the ankylosis is so severe that adjacent teeth begin to tip and create space loss. The last is when the exfoliation of the ankylosed tooth is significantly delayed.[31]

One aspect of ankylosed primary teeth that must be addressed differently in the mixed dentition is when the primary tooth is ankylosed and the permanent tooth is missing. If the vertical occlusal step becomes exaggerated, and the vertical bone level relative to adjacent teeth is exaggerated, intervention is indicated. This is the case because there is no permanent tooth to erupt and bring alveolar bone with it. If the primary tooth is allowed to remain, its eventual extraction will leave a bony defect adjacent to the remaining permanent teeth (Fig. 24.35). Timely removal of the primary tooth and further treatment will have to be considered. A second option for treatment is to decoronate the primary molar rather than remove it in cases where there is no permanent successor. There still is loss of vertical height of the alveolus but decoronation seems to maintain the alveolar width. Loss of bone due to extraction of a primary tooth without a successor is more

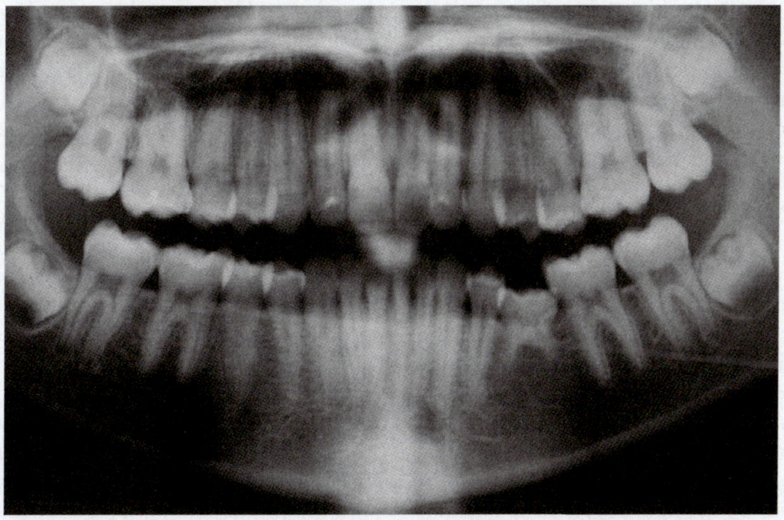

• **Fig. 24.35** The ankylosed primary mandibular second molar demonstrates the alteration of bone level that can occur when ankylosed primary teeth without successors are maintained too long. Timely removal of the ankylosed tooth and treatment planning for orthodontic movement of the adjacent teeth or prosthetic replacement is critical.

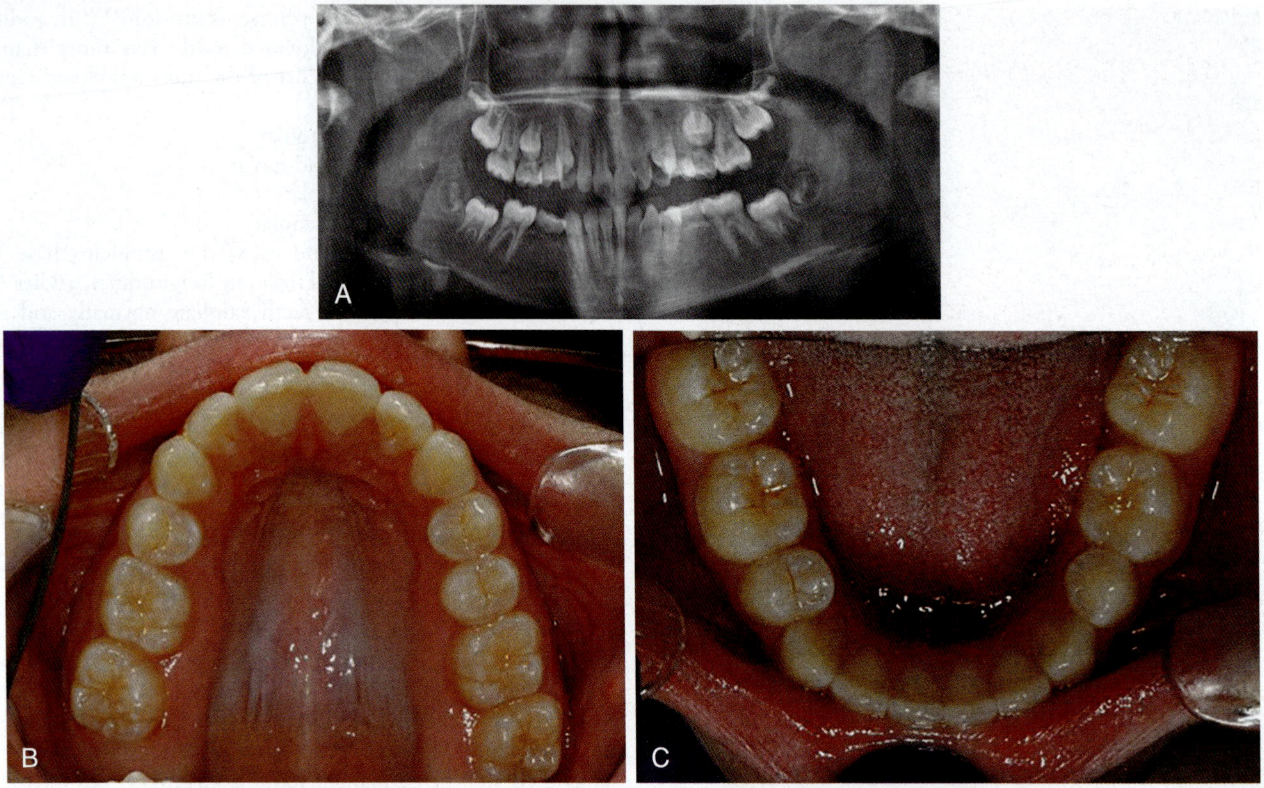

• **Fig. 24.36** The patient was missing both mandibular right first and second premolars (A). A maxillary second premolar was transplanted to the mandibular right position. This provides the patient with a lower right premolar and creates a class I molar and canine relationship on the right side (B–C)

rapid and severe in the anterior than in the posterior areas of the mouth. A missing posterior permanent tooth can also be treated with dental autotransplantation (Fig. 24.36).

Orthodontic Records and Diagnosis

A clinical examination followed by orthodontic records is necessary to complete a thorough diagnosis. The record-taking process and the interpretation of the records is discussed in *Contemporary Orthodontics,* Volume 7 (Elsevier). The reader is referred to this textbook to explain what records are obtained, the interpretation of the records, and the sequential development of a treatment plan or treatment plans. This process is critical for appropriate orthodontic management.

Skeletal Problems

Skeletal problems in the primary dentition are addressed if there is progressive asymmetry due to a functional disturbance.[32] The reason for treating these patients early is that treatment later may be more difficult and complex if the child continues to grow asymmetrically and dental compensation increases. The goal of early treatment is to prevent the asymmetry from becoming worse or to alter growth so that the asymmetry improves. Most progressive asymmetry patients are treated with removable functional appliances designed to alter growth by manipulating skeletal and soft tissue relationships and allowing differential eruption of teeth. Orthognathic surgery is a second treatment option for progressive asymmetry but is reserved for patients with severe asymmetry or those whose condition does not respond to functional appliance therapy. It may be necessary to operate a second time when the child is older because growth often tends to remain asymmetrical even after surgical correction. Because diagnosis and treatment of progressive asymmetry are difficult, it is recommended to refer these cases to a specialist for evaluation and treatment.

Orthodontic problems in the mixed dentition can be dental or skeletal in origin. The complexity of these problems varies tremendously. Skeletal problems, as diagnosed from the facial profile analysis and by supplemental records, are best managed by a specialist. However, the general practitioner should understand how skeletal discrepancies are treated.

There are three basic alternatives for treating skeletal discrepancies: growth modification, camouflage, and orthognathic surgery. Growth modification is a means to change skeletal relationships by using the remaining growth of the patient to alter the size or position of the jaws. Camouflage and orthognathic surgery usually are considered for adolescent patients with minimal or no growth remaining or nongrowing adult patients. Camouflage orthodontic treatment is aimed at hiding a mild skeletal discrepancy by moving teeth within the jaws so that the teeth fit together. The skeletal discrepancy still exists, but it is disguised by a compensated occlusion and acceptable facial esthetics. Orthognathic surgery places the jaws and teeth in a normal or near-normal position and improves facial esthetics using surgical procedures and presurgical and postsurgical orthodontic treatment.[33] For the mixed-dentition patient, only growth modification or no treatment are reasonable choices for skeletal problems.

Growth modification during the early mixed-dentition years rests on several assumptions that are not as clear as many would presume. First, a child must be growing for the growth to be modified. Most children in the 6- to 12-year age group are experiencing active statural growth, and their faces are also growing. Clinicians have thought that it is easiest to correct skeletal problems if a child is undergoing maximal facial growth during treatment. Although the data to support this contention are not voluminous or clear,[34] clinicians have long sought to predict maximum somatic growth and maximal facial growth from other indicators. There appears to be wide variation in the amount of facial growth occurring at one time and an equally wide variation in the correlation of facial growth with overall body growth and other indicators that have been chosen.[35–37]

It appears from the Mellion study that chronologic age works as well as hand-wrist films or cervical vertebral maturation scales in predicting the onset of the pubertal growth spurt and the maximum facial growth. Facial growth spurt in females starts around 9.5 years and peaks at 11.5 years. In males, the facial growth spurt begins around 11.5 years and peaks at 14.5.[38] Because of the always present variability, the clinician should use as many indicators as possible (personal growth history, secondary sexual characteristics, and onset of menarche) to make an educated decision about whether the child is growing at an acceptable rate. The data are not totally clear that one must treat children when they are at a certain rate of facial growth to be successful, and experience has shown that most moderate skeletal and dental problems can be managed in one phase during the transition from the mixed to permanent dentitions, capturing a segment of substantial growth and being able to manage the permanent teeth including the second molars. For these reasons a single stage of orthodontic treatment is most popular and adequately effective. This enables practitioners to successfully manage most problems with a more mature patient who is both reasonably cooperative and compliant. Asynchrony between dental development and rapid facial growth may create a situation in which the patient may be ready for growth modification but not for orthodontic dental treatment, or vice versa. These patients must be handled individually by balancing the dental and skeletal interventions.

The second assumption made when growth modification is undertaken is that the practitioner can accurately diagnose the source of the skeletal discrepancy and design treatment that will apply the appropriate amount and direction of force to correct the discrepancy. Diagnosis is not an exact science and may be confusing even with the use of cephalometric measures,[39] and the discrepancy may be due to several small skeletal problems rather than one easily identified discrepancy. It is important to remember that not all class II or class III malocclusions are equal or have only one skeletal feature at fault. Force delivery to dental and skeletal structures also is inexact, and the clinical impression and treatment response may dictate alteration in the amount and direction of force applied to modify growth. Certainly, orthodontic treatment for skeletal problems is not just a "see it" and "fix it" situation.

Third, growth modification is usually only one portion of a treatment plan. Most appliances used to modify growth (e.g., headgears and functional appliances) are designed to alter skeletal structures rather than precisely move teeth. Although these appliances cause tooth movement and camouflage, they are not as precise as fixed orthodontic appliances (braces) or clear aligners. Therefore most growth modification treatments are followed immediately or later by traditional fixed orthodontic appliances or clear aligners to move the teeth into a final position.

There are several theories offered to explain how growth modification works to achieve the desired results. The first theory suggests that growth modification appliances change the absolute size of one or both jaws. For example, a class II skeletal profile may be treated by making a deficient mandible larger to fit a normal-sized maxilla or by limiting the size of an oversized maxilla. Some clinical data show dramatic size changes, but there appears to be large variability in patient response to growth-modifying appliances, with modest changes in various structures being the rule rather than the exception. The dentoalveolar changes make up the difference.

Alternatively, growth modification may work by accelerating the desired growth but not changing the ultimate size or shape of the jaw. A deficient mandible may not end up larger than it ultimately would have been, but it may achieve its final size sooner. This requires the clinician to make some final dentoalveolar changes or compensations to establish an ideal occlusion after growth modification. This type of growth modification response also shows large individual variability. There is support for this interpretation of growth modification based on recent randomized clinical trials that demonstrate little difference between an early- and a late-treatment group of patients with skeletal class II malocclusion.[40]

A third possibility is that growth modification may work by changing the spatial relationship of the two jaws. The ultimate size of the jaw and its rate of growth are not changed, but by modifying the orientation of the jaws to each other a more balanced profile may result. For example, a convex profile and an increased lower facial height could be made more proportional to each other if the vertical growth of the maxilla could be inhibited and the mandible allowed to rotate upward and forward. The profile would then become less convex and the vertical relations more ideal. Jaw reorientation would be successful in a concave class III patient with a short face if the mandible could be rotated downward and backward (more vertical) to create a more acceptable profile. Reorientation does not work well in class II short faces or class III long faces because correcting one problem (e.g., the vertical) makes the other problem (e.g., the anteroposterior) worse. A review offered the following conclusions on growth modification with functional appliances: (1) functional appliances can accelerate forward growth of the mandible in the prepubertal and adolescent growth stages, (2) functional appliances restrain maxillary growth, and (3) functional appliances correct class II malocclusion with dental and skeletal changes.[41]

A number of studies have demonstrated early orthodontic treatment has a positive benefit on a patient's self-esteem and a reduction in negative social encounters.[42,43] However, there are some questions about early treatment and patient quality of life. Although it appears that orthodontic treatment has been found to enhance some aspects of quality of life (especially esthetics), it does not necessarily change social acceptance. In addition, treatment does not seem to improve oral health status or oral function compared with untreated populations.[44]

A Cochrane review on early orthodontic treatment and trauma prevention indicated there was a reduction in dental trauma, although there was a great deal of uncertainty regarding this finding.[45] Other studies question whether early treatment provides a protective benefit to incisal trauma.[46] The extent of overjet,[47] lip competence,[48] and previous trauma experience[49] can help direct treatment decisions. For many of these patients, dental retraction alone can be a satisfactory trauma prevention treatment and esthetic benefit, while leaving growth changes for a later, but still growing stage of treatment. A prudent approach may be to consider each individual patient and assess their psychosocial well-being and their risk factors for trauma. Otherwise, conventional late mixed-dentition treatment appears to be just as sensible.

Early evaluation of patients with dentofacial anomalies is also advocated. Dentofacial anomalies include several environmentally and genetically induced conditions that alter the relationship of the facial structures. Examples include cleft lip and palate, hemifacial microsomia, Crouzon and Apert syndromes, and mandibulofacial dysostosis (Treacher Collins syndrome). A specialist or interdisciplinary specialty team works to minimize the facial disfigurement through early surgical and orthodontic intervention.

Transverse Growth Modification

Facial growth can and does occur in all the planes of space, transverse, anteroposterior, and vertical, during adolescence. All occur simultaneously to some extent, and there is overlap of these dimensional changes,[32] When considering the preponderance of growth in portions of the face that are necessary and amenable to orthodontic treatment, it appears that the transverse growth ends first, anteroposterior second, and vertical third. That is why transverse dimension problems are usually considered and treated earlier than most others.

There are two basic approaches to the management of posterior crossbite in young children: (1) equilibration to eliminate mandibular shift and (2) expansion of the constricted maxillary arch. In a few cases, the mandibular shift is due to interference caused by the primary canines. These cases can be diagnosed by repositioning the mandible and noting the interference. Selective removal of enamel with a diamond bur in both arches eliminates the interference and the lateral shift into crossbite. This type of treatment has evidence-based support.[50]

The most common skeletal transverse problem in the preadolescent is maxillary constriction with a posterior crossbite. Management of maxillary constriction can begin as soon as the problem is discovered if the child is mature enough to accept treatment. Treatment has the potential to eliminate crossbites of the permanent teeth, increase arch length, and simplify future diagnostic decisions complicated by functional shifts. Most clinicians agree with the philosophy of early correction if there is a mandibular shift. In general, it is believed that long-term facial asymmetry attributable to soft tissue enlargement and in some cases mandibular asymmetry can result from untreated mandibular shifts.[51] Regardless of philosophy, treatment before adolescence and midpalatal suture interdigitation and bridging is recommended.

Three appliances can be used to correct the constriction, but the appliances are not interchangeable. The quad helix and W arch appliances provide both skeletal and dental movement in the 3- to 6-year-old child.[52] The W arch is constructed of 0.036-inch wire that rests 1.0 to 1.5 mm off the palate to prevent soft tissue irritation. The W arch is expanded approximately 4 to 6 mm wider than its passive width, or so that one arm of the W is resting over the central grooves of the teeth when the other arm is seated. To move teeth preferentially in the anterior region of the mouth, the appliance is activated by bending the palatal portion of the arm near the solder joint, as demonstrated in Fig. 24.37. If more correction is needed in the molar region, the appliance is activated via bending of the anterior palatal portion. The appliance expands the arch approximately 1 mm per side per month.

The patient should return monthly to allow the dentist to check the progress of treatment and to reactivate the W arch if needed. Usually, it is easier and more accurate to remove, activate, and recement the appliance. Expansion should continue until the crossbite is slightly overcorrected and the lingual cusps of the maxillary teeth occlude on the lingual inclines of the buccal cusps of the mandibular teeth. Most crossbites are corrected in 3 months, and the teeth are retained for an additional 3 months.

The quad helix is designed much like the W arch but incorporates more wire into the appliance, making it more flexible. It is constructed of 0.038-inch wire with two helices in the anterior palate and two helices near the solder joint in the posterior palate. The helices are wound away from the palate and can serve to remind the digit-sucking patient to refrain from the habit if they are positioned correctly where the patient places the finger or thumb. Therefore this is the preferred appliance for a patient with a finger habit and posterior crossbite. Because the quad helix has more wire than the W arch, it has a greater range of action and can be activated farther than the W arch while delivering an equivalent amount of force. Overcorrection and retention are also required for the quad helix.

Despite activation of the W arch or quad helix on one side only, teeth on both sides of the arch react to equivalent force. As the patient gets older, more dental change and less skeletal change occur. This is because the midpalatal suture, which was open at an early age, has developed bone interdigitation that makes it more difficult to separate. More force is required to separate the suture after initial interdigitation of the suture to obtain true skeletal correction than a quad helix or W arch can deliver. Realistically, most preadolescents can be treated with the lingual arch type appliances.

In the older preadolescent patient, in whom there is a chance that the midpalatal suture is closed, an appliance that can deliver large amounts of force is necessary to correct the skeletal constriction.[53] Rapid palatal expansion is the term given to the procedure in which an appliance cemented or bonded to the teeth is opened 0.5 mm/day to deliver 2000 to 3000 g of force (Fig. 24.38). In the active phase of treatment, there is a change in the inclination of the anchor teeth but little dental movement because the periodontal ligament has been hyalinized, which limits dental movement, and the force is transmitted almost entirely to the skeletal structures. However, during retention, the skeletal structures begin to relapse toward the midline. Because the teeth are held rigidly by the appliance, they move relative to the bones. Depending on the amount of expansion needed, active treatment normally takes 10 to 14 days. Another approach to skeletal expansion is slow rather than rapid palatal expansion.[54] Essentially the same appliance is used as in rapid palatal expansion, although force levels are calibrated to provide only 900 to 1300 g of force. Coupled with a slower activation rate, slow palatal expansion widens the palate by dental and skeletal movement. Although the final position of the teeth and supporting structures is approximately the same in rapid and slow expansion, proponents of slow expansion maintain that slower expansion is more physiologic and stable. There is some evidence that both rapid and slow maxillary expansion can result in loss of buccal bone (height and thickness).[55] These findings are from CBCT and should be viewed with some caution due to the resolution of the image.

Transverse growth modification can be accomplished by means of acrylic or wire buccal shields attached to functional appliances or lip bumpers. The buccal shields relieve the teeth and alveolar structures from the resting pressure of the cheek muscles and soft

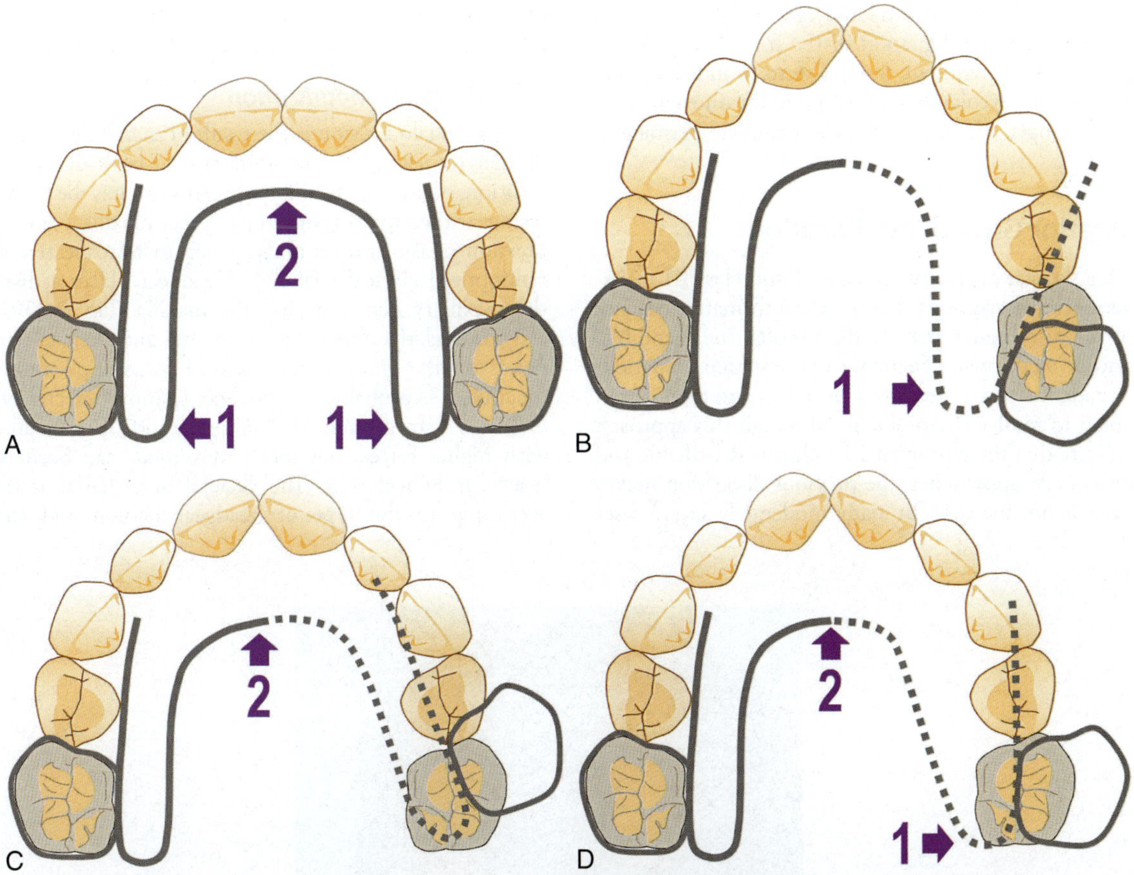

• **Fig. 24.37** (A) The W arch can be activated in two spots. (B) The preferred way to move teeth in the anterior region of the mouth is to activate the W arch by bending the arm of the W in the area marked location *1.* (C) If the clinician wants to obtain more movement in the molar region, the appliance is activated by bending the anterior portion of the W in the area marked location *2.* (D) In general, the appliance is activated 3 to 4 mm beyond its passive width or to a position where one arm of the W extends over the central grooves of the teeth when the other arm is seated in place.

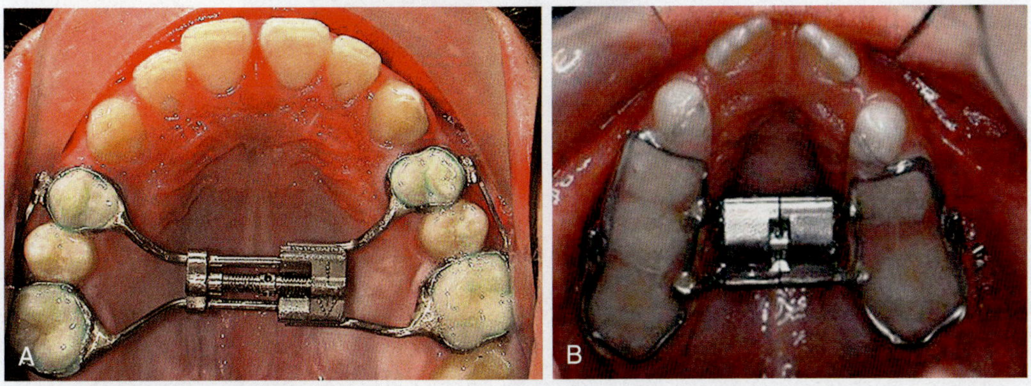

• **Fig. 24.38** Rapid palatal expansion is used to treat maxillary constriction and posterior crossbite when there is a chance that the midpalatal suture is partially closed. The jackscrew in the appliance provides approximately 2000 to 3000 g of force when it is opened 0.5 mm/day. Depending on the amount of expansion needed, the appliance is normally activated two times each day for 10 days to 2 weeks. The appliance can be either cemented on the teeth with orthodontic bands (A) or bonded to the teeth (B).

tissues. Transverse expansion of 3 to 5 mm can be achieved, although the changes vary considerably. Whether the movement is dental or skeletal and whether it will remain stable are still in question because there are no controlled experimental studies to provide answers.

Transverse expansion is also achieved by passive or active movement of teeth. Acrylic or wire buccal shields remove lip and cheek pressure to allow passive movement of both maxillary and mandibular teeth. Active expansion is performed with either a W arch–type appliance or a screw-type appliance. The decision to use one appliance or another is based on the age of the patient (an indirect measure of the interdigitation of the palatal suture) and the amount of expansion required. Studies seem to indicate there is less risk for buccal alveolar bone change if the movement is completed at a younger age rather than the complete permanent dentition.

Anteroposterior Growth Modification

Anteroposterior skeletal problems are class II and class III in nature. However, these descriptions are not very informative because the source of the discrepancy may be the maxilla, the mandible, or a combination of the two. Therefore the first step in patient evaluation is to identify the source of the problem and then design a treatment plan to resolve the problem. Although this approach appears to indicate that these problems are clearly identifiable and treatable with concise approaches, the previous discussion makes it clear that this is not the case. In many moderately severe cases of anteroposterior problems, several approaches may work that rely more on patient compliance than clinical expertise.

Class II Growth Modification

A class II malocclusion is the result of maxillary protrusion, mandibular retrusion, or a combination of both due to their size or position. Class II maxillary protrusion has been managed by headgear therapy to restrict or redirect maxillary growth by compression of the sutures and verified in retrospective studies and randomized clinical trials.[40,41] Headgear places a distal force on the maxillary dentition and the maxilla (Fig. 24.39). Theoretically, the relative movement of dental and skeletal structures depends on the amount and time of force application. In actual practice, it is probably not possible to move selectively only teeth or bones.[41] In general, skeletal and tooth movement are greater with higher forces, but tooth movement can occur with either heavy or light forces. The skeletal and dental response varies according to the type of headgear chosen and the resultant

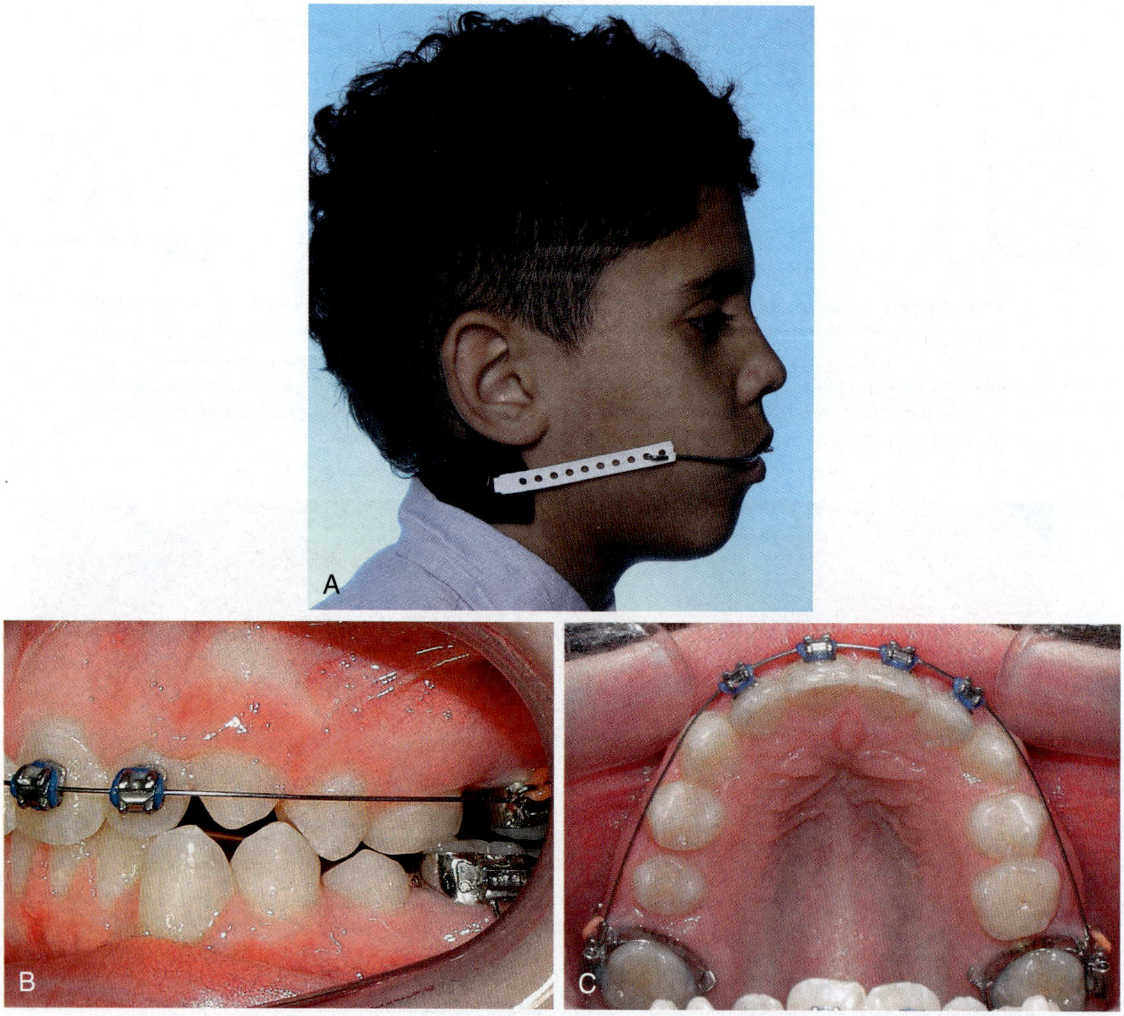

• **Fig. 24.39** The class II maxillary–protrusive patient is best treated by headgear therapy to restrict or redirect maxillary growth. (A) This patient is being treated with cervical headgear that places a distal and extrusive force on both maxillary skeletal and dental structures. The force is provided by a neck strap attached to the outer bows of the headgear. (B) The molar relationship is beginning to approach a class III dental position. (C) Space is beginning to open between the second primary molar and the first permanent molar. This type of change is not apparent for every patient because the amount of growth and the amount of cooperation can vary from patient to patient.

direction of force exerted by the headgear. The most common varieties, cervical and high pull, provide predominantly distal and occlusal or distal and apical forces, respectively. Traditionally, one avoids using a headgear that tends to extrude posterior teeth in a person with a long face or a limited overbite. On the other hand, a headgear that extrudes the molars is often useful in a patient with a short face and a deep bite.

Class II maxillary protrusion can also be managed with a removable functional appliance (Fig. 24.40). Although a functional appliance is primarily designed to stimulate mandibular growth, studies have indicated there are secondary effects of restricting forward maxillary skeletal and dental movement.[40,56,57] This happens because the mandible, which is postured forward, tends to return to a more distal position because of the distal muscle and

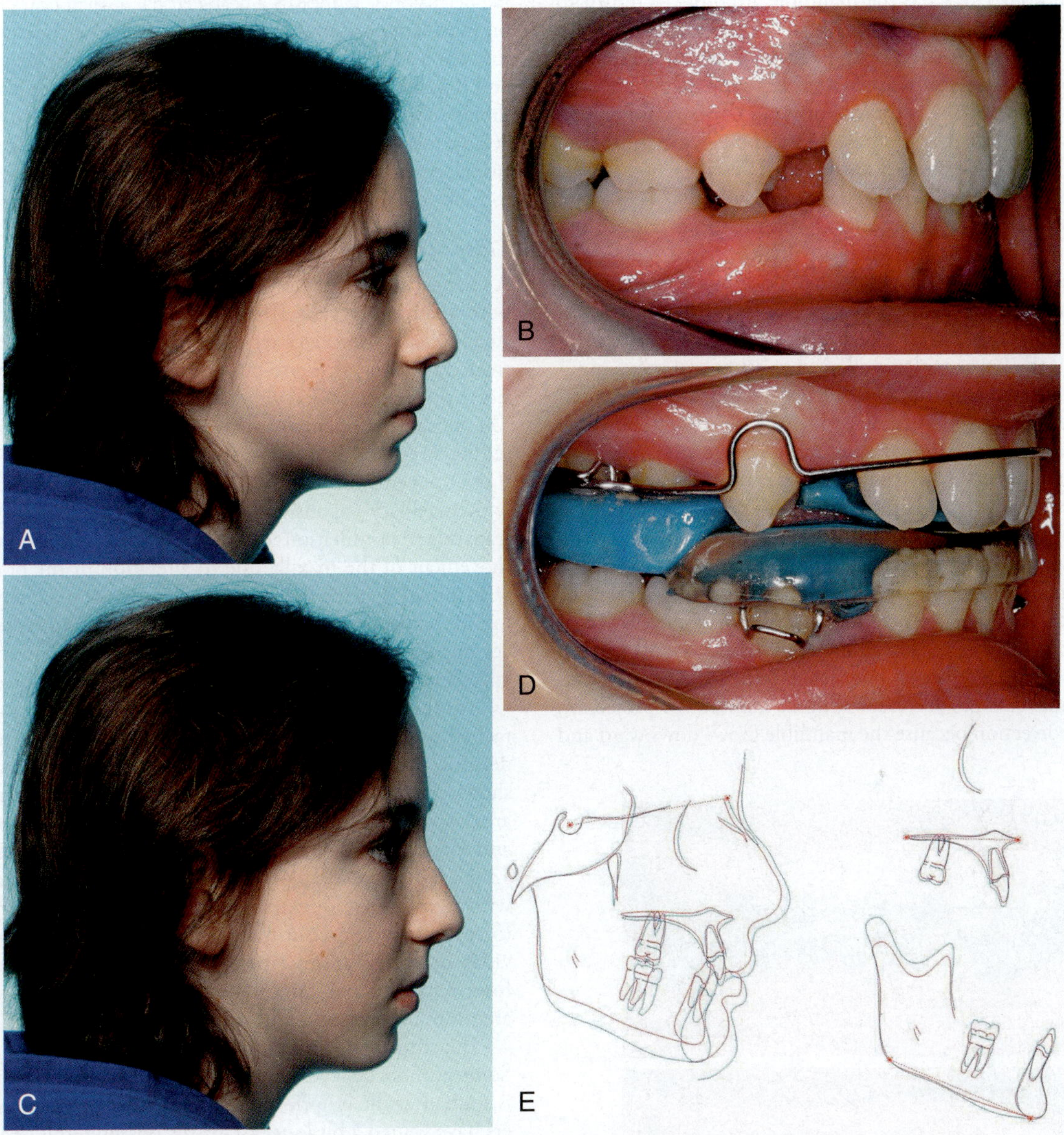

• **Fig. 24.40** The class II mandibular–deficient patient is usually treated with a functional appliance that positions the mandible forward in an attempt to stimulate, accelerate, or redirect mandibular growth. (A) This patient has a class II mandibular–deficient profile. (B) The patient's molar and canine relationships reflect the skeletal class II relationship. (C) The profile is immediately improved when the functional appliance is in place because the mandible is pushed forward into a class I relationship. (D) Because functional appliances (a twin block in this case) position the mandible forward using the upper and lower dental arches, there may be movement of the upper and lower teeth. Dental aspects of the malocclusion must be considered during treatment planning. (E) In this case the patient wore an appliance like that shown in (D) for approximately 1 year. In the overall superimposition the *blue lines* show there was slightly more change in the anteroposterior position of the mandible than in the maxilla. The maxillary superimposition shows the vertical position of the teeth was well controlled. In the mandibular superimposition, it is evident the patient grew favorably. In addition, the mesial and vertical eruption of the lower molar helped change the dental relationship to class I.

soft tissue forces. The distal force is transmitted through the appliance to the maxilla and its sutures and the maxillary teeth. The maxillary teeth tend to tip lingually rather than to move bodily while the mandibular teeth tip facially.

Another functional appliance is a fixed appliance used to reposition the mandible forward (Herbst). It is held in place with bands, stainless steel crowns, bonding, or a cemented cast framework (Fig. 24.41). A rod and tube apparatus forces the mandible forward and places constant force on the maxilla and the maxillary and mandibular teeth as the mandible attempts to return to a normal and more distal posture. Maxillary teeth tend to move distally, and mandibular anterior teeth move forward. This appliance has shown changes similar to other functional appliances in randomized clinical trials.[58] The use of temporary anchorage devices (TADs) combined with the Herbst appliance may reduce some of the lower incisor tooth movement.[59]

If the class II malocclusion is due to a mandibular deficiency, treatment options focus on changing the mandibular position. The mandibular-deficient patient is usually treated with a removable or fixed functional appliance that positions the mandible forward to stimulate or accelerate mandibular growth by unloading the condylar cartilage. Usually, upper molar eruption is restricted and the lower molar is allowed to erupt and move mesially. This rotates the occlusal plane clockwise. Retrospective clinical studies have shown that these appliances can produce a small average increase in mandibular projection (2 to 4 mm/year).[60,61] This has been confirmed by randomized clinical trials.[60,61] Patient response varies greatly, and in many cases the increased growth does not totally correct the class II skeletal problem for several reasons. First, the amount of growth is not enough to overcome the discrepancy. Second, all the available growth would have to be specifically directed to produce anteroposterior change. This is usually not the case because some dental eruption and vertical growth occur. This interaction between anteroposterior and vertical dimensional changes decreases ultimate mandibular projection and class II correction because the mandible grows downward and forward and not straight forward. The rest of the anteroposterior discrepancy is managed by restricting maxillary growth, tipping the maxillary teeth back, and tipping the mandibular teeth forward. Different appliances can be designed to exaggerate the secondary responses of maxillary restriction and dental movement if desired. Some studies indicate that headgear treatment may cause an increase in mandibular growth.[62,63]

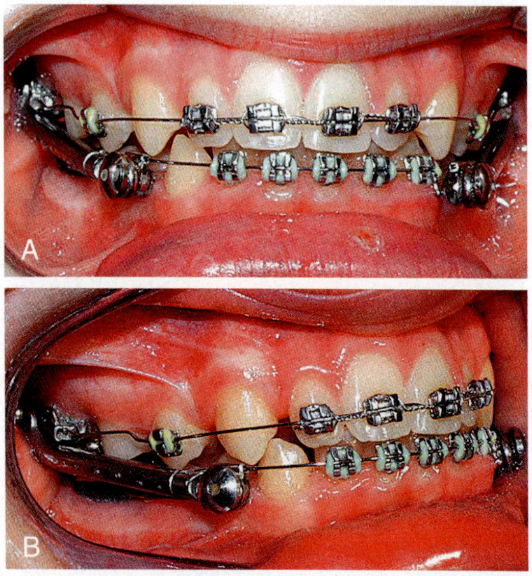

• **Fig. 24.41** The Herbst appliance is a fixed appliance that uses a pin and tube apparatus to reposition the mandible into a more forward position. (A) This class II patient demonstrates correction to a near class I occlusion. (B) Used in conjunction with fixed appliances, some of the dental effects can be more readily controlled.

In general, a review of class II treatments shows headgears and functional appliances are equally effective in treating the class II malocclusion.[64] It appears a headgear has a small restrictive influence on maxillary position, whereas functional appliances move B point forward leading to an ANB (the angle formed by A point, Nasion, and B point representing the relationship of the maxilla to the mandible) improvement of approximately 1 degree with either approach. A large portion of the change is dental in nature; headgears influence maxillary molar position distal, whereas functional appliances tend to move the lower molars mesial and procline the lower incisors.

Class III Growth Modification

A change in the position or size of the maxilla, the mandible, or both results in a class III malocclusion. The first possibility is a small maxilla (maxillary retrusion). True midface deficiency can be treated by using a reverse-pull headgear or facemask to exert anteriorly directed force on the maxilla and its sutures (Fig. 24.42).[65] The facemask applies force to the maxilla through an appliance (either a removable splint or fixed appliance) attached to the teeth; tooth movement also occurs. Some clinicians use the facemask with maxillary expansion (either rapid or slow) to enhance the transverse coordination of the arches and to facilitate anterior movement of the maxilla due to alteration of the bony interfaces with other skeletal structures. A comparison of clinical studies found that less maxillary incisor movement occurs when expansion accompanies protraction.[66] One prospective study found no difference between the expansion and nonexpansion approaches.[67]

Another approach is to use a facemask with miniplates attached to the maxilla. This method can be used in the late mixed dentition, probably at approximately 11 to 12 years of age, and shows greater skeletal change and movement in the zygomatic area as well.[68] Finally, miniplates can be attached to the maxilla and mandible, and intraoral elastics can be used at approximately 13 years of age and older. This has the effect of substantial change with no need for an extraoral appliance, which means the elastic force can be used continuously.[69] It appears this approach provides maxillary advancement and some mandibular restriction, fossa relocation, or ramus modeling. Both miniplate treatments are more invasive and require surgical placement and removal.

The timing of maxillary advancement has been controversial. Some authors believe that the ideal time to attempt this treatment is soon after the eruption of the permanent incisors, whereas others have waited a bit longer. Clearly, postpubertal treatment is not indicated for growth modification.[70] Data indicate that there is little anteroposterior difference in treatment effect whether treatment is applied early or late, if the treatment is completed before 10 to 11 years of age.[71,72] Unfortunately, the long-term success of maxillary protraction is not clear. One fact appears to be emerging: mistaken diagnosis or treatment in patients whose class III malocclusion is the result of mandibular protrusion will usually fail. Even with those who are correctly diagnosed, approximately one in four will require additional treatment to correct the skeletal malocclusion.[73] Another consideration is the amount of change that can be expected. If early facemask treatment yields 1 to 2 mm of maxillary change at A point and miniplates and a facemask

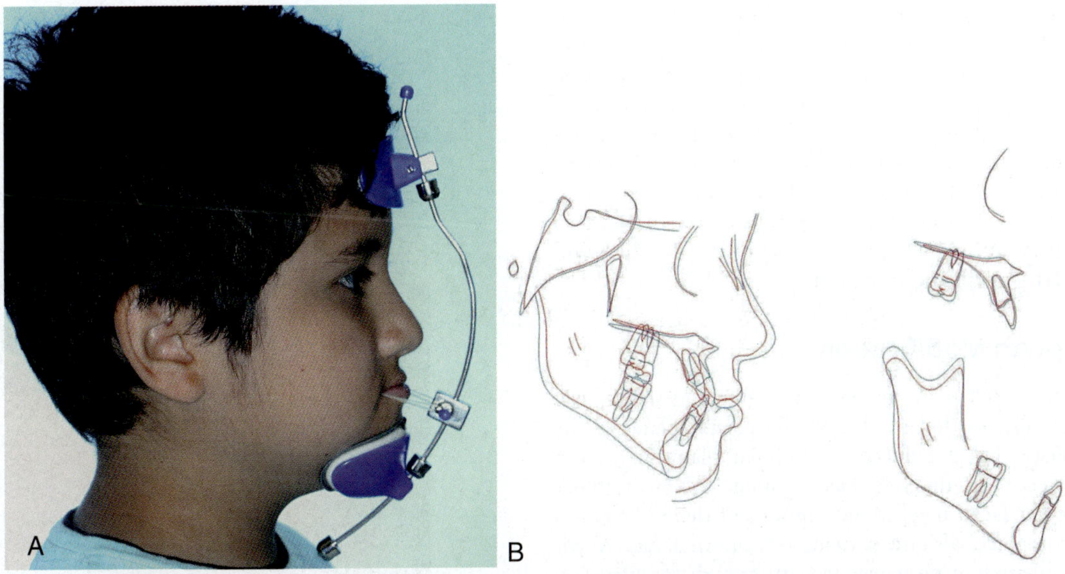

• **Fig. 24.42** (A) The class III maxillary–deficient patient is treated by using a reverse-pull headgear or facemask to exert anteriorly directed force on the maxilla. The force is provided by rubber bands extending from the facemask to intraoral hooks or wires. (B) These superimpositions show a successful case in treating a case of class III maxillary deficiency. The overall superimposition shows the maxilla has been moved forward to a greater extent than the mandible. The mandible was rotated down and backward somewhat, which helped with the anteroposterior change in the skeletal relations. There was little change in tooth position in both the maxillary and mandibular superimpositions, which suggests most of the change was skeletal in nature.

yield 2 to 3 mm, then a patient whose centric relation shows a 5-mm negative overjet will not be satisfactorily corrected unless the maxillary anterior teeth are proclined or the mandibular teeth retroclined. Pretreatment evaluation will reveal if tooth movement is possible and advisable.

Functional appliances designed to stimulate maxillary growth do not seem to be effective. The improvement in facial profile obtained by using these appliances in patients with very minor class III problems is usually the result of a downward and backward rotation of the mandible. The occlusion improves because of eruption of the maxillary molars, restricted eruption of the mandibular molars, facial tipping of the maxillary incisors, and lingual tipping of the lower incisors with a resulting counterclockwise rotation of the occlusal plane.

Class III mandibular protrusion has been historically managed with chin cup therapy (Fig. 24.43). The theory of chin cup therapy is to apply a distal and superior force through the chin that inhibits or redirects growth at the condyle. Again, studies in animals have shown some change in absolute mandibular size, but clinical application in humans routinely has been less successful.[74,75] The typical short-term treatment response to chin cup therapy is a distal rotation of the mandible and lingual tipping of the lower incisors. Therefore chin cup therapy is well tolerated in patients with mild mandibular protrusion and short to normal vertical proportions. However, it is contraindicated in a person with a long lower face because the anteroposterior correction would come at the expense of an increased vertical dimension.

In summary, treatment of class III malocclusion in the primary and mixed dentition is based on the diagnosis of maxillary deficiency or mandibular excess. In cases of mandibular excess, the clinician can choose between a chin cup or a class III type functional appliance. Both have been shown to restrict mandibular growth but have little influence on maxillary position.[76] Treatment is recommended before age 10. In maxillary-deficient patients a reverse-pull headgear can move the maxilla forward. If the headgear is attached to the maxillary teeth, there is some proclination of the upper incisors as well as downward and backward rotation of the

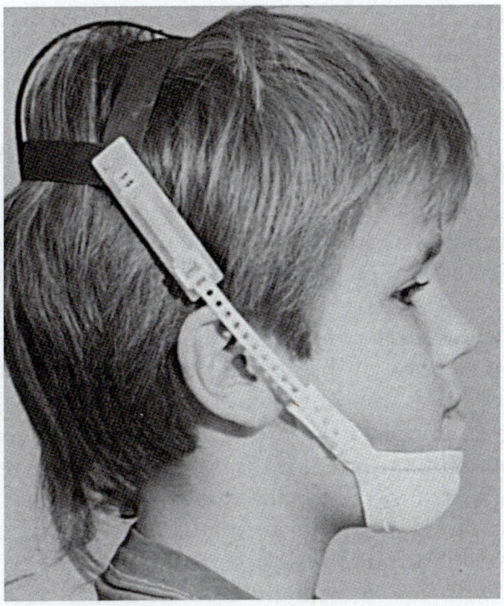

• **Fig. 24.43** The class III mandibular–protrusive patient has historically been treated with chin cup therapy. The chin cup was designed to apply a distal and superior force through the chin to inhibit growth at the condyle. In clinical practice, this device has not been proven to be routinely successful, although chin cup therapy does cause a distal rotation of the mandible. Therefore the chin cup may be useful for managing mild mandibular protrusion in which the vertical proportions are short to normal.

mandible. This results in an increased lower anterior facial height.[76] If treatment is delayed until the late mixed dentition when permanent teeth have erupted to a point where bone miniplates can be placed, a facemask or later a combination of upper and lower miniplates with continuous intermaxillary elastic traction has been shown to stimulate upper jaw growth and restrain lower jaw growth without dental compensations.[70] The issue seems to be the variable response from patient to patient. It is very difficult to predict how one individual will react to class III growth modification.

Vertical Growth Modification

Vertical skeletal problems are manifested as long and short facial heights and usually are located below the palatal plane.[77] The short-faced person has a reduced mandibular plane angle and undererupted teeth. In the long-faced patient the mandibular plane angle, lower facial height, and amount of dental eruption are increased compared with the patient with a normal face. Vertical skeletal problems can be managed with growth modification techniques, and some can be managed successfully; however, even when the treatment has been successful, maintaining the correction is extremely difficult. The face grows vertically for a long time, and there is a tendency for the original growth pattern and problem to recur.

Vertical Excess

Vertical skeletal excess may be managed with extraoral force or intraoral force. Extraoral force is delivered by means of a high-pull headgear through the maxillary first molars. The force is applied in a superior and distal direction and is designed to inhibit vertical development of the maxilla and eruption of the posterior maxillary teeth (Fig. 24.44). Because no force is applied to the mandibular teeth, they are free to erupt and compensate for the reduced vertical development in the maxilla. In some cases, this compensatory eruption can eliminate all the positive effects of the high-pull headgear and lead to downward and backward rotation of the mandible instead of forward mandibular projection.

An alternative method for controlling vertical development is to block the eruption of the maxillary and mandibular teeth. A functional appliance can be designed that will force the mandible open to an increased vertical rest position. The force of the mandible attempting to return to its original vertical rest position is transmitted to the maxilla and the teeth in both arches. This results in mandibular growth being directed forward because no dental eruption has occurred to increase the vertical dimension with less growth in lower and total face height (Fig. 24.45).[78]

TADs may prove to be of value in restricting vertical facial development. TADs are small-diameter titanium screws placed into cortical bone. They do not osseointegrate, so they can be removed easily without surgery after use. TADs provide the clinician with an anchor to apply force to teeth without causing other teeth to move because the screw is in bone. In theory, the screws should not move, although it appears they do move with force application. In cases of vertical excess, TADs are placed so an intrusive force can be applied to the maxillary posterior teeth.[79] Either small, closed coil springs or elastomeric chains are used to generate the force from the tooth to the TAD. Excellent patient cooperation is necessary because treatment must be continued or retained as long as the patient is growing.

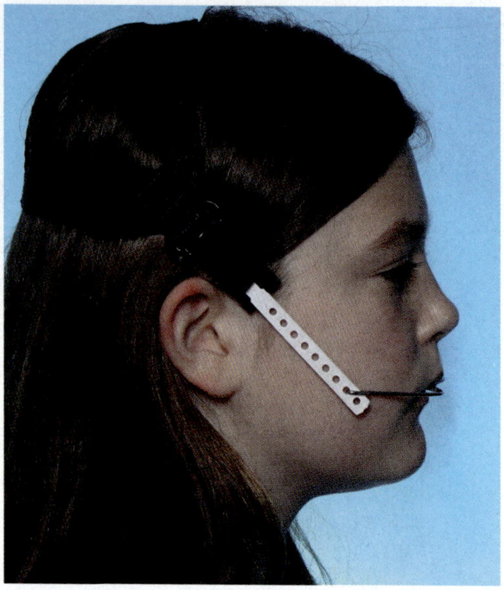

• **Fig. 24.44** The patient with vertical skeletal excess is often treated with high-pull headgear. The force, generated by the strap resting on the head, is applied in a superior and distal direction and is intended to inhibit vertical development of the maxilla and eruption of the maxillary posterior teeth.

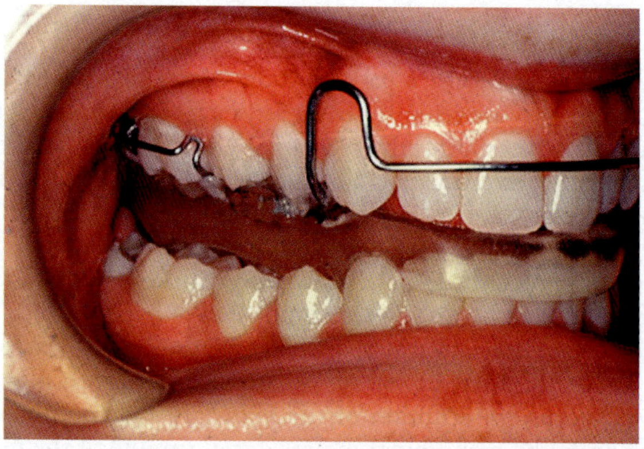

• **Fig. 24.45** Vertical skeletal excess also can be managed with a functional appliance designed to inhibit eruption of the maxillary and mandibular teeth. The appliance is constructed so that the mandible is placed in an open posture at an increased vertical position. The force of the mandible attempting to return to its normal, more closed vertical position is transmitted to the maxilla and to the teeth in both arches.

Vertical Deficiency

Vertical skeletal deficiencies can be managed with either headgear or functional appliances, depending on the accompanying anteroposterior relationships. The force vector from the headgear should direct the maxilla distally and extrude the maxillary posterior teeth, which would require cervical-pull headgear. Functional appliances are typically designed to inhibit or encourage eruption of upper and lower anterior and posterior teeth, depending upon the specific problem. For a vertically deficient patient, promoting eruption of the posterior teeth can also increase vertical facial height (Fig. 24.46). In addition, because there is a component of forward or mesial movement of teeth as they erupt, an astute clinician will encourage lower molar eruption in class II cases (lower

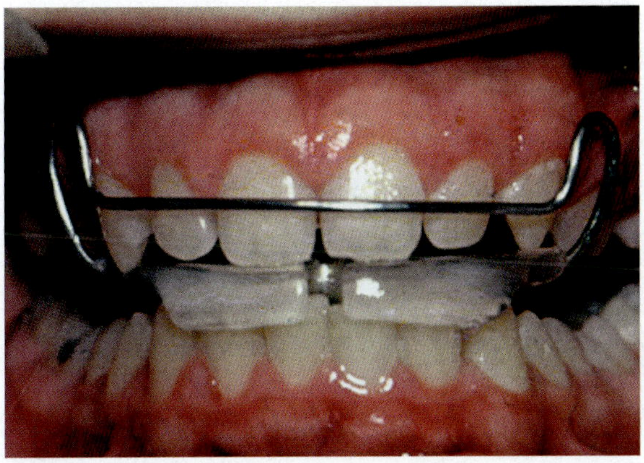

• **Fig. 24.46** This functional appliance is designed to allow the posterior teeth to erupt and, in this class II patient, drift anteriorly and aid in correction of the dental relationship. This type of appliance can open the bite and increase the dental and skeletal vertical dimensions.

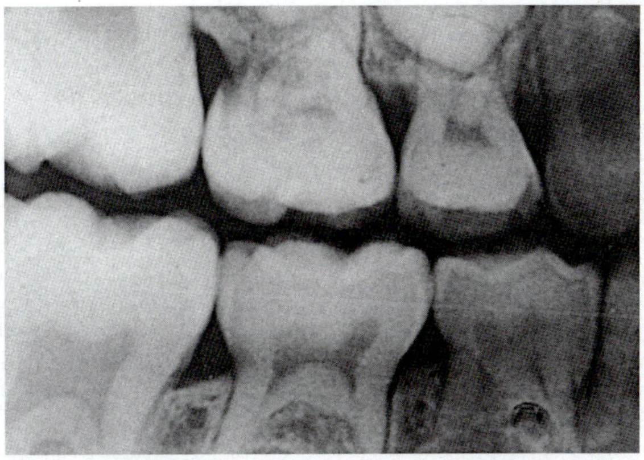

• **Fig. 24.47** This radiograph illustrates the ability of an ectopically erupting permanent first molar to self-correct spontaneously. Note that the distal root of the primary maxillary second molar has been resorbed. Usually, this type of resorption is the result of an erupting permanent molar that is caught on the distal aspect of the primary molar. If the resorption does not progress too far, the permanent molar usually "jumps" past the resorptive defect in 3 to 6 months.

molar moves forward into class I) and upper molar eruption in class III cases. As in vertical skeletal excess, the original growth pattern tends to recur until growth is complete, and retention should be designed to prevent this recurrence.

Dental Problems

Potential Alignment and Space Problems

Ectopic Eruption

When a permanent first molar is determined to be erupting ectopically, a 3- to 6-month observation period usually is the best initial therapy if the resorption is not too severe. There is a possibility that the molar will self-correct spontaneously or "jump" distally and erupt into its normal position (Fig. 24.47). Intervention is necessary if the molar is still blocked from erupting at the end of the observation period or if the permanent molar is severely impacted.[80] The goal of treatment is to move the ectopically erupting tooth away from the tooth it is resorbing, allow it to erupt, and retain the primary second molar.

If a small amount of movement is needed and little or none of the permanent molar is clinically visible, a piece of 0.022 to 0.028 inch brass wire can be passed around the contact between the permanent molar and the primary second molar and tightened. The periodontal ligament space is compressed, and the molar is forced distally until it can slip past the primary molar and erupt (Fig. 24.48). In some cases, a steel spring clip separator or an elastomeric separator may be used to dislodge the molar, but only in cases in which there is minimal resorption of the primary molar. It may be difficult to seat the spring if the contact point between the molars is below the cementoenamel junction of the primary molar. Elastomeric separators must be carefully supervised because they can dislodge in an apical direction and bury in the sulcus causing a periodontal abscess. Some elastomeric separators are not radiopaque and can be difficult to locate.

Another method of moving the permanent molar distal is to band the primary second molar and apply a distal force to the permanent molar through a helical spring or elastomer (Fig. 24.49). These methods require that the occlusal surface of the permanent molar is visible so that force can be applied to move the tooth distally. A small ledge of resin or a metal button can be bonded to the occlusal surface to serve as the point of force application, or the end of the spring can be bonded directly to the impacted tooth. However, salivary contamination of the occlusal surface sometimes makes bonding a frustrating and difficult procedure. Another effective technique is to bond a permanent first molar bracket on the primary second molar and a permanent second molar bracket on the permanent first molar; then a self-retained helical spring is constructed between the two teeth to move the permanent first molar distally. This can all be accomplished chairside in a few minutes by a proficient wire bender. Such a band and spring appliance should be evaluated every 2 weeks and can work effectively in a short time because of the minimal root development on the permanent molar.

Occasionally, the primary second molar must be removed if the permanent molar has caused extensive resorption of the primary root structure. In these cases, loss of arch length is certain, and some plan of treatment for the impending space deficiency should be considered in advance (Fig. 24.50). If there is a congenitally missing second premolar or premolar extraction is being considered because of the crowding, then reduction in arch length by mesial movement of the molars is advantageous. To manage the space after extraction of the primary molar, a distal shoe can be placed to guide eruption of the permanent molar. An alternative plan is to allow the permanent molar to erupt and then use the appropriate appliance to regain the space (described subsequently). After the space is regained, a space maintainer should be placed.

Ectopic eruption of lateral incisors is usually an early indication of crowding but may only be the result of aberrant tooth positioning. If a primary canine exfoliates prematurely because of ectopic eruption, the lower incisors typically drift to that side of the arch. A midline discrepancy may be present. If the laterals cause resorption and exfoliation of both primary canines, the incisors usually tip lingually and decrease arch length. When this happens and the incisors align, it appears that the space problem is corrected because the incisor alignment usually improves, but this is only temporary, and the space shortage will become apparent again when the permanent canines begin to erupt. Whether the loss of primary canines is unilateral or bilateral, the clinician should determine whether there is an arch length inadequacy and

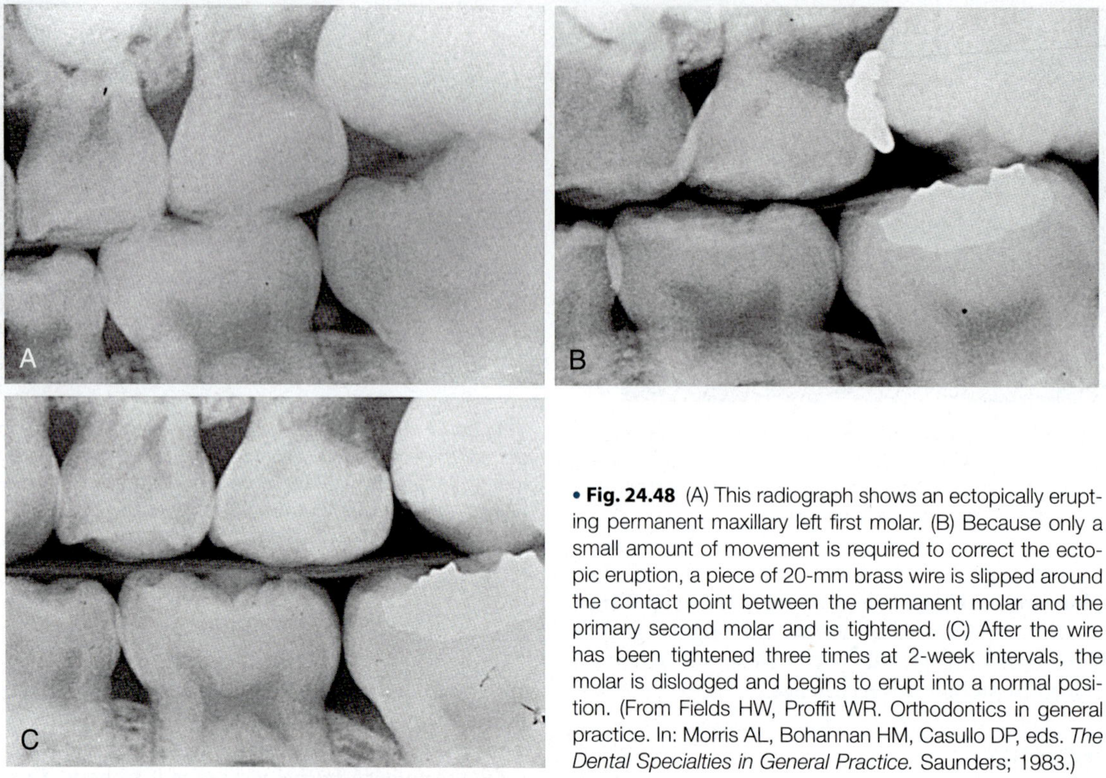

• **Fig. 24.48** (A) This radiograph shows an ectopically erupting permanent maxillary left first molar. (B) Because only a small amount of movement is required to correct the ectopic eruption, a piece of 20-mm brass wire is slipped around the contact point between the permanent molar and the primary second molar and is tightened. (C) After the wire has been tightened three times at 2-week intervals, the molar is dislodged and begins to erupt into a normal position. (From Fields HW, Proffit WR. Orthodontics in general practice. In: Morris AL, Bohannan HM, Casullo DP, eds. *The Dental Specialties in General Practice.* Saunders; 1983.)

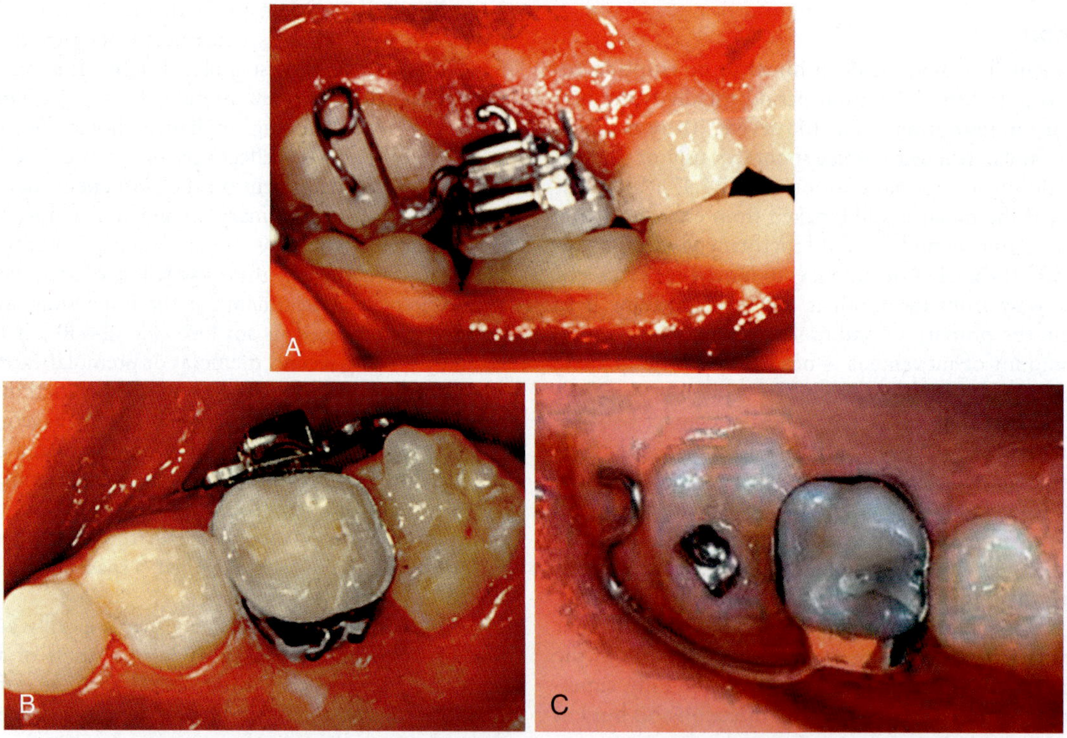

• **Fig. 24.49** (A–B) A band and helical spring appliance is used to treat an ectopically erupting permanent molar that requires a large amount of movement. The primary second molar is banded, and a helical spring is soldered to the band. A small ledge of composite resin, a metal button bonded to the occlusal surface of the permanent molar, or a small preparation can serve as a point of force application. The spring is reactivated at monthly intervals until the permanent molar is dislodged. (C) Another band and spring design with a metal button bonded to the occlusal surface of the erupting permanent molar. Elastomeric chain or thread is attached from the button to the distal hook on the wire and changed monthly to provide the distal force to dislodge the molar. ([A and B] From Fields HW, Proffit WR. Orthodontics in general practice. In: Morris AL, Bohannan HM, Casullo DP, eds. *The Dental Specialties in General Practice.* Saunders; 1983.)

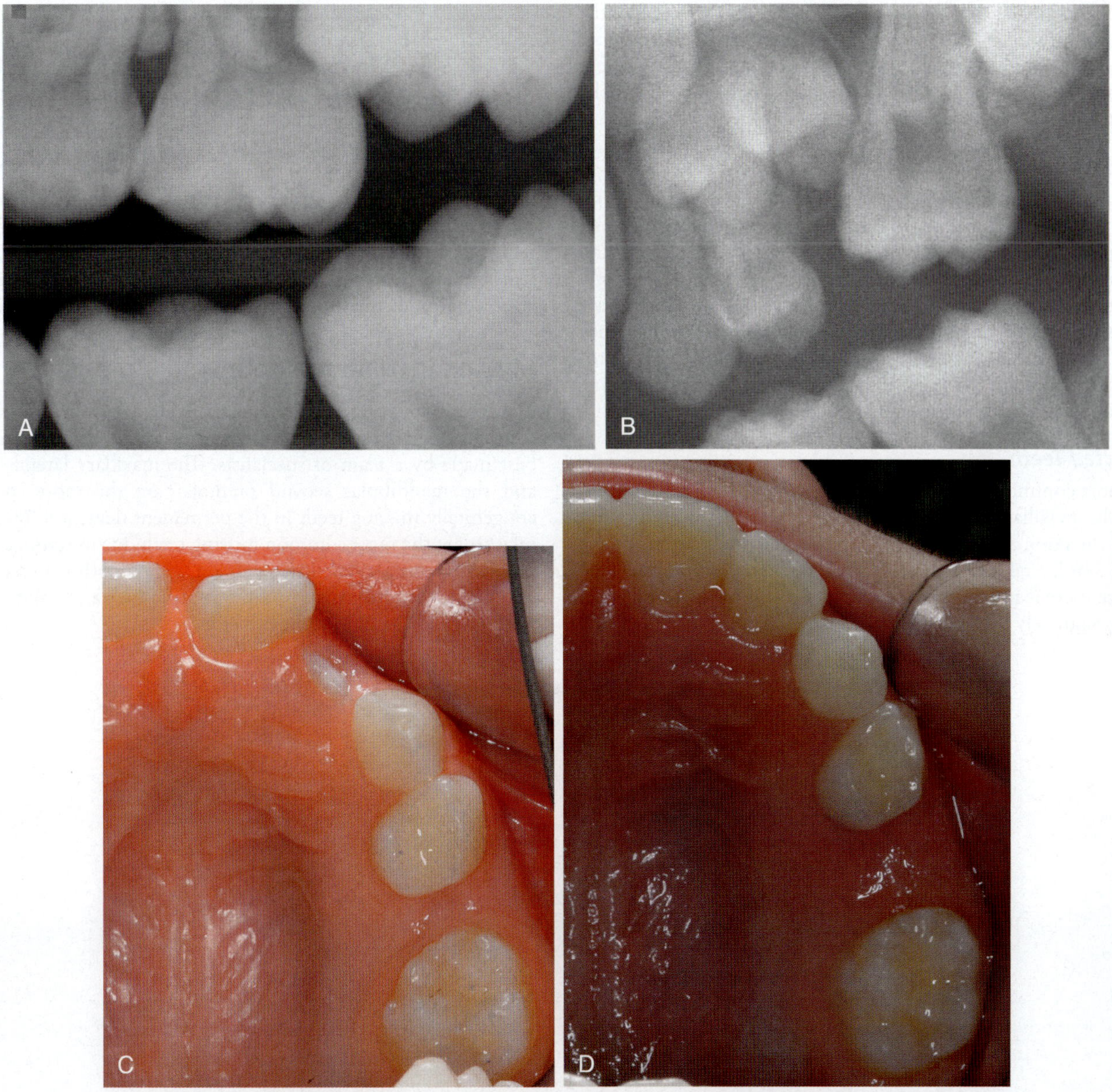

• **Fig. 24.50** (A) In some cases, ectopic eruption causes extensive resorption of the primary tooth root, and the tooth is lost prematurely. In some cases, the tooth may abscess due to communication with the oral environment. (B) When the primary second molar is lost, the clinician should anticipate mesial movement of the permanent molar and a reduced arch length. (C) This space loss occurred within the first 6 months of tooth removal. (D) The space was opened with braces and a coil spring. Space maintenance was necessary to hold space for the unerupted second premolar.

assess anteroposterior lip and incisor position. This information helps determine whether space maintenance, space regaining, or more extensive treatment is needed.

The goal of treatment should be to manage space according to the long-term plan. Past recommendations for treatment of crowding and lateral incisor ectopic eruption have included placing a lingual arch with a soldered spur distal to the lateral incisor to hold space and stabilize the midline. Some have recommended removal of the contralateral primary canine if the midline has shifted to promote spontaneous midline correction. However, there is no evidence in the literature that removal of the contralateral primary canine will result in spontaneous midline correction. There is also no evidence that the midline shift is progressive if the primary canine is not removed. A recent evaluation of growth study data confirmed there is no significant difference in the position of the lower dental midline after unilateral loss of a primary canine or normal exfoliation of both canines.[81] There are studies to show that removal of the mandibular primary canines will result in an improved irregularity index (a measure akin to crowding) compared with those that do not have primary canine removal. However, this tooth removal comes at the expense of nearly 3 mm in arch perimeter decrease.[82] Based on this evidence, the clinician should carefully consider whether to remove the contralateral canine when there is ectopic eruption of the lower lateral incisor. If there is sufficient crowding so that space maintenance is contraindicated, or if the incisors are considered too protrusive to be maintained in this position, no lingual arch should be placed after the extraction of the contralateral primary canine. In situations in which both canines exfoliate prematurely because of ectopic eruption, similar treatment decisions should be made, although the clinician does not normally have to worry about a midline shift.

Transposition

Early transposition can be addressed during the mixed dentition and provides an opportunity to intercept a developing problem. As mentioned earlier, the type of transposition amenable to early treatment is most commonly encountered in the mandibular arch. The lateral incisors resorb either the primary canine or primary canine and primary first molar (Fig. 24.51A). They rotate as they erupt, so treatment includes repositioning them mesially and derotating them (see Fig. 24.51B). If this is accomplished before canine eruption, transposition can be prevented (see Fig. 24.51C).

Impacted Teeth

The most common site of impacted teeth in the mixed dentition is in the maxillary canine region. These teeth often erupt in a mesial direction and become impacted in the palate or resorb the permanent lateral incisor roots.[83] This problem is often diagnosed because there is no bulge on the facial alveolus in the canine area at approximately 9 or 10 years of age.[84] Some type of radiograph is indicated to locate the canine. In most cases this is a panoramic radiograph. This may even merit the use of a small field-of-view CBCT image. If the permanent canine overlaps less than half of the lateral incisor root on a panoramic radiograph, there is a greater than 90% chance of redirecting the canine distally simply by timely extraction of the primary canines (Fig. 24.52).[85] If there is more than this amount of overlap, the chance of normal eruption diminishes. Other treatments have been proposed to prevent the maxillary canine from erupting into the palate. Besides removal of the primary canine, others have suggested palatal expansion and primary canine removal,[86] headgear treatment, and removal of both the primary canine and primary first molar.[87]

Missing Permanent Teeth

The absence of permanent teeth creates many treatment problems for the clinician, and most treatment decisions of this nature are best made by a team of specialists. The maxillary lateral incisor and the mandibular second premolar are the most common congenitally missing teeth in the permanent dentition. Maxillary incisors are the most common missing teeth due to trauma. Treatment decisions are based not only on which tooth is missing but also on arch length, adjacent tooth morphology and color, incisor position, and lip and profile esthetics.

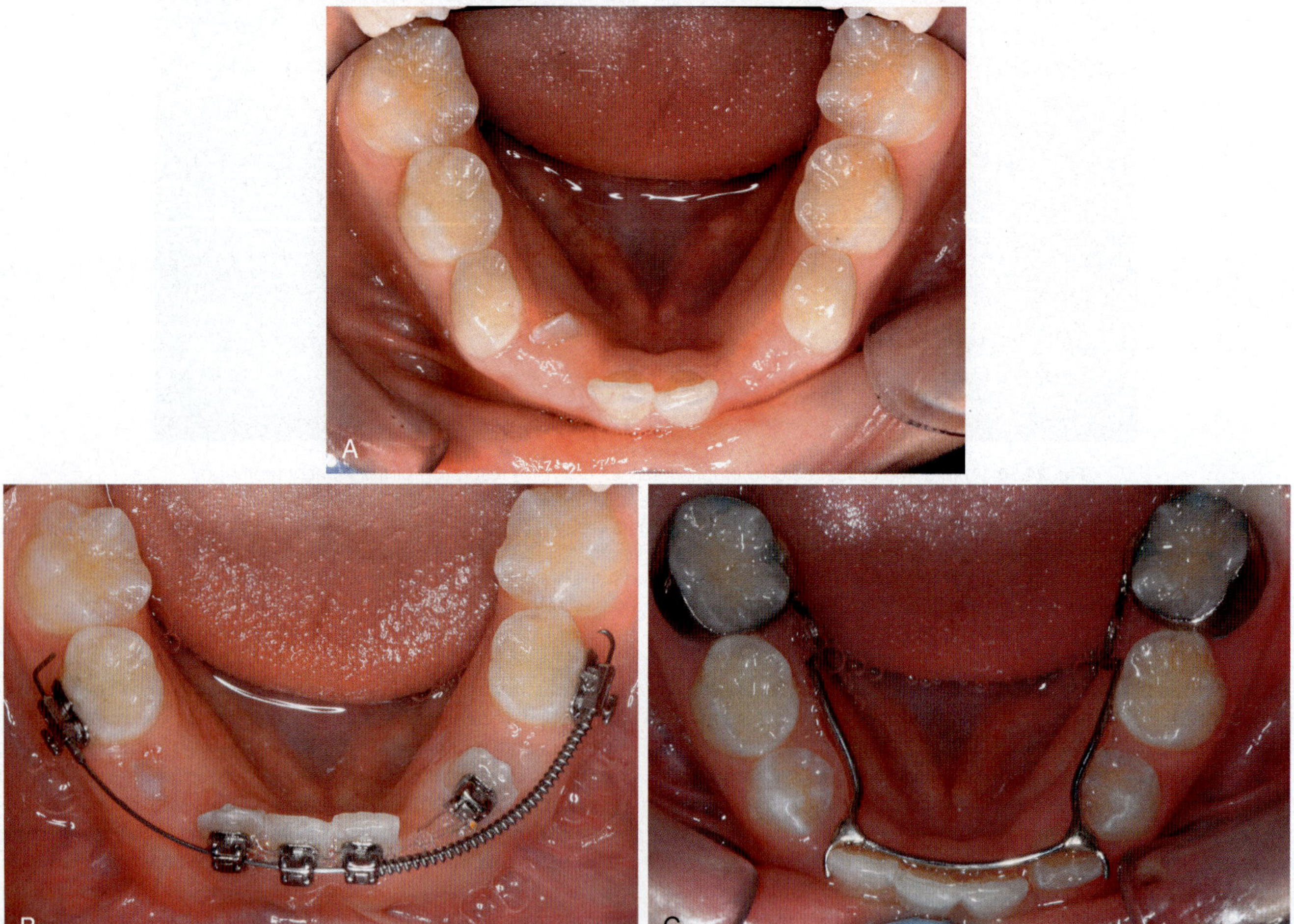

• **Fig. 24.51** (A) Early transposition can cause loss of the primary canine or primary canine and first molar. In this patient the lower left first primary molar was removed to allow the lateral incisor to erupt. (B) Often the lateral incisor will require mesial movement and rotation. (C) Correction with banded and bonded appliances has prevented true transposition.

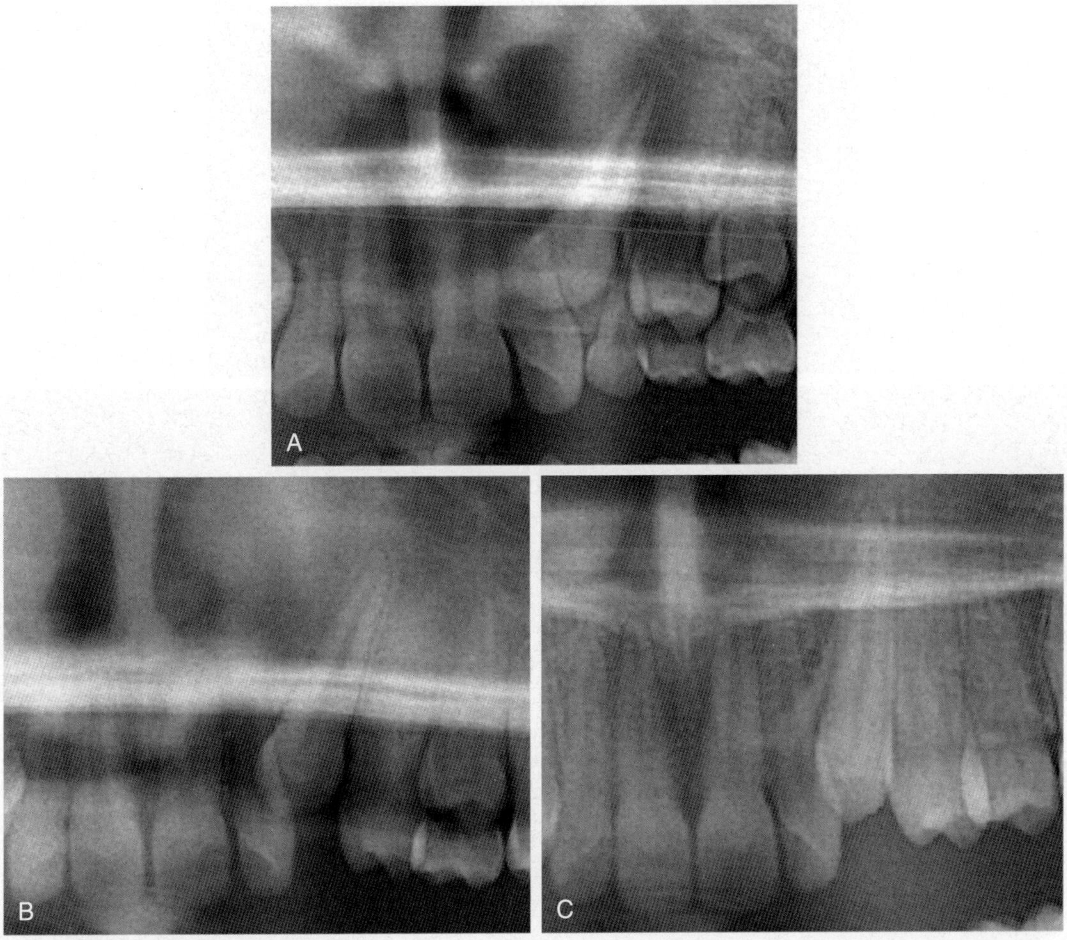

• **Fig. 24.52** (A) Even though this patient has considerable mesial migration of the permanent maxillary left canine and it overlaps the entire lateral root, the primary canine was extracted in an attempt to redirect its eruption path. (B) Note the distal and occlusal movement of the permanent left canine with reduced overlap of the lateral incisor. (C) Nearly 1 year later the permanent left canine will erupt into relatively normal position.

Treatment of congenitally missing maxillary lateral incisors varies depending on whether one or both incisors are absent and on the position of the permanent canine when it erupts into the arch. The canine either erupts into the normal canine position or resorbs the primary lateral incisor and spontaneously substitutes for the missing lateral incisor. If the canine erupts into its proper position, the primary lateral incisor will eventually have to be removed because it does not make an esthetically pleasing substitute for the permanent lateral incisor and because the root will eventually resorb. The missing lateral incisor can be replaced with a resin-bonded bridge or an implant. In general, prosthetic replacement of the missing lateral incisor is preferred when the occlusion, incisor position, and profile are nearly ideal (Fig. 24.53).[88] This approach should always be considered when the contralateral lateral incisor is present and has excellent size and shape. Until recently, this approach was also favored when the occlusion was near ideal because it was difficult to close the space without creating a midline discrepancy or retracting the incisors. The use of TADs has made space closure much easier and more predictable.

The clinician must also consider the long-term consequences of treatment. If the patient and clinician elect to open the space for prosthetic replacement of the lateral incisor, the placement of an implant or resin-bonded bridge must be delayed until the patient has stopped growing. This is often greater than 5 years between the finish of orthodontic treatment and a definitive restoration. Retention must be well planned, and the patient must be very compliant with retention, so the teeth remain in the ideal position for restorations. Even with good retention, studies have shown there is a 1 in 10 chance the roots of the central incisor and canine will converge and prevent implant placement.[89] Another long-term consequence of implant-supported restoration of the lateral incisor is the implant itself. Though the implant has a high success rate, there are implant failures. In addition, resorption of labial bone around the implant, a normal finding over time, causes the gingiva to appear blue. Lastly, the implant may show infraocclusion after several years. Because the implant does not erupt like teeth, any vertical growth change will result in a change in the vertical relationship of the implant and adjacent teeth.[90]

If the permanent canine erupts into the lateral incisor position, the primary canine can be extracted. Depending on the situation, the permanent canine can be moved back to the correct position, and a prosthetic solution for the missing lateral incisor can be determined as discussed previously. There are several factors to consider in canine substitution. The existing malocclusion, crowding, patient profile, crown shape and color of the canine, and smiling gingival display all influence whether this approach should be considered (Fig. 24.54). These canines require recontouring by enamel removal, bleaching to lighten the color, and resin addition to improve the esthetic appearance of the teeth.

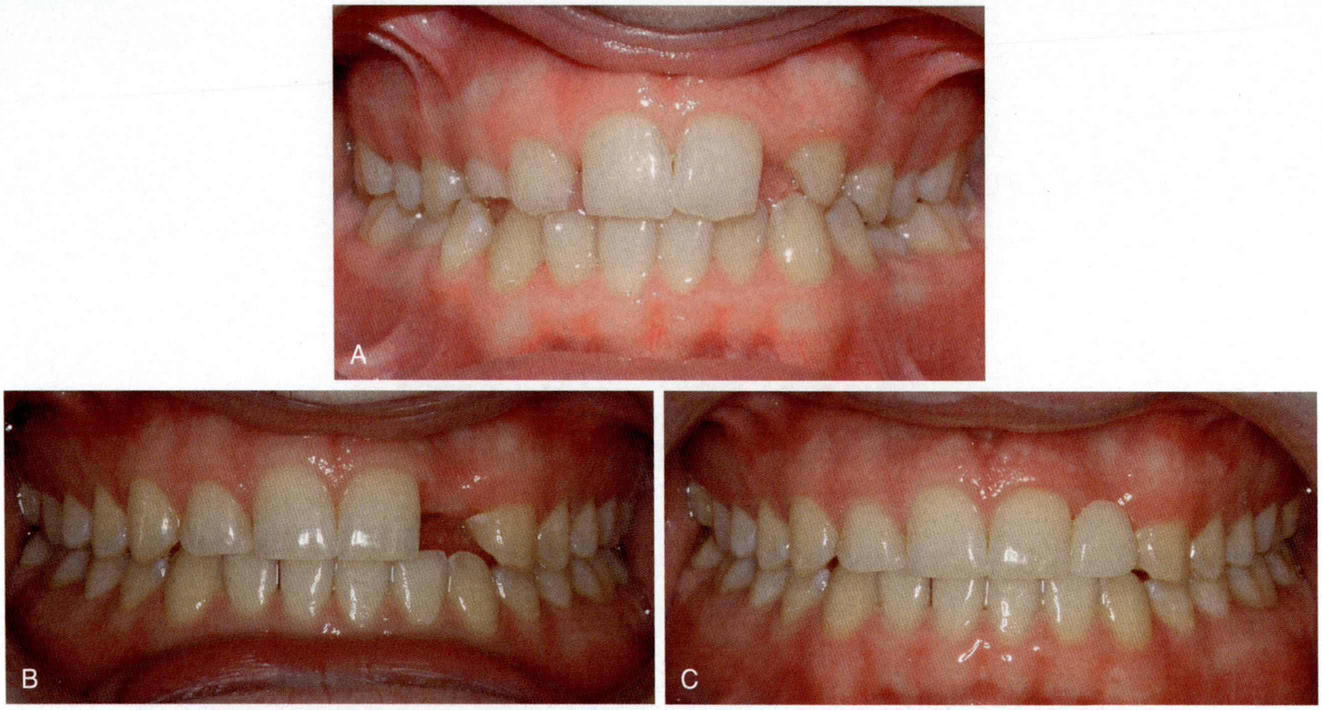

• **Fig. 24.53** (A) This patient is missing the maxillary left lateral incisor. Because the patient has class I molars and relatively good alignment, a decision was made to replace the missing lateral incisor prosthetically. (B) At the end of treatment, a space identical in size to the right lateral incisor was created to replace the left lateral incisor. (C) A dental laboratory created a left lateral incisor pontic with thin abutment wings. The abutment teeth were etched and composite resin was used to bond the abutment wings to each tooth. This type of restoration does not work with a deep bite because of the shearing force of occlusion on the lingual surface.

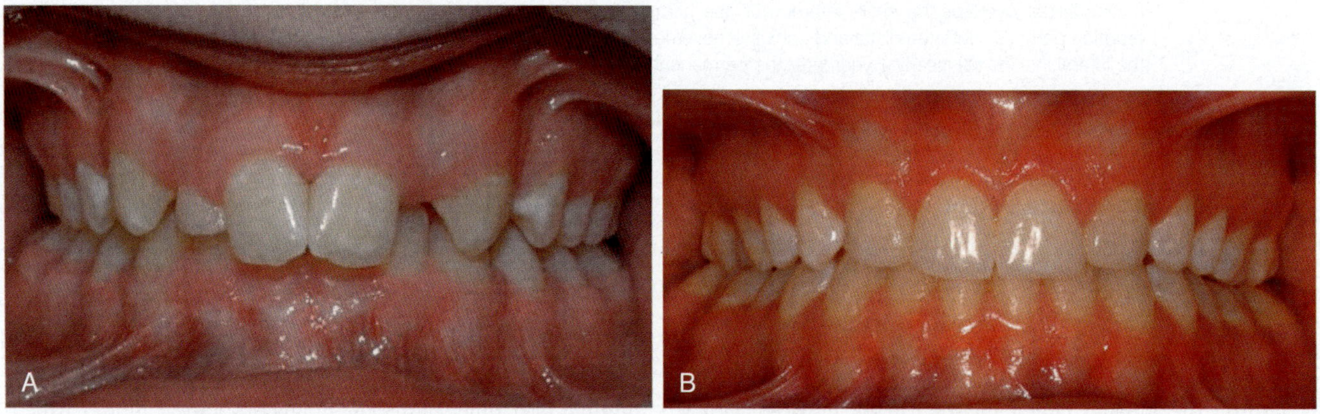

• **Fig. 24.54** (A) This patient was congenitally missing both upper lateral incisors. A decision was made to substitute the canines into the lateral position. (B) The central incisors and canines have been recontoured by adding resin and using a dental bur. If the first premolar is too small in shape, it is possible to recontour the first premolar with composite resin to mimic a canine.

The recommended treatment is to extrude the canine and intrude the first premolar to create gingival margins that match normal occlusions. The ideal case for canine substitution is a good profile, a class II dental relationship, no crowding in the lower arch, and small canines with color that matches the central incisors.[91] Canine substitution cases are considered difficult to treat well. A normal pretreatment occlusion favors canine retraction and prosthetic replacement, as does short or wide canine crown morphology and dark canine color. These elements reduce the chances of providing an esthetic canine substitution for the lateral incisor. Even if the canine must be retracted, this is not without some virtue. The canine brought bone with it during its eruption, and this bone will enhance future esthetics and potential implant placement in the lateral incisor position. The clinician should discuss all treatment options with the patient in missing lateral incisor cases. It is especially important when studies show patients are more satisfied with natural tooth replacement (canine substitution) than prosthetic replacement.[92,93]

A third option to consider when there is unilateral absence of the maxillary lateral incisor is dental autotransplantation. In most cases of unilateral absence, the contralateral lateral incisor is small in width.[93] This creates a Bolton tooth size deficiency in the maxillary arch. Depending on the size of the contralateral incisor, this deficiency can be up to 4 mm. A lower central incisor can be transplanted into the site of the missing lateral incisor and restored to match the small contralateral incisor. The removal of an approximate 5 to 6 mm lower incisor will shift the tooth size discrepancy from a maxillary deficiency to a maxillary excess of 2 mm. The case can be finished with class I molars and canines with a slightly increased overjet and overbite due to the tooth size issue. This type of solution favors patients with class I and class III malocclusions with missing teeth (Fig. 24.55).

When incisors are lost to trauma, the clinician must study the existing situation in a manner like congenitally missing lateral incisors. The age and growth status of the patient, the amount of crowding, and the skeletal relationship must be considered. The number of teeth lost, the status of the periodontium, and the injuries to adjacent teeth further complicate decisions. Not only is the clinician faced with the normal questions of conventional orthodontics, but the clinician is making decisions on teeth with uncertain prognoses and diminished or missing bony support. Traditional management of replacing incisors lost to trauma

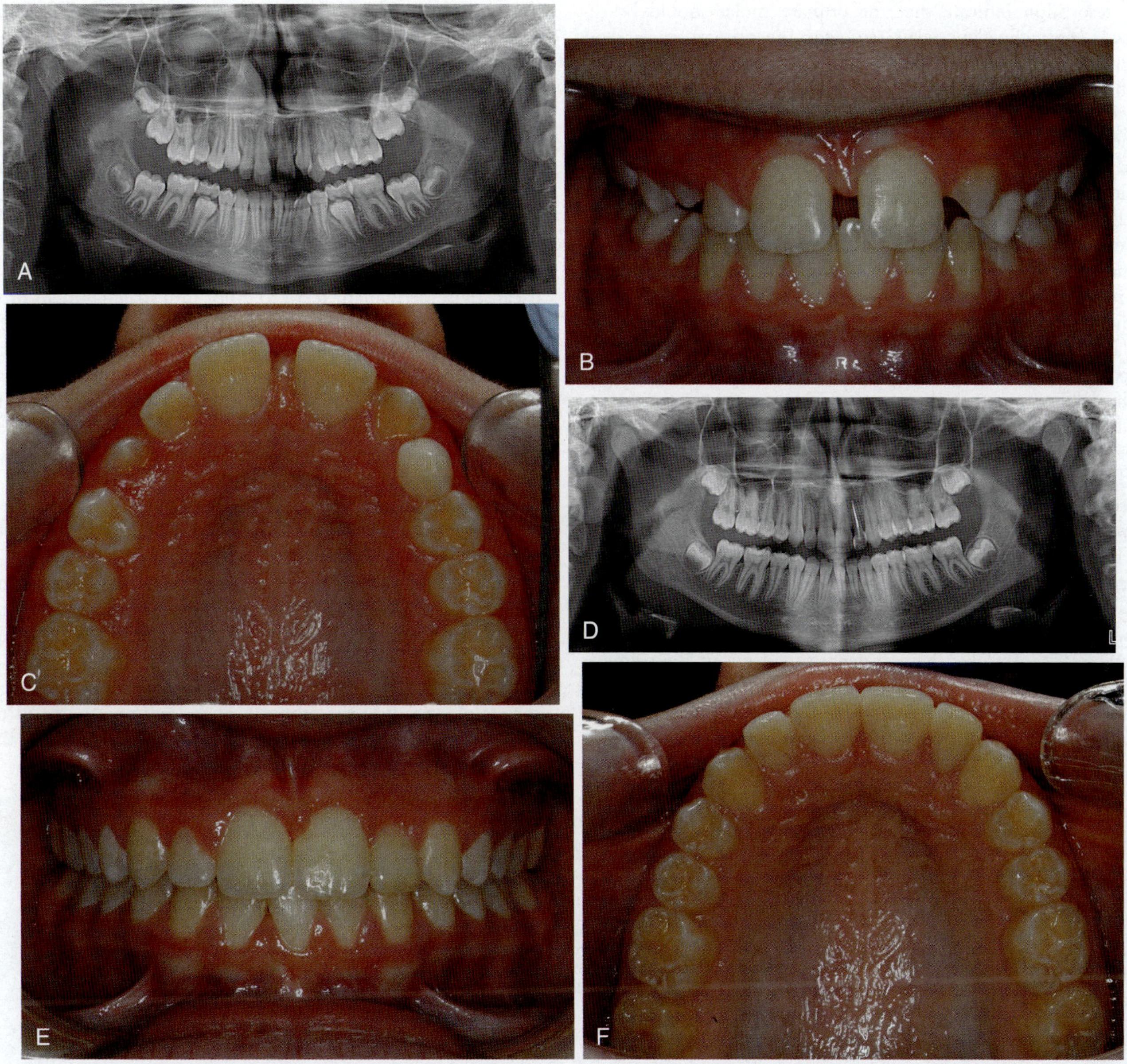

• **Fig. 24.55** (A) The panoramic radiograph showed this patient was missing the upper left lateral incisor. (B) The frontal view shows the missing lateral incisor and retained primary canine on the left. The right lateral incisor is small in size. (C) The occlusal view confirms the findings. (D) Panoramic radiograph of the case after treatment. A lower right central incisor was transplanted and restored to replace the missing maxillary left lateral incisor. (E) The frontal view of the transplanted mandibular central incisor. (F) The occlusal view of the finished case.

usually involves prosthetic tooth replacement or natural tooth replacement through substitution of teeth.

Another possibility is the use of transplanted posterior teeth, usually a premolar, into the position of the missing maxillary central incisor. With reshaping and either resin or veneer restoration, this option can be quite successful. Although not widely adopted in North America, posterior tooth transplantation is a real option in Europe, Japan, and South Korea.[94]

Arch length, incisor position, and facial appearance must be thoroughly evaluated before a treatment plan is generated when a premolar is congenitally missing. Unlike primary canines and laterals, a primary molar may be a reasonable substitute for a missing premolar. The size, shape, and restorative status of the primary molar give some indication of the possibility of maintaining the tooth for a period of time (Fig. 24.56). Ankylosis and advanced root resorption indicate that the primary molar should be removed. Most clinicians favor removing the primary molar and closing the space orthodontically (Fig. 24.57); but in certain situations, a resin-bonded bridge, conventional bridge, or implant may be a more ideal treatment (Fig. 24.58). Prosthetic replacement is more likely in class I skeletal and dental patients with ideal or nearly ideal occlusions or when a tooth is missing unilaterally. Again, the introduction of TADs allows the clinician to determine whether space closure is appropriate in a case where prosthetic replacement used to be automatic, such as when it would be difficult to move teeth without affecting the occlusion and relationship of the remaining teeth. The TAD can be used to move a posterior segment forward without causing the anterior teeth to shift (creating a midline deviation) because the movement of the teeth is pitted against the stability of the TAD within the bone and not the teeth. As a general guideline, use of TADs is contraindicated in children younger than 12 years because of bone density, the presence of unerupted teeth, and the inability to hold the miniscrew.

If the arch is so crowded that teeth must be extracted, or if the incisors are too protrusive or the profile too full, the retained primary molar should be removed and the case treated in a manner like that for a four-premolar extraction case. Typically, first premolars are removed in an extraction case, but most congenitally missing premolars are second premolars. If it can be determined that the second premolar is missing and that extractions are necessary to resolve the arch length inadequacy, the primary molar can be removed early, allowing the space to close by mesial drifting of the permanent first molar and distal drifting of the anterior teeth. Unfortunately, congenital absence of the second premolar may not be definitively determined at an early age, and this delays the extractions. The longer the extractions are delayed, the less drifting and spontaneous space closure will occur. Using the space of the missing second premolars to reduce protrusion is much more complicated and requires the teeth to be retracted into the space of the missing teeth. This precludes dental drifting and should be planned by the specialist.

One further word of caution. If the primary molars are ankylosed and the permanent successor missing, then the primary molars should be extracted before the vertical bony discrepancy of the alveolus becomes too great (Fig. 24.59). This may require subsequent space maintenance. Studies show that loss of bony ridge will be minimal, and the maintenance of good bony contours for the adjacent teeth without periodontal defects will be improved. There is a reduction of alveolar bone width of 25% to 30%, but the authors show that implant placement is still feasible without bone grafting.[95] Later, implants or restorations can be placed, and in some cases the space can be closed orthodontically. Some have suggested using decoronation of the ankylosed primary molar to maintain alveolar width, but this should be initiated before the growth spurt. A last alternative is to use dental autotransplantation of a premolar to another posterior position if tooth removal is being considered for orthodontic reasons.[96]

Supernumerary Teeth

A supernumerary tooth may create space and eruption problems. It can cause permanent teeth to erupt into malalignment or even prevent eruption. Treatment is directed at minimizing the effect of the supernumerary tooth by immediate removal or observation and later removal. Management of the supernumerary varies depending on the size, shape, number of supernumeraries, and the dental development of the patient. Typically, the supernumerary is detected on a panoramic radiograph or an anterior occlusal film unless there is clinical evidence of an extra tooth at an earlier age. If the supernumerary is conical and is not inverted, there is a reasonable chance that it will erupt, at which time it should be removed (Fig. 24.60). If the supernumerary is inverted, it may migrate superiorly away from the teeth and possibly into the nose. A tubercular-shaped tooth will not migrate but may, as with any supernumerary tooth, significantly impede eruption of the adjacent teeth. When multiple supernumerary teeth are present or if the supernumerary tooth fails to erupt, there is an increased chance of impeding the eruption of at least one tooth. In these cases, surgical removal makes sense. Ideally, the surgery is timed

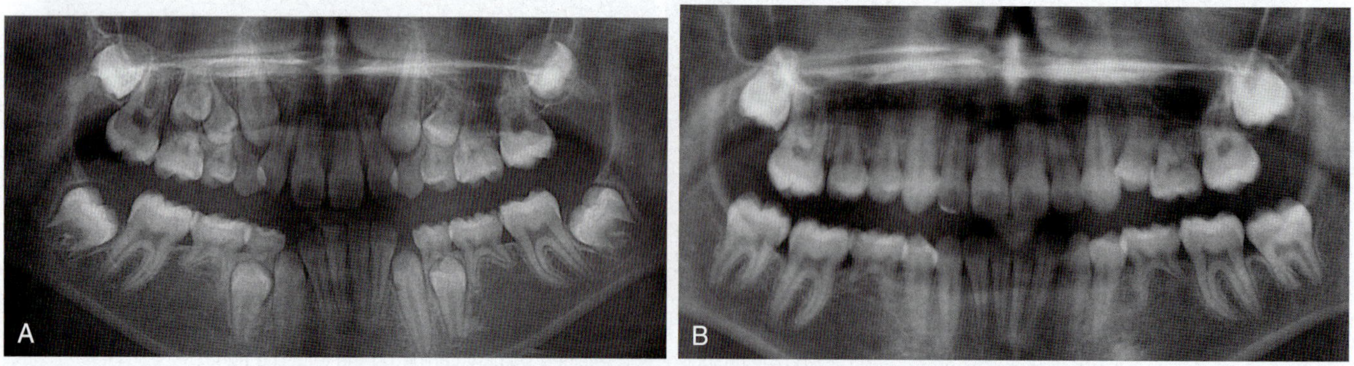

• **Fig. 24.56** In some cases, retaining primary molars as an interim replacement for missing premolars is acceptable. Usually, the primary molars ultimately will require replacement. (A) Patient with missing maxillary left second premolar and both mandibular second premolars. (B) The parents and patient did not want prosthetic replacement of teeth, so the orthodontic treatment was directed to the anterior teeth only.

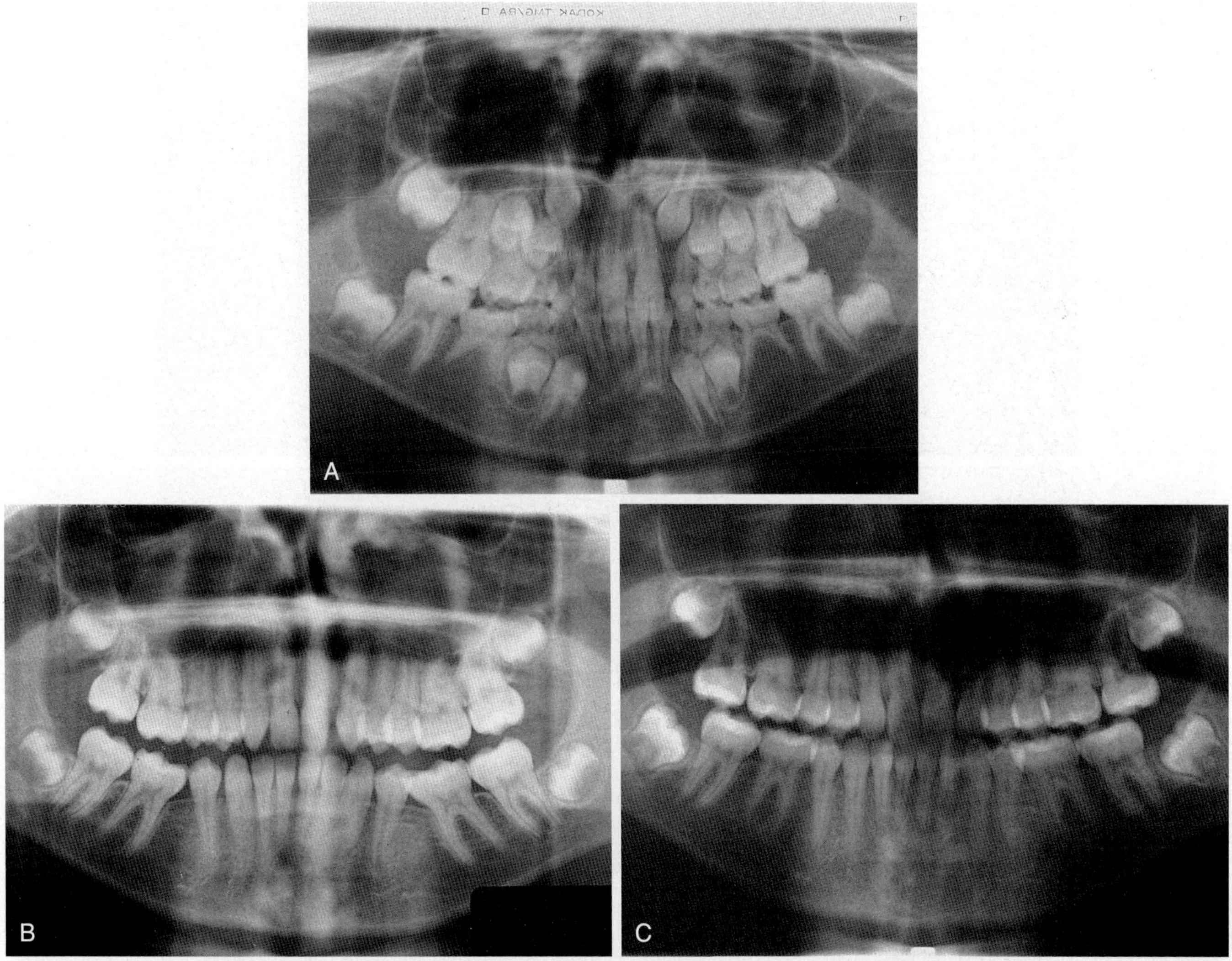

• **Fig. 24.57** Closing the spaces that accompany missing teeth and avoiding prosthetic replacements are sometimes advantageous. (A) This patient is missing maxillary lateral incisors and mandibular second premolars. (B) The remaining primary teeth were extracted and allowed to drift. (C) Orthodontics was completed, and the teeth were finally positioned.

so that removal of the supernumerary tooth does not interfere with permanent tooth development. However, the earlier the supernumerary can be removed, the more likely it is that the permanent teeth will erupt normally. Surgery to remove a supernumerary is often complicated, especially if there are multiple supernumerary teeth or if access to the supernumerary tooth is limited. These patients are appropriately referred to a specialist.

Tooth Size Discrepancies

Isolated tooth size discrepancies can cause alignment problems. The maxillary lateral incisor commonly creates this type of problem because it is undersized or has a pegged shape. Occasionally the lateral incisor can be restored to its normal size with composite resin and requires no other treatment. In some cases, the pegged lateral needs a combination of tooth movement and restorative dentistry to achieve normal occlusion. Depending on the size of the discrepancy, the pegged lateral can be treated in one of three ways.

If the lateral incisor is only slightly smaller than normal, the entire space can be closed. An alternative method for a marginally small incisor is to move the lateral incisor orthodontically until it contacts the central incisor and leave space distal to the lateral. This solution is generally not esthetically pleasing unless only a small space is left distal to the lateral. It also requires retention to hold the space. The canine usually is not brought forward to close the space because this would put the canine in an end-to-end relationship and disrupt the previously normal occlusion. An alternative to this approach is to use interproximal tooth reduction in the lower arch to make those anterior teeth narrower, so the upper space can be fully closed. A third solution, usually reserved for incisors that are considerably undersized, is a combination of orthodontic tooth movement and resin bonding to reshape the crown (Fig. 24.61). The lateral incisor should be positioned so that the resin addition will be cosmetically pleasing and will restore near-normal crown anatomy. In some cases, a diagnostic setup to plan the tooth movement and restorative requirements is suggested.

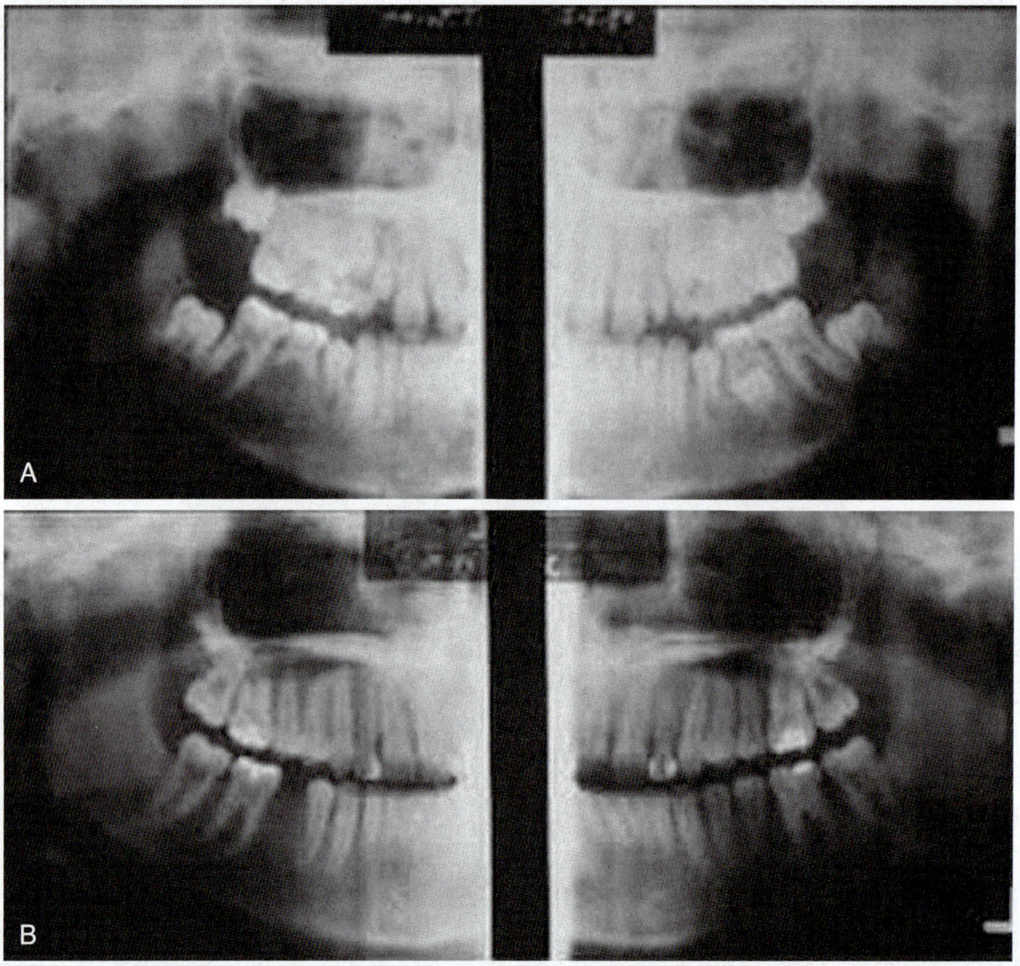

• **Fig. 24.58** When permanent teeth are missing, often unilaterally, the best solution is to adjust the space and plan for prosthetic replacement. (A) Because of the short roots and restorative status, the primary mandibular right second molar was extracted. (B) The space was adjusted to accommodate a prosthetic replacement.

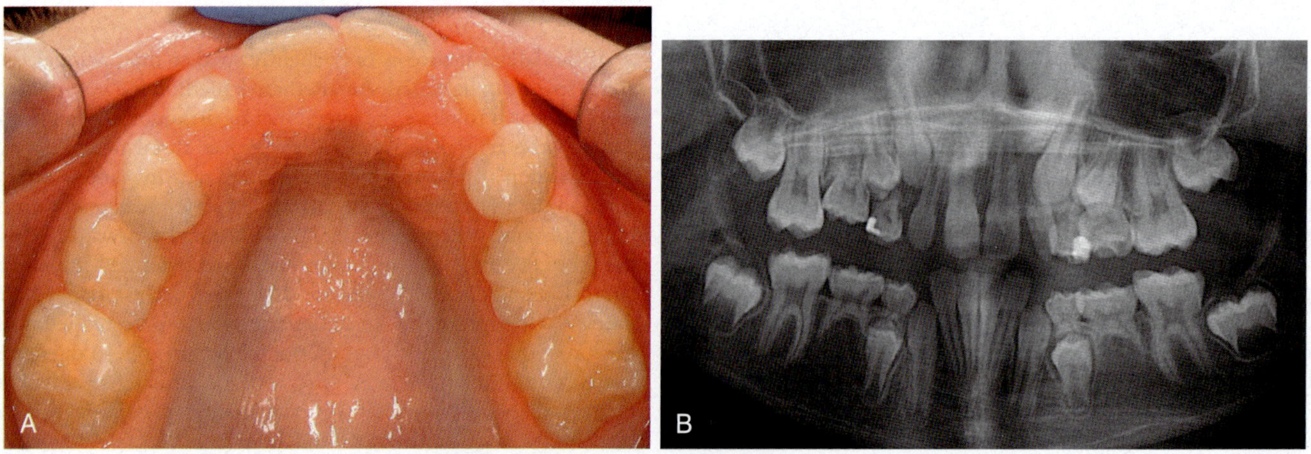

• **Fig. 24.59** (A) This patient has an ankylosed primary maxillary right second molar, as illustrated by the more apical marginal ridges of the tooth. (B) The panoramic radiograph shows that the maxillary right and mandibular second premolars are missing. Because of the developing vertical discrepancy in the bone levels, the primary molars should be removed as atraumatically as possible and the space either maintained or closed.

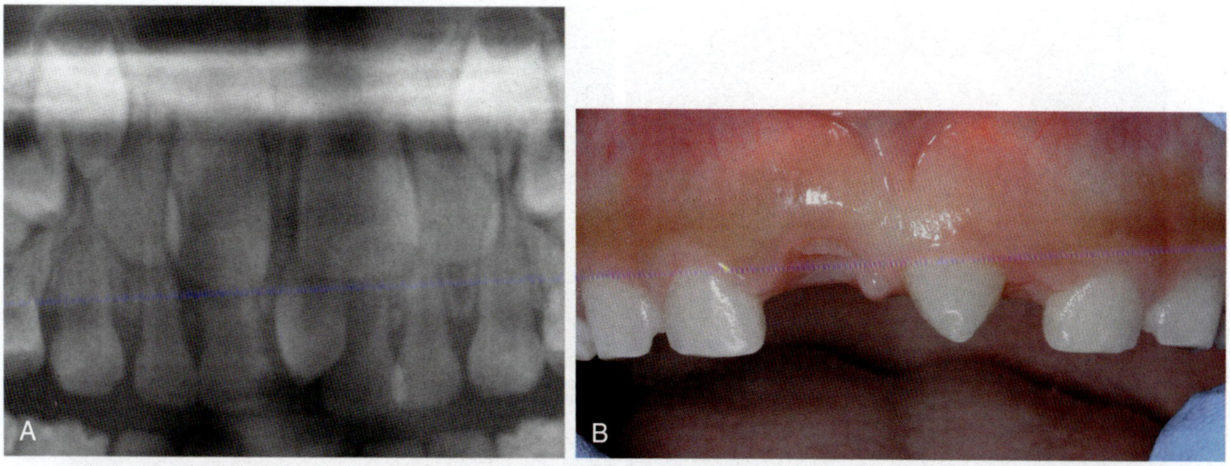

• **Fig. 24.60** (A) A conical supernumerary in the maxillary central incisor region was detected during a radiographic examination. This supernumerary was not interfering with the normal eruption of the permanent incisors. (B) The supernumerary was allowed to erupt before it was removed.

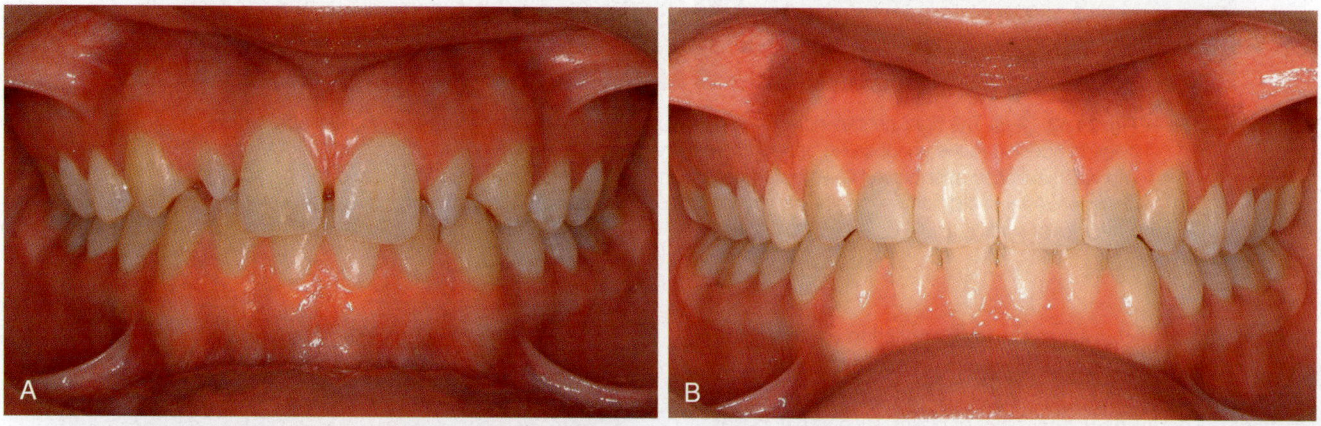

• **Fig. 24.61** (A) One possible solution to a small lateral incisor is a combination of orthodontic tooth movement and resin bonding to reshape the crown of the tooth. (B) This patient had bilateral small lateral incisors. The laterals were positioned so resin addition would make the teeth esthetically pleasing, restore near-normal crown anatomy, and provide good functional occlusion.

Occasionally a single tooth will be extremely large, which will result in crowding and malpositioning of the teeth. In these cases, the tooth often can be reduced to match the contralateral tooth and repositioned.

Fusion and gemination in the permanent dentition are even more difficult to treat. It is possible in some cases to divide fused permanent teeth, move one or both resulting teeth into good position, and then restore the remaining tooth or teeth.[97] Often endodontic treatment is required because the division violated the pulpal space (Fig. 24.62).

Dens evaginatus and incisor talon cusps provide interesting challenges in securing an ideal occlusion. In most cases of dens evaginatus a fine, threadlike pulp extends from the main pulp chamber into the evagination, and the location of this pulp tissue extension should be determined radiographically. Most such teeth in the posterior region do not require treatment because the force of mastication slowly wears the evagination down, and reparative dentin is formed. However, in the anterior region the attrition must be accomplished mechanically with a handpiece and bur. A small amount of tooth structure is removed at each appointment, and after each session calcium hydroxide paste is applied to the exposed dentin to stimulate the reparative process. Usually, the tooth can be treated at monthly appointments without permanent injury to the pulp. When treatment is complete, the exposed dentin is covered with a base and a resin restoration is placed.

Alignment Problems

Anterior and posterior tooth irregularities with adequate space should be regarded as different from anterior and posterior space shortages. Tooth irregularity alone consists simply of rotated and tipped teeth in which there is no shortage of arch length when the leeway space is considered. Arch length discrepancies (i.e., a true lack of space) also result in tooth irregularities but are a different situation and require different management and timing.

Appliance Considerations

Tooth irregularities can be managed with either fixed or removable appliances. If a simple tipping force and no rotation are required to align the tooth, a removable appliance with a finger spring is an appropriate choice. A great variety of removable appliances exist; however, several essential components must be included in the design.

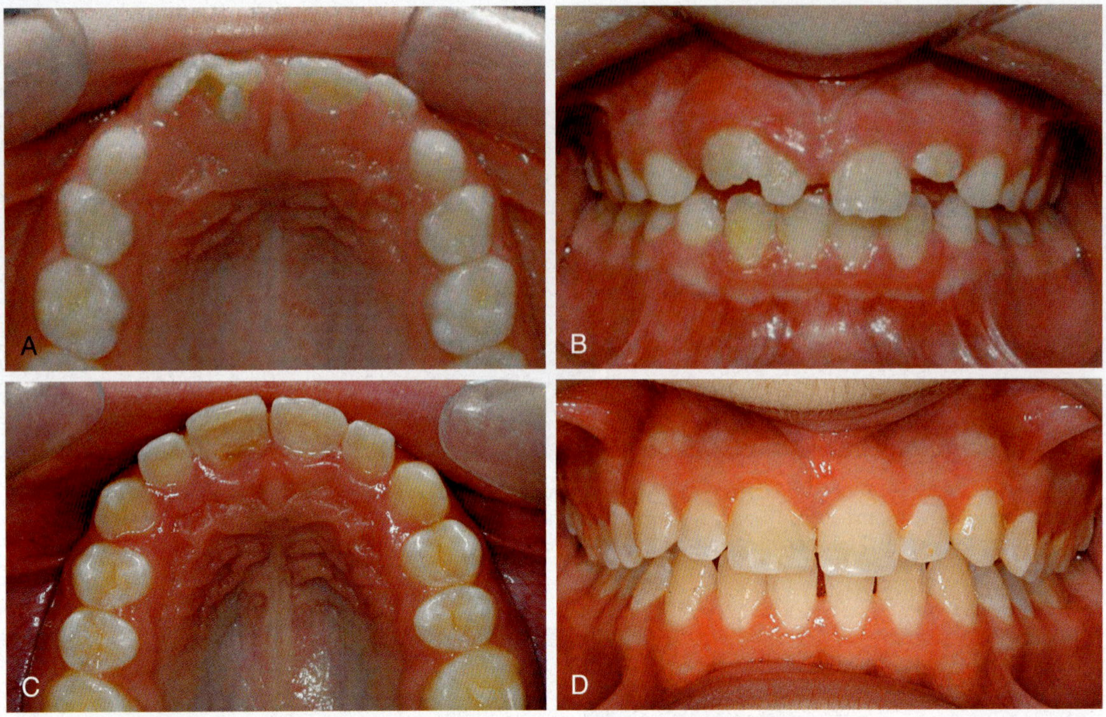

• **Fig. 24.62** (A–B) The right central incisor was fused to a supernumerary tooth creating a single large incisor. In addition to the unappealing appearance, there was no room for the lateral incisor to erupt. The tooth was sectioned after careful review of the canal anatomy with a cone beam computed tomography radiograph. After sectioning, the tooth was moved into correct position with orthodontics (C) and restored on the mesial surface (D).

The appliance must be retentive so the force applied to the tooth will not dislodge the appliance. Adams clasps are often prescribed and are very retentive, although they require careful adjustment and may interfere with the occlusion. Other types of clasps, such as ball clasps and "C" clasps, are also popular but provide distinctly less retention and flexibility. Multiple clasps should be used to enhance the retention. Additional retention and stability are gained from the palatal acrylic in maxillary appliances. A helical finger spring made of 0.022-inch stainless steel wire incorporated into the palatal acrylic delivers a light, continuous force. The spring should be activated 2 mm to move the tooth approximately 1 mm/month (Fig. 24.63).

Fixed appliances (braces) can be used to correct irregularities and are indicated when controlled tipping movements, bodily movement, or rotational control of teeth is necessary. Orthodontic appliances have evolved to a point in which specific brackets are designed for specific teeth. The brackets are constructed to provide proper crown and root positioning when they are precisely placed on the teeth and appropriate archwires are used.

Placement of fixed appliances and the different types of appliances should be reviewed in *Contemporary Orthodontics,* Volume 7 (Elsevier). It is also helpful to review archwires and archwire properties to select the appropriate orthodontic wire for each situation. Finally, retention strategies should be considered to pick the best retention plan for each patient.

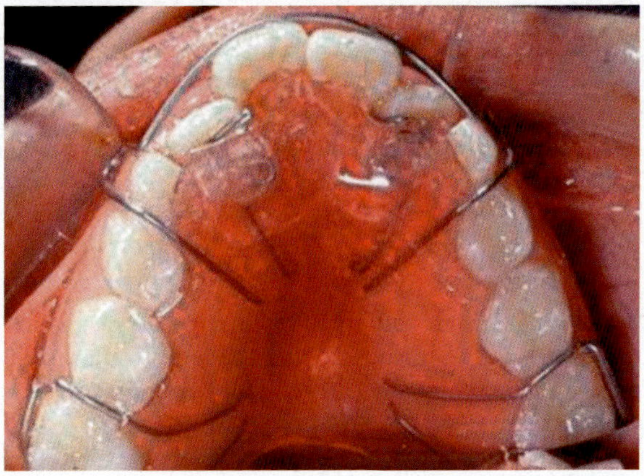

• **Fig. 24.63** Removable appliances can be used to manage alignment problems but are more effective for some problems than for others. Notice that the maxillary right lateral incisor can easily be tipped facially, but it is more difficult to rotate the left lateral incisor and requires use of the lingual finger spring and the labial bow in concert to create a movement. In general, this type of movement is more efficient with a fixed banded and bonded appliance.

Mild to Moderate Spacing

Many children have a midline diastema in the mixed dentition, and this is considered a normal stage of development. Occasionally, a large midline diastema is present that is due to a mesiodens or other midline intrabony pathologic process, protruding incisors, or a tooth size problem. A diastema caused by a midline supernumerary tooth or abnormality is managed by removal of the supernumerary tooth or the abnormality. The supernumerary tooth should be removed as early as possible without causing injury to the adjacent permanent teeth. Early removal of the mesiodens allows the permanent teeth to erupt normally, and the space usually closes spontaneously.

In some cases, a large diastema may be due to faciolingual rather than mesiodistal positioning of the incisors. Flared incisors are cosmetically unappealing and are at greater risk of traumatic injury.[98] If the teeth can be tipped back into an ideal position to close the diastema and if the overbite will not hinder tooth movement, a removable appliance may be selected.

Fixed orthodontic appliances are suggested if incisors are so protrusive that bodily movement is required to close the diastema or if the teeth are rotated. Orthodontic brackets are placed on the molars and incisors. The first step is to align teeth. After initial alignment, the teeth are retracted via a rectangular wire with closing loops or elastomeric chain (Fig. 24.64). Rectangular archwires are indicated to provide control of tooth position during retraction. If there are anchorage requirements, appliances such as headgear may be necessary to reinforce the molar anchorage. It is important to determine whether teeth should be tipped or bodily moved in the treatment planning phase. The decision on headgear is based on initial molar position, the amount of space to close, and vertical dimensions of the face.

If the diastema is due to a discrepancy in size between the upper and lower anterior teeth (the mandibular teeth are relatively larger than the maxillary), treatment usually requires the addition of resin to the interproximal surfaces of the maxillary incisors. Closing the space using orthodontics will result in a reduced overjet and overbite and possible anterior occlusal trauma due to occlusal interference of the anterior teeth. In addition, relapse is common because the occlusion will force the space open again.

Treatment to close a midline diastema is usually initiated if the diastema is greater than 2 mm and one of the following three situations exist. The first is if the diastema inhibits or disturbs the eruption of the lateral incisors. In general, treatment starts to coincide with the normal eruption time of the lateral incisor. If the diastema is large enough to be esthetically objectionable, a clinician can consider treatment if the patient is being teased or suffering psychological problems due to appearance. If the diastema is still present after the eruption of the permanent canines, treatment can be considered. The diastema is due to faulty mesiodistal positioning of the incisors, but the choice of appliance is still based on the tooth movement required to close the space. If the central incisors can be tipped together to close the diastema, a removable appliance can be used.

Brackets are bonded on the central incisors if the teeth require bodily mesiodistal movement or rotational control to close the diastema. After initial alignment, a large segmental or full rectangular archwire is placed in the brackets, and the teeth are moved together via elastomeric chain (Fig. 24.65). No matter which type of treatment is used to close a midline diastema, retention can be a problem and should be planned. In most cases a removable appliance maintains space closure. The appliance should be adjusted periodically if the diastema is closed before the lateral incisors and canines have erupted fully. If the diastema reopens during or after retention and the clinician determines the frenal attachment is contributing to the continued opening of the diastema, a surgical procedure called a frenectomy can be performed. If the diastema reopens after retention and the frenectomy, a small orthodontic wire can be bonded to the lingual surface of the incisors to keep the teeth together (Fig. 24.66). The only contraindications to a bonded wire retainer are an excessively deep bite (occlusion will dislodge the bonded wire) and poor oral hygiene.

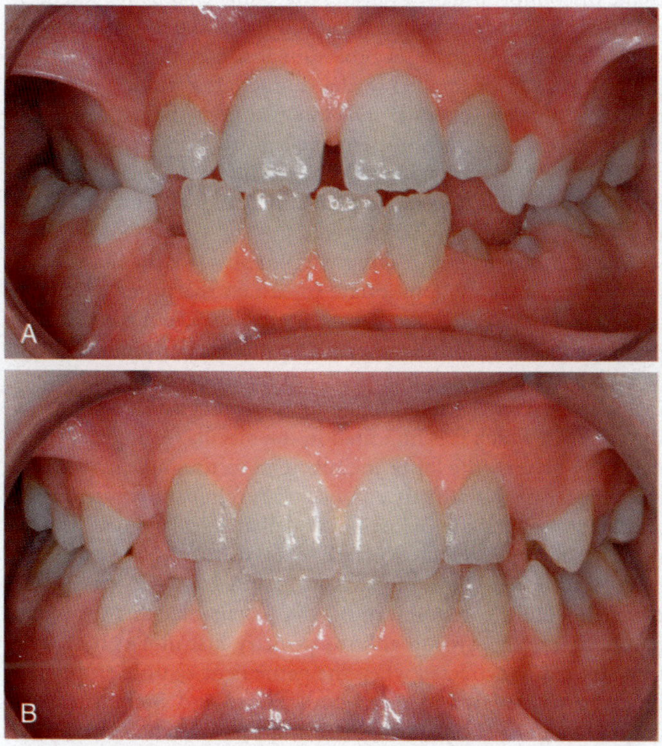

• **Fig. 24.64** (A) When rotations are present or bodily movement is required to close space and retract incisors, the best alternative is a fixed appliance. This patient required both transverse expansion and diastema closure to make room for the permanent canines. (B) The space closure was completed using fixed appliances and elastomeric chain.

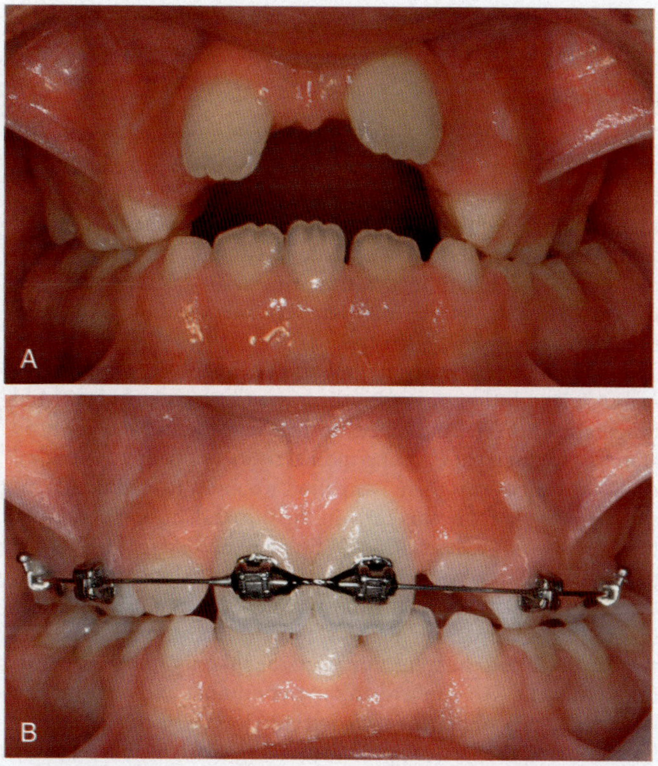

• **Fig. 24.65** (A) If bodily mesiodistal movement is needed to close a diastema, fixed appliances are placed on the teeth. (B) After initial alignment, either a segmental or a full archwire is placed in the brackets, and the teeth are moved together with an elastomeric chain.

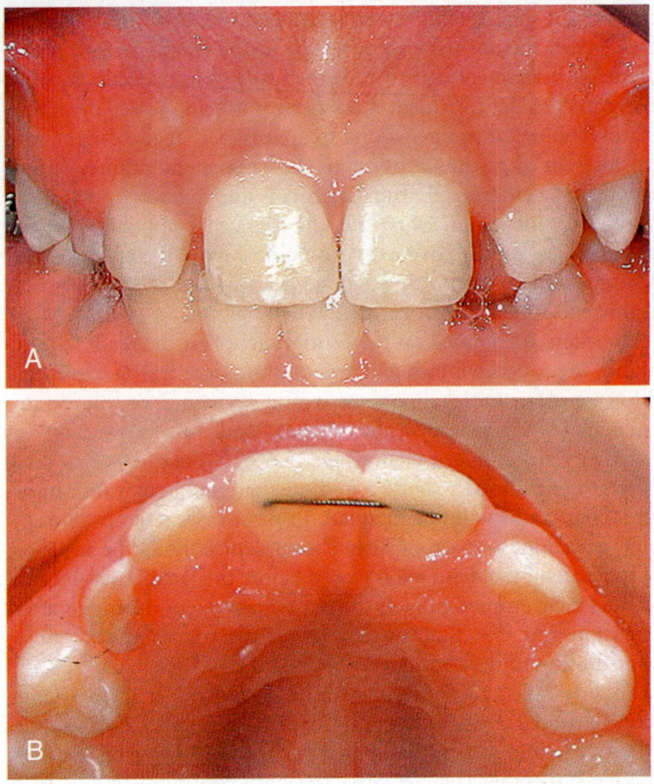

• **Fig. 24.66** (A) After diastema closure, retention is required. (B) One method that reduces the need for patient cooperation is the light, multi-stranded bonded wire. The wire must be placed far enough gingivally to prevent occlusal interferences. In addition, the patient must clean the area carefully and avoid direct contact with hard foods.

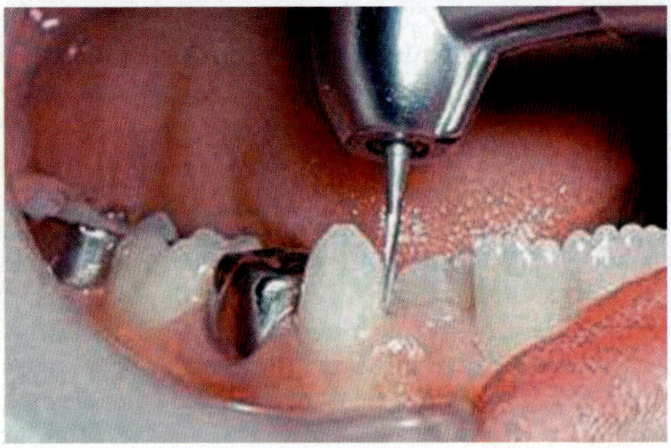

• **Fig. 24.67** When the arch length discrepancy is determined to be 2 mm or less and the lateral incisor is erupting lingual to its proper position, the primary canine can be disked with either a high- or low-speed handpiece or a handheld strip. In this case a tapered fissure bur in a high-speed handpiece is being used to disk the mesial surface of the primary canine.

Mild Crowding

The first sign of crowding in the mixed dentition usually coincides with eruption of the permanent incisors. Arch length insufficiency may manifest in several ways, ranging from slight incisor rotation and irregularity to gross incisor malalignment. The first step should be to perform a space analysis and determine the extent of the arch length inadequacy. This finding is then placed in the context of the facial profile analysis and posterior dental relationships.

Children can have various amounts of irregularity without any real arch length shortage when the leeway space is included. Mild irregularity is even considered normal in patients who have no arch length discrepancy. Longitudinal studies of people with ideal occlusions show that there is a period when up to 2 mm of transitional irregularity occurs early in the mixed dentition and eventually resolves.[99] Observation is usually the best course. Some patients have little or no overall arch length shortages and demonstrate noticeable crowding during incisor eruption. This is due to the larger permanent incisors and the transitional crowding they cause during the transition from the primary to mixed dentitions. Gianelly[100] has described these conditions and noted that a large percentage of patients with irregularity can be treated simply by protecting the leeway space with a lingual arch. If the leeway space is left unattended, the molars will move anteriorly into the leeway space and a true arch length shortage will exist.

The clinical management of irregularity without a true arch length shortage can take several forms depending on the amount of irregularity. In general, if the irregularity is minor, no treatment is indicated. If the irregularity is slightly more severe, interproximal stripping or disking of the primary teeth (usually the canines) can be accomplished to provide temporary space (Fig. 24.67). Disking may be accomplished with a handheld strip, a sandpaper disk in a low-speed handpiece, or a tapered bur in a high-speed handpiece. The enamel-reducing instrument must be held vertically to reduce the true mesiodistal dimension of the tooth even subgingivally to be successful. The procedure is performed without anesthesia so that the child can indicate any discomfort. Extreme discomfort usually indicates that sufficient enamel has been removed to cause the pulpal tissues to react. Careful disking can yield 2 to 6 mm of space. A professional-strength topical fluoride preparation can be applied to the canines after disking and may reduce postoperative sensitivity. Note that in the mixed dentition, interproximal reduction of permanent teeth before the eruption of the permanent canines and evaluation of the patient's tooth size is contraindicated. If teeth are prematurely reduced, an iatrogenic tooth size problem may be created.

If it is apparent that disking will not alleviate the anterior irregularity, it may be appropriate to extract the primary canines and place a lingual arch so that the available space can be used by the larger incisors for alignment, and the smaller premolars can erupt later in the remaining space. For the most part, this therapy is undertaken in the mandibular arch, although there are a few situations in which it is indicated in the maxilla. A lingual arch is necessary because the lower incisors tend to tip lingually without the support of the primary canines. This results in shortening of arch length and some reduction in dental alveolar bone. In this situation the lingual arch is placed in a passive state (i.e., the arch exerts no force to move the incisors and increase the space). The clinician should communicate to the parent that this treatment requires close supervision and the primary first molars may have to be disked or extracted when the permanent canines erupt. The lingual arch remains in place until the second premolars have erupted or until it is evident there will be sufficient space for all the permanent teeth to erupt. Essentially, one is using the leeway space and controlling all available arch length to achieve alignment of the teeth (Fig. 24.68). In some cases, this means the molars (those that are end to end) will not achieve a class I relationship because the mandibular mesial molar shift has been

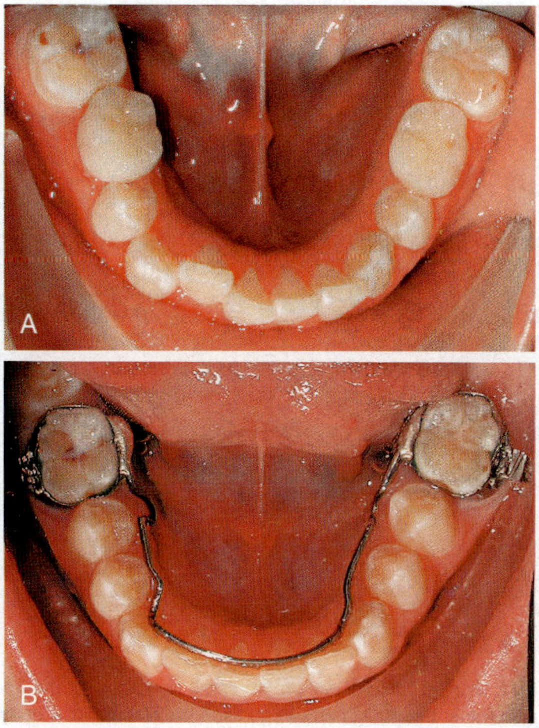

• **Fig. 24.68** Space that is available in the arches (leeway) can be used to alleviate crowding by maintaining space when crowding is present and allowing alignment when the larger primary second molars exfoliate or are extracted. (A) This patient shows some crowding with the primary second molars in place. (B) A lower lingual arch was placed so the leeway space could be used for spontaneous alignment.

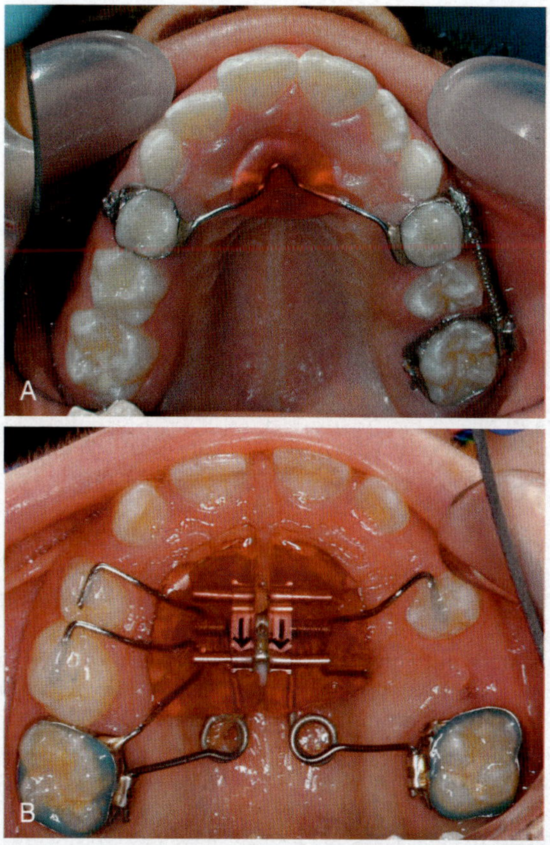

• **Fig. 24.69** A fixed appliance can be used to distalize molars in either arch. In the maxillary arch (A), a modified Nance palatal arch and nickel titanium springs on an archwire, or a Nance arch and helical springs can be used to distalize molars (B). Some anterior incisor movement also occurs.

prevented. Either headgear or interarch mechanics such as elastics will need to be used to achieve the correct occlusal relationships. In other situations, a class I molar relationship may have already been present and this is not a concern.

A true arch length discrepancy of 0 to 2 mm may not be apparent or may be manifested as a mild irregularity, most likely in the incisor region. Treatment may be indicated for these children if the lateral incisors erupt lingual to their proper position or in very irregular positions. If treatment is deemed necessary, interproximal stripping of primary teeth as described earlier may be used. With true, small arch length shortages, ultimately minor crowding will either be accepted, permanent teeth will have to be reduced in the mesiodistal dimension, or the arch will have to be expanded with fixed or removable appliances, as described in the next section.

Moderate Crowding

Treatment for a moderate arch length discrepancy of 5 to 9 mm is based on the facial profile, incisor position, crowding, and the amount of facial keratinized tissue. If the profile is straight, with good anteroposterior or slightly retrusive position of the lips and incisors, a small amount of expansion can be tolerated to accommodate all the teeth. Expansion is not a good treatment option if the incisors are already protrusive. The clinician should always keep in mind the interaction between crowding, incisor position, and profile because they are essentially all part of the same problem, just expressed in a different way.

Moderate crowding may be localized or generalized. Localized crowding may be the result of space loss after extraction or premature exfoliation of a primary tooth. If space loss is 3 mm or less, the adjacent tooth usually can be tipped into proper position with a removable appliance, an active lingual arch, or a fixed banded and bonded appliance. For example, a removable appliance with a finger spring can tip a permanent maxillary or mandibular first molar distally after removal of a primary second molar compromised by ectopic eruption. Numerous other fixed appliances such as lingual holding arches or a Nance lingual arch supporting segmental arches with compressed coil springs can be used (Fig. 24.69A). Alternatively, a Nance arch with compressed helical springs can be used to move posterior teeth distally (see Fig. 24.69B). Regardless of the appliance configuration, the method is basically the same, and these appliances can be used either unilaterally or bilaterally. For arch perimeter increases in the maxillary arch, the distal molar movement is accompanied by an anterior movement of the anchor or anterior segment.[101,102] Without additional anchorage, the anterior teeth move facially in a ratio of approximately one-third anterior and two-thirds posterior (Fig. 24.70). With additional anchorage, such as TADs in the anterior palate, distal molar movement of approximately 1 mm/month has been demonstrated with no change in the position of the anterior teeth.[103] The challenge then is to preserve the distal molar movement and retract and align the remaining teeth.

Alternatively, headgear can be used if bilateral space regaining is desired. After the space has been regained, arch length should be near ideal and should be maintained. A band and loop appliance or a lingual archlike appliance can be placed to maintain the space.

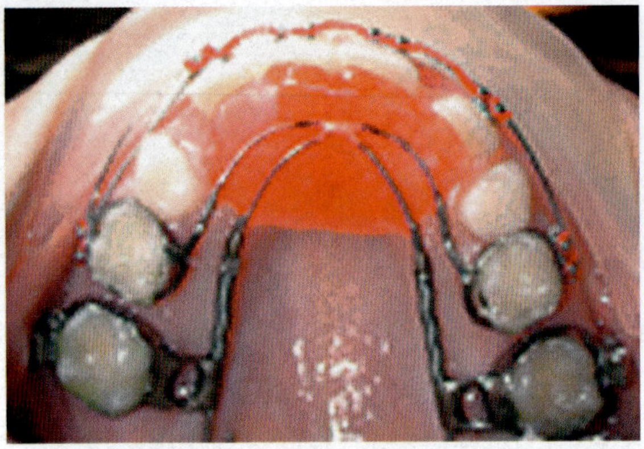

• **Fig. 24.70** Another approach to distalizing molars is to use palatal forces and springs supported by teeth and the palate. Even with this method, some anterior tooth movement is observed unless the appliance is supported with temporary anchorage devices.

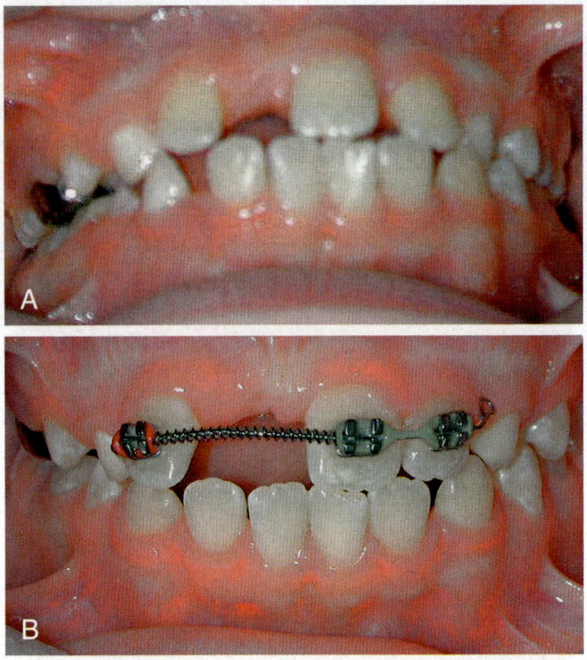

• **Fig. 24.71** Many situations rely on the same principles for treatment of crowding in the anterior segment. In general, the first step is to align and open space. (A) This patient lost the maxillary right central incisor to trauma and subsequently space redistributed. (B) The teeth were aligned with a segmental arch in the first phase of treatment, and then a coil spring was used to open the space for prosthetic replacement.

If localized crowding is not due to terminal molars drifting anteriorly but is in the anterior or midportions of the arch, permanent tooth impaction is likely. Orthodontic tooth movement is necessary to increase the space and allow room for eruption (Fig. 24.71). Fixed orthodontic appliances are placed on a portion or the entire arch, and the teeth are aligned. After alignment, a heavier archwire is placed to maintain good arch form during space-regaining movements. A compressed coil spring is the simplest means to open space and provides adequate force to open the space. After the space has been opened, the clinician should allow the tooth up to 6 months to erupt. If the tooth does not erupt within that time, it may be necessary to surgically expose the tooth. There are two surgical methods to expose a tooth. The first is a closed exposure. In a closed exposure a flap is elevated, and the tooth is located. An orthodontic attachment, often a bracket pad with a soldered gold chain, is bonded to the tooth. The gold chain is tied to the existing orthodontic appliances, and the flap is replaced. The clinician applies force to the gold chain by elastomeric thread, auxiliary wires, or loops from a continuous archwire to bring the tooth into position. Closed exposure is preferred when the tooth crown is located beyond the mucogingival junction. The other type of surgical exposure is an open exposure. In this type of exposure, the soft tissue is elevated and repositioned around the crown to provide adequate keratinized tissue around the impacted tooth. Open exposure is considered when the crown is below the mucogingival junction and minimal repositioning is required. Adequate attached gingiva is essential for good periodontal support and esthetic appearance. Closed exposure simulates the actual eruption of the tooth and usually results in better hard and soft tissue esthetics. In an open exposure the tooth can be allowed to erupt, or an orthodontic attachment is bonded to the crown and the tooth is moved into the arch (Fig. 24.72). Several methods can be used to generate the force to move the tooth occlusally, but using an overlay flexible wire (usually NiTi) is simple and effective. The overlay wire technique is an especially applicable technique for extruding traumatically intruded incisors so that they can be assessed and/or accessed for endodontic treatment. The method is simple, does not impinge on the adjacent tissue, permits easy cleaning, and allows reasonably efficient movement of teeth (Fig. 24.73).

Patients characterized by anterior or generalized crowding of less than 5 mm present difficult treatment decisions. As stated earlier, incisor and lip position provide important guides to whether arch length can be created by expansion as does the presence of adequate facial keratinized tissue. Upright or lingually inclined incisors may be moved facially into correct alignment if the lips are retrusive. However, the risk associated with generalized arch expansion is instability of the new position.[104,105] Movement of teeth facially may upset the existing equilibrium and cause relapse after the appliances are removed. Relapse does not occur in all cases; some patients maintain increased arch dimensions and remain stable after treatment is complete. However, there does not seem to be a good method for predicting stability.[106] Unfortunately, clinical judgment and long-term retention must be relied on in many cases.

If the clinician elects to alleviate arch length inadequacy by expansion (because the leeway space is inadequate), several approaches can be taken. An active lower lingual arch can be constructed with adjustment loops to tip the incisors facially if the overbite is not prohibitively deep to prevent movement of the incisors (Fig. 24.74); the lower lingual arch may also move the molars distally a small amount. When the appliance is activated, the wire contacts the tooth high on the cingulum of the incisors. The direction of force is apical, but it tips the incisors facially because of the inclination of the lingual surface of the teeth. In 4 to 6 weeks the appliance can be activated another millimeter. This process is repeated until the arch length is adequate for the permanent dentition. Primary canines may have to be disked or removed as discussed previously if the crowding is in the anterior region.

A lip bumper, a wire appliance inserted in tubes on the lower molars, may be used to decrease lower lip pressure and achieve generalized arch expansion in the incisor, canine, and premolar regions

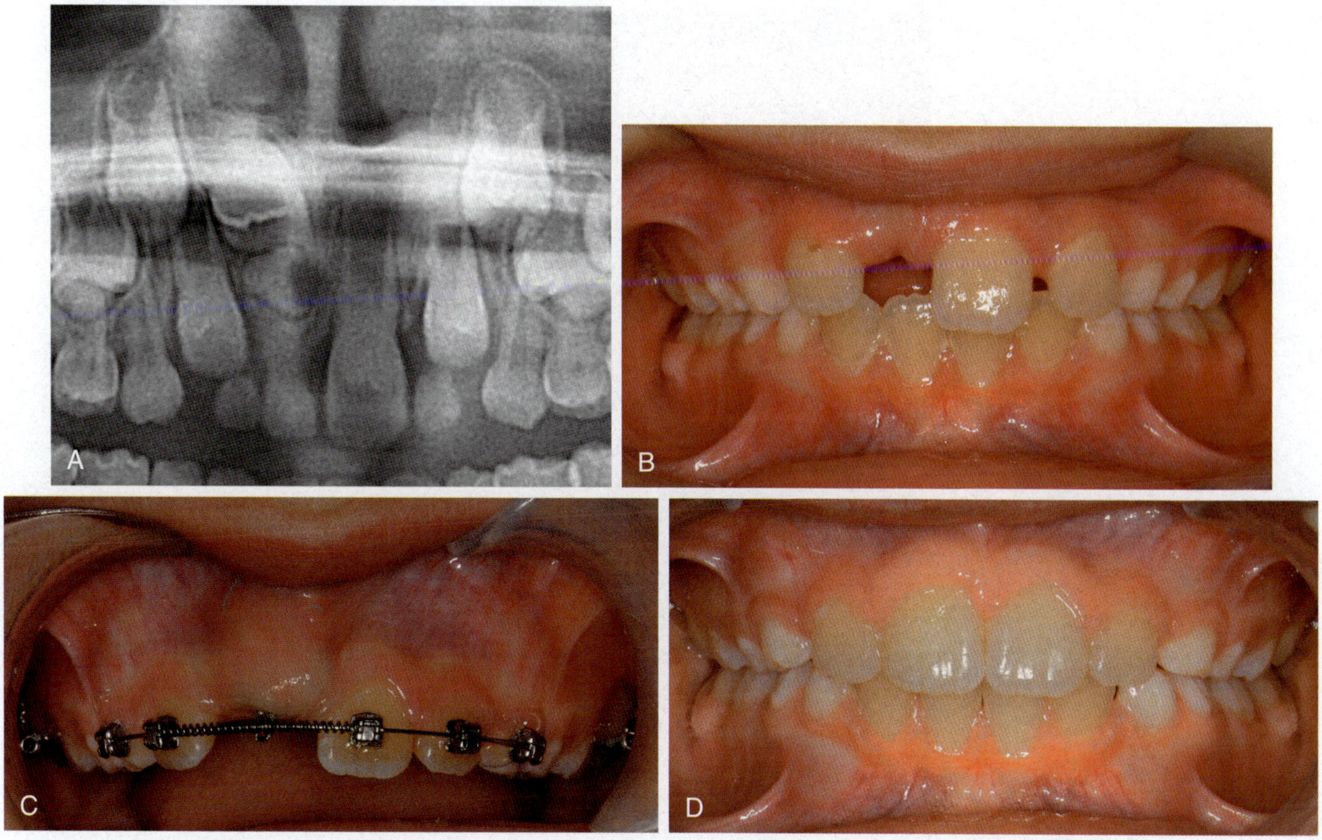

• **Fig. 24.72** (A) A panoramic radiograph was obtained on a patient who had an unerupted right central incisor. The radiograph showed that a supernumerary tooth was blocking the eruption of the central incisor. (B) The primary incisors and the supernumerary were removed to see if the central incisor would erupt. It was determined the central incisor would need to be exposed and a bonded bracket and chain attached so the tooth could be brought into alignment. (C) The space was opened for the unerupted central incisor, and it was brought into position with elastic thread tied to a base archwire. (D) The tooth is in the final position. Note the more gingival attachment on the extruded tooth. These levels should approximate one another with time.

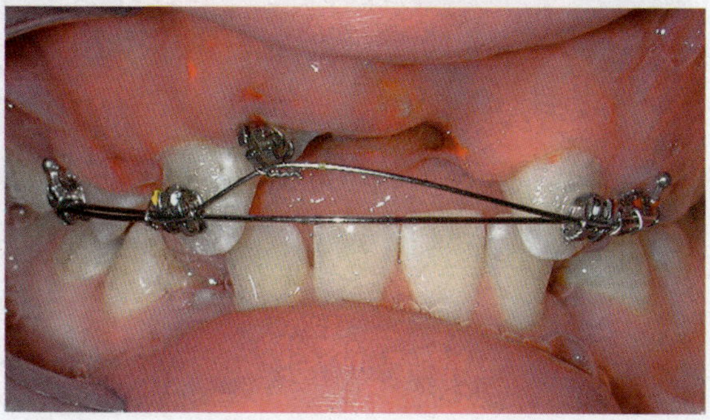

• **Fig. 24.73** Extrusion with overlay wires can be used successfully after traumatic intrusion injuries. The overlay archwire, which is a light and flexible wire and now usually nickel titanium, is ligated with a stiffer supporting archwire, usually stainless steel. The light wire is engaged in the bracket and provides light continuous forces over a large range to rapidly and physiologically extrude the tooth.

(Fig. 24.75). The location of the expansion depends on the location of the lip bumper. The lip bumper removes the resting pressure of the lips and cheeks from these teeth. The teeth move facially because of the lack of lip pressure and the force of the tongue pressure. The pressure from the lower lip may tip the molar distally.[107]

Arch expansion may also be accomplished via a functional appliance with buccal shields in the vestibule.[108] The buccal shields disrupt the equilibrium between the tongue and the cheek and allow the teeth to move facially (Fig. 24.76). Some investigators claim that properly constructed buccal shields stretch the underlying periosteum of the bone and cause skeletal remodeling in the transverse dimension. Although this claim has not been substantiated by careful investigation, there is no doubt that enough expansion can be created in this manner to relieve minor to moderate crowding.

Like removable appliances, fixed appliances can be used to tip teeth. Fixed orthodontic appliances are necessary to increase arch length when bodily movement of teeth is required to alleviate crowding and align the teeth. Banded and bonded appliances also offer the opportunity to efficiently control rotational problems of teeth. A variety of archwire designs can be used to expand the arch, depending on the number of teeth with attachments (Fig. 24.77). Clearly, any dimension of the arch can be altered with this method. After the expansion has been completed, a lower lingual arch is placed to retain the expansion.

In most cases, further treatment is necessary to align the remaining permanent teeth when they erupt (Fig. 24.78). In addition, distal movement of the maxillary molars may be required if some of the leeway space was used to align the mandibular teeth and cannot be used for the mesial molar shift. When a class I

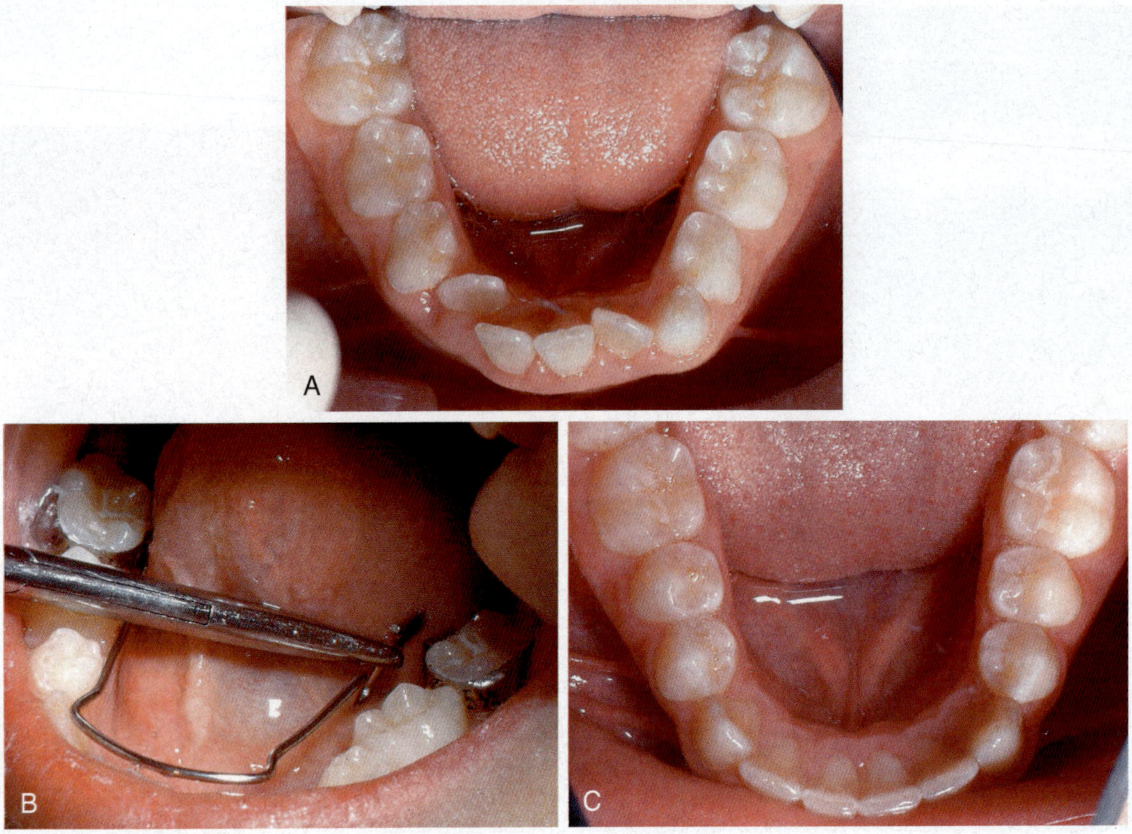

• **Fig. 24.74** (A) Generalized crowding of less than 5 mm is occasionally managed with an adjustable lingual arch if the overbite is not too deep to prevent facial movement of the mandibular incisors. (B) The appliance is activated on several occasions by opening the adjustment loops. (C) The same patient after treatment.

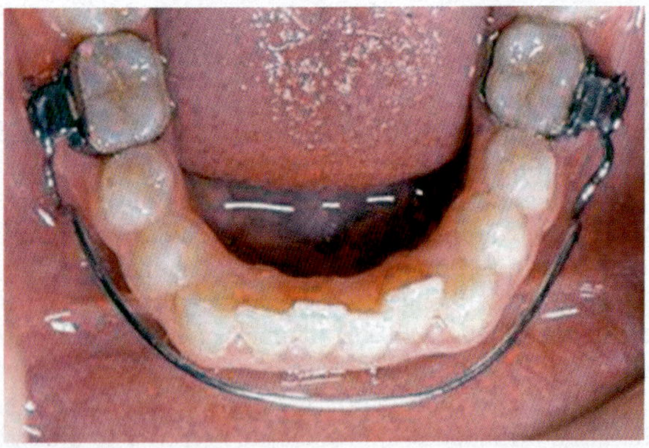

• **Fig. 24.75** A lip bumper is also used to treat generalized crowding of less than 5 mm. The lip bumper is designed to decrease lower lip pressure on the teeth and to allow generalized expansion by facial movement of the teeth.

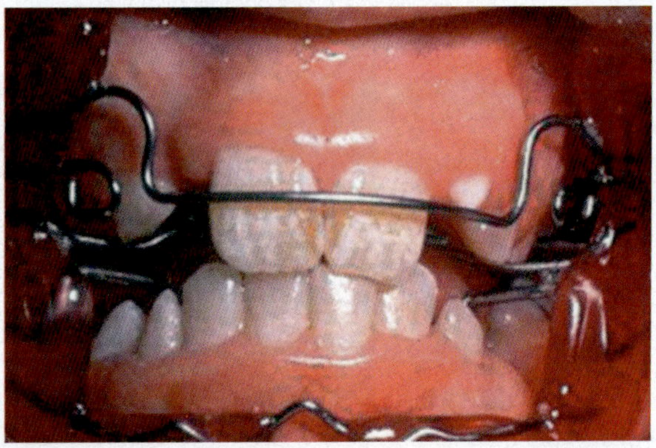

• **Fig. 24.76** Generalized arch expansion can also be accomplished via a functional appliance with buccal shields. The buccal shields disrupt the equilibrium between the facial musculature and the tongue and allow the teeth to move facially.

molar relationship is present initially, this is not an issue. Therefore multibonded appliances should be used sparingly in the lower arch, generally only in cases in which the molars are already class I and there is some increased overjet, unless one is prepared to complete the case appropriately by adjusting the interarch relationships. Regardless of which appliance is selected, expansion influences incisor position and profile.

Severe Crowding

Crowding of more than 9 mm is considered severe. This amount of crowding is managed either with generalized arch expansion or with removal of selected permanent teeth. This degree of generalized arch expansion can be accomplished with different appliances but usually requires bodily tooth movement with fixed appliances. Achieving considerable expansion often is difficult. Incisor position,

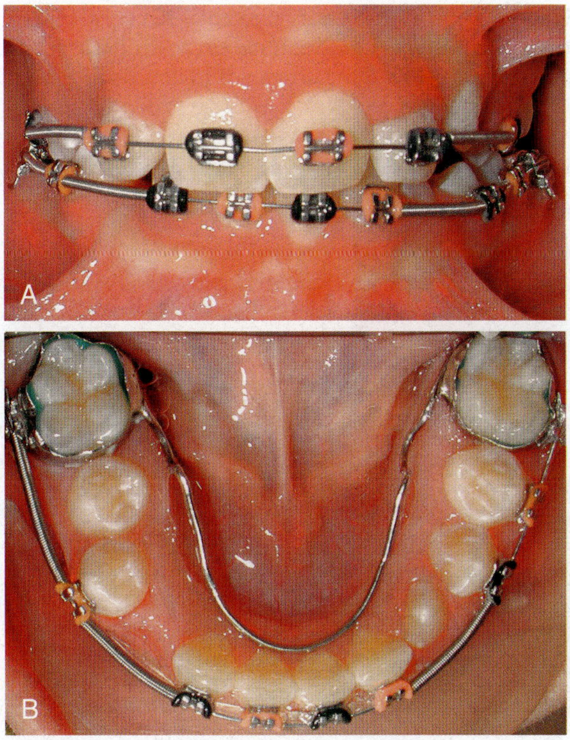

• **Fig. 24.77** Expansion of the dental arches to reduce crowding can be accomplished with fixed appliances and is usually indicated when there are rotations or bodily tooth movement is required. (A) Expansion during the mixed dentition using fixed appliances. (B) The mechanics often are a combination of coil springs and elastomeric chains to move teeth and increase arch dimensions. A lingual arch can be used for maintenance of the intermolar dimension. (From Proffit WR, Fields HW, Jr, Sarver DM. *Contemporary Orthodontics*. 5th ed. Elsevier; 2013.)

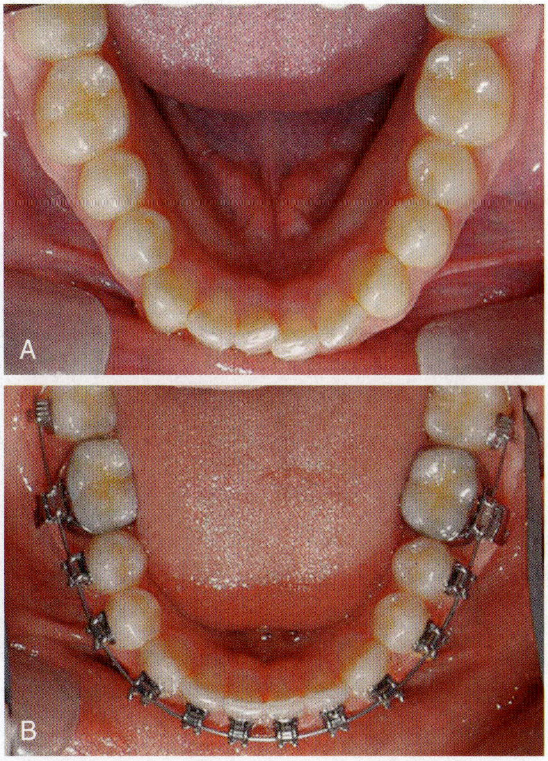

• **Fig. 24.78** (A) Arch expansion can be accomplished during the permanent dentition years too. (B) The anterior irregularities, mostly rotations, were managed with a fixed appliance. (From Proffit WR, Fields HW, Jr, Sarver DM. *Contemporary Orthodontics*. 5th ed. Elsevier; 2013.)

profile, and periodontal status all influence whether the patient should be treated without extraction. Patients with this degree of crowding are most appropriately referred to a specialist.

The decision to extract teeth is based on the same factors and is further influenced by the location of the crowding, the position of the dental midline, and the dental and skeletal relationships of the patient. After careful case analysis, appropriate teeth may be removed to make subsequent tooth movement easier to accomplish and to minimize the effects of extraction on the profile. The permanent first premolar is most often selected for extraction because it is located at a midpoint in the arch and because the space it occupies can be used to correct midline problems, incisor protrusion, molar relationship problems, or crowding. Other teeth can be removed depending on the specifics of the case and the type of therapy used.

In some children, crowding is so severe in the mixed dentition that expansion is not feasible, and extractions are necessary to obtain a suitable occlusion that is in harmony with the supporting structures and the facial profile. In these cases, a planned sequence of extractions of primary and permanent teeth can benefit the patient by reducing incisor crowding and irregularity in the early mixed dentition, which will make subsequent orthodontic treatment easier and quicker. The extractions also make room for teeth to erupt within the alveolus and through keratinized tissue rather than being forced buccally or lingually into positions that may affect the periodontal health of the teeth. Guidance of eruption and serial extraction are terms used to describe this sequence of extractions.[109,110] Guidance of eruption was originally developed to manage severe crowding without orthodontic appliances but now is viewed as the first step in treatment culminating in fixed orthodontic appliance therapy.

Guidance of eruption should be considered an option when crowding is greater than 10 mm per arch, a measurement that should be confirmed by space analysis after the permanent lateral incisors have erupted. In addition, the patient should have a class I dental and skeletal pattern with good lip and incisor position (unless one is prepared to address these problems) because guidance of eruption does not correct skeletal problems. Guidance of eruption begins in the early mixed dentition with the eruption of the lateral incisors (Fig. 24.79A). If a significant arch length discrepancy is predicted, the primary canines should be removed. This allows the incisors ample room to erupt and align (see Fig. 24.79B). Typically, the incisors also tip lingually and upright, causing the bite to deepen. Faciolingual incisor displacement usually improves, but rotations are more resistant to spontaneous correction.

The child is observed for 2 years or until it appears that the canines and premolars are ready to erupt. At that time, another space analysis should be completed to ensure that the arch length deficiency is still great enough to warrant permanent tooth extraction, and a radiograph should be obtained to determine the position of the unerupted teeth. The goal of treatment is to encourage the eruption of the permanent first premolar so that it can be extracted before the permanent canine erupts (see Fig. 24.79C).

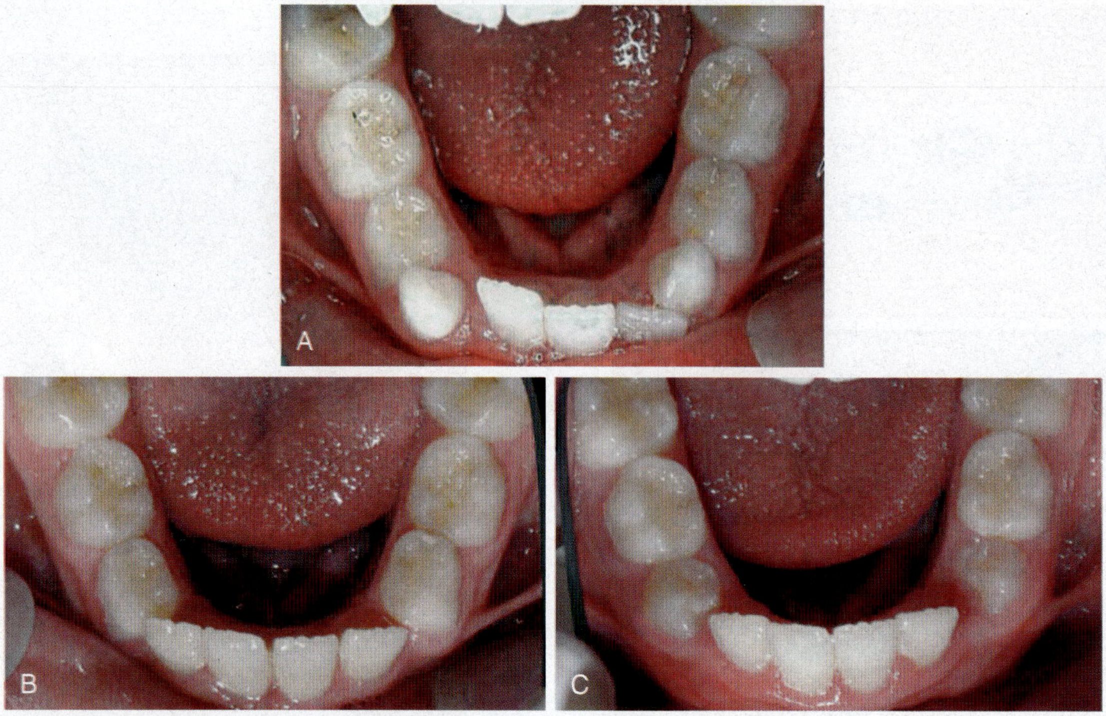

• **Fig. 24.79** The initial stages of serial extraction are described here. (A) Due to severe crowding and substantial overall arch length deficiencies, the primary canines require extraction. (B) This allows incisor alignment. (C) Extraction of the primary first molars speeds up the eruption of the first premolars that can then be extracted before permanent canine eruption.

Unfortunately, the mandibular canine erupts first nearly half the time in the mandibular arch. If it appears that the canine is ahead of the premolar and will erupt facially, the primary first molar can be removed when half to two-thirds of the first premolar root is formed. At this stage of root development, premolar eruption will be accelerated, and the premolar will erupt before the canine enters the arch. This makes removal of the first premolar much easier. In the maxillary arch the first premolar normally erupts before the canine, and this is not a problem. In some cases, the primary first molar is removed, but the permanent canine still erupts before the first premolar. This can lead to impaction of the first premolar, requiring surgical removal. Similarly, it may become apparent that the permanent canine will erupt before the first premolar regardless of the extraction sequence. In this situation the primary first molar and first premolar are removed at the same time. This procedure is called *enucleation* because the premolar is removed from within the alveolar bone.

Surgical removal of teeth from within the alveolar bone should be avoided if possible because it carries the potential for creating bone and soft tissue defects. These occur if the alveolar bone is fractured or removed. New alveolar bone will not be stimulated to form because no tooth will erupt through this area. Surgical soft tissue defects are resolved infrequently.

An alternative extraction sequence has been advocated to prevent lingual tipping of the lower incisors and the subsequent increase in overbite, but this sequence is recommended only when incisor crowding is limited. The primary canine is not removed when the lateral incisor erupts. Instead, the primary canine is retained, and the primary first molar is extracted to accelerate the eruption of the permanent first premolar. This allows some anterior crowding to resolve. The premolar is extracted when it erupts into the arch. The primary canine is often extracted at the same time as the premolar or is left to exfoliate when the permanent canine erupts. The drawback of this alternative is that substantial incisor crowding is not readily resolved, which somewhat defeats the goal of selective tooth removal to encourage good dental alignment.

Anteroposterior Dental Problems

Anterior Crossbite

Anterior crossbite in the mixed dentition is not an uncommon finding. The clinician should determine whether the crossbite is skeletal or dental in origin from the profile analysis and intraoral findings. The most common cause of nonskeletal crossbite is a lack of space for the permanent maxillary incisors to erupt. A space analysis verifies the space shortage. Anterior crossbite develops because the permanent tooth buds form lingual to the primary teeth. When space is inadequate, the incisors are forced to erupt on the lingual side of the arch. If it is apparent that the permanent incisors are beginning to erupt lingually, the adjacent primary teeth should be disked or removed to provide space for the permanent incisors. If space is provided as the incisors are just beginning to erupt, they may migrate facially out of crossbite, and appliance therapy may not be necessary.

If the incisor fails to erupt facially or if the anterior crossbite is not diagnosed early in the mixed dentition, appliance therapy is needed to correct the crossbite. Space for the incisors is gained by disking, extracting the adjacent primary teeth, or increasing the arch perimeter. At this point a decision must be made as to whether the teeth should be tipped into position or moved bodily into place. If tipping will accomplish treatment goals, the dentist can use either a removable appliance or a fixed appliance to correct the crossbite. As described earlier, a removable appliance can be used to tip one or more teeth into proper alignment. The appliance is constructed of palatal acrylic with at least two Adams clasps for retention and a finger spring to move the teeth (Fig. 24.80). The spring is a double helix design that provides a physiologic amount of force over an extended range of action. The spring is activated 2 mm to provide 1 mm of tooth movement per month. As with most removable appliances, full-time wear (except for eating and brushing) is necessary to accomplish the desired tooth movement.

An anterior crossbite with an accompanying deep overbite does not necessarily require a bite plane or bite-opening device during treatment. Most people habitually keep the mandible open and occlude only during swallowing and parafunctional movements. If the crossbite has not improved after 3 months of active treatment, it may be necessary to open the bite by adding acrylic to the appliance to cover the occlusal surfaces of the posterior teeth. This limits closure and keeps the anterior teeth apart, which allows uninhibited incisor movement. In most cases the crossbite will correct quickly and the bite plane can be removed. Extended use of a bite plane is discouraged because the teeth not in contact with the appliance will continue to erupt, creating a vertical occlusal discrepancy.

Fixed appliances also can tip teeth out of crossbite and do not require as much cooperation from the child. A fixed appliance also provides precise control of tooth movement in all three planes of space by using rectangular wires (Fig. 24.81). The disadvantage of either a labial or a lingual fixed appliance is the patient's inability to clean around the teeth and appliance thoroughly, which can result in marginal gingivitis and caries. A maxillary lingual arch is a suitable appliance to correct an anterior crossbite if the teeth require tipping. The maxillary arch is constructed of 0.036-inch wire and has adjustment loops like those used in a lower lingual arch. Finger springs made of 0.022-inch wire provide the tooth-moving force. The springs are usually soldered on the opposite side of the arch from the tooth being moved to increase the length and range of the spring (Fig. 24.82). The springs are activated approximately 3 mm before the appliance is cemented in place. During cementation, the springs are tied with steel ligatures to the lingual arch so that they will not interfere with the seating of the appliance. After the excess cement has been cleaned away, the ligature is cut away to activate the springs. In some cases, the spring slips over the incisal edge of an incisor that is not fully erupted. In these cases, additional retention is needed to keep the spring in place. The retention can come from bonding a stainless steel button or a composite ledge to the lingual surface of the tooth. Conversely, a stainless steel guidewire can be soldered to the lingual arch at the midline to prevent the spring from slipping incisally. Three millimeters of activation provides 1 mm of tooth movement per month. The appliance should be removed, reactivated, and recemented at 4- to 6-week intervals until the crossbite is corrected.

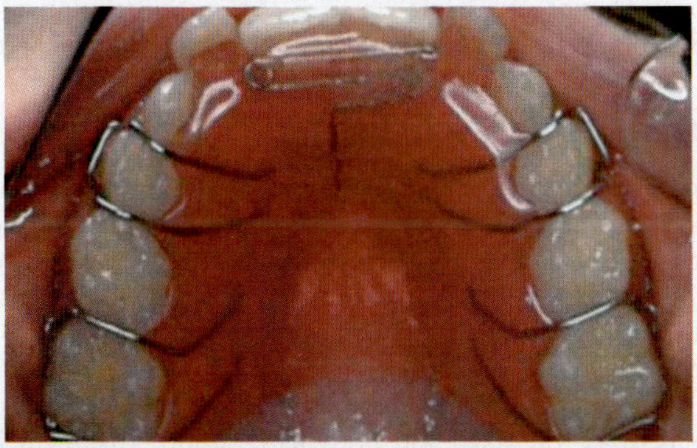

• **Fig. 24.80** If an anterior crossbite can be corrected by tipping the teeth facially, a removable appliance will accomplish this goal. In this case a single finger spring is tipping both maxillary central incisors out of crossbite.

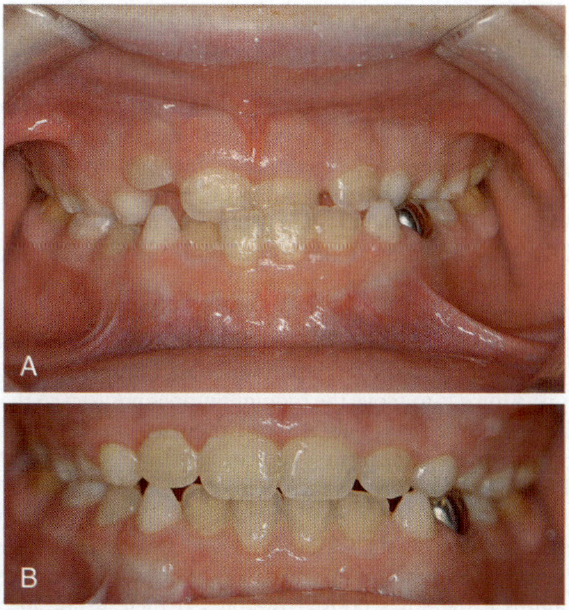

• **Fig. 24.81** (A) Fixed appliances also can be used to tip teeth out of anterior crossbite. In this patient, both maxillary lateral incisors were in anterior crossbite. (B) After the brackets were placed, progressively larger round wires were used to tip the teeth out of crossbite. A rectangular archwire will be used to achieve proper crown and root position.

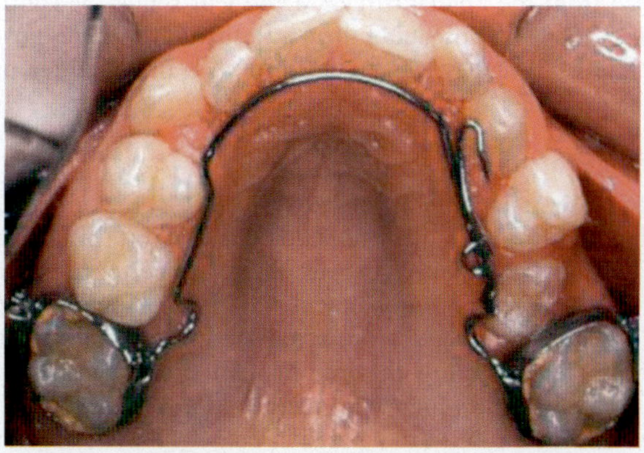

• **Fig. 24.82** Fixed lingual appliances can be used to tip the teeth out of anterior crossbite. This patient required facial movement of the maxillary left canine to correct the crossbite. A small finger spring was soldered to the base lingual arch and was activated to provide the force necessary to move the tooth.

In older patients, space may need to be created for crossbite correction by arch expansion because there are no primary teeth to disk or extract. In this situation the permanent molars should be banded and the incisors bonded with orthodontic brackets.

An anterior crossbite that requires bodily movement of teeth to correct the problem is best managed with bonded brackets and a planned sequence of archwires. Initially, teeth can be tipped out of crossbite. Usually, an archwire is selected that is strong enough to withstand the force of occlusion in the posterior segments yet flexible enough in the anterior region to engage the brackets of the malaligned teeth. If posterior strength is a requirement, a stainless steel archwire with loops bent mesial and distal to the tooth in crossbite is placed. Loops in the anterior region are designed to provide horizontal or vertical tooth movement and exert optimal force to move the teeth out of crossbite while stabilizing those that are in the correct position. Alternatively, a flexible titanium alloy wire can be used for alignment. This requires no wire bending or loop forming but moves both the teeth in crossbite and those not in crossbite.

After alignment is completed by either method, a rectangular archwire is inserted into the brackets that can deliver a root-positioning force to the tooth previously in crossbite. The purpose of such a force is to move the root into proper position so that the entire tooth essentially moves forward out of crossbite, and the angulation of anterior teeth is similar.

Retention must be planned in all cases, regardless of the selected appliance. Active tooth movement is usually continued until the crossbite is slightly overcorrected. The correction should be retained with a passive fixed or removable appliance for 2 months if there is a positive overbite. If there is not adequate overbite, retention should be continued until adequate overbite develops. In a small number of cases the anterior crossbite is caused by excessive spacing and flaring of the mandibular incisors. A removable appliance can be constructed with an adjustable 0.028-inch labial bow to retract the lower incisors and close the space. The appliance is activated 2 mm/month and acrylic removed from the lingual surface. Treatment should be continued until the space is closed and there is positive overbite and overjet. The tooth movement can be retained with the same removable appliance, which is made passive.

Incisor Protrusion

Incisor protrusion in the mixed dentition is a serious esthetic problem for the preadolescent patient. Spaced, protrusive incisors are not only unattractive but also more prone to dental injury than incisors with a normal angulation. For these reasons, treatment is usually undertaken to move the incisors lingually into a more suitable position if the overbite is not prohibitively deep and the overjet will allow lingual movement. This treatment is used for a dental problem but can be used in cases with skeletal problems if the anterior teeth are spaced and or flared. Then, the teeth can be retracted and the skeletal treatment implemented later when growth modification may be limited to one stage with comprehensive orthodontic care.

If bodily movement of teeth is necessary to correct incisor protrusion, the maxillary first molars should be banded, and brackets bonded to the anterior permanent teeth. A small, round, flexible archwire is placed in the brackets to align the teeth initially. Anterior tooth retraction is accomplished by either a round or rectangular archwire with a closing loop or elastomeric chain, depending on whether tipping or bodily tooth movement is required. A headgear or a transpalatal arch is usually used during retraction to supplement anchorage. The choice between cervical or high-pull headgear is based on the patient's vertical facial dimensions, although this is not as simple as one might imagine. Cervical headgear is generally used when the patient has normal vertical facial proportions, whereas high-pull headgear is indicated when the patient has increased lower facial height. The clinician should follow cases of incisor retraction carefully to prevent problems associated with retraction. A complication encountered during incisor retraction is movement of the root of the permanent lateral incisor into the path of the unerupted permanent canine. The lateral incisor root either impedes eruption of the canine or may be resorbed. To avoid this complication, the wire should be bent, or the bracket placed so that the lateral incisor root is upright or even tipped slightly to the mesial.

Transverse Dental Problems

Posterior crossbite correction in the mixed dentition can be difficult and confusing. The clinician must rely on a well-documented database to determine whether skeletal or dental correction is necessary. The presence of a mandibular shift also is an important finding. A posterior crossbite with an associated mandibular shift should be managed as soon as possible to prevent soft tissue, dental, and skeletal compensation. Crossbites can be corrected with a W arch or a quad helix in the primary and early mixed dentitions. Both skeletal and dental movements occur with these appliances, and it is difficult to affect only one or the other. In the late mixed dentition, the midpalatal suture may be more interdigitated, and the clinician can make primarily dental or skeletal changes depending on the appliance selected to treat the patient. It is infrequent that a patient requires skeletal crossbite correction and has no other orthodontic issues.

Posterior dental crossbites are either generalized or localized. Localized crossbites are usually due to displacement of single teeth in one or both arches. For example, a maxillary lingual crossbite involving the permanent first molars is usually the result of lingual displacement of the maxillary molar or the facial displacement of the mandibular molar. If teeth in opposing arches are both at fault, it is easy to correct the problem using a simple crossbite elastic. The offending teeth are fitted with orthodontic bands without attachments. After the bands are fitted, they are removed, and a button is welded to the opposite surface of the band from the direction in which the tooth is to be moved. Another method is to bond the teeth with buttons attached to bondable pads. There is a greater risk of bond failure than band loosening. Whether the buttons are bonded or banded, the technique to correct the crossbite is identical.

In the example just noted, a button is welded to the lingual surface of the maxillary band and to the buccal surface of the mandibular band. After the bands have been welded and cemented, a medium weight ($^{3}/_{16}$-inch, 6-ounce elastic) is attached from button to button through the occlusion (Fig. 24.83). The elastic should be worn full time, except when the patient is eating, and should be changed at every meal. The elastic should be worn until the crossbite is slightly overcorrected. It may be prudent to leave the bands in place and discontinue the use of elastic for 1 month to ensure that the teeth do not relapse into crossbite. When the occlusion is stable after 4 to 6 weeks without elastic force, the bands can be removed.

Vertical Dental Problems

Vertical problems in the mixed dentition are primarily open bite or deep bite malocclusions. Vertical problems are difficult to diagnose. Treatment is based on which teeth should be encouraged or discouraged from erupting. Dental open bite is most often the result of an active digit habit that has impeded eruption of the anterior teeth. In some cases, the digit habit has been discontinued but the open bite has been maintained because the tongue rests between the teeth and prevents eruption. Treatment is essentially the same as that described for digit habits in the late primary and early mixed dentitions. If therapy without an appliance is unsuccessful, a palatal crib (see Fig. 23.8) is effective if the patient desires to stop the habit. The crib reminds the child to

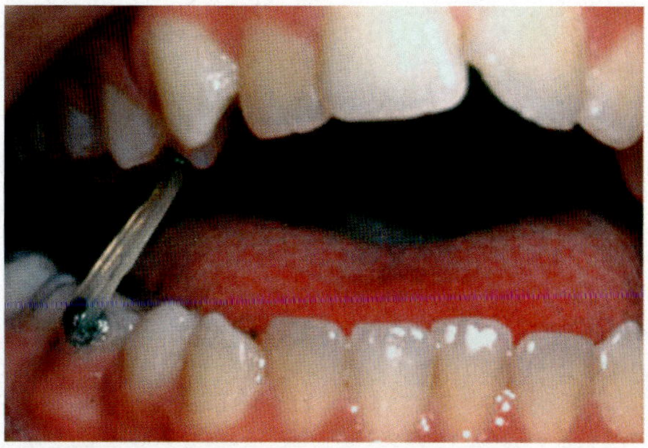

• **Fig. 24.83** If teeth are at fault in both arches, a simple crossbite elastic is used to correct the crossbite. Bands can be placed on both permanent right first molars, and buttons can be welded to the lingual side of the maxillary band and to the facial side of the mandibular band. A medium-weight (4- to 6-ounce) elastic is attached from one button to the other to provide the force required to correct the crossbite.

refrain from the habit and blocks the tongue from being placed forward. Therapy is successful in most cases, unless the child is unwilling to abandon the habit.

In some cases of open bite and minimal incisal display, the anterior teeth are encouraged to erupt. This is accomplished by opening the bite and preventing the posterior teeth from erupting with acrylic stops between the teeth while allowing the anterior teeth to erupt (Fig. 24.84).

Crowding Problems

Dental deep bite is caused by overeruption of the anterior teeth or undereruption of the posterior teeth. It should be distinguished from skeletal deep bite, which is characterized by a flat mandibular plane angle and a short vertical dimension as well as by overerupted and undererupted teeth. In a normal incisor-to-lip relationship, 2 mm of the maxillary central incisor is exposed when the lip is at rest. If more than 2 mm of incisor is exposed, maxillary anterior overeruption should be considered. In the mandibular arch, overeruption is difficult to diagnose; however, the curve of Spee may provide some clue. An excessive curve of Spee (2 mm or more) suggests mandibular incisor overeruption.

Management of deep bite in a growing patient can usually be incorporated into comprehensive orthodontic treatment. Occasionally, treatment in the mixed dentition is aimed at preventing further anterior eruption and encouraging or allowing posterior eruption. This is usually only indicated when the mandibular anterior teeth are impinging on the maxillary lingual gingiva and causing tissue irritation or gingival recession. In these cases, the incisor teeth are placed in contact with a bite plane, and the appliance is constructed so that acrylic touches the upper and lower incisors but allows the posterior teeth to erupt. This is a variation of the appliance shown in Fig. 24.83. The appliance must be worn full time to enable correction and then must be worn as a retainer to maintain the correction until the patient stops growing vertically.

If the deep bite is deemed to be the result of maxillary incisor overeruption or a combination of maxillary and mandibular incisor overeruption, fixed orthodontic appliances are placed on the teeth. An intrusion arch, a wire that connects the permanent first molars to the incisors, is constructed to exert a light intrusive force on the incisors (Fig. 24.85). An alternative is a continuous archwire with a V bend near the molars and a 2 × 4 appliance.

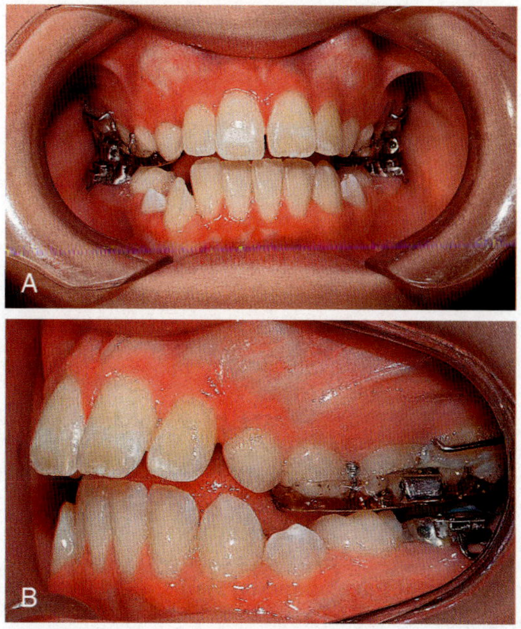

• **Fig. 24.84** A removable bite plane can allow eruption of posterior teeth or anterior teeth to increase or reduce overbite. (A) This bite plane prevents eruption of posterior teeth while encouraging anterior teeth to erupt. (B) The bite plane is retained with the clasps around the molar tubes. For posterior eruption to occur, the acrylic would open the bite and be placed between the anterior teeth.

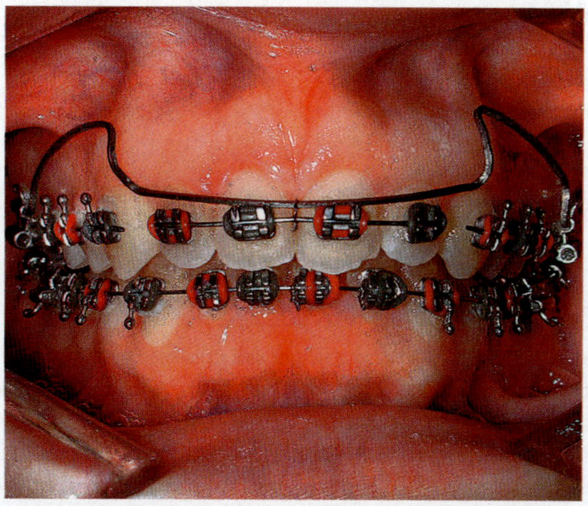

• **Fig. 24.85** The intrusion arch can be used to lift the maxillary teeth and reduce overbite. The auxiliary arch, shown here extending from the molars to the incisors gingival to the brackets, is inserted in the auxiliary molar tube. The molar is tied to the segmental archwires so it uses the anchorage of the molars, premolars, and canines.

Because there is an equal and opposite reaction to every force placed on the teeth, the molars experience an extrusive force by either means. Specifically, the molar erupts and tips distally and facially. Facial movement of the molars can be counteracted by a transpalatal arch or a lower lingual arch, but neither will prevent distal crown tipping. In the maxillary arch, headgear that delivers distal root tip to the molars can offset the extrusive and distal crown tipping forces of intrusion arches. Often overbite reduction is the first phase of comprehensive orthodontic treatment, and consultation with a specialist is appropriate.

Visit eBooks.Health.Elsevier.com to see full list of references.

25

Orthodontic Treatment in the Permanent Dentition

JOHN R. CHRISTENSEN AND HENRY FIELDS

CHAPTER OUTLINE

Determination of Developmental Status

Patients in the preadolescent stages are growing rapidly, and many clinicians prefer to attempt orthodontic growth modification then. If that can be tied to the transition to the permanent detention, then one stage of orthodontic treatment can be sufficient to complete the care. For others, growth modification must start before the eruption of all permanent teeth so there are two phases of treatment; growth modification is followed by a final phase of comprehensive treatment. After peak growth, statural and facial growth decrease dramatically. At that point, the only logical options for care of a skeletal discrepancy are camouflage or surgical orthodontic care.

The most important question is whether patients have remaining facial growth. It determines when surgical care can be instituted for those with excess growth issues like mandibular protrusion or vertical facial excess. The most reliable and sensible method, which speaks directly to this issue, is taking serial cephalometric radiographs and superimposing their tracings (see Fig. 25.4). Other growth indicators such as growth charts, hand wrist films, and cervical vertebral matureations should be assessed to help determine remaining growth. These methods are helpful not only for orthodontic treatment planning but also for determining when implant and other prosthetic work is feasible.

Head and Neck Examination

The principles of the head and neck examination of the teenager are like those applied to the adult or child. Variations from normal can be caused by a variety of factors, the most notable of which are growth and developmental changes and the effects of the adolescent's environment.

The physical changes and habits in the teen require modification of the procedures used in children. On the positive side, the loss or redistribution of body fat and the elongation of the neck allow one to perform a better lymph node evaluation. These changes facilitate a thorough head and neck and cancer examination.

Facial Examination

In the facial examination the dentist analyzes the soft tissue profile and the frontal face. During adolescence the face is beginning to assume adult-like features, and treatment decisions can be based more on current rather than projected facial appearance. This does not mean that growth is complete, only that it has slowed considerably from its previous pace during the early adolescent growth spurt. The adult profile tends to be straighter than the adolescent's because of continued mandibular skeletal growth. In addition, the soft tissue of the chin increases slightly in thickness. The nose continues to grow in horizontal and vertical directions. Most of this growth is horizontal, but the nasal tip tends to drop a small amount. The lips are less protrusive in adults because of these nasal and chin changes combined with a slight thinning of the soft tissue thickness of the lips.

For patients with class I skeletal and dental characteristics, the facial profile examination should provide an adequate basis for analysis when minor orthodontic treatment is considered. For the patient with a skeletal problem, additional information (e.g., a cephalometric radiograph and analysis) is suggested to diagnose the problem definitively and prescribe treatment.

Treatment of skeletal orthodontic problems during preadolescence or early adolescence, when the adolescent growth spurt is still active, can result in growth modification. The preadolescent patient is assumed to be growing and is expected to experience a pubertal growth spurt. The young adolescent, especially the male, still has enough growth remaining to allow significant skeletal changes to occur with treatment. Once the adolescent has experienced the pubertal growth spurt, growth remains but is significantly slower, and equal to the downside of the growth rate curve. Adults have such limited facial growth it is of little therapeutic potential.

These differences in growth potential have a large effect on how skeletal malocclusion is managed in adolescents. As the individual becomes more skeletally mature, less skeletal growth modification can be accomplished. Therefore, as noted earlier, it is essential to establish the growth or developmental status of the patient to plan sensible treatment.

Intraoral Examination

The larger size of the adolescent oral cavity permits good visualization. Normal intellectual status and reasonable behavior provide cooperation in functional assessment of the occlusion and the temporomandibular joint (TMJ). There are more teeth to evaluate, and gingival and periodontal issues are present that were not critical in early childhood. The clinician should approach the adolescent as an adult, especially in the later teen years. For the first visit, the dentist may choose to "walk" the adolescent through the examination, using a hand mirror or computer images to explain procedures and normal findings.

Periodontal Evaluation

In adolescents more emphasis is placed on the periodontal examination. The prevalence of periodontal disease begins to increase in this age group.[1] Although usually minor, loss of periodontal support due to periodontitis is common in the teenage population.[2] Therefore a thorough evaluation of the supporting structures is necessary. A periodontal probe is used to measure pocket depths, the width of keratinized gingiva, and the amount of attached gingiva and to establish a bleeding index (Fig. 25.1). Periodontal probing should be confined to fully erupted teeth. Mobility tests may reveal slightly increased mobility in erupted teeth without complete root formation. The use of disclosing agents to reveal plaque may be helpful. If a panoramic radiograph is used for diagnosis, selected periapical films may be needed if the clinical examination exposes any unusual periodontal findings. Referral to a specialist is suggested if significant periodontal disease is evident. During orthodontic treatment, gingival, plaque, and bleeding indices should be established at regular intervals to detect newly active periodontal disease. With the increase in childhood and adolescent obesity there has been an increase in the number of adolescents with diabetes mellitus type 2 (non–insulin-dependent diabetes).[3] Approximately one-third of children and adolescents are now categorized as overweight or obese, so it is more likely to see adolescent patients exhibit many of the comorbidities associated with diabetes, such as periodontal disease and bone loss. Studies support a strong correlation between glycemic control and severity of periodontitis.[4]

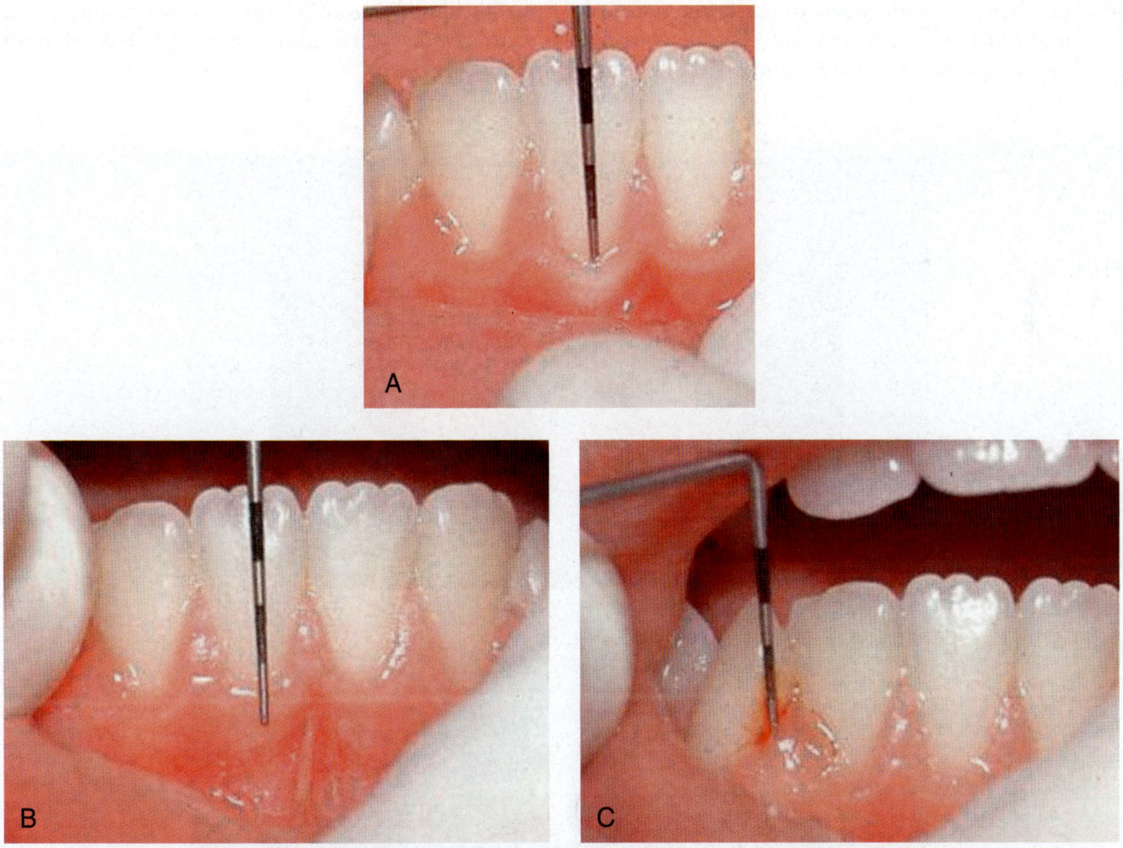

• **Fig. 25.1** The prevalence of periodontal disease begins to increase in the adolescent patient; therefore a thorough evaluation of the periodontium is absolutely necessary. A periodontal probe is used to measure pocket depth (A) and the width of the keratinized gingiva (B). Probing is also done to establish a bleeding index (C). The amount of attached gingiva is determined by subtracting the pocket depth from the width of the keratinized gingiva.

Related Hard and Soft Tissue Problems

Several pathologic conditions may occur in adolescence and be first noticed in this period. One is temporomandibular disorder (TMD), as described in Chapter 45. An eating disorder can manifest as enamel erosion of all teeth if vomiting is a regular component of this psychiatric disorder.[5] *Bulimia* is the term given to characterize those who vomit regularly to purge themselves of food in a misdirected attempt to control their weight. Bulimia affects far more girls than boys, but boys can exhibit similar behavior. The regurgitated stomach contents, which are highly acidic, erode the enamel of teeth in a process called perimolysis. Dentin is exposed, making teeth sensitive and encouraging decay. Enamel flakes off, leaving sharp edges. Restorations may appear to have grown out of their preparations as enamel and dentin dissolve around them. In the early bulimic, these clinical signs may be absent. Pulpal pathosis, elongated clinical crowns, gingival recession, and loss of vertical dimension are a few of the treatment issues noted in bulimia. Unless the vomiting is stopped, extensive treatment may be futile. The dentist should work with a psychotherapist to deal with this problem. Dental erosion may have a variety of etiologies aside from bulimia in this age group, such as sports and carbonated beverage intake[6] or gastroesophageal reflux.[7] The dentist should investigate the cause of erosion carefully before making treatment recommendations and referrals.

Another pathologic problem is dental trauma. The clinical and radiographic examinations should address tooth crazing, chips, or discoloration with adjunctive radiographs to clarify the status of teeth. Not all teeth that appear sound are clinically healthy (Fig. 25.2), and not all trauma is to hard tissues. It is important to obtain a thorough trauma history during the patient interview process. The effects of smoking and oral sexual activity may also be identified during the examination. Oral piercing has become popular among teenagers and young adults. It is associated with risks of systemic infection and tissue damage during placement as well as tooth fracture, gingival recession, and localized infection while the item is being worn.[8]

Evaluation of third molars is usually completed during mid to late adolescence. Parents commonly ask about treating these teeth. The reasons for extraction of third molars include but are not limited to impaction or failure to erupt, periodontal disease, cysts or tumors, decay, posteruption malposition, nonfunction because of an absent opposing tooth, difficulty with hygiene, and recurrent pericoronitis. If any of these conditions are present, the clinician should discuss removal with the parent and patient. The American Association of Oral and Maxillofacial Surgeons has conducted trials on third molars and oral health.[9] They have recommended advising patients and parents about the odds of a third molar remaining free of symptoms and pathology and then decide about removal. The discussion must also include the risks of surgery to remove the third molar.

The concept of anterior crowding as the result of forward pressure from third molars is currently unproven and is not a reason to extract. Surgical access and root development are important issues in determining when to extract. Some root development is desired to stabilize teeth, but complete root development can make extraction more difficult and may increase the likelihood of root fractures. Smokers, and females using oral contraceptives, may also run a high risk of postsurgical dry socket.[10]

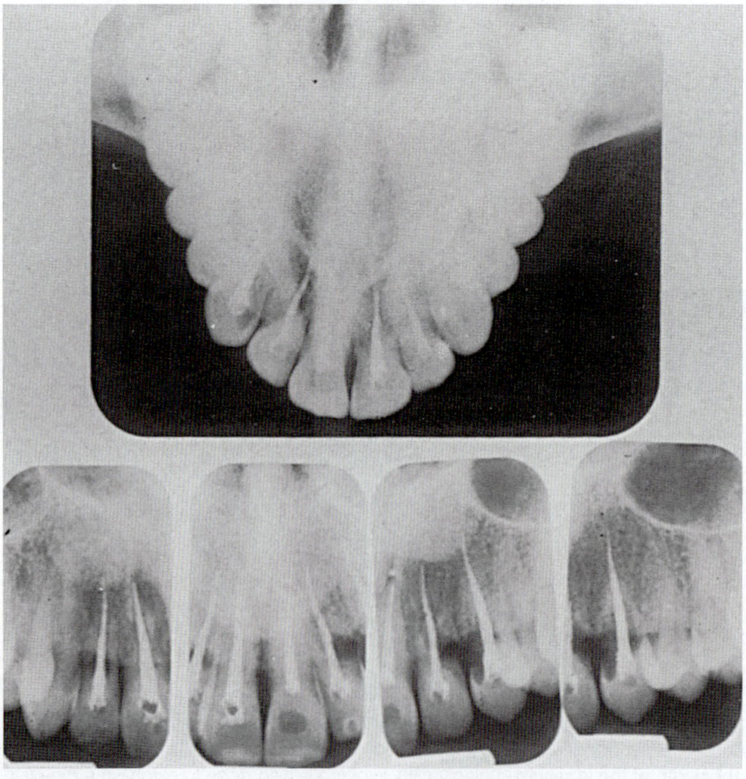

• **Fig. 25.2** Severe resorption of roots secondary to trauma is evident on radiographic examination. These teeth were remarkably clinically stable despite the amount of root resorption.

Occlusal Evaluation

The anteroposterior, transverse, and vertical components of the occlusion should be evaluated. The major difference from the mixed dentition is that arch length deficiencies are no longer predicted from space analyses but are measured directly from the casts because all permanent teeth have erupted by this age (Fig. 25.3).

Careful attention should be paid to teeth adjacent to edentulous areas because the adjacent teeth may need to be repositioned with orthodontics before restorative treatment. The position of the teeth, the amount of supporting bone, the health of the teeth, and the number of missing teeth will determine the direction of treatment.

Once again, the interaction between the facial profile and dental crowding should be considered. Committing the patient to treatment based solely on dental characteristics can have a disastrous effect on the facial profile. The nose and chin will continue to grow and the lips thin over time so the clinician must factor these changes into decisions on how to manage the crowding.

Treatment Planning and Treatment for Orthodontic Problems

Adolescent orthodontic problems create difficult treatment decisions for the general practitioner and the specialist. The nature of the malocclusion heavily influences how the problem will be managed.

Skeletal Problems

If the malocclusion is skeletal, treatment is aimed at altering the relationship or orientation of the jaws and teeth. This can be accomplished by growth modification, camouflage, or orthognathic surgery. Because the physical maturity of the adolescent patient varies among persons of the same age, any one of three treatments may be appropriate. If the developmental assessment of the patient suggests that the patient is actively growing, growth modification is a viable treatment alternative. Growth modification attempts to change the actual size, shape, or orientation of the jaws to obtain an acceptable occlusion. Functional appliances and extraoral traction are used to secure these changes. The clinician may lean toward more noncompliant appliances in this age group because the remaining growth potential is so small there can be no wasted time not wearing appliances.

In the nongrowing, physically mature adolescent, which is most likely the case, skeletal malocclusion in the anteroposterior dimension is appropriately treated by camouflage or orthognathic surgery. Camouflage is the orthodontic movement of teeth without changing the underlying skeletal malocclusion. Camouflage should be considered only when the soft tissue profile is acceptable and when tooth movement will not change or compromise the profile. Teeth are tipped or bodily moved on the denture base to positions considered less than ideal but acceptable for normal occlusion. For example, a mild class II mandibular deficiency with a relatively prominent bony pogonion can be managed by camouflage (Fig. 25.4). To camouflage this type of problem, the upper teeth are moved backward, and the lower teeth are tipped forward to bring the teeth together and disguise the skeletal problem. In conjunction with the tipping of teeth for camouflage, often teeth in the maxillary arch are extracted to provide space in which to move the upper teeth backward. Although a small amount of soft tissue change may occur and the final position of the mandibular incisors may be less than ideal, functional occlusion can be

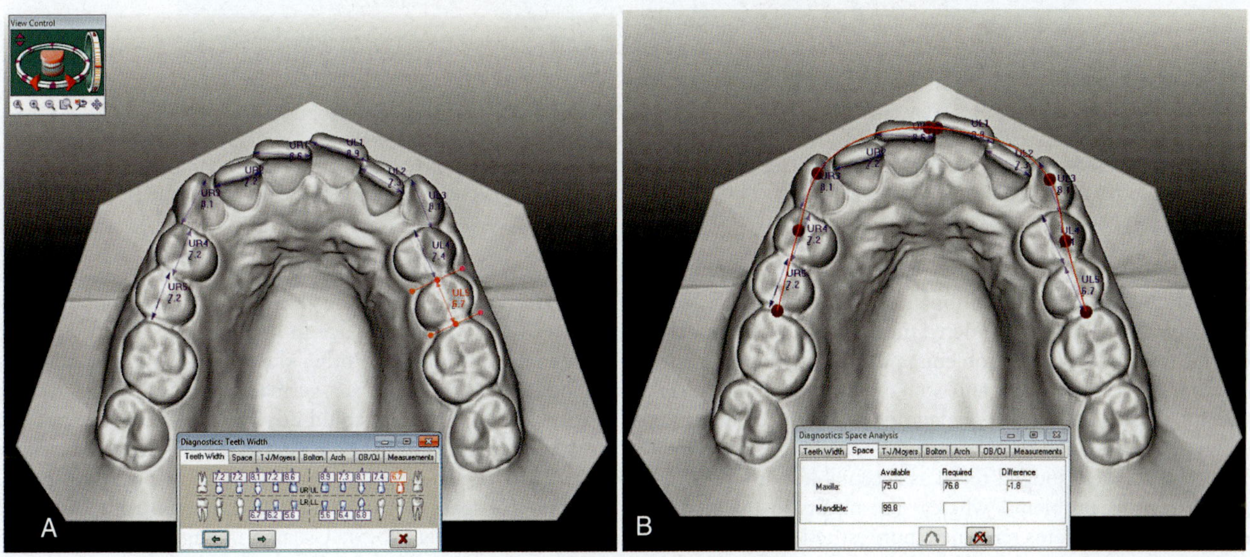

• **Fig. 25.3** (A) Arch length analysis in the adolescent patient is measured directly from casts rather than by using prediction tables of mixed dentition space analysis because all permanent teeth usually have erupted by this age. The first step is to measure the mesiodistal width of each individual permanent tooth. Depending on the software, the tooth widths are added together to get a sum of the mesiodistal widths in the arch. (B) Next, the arch circumference is determined by digital placement of the measuring tool from the mesial of the permanent first molar to the mesial of the contralateral first molar. The difference between the arch circumference and the sum of the mesiodistal width indicates the amount of crowding or spacing within the arch. If one or two primary teeth have not exfoliated, the width of the contralateral erupted permanent tooth can be substituted for the unerupted permanent tooth.

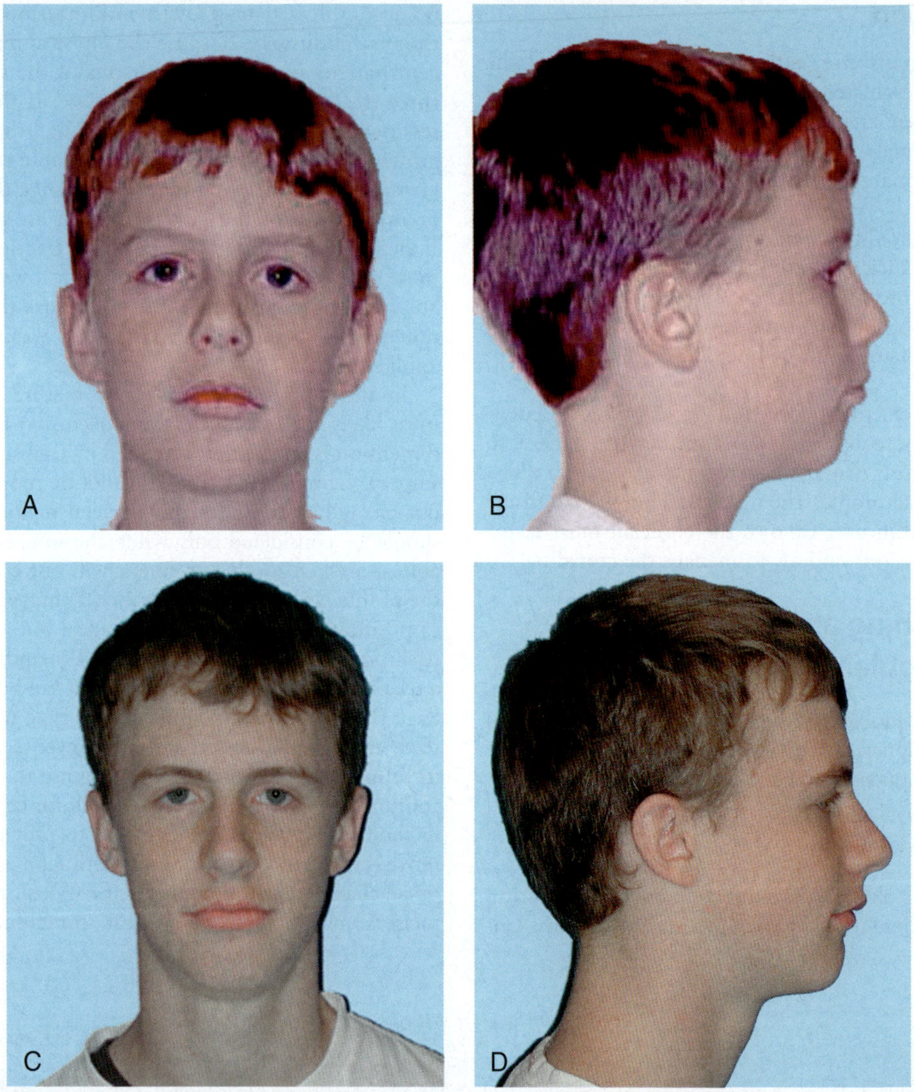

• **Fig. 25.4** (A) This preadolescent patient has a convex facial profile (B) due to maxillary protrusion. Because the facial profile is acceptable even though the skeletal relationships are not ideal, the teeth were moved to reduce the overjet and obtain a functional occlusion by retracting the maxillary teeth and proclining the mandibular teeth. (C) At the adolescent posttreatment stage, the facial profile (D) remains convex but acceptable with continued maxillary protrusion.

achieved without surgery. Traditionally, camouflage of class II skeletal problems has been considered more acceptable in females and camouflage of class III problems more acceptable in males because the respective convex and straight profiles are more acceptable for these groups. Recent data indicate more acceptance among laypeople.[11] The esthetic results in males with moderately class II problems were judged to be as acceptable as those in females with class II problems, whereas the results in males with moderate class III problems remained more esthetically acceptable than those in females with class III problems. Camouflage of class III problems usually is addressed with lingual tipping of mandibular anterior teeth to obtain an acceptable overbite and overjet while at the same time moving the upper dentition anteriorly. Often, mandibular tipping is more easily accomplished when extractions are performed in the lower arch. At least for class II patients, most consider treatment by camouflage extremely acceptable even though they realize they have somewhat smaller or more retrusive chin points.[12]

With the maturity of the alveolar bone, temporary anchorage devices (TADs) have a place in orthodontic treatment planning for the adolescent, as do other skeletal anchorage methods, such as bone plates. TADs are germane to camouflage treatment. Patients who previously could not lose any anchorage can now be treated with near absolute anchorage when TADs are placed. This opens new dimensions of treatment in many planes of space. The direction of space closure can be carefully controlled as can absolute intrusion (Fig. 25.5). Usually, the age of 12 years is a safe time to begin skeletal anchorage considerations due to bone maturation.

The use of TADs in the transverse dimension has become more prevalent in recent years. Up until the development of miniscrew-assisted maxillary rapid palatal expansion (MARPE), transverse constriction or posterior crossbite was treated before 15 years of age because the midpalatal suture and adjacent articulations start to fuse and become more rigid. Forces exerted by traditional palatal expanders were not sufficient to open the suture and make

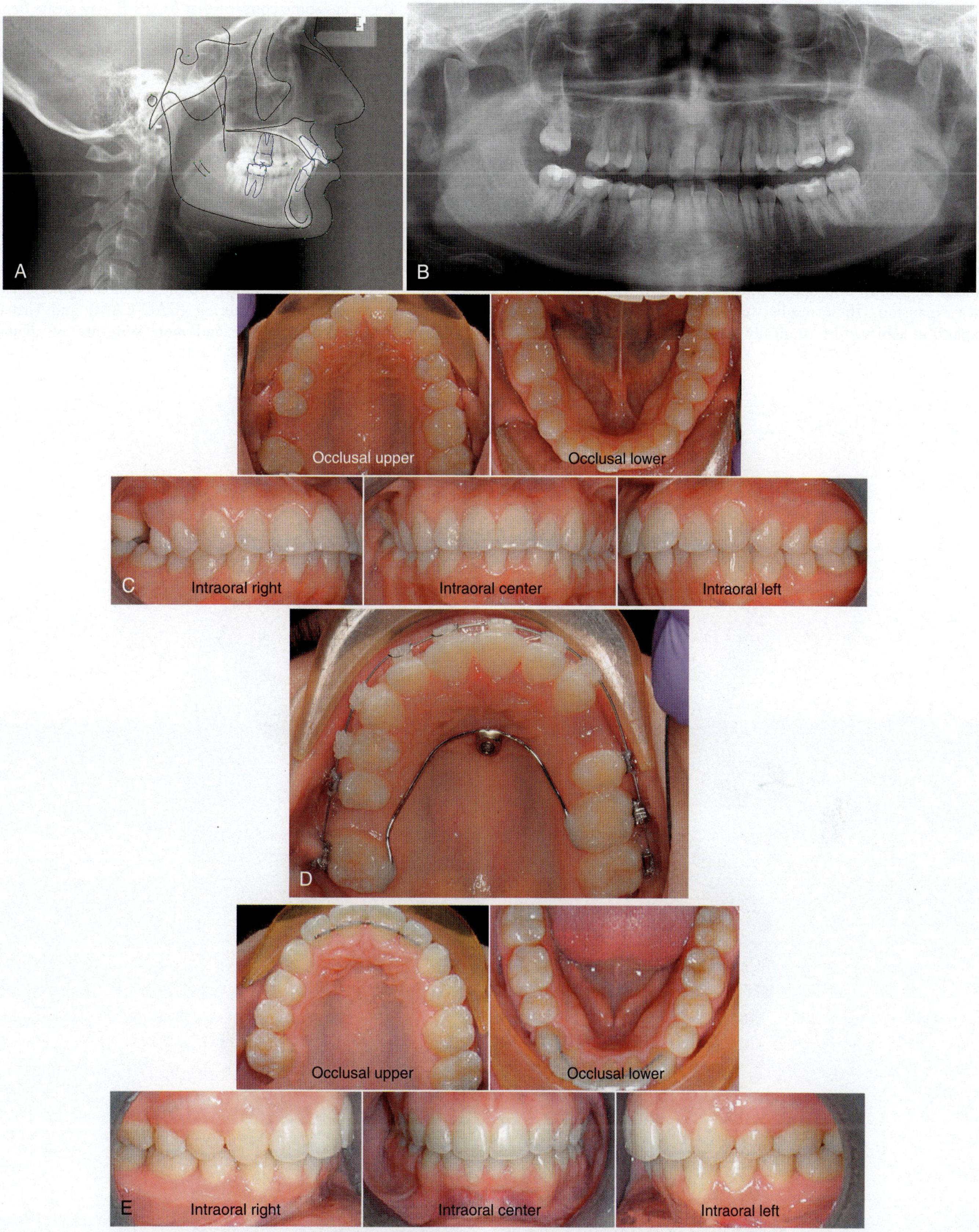

• **Fig. 25.5** (A–C) This patient has a class II malocclusion, increased overjet, and missing teeth. In an attempt to reduce the malocclusion and the class II skeletal tendency, she was treated with extractions and space closure. (D) An osseointegrated implant was placed in the palate and used to control the space closure and retraction. (E) The problems were successfully addressed using this implant-supported camouflage treatment. Subsequently, the implant was removed.

skeletal change. As a result, the clinician would see buccal crown tipping of posterior teeth, increased bite opening, and development of hard and soft tissue loss (gingival recession and alveolar bone dehiscence). Surgery and RPE were used to overcome this problem by surgically releasing the suture before maxillary expansion. However, there was the risk of the surgical procedure and associated financial costs that created some reluctance to undergo this treatment. MARPE was introduced to open the palatal suture without surgery. Rapid palatal expansion devices were designed to attach solely to the palatal bone or to the palatal bone and teeth that provided enough force to the basal bone to open the suture. A systematic review found that MARPE had a high success rate for maxillary expansion (mean 92.5%) and created both skeletal (mean 2.33 mm) and dental (mean 6.55 mm) transverse maxillary expansion. These results were clinically comparable to the expansion achieved by surgically assisted rapid palatal expansion (SARPE). There was some concern that MARPE may create dental and periodontal side effects and affect perioral soft tissues.[13]

Skeletal malocclusion in the nongrowing patient can also be managed with orthognathic surgery.[14] The specialist works with an oral and maxillofacial surgeon to surgically reposition one or both jaws into proper alignment (Fig. 25.6). Typically, the orthodontic treatment plan calls for a presurgical period of orthodontic tooth movement to align teeth in both arches and position the teeth over the bony bases so that they will fit together after surgery. Orthognathic surgery is planned to accurately move and position the mandible and maxilla. With the development of three-dimensional (3D) computerized technology, the planning of orthognathic surgery has changed from conventional clinical assessment with cephalometric head films and plaster model surgery to the use of computer-aided design/computer-aided manufacturing (CAD/CAM) and virtual surgical planning (VSP).[15] More and more surgeons use digital

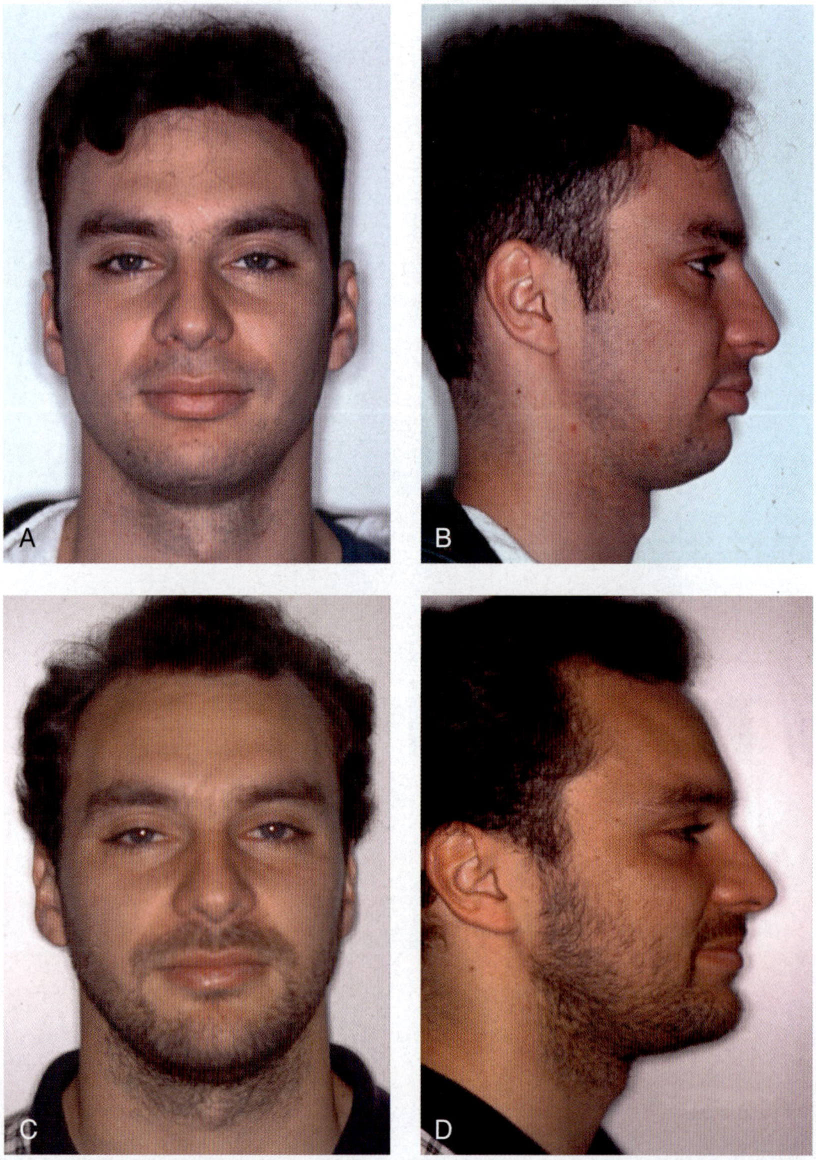

• **Fig. 25.6** (A) This nongrowing patient has a severe class II malocclusion and convex facial profile (B) due to mandibular retrusion. The teeth cannot be moved together to provide a stable, functional occlusion, so orthognathic surgery was performed to advance the mandible. (C) After surgery the patient demonstrated more mandibular prominence (D) and facial height.

planning software to increase accuracy and predictability. Orthognathic surgery is performed under general anesthesia, and the maxilla, mandible, or both jaws are repositioned and held in the new position by surgical screws or bone plates and screws. It is possible to move the entire jaw or individual segments of the jaw in almost any direction within the constraints of the soft tissue covering. There is some restriction on the amount of change that can be achieved, and some types of change are more stable than others. After the surgical procedure, jaw function is reduced with elastic traction. After healing is demonstrated, a short period of postsurgical orthodontic tooth movement is necessary to settle the teeth into the final occlusion.

Dental Problems

If the orthodontic problem in the adolescent is strictly dental, conventional orthodontic treatment can be used to manage the malocclusion. Identification and management of dental orthodontic problems have already been discussed and basically do not change with the age of the patient. However, there are several aspects of dental orthodontic treatment that have not been discussed and should be mentioned here. Despite the preventive efforts of the dental profession, some people continue to lose permanent teeth to decay or trauma. Other patients lose primary teeth during adolescence and have no successors. When this occurs, a combination of orthodontic tooth movement and restorative dentistry is recommended to obtain optimal esthetic and functional results.

In the anterior region, orthodontic treatment is often designed to move teeth to simplify restorative or prosthetic treatment. To provide precise control of tooth movement, orthodontic brackets should be placed on the anterior teeth and the permanent first molars. Treatment must be carefully planned so that only the teeth that require movement are affected, and the other teeth remain stationary. This means that molar, canine, and midline relationships should be carefully studied and controlled during treatment. The advent of clear aligners to move teeth aids in controlling individual tooth movement as the practitioner can request some teeth to move and hold others from movement.

In cases of missing or small teeth, a diagnostic setup is performed so final tooth position and dental relationships can be defined for the best result. The widespread development of dental scanners has made this much easier than past exercises. Often, multiple setups are required for a single patient to represent different treatment approaches. Digital study casts can be manipulated so several treatment alternatives can be examined by the patient and dentist (Fig. 25.7).

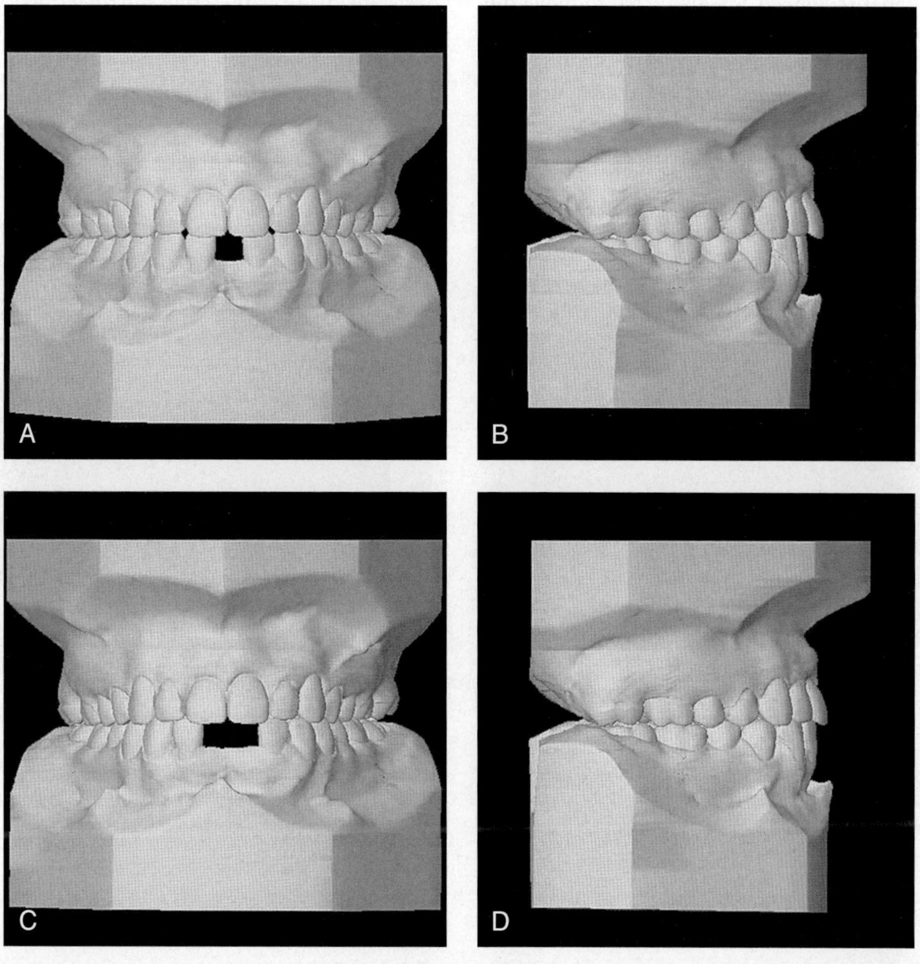

• **Fig. 25.7** It is now possible to produce digital casts and manipulate the images to simulate setups. This series of images demonstrates options for this patient with missing lower central incisors using this technology. (A) An alternative is to make space for one incisor implant. (B) This solution positions the anterior teeth with more overbite and overjet than a setup with space for two mandibular central incisors implants (C), which reduces the overbite and overjet when the posterior dental relationships are identical (D). (Courtesy OrthoCAD by Cadent, Inc., Carlstadt, NJ.)

Coil springs, elastomeric chains, and intraoral elastics can be used to open and close space for the best potential result. It is also an excellent opportunity to consider the use of a TAD because the adolescent has dense enough bone to support this type of anchorage. These opportunities can be used for solutions to anterior problems (Fig. 25.8) and posterior problems (Fig. 25.9). Once the space has been established and is nearly ideal, a closed coil spring or loops bent into the archwire are used to hold or maintain the space until the restorative or prosthetic treatment is completed. Although this type of treatment sounds simple, close attention to detail is necessary. Uncontrolled tooth movement can result in unanticipated changes in the midline, overjet, and overbite.

In certain cases, treatment can be accomplished with clear aligners. This approach to tooth movement was initially considered when there was generalized malalignment and good skeletal relations. The development of new materials and a more complete understanding of how aligners move teeth has expanded the types of cases being treated. The clinician uses a removable tray to exert force on the tooth to move it rather than using traditional orthodontic brackets and wires. An accurate impression or intraoral scan is made of the patient. The result is a digital representation of the malocclusion. Computer software has been designed to move the teeth individually in approximately 0.25 mm increments (Fig. 25.10). A series of aligners is constructed to move the teeth into position as determined by the doctor. Aligner construction can be done in the dental office or at specially configured dental laboratories. The patient is scheduled for aligner delivery and wears one tray after another until the tooth movement is complete. The aligners are more esthetic than traditional braces and more comfortable; however, there is still discomfort associated with tooth movement. The major drawback to removable aligners is that certain precise tooth movements are not as easy to make as with braces, so tooth movement can be less predictable. Obviously, to be successful, the patient must be thoroughly cooperative to wear the appliances as instructed. Clear aligner therapy continues to evolve, and more and more challenging cases are being successfully treated. The overall accuracy for all tooth movement using clear aligners is around 50%[16] and significant differences between predicted and actual tooth movement should be expected. These differences in predictability depend on the type of tooth movement, the tooth being moved, and the cooperation of the patient.[16–18]

Adolescent orthodontic treatment is a challenging exercise in problem solving. A good database and growth assessment are necessary to allow proper decisions about treatment alternatives. Unless the orthodontic problem is obviously the result of dental malalignment, the patient should be referred to a specialist because of the difficulty in managing skeletal discrepancies in patients of this age. The unknowns of how much more a patient may grow and the direction the growth that may occur make treatment decisions very difficult. It is not an overstatement to say decisions made at this time can affect how an individual will appear for life.

Visit eBooks.Health.Elsevier.com to see full list of references.

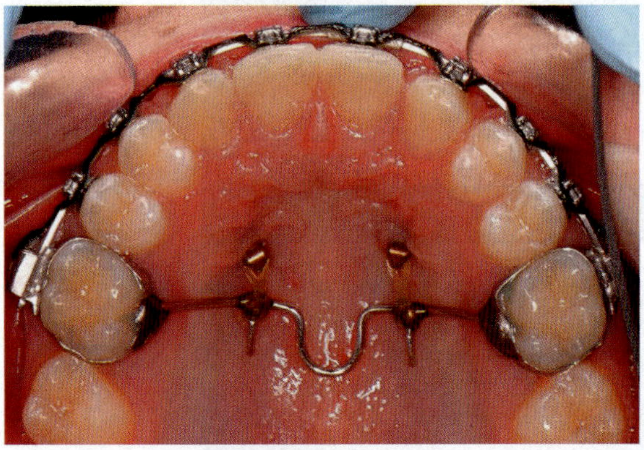

• **Fig. 25.8** This patient had missing maxillary lateral incisors, and the canines were substituted for them. The canines have already been recontoured to mimic a lateral incisor, and further reduction is anticipated. Palatal temporary anchorage devices (TADs) were placed before space closure. A transpalatal arch with hooks was constructed so elastomeric chains could be stretched from the hooks to the TADs. This allows the posterior teeth to come forward without lingual movement of the upper incisors.

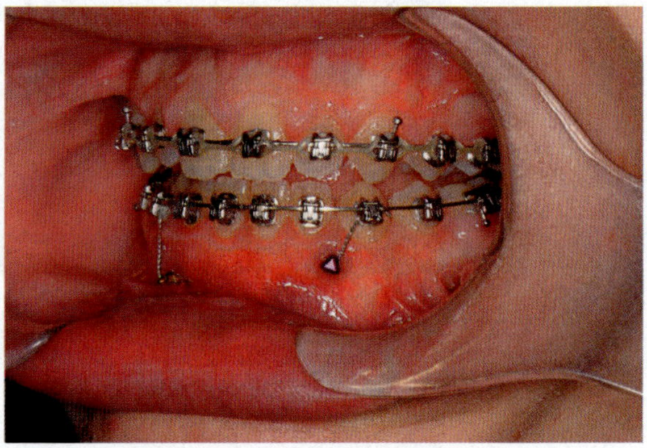

• **Fig. 25.9** The advent of temporary anchorage devices (TADs) has made closure of posterior space feasible when posterior permanent teeth are missing. In this case the patient was missing both second premolars, and the clinician elected to close all the space without prosthetic replacement of teeth. The TADs anchor the anterior segment and the posterior teeth to move forward with minimal posterior movement of the lower incisors. This is an example of indirect anchorage. In some cases, the TAD is used to directly bring the posterior teeth forward, in which case it is called direct anchorage.

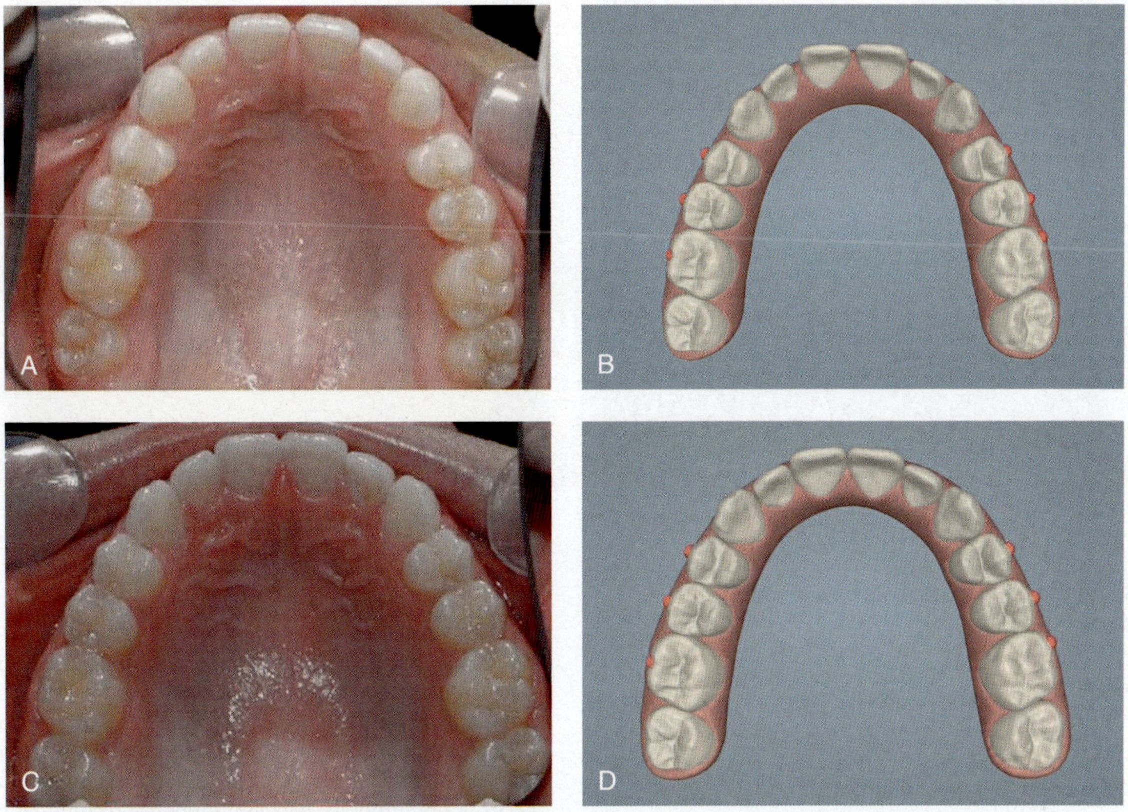

• **Fig. 25.10** Orthodontic treatment for adolescents can be accomplished with removable aligners. The clinician submits a polyvinylsiloxane impression of the original malocclusion (A) to the dental laboratory to create a digital representation of the malocclusion (B). A series of aligners is created by the software and then constructed on actual models. The series is sent to the clinician who monitors the progress of the case and compares the actual tooth movement with the predicted movement. At the end of treatment, the clinician can compare the actual tooth movement (C) with the predicted movement (D).

26

Behavior Guidance of the Pediatric Dental Patient

MARTHA H. WELLS AND JANICE A. TOWNSEND

CHAPTER OUTLINE

Understanding the Child Patient: Review of Child Development

To understand behavior guidance is to understand the child and potential sources of poor cooperation and fear. Children are not little adults, and children at different states of cognitive development have a unique understanding of the world around them. Communication must be adapted to meet their developmental needs. Contemporary behavior guidance techniques are based on developmental theories.

Cognitive Development

The term *cognitive development* describes the evolving ability of children to think, understand, and assign meaning to their experiences.[1] Developmental theory is often presented in stages or periods of relatively stable behavior. The age that children reach a stage is variable, but the sequence is constant among typically developing children. Jean Piaget's stages of child development can help the dentist understand the perspective of the child patient, as summarized in eBox 26.1.

Learning Theory

Early learning theory asserts behavior is learned; the response to past behaviors influences future behaviors.[2] This theory can explain how undesirable behavior can be unintentionally reinforced. For example, young children may perceive any adult attention as a type of positive reinforcement. The parent and/or dentist may inadvertently reinforce inappropriate behaviors by verbally correcting the child.[2,3] The American Academy of Pediatrics recommends active ignoring of minor infractions, and the dentist may consider disregarding small movements or intentional misbehavior instead of drawing attention to them.[4] Conversely, the dentist can specifically praise good behavior telling a child, "I love it when you . . .," which reinforces desired behavior.[5]

Temperament

Child behavior can vary widely in families with shared environment and genetics, and this additional influence is thought to be temperament. Temperament is used to describe traits that manifest early in life and are stable and consistent across different settings.[6] Chess and Thomas classified children according to nine temperament categories and formulated three higher-level categories, or constellations, made up of various combinations of the individual categories that had significance: easy temperament, difficult temperament, and slow-to-warm-up temperament, as described in eBox 26.2.[7]

Studies have shown that temperament, as measured by established psychological tools, can be significantly associated with behavior at a dental visit. Tsoi et al. found a correlation between uncooperative dental behavior in children ages 4 to 12 and temperamental characteristics of emotionality, activity, and shyness.[8] Impulsivity and negative emotionality have also been more commonly found in children with behavior management problems.[9] These temperament profiles (impulsivity and negative emotionality) are a poor fit with the demands and formal structure of a dental visit. Patients with dental behavior management problems are less likely to have a balanced temperament profile than control groups.[10]

Coping

Coping is the ability to manage threatening, challenging, or potentially harmful situations and is crucial for well-being. Coping is a goal-directed process that uses intentional physical or mental actions to resolve a course of stress.[11] An example of behavioral coping is the use of self-statements focusing on competence, such as "I am brave," which can help children tolerate uncomfortable situations for a longer period of time.[12] Effective coping strategies enable the individual to perceive some sense of control over the stressful event. Typically, older children have a more extensive coping repertoire than younger children. Girls have also been reported to use more emotional and comfort-seeking strategies when faced with a stressful event, but boys use more physical aggression and stalling techniques. However, coping skills vary greatly among individuals. Studies involving venipuncture show that lower pain scores were associated with children who reported using behavioral coping strategies.[11] Coping skills in patients with dental anxiety can be improved through cognitive behavioral therapy (CBT).[13]

Factors Influencing Child Behavior

Child behavior in pediatric dentistry is typically studied in terms of dental fear and/or anxiety (the feeling the patient has regarding dentistry) and dental behavior management problems (the patient's reaction to the dental procedure often defined in terms of the dentists' experience). Pediatric dental behavior management problems and fear are different entities, but because of their significant association, they will be discussed together as we explore variables related to uncooperative behavior.[14] Child behavior is a complex manifestation of cognitive status, anxiety, temperament, culture, socioeconomic status, and past experiences.[15]

Dental Fear

The relationship between dental fear and negative behavior is not straightforward, and it would be an oversimplification to attribute all misbehavior to dental fear. The etiology of dental fear in children is multifactorial and a product of previous experience, generalized fear, and familial anxiety.[16]

Dental anxiety ranges from 10% to 29.3% worldwide, and in the United States anxiety is on the higher end of this range.[17] Although the odds are increased that children who exhibit negative behavior have dental fear, and children who have dental fear may exhibit negative behavior, not all uncooperative children report dental fear.[9,18] Children who report being fearful by various measurement tools are twice as likely to behave negatively than children who are not fearful.[9]

Anxiety is a generalized response to an unknown threat or the response to a stressful stimulus specific to the dental environment.[16] It is helpful for the dentist to determine whether this is a state condition (anxiety about dentistry only) versus a psychiatric disorder such as generalized anxiety, which would be categorized as a trait condition.[16] Anxiety may manifest as worries about future encounters. In contrast fear is an "in the moment" emotional response to a dangerous situation and is much more physically robust than anxiety.[15] Fear may be in response to a past traumatic dental experience or generalized fear from a different medical procedure. Dental fear can be learned socially from elders, media, and friends with personal experience via the informative pathway.[19,20] One of the most common initial responses is to try to avoid the dental setting.[16] Irregular dental visits and increased length of time since the last dental visit are significantly associated with increased dental anxiety.[20] Unfortunately, the vicious cycle of avoiding dental care, having increased need for invasive and emergent dental needs, and having a painful experience that reinforces avoidance can be observed in childhood and adolescence.

Phobias are a distinct entity and are an exaggerated response that persists in nondental, "safe" settings.[16] The phobia response is disproportionately strong and may benefit from referral to a mental health specialist.[15] Patients with dental fear and anxiety may be more prone to other psychological disorders.[21]

Demographics

Studies largely find that negative behavior in the dental office is most intense in younger children and decreases as children grow older.[22] Dental anxiety also decreases as the child grows older, most likely due to maturing communication and coping skills.[17,21,23,24] Female sex is likely a risk factor for increased dental fear and anxiety.[17,21,23,24] This may be due to increased willingness for female patients to verbalize fears because of conditioning secondary to gender culture norms.[24,25]

Environment

In recent decades, research has overwhelmingly shown that the social determinants of health (the social, economic, environmental, and community conditions where people live) have a significant effect on outcomes.[26] Early childhood adversities have devastating lifelong effects as a result of toxic stress, which is strong, frequent, or prolonged activation of the body's stress response systems in the absence of the buffering protection of a supportive adult relationship.[27–29] This type of stress may be a result of child abuse and neglect, exposure to violence, poverty, or maternal depression.[28] Exposure can begin prenatally and can result in lasting changes to the brain and immune system resulting in persistent developmental and physiologic harm and increasing risks for lifelong chronic diseases.[28]

Studies have linked dental anxiety and resultant behavior management problems to socioeconomic status and household characteristics.[9,30,31] Lower socioeconomic status has been associated with increased caries risk in children, and individuals with lower levels of education typically have higher levels of dental anxiety.[21] Increased anxiety and behavior management problems may be the result of invasive treatment and/or lack of access to dentists with experience treating children.[32] Behavior management problems have also been linked to single-parent homes, possibly due to increased economic and social pressures in these environments.[9] Preliminary research shows that adverse childhood experiences are associated with increased dental anxiety in adults[33] (see Chapter 43).

Culture may be defined as a system of beliefs, values, traditions, and behaviors that are shared with a group and distinguish this group from others.[24] Precooperative children are not affected by culture as children typically act the same at younger ages.[24] However, children are increasingly influenced by culture once they reach the formal operations stage of cognitive development. Although cooperation may be greater in cultures that stress obedience or bravery, dental anxiety, if assessed by behavior, may be overlooked.[24]

Pain

Previous painful or traumatic dental experiences undoubtedly contribute to anxiety and fear. However, not all fearful patients have had traumatic or painful experiences and not all people with painful past experiences are fearful.[34] The child in pain will almost always exhibit behavior guidance challenges. Uncontrolled pain increases dental anxiety and unmanaged anxiety upregulates pain, creating a vicious cycle. Pain is an inherently subjective experience and should be assessed and treated as such. Pain has sensory, emotional, cognitive, and behavioral components that are interrelated with environmental, developmental, sociocultural, and contextual factors.[35] Tissue damage is not required to provoke pain, and reports of pain should not be casually dismissed. It is counterproductive to argue with the child that a sensation is "uncomfortable but does not hurt," especially in young children who are unable to describe levels of pain and experience noxious stimuli dichotomously (i.e., either "yes, it hurts" or "no, it does not hurt"). Patient self-report of pain is the gold standard, and validated scales such as the Wong-Baker FACES, Faces Pain Scale (Revised), and visual analog scale are valuable tools that are effective in all but very young children. Additionally, observational pain scales such as the Faces, Legs, Activity, Cry, and Consolability score can be used by trained observers to quantify pain. See Chapter 28 for a discussion of pain perception.

Children may describe any new sensation as painful. Introduction to new stimuli at the dental office through the tell-show-do (TSD) technique can help the dentist redefine the perception. The potentially unpleasant sensation of the slow speed handpiece can be described as feeling like riding a bike on a bumpy road. Using a slow speed on intact enamel can help gauge the child's reaction. If they exhibit an exaggerated reaction to this painless sensation, they are at higher risk for poor behavior.

Influence of the Parent

The dental anxiety of children is influenced by their family.[23,36,37] Parental anxiety, especially maternal anxiety, is influential on the child's development of anxiety. Although the mother has been attributed as the primary source of fear, recent studies have suggested fathers can also affect their children.[38] Asking about the parents' anxiety about dentistry may be of value, such as "How would you rate your own nervousness about being at the dentist?"

Parenting styles may also affect child behavior. Baumrind defined three specific parenting styles—(1) authoritative, (2) authoritarian, and (3) permissive—and a fourth, neglecting, has since been added (Table 26.1).[39,40] Positive behavior has been associated with children of authoritative parents compared with children of authoritarian and permissive parents.[41] Most likely, this parenting style is associated with improved behavior because it reinforces adult authority so that a child will follow commands of the dentist, but the style also offers parental nurturing and support for any anxiety the child may have about the dental visit. Changes in parenting norms are discussed later in the chapter (see "Changes in Society and Parenting").

Validated questionnaires to determine parenting styles are available,[42] but they are usually too lengthy to be of great clinical value. However, a short interview with the parent at an initial visit may give insight into a parent's preferences on rules, discipline, communication, emotional support, and child independence. For example, the practitioner might have the following conversation: "It would help me to know more about your family to hear you tell me a little bit about what it is like to be Charlie's parent. There are no right answers; I just want to know more about how you prefer to parent him. It helps our office know how best to work with our children and families. What kind of rules do you set at home (i.e., bed time or screen time)? How do you typically respond if Charlie breaks the rules? When Charlie asks 'why' he can't do something, how do you usually respond? When Charlie is upset, what do you do to comfort him? How do you decide what Charlie wears or eats each day? Do you let him choose?" Answers to these questions may give deeper insight into the level of boundaries and warmth in the home.

Setting the Stage for Successful Behavior Guidance

The Dental Office

Offices that exclusively treat children have a wide array of decor, from a child-friendly theme to office artwork or the presence of

TABLE 26.1 Parenting Styles

Parenting Style	Description
Authoritative	High parental responsiveness/affection and high parental demand for obedience; warmth and involvement, reasoning/induction, democratic participation
Authoritarian	Low parental responsiveness/affection but high parental demand for obedience; clear parental authority, unquestioning obedience, and punitive strategies
Permissive	High parental responsiveness/affection but low parental demand for obedience; tolerance, tendencies to ignore child's misbehavior; child shares in the decision-making process with parent generally accepting child's decisions
Neglectful	Low parental responsiveness and low parental demand

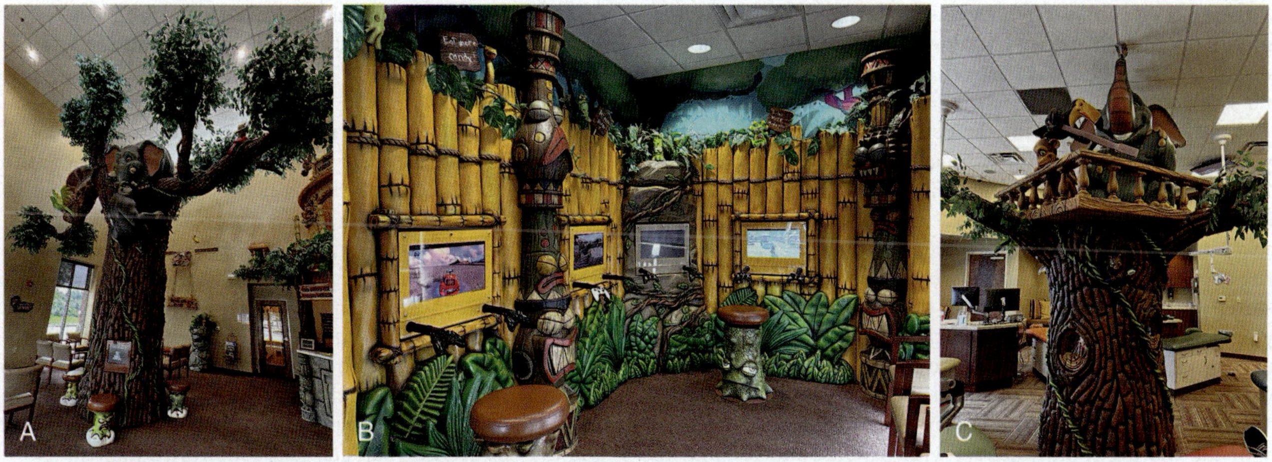

• **Fig. 26.1** (A) Child-friendly waiting room. (B) Audio-visual distraction and child-friendly decor. (C) Child-friendly open-bay and operatory. (Photos courtesy of Chuck Hughes.)

video games (Fig. 26.1). Creating the child-friendly environment in an office that treats both children and adults can be more challenging, but a poster on the ceiling of the operatory or a few stuffed animals can make the child patient more at ease. Sending the message that this is a place where children have been before and are warmly welcomed is important.

Preparing the Child for the Dental Visit

Uncertainty about what to expect is associated with anticipatory anxiety in children. Many offices have new patient packets or websites that familiarize parents with office policies and set expectations that may include letters directly to the children or activities for the children to prepare them for the visit. Parents can be encouraged to help prepare their children for the dental visit. Parents should be educated about what kind of information to give and how to present it because inadequately presented information can lead to negative stress (Case Study: Prepared Parents, Prepared Children, Positive Coping). See "Previsit Preparation" later in the chapter for a more in-depth discussion of techniques.

Scheduling

Conventional wisdom states that very young children are usually at their best early in the day. They may be able to tolerate a prophylaxis visit that is minimally demanding in the afternoon, but they may be too tired later in the day for an operative appointment with higher levels of stress. There are no studies to support this view, and one historical study found decreased negative behavior for restorative treatment in afternoon visits versus morning.[43] However, the dentist may want to schedule these patients when staff have the most energy, and if a patient does have a difficult operative visit, reappointing for a morning visit might be beneficial before resorting to advanced behavior guidance techniques.

Typically, dentists believe that a child needs an introductory visit to the office before performing an invasive procedure. Feigal refers to this examination appointment, with or without a prophylaxis, as a "preconditioning appointment" and claims it helps ease children into the dental experience with as little stress as possible.[44] However, Brill[45] showed no difference in behavior between children who had an initial nonthreatening dental visit and those who had a first restorative treatment visit. Thus emergent or urgent treatment should not be delayed on these grounds alone. However, an examination appointment allows the dentist to build rapport with the child and the family to build a trusting relationship before performing invasive treatment.

The Dentist and the Dental Team

The successful behavior guidance of a child is dependent on the dentist's ability to communicate with the parent, child, and staff.[46] Dentists who treat children can have a variety of personalities and still be effective. Some are very extroverted and emotive, providing an energetic atmosphere that makes children feel included and special. Other dentists tend to be quiet and gentle to put patients at ease. This flexibility is beneficial because some children need upbeat encounters, and others need quiet ones.[47] As long as the underlying message is kindness and regard for the child's well-being, dentists with almost any personality type can be successful at treating children.

The dentist's appearance should be neat and professional. Traditional attire such as a white coat need not be avoided, because a few studies have shown parents and children to prefer it.[48,49] In addition, protective gear required for universal precautions has not been shown to increase fear in children.[50] However, it is ideal to greet children without a mask when possible to convey nonverbal communication, such as smiling.

The dental team should reflect the office philosophy. The entire team should display a positive, friendly attitude toward the patient. Training in communication, multicultural awareness, child development, behavior guidance, and informed consent for auxiliaries can help them become an integral part of successful behavior guidance.[51] Using the same euphemisms and terms by staff can help provide consistency for the child.

Patient Assessment

To enhance the child's experience, the dentist should establish familiarity with the child before treatment. At a minimum, the dentist should inquire about previous dental visits and the patient's behavior at these visits. Previous disruptive behavior for a dental appointment and previous extraction is significantly associated with dental anxiety status.[52,53] Generally, it is helpful to ask parents how they feel the child will cooperate today, and it may also be helpful to ask how the patient copes with medical visits. Although this assessment is not always correct, it can help the dentist get a better sense of the child and parental expectations.

A number of questionnaires and surveys are available that can help the dentist gather more information about the fear, anxiety, and temperament of the child patient, although their clinical efficacy is unknown. A simple facial images scale with smiling, neutral, and frowning faces has been validated in children as young as 3 years to assess dental anxiety.[54] The dental subset of the Children's Fear Survey Schedule has been used to determine fear in younger children,[55] and the Emotionality, Activity, and Sociability (EAS) Temperament Survey can gauge for temperament types more prone to distress, particularly shyness.[56]

Often much can be learned from observing patients as they play in the waiting room, interact with parents, and respond to the initial approach of dental personnel.[57,58]

Parents in the Operatory

Studies in medicine and dentistry show that contemporary parents overwhelmingly prefer to accompany their children in the operatory.[59,60] The most recent survey of pediatric dentists found that the majority of respondents routinely had parents in the operatory, although they have varying opinions as to the benefits.[61]

A systematic review of 16 studies examining parental presence in the dental operatory found no effect on behavior, anxiety, or fear in children.[60] Having parents in the operatory provides an opportunity for immediate communication on changes in treatment plan, oral hygiene instructions, and postoperative instructions from the dentist rather than an intermediary. It fosters a relationship with the parent to establish trust and reduces the possibility of a parental misunderstanding or disagreement regarding how the child was treated.

If parents are to remain in the operatory, then the dentist should prepare them to best assist with treatment. Giving parents a formal role in the psychological aspects of anxiety and pain management may give them a sense of control and improve their satisfaction with the dental experience. Parents should be informed that natural parent behaviors such as reassurance and apologizing can contribute to child distress and should be avoided[62] (Table 26.2). Instead, modeling, teaching, and supporting children in using active coping skills will prepare them to manage distress that comes with novel experiences. (Case Study: Prepared Parents, Prepared Children, Positive Coping). The online case study details some of the ways that parents can teach their child coping skills to be successful during the visit. During the visit, a dentist may ask a parent to be a "silent observer" so that the child can focus on the dentist's voice and requests. In historic studies, no increase in negative behavior was noted when parents were present as passive observers.[63,64] Most parents are compliant with written and verbal instructions to remain a silent observer during dental procedures,[65,66] and most dentists report that they do use parental help with basic communication, reinforcement, and occasional stabilization.[67] Rodriguez and colleagues found a simple preparatory statement to be effective and did not decrease parental satisfaction with the visit[66]:

> *"We always like parents to support their children by being here. We ask parents to remain a passive observer while the dentist treats their child. A passive observer parent stays in their seat and watches their child and the dental procedure. It is best if you help us by letting us explain things to your child using easy-to-understand, non-threatening, and age appropriate language. The passive observer parent plays an important role by allowing the dental staff to develop a positive relationship with your child and focus our attention on their treatment while minimizing distractions. We like to have the parents in the room with their children during treatment."*

The dentist should use caution in determining whether siblings should observe an operative visit, especially one with local anesthesia. Also, it is best to have only one parent in the operatory to reduce distraction and the occasional disagreement between parents. Dentists must have clear policies that are communicated to parents before treatment about their presence in the operatory and their role. Parents can use this information to decide if the practice is best for their needs.

Setting Parent Expectations

Before any procedure, the dentist should inform the parent of reasonable expectations of the child's behavior based on their assessment and

TABLE 26.2 Distress-Promoting Behaviors Often Employed by Parents

Distress-Promoting Behavior	Example	Alternative
Uninformative reassuring	"Don't worry, Billy. Everything will be okay."	"You are a brave boy! Going to the dentist will be easy for such a brave boy."
Giving control to the child when there really is not a choice	"Are you ready to start now?"	"It is time to get your teeth counted!"
Apologizing	"I'm sorry this is taking so long, honey."	Use distraction: "What do you want to do when we leave? Would you like to go to the park? I know the slide is your favorite!"
Displaying empathy	"I know it hurts."	Reframe it: "Let's play a game! It's called the tooth dance. Your tooth is going to wiggle, wiggle, wiggle—look, it's dancing!"
Making confusing statements	"Bonnie, you can do anything but move."	Use clear directions: "Bonnie, keep your hands in your lap."
Making demands to the provider	"Johnny does better if you give him choices. Don't just tell him what to do." "Don't lie to my child; he knows he's going to get a shot."	Parent is encouraged to observe quietly without participating and to allow the team to lead the visit.

discuss how this behavior will be managed. Gaining a valid informed consent from the parents before treatment is critical. See "Informed Consent" later in this chapter. Parents should also be warned that behavior at the examination visit may deteriorate with the added demands of restorative procedures. Positive acceptance of operative treatment by preschool children tends to decrease over the appointments, indicating a negative "appointment effect" in younger children.[55] This means that sometimes more urgent needs should be treated first instead of starting with simple procedures and completing complex procedures at subsequent visits. In addition, children who have invasive procedures may exhibit more negative behavior at recall visits than those who do not receive restorative treatment in between recall visits.[68]

Review of Behavior Guidance Techniques

Discrete behavior guidance techniques have been described in the literature and are listed in the American Academy of Pediatric Dentistry (AAPD) guidelines[69] but are rarely used in isolation. The experienced practitioner weaves many of them into a visit to help guide the patient through challenges and to reward cooperative behavior. Although these techniques seem intuitive and may be used by the dentist not instructed in behavior guidance, consciously practicing them can help improve skills and success with children. The dentist should formulate a behavior guidance treatment plan for the total patient's well-being, including short-term and long-term goals of this treatment.[70]

Basic Behavior Guidance

Communication and Communicative Guidance

The foundation for all basic behavior guidance is communication. The dental appointment involves a series of requests from the dentist and responses from the child. Requests and commands for the child patient are best when they are direct, brief, literal, and appropriate for the child's level of understanding. Avoid "don't" commands in toddlers and preschoolers as they have less developed language processing skills and are more likely to make impulse errors in communication.[3,71] These commands may prompt the unwanted behavior they are intended to avoid. Extensive explanations are ineffective and can erode the authority of the dentist. Sarcasm and belittling of patients are inappropriate in pediatric dentistry.

To achieve cooperation and success, the dentist should establish open lines of communication with the child and preserve them throughout the appointment. When communicating with children it is important to use a relaxed tone of voice, acknowledge their interests, and talk to them at an appropriate developmental level.

Communication should come primarily from the dentist who must establish a relationship of trust through verbal and nonverbal techniques. All dental team members should be aware of any off-putting nonverbal habits they have, such as sighing or avoiding eye contact, because patients and parents quickly perceive and interpret them negatively.[51] The exercise of video recording oneself during patient interactions can alert the practitioner to undesired habits that may interfere with the message.

Requests should be phrased so that they encourage compliance and give the child choices only when choices are possible. For example, when applying topical anesthetic, the dentist should not ask, "Can I put on the sleepy jelly now?" Instead, the dentist may state the following: "I am going to rub some tickle jelly on your tooth. Would you like strawberry or bubble gum flavor?" This choice preserves a sense of control for the patient.[72]

The focus of all conversation should be the child. A discussion with the dental assistant or parent does nothing to encourage cooperation from the child and may provoke undesired behavior for attention. A child-focused conversation provides distraction for the child.

One challenge often encountered is how truthful to be when the dentist is fearful that the truth may cause the child to object to a procedure that is safe. The obvious example of this is when the child patient asks, "Am I getting a shot?" One way to cope with a difficult question like this may be to use a euphemism, such as "Oh, at my office I use sleepy juice by your tooth so it doesn't bother you. I even put a little numbing gel on your cheek first to make you comfortable." Other dentists are more direct in explaining the need for the local anesthetic, and in one study, showing the syringe was associated with similar behavior outcomes as concealing it.[73] Table 26.3 contains some possible responses to difficult statements or questions. Clinicians must use their best judgment to honor the trust of the child while helping them cope with the procedure as much as possible. eTable 26.4 is a summary of guidance techniques and examples of their implementation.

Previsit Preparation

Studies in medicine and dentistry generally show that providing developmentally appropriate preparatory information to child patients has a positive effect on their anxiety and experience. Preparation gives children the opportunity to process information and to think about and rehearse coping strategies before the appointment.[74,75] Children should receive procedural, sensory, and self-regulatory information about the visit[74] (Fig. 26.2). Children are active knowledge builders and problem solvers. Preparatory information allows children the opportunity to practice coping skills and have a plan for any distress they may feel. See Case Study: Prepared Parents, Prepared Children, Positive Coping

Techniques for preparing a child include positive previsit imagery, which has its foundation in social learning theory and involves showing children positive images of dentistry before the visit.[76] Two studies have shown that exposing children to positive images of dentistry reduced anxiety compared with neutral pictures.[76,77] Storytelling, interactive computer illustrations, and videos of children receiving dental treatment that are watched at home have all been shown to improve patient behavior.[78] A pre-exposure visit to the office is not usually necessary for healthy children[79] but should be considered for children with disabilities such as autism spectrum disorder (see Chapter 36).

Tell-Show-Do

The technique known as tell-show-do (TSD) is a key behavior guidance technique when working with children. In TSD, the patient is introduced to the dental environment in a nonthreatening, child-friendly manner. The child is shown what will happen or what will be used, and allowed to see, touch, or smell the material or instrument, or watch a demonstration of the procedure. For example, the rubber dam may be called a "trampoline," and once the child is told about the explorer, the dentist may use it to feel the child's fingernail (Fig. 26.3). Finally, the child experiences the procedure, instrument, or material. This technique works best with children capable of communication and is very successful in all but very young toddlers. This technique is universally adopted by dentists[80] and is universally acceptable to children and parents.[61,81,82]

Many of a dentist's actions are psychologically neutral. The sensation is present, but their pain- or fear-inducing qualities are interpretations added onto the sensation, usually through previous

TABLE 26.3 Parent or Provider Responses to Difficult Statements/Questions

Child Statement or Question	Possible Parent or Healthcare Provider Response	Statements to Avoid	Rationale for Avoiding Statements
I don't want to go. I don't like it. I'm scared.	It's okay to feel scared, you don't know Dr. Jones. She's very kind and will help take care of your teeth.	Don't be scared. Don't worry. It will be okay. If you don't go, you will lose your teeth.	Parents reassure children because they think it will make them feel better. However, research shows that denying a child's concerns or reassuring them "not to worry" has been shown to increase child distress.
Am I going to get a shot?	Dr. Smith will put some numbing medicine by your teeth. This is a great way to help you feel more comfortable. Some children say it makes their cheek feel heavy and tingly.	Dr. Smith will give you a shot but it won't hurt. Dr. Smith will numb your teeth and it will feel like a sharp scratch or little bee sting.	Using more neutral terms like "medicine," "numb," "pressure," or even "poke" can decrease anxiety. Negative suggestions like "sharp scratch" can increase the pain experience.
Will it hurt?	It's okay if you're a little scared. It's normal. Some kids are bothered by it and others think it is okay. We are going to do some things to make it bother you less. It may feel a bit hot or tingly, but they'll be careful to do it really gently. We're going to make a plan to make you feel more comfortable and in control.	It won't hurt. This is going to hurt. Don't be a baby. Big kids don't cry.	Pain is an individualized experience, and some children will experience sensations they interpret as pain. Encourage child to use coping skills. Remind them of what they can do to stay calm and relaxed like bring a stuffed animal or listen to a favorite song. Praise brave behaviors.

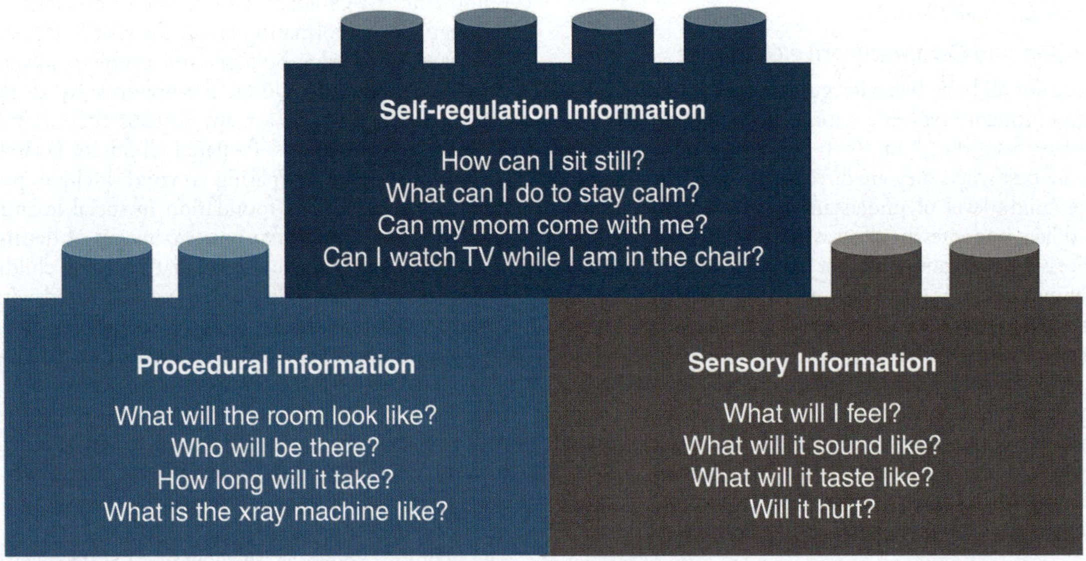

• **Fig. 26.2** Building blocks of procedural preparation and information needs of children in order to cope with treatment. (Adapted from: Bray L, Appleton V, Sharpe A. The information needs of children having clinical procedures in hospital: will it hurt? Will I feel scared? What can I do to stay calm? *Child Care Health Dev.* 2019;45[5]:737-743.)

experience or by influencing figures such as parents and siblings. TSD and euphemisms, such as those shown in Table 26.5, allow the dentist to define new sensations.

Some children have expressed concern that seeing the tools could increase anxiety.[83] One way to avoid anxiety over seeing the instruments is to cover all of the tools with the patient napkin, except nonthreatening items like the mirror and a toothbrush. A common mistake that novice clinicians make is showing the child several different instruments and materials before starting any procedure. This can overwhelm the patient, increase anxiety, and delay treatment. It is best for the practitioner to apply TSD to one procedure at a time and work through the various steps of the procedure.

Nonverbal Behavior Guidance

Nonverbal communication is the reinforcement and guidance of behavior through appropriate contact, posture, facial expressions, and body language.[69] Children constantly receive nonverbal cues

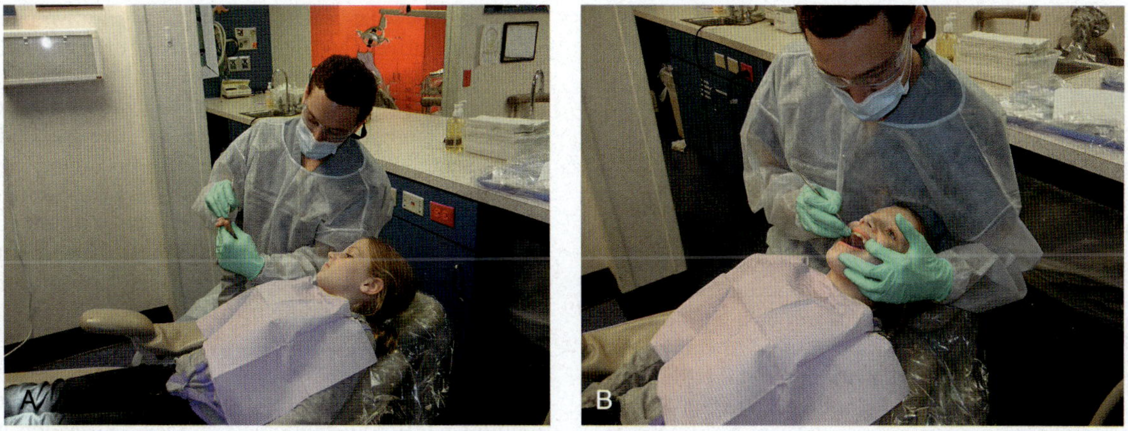

• **Fig. 26.3** Tell-Show-Do. (A) The patient is told about the explorer and shown how it will be used on the teeth in a nonthreatening manner. (B) The explorer is immediately introduced into the mouth and the teeth are examined.

TABLE 26.5 Common Euphemisms for Tell-Show-Do

Device	Euphemism
Rubber dam	Trampoline, raincoat with tooth ring
Isolation system	Whale tail
High-speed handpiece	Mr. Whistle
Slow-speed handpiece	Mr. Bumpy
Fluoride varnish	Bubble gum tooth vitamins
High-volume suction	Mr. Thirsty
Saliva ejector	Bubble straw
Stainless steel or zirconia crown	Princess crown; superhero hat
Cement for crowns	Lemon cupcake icing; tooth glue
Curing light	Flashlight
Etch	Blue shampoo
Sealant or composite	Tooth paint
Nitrous hood	Astronaut mask

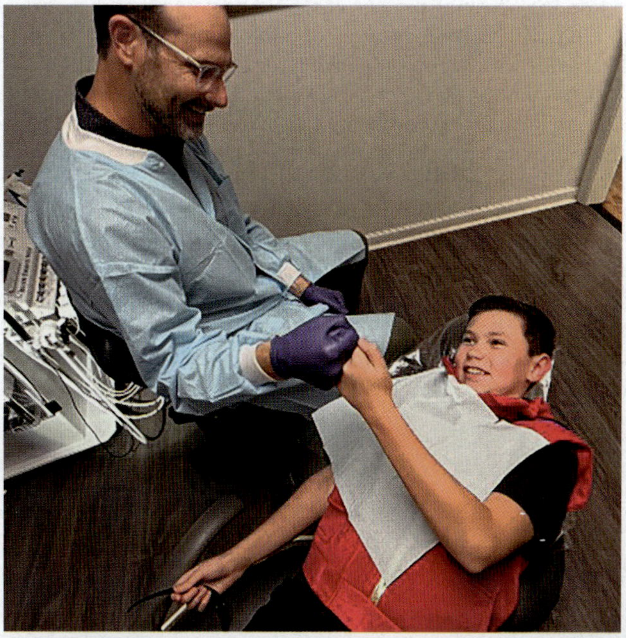

• **Fig. 26.4** Example of Nonverbal Communication. The dentist is conveying that the child will have a great visit.

to interpret the world around them, and these cues work synergistically with words and style to communicate with children.

The conscientious practitioner can use this form of communication to help shape ideal behavior in the child patient.[84] Smiling, making eye contact, and an upbeat tone of voice convey to the child that the practitioner is confident that the child will enjoy the visit (Fig. 26.4). A practitioner must remember that personal protective equipment (PPE) such as a mask and eye protection may hide the practitioner's facial expressions, and practitioners should not walk into the operatory to greet a patient in PPE. Nonverbal cues are important for the young child, and smiles and a friendly pat on the arm may help the toddler with limited verbal skills feel more comfortable. In a classic study on nonverbal behavior guidance, children between the ages of 7 and 10 years who were patted on the upper arm or shoulder during the visit displayed less fidgeting behavior than their counterparts who did not receive this touch; they also reported greater enjoyment of the visit.[85] Alternatively, if a child is misbehaving, a stern facial expression and more upright posture can convey authority and regain the child's attention and compliance.

The dentist may choose to sit down and let the preschool patient approach, reducing the risk of being intimidating because of height. This technique is called "leveling" and aims to reduce the physical height difference between the dentist and the patient, creating a more relaxed and less intimidating environment.

One must recognize that very young patients may misinterpret nonverbal cues. Wilson and associates[86] found that 3-year-old patients were significantly less accurate than 6- and 9-year-olds at correctly identifying emotions associated with facial expressions depicted in photographs. Three-year-old patients were significantly more likely to confuse happy and angry for sad.[86] The dentist should be especially careful with patients of this age to make verbal and nonverbal communication as clear as possible.

Positive Reinforcement

Positive reinforcement is a way to recognize the cooperation of the child patient and promote future positive behavior through rewards. Positive reinforcement is universally accepted[61,83,84] and contributes to the child's overall sense of accomplishment with successfully completing a dental procedure. Social positive reinforcement is most effective and best when it is specific to the behavior that is cooperative. While the patient will be pleased by a comment such as "You are being such a great patient today," children are more likely to continue desired behaviors if the praise is specific, such as "You are sitting so still and opening so wide!" Such a focused comment often motivates a child to continue to sit still and open a bit wider. Complimenting the child in front of parents and dental assistants, again being specific to the positive behaviors the child exhibits, is a great way to boost the child's self-esteem and memories of the visit.

Rewards such as a small toy or sticker also provide positive reinforcement, as shown in Fig. 26.5. These items are concrete, and the child can take them home and show them off as a source of pride and accomplishment. It should be noted that these prizes will not have the same meaning or reinforcement of positive dental behavior without accompanying social reinforcement.

Some question whether positive reinforcement is appropriate in all circumstances. For example, should children receive a reward if they do not exhibit cooperative behavior, or will this reinforce bad behavior? This is determined by the individual philosophy of the practitioner and should be consistently enforced. A practitioner may find one positive aspect of the child's behavior during the appointment and give a sticker for that aspect. For example, "Thank you for coming to see me today. I appreciate you sitting in the chair and opening your mouth wide for me, and this sticker is for being so good at that. I think next time if you can sit still the entire time, you'll get two stickers."

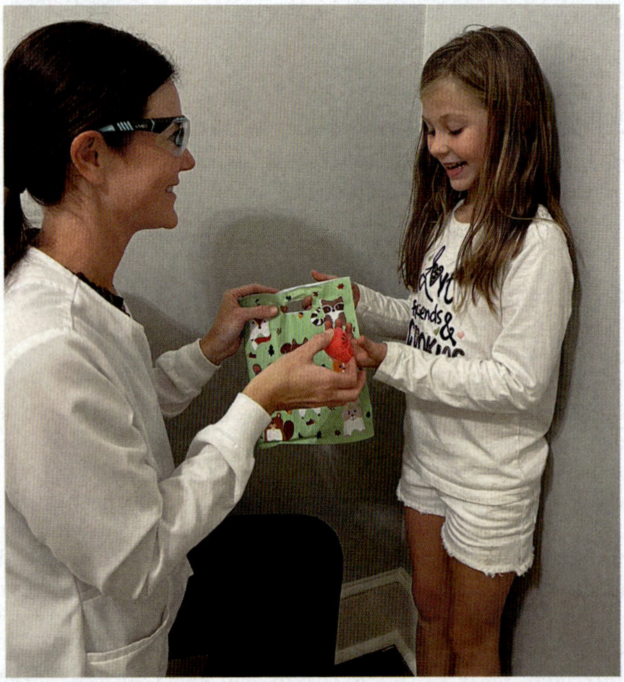

• **Fig. 26.5** Social and tangible positive reinforcement at the end of the appointment.

Sometimes what parents intend to be positive reinforcement becomes negative. They may preemptively offer children multiple, large rewards, such as going to a fast-food restaurant and getting a prize at a toy store. The notion that the ordeal they are going to experience merits these rewards can increase the anxiety of the children and cause them to view the upcoming treatment as threatening. Preparing the parent before the operative appointment and asking them not to make large promises to the child before the visit can avoid this situation. At the end of the visit, if the child indeed did cooperate, the parent can surprise the child with such a treat, providing irregular reinforcement.

Distraction

Of all the pediatric behavior guidance techniques, distraction has the most research to support its efficacy. Distraction is the most widely studied cognitive strategy for needle-related procedural pain in children, and a Cochrane review found strong evidence supporting its use.[87]

Dental visits are challenging, and all forms of distraction (verbal, audiovisual, physical) are effective in promoting coping. The majority of pediatric dentists report using distraction routinely and having high parental acceptance of the technique.[61]

Traditional distraction techniques include conversation with the dentist, toys, books, stories, and distraction by imagination. Storytelling can be related to the procedure, such as telling a child you are chasing "sugar bugs" while using the high-speed handpiece. One former student would chase away all the different colors of sugar bugs and then knock down their house. Other stories may be completely unrelated to dentistry to take them away from the experience, such as a shopping trip with a cartoon character or a story about pets. Counting is also a very popular form of distraction for some children.[84] Games such as guessing favorite colors or teachers' names are a fun way to take a child's mind off the procedure. The dentist may enlist the help of an auxiliary in distracting the patient, either by telling a story or playing a game. Physical distraction is also helpful, such as asking a child to rotate different feet during the injection or shaking the cheek.[88,89] Parents may also be utilized during distraction as they know their child's interests best. When trained properly to avoid distress-promoting behavior, parents can make a strong contribution to coping strategies, as shown in Tables 26.2 and 26.3 and Case Study: Prepared Parents, Prepared Children, Positive Coping.[41,62,80,82]

Technology-based distraction includes audiovisual, music, mobile applications, and/or virtual reality (VR). The use of mobile applications, songs, and three-dimensional glasses has shown varying levels of reduction in anxiety and pain perception and improvement in behavior.[90] A number of studies have shown that wraparound eyewear is effective in reducing uncooperative behavior and may be because of the ability of this type of eyewear to block out upsetting stimuli and to use popular and engaging programs.[91–93] However, in a survey of pediatric dentists only 2.1% use VR in their practices, which highlights that VR may have more research interest than clinical application.[90]

The use of mobile applications (apps) or games during a dental restorative visit has been shown to reduce anxiety in children, and dental-specific apps such as "Lovely Little Dentist" are available.[78,94] The digital health app market continues to grow and may be beneficial for patients. For example, in adults, a study showed that a mobile app was able to help with needle phobia.[95] As healthcare mobile apps continue to be developed, providers may benefit from interactive apps that can assist children in coping with dental treatment.

Direct Observation/Modeling

Direct observation uses social learning theory and the concept of modeling to improve behavior by allowing a child to observe a cooperative patient undergoing dental treatment. *Modeling* refers to learning by observation. In addition to helping children acquire new behaviors, it can help extinguish fear behavior through the process of "vicarious extinction," where children observe other children undergoing experiences that they fear and become less afraid. For example, a younger or fearful patient typically watches a cooperative sibling undergo a procedure to extinguish fears and this may be useful for children who have had no prior exposure to dental treatment. This observation can be live or in video form. Systematic reviews evaluating multiple randomized clinical trials of modeling suggest that it may be useful for anxiety reduction and improved behavior, particularly when the modeling represents a coaching model or displays stress coping skills.[78,96] For example, an especially useful video might show the following: gradual exposure to the dental appointment for the child, the child employing deep breathing, the child reciting a coping statement like "I am a little nervous but I can do new things," and the child finishing the appointment feeling brave and receiving a small reward (positive reinforcement) for coping with a new experience.

Desensitization

Desensitization is exposure to fear-invoking stimuli in a progressive manner, beginning with the least disturbing.[97] Patients self-identify their fears, are taught relaxation techniques, and are gradually exposed to the situations that they identify. Studies and case reports have described this technique to be successful in reducing dental fear in adolescents, adults, and patients with special healthcare needs.[98–101] The desensitization process can be time consuming, depending on the patient's level of anxiety. For those with severe anxiety, a psychologist can assist in implementing this approach.

Enhanced Control

Enhanced control allows the patient, especially an anxious one, to assume an active role in the dental appointment.[69] Control in this sense does not imply the possibility of avoiding the situation but rather the possibility of influencing how it is experienced.[102] The dentist tells patients that if they become uncomfortable or want to pause treatment, they should give the dentist a signal (e.g., raising a hand). The signal is practiced before beginning treatment. If the patient displays the gesture, the dentist should respond immediately and acknowledge the concern. The object of the technique is to allow the patient to feel a sense of control and to build trust for the patient that the dentist will acknowledge concerns. At first, a child may pause treatment several times to test if the dentist will respond. Generally, the interruptions will become more and more infrequent as the child learns to trust that the dentist will acknowledge his or her concern. This technique may deter disruptive behaviors later into the appointment or at future visits.

Parental Presence/Absence

As discussed previously, parents prefer to be present in the operatory for their child's dental visit. However, parental presence can be used as a guidance tool.[69] The child's desire for parental presence can become an important adjunct to cooperative behavior. For this technique to work properly, parents should be informed of the technique, consent before its use, and must be willing to comply when they are asked to leave the operatory. If a child is behaving poorly, then the dentist requests that the parent leave until the child becomes cooperative. This is an effective way to encourage communication for the child unwilling to interact with the dentist. A child must have the appropriate cognitive development to understand contingency (i.e., parent's presence is contingent on cooperative behavior). Parents may feel more comfortable with this technique if they are told that they do not have to leave the room; moving just out of the line of vision of the child is sufficient. When the child cooperates, the dentist should offer praise, and the parent should return promptly. This technique demands the trust of the parent, highlighting the importance of establishing a positive relationship with the family before an invasive procedure.

Memory Restructuring

A child's memory of an event is influenced by the information he or she receives after the event.[103] As children share their memories with others, those individuals' language and interaction play a powerful role in shaping what and how experiences are remembered.[104] If a parent reminds the child of an unpleasant dental experience, memories of the visit can become more negative. Memory reframing has been suggested as a tool to prevent dental fear and memory distortion (i.e., recalling higher pain compared with the initial report).[105] Few clinical trials have evaluated memory restructuring after needle-involved procedures, and only one has evaluated it in dentistry.[105]

In dentistry, this technique has four specific elements. At the first appointment a happy picture of the child smiling in the chair is taken. At the second appointment, that *visual reminder* (i.e., happy picture) is shown to the child. The child is asked if the parent was told how brave the child was during the dental visit. The child is enlisted in role-play to tell the dentist what the parent was told. This is the *verbalization* component where the child reports behaving well. Then the dentist praises the child with specific, *concrete examples* of the cooperative behavior, such as sitting very still. Finally, the child is asked to demonstrate the behaviors again (i.e., show us how wide you can open) to satisfy the *sense of accomplishment.* Pickrell et al., in a study of 6- to 9-year-old patients, found this technique improved child behavior and changed memories of fear.[105]

Additional memory-reframing interventions include telling children they were brave and that they did not cry, correcting exaggerations in memory, and praising them for using adaptive coping skills.[104] In medicine, research has shown that poorly managed needle procedures in children can result in distressing memories that lead to needle fears, phobias, and avoidance of medical care.[104] Given that memory reframing can be a simple intervention and that parents may be particularly influential in altering memory, parent education on reframing may be valuable and can be quickly taught by team members.

Voice Control

Voice control is a deliberate alteration of voice in volume, tone, or pace to influence a patient's behavior.[69] The volume may sometimes be reduced to a whisper to get the patient's attention; however, in classic voice control, instructions are firm, definite, and convincing with the facial expression mirroring the message.[106] Typically, the practitioner will make a request in a normal tone. If this request is not honored, the dentist can rephrase it in a firmer, louder tone. More importantly, the command should be repeated slowly and clearly. This technique is most acceptable to the child, dentist, and parent when it is discussed at the beginning of the appointment and is followed by positive reinforcement for improved behavior and the previously positive tenor of the appointment is reestablished. This reinforces the dentist as the coach who helps guide the patient to proper behavior.

Voice control can be considered an aversive technique because parents may interpret this as punishing the child by "yelling at him or her." This is not an accurate reflection of the true intent of voice control. Human nature values the approval of others, and a change to a negative tone signals disapproval with an intent to gain the patient's attention. Although voice control can be effective at normal and reduced volume, Greenbaum and colleagues[107] found that the loud voice was most effective at minimizing disruptiveness. Furthermore, Greenbaum and colleagues found that children who received voice control did not rate their experience as negative but reported a more positive experience than those who only experienced normal voice. However, parental acceptance of classic voice control has steadily declined throughout the past several decades[78] and has variable acceptance across parental cultures and socioeconomic statuses.[82,108]

Given parental reluctance toward the technique, parents should be informed of the possibility of its use before the appointment. Multiple studies have shown that a thorough explanation of techniques before their use greatly affects parental acceptance.[108–110] One explanation might be "I would like to keep your child as safe as possible and provide the best quality dentistry. If your child begins behavior that will interfere or be unsafe, like reaching up to grab instruments, I will change my tone to sound firmer to get his attention, just like you would if he were about to do something that would hurt him."

Nitrous Oxide

The use of nitrous oxide/oxygen (N_2O/O_2) is a form of pharmacologic behavior management, and the technique of administration is discussed in detail in Chapter 27. N_2O/O_2 is discussed in this chapter as well because it is considered a basic behavior guidance technique by the AAPD.[69] Box 26.3 lists the objectives of N_2O/O_2. It has been found to have a significant effect on reducing mild to moderate anxiety and uncooperative child behavior, and facilitates coping at subsequent visits, even if it is not used at those visits.[111,112] It is important to understand that the use of N_2O/O_2 is only effective if accompanied by communicative behavior guidance techniques. N_2O/O_2 is used to improve the child's ability to cope so that they are more receptive to techniques such as TSD, positive reinforcement, and distraction. The child must have some coping skills and an appropriate temperament to be receptive to N_2O/O_2 sedation. Nelson et al. found that children with high effortful control (the ability to inhibit negative reactions and focus on a task and persist even if it is difficult) were more successfully sedated with N_2O/O_2.[113] Generally N_2O/O_2 is readily accepted by parents.[114,115]

• BOX 26.3 Goals of Nitrous Oxide Administration

1. Decrease or eliminate anxiety
2. Enhance patient cooperation and reduce untoward movement
3. Raise the pain threshold (due to analgesic effects)
4. Reduce gagging
5. Enhance patient's tolerance for longer appointment

Additional Techniques to Consider

Humor

Humor supports relationships, emotional health, and cognitive function by easing social tension and reducing stress. A child's humor appreciation evolves with development, from recognizing incongruities in toddlerhood to enjoying jokes by age 7.[116] Though underexplored in pediatric dentistry, humor has proven benefits in medicine, such as reducing anxiety through medical clowns.[117] Dentists should understand humor development to enhance communication and create a positive experience for patients and families.

Mind-Body Therapies

Mind-body therapies in children, including biofeedback, breathing exercises, and hypnosis, may help decrease pain and reduce anxiety in the clinical setting.[69] The objective of mind-body therapies is to replace negative thoughts or maladaptive behaviors with more positive attitudes and adaptive behaviors. Cognitive strategies target thoughts such as positive coping statements (e.g., "I've been brave before, and I can be brave again"). Behavior therapies attempt to provide appropriate copings skills. For example, breathing exercises such as deep inhalation and slow exhalation can be taught to very young children as bubble breathing and have been shown to reduce anxiety and pain for needle-related procedures.[87] Often therapies are combined as cognitive and behavior therapies (i.e., CBT) and include distraction, relaxation training, deep breathing, hypnosis, preparing for and rehearsing the procedure in advance, using positive reinforcement for adaptive behaviors, making positive coping statements, and receiving coaching to use adaptive strategies.[87] CBT can reduce physiologic responses to stress, distress, and perceived pain.

Escape

Escape is a brief (e.g., 10 seconds) break from dental "treatment" and is the cessation of activity in the mouth, not getting up from the chair. Two different types of escape have been discussed: contingent and noncontingent. Contingent escape is given when a patient complies with a request or exhibits cooperative behavior. An example of this is "If you can hold still until I count to 10, we can take a break." Contingent escape requires the dentist to respond to the cooperative behavior and cease treatment. If the handpiece is stopped for any reason, it can be rephrased as a break. This technique is nonaversive and generally takes no more time than other behavior guidance techniques.[118,119]

Noncontingent escape is given regardless of behavior; it is granted at a predetermined interval (e.g., every 3 to 5 minutes by use of a timer). Escape is given more frequently at the beginning of an appointment, and as anxiety decreases and behavior improves, the intervals between breaks can increase. Studies have shown similar improvements in behavior with contingent and noncontingent escape.[120] Practically, noncontingent escape can be difficult to carry out consistently because breaks may be required when it is inconvenient, but the concept of breaks is very effective with children.

Animal-Assisted Therapy

Animal-assisted therapy (AAT) has been beneficial in a variety of healthcare settings including dentistry. AAT is goal oriented, complementary to other basic guidance techniques, and utilizes a trained animal (typically a dog) to assist the patient in alleviating anxiety, pain, or distress.[69] It can promote better interaction between the patient and the dental team and distract the child from a stressful situation (Fig. 26.6).

No centralized agency offers standardized training requirements, though the American Animal Hospital Association has released guidelines and recommendations regarding temperament, behavior, and dog health.[121] Practitioners should bear in mind the risks involved with the presence of animals in the dental environment: zoonotic diseases, dog allergens, fall/trip hazards, and animal bites.[122] There is a need for high-quality research to substantiate the effects of AAT in the dental environment, but low-quality evidence suggests that AAT may reduce anxiety and improve cooperation in children and adolescents who need dental treatment.[90]

Treatment Deferral

Deferring treatment is a viable option when behavior hinders safe, quality care, and treatment is not urgent.[69] Although pain, infection, and advanced caries require prompt care, minor lesions, sealants, and space maintenance can often wait. Interim therapies like silver diamine fluoride, Hall crowns, and fluoride varnish can manage caries until definitive treatment.[69] Parents must understand the delay, its risks, and the need for ongoing observation, known as "active surveillance." See Chapter 14 for more on therapeutic interventions.

Behavior Guidance for the Child With Previous Negative Dental Experiences

Negative experiences unfortunately occur in dentistry for children. If the experience occurred at another office, separate the child and parent or ensure the child cannot hear the re-telling of the negative experience, and gather as much information from the parent about the previous experience as possible to get a sense of the child's temperament, coping skills, and parent expectations and to avoid past triggers.

The negative experience may have occurred at your office due to the need for time-sensitive treatment, a challenging procedure, or unexpected uncooperative behavior in the middle of an appointment. Negative appointments should be discussed with the caregiver as soon as feasible whether that be in person or in a follow-up phone call. The dentist should address any concerns empathetically, taking into consideration that it is distressing to parents to see their child struggle. Then the dentist and parent should partner to minimize the impact of the negative experience.

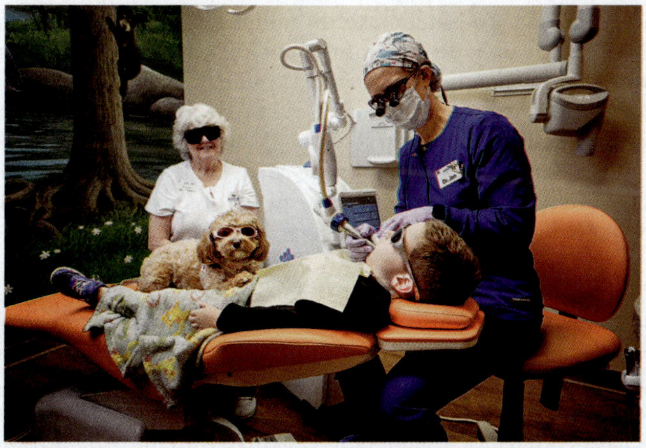

• **Fig. 26.6** Animal-assisted therapy in the dental setting. (Courtesy Dr. Jen Bryk Hechko and photographer credit to Seth Kerechanin.)

Parents should be discouraged from reminding the child of previous difficult dental experiences, because the memories are not always easily recalled by the child. If parents repeatedly tell the story of a child crying or being "held down," they will vicariously obtain this "memory." At the next dental visit, the dentist and parent should focus on positive aspects of the present dental visit that distinguish it from previous ones. The parent may compliment how child friendly the office is and how you enjoy treating children. Or the dentist may emphasize that is great to see the child on a day their teeth are happy. Even if the child has no dental needs, reintroducing them to the dental environment with an examination and prophylaxis can help extinguish fears and promote positive memories using the previously discussed memory-restructuring techniques.[105]

Advanced behavior techniques may not be needed solely on the basis of a previous bad experience. Sometimes the child can be treated successfully by a compassionate dentist using communicative techniques in a new environment, and N_2O/O_2 can be a helpful adjunct in retraining fearful patients. For other children, advanced guidance techniques may be appropriate if urgent treatment needs remain.

Advanced Behavior Guidance Techniques

For some children, basic behavior guidance is inadequate to permit safe, high-quality dental care. This may be because of the lack of psychological or emotional maturity or a disability.[69] In these cases it is important to engage the parents to discuss risks, benefits, and alternatives of advanced behavior guidance so that they can make an informed decision for their child. These techniques are accompanied by an increased risk of physical and emotional harm and require advanced training and informed consent.

Protective Stabilization

Protective stabilization, also known as medical immobilization, is defined as "any manual method, physical or mechanical device, material, or equipment that immobilizes or reduces the ability of a patient to move his or her arms, legs, body, or head freely."[123] It is used to decrease risk of injury during treatment and may be classified as either active or passive. (See Case Study Protective Stabilization).

In active stabilization, the parent, dentist, or assistant helps stabilize the patient; typically this is carried out only for a very short period of time or in times of unexpected, physically uncooperative behavior.[124] Passive protective stabilization is the use of a device to restrict patient movement for safety. Commonly used devices are Papoose Boards (Olympic Medical Corporation, Seattle, WA) or Rainbow Wraps (Specialized Care Co Inc., Hampton, NH), as shown in Fig. 26.7, Table e26.6. These devices have fabric wraps to help reduce the movement of arms and legs. Often this technique is employed when patient behavior unexpectedly deteriorates during an appointment, and the procedures must be brought to a safe conclusion or in emergency settings.[124] Passive protective stabilization may also be used during a sedation appointment to minimize movements interfering with safe care and monitoring. Finally, these devices may be used in nonemergency settings to provide limited treatment (i.e., examination and prophylaxis) for patients with intellectual disability when the risk or barriers to sedation or general anesthesia make these alternatives impractical. The American Academy of Developmental Medicine and Dentistry states that individuals with intellectual disability deserve high-quality dental care and that when used appropriately, protective stabilization is indicated to ensure successful procedure completion.[125]

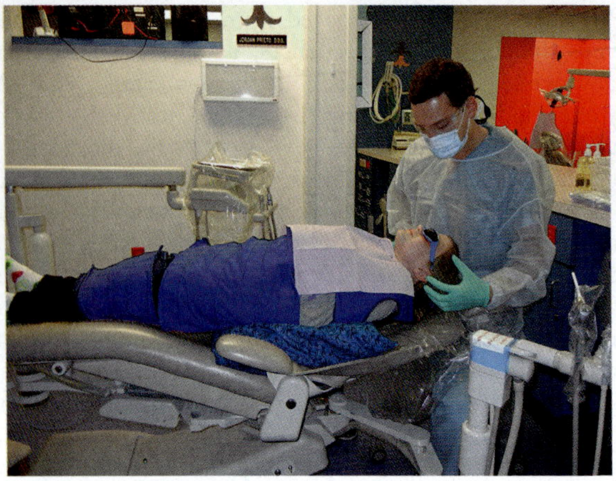

• **Fig. 26.7** Medical stabilization with a papoose board.

Generally, the least restrictive stabilization is indicated, which would suggest active immobilization is preferred. However, active stabilization is less effective in preventing untoward movement, especially in large patients. In one study of adult patients with intellectual disability, active stabilization was associated with more injuries compared with passive immobilization.[126]

The risks of protective stabilization are physical or psychological harm, loss of dignity, and violation of patient's rights. Contraindications include patients who cannot be immobilized safely due to medical, psychological, or physical conditions.[124] Examples include patients with bone fragility, thermoregulation disorders such as anhidrotic ectodermal dysplasia, or previous child abuse.

Any dentist using this technique should review the AAPD guidelines for protective stabilization and should have training beyond the predoctoral dental school curriculum where this skill is rarely practiced.[127] Protective stabilization is the most contentious of the behavior guidance techniques. Parents tend to rate both active and passive immobilization as unacceptable,[81,82,128] and many pediatric dentists find its use rarely acceptable for routine dental treatment.[80,129] International views vary widely, and it is not considered professionally acceptable in some countries.[129] It is important to note that in studies where parents were asked to rate acceptability of various techniques, they were shown videos of procedures with little or no explanation. Kupietzky found that parents are more accepting of passive stabilization use during sedation after a positive explanation and were more likely to attribute child crying to fear, not the device.[130] Protective stabilization should be used compassionately and in a way that gives a child boundaries and can instill confidence in accepting dental treatment.

Specific informed consent should be obtained, documented, and reviewed at each appointment, and child assent should be obtained when possible.[124] Use of protective stabilization should be documented, including type of stabilization, duration, indication, presence of parent or reason for their absence, behavior in the device, and untoward outcomes. A caregiver should remain in the operatory with the child, unless they expressly choose otherwise, so they can provide psychological support and so, if they withdraw consent, the patient can be released from stabilization as soon as it is safe. If it is likely that a patient may become uncooperative during a procedure that the dentist and caregiver feels must be completed that day, treatment can be performed on an unwrapped stabilization device. Before initiation of treatment, the parent and dentist should discuss critical steps during the procedures (i.e., local anesthesia administration) and what behaviors would prompt aborting treatment. The dentist should inform parents in advance when procedures cannot be stopped immediately without risk for pain and infection. Use of protective stabilization can be stressful to the dental team and the family, but it is an important skill for the pediatric dentist. Providers who care for children who do not have access to sedation or operating rooms use protective stabilization to humanely relieve pain, address infection, or treat time-sensitive emergencies.[131] (See Case Study: Protective Stabilization.)

Mouth Props in Dentistry for Children

Mouth props are routinely used in both general and pediatric dentistry to improve the quality of dental care and the comfort and safety of the patient. They can help prevent fatigue from the mouth staying open during long visits, improve visualization, and prevent accidental closing that may cause trauma or moisture contamination. Use of a mouth prop by a compliant child is not considered protective stabilization.[124] However, use for an uncooperative patient should be discussed in advance with the guardian to set appropriate expectations and to review risks and benefits.

Multiple types of mouth props are used in pediatric dentistry, as shown in Fig. 26.8, and they all have specific indications, advantages, and disadvantages. The McKesson style of mouth props (Hu-Friedy, Chicago, IL) is a rubber, wedge-shaped device and is generally well accepted by patients. It is not adjustable, and the correct size should be used to prevent discomfort. Uncooperative patients may easily dislodge this device. These mouth props can also make the approach for an inferior alveolar nerve block difficult. They can fall to the back of the mouth and should be tied with a long piece of floss to facilitate easy retrieval.

Molt mouth props (Hu-Friedy, Chicago, IL) are an alternative device that is adjustable. Their appearance may intimidate children, but with TSD they are well accepted. The child can be told that they have a "popcorn popper" in their mouth to explain the clicking noise of opening the mouth prop. The practitioner must use caution because rapid opening of the mouth prop can result in luxation or avulsion of anterior teeth. If the patient removes the appliance from the mouth before it is released, the anterior teeth can be traumatized.

Soft foam mouth props (Specialized Care Co., Hampton, NH) may be used for children with intellectual or physical disabilities who cannot comply with opening. They are less rigid and less likely to damage anterior teeth compared with other mouth props. The foam is easily deformed and may not prevent a patient from injuring themselves with an instrument. If a patient is biting through the foam mouth prop, it can be used to initially support opening and then be replaced with a McKesson rubber prop.

Before using a mouth prop, it is advisable to check for any loose teeth. Loose primary teeth can be dislodged and possibly swallowed or aspirated with any type of mouth prop.

Sedation and General Anesthesia

Sedation is a pharmacologic behavior management technique described in depth in Chapter 27. As with N_2O/O_2, sedation is an adjunct to the child's innate coping. Children under sedation should be arousable, interactive, and benefit from communicative behavior guidance techniques. Children with no coping skills (such as those who are very young or who have medical or developmental disabilities) and/or those with extensive needs that

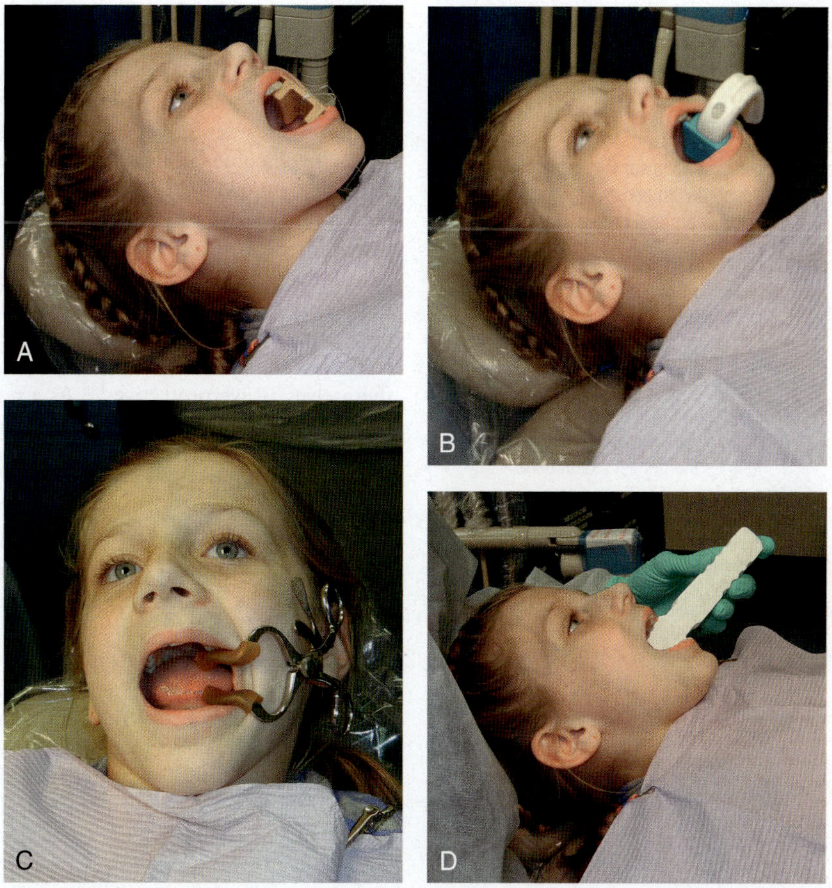

• **Fig. 26.8** Mouth Props. (A) McKesson style mouth prop. (B) Mouth prop with extraoral handle. (C) Molt mouth prop. (D) Disposable foam mouth prop.

would warrant multiple sedation visits may benefit from general anesthesia. Children with shy temperament (see eBox 26.2), high impulsivity, and lower self-control have tended to have less successful sedations than those who exhibit easy temperament, effortful control (i.e., "can easily stop an activity when he/she is told no"), and soothability (i.e., "is easy to sooth when he/she is upset").[132,133]

Research examining behavior at subsequent appointments after these modalities affirms pharmacologic management's effectiveness in safeguarding the developing psyche of patients. McComb and colleagues concluded that treatment with oral sedation had no significant effect on future dental behavior at a recall examination performed 2 to 34 months later.[134] Other studies have shown that children exhibit more positive behavior after treatment under general anesthesia compared with conscious sedation.[135,136]

Although parents have previously expressed poor acceptance of sedation and general anesthesia for their children's dental care, this view has changed dramatically in the past two decades.[128] In the past, pharmacologic management was the least acceptable behavior technique, even with explanation of the need for the procedure.[110] Contemporary data suggest that parents prefer sedation or general anesthesia over more aversive techniques such as active or passive stabilization or voice control.[81,82,108] In general, parents view sedation as safe, though they may have misconceptions about the sedation experience (e.g., thinking their child will be asleep or will not need local anesthetic).[137] Additionally, parental acceptance of behavior guidance techniques vary by parent background and culture.[108] The dentist must take into account the health and airway status of the patient (see Chapter 27), the risks of sedation, the extent of treatment needs, and the temperament and potential cooperation of the patient before deciding to use an advanced behavior guidance technique.

Documenting Behavior and Use of Behavior Management Techniques

The behavior of the child patient is an important component of the visit that must be documented. A variety of scales for behavior exist, and a commonly used one is the Frankl score, as shown in Table 26.7.[138]

Qualitative comments, in addition to a quantitative score to record behaviors, can help in planning future management strategies for a child. The comments should be objective and nonjudgmental about the child and parents. Words like "overindulged" or "spoiled" are subjective, should be avoided, and may offend parents on review of the record. Electronic health records (EHRs) are becoming more integrated to allow interoperability and portability for patients to have access to and control of all of their healthcare records.[139] Dentists need to be mindful that EHRs will be available to patients and documenting pertinent information appropriately will help ensure the relationship with the parent is not adversely affected. Appropriate verbiage might include the following: patient

TABLE 26.7 Frankl Behavior Rating Scale

Behavior Score	Classification	Description
Pre-Coop	Precooperative	Cooperative behavior is not routinely expected with consistency at this age (3 years and under)
Frankl 4	Definitely positive	Good rapport with the dentist Interested in the dental procedures Laughing and enjoying the situation
Frankl 3	Positive	Accepting of treatment but at times cautious Willing to comply with the dentist, at times with reservation, but patient follows the dentist's directions Cooperative
Frankl 2	Negative	Reluctant to accept treatment Uncooperative Sullen, withdrawn
Frankl 1	Definitely negative	Refusal of treatment Crying forcefully Fearful

From Frankl SN, Shiere FR, Fogels HR. Should the parent remain with the child in the dental operatory? *ASDC J Dent Child*. 1962;29(2):150-163.

was active in chair, inquisitive, reached up to grab instrument, kicked feet, or had tears for local anesthetic.

Behavior guidance techniques should be documented. Typically communicative techniques do not need to be recorded, but it is helpful to include particularly effective techniques as a reminder for future visits. Pharmacologic and advanced techniques must be recorded specifically. The monitoring and recording requirements for N_2O/O_2, sedation, and general anesthesia should comply with state regulations. If active immobilization is used, it is important to record who immobilized the patient, what body part was immobilized, for what part of the procedure, and for how long (e.g., Tiffany stabilized patient's arms during local anesthesia). If passive immobilization is used, the type of device and the approximate time it is used should be recorded.[124] It is also prudent to document that an updated verbal consent was obtained in addition to the written consent obtained before use.

Role of Behavior Management in Society

Dentists do not care for children in a vacuum. Society, parents and their children, the insurance industry, regulatory bodies, the legal system, dental staff, and the education, expectations, and choices of dentists all influence the options available for child patient management.[51]

Changes in Society and Parenting

Many societal changes in the past two decades have impacted the nature of parenting in America. The changing economic and social climate has produced different types of families (e.g., multicultural, blended, single-parent). Families tend to live increasingly isolated and disconnected lives because of young families moving away from extended family members. There has been an increased incidence of single parents and free-time limitations caused by the work schedules of dual-income or single parent families.[140] Economic stress has added to the loss of emotional and practical support. Thirty seven percent of children under age 9 in America live in low income families.[141] Stressed parents have been reported to implement inconsistent (sometimes lax or overreactive) parenting, more negative communications, and unclear rules and limits on children's behavior.[142] The cultural norm of parenting is a child-centered, time-intensive parenting in which parents invest heavily in each child even at the expense of the collective family.[143] This parenting style is characterized by overprotection and control with almost half (45%) of American parents describing themselves as overprotective.[144] As a result there has been a continuous decline in opportunities for children and adolescents to engage in independent activity (e.g., unstructured play, roaming, walking, or riding a bicycle around the neighborhood) without direct oversight by adults.[145] Independent activity allows children the opportunity to problem solve, practice social interactions, and make decisions on their own. It promotes a strong locus of internal control (the belief that one has control over his/her life and can solve problems if they arise), increases resiliency, and develops coping skills.[145] Another aspect of contemporary culture that is correlated with decreased coping skills and resiliency in children is the increase of screen time and digital media.[146] In a survey of the AAPD on behavior management techniques, 85% of practitioners indicated that they believed that parenting styles have changed during their years in practice. They most frequently indicated parents are "less willing to set limits for their children" and are "less willing to use physical discipline."[147] A survey of millennial parents revealed that 75% practice gentle parenting. Educators and school administrators also report a growing urgency to prepare teachers to manage the rise in problem behaviors in children.[148] The changes in parenting culture suggest that clinicians treating children will need a wide array of behavior guidance skills to help today's children cope with dental treatment and will need to hone excellent communication skills to partner with parents to help guide them and their children through the dental experience.

Changing Parental Perspectives of Behavior Management

Parental acceptance of behavior guidance techniques has shifted, with physical restraints declining and pharmacologic methods and minimally invasive/caries-arresting therapies gaining favor.[81,149] Positive reinforcement, rapport-building communication, and TSD remain widely accepted.[61] Caregivers often resist restraints, parental absence, or voice control, accepting them only for urgent procedures like injections or extractions.[90] These techniques should be discussed in advance to support shared decision making.

Third-Party Reimbursement

A concern for dentists is lack of reimbursement for the time and skill needed to manage the behavior of a child patient effectively. Third-party insurers lack shared standards and coverage for codes related to dentistry, specifically behavior management techniques, N_2O/O_2, sedation, and general anesthesia.[150–152] As a result, dentists may be less willing to attempt time-consuming nonpharmacologic behavior guidance techniques for children who may be uncooperative. Pharmacologic alternatives may not be covered by third-party insurers, or these insurers may have stipulations that make these options impracticable such as requiring multiple failed attempts with N_2O/O_2 sedation before general anesthesia is covered.

General anesthesia is typically too expensive for families without insurance, and third-party providers may not cover this service. In addition, low reimbursement rates have resulted in hospitals reducing or eliminating access for dentists.[150] Third-party reimbursement for general anesthesia for dental procedures for young children is largely dependent on state regulations. The majority, but not all, states require medical insurance to cover general anesthesia for dental procedures when deemed medically necessary.[153]

Informed Consent

Informed consent is essential so the parent or guardian understands the proposed treatment and its risks, benefits, and alternatives, and can actively participate in the oral care plan.[154] With rare exceptions, only a parent or legal guardian can provide informed consent for a minor patient. Adult patients with intellectual disability should be included in the consent process but may need the assistance of trusted caregivers and legally may be unable to give consent.[155] The dentist should ascertain who is the legal guardian of a minor and, if guardianship is held by anyone other than the birth parents of a minor, it is appropriate to ask for relevant legal documents. When possible, assent should be obtained by the patient.[156] Adolescents have the capacity to make appropriate healthcare decisions and should be intimately involved in any treatment planning conversation.

Written informed consent is required before patient treatment in most states.[154] Preprinted forms can provide a framework for discussion and to document the conversation took place but are not a substitute for communication that includes benefits, risks, and reasonable alternatives. Informed consent is a process that relies on honest communication from the practitioner and willingness to understand by the parent. eBox 26.4 is an example of describing various guidance techniques for parent education, discussion, and consent. Dentists should convey what level of cooperation is required for treatment and come to an agreement with parents regarding acceptable behavior guidance techniques. Misrepresentations regarding behavior guidance techniques can cause conflict in the parent-dentist relationship and have legal consequences.[157]

The informed consent discussion should allow time for the caregivers to ask questions and may be supplemented by photos, videos, or models.[154] An interpreter should be available if needed, and audio or tablet interpretation is an acceptable alternative.[158] When possible, caregivers should have time to consider significant treatment decisions. They should be given sources of accurate information for reference. Families today are overwhelmed with the amount of information available to them about medical care. Exposure to health misinformation, whether intentional or not, is increasing.[159] For example, most internet posts regarding fluoride on a popular social media platform were misinformation with links to commercial interests.[160]

Informed consent is an area where the investment of time and patience can prevent future problems, because malpractice complaints have been reported to occur more frequently when a good relationship between the provider and patient is lacking.[161] Sometimes a parent will not accept recommended treatment, which is known as informed refusal.[158] Providers should work to understand the reasoning behind the decisions and to be open to reasonable alternatives.[162] If no alternative exists and a parent still refuses to provide informed consent, the consequences of no treatment should be discussed, and the refusal should be documented. These parents should be encouraged to seek a second opinion.

Conclusion

Sheller nicely summarizes the demands of dentistry for children by stating that "the task of pediatric dentists is the same as it was a generation ago: to perform precise surgical procedures on children whose behavior may range from cooperative to hostile to defiant."[51] Behavior guidance will remain the art of recognizing the complexities of children's and dentists' temperaments, parental attitudes, and varying treatment needs and creating an optimal treatment plan to best address the child's needs.

Visit eBooks.Health.Elsevier.com to see full list of references.

27

Behavior Guidance-Pharmacologic

THOMAS TANBONLIONG, TRAVIS NELSON, AND SARAT THIKKURISSY

CHAPTER OUTLINE

Introduction

Most children can be treated safely in the dental setting by using only local anesthesia and basic behavior guidance techniques (see Chapter 26). For those who are unable to tolerate dental procedures comfortably despite such efforts, procedural sedation or general anesthesia (GA) may be necessary to safely and effectively complete dental treatment.

The primary purpose of pharmacologic management of young patients is to minimize or eliminate anxiety and protect the developing psyche. Procedural sedation produces depth-dependent anxiolysis, which reduces pain reaction and facilitates coping. In contrast, a patient treated with GA is cognitively unaware, eliminating the need for bidirectional communication during most of the treatment process. Although these strategies convey many advantages, there are risks inherent with all pharmacologic techniques. Therefore risk/benefit analysis is required whenever procedural sedation or GA is considered. This may include assessing drug factors (e.g., medication, dose, route, and rate of administration), patient characteristics (e.g., age, health status, and physical characteristics such as body mass index), operator characteristics (e.g., comfort with procedure, estimated working time, and access to emergency support), depth of sedation, and dental needs (Fig. 27.1).

Procedural sedation ranges from minimal (previously termed *anxiolysis*) to moderate (previously termed *conscious sedation*) to deep sedation and GA. Dental schools typically teach minimal sedation, focusing on nitrous oxide/oxygen and sometimes oral sedation. Moderate sedation, when taught, is often an elective for select students and is primarily taught for adults. Pediatric sedation (for those aged 12 years and younger) requires specialized training due to anatomical and physiologic differences (See Chapter 7, Table 7.2), and deep sedation and GA necessitate Commission of Dental Accreditation (CODA)–accredited postdoctoral training.

In 1985, the American Academy of Pediatrics (AAP) and the American Academy of Pediatric Dentistry (AAPD) jointly endorsed "Guidelines for the Elective Use of Conscious Sedation, Deep Sedation, and General Anesthesia in Pediatric Patients."[1] These guidelines, and their subsequent revisions, established the standard of care for pediatric dental sedation. The most recent cosponsored guidelines were published in 2016 and are broadly summarized in Table 27.1.[2]

The AAP/AAPD joint guidelines emphasize the goals of sedation, which are the following: (1) guard the patient's safety and welfare; (2) minimize physical discomfort and pain; (3) control anxiety, minimize psychological trauma, and maximize the potential for amnesia; (4) control behavior and/or movement, which allows the safe completion of the procedure; and (5) return the patient to a state in which safe discharge from medical supervision, as determined by recognized criteria, is possible.[1]

Sedation exists on a continuum, with overlap between levels. This chapter focuses on pediatric minimal and moderate sedation, but understanding all levels is crucial for safe practice within one's training and licensure. Providers must be prepared

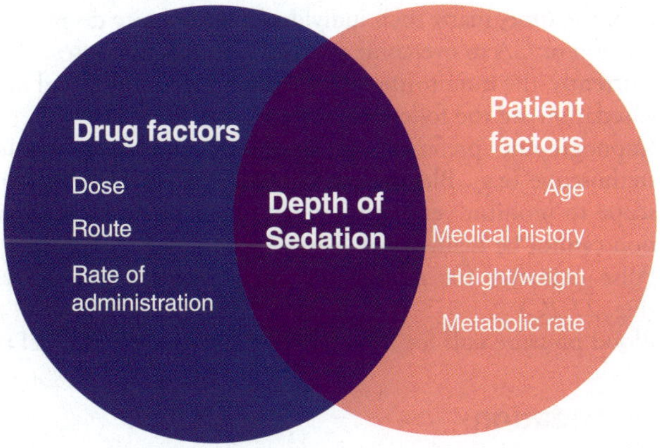

• **Fig. 27.1** Depth of sedation based on drug and patient factors.

to rescue patients from deeper sedation than intended, such as responding to deep sedation when targeting moderate sedation.

Levels of Sedation

Minimal and Moderate Sedation

Minimal sedation is a drug-induced state in which a patient responds normally to verbal commands. Although cognitive function and coordination may be impaired, ventilatory and cardiovascular functions are unaffected.[1] Moderate sedation is a drug-induced depression of consciousness during which patients respond purposefully to verbal commands (e.g., "open your eyes," either alone or accompanied by light tactile stimulation—a light tap on the shoulder or face, not a sternal rub).[1] In moderate sedation a patent airway is continuously maintained without

TABLE 27.1 Definitions and Characteristics for Levels of Sedation

	Minimal Sedation	Moderate Sedation	Deep Sedation
Definition	Drug-induced state during which patients respond normally to verbal commands	Drug-induced depression of consciousness during which patients respond purposefully to verbal commands or light tactile stimulation The caveat that loss of consciousness should be unlikely is a particularly important aspect of the definition of moderate sedation The drugs and techniques used should carry a margin of safety wide enough to render unintended loss of consciousness highly unlikely	Drug-induced depression of consciousness during which patients cannot be easily aroused but respond purposefully after repeated verbal or painful stimulation
Cognitive and physiologic functions	Although cognitive function and coordination may be impaired, ventilatory and cardiovascular functions are unaffected	No interventions are required to maintain a patent airway (i.e., patients should be able to maintain their airway without assistance), and spontaneous ventilation is adequate Cardiovascular function is usually maintained	The state and risks of deep sedation may be indistinguishable from those of general anesthesia
Personnel needed	2	2	3
Monitoring	Children who have received minimal sedation generally will not require more than observation and intermittent assessment of their level of sedation	There should be *continuous* monitoring of oxygen saturation and heart rate and *intermittent* recording of respiratory rate and blood pressure; these should be recorded in a time-based record	In addition to the equipment previously cited for moderate sedation, an ECG monitor and a defibrillator for use in pediatric patients should be readily available These vital signs must be documented every 5 minutes in a time-based record
Other considerations	Some children will become moderately sedated despite the intended level of minimal sedation; should this occur, the guidelines for moderate sedation will apply	Restraining devices should be checked to prevent airway obstruction or chest restriction If a restraint device is used, a hand or foot should be kept exposed The child's head position should be checked frequently to ensure airway patency A functioning suction apparatus must be present	One person must be available; their only responsibility is to constantly observe the patient's vital signs, airway patency, and adequacy of ventilation and to either administer drugs or direct their administration Patients receiving deep sedation should have an intravenous line placed at the start of the procedure or have a person skilled in establishing vascular access in pediatric patients immediately available

From Coté CJ, Wilson S. American Academy of Pediatric Dentistry, American Academy of Pediatrics. Guidelines for monitoring and management of pediatric patients before, during, and after sedation for diagnostic and therapeutic procedures. *Pediatr Dent.* 2019;41(4):E26-E52.

intervention. When moderate sedation is the intended outcome, the drugs and techniques used should carry a wide enough margin of safety to render unintended loss of consciousness unlikely.[1]

In moderate sedation a child may be in a state wherein their eyes are temporarily closed. However, they should be easily arousable after a verbal prompt (i.e., "open your eyes") or respond with withdrawal *and* crying after a mildly painful stimulus, such as injection of local anesthetic. Purposeful withdrawal from painful stimuli and crying are prominent at this level of sedation, whereas deeper levels of sedation may result only in reflex withdrawal or reflex withdrawal and moaning. See Case Study: Considerations for Sedating the Pediatric Patient, eVideo 27.1 If arousal does not occur, especially after a repeated painful stimulus (e.g., trapezius muscle pinch, sternal rub), then the child is in a state of deep sedation and must be managed accordingly. This frequently entails stopping the procedure and focusing on returning the patient to minimal or moderate sedation level. Very young patients (e.g., under 36 months of age) and those with intellectual or physical impairments may be incapable of typical bidirectional verbal communication with the dental provider. Therefore for safety reasons, it is preferable to maintain a minimally depressed level of consciousness for these individuals. Most of the time, many such individuals may require deeper levels of sedation or GA to overcome primal emotional responses.[1–3]

Currently, the monitoring requirements for minimal and moderate sedation are the following:

- Capnography, preferred or amplified, audible pretracheal stethoscope (e.g., Bluetooth technology) or precordial stethoscope to monitor ventilation when bidirectional communication cannot be maintained (Fig. 27.2A–B)
- Pulse oximeter for monitoring oxygenation and pulse rate (Fig. 27.2C)
- Blood pressure cuff for monitoring circulation (Fig. 27.2D)

Deep Sedation

Deep sedation is a controlled state of depressed level of consciousness or unconsciousness from which the patient is not easily aroused. Deep sedation may be accompanied by a partial or complete loss of protective reflexes, including the ability to maintain a patent airway independently and respond purposefully to physical stimulation or verbal commands. Young patients in deep sedation may respond minimally or with only a reflex withdrawal

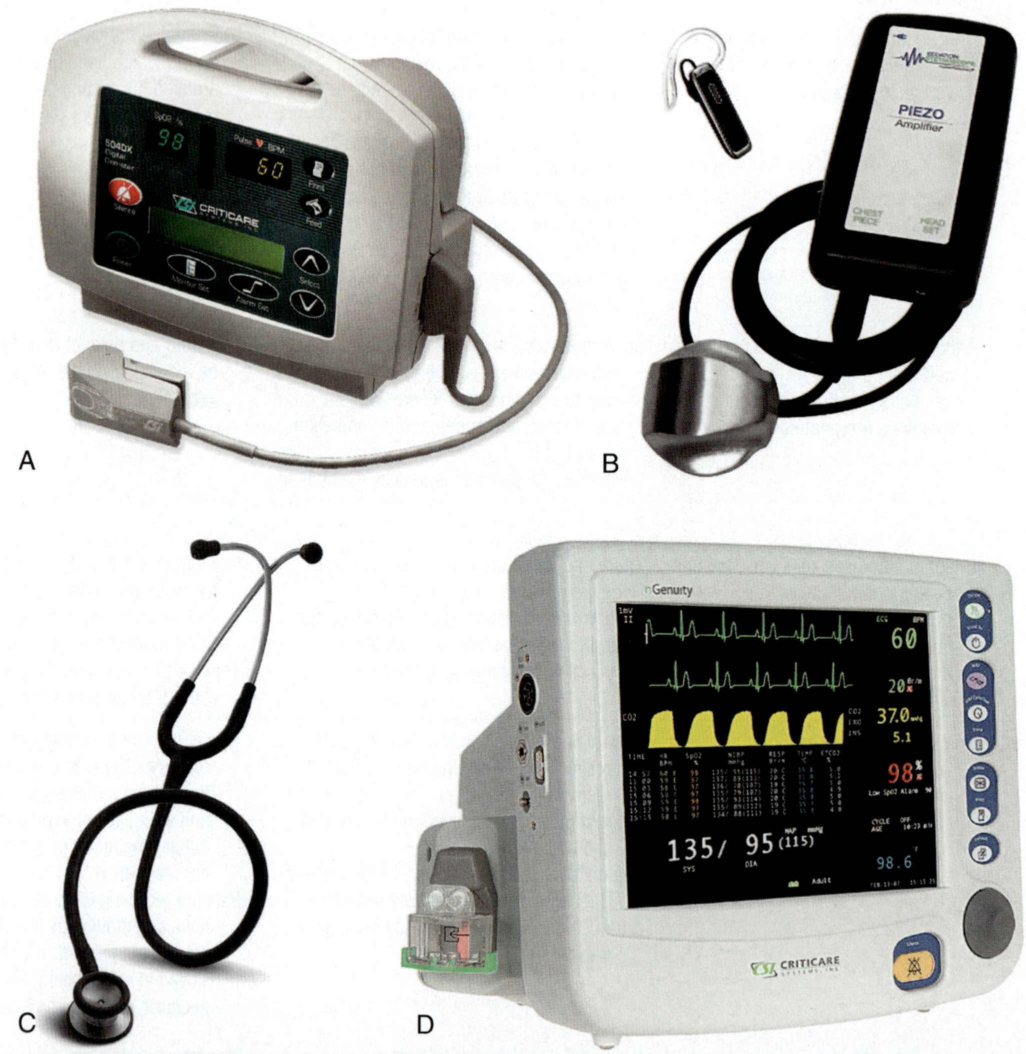

• **Fig. 27.2** (A) Capnograph. (B) Bluetooth precordial stethoscope. (C) Pulse oximeter. (D) Blood pressure cuff. (A, Courtesy Criticare Systems, Inc., Waukesha, WI; B, https://sedationresource.com/; C, Courtesy 3M Littman Stethoscopes, St Paul, MN.)

to an intensely painful stimulus. Monitoring of deep sedation must include pulse oximetry, capnography or precordial stethoscope, electrocardiography, and use of blood pressure cuff. (See Case Study: Considerations for Sedating the Pediatric Patient for videos of the sedation depth continuum.)

General Anesthesia

GA is a controlled state of unconsciousness accompanied by a total loss of protective reflexes, including the inability to maintain an airway independently and respond purposefully to physical stimulation or verbal commands.

Minimal and Moderate Versus Deep Sedation: A Critical Question

The distinctions between minimal, moderate, and deep sedation must be well understood by those who sedate pediatric dental patients. At the intended endpoint of minimal and moderate sedation the patient is not unconscious or unresponsive to verbal or minimally painful stimuli. A reflex withdrawal response alone to repeated minimal or moderately painful stimuli indicates deeper levels of sedation beyond minimal and moderate sedation. In minimal and moderate sedation, the patient's cardiovascular and respiratory functions are unaffected and should fall within the expected physiologic parameters for the age of the child (See Chapter 7, Table 7.2).

There is a higher chance of respiratory and cardiovascular complications occurring as depth of sedation increases. Although protective reflexes are maintained in minimal and moderate sedation, coughing and maintaining a patent airway independently may be lost in deep sedation. The resulting laryngospasm, aspiration, hypoxemia, or apnea (absence of breathing) can be life-threatening.[2] Accordingly, providers who practice deep sedation and GA are required to have additional training that enables them to swiftly address such issues and return the patient to a safe and controlled state.

Rescue

Rescue is an essential sedation concept. Because the sedation level is not always predictable, especially with oral routes of administration, the practitioner must be trained and capable of rescuing a child who enters a deeper level of sedation than originally intended or planned for the procedure.[3,4]

Often, the first action in an emergency is activating emergency medical services (EMS). However, children decompensate rapidly, so the practitioner cannot rely solely on the arrival and intervention of the EMS personnel. They must master the skills of ventilation and airway management to support life while awaiting EMS arrival.

The standards of care specified in the guidelines are stringent for practitioners who practice deep sedation. Additional educational training and experience are necessary to ensure patient safety and reduce patient morbidity and mortality. Specifically, administration of deep sedation requires a higher level of personnel training, increased vigilance in monitoring, additional dedicated personnel, intravenous access, and equipment.[1–3]

The Guidelines as the Standard of Care for Minimal and Moderate Sedation

In the appropriate context, procedural sedation is safe and effective, but when the appropriate safety measures are not implemented, it can also result in significant morbidity and mortality.[5–8] Perhaps the most significant advances in patient safety have been achieved by implementing the joint AAP/AAPD guidelines, which establish a standard of care for minimal and moderate sedation of pediatric patients. The guidelines focus on preoperative parental instructions, dietary precautions, and in-depth health and physical assessment. They include specific requirements for documentation of the patient's vital signs, medications administered, and responsiveness throughout the procedure. Thorough preparation reduces the possibility of sedation adverse events, and to our knowledge, death has never occurred when the practitioner has faithfully followed the guidelines.

The three elements of the guidelines that most dramatically impact the way pediatric sedation is practiced in the office setting relate to (1) personnel, (2) patient monitoring, and (3) preprocedural prescriptions.

Personnel: This assistant must be trained to monitor appropriate physiologic parameters and assist in any support or resuscitation measures required.

A trained individual must continuously monitor patient vital signs. A precordial stethoscope, blood pressure cuff, and pulse oximeter are essential for obtaining continuous heart rate, oxygen saturation, and respiratory rate information.[9,10]

Preprocedural prescription: All patients exist within a bell-shaped curve of response; although most patients will have an expected dose-response, the ends of the bell curve represent children with atypical dose responses. Some of these children will be "hyperresponders" suggesting that their metabolic factors may induce a more rapid sedation, or an increased depth than what was targeted. With this in mind, writing preprocedural prescriptions for parents to administer sedative agent(s) outside of the treatment facility is not appropriate in pediatric sedation. Drugs intended for sedation should not be administered at home by parents or guardians on the night before or during the day of sedation before transporting a child to a facility where the procedure will be performed. This eliminates the possibility of a child becoming oversedated outside the supervision of trained medical personnel.

Routes of Administration

Sedative medications can be administered through several routes. The primary routes of administration for minimal and moderate sedation are (1) inhalational; (2) enteral (e.g., oral or rectal); and (3) parenteral (e.g., intramuscular, subcutaneous, submucosal, intranasal, or intravenous). Medication latency, half-life, and duration can vary according to administration route. The sedation practitioner must understand the operational advantages and disadvantages of these routes.

Inhalational Route

Nitrous oxide/oxygen (N_2O) is the primary inhalational sedative in dentistry, providing minimal to light moderate sedation without risking loss of consciousness or airway control. Its low blood:gas solubility (blood:gas coefficient 0.48) allows for rapid onset and quick elimination, enhancing efficiency and safety. Lobo notes that the mean alveolar concentration (MAC) provides "a correlation between anesthetic dose and immobility. It can be applied to all inhalational anesthetics and is used to compare anesthetic potency."[11] It is commonly defined as the concentration of inhaled anesthetic at which 50% of the population would not move in response to a surgical stimulus.[14] The MAC for nitrous oxide is often listed as 104% to 105%, meaning it is mathematically impossible to place a patient under GA with nitrous oxide alone. Fail-safe dental delivery systems further ensure safety by limiting nitrous oxide to a maximum of 70% in nongeneral anesthesia cases.

One advantage of nitrous oxide is that it is titratable. There are two ways to administer nitrous oxide to children. One is the standard titration technique used on adults, and the other is the rapid "induction" technique. The standard titration technique involves nitrous oxide being initially administered at 10%. It is then increased in increments ranging from 5% to 10% until the patient becomes comfortable and clinical signs of optimal sedation are noted. The signs of optimal sedation include slight relaxation of the limbs and jaw muscles, ptosis of the eyelids, a blank stare as if looking up at a star-filled evening sky, palms open, warm, and slightly moist, a slight change in the pitch of the patient's voice, a lowered heart rate, and patient reports of being comfortable and relaxed.[14] Each time the clinician increases the concentration, they should wait at least 30 to 60 seconds while talking with the child and watching for signs of optimal sedation before adjusting the concentration again. When minimal sedation is the target sedation endpoint, the maximal concentration of nitrous oxide should not exceed 50%. Most children seem comfortable and demonstrate optimal signs of sedation in the concentration range of 35% to 50% nitrous oxide (Fig. 27.3). The standard titration technique is primarily used for mildly to moderately anxious but cooperative children and teenagers.

A second nitrous oxide administration approach is the rapid "induction" technique. It is usually indicated for the mild to moderately anxious, potentially cooperative child who may be on the edge of losing coping abilities and needs to be controlled quickly by the clinician. The technique involves administering up to 50% nitrous oxide immediately to the patient without titration.

In either technique, nitrous oxide should be discontinued if the child becomes disruptive or no longer breathes through the nitrous oxide hood. Gas flow should also be terminated if the child becomes nauseated or vomits. In addition, good nitrous oxide hygiene is imperative. This includes using a scavenging system, large operatories, rapid room air exchanges, supplemental movement of air (i.e., fans, air filtration units), and a nasal hood that adapts closely to the face. Nitrous oxide is physiologically safe for the patient when administered with adequate oxygen. The most common adverse effect is nausea, which should be very rare unless high concentrations (i.e., >50%) are administered or fluctuations of nitrous oxide are used. Poor technique with high concentrations may also result in an "excitement phase" in which the patient may become uncomfortable, uncooperative, and delirious, resembling a transitional stage to GA.

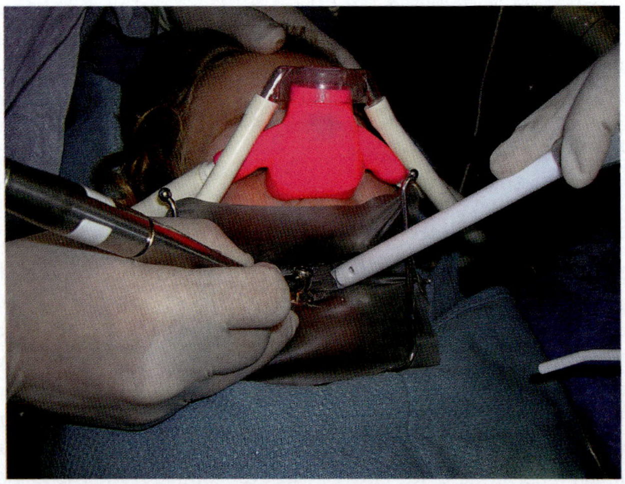

• **Fig. 27.3** Patient receiving inhalation sedation with nitrous oxide during restorative treatment.

Despite the significant advantages of using nitrous oxide in dentistry, it is not without side effects. Some adults and children do not find the effects of nitrous oxide pleasant. These patients may become overtly noncompliant, remove the nasal mask, or otherwise become uncooperative. Attempts to increase the concentration of nitrous oxide to control *moderately or severely* anxious patients are often fraught with failure. They may result in poor inhalation and increased anxiety, which may be unpleasant for the operator and the patient. Additionally, using a nitrous oxide nasal mask may hinder access to the operative field in some areas, such as the maxillary anterior teeth. This is especially true in small children. The nasal hood may also obstruct the view of the parent or caregiver, resulting in increased anxiety for those susceptible to separation anxiety.

The only absolute contraindication for nitrous oxide is lack of consent. All others can be considered "relative contraindications," typically indicating additional medical subspecialty consultation. These conditions include acute otitis media (middle ear infection), which may allow nitrous oxide to enter the closed tympanic space and rupture the eardrum. Children with active pulmonary infection are generally not good candidates for nitrous oxide but are usually not seen in the dental office until their disease resolves. Children who have nasal obstructions or are uncooperative when directed to breathe through the nose are poor candidates for nitrous oxide administration. Asthma is not a contraindication to nitrous oxide use. The anxiolytic effect of nitrous oxide may supersede anxiety-related asthma triggers. However, children with moderate persistent asthma may be more prone to exacerbations during nitrous oxide inhalation sedation. The extent of disease and triggers should always be documented and assessed before treatment and may be cause for medical consultation. Children with behavioral diagnoses/psychoses that are refractory or poorly responsive to medications may respond inappropriately to the psychogenic effects of nitrous oxide and other sedatives. This may result in a paradoxical reaction, and it is advised to consult the medical team managing behavioral issues before the use of nitrous oxide. Children undergoing bleomycin sulfate should consult their oncologist before nitrous oxide is administered.[12]

Evaluations by the National Institute for Occupational Safety and Health (NIOSH) found that personal nitrous oxide (N_2O) exposures among dental personnel occasionally exceeded recommended occupational exposure limits. These elevations were attributed primarily to patient mouth breathing, crying during pediatric procedures, and inadequately fitting nasal scavenging masks. Although staff adhered to dental industry best practices—most notably the use of scavenging systems shown to significantly reduce ambient N_2O levels—exposures still occurred. In addition, the facility's ventilation system, last tested and balanced in 2009, may not have provided sufficient outdoor air exchange. Employees also reported symptoms potentially consistent with nitrous oxide exposure, underscoring the importance of optimized scavenging, mask fit, and ventilation when using inhalation sedation in dentistry.[13,14] In crying or uncooperative children, the vacuum scavenger located in the nasal hood is not optimally effective because significant amounts of nitrous oxide are exhaled through the mouth.

Although nitrous oxide/oxygen sedation is relatively mild and safe when used as a sole sedative, moderate sedation, deep sedation, or even GA may be produced if nitrous oxide is combined with other sedative drugs. Although nitrous oxide's exact mechanism of action is not well understood, the most accepted theory is that nitrous oxide interacts with Gamma-aminobutyric neurotransmitter (GABA) receptors in the brain and mimics a benzodiazepine-like effect. This leads to a potentiation effect, which results in exacerbated and prolonged effects of other sedatives.[15] Therefore the combination of nitrous oxide with other sedation agents must be undertaken with extreme care and by an individual who has the proper training and experience.

Practical Use of Inhalation Sedation Techniques

Nitrous oxide is both an anxiolytic and an analgesic. Its analgesic properties help raise the pain threshold and may be used to lessen discomfort during a local anesthetic injection. However, nitrous oxide will not eliminate the need for local anesthetic pain control in most children, except for minor dental procedures (e.g., small class V preparations).

Nitrous oxide changes the patient's perception of the environment and the passage of time. This makes it helpful in managing children, especially those with short attention spans. These effects may occasionally be perceived by some children as unpleasant, in which case the level of nitrous oxide concentration should be decreased, or the administration should be discontinued.

The initial gas flow rate should be established first with 100% oxygen. It should ideally match the baseline minute ventilation rate of the patient. An adult will require 5 to 7 L/min, whereas a 3- to 4-year-old will require 3 to 5 L/min. The nasal hood should be introduced, and instructions should be given for breathing through the nose. While adjusting the controls, the dentist should use the "tell-show-do" technique with terminology appropriate for the age level of the child (e.g., "smell the happy air"). Light finger pressure under the lower lip to produce a seal and gentle tapping of the nosepiece can be helpful to encourage nasal breathing in the young child.

After stabilization of the nosepiece and delivery of 100% oxygen for 3 to 5 minutes, the nitrous oxide level should be increased to 30% to 35% and administered for 3 to 5 minutes for the induction period. While administering the nitrous oxide, the dentist should talk gently to the child to promote relaxation and reinforce cooperative behavior. Although asking older children and adults if they feel tingling sensations in the fingers and toes is appropriate for verification of early signs of central nervous system (CNS) effects from the nitrous oxide, these suggestive questions to the young child may lead to undesirable body movements. An indication of such CNS effects would be minimal or continual movements of the fingers and toes in the young child.

Many dentists prefer to increase the level of nitrous oxide to 50% for 3 to 5 minutes to provide maximum analgesia for the local anesthetic injection; however, concentrations of nitrous oxide over 50% are not indicated when minimal sedation is the intended endpoint. Moderate sedation monitoring guidelines must be implemented if >50% nitrous oxide is administered. When the dental injection is completed, the nitrous oxide level can be reduced to 30% to 35% for a maintenance dose during the dental treatment; alternatively, 100% oxygen may be administered when the nitrous oxide is needed only for behavior management related to the dental injection.

Upon termination of nitrous oxide administration, inhalation of 100% oxygen for 3 to 5 minutes is recommended to prevent diffusion hypoxia. This allows rapid diffusion of nitrous oxide from the venous blood into the alveolus while maintaining oxygenation. It also facilitates the scavenging of exhaled nitrous oxide and enables the patient to return without incident to pretreatment activities. Inadequate oxygenation may produce postoperative side effects such as nausea, light-headedness, or dizziness, which can be reversed with continued oxygen administration. Patients susceptible to adverse events associated with minor arterial/venous oxygen pressure drops, such as sickle cell disease, should be monitored closely during this phase.[15]

It is important for the dentist to recognize that nitrous oxide analgesia should not be used as a substitute for nonpharmacologic behavior guidance. It is most effectively administered as an adjunct to other communicative techniques to aid in managing minimal anxiety in the child capable of cooperating in the dental chair.

Oral Route

The oral route of administration is commonly used for minimal and moderate sedation in pediatric dentistry. It is desirable in this patient population because it is generally well tolerated and eliminates the need for intravenous access. This is especially true if the medication tastes good and can be delivered in low volume (Fig. 27.4). Additionally, the barriers to implementation are relatively low. Aside from physiologic monitors, no other special office equipment must be purchased or maintained to administer oral sedative medications aside from those required from emergency preparedness. Usually, it is best to administer oral sedative medicines in a separate, quiet area of the office. This allows the parent and child to focus on taking the medication in a calm and relaxing environment.

The oral route of sedation is extremely safe when minimal therapeutic doses of single drugs are administered in single doses. However, if multiple drugs or routes are combined (e.g., oral premedication followed by intravenous or inhalational medications), the chances of adverse side effects significantly increase.[1] For this reason, many states now require a special sedation permit to administer moderate sedation to children 12 years or younger.

The biggest disadvantages of the oral route of administration are that it cannot be titrated and the hepatic first-pass effect. In pediatrics, dosing is generally weight based. However, because of individual variations in the metabolism of drugs, children of the same weight may respond quite differently to the same dose of medication (see the previously mentioned "hyperresponder"). Several factors, such as the presence of food, autonomic tone, fear and anxiety, emotional makeup, fatigue, medications, and gastric emptying time can also alter absorption of the drug from the gastrointestinal tract. Sometimes, the patient may not cooperate in ingesting the medication or may vomit, making it impossible to estimate the actual dose received. In such cases, a second dose of oral medication should *never* be given. If absorption of the initial dose has been delayed for any reason and a second dose is subsequently given on the assumption that the first dose was inadequate or ineffective, both doses will eventually be absorbed, possibly resulting in a high serum level of the CNS depressant drug, potentially leading to serious consequences such as respiratory arrest, cardiovascular collapse, and death.[1,5,6]

Oral drug administration has the longest time of onset of any administration route used for sedation. The latent period required to reach peak plasma concentration varies from 15 to 90 minutes, depending on the drug. For optimal results, it is important to allow adequate time between administration and initiation of treatment.

Intranasal Route

The intranasal route is occasionally used in pediatric dentistry, especially for young children who may have difficulty drinking unpleasant tasting medication. In this situation, the medication is sprayed or dripped into the nostrils. The intranasal route of administration requires little to no cooperation from the child, and the total calculated dose is given with a high degree of certainty. A mucosal atomization device (Fig. 27.5) creates a seal around the nares and improves patient comfort during the administration of a fine particle "mist" that is readily absorbed into the bloodstream. The intranasal route bypasses the gastrointestinal tract and forgoes hepatic metabolism; thus doses are generally lower than those given orally for safety. Intranasally administered CNS drugs are rapidly absorbed through the nasal mucosa in the region of the cribriform plate into the systemic circulation, after which they cross the blood–brain barrier to exert central effects. This results in a more rapid onset than the oral route. Unfortunately, delivery of medications with low pH (e.g., midazolam) is associated with a burning sensation that can upset a pediatric patient. Although using a topical anesthetic spray before drug administration may minimize this disadvantage, this technique requires a young child to endure two drugs delivered intranasally and increases risk due to the toxicity of topical/local anesthetics. As with the oral route, the drug effect cannot be titrated with intranasal delivery.

Intramuscular Route

The intramuscular (IM) route of drug administration involves the injection of the sedative agent into skeletal muscle (Fig. 27.6).

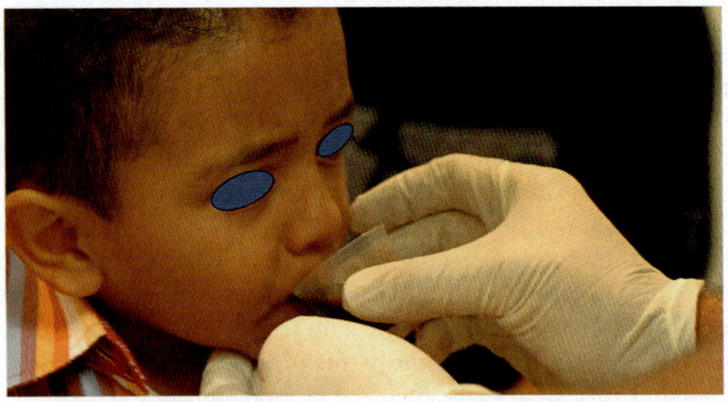

• **Fig. 27.4** Oral route of drug administration.

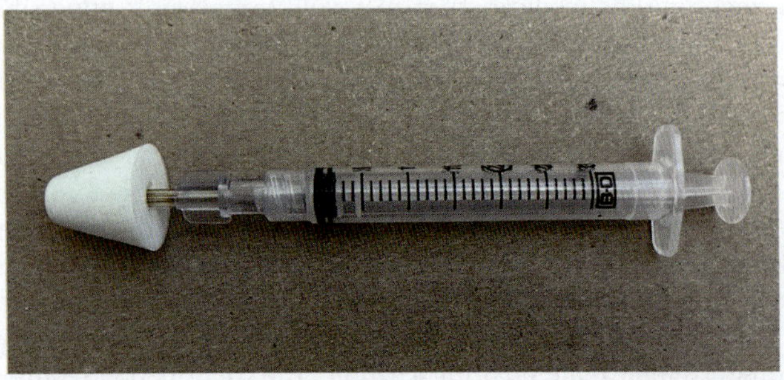

• **Fig. 27.5** Mucosal atomizer device for intranasal sedation.

The IM route is generally used to achieve a deeper level of sedition. As with other techniques, this route conveys certain advantages and disadvantages. Absorption from an injection deep into a large muscle is much faster and more dependable than absorption from the oral route. IM administration is also relatively simple, requiring minimal technical skill and no special equipment except a syringe and needle. Little or no patient cooperation is needed; therefore the total calculated dose is given with a high degree of certainty. Even when a child requires restraint, IM injections are easier to accomplish technically than the placement of an intravenous cannula, though it may be momentarily painful.

Absorption of the injected drug can be decreased or delayed by several factors. A patient who is cold or very anxious may experience peripheral vasoconstriction in the area of the injection, significantly reducing the absorption rate. Perhaps the biggest variable in onset is related to where the drug is actually deposited. If the drug is deposited deep into a large muscle mass, the high degree of vascularity there will allow rapid uptake. However, absorption may be quite unpredictable if some or the entire drug is deposited in fat or between muscle layers (distinct possibilities in small, struggling children). Injection sites devoid of large nerves and vessels are used for IM injections, such as the mid deltoid region, the vastus lateralis muscle of the thigh, and the gluteus medius muscle. Proper selection of the injection site and thoughtful technique minimize the possibility of tissue trauma. However, in all cases, it is important to inform parents that a hematoma may occur at the injection site.

Intravenous Route

The intravenous (IV) route is the gold standard for the administration of sedative agents, which is solely used in deep sedation and GA in pediatric dentistry. Among the parenteral routes, only the IV route allows titration to a desired drug effect. Because the drug is injected directly into the bloodstream, the effect is experienced within minutes, and bioavailability is nearly 100%. Small, incremental doses may be given over a relatively short period until the desired level of sedation is achieved, thus avoiding underdosing or overdosing (unlike oral or IM routes that dose with a standardized, weight-based single bolus) (Fig. 27.7).

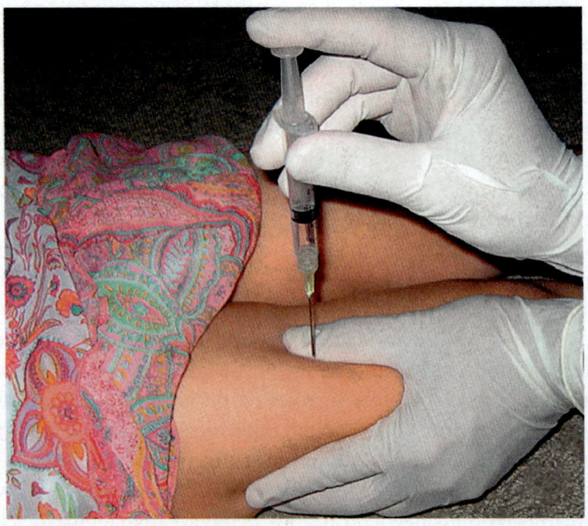

• **Fig. 27.6** Intramuscular route of administration.

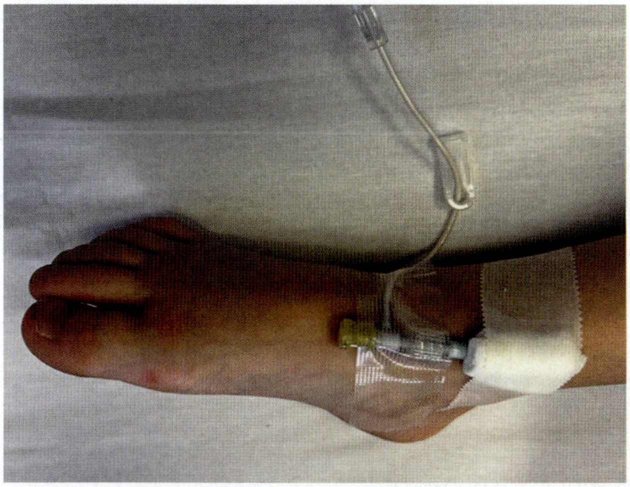

• **Fig. 27.7** Intravenous route of administration.

Because potent drugs are injected directly into the bloodstream, the IV route carries an increased potential for complications. Extravasation of drug into the tissues, hematoma formation, and inadvertent intraarterial injections are possible complications of a misplaced IV catheter. Thrombophlebitis is another rare complication that is attributable directly to the IV cannula or irritating IV medications. If the medication is injected too rapidly, exaggerated effects may be produced. An immediate anaphylactic allergic reaction may become life-threatening more rapidly if it is caused by an IV bolus of a drug than if it is caused by an oral or IM dose. All these complications can be avoided by using a test dose and careful technique.

Intravenous Access

In the event of a medical emergency, the administration of emergency drugs is always best accomplished through the IV route. However, establishing IV access after an emergency has occurred can be difficult and can consume precious time. Therefore some drugs may be better administered via the intranasal route (e.g., naloxone for opioid reversal). Others may be best administered intramuscularly (e.g., epinephrine via autoinjector for anaphylaxis).

Some state laws consider the intranasal route parenteral. The IM and IV routes are also considered parenteral and are generally used to induce moderate or deep sedation. As a result, these techniques have a greater risk profile, and many state boards require a higher level of sedation permitting.

Preoperative Assessment

Preoperative assessment is key to selecting patients optimally suited for pharmacologic behavior guidance. Obtaining a complete medical history and performing a directed physical examination facilitate determining the patient's overall risk profile[16] (Box 27.1). This information allows the clinician to make an informed decision about whether it is safe to proceed with sedation and aids in selecting the appropriate care venue (e.g., dental office, outpatient surgery center, hospital).

• BOX 27.1 Medical Assessment: Review of Systems

Medical History: A Review of Systems

- **Age and Birth History**: Patient age is considered an independent risk factor, because the risk of complications with sedation and general anesthesia is greatest for the youngest patients. Many experts recommend avoiding procedural sedation of children under 24 months old, except in the hospital setting. Children born prematurely may also have significant pulmonary and airway complications that make them poor candidates for in-office sedation.[24]
- **Cardiovascular**: Most drugs used for sedation and analgesia can cause vasodilation and hypotension. Therefore patients with known cardiovascular disease (e.g., congenital cyanotic heart disease, heart failure, dysrhythmias) are generally not good candidates for in-office sedation.[25]
- **Respiratory**: The risk of respiratory complications, including laryngospasm, is elevated in patients with active respiratory illness.[26] Respiratory disorders (e.g., poorly controlled asthma, bronchopulmonary dysplasia) are relative contraindications because these conditions may impair the patient's ability to maintain adequate oxygenation during the procedure.[27]

  Patients with sleep-disordered breathing/obstructive sleep apnea should not be sedated in the office. They may have decreased brainstem sensitivity to carbon dioxide, leading to a decreased respiratory drive. Many also experience an up-regulation of opioid receptors in the central nervous system that leads to increased sensitivity to medications like opioids.[28,29]

  Patients who are diagnosed with craniofacial anomalies that affect their airway are also contraindicated for in-office sedation. Examples of these are Pierre Robin sequence, Down syndrome, and hemifacial microsomia[30].
- **Neurologic/Developmental**: A psychiatric diagnosis such as autism or attention-deficit/hyperactivity disorder can make sedation unpredictable and should be weighed in the risk/benefit analysis. Neurologic conditions such as seizures require consultation with the patient's physician, because medications used for sedation may alter the patient's neurologic status, and medications that the patient takes for neurologic management may increase depth of sedation.
- **Gastrointestinal**: Abnormalities of the gastrointestinal system should be investigated thoroughly because they may affect absorption and distribution of oral medications. Patients with gastroesophageal reflux disease or feeding tubes (g-tube, j-tube) may also be at higher risk for aspiration during sedation.
- **Hepatic and Renal:** The presence of a hepatic or renal abnormality may affect metabolism and excretion of oral medications. These conditions are therefore relative contraindications to procedural sedation in the office setting.[31]
- **Hematologic Disorders:** Anemia and sickle cell disease may impair the oxygen-carrying capacity of the blood. Patients with sickle cell disease are at high risk of sickle cell crisis if they experience a hypoxic event during sedation.[32] Patients with bleeding disorders such as hemophilia and Von Willebrand disease may not be able to tolerate invasive dental procedures safely. They also pose greater bleeding risk during intubation, should it be required in an emergency.
- **Endocrine/Metabolic:** Patients with diabetes, hypo/hyperthyroidism, adrenal disorders, and inborn errors of metabolism present unique challenges that generally make them poor candidates for in-office sedation.[30]

Prior History of Sedation or General Anesthesia (GA): A thorough history of the patient's experience with sedation and/or GA will determine whether any adverse events have occurred in the past. This information will elucidate factors that should be considered in the future.

Of all the items in the health history, the most significant risk factors for adverse sedation events are young age, premature birth, chronic reactive airway disease, current upper respiratory infection, and obstructive sleep apnea. It should also be noted that children with developmental delay/intellectual disability have been shown to have a significantly greater incidence of desaturation during sedation compared with children who do not have disabilities.[17] The American Society of Anesthesiologists (ASA) has created a physical status classification system that should be used for every sedation patient. ASA I or II children are appropriate candidates for treatment in the outpatient setting (Table 27.2). Those classified as ASA III or greater are more appropriately cared for in the hospital setting.[18]

Along with a review of systems, a physical assessment of the patient is necessary to identify high-risk patients and reduce the risk of adverse events (see Box 27.2, Fig. 27.8, Table 27.3). Using a standard form for preoperative assessment eliminates guesswork and improves patient selection (eFig. 27.9). Additional documentation that must be included in every sedation visit includes the signed informed consent, the sedation record, and written postoperative instructions.

TABLE 27.2 American Anesthesiology Risk Assessment Classification

Classification	Definition	Examples
ASA I	Healthy patient	Healthy, nonsmoking, no or minimal alcohol use
ASA II	Patient with mild systemic disease	Mild diseases only without substantive functional limitations. Examples include (but are not limited to) the following: current smoker, social alcohol drinker, pregnancy, obesity (30< BMI <40), well-controlled DM/HTN, mild lung disease
ASA III	Patient with severe systemic disease	Substantive functional limitations: One or more moderate to severe diseases. Examples include (but are not limited to) poorly controlled DM or HTN, COPD, morbid obesity (BMI ≥40), active hepatitis, alcohol dependence or abuse, implanted pacemaker, moderate reduction of ejection fraction, ESRD undergoing regularly scheduled dialysis, premature infant PCA <60 weeks, history (>3 months) of MI, CVA, TIA, or CAD/stents
ASA IV	Patient with severe systemic disease that is a constant threat to life	Examples include (but are not limited to): recent (<3 months) MI, CVA, TIA, or CAD/stents, ongoing cardiac ischemia or severe valve dysfunction, severe reduction of ejection fraction, sepsis, DIC, ARD, or ESRD not undergoing regularly scheduled dialysis
ASA V	Moribund patient who is not expected to survive without the operation	Examples include (but not limited to): ruptured abdominal/thoracic aneurysm, massive trauma, intracranial bleed with mass effect, ischemic bowel in the face of significant cardiac pathology, or multiple organ/system dysfunction
ASA VI	A declared braindead patient whose organs are being removed for donor purposes	—

ARD, Acute respiratory distress; *ASA*, American Society of Anesthesiologists; *BMI*, body mass index; *CAD*, coronary artery disease; *COPD*, chronic obstructive pulmonary disease; *CVA*, cerebro vascular accident; *DIC*, disseminated intravascular coagulation; *DM*, diabetes mellitus; *ESRD*, end stage renal disease; *HTN*, hypertension; *MI*, myocardial infarction; *PCA*, patient controlled analgesia; *TIA*, transient ischemic attack.
From American Society of Anesthesiologists Physical Status Classification. ADA Council on Dental Education and Licensure. *Guidelines for Teaching Pediatric Pain Control and Sedation to Dentists and Dental Students.* American Dental Association; 2021.

• BOX 27.2 Physical Assessment of the Sedation Candidate

- **Airway:** Airway patency is a critical aspect of the presedation physical assessment. The relative percentage of tonsillar obstruction, as evaluated by Brodsky's classification, is a good predictor of potential airway obstruction. Patients with tonsillar hypertrophy, rated as III + or greater, are generally not good sedation candidates (see Table 27.6 and Fig. 27.8).[1] The Mallampati grading scale, originally used by anesthesiologists to grade intubation difficulty, can also be used to assess the airway before sedation[16,33,34].
- **Weight/Obesity:** In the past several decades the prevalence of obesity has increased worldwide, and today in the United States approximately 20% of children and adolescents are obese.[35,36] Sedation in the office is relatively contraindicated in children with obesity. Obese patients may have underlying respiratory issues, obstructive sleep apnea, limited intravenous access (needed in the event of an emergency), altered drug metabolism and distribution, and prolonged recovery.[37,38] Weight also complicates the dosing of sedation medications because the patient's ability to metabolize medications does not correlate linearly with their actual weight, so they should be dosed at an ideal body weight for their age group.[39]
- **Cardiovascular System:** Assess the heart by auscultation for murmurs, which could indicate structural abnormalities. The patient's heart rate, blood pressure, and blood oxygen saturation should also be verified as within normal limits See Chapter 7, Table 7.2. A history of cardiac surgery, murmur, heart failure, irregular heartbeat, or high blood pressure is cause for further investigation/medical consultation.
- **Respiratory System:** Verify that respiratory rate is within normal parameters for the patient's age (See Chapter 7, Table 7.2). The patient should have clear lung sounds on auscultation and no history of recent respiratory illness.
- **General Impression:** Make a general assessment of the child. They should appear healthy and without any unusual facial or physical characteristics. These observations may not otherwise be reflected in the physical examination but could prove to be important.
- **Fasting Status:** Adherence to the American Society of Anesthesiologists nil per os (NPO) guidelines ensures that food does not interfere with the absorption of sedation medications and minimizes the chance of emesis and subsequent aspiration during the procedure.[40] For children who take daily medications (e.g., stimulants for attention-deficit/hyperactivity disorder), it is usually permissible for them to take their medication with a small sip of water. Refer to Table 27.7 for the American Society of Anesthesiology Fasting Recommendations for Patients Undergoing Preprocedural Sedation.

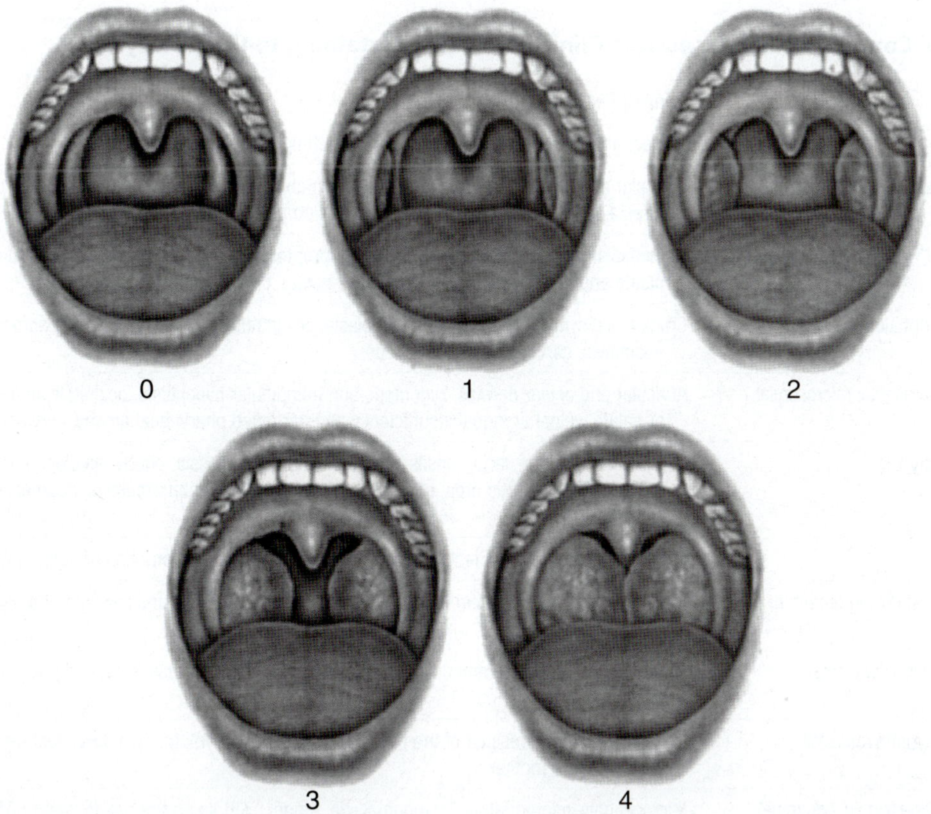

• **Fig. 27.8** Brodsky's Tonsil Classification.

Common Pharmacologic Agents Used for Sedation

Many drugs are available for use in sedation. This section provides an overview of those most commonly used in pediatric patients: antianxiety agents, antihistamines, and opioid analgesics (Tables 27.4 and 27.5). Each group acts primarily in a different area of the brain and produces a distinctive primary effect. Safe and effective sedation requires an understanding of the specific effects of each medication in the context of pediatric-specific medication dosing.

Antianxiety Agents

Benzodiazepines

Anxiety is often the primary problem in people with dental phobias. Drugs in this category have the primary effect of alleviating or decreasing anxiety. Their primary site of action is the limbic system, which is the "seat of the emotions." Theoretically, a dose exists for each antianxiety agent at which anxiety will be decreased without producing significant sedation. However, as doses are increased, the reticular activating system and cortex are affected, producing sleep and sedation. Antianxiety drugs possess a flatter dose-response curve, pharmacologically, allowing for a relatively safe therapeutic index. This means that for most antianxiety drugs (e.g., diazepam), a larger difference exists between the dose that will produce loss of consciousness than is the case with a rapidly acting drug, which has a steep dose-response curve (i.e., the difference between a minimally sedating dose and a general anesthetic dose is smaller). Drugs such as fentanyl or remifentanil should not be used for sedation for this reason. A disadvantage of benzodiazepines is the absence of analgesic properties.

The antianxiety agents consist primarily of the benzodiazepines, such as diazepam (Valium), midazolam (Versed), and triazolam (Halcion). They are principally used for minimal and moderate sedation in adults. Midazolam is the only agent extensively studied in children and is the most frequently used agent for pediatric oral sedation in medicine and dentistry.[19] Midazolam possesses some positive characteristics, such as rapid onset, a wide margin of safety with a decreased likelihood of inducing loss of consciousness, anterograde amnesia, and a reversal agent. However, it has some characteristics that are not always beneficial to the practitioner for some operative procedures. These include short duration of action and the potential for increased patient irritability, including paradoxical reactions. Flumazenil is a benzodiazepine antagonist that can reverse the effects of benzodiazepine-related sedation and overdose. As with many reversal agents, the practitioner must be aware that the duration of action of a reversal agent may not last as long as the effects mediated by the drug being reversed. Consequently, the reversal agent, flumazenil, may have to be given parenterally in repeated doses. Vigilant monitoring postoperatively is essential to avoid resedation.

Antihistamines

Some antihistamines, such as hydroxyzine (Vistaril and Atarax), diphenhydramine (Benadryl), and promethazine (Phenergan), possess both antianxiety and sedative-hypnotic properties. They are often classified as antianxiety agents. These drugs have limited efficacy when used alone but are more efficacious when combined with other medications, such as opioids (discussed later), as potentiating

TABLE 27.3 Congenital Conditions and Associated Clinical Features Pertaining to the Airway

Condition	Clinical Feature
Pierre Robin sequence	Micrognathia, macroglossia, glossoptosis, cleft lip and palate
Treacher Collins syndrome (mandibulofacial dysostosis)	Auricular and ocular defects, zygomatic and mandibular hypoplasia or aplasia, microstomia, choanal atresia, palatopharyngeal incompetence, cleft palate
Crouzon syndrome	Craniofacial synostosis, towering skull with proptosis, maxillary hypoplasia, beaked nose, high arched palate and malocclusion, cleft lip and/or palate, cervical vertebral fusions
Apert syndrome (acrocephalosyndactyly)	Craniofacial synostosis, maxillary hypoplasia, prognathism, cleft palate, tracheobronchial cartilaginous anomalies, cervical vertebral fusions
Goldenhar syndrome (hemifacial microsomia)	Auricular and ocular defects, zygomatic and mandibular hypoplasia, occipitalization of atlas, cleft lip and/or palate, velopharyngeal insufficiency and narrowed pharyngeal airway, cervical vertebral fusions
Down syndrome (trisomy 21)	Narrow nasopharynx, large tonsils and adenoids, macroglossia, poorly developed or absent bridge of the nose, small subglottic area, microcephaly, cervical spine abnormalities, atlantoaxial subluxation, broad short neck, obesity
Klippel-Feil syndrome	Congenital fusion of a variable number of cervical vertebrae, restriction of neck movement, cleft palate
Beckwith-Wiedemann syndrome (infantile gigantism)	Macroglossia, predisposition for development of various neoplasms involving the head and neck
Cherubism (familial fibrous dysplasia)	Tumorous lesions in the mandible and maxilla with intraoral masses, limited jaw closure and tongue displacement
Cretinism (congenital hypothyroidism)	Macroglossia, compression of the trachea, deviation of larynx/trachea, laryngeal nerve palsies, paradoxical vocal cord motion
Cri-du-chat syndrome (deletion 5p syndrome)	Microcephaly, micrognathia, laryngomalacia, stridor, cleft lip and/or palate, short neck, hemivertebrae
Von Recklinghausen disease (neurofibromatosis)	Tumors may occur in the larynx and right ventricle outflow tract, cervical spine abnormality, tongue lesions, and macroglossia
Hurler syndrome (mucopolysaccharidosis I)	Gargoyle facies, enlarged tongue, small mouth, profuse and thick secretions, upper airway obstruction caused by infiltration of lymphoid tissue, abnormal tracheobronchial cartilages, stiff joints, kyphoscoliosis
Hunter syndrome (mucopolysaccharidosis II)	Similar but less severe than effects seen with Hurler syndrome
Pompe disease (glycogen storage disease II)	Macroglossia, muscle deposits, respiratory muscle weakness
Prader-Willi syndrome	Severe obesity, hypotonia
Osteogenesis imperfecta	Long bone and spine deformities, short neck, joint hyperextensibility, hypoplastic maxilla, occipitalization of upper cervical vertebrae
Moebius syndrome (congenital facial diplegia)	Hypoplasia of tongue and mandible, upper midfacial protrusion, high or cleft palate, microstomia, and hypotonia creating swallowing difficulty, lack of facial expression, drooling, aspiration risk
Saethre-Chotzen syndrome	Craniosynostosis, facial asymmetry, maxillary hypoplasia, narrow highly arched palate, cleft palate, cervical vertebral fusions
Rubenstein-Taybi syndrome	Facial deformation, highly arched palate, micrognathia, bifid uvula, palatal clefting, macroglossia, joint hyperflexibility, high potential for collapse of laryngeal wall
de Lange syndrome (Brachmann–de Lange syndrome)	Severe growth deficiency, recurrent respiratory infections, depressed nasal bridge, highly arched palate, short muscular neck, micrognathia, cleft palate, prone to regurgitation and aspiration

From Waage NS, Baker S, Sedano HO. Pediatric conditions associated with compromised airway: part I—congenital. *Pediatr Dent.* 2009;31(3):236-248.

agents. Antihistamines also possess antiemetic properties. They help alleviate nausea and vomiting, which can be common when coadministering other sedatives like narcotics.

Analgesic Agents

Opioids (Narcotics)

Opioids are sometimes referred to as narcotics. These drugs are used in sedation for their primary action of analgesia and euphoria. The site of action of the narcotics is the mu receptors of the CNS. These drugs modify the interpretation of the pain stimulus in the CNS, raising the pain threshold. The analgesia obtained with narcotics cannot be used as a substitute for adequate local anesthesia. As the narcotic dose is increased, other effects, such as sedation, will occur. It should therefore be recognized that sedation is not the principal intent when administering narcotic medications in most medical settings. However, opioids strongly potentiate other CNS depressant drugs, so they are used to augment the effects of the sedative-hypnotic or antianxiety agents

TABLE 27.4 **Most Common Sedative Regimens Used in Minimal and Moderate Sedation of Pediatric Dental Patients**

Sedative Regimens	Route of Administration	Commonly Used Dosages	Max Dose	Peak Effect	Working Time
Midazolam	Intranasal	0.3 mg/kg	10 mg	5 min	10 min
Midazolam	Oral	0.5 mg/kg	20 mg	10 min	30 min
Diazepam	Oral	0.25–0.5 mg/kg	10 mg	40 min	45 min
Midazolam + Hydroxyzine	Oral	Midazolam: 0.3 mg/kg + Hydroxyzine: 0.6–2 mg/kg	Midazolam: 10 mg Hydroxyzine: 50 mg	30 min	40 min
Meperidine + Hydroxyzine	Oral	Meperidine 1–2 mg/kg + 0.6–2 mg/kg	Meperidine: 50 mg Hydroxyzine: 50 mg	30 min	45 min
Morphine + Hydroxyzine	Oral	Morphine: 0.5 mg/kg + Hydroxyzine: 0.6–2 mg/kg	Morphine: 50 mg Hydroxyzine: 50 mg	30 min	45 min
Midazolam + Meperidine + Hydroxyzine	Oral	Midazolam: 0.3 mg/kg + Meperidine: 1–2 mg/kg + Hydroxyzine: 0.6–2 mg/kg	Midazolam: 10 mg Meperidine: 50 mg Hydroxyzine: 50 mg	30 min	45–60 min
Diazepam + Meperidine + Hydroxyzine	Oral	Diazepam: 0.25 mg/kg + Meperidine: 1–2 mg/kg + Hydroxyzine: 0.6–2 mg/kg	Diazepam: 10 mg Meperidine: 50 mg Hydroxyzine: 50 mg	30 min	45–60 min
Morphine + Midazolam + Hydroxyzine	Oral	Morphine: 0.5 mg/kg + Midazolam 0.3 mg/kg + Hydroxyzine: 0.6–2 mg/kg	Morphine: 30 mg Midazolam 10 mg Hydroxyzine: 50 mg	30 min	45–60 min

TABLE 27.5 **Cardiopulmonary Effects of Common Procedural Sedative/Anesthetic Medications in Dentistry**

Drug	Cardiac Effects	Pulmonary Effects
Meperidine *(Demerol)*	↓BP, ↓PVR, myocardial depression, ↑HR	Respiratory depressant, possible chest wall rigidity
Morphine	↓HR, ↓BP	Respiratory depressant, ↑ airway resistance, apnea
Ketamine	↑BP, ↑HR, ↑CO (unless depleted catecholamine stores), ↑ myocardial O_2 consumption, possible arrhythmias	↑ airway secretions, slight ↓RR, bronchodilation
Nitrous oxide	↑LV filling pressure, ↓PAP, ↓PVR, ↓CVP	Pulmonary vasodilation, rebound hypoxemia
Chloral hydrate	↓BP, ↓HR, possible arrythmias	Respiratory depressant
Midazolam *(Versed)*	↓BP, ↓SVR, ↓CO, ↑HR	↑RR (at low doses), ↓RR (at high doses), ↑ upper airway obstruction, ↓VT, hypoxic respiratory drive
Diazepam *(Valium)*	↓BP, ↓HR, ↓SVR	↓VT, ↓ minute volume, ↓$Paco_2$, hypoxic respiratory drive
Triazolam *(Halcion)*	Minimal effects on HR and BP	Slight ↓RR, ↓VT
Hydroxyzine *(Vistaril)*	Minimal effects on BP and HR, arrhythmias	Minimal effects on RR
Diphenhydramine *(Benadryl)*	↓BP, possible palpitations	Bronchodilation, nasal congestion, thickened secretions
Propofol *(Diprivan)*	↓CO, ↓BP, ↓HR, myocardial depressant	↓RR, ↑$etCO_2$, $Paco_2$, transient apnea

BP, Blood pressure; *CO,* cardiac output; *CVP,* central venous pressure; *$etCO_2$,* end-tidal carbon dioxide; *HR,* heart rate; *LV,* left ventricular; O_2, oxygen; $Paco_2$, partial pressure of carbon dioxide; *PAP,* pulmonary artery pressure; *PVR,* peripheral vascular resistance; *RR,* respiratory rate; *SVR,* systemic vascular resistance; *VT,* tidal volume.

Data from Tobias JD, Leder M. Procedural sedation: a review of agents, monitoring, and management of complications. *Saudi J Anaesth.* 2011;5(4):395-410; White P. *Perioperative Drug Manual.* 2nd ed. Saunders; 2005.

and provide analgesia that other agents do not offer. It is important to recognize that narcotics potentiate respiratory depression when combined with sedative-hypnotics or antianxiety agents. This means that the respiratory depressant effect of the combined agents is much greater than the respiratory depressant effects of a single agent. As the opioid dosage is increased to achieve sedation, serious adverse effects may be encountered, the most common of which are respiratory depression leading to apnea that leads to hypoxia and death. Opioids also have a high propensity to produce nausea and vomiting, especially when used alone without an antiemetic.

TABLE 27.6 Brodsky Tonsil Classification (see eFig. 27.8)

Classification	% Tonsillar Obstruction
0	Absent Tonsils
1+	<25%
2+	25%–50%
3+	50%–75%
4+	>75%

TABLE 27.7 American Society of Anesthesiology Fasting Recommendations for Patients Undergoing Elective Procedures[1]

Ingested Material	Minimum Fasting Period (Hours)
Clear liquids: water, fruit juices without pulp, carbonated beverages, clear tea, black coffee	2
Breast milk	4
Infant formula	6
Nonhuman milk: because nonhuman milk is similar to solids in gastric emptying time, the amount ingested must be considered when determining an appropriate fasting period	6
Light meal: a light meal typically consists of toast and clear liquids. Meals that include fried or fatty foods or meat may prolong gastric emptying time.	6[a]

[a]Additional fasting time (e.g., 8 or more hours) may be needed in these cases. Both the amount and type of foods ingested must be considered when determining an appropriate fasting period.

When considering the use of opioids in pediatric dentistry, it is essential to recall that in minimal and moderate sedation, loss of consciousness is more likely in drugs that have steep dose-response curves, so they must be used with extreme caution. Opioids carry a high risk of producing respiratory depression and loss of consciousness, especially if they are combined with other agents such as nitrous oxide and local anesthesia. The narcotic most used in pediatric sedation techniques is meperidine, which has been used and studied in pediatric dental sedations for several decades. Its safety track record is well established. Recently most pediatric medical institutions have abandoned meperidine as a pain medication due to its side effects. Morphine sulfate is emerging as another agent used in pediatric dental sedation. However, limited pediatric oral sedation studies investigating its use have been published in the literature.[20]

Naloxone is an opioid antagonist that can be administered parenterally to reverse the adverse effects of opioid-related sedation (e.g., respiratory depression). Like flumazenil, naloxone necessitates close postoperative monitoring to ensure the patient returns to baseline and can safely be discharged.

Balanced Technique

Balanced anesthesia is a concept designed to minimize risk and maximize benefit. A balanced protocol requires an assessment of the patient and the dental procedure. The technique pairs decreased dosages of concurrent mixtures and takes advantage of different sedatives' additive and synergistic effects. It should be appreciated that all medications have two maximums that must be considered—a milligram/kilogram max (dosing max) as well as an overall milligram (total dose) max. This is particularly important in children where a weight-based dosing method is used. Milligrams' maximum dosages are always lower when drugs are used in combinations. Table 27.4 illustrates the most common sedative combinations and dosages used in minimal and moderate sedation of pediatric patients.[4]

Monitors

Physiologic monitoring is an essential and required element of procedural sedation. By assessing and interpreting patient vital signs, the operator can determine the patient's physiologic stability. It should be noted that it is the responsibility of the sedation operator to use the information provided by the monitoring equipment to establish the following: (1) the level of sedation, (2) overall patient stability, and (3) reactions to administered medications. Various monitoring equipment may be used during procedural sedation and GA.[10] Fig. 27.2 The most common physiologic monitors are pulse oximeters, capnography, automated blood pressure cuffs, precordial stethoscopes, electrocardiographs, and temperature probes. The monitors required for sedation, and recording their measurements at specific time intervals, are dictated by the intended level of sedation, recognizing that patients may drift between levels of sedation. As mentioned previously, practitioners should refer to their state dental practice acts and the AAP/AAPD joint guidelines to establish specific monitoring requirements.

A key concept in the monitoring of procedural sedation is oxygenation versus ventilation. Oxygenation refers to the attachment of oxygen to hemoglobin and successful transport to tissues. Ventilation refers to the movement of air through all elements of the respiratory tract. This is clinically significant because, in a sedation emergency, patients will always have a ventilation issue before having a problem with oxygenation. The most common monitors for minimal and moderate sedation are briefly described in this chapter. It is important to recognize that they are intended to detect ventilatory irregularities (e.g., respiratory distress, apnea) or later signs of hypoxia (e.g., low blood oxygen levels).

Pulse Oximeter

A pulse oximeter noninvasively monitors the degree of oxygen saturation of the patient's hemoglobin and the patient's pulse rate. Oxygen sensors placed across perfused tissue beds where a pulse can be detected (e.g., the fingertip, toe, earlobe) determine oxygen saturation by measuring differences in the absorption of red and infrared light emitted by the sensors. Normally, the hemoglobin in arteries of healthy children and adults is 97% to 99% saturated, though at these optimal levels, it is frequently displayed as 100% on pulse oximeters. The pulse oximeter is generally quite accurate, but factors such as patient movement, nail polish in the nail beds, mismatched sensor/tissue bed size, and poor perfusion of tissue beds may cause "false alarms" that incorrectly indicate low oxygen levels. When interpreting pulse oximetry, it is critical to recognize that there is a lag time associated with readings. Stated simply, the number displayed on the digital monitor may reflect the patient's oxygenation seconds or even minutes in the past.[21]

Precordial Stethoscope

A precordial stethoscope is a device that may be temporarily attached to the chest wall or neck to auscultate the patient's breathing and ventilation. By listening through the stethoscope, the clinician can determine the respiratory rate, quality of air movement, and heart sounds. The closer the bell of the stethoscope is placed to the precordial notch (the soft tissue area immediately above the manubrium of the chest), the louder the breathing sounds compared with the heart sounds (Fig. 27.10). Partially occluded or restrictive airways have different sound qualities, including wheezing, stridor, and crowing.[10] Because the precordial stethoscope is especially sensitive to competing operatory sounds (e.g., the pitch of the high-speed handpiece, crying), the operator must frequently rely on other clinical signs (e.g., chest excursions, tissue color) or physiologic monitors (e.g., capnograph, pulse oximeter) to determine the status of the patient.

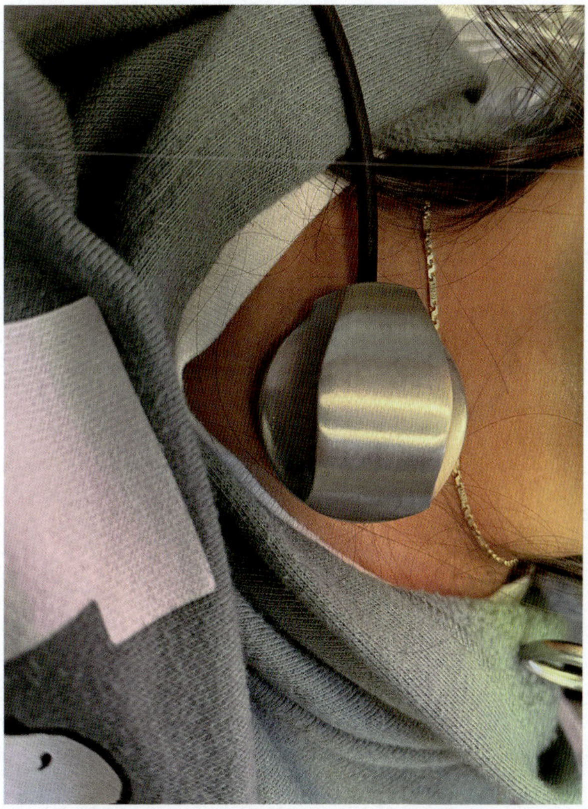

• **Fig. 27.10** Placement of precordial stethoscope.

Capnography

Capnography measures end-tidal carbon dioxide, the peak exhaled CO_2 before inhalation. Brady et al. noted in 2017 that patients monitored with capnography in addition to standard monitoring (pulse oximetry) had a reduced risk of hypoxemia compared with those with only standard tracking. Pulse oximetry is noted to have a time lag, but capnography displays ventilatory rate and depth in real time. Therefore it can be used to quickly determine whether the patient has entered a state of apnea or respiratory distress[22] (Fig. 27.11).

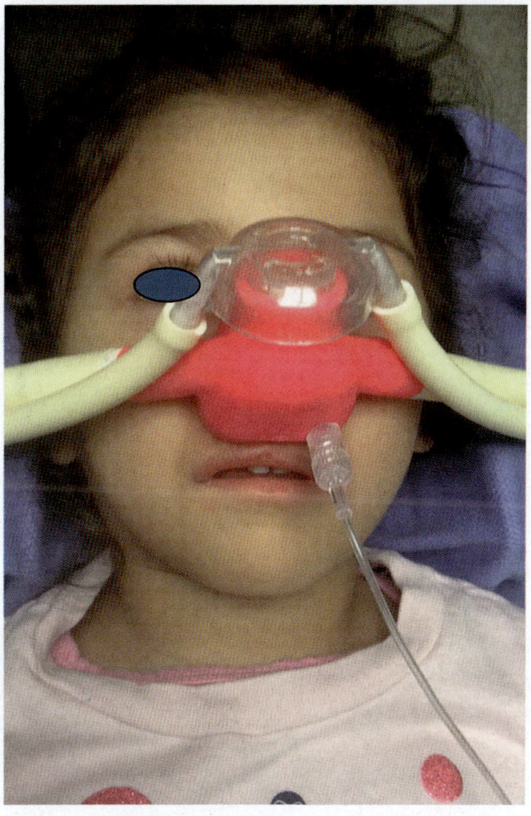

• **Fig. 27.11** Capnography utilization via nitrous oxide nosepiece.

Recovery and Discharge

The dental provider is responsible for returning the child to a state in which safe discharge is possible. Postoperative vital signs and level of alertness and consciousness should be recorded. The AAP/AAPD guidelines have recommended the following discharge criteria for pediatric patients after preprocedural sedation is completed: (1) cardiovascular function and airway patency are satisfactory and safe; (2) the patient is easily arousable, and protective reflexes are intact; (3) the patient can talk (if age appropriate); (4) the patient can sit up unaided; (5) adequate state of hydration; and (6) for a child with a disability who is incapable of the usually expected response, the presedation level of responsiveness or a level as close as possible to the normal level for that child should be achieved.[1]

A responsible adult caretaker familiar with the child and capable of following the postoperative instructions given by the provider must accompany the child out of the facility en route home. A follow-up phone call should be made before the end of the day to ensure the proper disposition of the child.

The Future

The level of training required for a dentist to administer sedation or anesthesia has long been debated. Today, throughout the United States, it is frequently possible to administer minimal sedation with only a dental license. However, special permits are generally required by most state dental practice acts to administer moderate sedation, deep sedation, or GA. Because of the increased risk associated with the care of child patients, it is now increasingly common for states to require an additional level of permitting for pediatric sedation.

Deep sedation and GA are grouped together for training requirements, medicolegal reasons, and purposes of malpractice insurance. The suggested educational requirement for the administration of deep sedation or GA is the completion of a CODA-accredited residency training program that provides comprehensive training in GA. All states have adopted requirements for administering deep sedation and GA by dentists.

Summary

Many pediatric dental patients can be treated using basic behavior guidance techniques, but some children require advanced pharmacologic strategies. In these situations, procedural sedation may be used to facilitate the provision of high-quality dental care. Although sedation conveys many benefits to the patient and dental team, it also carries significant risks. As with any area of healthcare, the provider must be guided by the Hippocratic principle, "do no harm." In sedation, this is best reflected by establishing a culture of safety in the dental office. That entails thorough training of the dental provider and staff, adherence to published sedation guidelines, utilization of appropriate equipment, and selection of medications suited to the experience level of the provider and patient needs.

Visit eBooks.Health.Elsevier.com to see full list of references.

28

Assessment and Management of Pain in the Pediatric Patient

ELIZABETH S. GOSNELL, PATRICK T. RUCK, AND THOMAS R. STARK

CHAPTER OUTLINE

The Impact and Management of Pain

Pain is one of the most common reasons patients seek dental care.[1] Pain characteristics depend on symptom duration and tissue type. For example, dental pain differs from gingival pain, and alveolar bone pain differs from pain related to a temporomandibular disorder. Pain may be acute (seconds to days) or chronic (months to years). Acute pain signals injury, inflammation, or infection, indicating the need for healing or treatment to prevent further damage. Thus pain signaling serves as a valuable guide for maintaining health and guiding a person's activities in life.

The impact of pain goes beyond the mere processing of noxious stimuli. Pain perception involves a complex, multifaceted interaction of biologic, psychological, and social elements. Several factors determine how an individual interprets and reacts to painful stimuli. The persistence of pain may be associated with comorbid symptoms, including increased suffering, reduced quality of life, and delayed recovery from the initial insult.[2]

A related clinical observation is that pain often leads to learned behaviors and anticipatory responses. Pain often triggers stress and fear, leading to anticipatory behaviors. For example, a 4-year-old with painful abscessed maxillary anterior teeth who poorly endures local anesthesia and extractions may develop strong negative reactions. These reactions—crying, covering the mouth, refusal to cooperate, kicking, screaming, shaking the head, spitting, or biting—can persist in later dental visits.

Most pharmacologic agents used in dentistry are administered to manage anxiety and pain. Generally, eliminating pain in the dental setting requires blocking pain sensation either peripherally using local anesthesia or centrally with general anesthesia. Anxiety is managed by nonpharmacologic and/or pharmacologic techniques. Anxiety and pain and their management in clinical practice overlap to a significant degree.

There is no single *best* technique for managing anxiety and pain. A practitioner may have a preferred method, but one technique is not helpful for all dental patients in all situations. A working knowledge of several techniques enables practitioners to select the most appropriate method for a particular patient or may sometimes necessitate referral for advanced care.

Definition of Pain

Pain is defined by the International Association for the Study of Pain as "an unpleasant sensory and emotional experience associated with or resembling that associated with actual or potential tissue damage," and the perception of pain varies from person to person based on biologic, psychological, and social influences.[3] In dentistry, pain can be viewed as a highly personal experience in response to either actual tissue damage (e.g., trauma, pulpitis) or potential tissue damage (i.e., the anticipation of a dental procedure).[3] Pain is influenced by life experiences, making each person's pain unique; it is essential to respect an individual's report of pain.[3]

Pain Neuroscience

Understanding neuroanatomy and neurophysiology can help providers better comprehend contemporary principles of pain management. Pain characteristics vary depending on the types and distributions of sensory nerves in the target tissues. Sensory nerves can be categorized based on spatial, biochemical, size, and shape characteristics. Further classification can be made based on the degree of myelination and conduction speed. There are three main types of sensory nerve fibers: A-beta, A-delta, and C fibers. The A-beta fibers are the largest and most heavily myelinated fibers. The A-beta fibers also have the fastest conduction velocity at 85 m/s.[4] Under normal conditions, A-beta fibers code for light touch sensation.[5] Thinly myelinated A-delta fibers are the second fastest at 30 m/s.[5] The A-delta fibers transmit signals for both temperature and pain, particularly brief, sharp pain.[5] Unmyelinated C fibers are the smallest fibers with the slowest conduction velocity at 2 m/s.[5] C fibers carry signals for lingering dull, burning, and aching pain.[6] The conduction velocity and actions of these sensory nerves can be explained by considering what happens during a common injury, such as stubbing a toe on a coffee table. A-beta fibers first detect contact with the table, without pain. Next, A-delta fibers transmit a sharp pain, signaling injury. Finally, C fibers carry a lingering dull ache. Specific nerve fibers can account for dental pain as well. For dental pain, the sharp, shooting pain experienced when exposed dentin is stimulated by cool air can be explained by the action of rapidly firing A-delta fibers.[6] On the other hand, the slow-firing C fibers are responsible for the poorly localized, achy, throbbing sensation of a lingering toothache.[6] Pulp tissue contains a significant quantity of high-threshold nerve fibers, which require a considerable stimulus to elicit a response. This explains why slight temperature changes do not cause dental pain, but very cold beverages can result in a painful dental response.[7]

Pain Processing

Pain processing describes a sequence of events involving the activation of peripheral and central pathways resulting in the perception of pain.[8] The process begins in the peripheral nervous system (PNS) with the transduction of a noxious stimulus (e.g., dental abscess or pulpitis). A subset of sensory nerves (i.e., nociceptors) detects noxious mechanical, thermal, or chemical stimuli with specialized receptors on their terminal endings. In response to the noxious stimuli, activated nociceptors (i.e., sensory neurons) transmit an electrical impulse along the axon toward the central nervous system (CNS). Within the CNS, the **presynaptic** primary afferent neurons release excitatory neurotransmitters (e.g., glutamate), which activates receptors (*N*-methyl-D-aspartate [NMDA] receptors) on **postsynaptic** projection neurons involved in transmitting electrical signals to the thalamus. Further processing occurs at the level of the thalamus, and signals are eventually transmitted to the higher regions of the brain where pain is perceived. Although the term "pain" is often used to describe all levels of sensory processing, the perception of pain only occurs in the supraspinal brain centers (e.g., primary somatosensory cortex, anterior cingulate cortex). Thus the processing and encoding of noxious stimuli along a multitude of pathways is more appropriately termed nociception.[3]

Disrupting Pain Signaling

Pain is managed by blocking signals in the PNS and CNS. In the PNS, agents like nonsteroidal antiinflammatory drugs (NSAIDs) reduce noxious chemical mediators (prostaglandins, substance P) at the injury site. In the CNS, pain signaling is regulated by ascending and descending pathways. Opioid receptor agonists (i.e., mu receptor agonists) reduce pain by blocking pain signaling in the CNS,[9] whereas GABA-activating agents like nitrous oxide and diazepam inhibit synaptic transmission.[9] Other sensory systems involved include proprioception, motor reflexes, and immune response.

The limbic system, including the amygdala, basal ganglia, and cingulate gyrus, influences pain through emotion, behavior, motivation, and memory.[10] Awareness, fear, anxiety, and self-regulation shape the pain experience.[10,11] The interaction between limbic and cortical structures explains cognitive pain processing and control.[10] Techniques like cognitive reframing and relaxation can help reduce *perceived* pain.[12–14]

Theories of Pain

Gate Control

The gate control theory of pain describes how pain signaling can be modulated at the level of the CNS by nonpainful stimuli. The theory proposes that spinal cord neurons function as gates, either allowing or preventing pain signals from reaching the brain.

When the gates are open, pain signals are allowed to travel freely to the brain. However, when the gates are closed, pain signaling is blocked (Fig. 28.1). The theory proposes that signals from noxious input normally transmitted to the CNS via A-delta fibers can be modulated within the spinal cord by large-fiber neurons. Postulated mechanisms for the gates include presynaptic inhibitory effects on secondary projection neurons in the spinal cord. This implies that large A-beta fibers can excite the inhibitory interneuron, which decreases the likelihood that projection neurons will transmit pain signals to the brain.

A simple example is a parent rubbing a child's knee after a fall, which helps reduce pain by blocking pain signals. The light rubbing disproportionately activates greater numbers of large fibers that inhibit previously activated small fibers. Shaking the lip during delivery of local anesthesia is an example of gate control theory in dentistry. When the lip is jiggled, large A-beta fibers, normally responsible for transmitting light touch and vibration sensations, become active and transmit signals to the brain more rapidly than the smaller A-delta fibers and C fibers responsible for pain signaling.

Transcutaneous electrical nerve stimulation (TENS), or the use of low-intensity electrical stimulation at peripheral sites, relies on the gate control theory to relieve pain.[15] TENS-mediated pain relief is due to activation of large-diameter, primary afferent fibers that in turn inhibit small-fiber transmission as previously described by the gate theory. TENS has been shown to produce partial analgesia due to the electrical stimulation of tooth pulp in school-aged children.[16]

Conditioned Pain Modulation

The conditioned pain modulation theory is best described as "pain inhibits pain." When two different parts of the body are injured, the brain focuses on one pain, lessening the other. This theory can be tested by placing a hand in a bucket of ice water during a painful procedure. The neurons that carry sensory information from the spinal cord to the brain are temporarily inhibited. This is thought to result from descending inhibition from areas of the midbrain, specifically the periaqueductal gray and dorsal raphe. Conditioned pain modulation may be related to the endogenous pain modulation system.[17] Endogenous opioid and dopaminergic pathways are examples of "top-down" or descending pathways that modulate pain perception.[18] Endogenous opioids are peptides that are naturally synthesized in the body and cause effects similar to those of opiates (e.g., morphine). Similarly, endogenous dopamine, released in response to surprise and novelty seeking, can relieve pain.[18] Thus pain modulation from the level of the midbrain can disrupt pain signals before they reach the higher regions of the brain. Emphasis has been placed on the role and influence of higher CNS influence of pain perception and reactivity.[11,19–21] This reorientation is partially the result of more sophisticated studies suggesting the need for a more comprehensive explanation of cognitive, behavioral, and emotional influences in pain perception and control.[22]

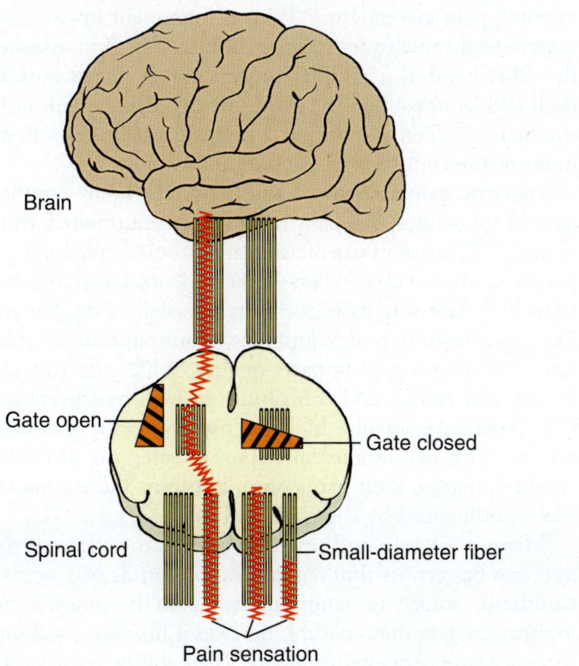

• **Fig. 28.1** The gate control theory of pain. (From deWit SC. *Medical-Surgical Nursing: Concepts and Practice*. Saunders; 2009.)

Neuromatrix

The components of the CNS, generally referred to as higher levels of CNS functioning (i.e., above the midbrain), are key components of the neuromatrix pain theory.[23] In this model, a highly complex neuronal network or matrix within the brain affects pain signaling (eFig. 28.2). Fear, emotional response, memories, and associations with reward and consequences are incorporated into the neuromatrix theory.[24]

Biopsychosocial

Modern pain management follows the biopsychosocial model, recognizing that pain is more than a sensory response.[3] This approach considers biologic, psychological, and social factors.[24] Biologic aspects, like genetics, influence inflammatory mediators and medication effectiveness (i.e., hepatic enzyme metabolism). Psychological factors, such as emotions and behavior, affect how the brain processes the pain experience. Social elements, including stress and environment, also shape pain perception. Although treating acute pain at the sensory level is essential, this model helps practitioners address pain comprehensively.[24]

Peripheral and Central Nervous System Effects on Pain Perception and Control

Sensitization can occur in various situations when the nervous system produces an exaggerated pain response. When sensitization is present due to biologic changes in the region of the injury, it is termed **peripheral sensitization.** Proinflammatory mediators in the region of the injury sensitize the neighboring peripheral nerves. In this situation, a normally painful insult will result in an exaggerated response called **hyperalgesia.** Consider a patient with a painful oral ulcer. The tissue around the ulcer has become more sensitive due to the presence of inflammatory cytokines and pain mediators. Inserting a needle into this area would result in an excessively painful or "hyperalgesic" response due to the sensitization of the peripheral sensory nerves. In contrast, central sensitization is a phenomenon that occurs when the CNS is sensitized.[25] When a nonpainful stimulus, such as light touch, becomes painful, it is referred to as **allodynia.** In this scenario, the activation of low threshold, myelinated nerve fibers (A-beta), normally responsible for light touch sensation, results in a painful response.

Central sensitization occurs in dentistry in cases where there is significant, sustained pain in the orofacial region.[25] For example, if a patient has an inflamed tooth, lightly touching the cheek may elicit a painful reaction. Sensitization can negatively affect the delivery of dental care if profound analgesia or anesthesia cannot be obtained.

Cognitive Elements of Pain Perception

Cognition is a complex process that results in an appreciation and often subsequent recognition of potential consequences as a function of "knowing." Knowing involves a multitude of processes, including, but not limited to, perceiving, organizing, judging, meaning, reasoning, and responding.

Cognition involves recognizing and understanding potential consequences through processes like perception, reasoning, and response. It includes awareness of internal and external influences and the ability to control responses (e.g., coping), such as using mental techniques to reduce discomfort. Coping strategies for stress and pain vary based on perception, timing, and personal resources. Techniques like hypnosis, relaxation, distraction, and reconceptualization help manage pain. Effective coping typically involves assessing the issue, reshaping perspective, developing skills (e.g., breathing, relaxation), maintaining these skills, and measuring success.[26] (See Chapter 26 for a more detailed discussion of techniques.)

Evidence supports the notion that coping skills in the context of pain and anxiety can be taught even to children, and the effectiveness of cognitive training can be evaluated through self-report or physiologic/behavioral measures. In one study, children who were undergoing restorative procedures were taught distraction and self-support techniques before undergoing dental procedures; they were subsequently compared with a group of children who were read stories. Self-report of anxiety for specific procedures (e.g., the injection) was less in those who received the cognitive training than in those who did not.[27] School-aged children who have had opportunities to exercise self-control in anxiety-provoking circumstances may be able to invoke their personalized coping skills in preparation for an anticipated event during a dental appointment.

However, knowing ahead of time about impending discomfort can have a detrimental effect under certain conditions. For instance, the less time between informing a young child, who cognitively is incapable of significant coping strategies (i.e., 3 years or less), of a procedurally related painful stimulus (e.g., injection) and doing it allows correspondingly less time for interference behaviors to occur. It is even possible that the length of emotional outbursts before and following the procedure may be reduced under these circumstances. In contrast, in school-aged children, knowing ahead of time offers children the opportunity to process, develop a coping plan, and even practice coping skills for the experience.[28] See Case Study in Chapter 26: Prepared Parents, Prepared Children, and Positive Coping.

Cognitive development and maturation are keys to the success of cognitive strategies. Anxiety reduction can be attained in the medical and dental environment as a function of age in school-aged cohorts. The extent to which these strategies can be successfully applied to preschoolers is yet to be determined. However, younger children are capable of significant pain modulation through processes resembling cognitive strategies. In one study, play therapy with needles and dolls before venipuncture resulted in a significantly more rapid return of heart rate and less body movement within 5 minutes of blood drawing compared with controls. This finding was interpreted as evidence of reduced anxiety in the children.[29]

Emotional Elements of Pain Perception

Although pain and the anticipation of painful stimuli (i.e., anxiety) invoke a personalized emotional experience, most humans have a common understanding of the attendant emotions of such experiences. Certainly, we are adept at recognizing another's suffering and possibly even better attuned to appreciating another person's anticipation of discomfort.

The expression of emotional content during or preceding painful experiences is most likely a complex combination of a partially inherited yet learning-tempered phenomenon that occurs early in life. An infant's expression of discomfort resulting from inoculations changes with aging from a more diffuse, crying, and reflexive response to one of anticipation, attentiveness toward the noxious object, and sometimes expression of anger.[30,31]

The social response to pain can be a commanding and attention-gathering entity.[32] For example, the toddler who skins a knee during a fall initially may not react as if in pain until the parent secondarily reacts to the injury. Depending on the parental response, the child may burst into tears if the parent looks upset or does not respond at all, based on the support of the parent's verbal encouragement.

Emotions play a key role in pain perception. Although pain itself is primary, emotions can modulate it (amplify or lessen). Some drugs (e.g., nitrous oxide, benzodiazepines) target CNS areas responsible for emotions; a person feels pain but is not particularly annoyed by it. Conversely, emotional distress in anticipation of discomfort lowers pain tolerance. Positive emotions, like humor, can reduce anxiety and pain sensitivity. (See Chapter 26 for coping strategies.)

Pediatric Pain Assessment

Perception of pain in children is complex and multifactorial, including physiologic, psychological, behavioral, social, and developmental factors.[33,34] There are reliable, valid, and clinically sensitive pain assessment tools for infants through adolescence for ongoing pain assessment.[35] Pain measurement involves assigning a numerical value to represent pain intensity. Pain assessment, on the other hand, is a complex process that evaluates both the pain itself and its impact on the child, incorporating quantitative measurements.[33] Dentists should anticipate painful experiences and monitor the condition of patients accordingly.

Pediatric pain assessment and management are emphasized in clinical guidelines, yet pain remains underestimated and undertreated.[36] Consistent use of assessment tools can help, but current practices often fail to align with evidence-based recommendations.[37–39] Assessing pain in children is challenging due to factors like age, cognitive development, communication skills, and fears.[33] Pediatric pain impacts quality of life, affecting sleep, behavior, and eating, and contributes to high healthcare costs.[38–41] Pain experiences involve biologic, psychological, and social interactions, with developmental responses emerging in infancy.[42] As children mature, their pain communication and coping strategies evolve, influenced by cognitive and social factors.

Memory of pain and resultant anticipatory fears of sharp objects can be seen in children around 6 months to 1 year of age.[42] Children's ability to communicate pain becomes increasingly sophisticated as they mature, develop a broader vocabulary, and witness a variety of environments. Their ability to use various coping strategies is influenced by their cognitive development. Children as young as 18 months old are aware of ways to alleviate pain, such as asking for hugs and medicine. Children aged 3 to 4 years old can use distraction to cope with pain when directed. Children are unable to initiate control strategies such as relaxation before the age of about 5 years.[42] The development of self-management strategies results from the interactions of multiple factors, including the maturation of coping skills, appreciation of self-control, and social influences. Dental procedures can cause pain and distress in children. Recognizing behaviors that indicate anxiety or pain and implementing coping strategies can foster positive treatment experiences. Various management techniques support children in developing and utilizing coping skills to handle pain and distress[43] (see Chapter 26).

Studies have shown that healthcare providers tend to underestimate the pain experienced by children.[33,35] A pain assessment tool, or pain scale, should be utilized to provide the practitioner with a more objective method of assessing and adequately managing pain in pediatric patients.[33,35]

Pain assessment tools include self-report, observational/behavioral, and physiologic measures, depending on age and communication ability. Self-report is the most valid and preferred method because pain is subjective, but behavioral observation complements it and serves as an alternative when self-reporting is not possible. Verbal and nonverbal self-report tools require cognitive and language development for accuracy.[33,35] It has been reported that proxy judgments underestimate the pain experienced by others. When possible, use parental reporting in addition to the assessment tools presented here.[35]

An *observational/behavioral assessment tool* is used for those patients who are very young or cognitively impaired; for example, preverbal children or those who are unable to understand the self-report scale. The *self-report assessment tool* is ideal but requires the child to be able to understand instructions and point to or verbalize his or her response. Certain *physiologic measurements,* especially heart rate, in conjunction with self-report of discomfort, add another important dimension to the characterization of response specificity to painful stimuli.[33,42] Many reliable and valid assessment tools exist; those presented here are the most reliable and valid. The appropriate scale should be chosen based on developmental age, with chronologic age serving only as a guide.[40,44]

It may appear difficult to measure the degree of pain or discomfort experienced by young children, especially preschool children, because of their level of cognitive and language development. Most 2-year-old children can report the presence and location of pain, but they are not able to describe pain intensity until around age 3 to 4 years of age. A 3-year-old child can start to differentiate pain severity and can use a three-level pain intensity scale with simple terms such as, "no pain, little pain, or a lot."[33]

Self-report measures of pain intensity are not sufficiently valid for children less than 3 years of age. An observational measurement tool may be used to assess pain intensity in this age group.[44] The Face, Legs, Activity, Cry, Consolability (FLACC) scale is valid for children aged 1 and older and is a five-item scale in which raters score each of five categories from 0 to 2 with a total score range of 0 to 10 (Table 28.1).[45,46] Examples of observational tools include the FLACC, revised FLACC (r-FLACC), and the Observational Scale of Behavioral Distress (OSBD).[33]

Children aged 4 can use a 4- to 5-item pain scale, and 5-year-olds can rate pain intensity. Self-report and facial expression scales are commonly used starting at age 4. For children 4 to 16 years of age, the *Faces Pain Scale–Revised* (FPS-R) is a valid pain measurement tool. This self-report ordinal scale consists of six gender and ethnicity-neutral line drawings of faces that are scored 0 to 10 (Fig. 28.3); it has been translated into over 40 languages. The faces in this revised scale do not show a smile or tears at the extremes to avoid evoking the emotions or fear that may coincide with pain but do not directly correlate with the pain experienced. It was adapted from the Faces Pain Scale to have a pain rating on the 0-to-10 scale. It is important for the person implementing the scale to use appropriate language, such as, "These faces show how much something can hurt. This face [point to face on far left] shows no pain. The faces show more and more pain [point to each from left to right] up to this one [point to face on far right]—it shows very much pain. Point to the face that shows how much you hurt [right now]." It is imperative to avoid using the words *happy* and *sad.* In addition, this scale is intended to measure how the child feels; this will not necessarily correlate with his or her facial expression.[33,34,47,48]

TABLE 28.1 The Face, Legs, Activity, Cry, Consolability Behavioral Pain Assessment Scale

	SCORING		
Categories	0	1	2
Face	No particular expression or smile	Occasional grimace or frown; withdrawn, disinterested	Frequent to constant frown, clenched jaw, quivering chin
Legs	Normal position or relaxed	Uneasy, restless, tense	Kicking or legs drawn up
Activity	Lying quietly, normal position, moves easily	Squirming, shifting back and forth, tense	Arched, rigid, or jerking
Cry	No cry (awake or asleep)	Moans or whimpers, occasional complaint	Crying steadily, screams or sobs; frequent complaints
Consolability	Content, relaxed	Reassured by occasional touching, hugging, or being talked to; distractible	Difficult to console or comfort

This is a five-item scale in which raters score each of five categories from 0 to 2 with a total score range of 0 to 10.

The FLACC scale was developed by Sandra Merkel, MS, RN, Terri Voepel-Lewis, MS, RN, and Shobha Malviya, MD, at C.S. Mott Children's Hospital, University of Michigan Health System, Ann Arbor, Michigan. © 1997 The Regents of The University of Michigan. From Merkel SI, Voepel-Lewis T, Shayevitz JR, Malviya S. The FLACC: a behavioral scale for scoring postoperative pain in young children. *Pediatr Nurs.* 1997;23(3):293-297. The FLACC scale was developed by Sandra Merkel, MS, RN, Terri Voepel-Lewis, MS, RN, and ShobhaMalviya, MD, at C.S. Mott Children's Hospital, University of Michigan Health System, Ann Arbor, Michigan.

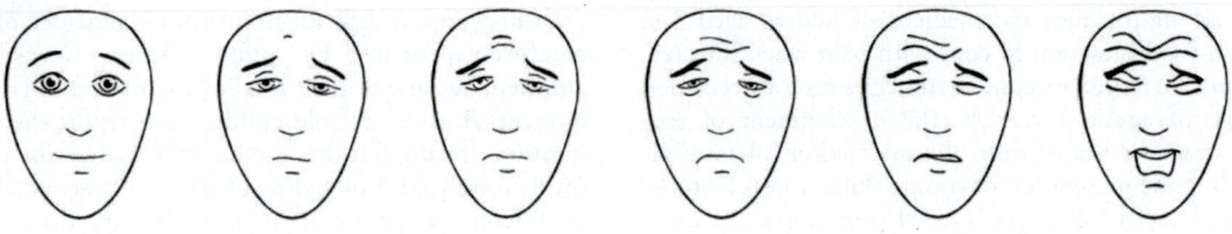

• **Fig. 28.3** Faces Pain Scale—Revised. This is a self-report scale consisting of six line drawings of faces, scored 0 to 10 in pain intensity. (From International Association for the Study of Pain Copyright 2001; Hicks CL, von Baeyer CL, Spafford P, et al. The Faces Pain Scale—Revised: toward a common metric in pediatric pain measurement. *Pain*. 2001;93[2]:173-183.)

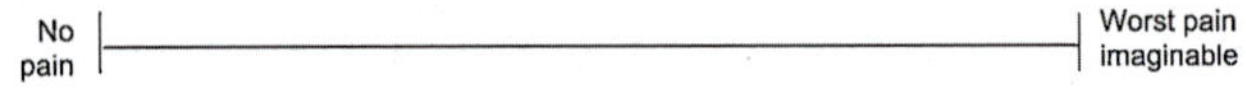

• **Fig. 28.4** Visual Analog Scale. This is a self-report scale. The patient marks a line signifying the intensity of pain experienced. (From Heller GZ, Manuguerra M, Chow R. How to analyze the visual analog scale: myths, truths, and clinical relevance. *Scand J Pain*. 2016;13:67-75.)

Other nonverbal self-report techniques include the number of poker chips selected (Hester Poker Chip Tool), the Thermometer pain scale, the Colored Analog Scale, and the Oucher scale.[33,49]

For children aged 8 and older, the *visual analog scale* (VAS) is appropriate. Children approximately 8 years of age are able to rate the quality of pain.[33] A VAS is a continuous scale consisting of a line approximately 100 mm in length, with each end anchored by extreme descriptors (e.g., *no pain* versus *severe pain*). The patient indicates the degree of perceived *pain intensity* by making a mark on the line. The length of the line from the left-hand margin to the mark determines the magnitude of pain for that individual (Fig. 28.4). Physiologic measurements, especially heart rate, in conjunction with self-report of discomfort, also help characterize the response to pain.[33,34] In addition, a qualitative pain assessment history can be obtained, for example, the OPQRSTU assessment (see Chapter 45 and Table 45.1).

For children and adolescents with cognitive impairment (CI), self-report tools may not be applicable. Healthcare providers must be able to observe and assess the presence and intensity of pain to effectively manage pain for children with CI. For this population, the r-FLACC is valid and reliable for postoperative pain assessment (Table 28.2). This observational scale considers the various facial expressions or bodily movements that may be exhibited. It incorporates additional behavioral descriptors including tremors, increased spasticity, jerking movements, changes in respiratory pattern, and verbal outbursts. Parents also can input their individual responses with open-ended descriptors in each category to include typical and atypical individual pain behaviors.[50,51]

Family and cultural elements are apparent in the mediation of pain-related expressions and their effects. An infant's cry may elicit protective and indulging types of behavior or, sadly, abusive behaviors in adult caretakers. Parental reaction to pain influences the child's pain experience. For example, parental anxiety can inadvertently teach the child to be fearful of procedures. A parent's denial of pain can fail to prevent or manage a child's pain adequately.[42] Some societies/cultures are highly sensitive to infant distress whereas others are less sensitive. In addition, behavioral manifestations of pain as well as self-report measures are subject to effects of minimization, exaggeration, and the influence of social and contextual variables.[42] There are strengths and flaws in any assessment method. For example, patients tend to choose the extreme facial expressions in the FPS-R. When appropriate, composite measures can be used, which is a combination of behavioral observation and self-report methods in conjunction with physiologic measures (eTable 28.3).[33,50]

In summary, many factors may contribute to a child's perception of pain. McGrath and colleagues have listed intrinsic and extrinsic factors that tend to exacerbate pain in children with cancer and suggest developmental considerations for the assessment of pain (eBox 28.1).[52]

Pain Control With Analgesics

The agents used for pain relief are termed *analgesics.* Ideally, analgesic drugs should relieve pain without significantly altering consciousness. Analgesics act either in the peripheral tissues, centrally in the brain and spinal cord, or both. Opioid analgesics are thought to act primarily in the CNS. Nonopioid analgesics (e.g., NSAIDs like ibuprofen) reduce pain by decreasing peripheral inflammation and inhibiting sensitization of the CNS. Most dental pain in pediatric patients can and should be managed using nonopioid agents. Refer to Table 28.4 for an overview of analgesics used in children.

Nonopioid Analgesics

Generally, nonopioid analgesics are useful for mild to moderate pain, which includes the vast majority of dental procedural pain. Nonopioid analgesics differ from opioids in their site and mechanism of action, their adverse effect profile, and their analgesic ceiling effect, which is the dose at which maximum pain relief can be achieved. Nonopioid analgesics should be considered first-line therapeutic agents for pediatric pain management.

Acetaminophen

Acetaminophen (e.g., Tylenol) is the most common analgesic used in pediatrics in the United States today. It is an effective antipyretic (fever reducer) and analgesic for the management of mild to moderate pain. Unlike NSAIDs, acetaminophen does not inhibit coagulation or cause gastric upset.[53] The primary disadvantage of acetaminophen is that it lacks antiinflammatory properties.[54] Acetaminophen is a good alternative analgesic in patients who do not require an antiinflammatory effect. See Table 28.4 for dosing information. Although allergic reactions and drug interactions are rare, excessive use of acetaminophen can be problematic.

Many over-the-counter and combination medications contain acetaminophen, which has led to an increase in unintentional overdose.[55] Acute liver failure or fatal hepatic necrosis can be a result of acetaminophen overdose.

TABLE 28.2 Revised Face, Legs, Activity, Cry, Consolability Scale

	Individual Behavior
Face 0 No particular expression or smile 1 Occasional grimace/frown; withdrawn or disinterested; appears sad or worried 2 Consistent grimace or frown; frequent/constant quivering chin, clenched jaw; distressed-looking face; expression of fright or panic Individualized behavior:________	"Pouty" lip; clenched and grinding teeth; eyebrows furrowed; stressed looking; stern face; eyes wide open—looks surprised; blank expression; nonexpressive
Legs 0 Normal position or relaxed; usual tone and motion of limbs 1 Uneasy, restless, tense; occasional tremors 2 Kicking, or legs drawn up; marked increase in spasticity, constant tremors or jerking Individualized behavior:________	Legs and arms drawn to center of body; clonus in left leg with pain; very tense and still; legs tremble
Activity 0 Lying quietly, normal position, moves easily; regular, rhythmic respirations 1 Squirming, shifting back and forth, tense or guarded movements; mildly agitated (e.g., head back and forth, aggression); shallow, splinting respirations, intermittent sighs 2 Arched, rigid, or jerking; severe agitation; head banging; shivering (not rigors); breath holding, gasping or sharp intake of breaths, severe splinting Individualized behavior:________	Grabs at site of pain; nods head; clenches fists, draws up arms; arches neck; arms startle; turns side to side; head shaking; points to where it hurts; clenches fist to face, hits self, slapping; tense, guarded, posturing; thrashes arms; bites palm of hand; holds breath
Cry 0 No cry/verbalization 1 Moans or whimpers; occasional complaint; occasional verbal outburst or grunt 2 Crying steadily, screams or sobs, frequent complaints; repeated outbursts, constant grunting Individualized behavior:________	States, "I'm okay" or "All done"; mouth wide open and screaming; states "Owie" or "No"; gasping, screaming; grunts or short responses; whining, whimpering, wailing, shouting; asks for medicine; crying is rare
Consolability 0 Content and relaxed 1 Reassured by occasional touching, hugging or being talked to; distractible 2 Difficult to console or comfort; pushing away caregiver, resisting care or comfort measures Individualized behavior:________	Responds to cuddling, holding, parent, stroking, kissing; distant and unresponsive when in pain

This revised scale is useful for patients with cognitive impairment. The additional descriptors include facial expressions, bodily movements, and vocalizations that may signify behavioral changes. There are also open-ended descriptors for the parent to input information.

From Malviya S, Voepel-Lewis T, Burke C, et al. The revised FLACC observational pain tool: improved reliability and validity for pain assessment in children with cognitive impairment. *Paediatr Anaesth.* 2006;16(3):258-265.

The pathophysiology of hepatotoxicity is related to the buildup of the metabolite, *N*-acetyl-para-benzo-quinone imine.[56] Acetylcysteine, commonly stocked in hospitals, is used to treat acetaminophen overdose.[57]

Nonsteroidal Antiinflammatory Drugs

NSAIDs exert their analgesic effects by inhibiting cyclooxygenase (COX) enzymes, which are involved in the synthesis of prostaglandins and thromboxane. COX inhibitors possess antipyretic, analgesic, and antiinflammatory properties and are effective for the management of acute pain and swelling after minor surgery or trauma. Different NSAIDs have varying potencies, absorption rates, oral bioavailability, and elimination half-life. They are thought to act primarily in the PNS and produce fewer bleeding problems than aspirin because of their *reversible* inhibition of platelet aggregation. Reported side effects include gastrointestinal upset, cardiovascular effects, rash, headache, dizziness, eye problems, hepatic dysfunction, and renal dysfunction. NSAID use has the potential to worsen hypertension and induce thrombosis in patients at risk for stroke. There are relatively few clinical drug trials evaluating NSAIDs in children, but common agents approved by the US Food and Drug Administration (FDA) for children are ibuprofen, naproxen, and tolmetin. Both ibuprofen and naproxen are available in oral suspension form.[58] Ibuprofen has a rapid onset, low potency, and a short elimination half-life; naproxen also is low in potency, but has a slow onset and long half-life. Ketorolac is a high-potency NSAID that is commonly administered intravenously for surgical patients for postoperative pain management.[59]

TABLE 28.4 **Commonly Used Analgesics for Children**

	Drug	Class	Generic Name	Trade Name	Dose
Mild to moderate pain	Acetaminophen	Nonopioid analgesic	Acetaminophen	Tylenol	10–15 mg/kg/dose q4–6h as needed; **DO NOT** exceed 5 doses in 24 h
	Ibuprofen	NSAID	Ibuprofen	Advil; Children's Motrin	4–10 mg/kg/dose q6–8h; maximum daily dose: 40 mg/kg/day
Moderate to severe pain	Acetaminophen and ibuprofen	Nonopioid analgesic	Acetaminophen and ibuprofen		Acetaminophen: 10–15 mg/kg/dose q4–6h as needed; **DO NOT** exceed 5 doses in 24 h Ibuprofen: 4–10 mg/kg/dose q6–8h; maximum daily dose: 40 mg/kg/day Take dosages at same time or alternate each drug every 3 h

NSAID, Nonsteroidal antiinflammatory drug.

It has been reported that children undergoing invasive restorative treatment require postoperative analgesia.[60,61] Because most cases of postoperative pain include an inflammatory component, NSAIDs are considered first-line agents in the treatment of mild to moderate postoperative pain.[62] It is rare that the recommended doses of acetaminophen or NSAIDs alone or in combination will not manage dental pain.

Aspirin

Aspirin, a salicylate, was widely used for its analgesic, antipyretic, antiplatelet, and antiinflammatory properties. Aspirin affects coagulation by *irreversible* inhibition of platelet aggregation and is rarely prescribed as an analgesic for pediatric patients because other NSAIDs have a more favorable side effect profile. However, aspirin is sometimes used for its anticoagulant properties in some pediatric patients (e.g., Kawasaki disease) at risk for forming blood clots.[63] Due to aspirin's association with viral infection and Reye syndrome (a serious condition characterized by swelling in the liver and brain), it should be avoided for most patients under 16 years old.[64]

Opioid Analgesics

Opioid analgesics act centrally to inhibit pain by interacting with opioid receptors in the brain and spinal cord.[65] Opioids are effective for severe pain, sedation, and cough suppression. However, they can produce serious adverse effects such as oversedation, respiratory depression, cardiac depression or arrhythmias, histamine release, constipation, opioid hyperalgesia, euphoria, dependence, and addiction. Extreme caution should be used when considering the use of opioids in pediatric and adolescent patients. The use of opioid analgesics for pain management in pediatric and adolescent patients carries risks, and an evidence-based approach is recommended.[58,66]

Opioid analgesics include morphine, meperidine (Demerol), fentanyl, codeine, hydrocodone (e.g., Norco, Vicodin), oxycodone (e.g., Percocet), and hydromorphone (Dilaudid).

Due to individual variance in cytochrome P450 family 2 subfamily D type 6 (CYP2D6) metabolism,[67] some opioids (e.g., tramadol, codeine) may be rapidly broken down into by-products that can lead to serious adverse effects. The FDA does not recommend codeine or tramadol use in pediatric patients due to the potential for slowed or difficult breathing and death, which appear to be a greater risk in children under the age of 12. Hydrocodone and oxycodone are more potent analgesics with a greater affinity for opioid receptors than codeine. However, the safety and effectiveness of these drugs in patients under the age of 18 have not been established. Opioids are not first-line agents for pain management and should be reserved for moderate to severe "breakthrough" pain. In the uncommon situation where dental pain is refractory to nonopioid analgesics, a more potent agent such as hydrocodone or oxycodone may be considered. Practitioners should be careful to distinguish physiologic pain from a behavioral response. The duration of such drug usage should generally be brief, and a prolonged perceived need for analgesics should prompt reevaluation or further consultation to determine the etiology of persistent reported pain. Additionally, state regulations/mandates should be considered when prescribing an opioid to a minor. Many states require specific consent to be obtained with the legal guardian and verification to ensure the patient has no open opioid prescriptions.[65]

Dosing Schedule

Analgesics should be administered on a regular timed schedule if moderate to severe pain is expected. This is called *around-the-clock dosing* and has been consistently shown to be the most effective way to decrease breakthrough pain because it keeps the plasma levels of analgesics stable. Advising parents to give a pain medicine "as needed" sometimes means that the child will not receive any medicine unless they are vocal in their complaints.[68] For dental pain, using an analgesic as prescribed (e.g., every 4 to 6 hours) for the first 36 to 48 hours is recommended.[62]

Multimodal Therapy

Multimodal pain management involves the use of medications with different mechanisms of action along with adjunctive strategies (ice, local anesthesia, nonpharmacologic techniques).[58] NSAIDs alone or in combination with acetaminophen should be considered as first-line therapy for managing acute dental pain.[58] Prescribing medications that work on multiple pathways can improve pain management. When one agent is ineffective in controlling postoperative pain, an alternation between acetaminophen and ibuprofen may be used. For example, if ibuprofen is given at 9:00 AM, acetaminophen is given at 12:00 PM, ibuprofen is given at 3:00 PM, acetaminophen is given at 6:00 PM. Alternation allows adequate spacing between doses of the same drug but also ensures continuous adequate plasma levels of pain medication. Parents should write down the time when medication is given, or mobile healthcare applications for phones can help a parent keep track of correct dosing. Acetaminophen can be alternated or given alongside ibuprofen because these agents target different receptor sites.[52]

Generally, the use of opioids should be avoided. However, a brief course of opioids (e.g., oxycodone) may be considered for adolescents with severe pain if first-line therapy is determined to be ineffective.[66] Given the complex nature of pain, a multimodal approach can be beneficial for managing both acute and chronic pain.[69]

Pain Control With Local Anesthesia

Profound local anesthesia facilitates the successful treatment of patients, especially pediatric patients, by relieving their anxiety and discomfort during restorative and surgical procedures. Good operator technique in obtaining local anesthesia in pediatric patients is essential and requires mastery of (1) child growth and development (physical and mental), (2) behavior management, (3) sound technique, and (4) pharmacology of local anesthetics. As with any anesthetic administration, a thorough preoperative medical evaluation must be conducted before selection of technique and agent (see Chapter 35, Figure 35.2). This should include but not be limited to review of medical history, evaluation of the patients' weight and body mass index, potential for adverse drug interactions, and completion of medical consults as needed.[70]

Mechanisms of Action

Local anesthesia is used to block the flow of impulses from the painful part of the body (the tooth) to the CNS. The initial process of odontogenic pain perception involves the production of nerve impulses by noxious stimuli that stimulate specialized myelinated and unmyelinated nerve fibers—termed *nociceptors* and are classified as A-delta and C fibers. These impulses transmit pain information via a generator potential, and if large enough, a propagated action potential. This propagated action potential travels to the CNS via the trigeminal nerve. The trigeminal nerve has three branches: the ophthalmic (V1), maxillary division (V2), and mandibular division (V3). The cell bodies of the three branches of the trigeminal nerve are in the trigeminal ganglion and project to the spinal trigeminal tract to synapse with second-order neurons. This information travels through the spinal nucleus of the trigeminal nerve situated in the caudal pons and medulla of the brainstem and then travels to the thalamus and then to the somatosensory cortex of the brain. The somatosensory cortex is responsible for processing sensations like touch, temperature, pain, and proprioception.[71]

The myelinated A-delta fibers are activated by high-intensity stimuli such as air blasts, heat/cold, drilling, probing, hyperosmotic solutions, and inflammatory mediators. The characteristics of this pain stimulation would be described as fast, sharp, short-lasting, nonlingering, and well localized. The unmyelinated C fibers are activated by low-intensity stimuli. The C fibers are polymodal nociceptors and have high thresholds for activation. They are insensitive to hydrodynamic stimulation, activated by intense heat/cold stimuli, and are more likely to become activated by inflammatory mediators. The characteristics of this pain stimulation would be slow, dull, aching, throbbing, long-lasting, lingering, spontaneous, and poorly localized. These nerve impulses travel along the nerve fibers via a process involving ion transport across the neuronal membrane.[72–75]

The primary effect of local anesthetic agents is to penetrate the nerve cell membrane and block receptor sites that control the influx of sodium ions associated with membrane depolarization.[75] The sequence of events involved in a local anesthetic block consists of (1) intraneuronal penetration of the local anesthetic and subsequent binding to a receptor site that exists on the inside of the cell membrane, (2) blockade of the sodium channels through which the sodium ions would normally enter during depolarization, (3) a decrease in sodium conductance, (4) depression of the rate of electrical depolarization, (5) failure to achieve threshold potential, and (6) lack of development of a propagated action potential and thus *blockade of conduction* of the nerve impulse.[75] Fig. 28.5 illustrates the local anesthetic mechanism. The net result is inhibition of neuronal excitability, which reduces the likelihood of action potential transmission. Therefore local anesthetics alter the reactivity of neural membranes to propagate action potentials that may be generated in tissues distal to the anesthetic block. Action potentials that enter an area of adequately anesthetized nervous tissue are blocked and fail to transmit information to the

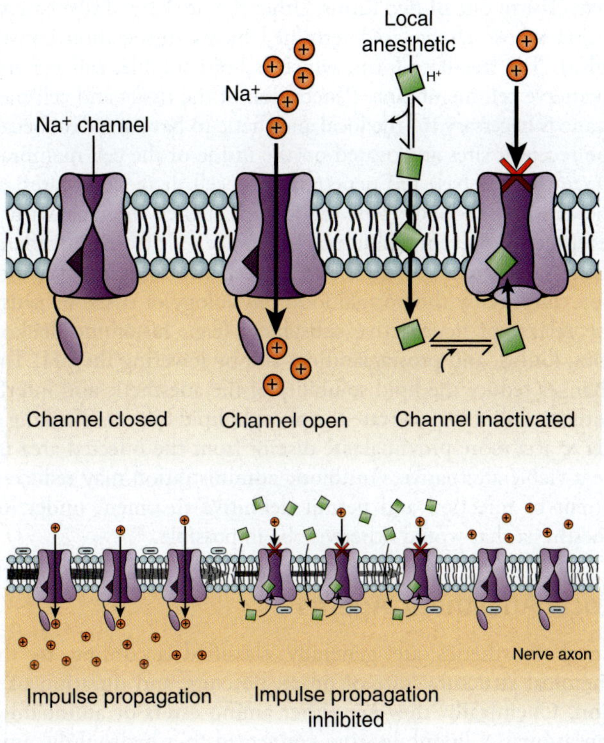

• **Fig. 28.5** This sequence is a proposed mechanism of action of local anesthetics: (1) Displacement of calcium ions from the sodium channel receptor site, which permits (2) binding of the local anesthetic molecule to this receptor site, which produces a (3) blockade of the sodium channel and a (4) decrease in sodium conductance, which leads to (5) depression of the rate of electrical depolarization and (6) failure to achieve the threshold potential level, along with (6) lack of development of propagated action potentials, which is called a (8) conduction blockade.[58] (Image from Shaikh H, Chumpitazi C. *Rosen's Emergency Medicine: Concepts and Clinical Practice,* 157, 2016–2029.e2.)

CNS.[75] In general, nerve fiber susceptibility to the onset of action of local anesthetics is greater for neural fibers that have more rapid firing rates, have smaller diameters, and are myelinated. The following considerations are presented:

1. Firing rate: Local anesthetics have a greater affinity for receptors within sodium channels during their activated and inactivated states than when they are in their resting states, meaning that neural fibers having more rapid firing rates are most susceptible to local anesthetic action.
2. Diameter of nerve fiber: Larger-diameter myelinated fibers have a greater internodal distance than smaller myelinated fibers. Smaller fibers are generally more susceptible to local anesthetics solution, because a given volume of solution can more readily block the requisite number of sodium channels for impulse transmission to be entirely interrupted.
3. Myelinated versus unmyelinated fibers: In myelinated fibers, local anesthesia only needs to act at the nodes of Ranvier to inhibit nerve conduction. However, profound local anesthesia could be more related to needle placement and technique than fiber type, as free nerve endings are easily anesthetized. Nerve blocks can be more challenging than local infiltrations due to the anatomical barriers that may prevent ideal needle and anesthetic placement. Additionally, certain local anesthetics have pharmacologic properties that allow them to diffuse through neuronal membranes more effectively than other agents.[70,74–76]

Local anesthetic agents are weak chemical bases and are supplied generally as salts, such as lidocaine hydrochloride. The salts may exist in one of two forms, either the uncharged free base or a cation whose charge is determined by its dissociation constant (pKa). The free-base form, which is lipid soluble, can penetrate the nerve cell membrane. Penetration of the tissue and cell membrane is necessary for the local anesthetic to have an effect because the receptor sites are located on the inside of the cell membrane. Once the free base has penetrated the cell, it reequilibrates, and the cation is thought to be the form that then interacts with the receptors to prevent sodium conductance.[75] Infected or inflamed tissues are harder to anesthetize. Local infection and inflammation can modify the normal local physiology of tissue by causing the release of neuroactive substances (e.g., histamine, leukotrienes, kinins, and prostaglandins) and by lowering the pH. These changes reduce the lipid solubility of the anesthetic and interfere with its ability to penetrate the phospholipid bilayer. Blocking the nerve at a more proximal site distant from the infected area may be a viable alternative. Antibiotic administration may reduce the extent of infection and permit definitive treatment under local anesthesia that would otherwise be impossible.[75]

Local Anesthetic Agents

Local anesthetics are generally classified according to their chemical structure, rate of onset, potency, and duration of action. Chemically, they are either amino esters or aminoamides (an aromatic, lipophilic ring connected to a hydrophilic amine group by an intermediate chain containing either an ester or amide linkage).[70]

Esters

Benzocaine, the only commonly used ester, is a topical anesthetic and may cause allergic reactions. Ester anesthetics are hydrolyzed by pseudocholinesterase in the plasma and metabolized to para-aminobenzoic acid (PABA), which has been associated with allergic sensitization.[70,75,77]

Amides

Amides, introduced with lidocaine in 1943, are amide derivatives of diethylamino acetic acid and have fewer allergic reactions. They are more commonly used than esters due to lower allergenic risks and greater potency. Amides are metabolized in the liver, so liver function can affect metabolism rates. Significant liver dysfunction may result in slower metabolism and increased risk of local anesthetic toxicity. The amides commonly used include lidocaine, mepivacaine, prilocaine, bupivacaine, and articaine.[70,75,77]

The selection of a local anesthetic should be based on the patient's medical history, treatment invasiveness, and the anesthesia duration. In pediatric dentistry, 2% lidocaine has been considered a gold standard local anesthesia and the most efficacious anesthetic agent since its debut in the 1940s for pediatric patients.[78] However, 4% articaine, introduced in 1976 in Europe and 2000 in the United States, is gaining interest in pediatric dentistry.[79] Due to its unique physical and chemical properties, low-quality evidence suggests that articaine is more effective at achieving a more profound anesthetic than lidocaine, particularly for mandibular *infiltration*.[80,81] Other local anesthetics without epinephrine, like mepivacaine, are appropriate for certain patients such as those with cardiac concerns or in procedures where epinephrine should not be utilized, like regenerative endodontics.[82]

Articaine

Articaine is an amide, but its structure is unique among this group in that it does not contain a benzene ring; instead, it contains a thiophene ring. This thiophene ring increases its liposolubility, making it a more effective anesthetic in crossing lipid barriers. It also contains an additional ester group, which enables articaine to undergo biotransformation in the plasma as well as in the liver. These properties allow the quick hydrolysis of articaine in the blood and minimize the risk of systemic toxicity. Compared with lidocaine, articaine is 1.5 times more potent and 0.6 times less toxic. It had been previously reported that the use of articaine HCl, specifically in inferior alveolar nerve blocks (IANBs), resulted in a higher incidence of persistent paresthesia of the oral tissues with incomplete or no recovery. Currently there exists conflicting evidence about associating articaine with a higher incidence of paresthesia. A 2011 publication from Yapp and colleagues found existing publications on the matter to be of low-level evidence with biases in data recruitment and protocols, resulting in the inability to derive any clinical recommendations.[83] When adjusted for market share, articaine has a higher percentage of paresthesia cases from IANBs compared with other commonly used local dental anesthetics.[75,84] Uncertainty still surrounds the probability of articaine to cause paresthesia, with multiple studies available offering conflicting results and opinions on this matter.[79] In 2000, the FDA issued that Septocaine (Septodont, Lancaster, PA) was indicated for local, infiltrative, or conductive (i.e., block) anesthesia in both simple and complex dental procedures in adults and pediatric patients 4 years of age or older. Safety and effectiveness of Septocaine in pediatric patients younger than 4 years had not been established. Safety of doses greater than 7 mg/kg (0.175 mL/kg) in pediatric patients have not been established.[85] Conversely, there have been several reports documenting the safety and efficacy of articaine in children of all ages, including those under age 4.[82,86] No difference between articaine and lidocaine in frequencies of anesthetic-related adverse events in children has been reported.[87,88]

As articaine is becoming more popular with new graduates and showing potential market share growth, further studies, especially randomized controlled trials, are required to increase the strength of the evidence and help clinicians make an informed decision as to which local anesthetic to choose when carrying out an IANB.[75–89]

Excretion of Local Anesthetics

For both ester and amide local anesthetics and their metabolites, the kidneys are the primary organ for excretion. Significant renal impairment may result in an inability to eliminate the local anesthetic, thus resulting in increased risk for toxicity.[70,76]

Local Anesthetic Properties

Individual local anesthetic agents differ from one another in their pharmacologic profiles (Table 28.5).[90] The reader may refer to additional readings for more in-depth information on local anesthetics that are rarely used in children. They vary in their potency, toxicity, onset time, and duration of action. All these characteristics may be clinically significant, and all vary as a function of the intrinsic properties of the anesthetic agent itself and the regional anesthetic procedure employed. Furthermore, these characteristics may be modified by the addition of vasoconstrictors.[75]

Potency

The intrinsic potency of a local anesthetic is the concentration required to achieve the desired nerve blockade and is best predicted by its lipid solubility. Greater lipid solubility, which is 90% lipid, allows the anesthetic to penetrate the nerve membrane more readily.[75] Lidocaine, prilocaine, mepivacaine, and articaine have intermediate potency, and bupivacaine has the highest potency.[75] The efficacy of local anesthesia depends on the concentration of the anesthetic on a segment of the nerve. Beyond the fixed amount of local anesthetic necessary to block neuronal impulses, any excess is wasteful and potentially dangerous. Failure to obtain anesthesia is likely due to operator error in depositing the solution sufficiently close to the nerve or anatomical aberrations (e.g., accessory innervation). Inflammation and infection are additional obstacles to anesthetic performance.[75,89]

In pediatric dentistry, appropriate dosage (based on body weight) will minimize the chance of toxicity, especially when used in combination with other agents affecting the cardiovascular system and the CNS (e.g., sedatives). Neurologic complications after local anesthetic injection are complex and often multifactorial. They can be caused by mechanical injury, ischemia, the neurotoxicity of local anesthetic, or a combination of these factors. Drug errors occur when the patient receives too large a dose of local anesthetic, or an intravascular administration of local anesthetic occurs, and the patient demonstrates an abnormal reaction of systemic toxicity despite no preexisting medical conditions.[70,72,90]

Onset Time

Onset time is the time required for the local anesthetic solution to penetrate the nerve fiber and cause complete conduction blockade. The pKa, which measures a molecule's affinity for hydrogen ions, is the most important factor in determining onset time. Anesthetics with a high pKa value will have fewer molecules available in the free-base form. Thus it is slow to diffuse through the

TABLE 28.5 Local Anesthetic Agents and Pharmacologic Properties

INJECTABLE LOCAL ANESTHETICS								
	DURATION OF ACTION IN MINUTES[a]							
Anesthetic	MAXILLARY INFILTRATION		INFERIOR ALVEOLAR BLOCK		MAXIMUM DOSAGE[b]		Anesthetic/ 1.7 mL	Vasoconstrictor/ 1.7 mL
	Pulp	Soft Tissue	Pulp	Soft Tissue	mg/kg	mg/lb	mg	mg
Lidocaine[c]	60	170	85	190	4.4	2		
2%+ 1:50,000 epinephrine							34	0.034
2%+ 1:100,000 epinephrine							34	0.017
Articaine[d] 4%+ 1:100,000 epinephrine	60	90	90	230	7	3.2	68	0.017
Mepivacaine								
3% plain	25	90	40	165	4.4	2	51	
2%+ 1:20,000 levonordefrin	50	130	75	185			34	
Bupivacaine[e] 0.5%+ 1:200,000 epinephrine	40	340	240	440	1.3	0.6	8.5	0.085

[a]Duration of anesthesia varies greatly depending on concentration, total dose, and site of administration; use of epinephrine; and the patient's age.
[b]Use the lowest total dose that provides effective anesthesia. Lower doses should be used in very vascular areas or when providing local anesthesia without vasoconstrictor. Doses of amides should be decreased by 30% in infants younger than 6 months. For improved safety, American Academy of Pediatric Dentistry, in conjunction with the American Academy of Pediatrics, recommends a dosing schedule for dental procedures that is more conservative that the manufacturer's recommended dose (MRD).
[c]This table lists the long-established pediatric dental maximum dose of lidocaine as 4.4 mg/kg; however, the MRD is 7 mg/kg.
[d]Use in pediatric patients under 4 years of age is not recommended.
[e]Use in patients under 12 years of age is not recommended.
Adapted from the American Academy of Pediatric Dentistry. *Use of Local Anesthesia For Pediatric Dental Patients.* The Reference Manual of Pediatric Dentistry. American Academy of Pediatric Dentistry; 2024:386-393; and Haas DA. An update on local anesthetics in dentistry. *J Can Dent Assoc.* 2002;68(9):546-551.

membrane and has a slower onset of action. Hence, drugs with a lower pKa have a more rapid onset of action.[75] The rates of onset time for local anesthetics are as follows: mepivacaine is the fastest; articaine, lidocaine, and prilocaine have moderate onset times; and bupivacaine has the longest onset time.[70,75] The clinician must understand that conduction blockade requires time to become effective; otherwise, unnecessary pain may result from beginning a procedure too soon.

Duration

The duration of anesthesia is crucial in choosing a local anesthetic and is largely determined by protein-binding properties. After penetrating the nerve sheath, the anesthetic equilibrates between base and cationic forms, with the cationic form binding to sodium channels. Vasodilatory properties affect the duration, and adding a vasoconstrictor slows absorption into the bloodstream (away from the injection site), prolonging the effect. Thus anesthetics with higher protein binding and a vasoconstrictor have longer durations. See Table 28.5 for commonly accepted anesthetic durations.[73,88]

Regional Technique

The type of regional (local) anesthetic procedure employed is a significant factor in determining drug characteristics. Depending on whether topical, infiltration, or a major or minor nerve block is employed, the onset and duration of the various agents will vary. Potency is not affected.

Onset

Local anesthesia of the soft tissues by the infiltration technique occurs almost immediately with all the local anesthetics. As more tissue penetration becomes necessary, the intrinsic latency of onset previously discussed plays a more significant role. Generally, in dentistry, for any given drug, the onset time required is shortest with an infiltration and longer for a peripheral nerve block.[70,75]

Duration

The duration of anesthesia varies significantly with the regional technique performed. See Table 28.5 for differences in pulpal and soft tissue duration of anesthesia by injection type.[75] Duration of soft tissue anesthesia is important when considering potential postoperative complications, particularly trauma. Young children are more prone to self-induced soft tissue injuries (e.g., lip and cheek biting) as a common complication of local anesthetic use. Most lesions of this nature are self-limiting and heal without complications, although bleeding and infection are possible.[90] Using an anesthetic without epinephrine has not been shown to reduce soft tissue anesthesia duration.[90]

Other Factors

Dose

For consistently effective local anesthetic blocks, an adequate concentration and volume must be administered. However, increases in dosage must be limited by toxicity concerns. To calculate the maximum dosage of an anesthetic, the child should be weighed in kilograms. The maximum recommended dosage of local anesthetics is listed in Table 28.5.[90] See Box 28.2 for an example of local anesthetic calculation.

• BOX 28.2 Calculating Maximum Allowable Local Anesthetic

Example of 2% Lidocaine With 1:100,000 Epinephrine

Step 1
- Weight of child in kilograms (kg)
- Weight calculation from pounds to kilogram (44 lb/2.2 = 20 kg)
- Weight (for example) = **20 kg**

Step 2
- Multiply weight by maximum allowable dose of anesthetic
- 20 kg × 4.4 mg/kg = **88 mg maximum allowable lidocaine**

Step 3
- Divide maximum mg allowable of local anesthetic by mg of local anesthetic per carpule of local anesthetic
- Result is maximum allowable number of carpules
- 88 mg × 1 carpule/34 mg per carpule = **2.5 maximum allowable carpules**

Vasoconstrictors

The addition of vasoconstrictors like epinephrine affects onset, duration, and quality of a block. Vasoconstrictors reduce systemic absorption by constricting blood vessels, which maintain higher anesthetic concentration at the injection site. This prolongs anesthesia, improves effectiveness, and reduces toxic effects by delaying systemic absorption. It may also shorten the onset time.

A vasoconstrictor is generally indicated in pediatric dental patients because of the potential for increased systemic uptake in pediatric physiology. Increased uptake will produce a shorter duration of action and a more rapid accumulation of toxic levels in the blood. Finally, vasoconstrictors produce local hemostasis after local anesthetic infiltration into the operative field. This assists in postoperative hemorrhage control—an advantage in the management of young children undergoing dental extractions.

Vasoconstrictors are all sympathomimetic agents that carry intrinsic toxic effects including tachycardia, hypertension, headache, anxiety, tremor, and arrhythmias. It has been shown that 2% lidocaine containing a concentration of 1:200,000 epinephrine is as effective in increasing the depth and duration of local anesthesia block as higher concentrations of epinephrine, such as 1:100,000 or 1:50,000.[74] To prevent vasoconstriction toxicity in children, a concentration of 1:100,000 epinephrine should not be exceeded. For healthy patients, the maximum recommended dosage is limited by the dosage of the local anesthetic drug. In patients with cardiovascular disease, a medical consultation before local anesthetic with vasoconstrictor administration is warranted. Generally, the maximum recommended epinephrine dose of 0.04 mg should not be exceeded for patients with cardiovascular disease.[74] In addition, caution should be taken in patients taking medications with drug interactions, for example, β-adrenergic blockers and tricyclic antidepressants.[70,75,91] The reader is referred to textbooks of local anesthesia for a comprehensive discussion of vasoconstrictors in patients with cardiac disease.

Toxicity

Local anesthetic toxicity in dentistry is often overlooked. Toxic reactions can result from overdose, accidental intravascular injection, idiosyncratic response, allergic reactions, or interactions with other drugs (e.g., sedatives).[58,71] To avoid overdose in pediatric patients, dental practitioners must know the maximum recommended dose for each anesthetic based on body weight, not just the milligram dosage for an average adult.

Children's pharmacokinetics require careful consideration when using local anesthetics. Due to higher cardiac output, metabolic rate, and tissue perfusion, anesthetics are absorbed more rapidly. The less mature liver enzymes in young children may slow detoxification, and altered kidney function and immature nervous and cardiovascular systems make them more susceptible to toxicity than adults. Therefore precise technique with aspiration, the use of a vasoconstrictor, and knowledge of anesthetic properties are essential. *Above all, the recommended maximal safe dose of local anesthetic should be calculated precisely for each patient and must never be exceeded.* Maximal safe doses for local anesthetics are listed in Table 28.5.[75,92]

Central Nervous System Reactions

No CNS effects of clinical significance have been noted at safe, therapeutic dosages of local anesthetic.[75] At higher doses, adverse reactions may occur. The initial signs of overdose are seen in the CNS. Local anesthetic agents cause a biphasic reaction in the CNS as blood levels increase (excitation followed by depression). Although local anesthetics have depressant effects in general, they are thought to selectively depress inhibitory neurons initially, producing a net effect of CNS excitation. Subjective signs and symptoms of early anesthetic toxicity include circumoral numbness or tingling, dizziness, tinnitus (often described as a buzzing or humming sound), cycloplegia (difficulty in focusing the eyes), and disorientation. Depressant effects may be evident immediately. These include drowsiness, sedation, or even transient loss of consciousness. Objective signs may include muscle twitching, tremors, slurred speech, and shivering, followed by overt seizure activity. Generalized CNS depression characterizes the second phase of local anesthetic toxicity, sometimes accompanied by respiratory depression.[70,75,92,93]

Cardiovascular System Reactions

The cardiovascular response to local anesthetic toxicity is also biphasic. The heart rate and blood pressure may increase during CNS stimulation because of increased sympathetic activity. When plasma levels of the anesthetic increase, vasodilation followed by myocardial depression occurs, and a subsequent fall in blood pressure occurs. Bradycardia, cardiovascular collapse, and cardiac arrest may occur at higher levels of the agents. The depressant effect on the myocardium is essentially proportional to the inherent potency of the local anesthetic.[75]

Operator Technique

Local anesthesia may be obtained anatomically by one of three means:

1. *The nerve block* is the placement of anesthetic on or near a main nerve trunk. This results in a wide area of tissue anesthesia.
2. *The field block* is the placement of anesthetic on secondary branches of a main nerve.
3. *Local infiltration* is the deposition of the anesthetic on terminal branches of a nerve. Adequate diffusion of local anesthetic from local infiltration readily occurs in children because their bones are less dense than those of adults.[72]

Topical Anesthesia

Topical anesthesia is used to decrease discomfort from needle insertion. Its effectiveness has been debated, although studies have shown it is more effective than placebo.[72] Disadvantages include the taste, anticipatory anxiety before the needle, and establishment of conditioned responses.[94] However, effective distraction and coping strategies may outweigh these issues. A benzocaine gel is recommended for its ease of use. The best results behaviorally and physiologically occur when the gel is used sparingly and applied to a *dry* mucosal surface for at least *2 minutes.*

A small amount of topical anesthetic should be applied with a cotton-tipped applicator to a mucosa that has been adequately dried and isolated with a 2 × 2-inch cotton gauze pad (Fig. 28.6). The topical anesthetic should be applied to the tissue for 2 minutes. When applied appropriately, topical anesthetics are effective for surface tissues up to 3 mm in depth.[75] This allows for atraumatic needle penetration of the mucous membrane. Although a toxic response to topical anesthesia is rare, as it is poorly absorbed into the cardiovascular system, the application of an excessive amount should be avoided.[75] Topical anesthetics typically used in dentistry are 20% benzocaine, and less frequently 5% lidocaine. Compounded topical anesthetics have become popular; however, these should be used with caution as compounded topicals may differ in their composition, the quality of the mixture, and the strength of anesthesia potentially adding to the local anesthesia overall dose.[75] The most common compounded topical anesthetic formulations consist of 20% lidocaine, 4% tetracaine, and 2% phenylephrine.

Complications of Topical Anesthesia

Benzocaine, an ester anesthetic, can potentially cause an allergic reaction. In addition, benzocaine may result in methemoglobinemia,[95,96] which is a condition that the typically ferrous (Fe^{2+}) state of iron, which is functional for oxygen transport, is oxidized to the ferric (Fe^{3+}) state (estimated to occur 1 in 7000 exposures). This results in a nonfunctional hemoglobin incapable of binding to oxygen and may cause hypoxemia.[97] Overdosage (physiologic concentrations typically near or above 8% vs. the recommended 1%) may result in methemoglobinemia and tissue hypoxia, which in its initial stages is not detectable by pulse

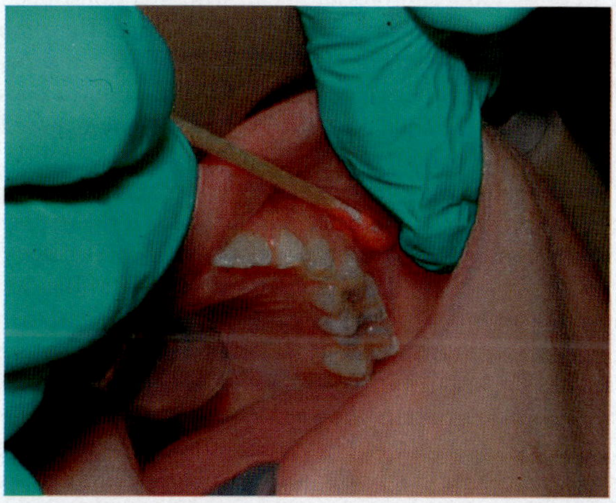

• **Fig. 28.6** Application of Topical Anesthetic to Maxillary Vestibule for Buccal Infiltration. Note a minimum amount of anesthetic on the cotton-tip applicator. Technique: (1) Reflect tissue to expose injection site. (2) Dry soft tissue with 2 × 2 gauze. (3) Apply topical anesthetic gel with cotton-tipped applicator, slowly burnishing into tissues for 30 seconds (see manufacturer's recommendations). Remove applicator and proceed with injection.

oximetry. It is imperative that clinicians use the minimal clinically effective required dose of benzocaine.[98] Given these risks, the FDA issued a warning in 2018 directing parents not to use benzocaine for teething in infants and children younger than 2 years.[99]

Alternative Topical Anesthetics

Studies show that cooling the injection site before administering local anesthetic reduces pain perception. Methods include refrigerant spray (5 seconds), ice sticks, or an ice-filled glove finger (1 to 2 minutes). This simple, reliable technique offers an alternative to topical anesthetic gel.[100–102]

Needle Selection

The needle gauge should be determined by the injection required. A short (20-mm) or long (32-mm) 27- or 30-gauge needle may be used for most intraoral injections in children, including mandibular blocks. Very little difference in discomfort level has been noted between the 25-gauge, 27-gauge, and 30-gauge needles for inferior alveolar injections; thus the 27-gauge needle would seem less likely to break or bend during injections and is preferred.[75] An extra short (10-mm) 30-gauge needle is appropriate for maxillary anterior injections.

To prevent needlesticks, alternative systems like retractable covers and self-sheathing needles are available. Injection delivery systems shield needles, eliminating risks from resheathing. If retractable needles are not used, a needle holder should be in place to avoid two-hand resheathing.[75]

Injection Technique

Communicating at a level appropriate to the child's development is necessary to accommodate the level of the child's understanding when discussing the injection. (See Chapter 26 for a detailed discussion of behavior guidance techniques.)

The discomfort of the injection may be lessened by counterstimulation, distraction, and a slow rate of administration. Counterstimulation is the application of vibratory stimuli (e.g., shaking the cheek) or moderate pressure (e.g., with a cotton-tipped applicator) to the area adjacent to the injection site. These stimuli have a physical and psychologic basis for modifying noxious input. Distraction can be accomplished by maintaining a constant monologue with the child and keeping their attention away from the syringe. The operator should always aspirate (i.e., gently pull back on the plunger of the dental syringe to cause negative pressure; aspiration of blood into the carpule occurs if the needle is in the blood vessel) and alter the depth of the needle if necessary and reaspirate before slowly injecting the anesthetic. The recommended rate of injection is 1 mL/min. Rapid injections are more painful because of rapid tissue expansion. They also potentiate the possibility of a toxic reaction if the solution is inadvertently deposited in a blood vessel.[75]

The dental assistant's role is important during the transfer of the syringe and in anticipation of patient movement. During the transfer of the syringe from the assistant to the dentist, the child's eyes tend to follow the dentist. The dentist's eyes should be focused on the patient's face (Fig. 28.7). The hand that receives the syringe is extended close to the head or body of the child. The body of the syringe is placed between the index and middle fingers, with the ring of the plunger slipped over the dentist's thumb by the assistant. The assistant then removes the plastic sheath protecting the needle. The dentist's peripheral vision guides the syringe to the patient's mouth in a slow, smooth movement.

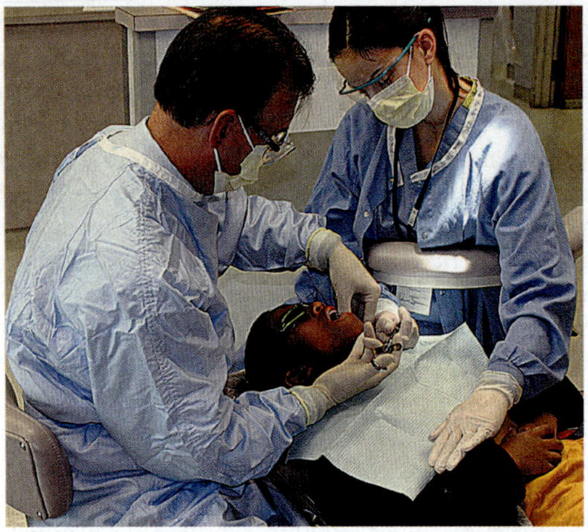

• **Fig. 28.7** Preparing for the Injection. Note the hand positions of the dentist and assistant in stabilizing the child's head and body during the injection.

Reflexive movements of the child's head and body should be anticipated.[75] The head can be stabilized by being held firmly but gently between the body and arm or hand of the dentist. The assistant passively extends his or her arm across the child's chest to intercept potential arm and body movements. The area of soft tissue to receive the injection is reflected by the free hand of the dentist and held taut, allowing the needle tip to penetrate the mucosa easily.[75] This hand can also block the child's vision as the syringe approaches the mouth. Once tissue penetration by the needle has occurred, the needle should not be retracted in response to the child's reactions. Otherwise, if the child anticipates reinjection, his or her behavior may deteriorate significantly. The use of finger rests is strongly advocated. After administering a local anesthetic, the syringe is carefully withdrawn, and the needle is recapped using a needle holder. After administration, the patient should never be left unattended.

Maxillary Primary and Permanent Molar Anesthesia

The innervation of maxillary primary and permanent molars arises from the posterosuperior alveolar nerve (permanent molars) and middle superior alveolar nerve (mesiobuccal root of the first permanent molar, primary molars, and premolars).

In anesthetizing the maxillary primary molars or permanent premolars, a supraperiosteal injection is indicated. The needle should penetrate the mucobuccal fold and be inserted to a depth that approximates the apices of the buccal roots of the teeth (Fig. 28.8). The solution should be deposited adjacent to the bone. The maxillary permanent molars may be anesthetized with a posterosuperior alveolar nerve block or by local infiltration.

Maxillary Primary and Permanent Incisor and Canine Anesthesia

The innervation of maxillary primary and permanent incisors and canines is by the anterosuperior alveolar branch of the maxillary nerve. Labial infiltration, or supraperiosteal injection, is commonly used to anesthetize the primary anterior teeth. The needle is inserted in the mucobuccal fold to a depth that approximates the apices of the buccal roots of the teeth (Fig. 28.9). Rapid deposition of the solution in this area is contraindicated because it

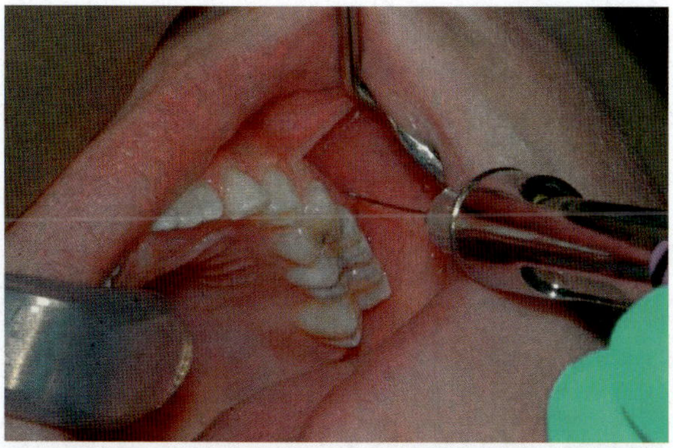

• **Fig. 28.8** Buccal Infiltration for Anesthetizing Maxillary Primary Molars. Technique: (1) Reflect tissue to expose injection site. (2) Orient bevel of needle parallel to the bone. (3) Insert needle in mucobuccal fold. (4) Proceed to depth that approximates the apices of the buccal roots of the molars. (5) The bevel of the needle should be adjacent to the periosteum of the bone. Aspirate. (6) Deposit the bolus of anesthetic slowly. (7) Remove needle and apply pressure with 2 × 2-inch gauze for 1 minute to obtain hemostasis.

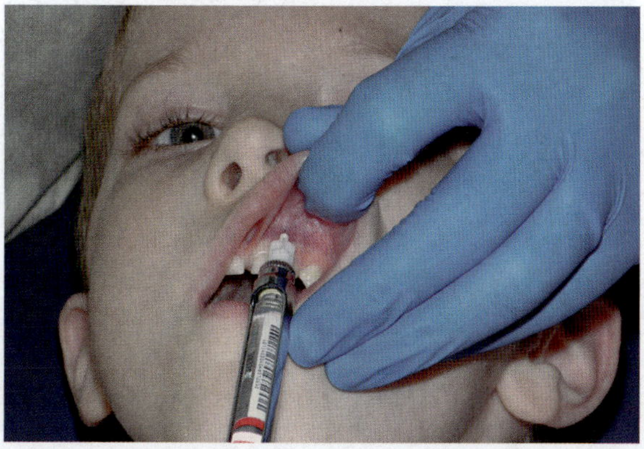

• **Fig. 28.9** Labial Infiltration of Maxillary Incisor Area. Technique for maxillary primary and permanent incisors and canines: (1) Reflect tissue to expose injection site. (2) Orient bevel of needle parallel to the bone. (3) Insert needle in mucobuccal fold. (4) Proceed to depth approximating that of root apices. This depth is less in the primary dentition than in the permanent dentition. (5) The bevel of the needle should be adjacent to the periosteum of the bone. Aspirate. (6) Inject the bolus of anesthetic very slowly. (7) Remove needle and apply pressure to area with 2 × 2-inch gauze for hemostasis.

produces discomfort during rapid expansion of the tissue. The innervation of the anterior teeth may arise from the opposite side of the midline. Thus it may be necessary to deposit some solution adjacent to the apex of the contralateral central incisor.

Palatal Tissue Anesthesia

The anterior palatine and nasal palatine nerves innervate the tissues of the hard palate. Surgical procedures involving palatal tissues usually require a nasal palatine nerve block or anterior palatine anesthesia. These nerve blocks are painful, and care should be taken to prepare the child adequately. These injections are not usually required for routine restorative procedures unless the procedure involves palatal tissue. However, if it is anticipated that the rubber dam clamp will impinge on the palatal tissue, a small amount of anesthetic solution should be deposited into the marginal tissue adjacent to the lingual aspect of the tooth. Adequate topical anesthesia at the injection site should be applied. Pressure anesthesia can be produced by applying pressure with a cotton applicator stick. It should be held firmly adjacent to the injection site and should produce blanching of the tissue. This should be maintained throughout the administration. The palatal tissue is tightly bound to bone, so a slow deposition will limit the discomfort the patient feels during tissue expansion. Blanching of the tissue will be observed (Fig. 28.10).

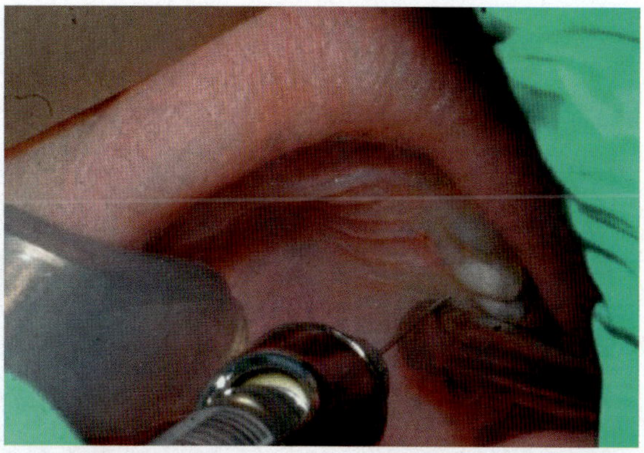

• **Fig. 28.10** Palatal Infiltration of Primary Molars Anesthetizing the Anterior Palatine Nerve. The cotton-tipped applicator is held firmly against the palatal tissue. The needle is inserted in the area between the applicator and tooth. The applicator may provide a masking or distracting effect. Technique: (1) Apply pressure with cotton-tipped applicator to the site to receive the needle. (2) Insert needle with bevel oriented parallel to the bone immediately adjacent to the applicator. (3) Proceed to depth at which the bevel of the needle is adjacent to the periosteum and aspirate. (4) Inject the bolus of anesthetic very slowly. (5) Remove needle and apply pressure to area with 2 × 2-inch gauze for hemostasis.

Mandibular Tooth Anesthesia

The IAN innervates the mandibular primary and permanent teeth. This nerve enters the mandibular foramen on the lingual aspect of the mandible. The position of the foramen changes by remodeling more superiorly from the occlusal plane as the child matures into adulthood. The foramen is at or slightly above the occlusal plane during the primary dentition period.[103] In adults, it averages 7 mm above the occlusal plane. The foramen is approximately midway between the anterior and posterior borders of the ramus of the mandible.

For the IANB, the child is asked to open his or her mouth as wide as possible. Mouth props may aid in maintaining this position for the child. The ball of the thumb is positioned on the coronoid notch of the anterior border of the ramus, and the fingers are placed on its posterior border. The needle is inserted between the internal oblique ridge and the pterygomandibular raphe (Fig. 28.11). The barrel of the syringe overlies the two primary mandibular molars on the opposite side of the arch and parallels the occlusal plane. The needle is advanced until it contacts bone, aspiration is completed, and the solution is slowly deposited.[75,104] (See Case Study: Local Anesthesia, eVideo 28.1).

Occasionally, the IANB is not successful. A second try may be attempted; however, the needle should be inserted at a level higher than that of the first injection. Care must be taken to prevent an overdose of anesthetic (see Table 28.5).

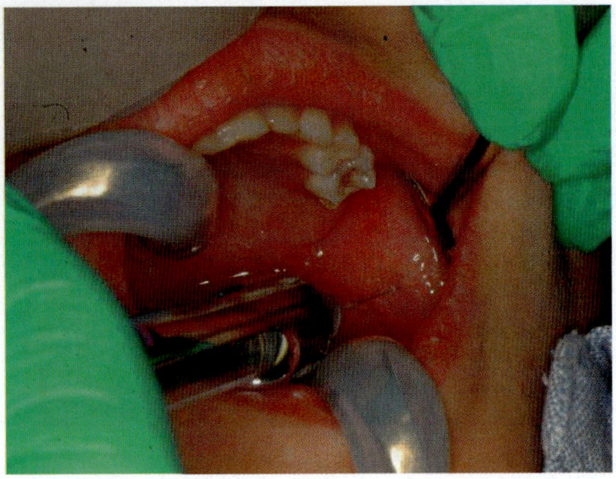

• **Fig. 28.11** Inferior Alveolar Block. Technique: (1) With patient's mouth opened as wide as possible, place the ball of the thumb on the coronoid notch on the anterior border of the mandible. (2) Position the index and middle fingers on the external posterior border of the mandible. (3) Insert the needle with the bevel oriented parallel to the bone and at the level of the occlusal plane between the internal oblique ridge and the pterygomandibular raphe. The barrel of the syringe will be exiting the mouth adjacent to the lip commissure contralateral to the side that is to be anesthetized. (4) Insert the needle to a depth adjacent to the bone. Aspirate. (5) Slowly inject the bolus of anesthetic. (6) Remove the needle and apply pressure to the area with 2 × 2-inch gauze for hemostasis.

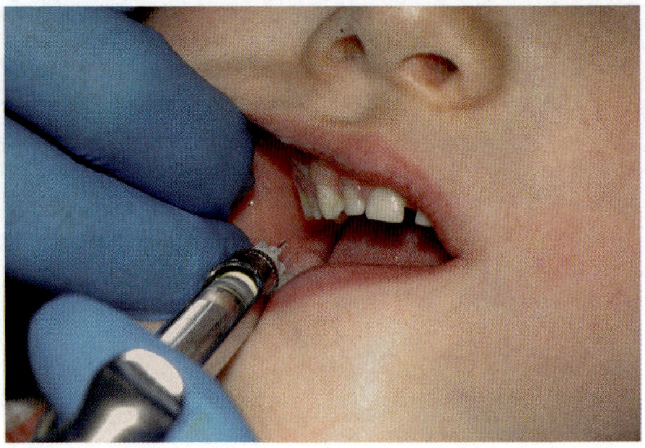

• **Fig. 28.12** Long Buccal Nerve Block. Technique: (1) Reflect tissue to expose the site of injection. (2) Insert needle in the mucobuccal fold at a point distal and buccal to the most posterior molar. The bevel of the needle should be oriented parallel to the bone. (3) Insert needle to a depth adjacent to the bone. Aspirate. (4) Slowly inject the bolus of anesthetic. (5) Remove the needle and apply pressure to the area with 2 × 2-inch gauze for hemostasis.

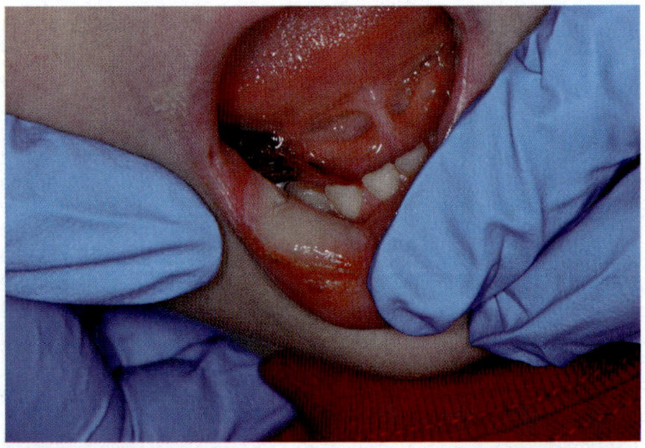

• **Fig. 28.13** Masticatory trauma to lower lip that has been anesthetized with an inferior alveolar block.

Local infiltration in the mandibular buccal vestibule adjacent to teeth requiring treatment has been explored and found to be an effective alternative to IANBs in pediatric patients.[79,105,106] Additionally, the effectiveness of articaine as a local anesthetic in pediatric dentistry was better than the gold standard lidocaine, but the difference was small.[79] The mandibular infiltration has been advocated as a less painful and more simplistic injection technique that may diminish soft tissue anesthesia and possible soft tissue injury associated with an IANV.[79,105,106]

The long buccal nerve supplies sensory innervation to the molar buccal gingivae. It should only be anesthetized if manipulation of these tissues is anticipated. This may be done along with the IANB after confirming the success of the block. A small quantity of solution is deposited in the mucobuccal fold at a point distal and buccal to the most posterior molar (Fig. 28.12).[75]

Some operators advocate the use of a periodontal ligament (PDL) injection for anesthetizing singular teeth.[75] An advantage of this method is that limited soft tissue is anesthetized, which may prevent inadvertent tissue damage resulting from chewing after dental procedures. However, there is some evidence that this type of injection may produce areas of hypoplasia or decalcification on succedaneous teeth.[107]

Complications of Local Anesthesia

The complications of local anesthesia may include local and systemic effects.[75] Local complications may include masticatory trauma (Fig. 28.13), hematomas, infections, nerve damage by the needle, trismus, and, rarely, needle breakage in the soft tissue. These types of complications may be minimized by aspirating, decreasing needle deflection, never "burying" the needle to its hub in soft tissue, and warning the parent and child that the soft tissue will be anesthetized for a period of up to 1 to 2 hours after the restorative procedure. Paresthesia is persistent anesthesia beyond the expected duration. Potential etiologies may include trauma to the nerve, hemorrhage in or around the nerve, or trauma by the needle. Deposition of local anesthetic directly on a nerve trunk or too near a nerve trunk in a susceptible patient may result in long-term or permanent paresthesia. Local anesthetic neurotoxicity generally increases as potency increases.[75,90]

Phentolamine mesylate (PM) is a nonselective competitive α-adrenergic antagonist and a vasodilator indicated for adult and pediatric patients ages 3 years and older for the reversal of soft tissue anesthesia. When PM (OraVerse; Septodont, Lancaster, PA) is injected in the same area as a previous injection of local anesthetic, it facilitates the clearance of local anesthetic from the area via vasodilation, thus reducing the duration of soft tissue anesthesia. Research indicates a reduction in the duration of soft tissue anesthesia by approximately 45 minutes in children as young as 4 years of age.[108–110] PM is not a true local anesthetic reversal agent (as naloxone is to opioids), which means that it cannot be used to treat local anesthetic toxicity.

Systemic complications of local anesthetics include allergic reactions and cardiovascular and CNS dysfunction. Local anesthetic cartridges contain preservatives, organic salts, and vasoconstrictors. The preservative sodium bisulfite may be a source of allergic reactions and should be considered in the medical evaluation of the patient before its use. The concern about rubber products in local anesthetic cartridges being a source of allergic reactions has not been supported by any studies or case reports.[75] An allergic reaction can manifest in various ways, including urticaria, dermatitis, angioedema, fever, or anaphylaxis.[75] The practitioner should be prepared to manage emergencies as they arise (see Chapter 35).

As discussed earlier, the CNS responses to local anesthetics are complex and depend on plasma concentrations. Significant adverse events can occur when dose limits of local anesthetics are exceeded in the presence of sedatives, especially opioids. Management of overdoses may require oxygen supplementation, ventilatory support, and possible hospitalization. As discussed in Chapter 36, the dentist should be skillful in the management of emergency events.

Alternative Anesthesia Systems

Conventional anesthesia and behavioral techniques work for most children but can be overwhelming for some. In recent years, alternative delivery systems of dental anesthesia have been made available.

Buffered Local Anesthesia

The pH of an amide anesthetic with vasopressor is very low, approximately 3.5, which results in a burning sensation during administration. Increasing the pH of the cartridge of lidocaine HCl with epinephrine raises the pH to 7.4 and results in (1) increased patient comfort, (2) more rapid onset of anesthetic, and (3) decreased potential for postinjection injury. To buffer the local anesthetic, sodium bicarbonate ($NaHCO_3$) solution is mixed with the local immediately before administration. A system is available in which the local anesthetic cartridge is inserted into a mixing pen to buffer the local solution consistently. Existing studies have shown that buffered lidocaine had decreased onset time and injection pain and was beneficial for patients with difficulty achieving profound anesthesia compared with nonbuffered solutions.[111] Another systematic review and meta-analysis found no appreciated reduction in onset time when alkalinized lidocaine was administered with terminal infiltration techniques in normal tissues. However, there was an accelerated onset of time for IANBs (−1.26 minutes) and inflamed tissues (−1.37 minutes).[109]

Intranasal Anesthetic Spray

Intranasal delivery is a novel technique for achieving local anesthesia of maxillary teeth by infiltration of an anesthetic solution through the nasal mucosal walls by a metered device.[109,112] It constitutes a mixture of 3% tetracaine hydrochloride and 0.05% oxymetazoline, and is FDA-approved as Kovanaze (St. Renatus LLC, Fort Collins, CO) for use in adults and children weighing more than 40 kg (88 lb). Previous reports have shown that nasal spray afforded less pulpal anesthesia than infiltration with lidocaine and undesirable effects like nasal drainage, burning, pressure, severe respiratory depression, seizures, convulsion, and disorientation.[109,112] However, other publications suggest that this anesthetic solution was successful and well tolerated by adults.[109,112] There is limited published information on the use of intranasal anesthetic spray in pediatric populations. More studies on its efficacy and safety of administration, especially for pediatric patients, are necessary.

Computer-Controlled Intraligamentary Anesthesia

Computer-controlled local anesthetic delivery (C-CLAD) systems ensure a consistent, computer-controlled anesthetic flow rate. A series of clinical studies have demonstrated the efficacy of C-CLAD devices in decreasing subjective pain and disruptive behavior in children undergoing dental treatment compared with a conventional syringe.[75] The Wand STA (single tooth anesthesia) system (Milestone Scientific, Livingston, NJ) is an intraligamentary C-CLAD system with an additional function for dynamic pressure sensing (DPS), providing real-time feedback to the practitioner. This DPS technology permits a guided PDL injection that safely and effectively absorbs greater volumes of anesthetic solution through the intraligamentary tissues[75,109,112] (Fig. 28.14). See Case Study: Local Anesthesia, eVideo 28.2.

Computer-Assisted Intraosseous Anesthesia

The SOAN and SleeperOne (Dentalhitec, Cholet, France) are computer-assisted intraosseous (CAIO) anesthesia devices that utilize a specialized syringe needle, Effitec (Dentalhitec, Cholet, France), that possesses the distinctive feature of a double-beveled cutting edge resembling a scalpel blade. The Effitec needle provides easier mucosal entry and painless penetration with proper technique. The unique needle's tip structure allows penetration by incising the tissue without tearing. These devices can be utilized for traditional anesthetic delivery (attached and free mucosal gingiva infiltration, palatal, inferior alveolar block), intraligamentary (PDL), intraseptal, and intraosseous (IO) injection for pediatric patients. When utilized for IO anesthesia, the CAIO devices deliver an anesthetic solution with computer-controlled, increasing velocity and pressure directly into the cancellous bone in the region of the tooth being treated. The IO injection technique can provide anesthesia for a single tooth or multiple teeth in a quadrant and is found to eliminate injection pain, and the onset of the anesthetic effect is immediate. An additional benefit, because of the IO placement of anesthetic solution, is a lack of peripheral soft tissue anesthesia and a lack of the potential

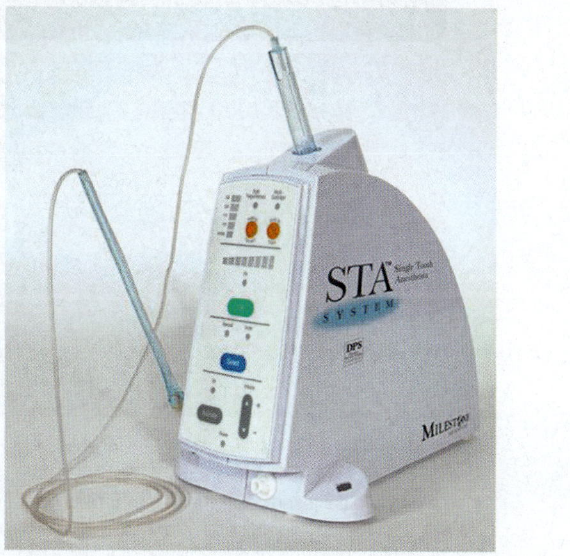

• **Fig. 28.14** Single Tooth Anesthesia (STA) System, a computer-controlled local anesthetic delivery system including the wand hand piece. (Courtesy Milestone Scientific, Livingston, New Jersey, Copyright 2010.)

experience for self-induced soft tissue trauma (e.g., lip and cheek biting). Existing publications find that C-CLAD systems could be preferred in pediatric patients because of reduced pain and anxiety. More specifically, these systems offer the provider the ability to utilize IO techniques in pediatric populations as a routine, first-choice anesthetic technique rather than as a supplemental technique when other injection methods have failed to provide adequate anesthesia[75,109,112,113] (Fig. 28.15).

Vibrotactile Devices

Vibratory devices attached to dental syringes or adjacent to the dental syringe are available. Examples include VibraJect (Newport Coast, CA) and DentalVibe (BING Innovations LLC, Boca Raton, FL). Their purported effectiveness is based on the gate control theory of pain and possibly auditory distraction. The VibraJect is an attachment to a traditional syringe that is intended to activate large A-beta fibers consistent with the gate theory of pain. Studies have been limited in the pediatric population, and there is inconclusive evidence to support a vibratory device over a conventional technique.[109,114,115]

Cryo-vibrotactile Devices

Buzzy (Pain Care Labs, Atlanta, GA) is an external cryo-vibrotactile device that is composed of two components: an external vibrating body that resembles a bee's body and a cold component in a frozen ice pack that is designed in the form of a bee's wings

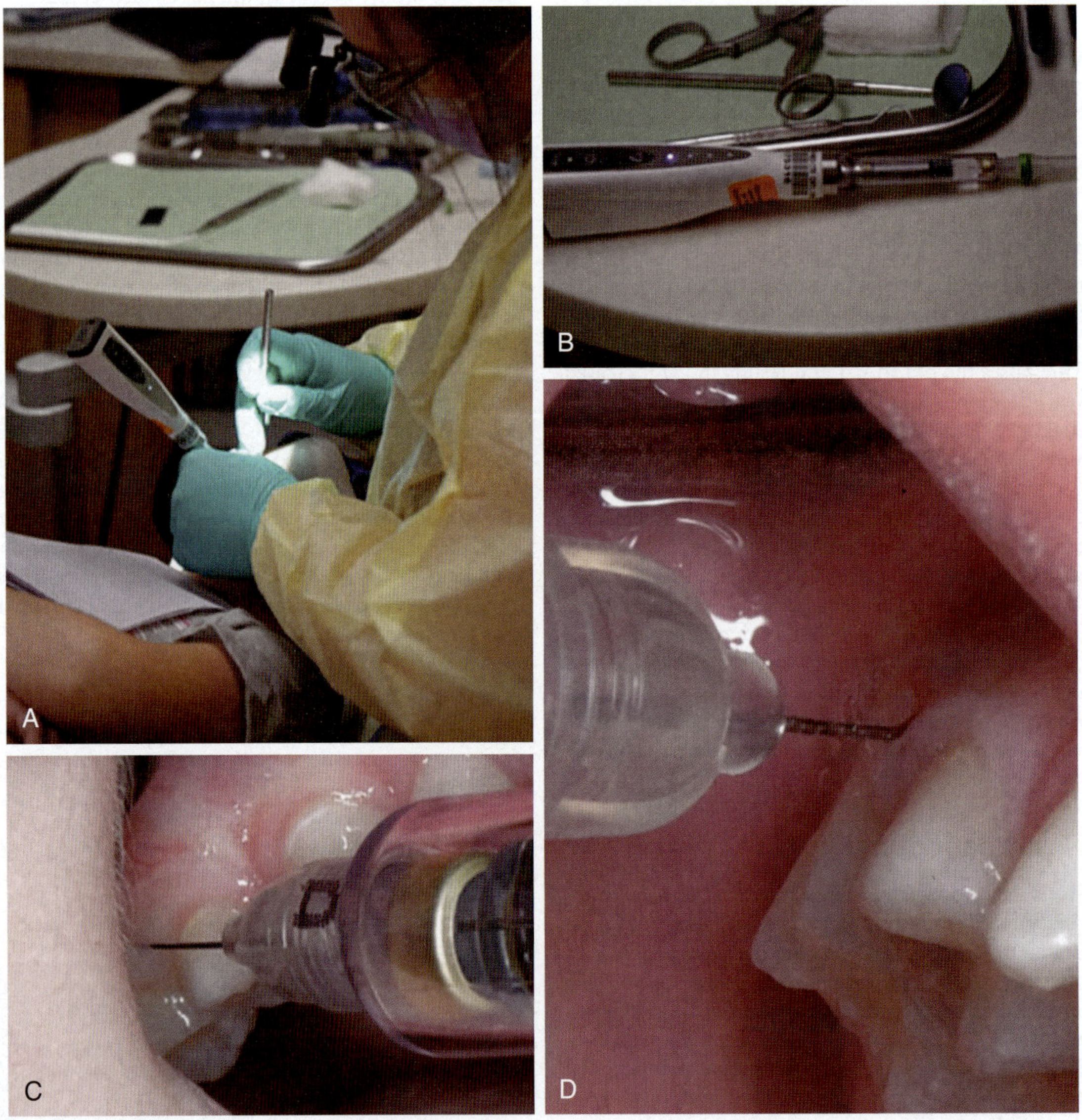

• **Fig. 28.15** (A) The SOAN (Dentalhitec, Cholet, France) a computer-assisted intraosseous (CAIO) anesthesia device. (B) Armamentarium of the SOAN showing the 9-mm Effitec needle (Dentalhitec, Cholet, France). (C) Initial insertion of the 9-mm Effitec needle at the base of the papilla of about 0.5 mm. The *D* indicator of the Effitec needle must be visible and on the opposite side of the gingiva. A small amount of anesthetic is delivered blanching the papillary tissue. (D) The Effitec needle should then be positioned 20 to 45 degrees relative to the long axis of the tooth/teeth being anesthetized. Penetration of interdental septum may correspond to a dropping sensation as the needle enters the spongy bone. Before proceeding with the anesthetic injection, the needle is slightly drawn back.

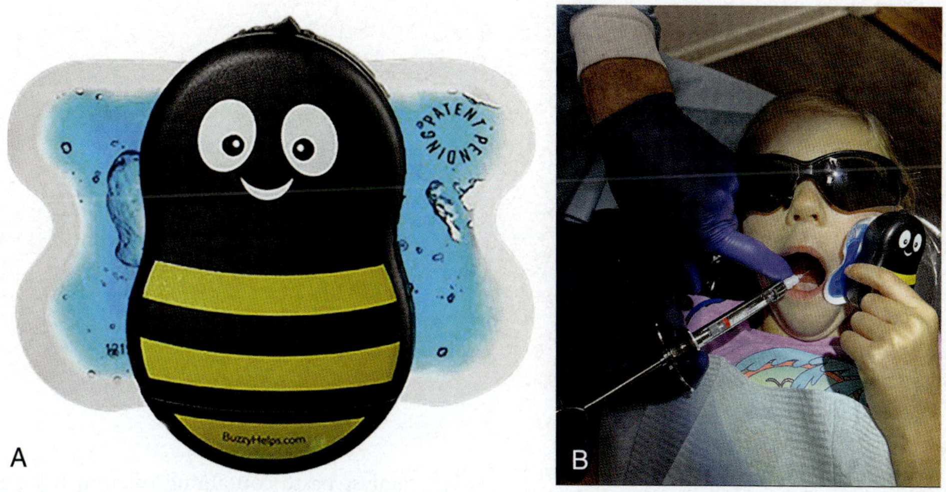

• **Fig. 28.16** (A) Buzzy (Pain Care Labs, Atlanta, GA) an external cryo-vibrotactile device that is composed of two components: an external vibrating body that resembles a bee's body, and a cold component in a frozen ice pack that is designed in the form of a bee's wings. (B) Buzzy applied to patient's cheek adjacent to injection site.

(Fig. 28.16). The vibration may stimulate A-beta fibers and cooling of the tissue may slow nerve conduction and pain signaling by activating C fibers.[109] Existing literature has demonstrated that cryo-vibrotactile devices have significantly reduced pain perception during local anesthetic infiltration in pediatric patients. These devices may be incorporated as an adjunct in the routine dental practice while administering local anesthesia to children.[109,116,117]

Conclusion: Local Anesthetics

Profound local anesthesia is crucial for safe, effective dental care. Pediatric patients pose challenges due to immature physiology, communication limits, and behavior. The dental team must ensure proper anesthetic delivery for a comfortable treatment experience.

Visit eBooks.Health.Elsevier.com to see full list of references.

29 Dental Materials

JAYAKUMAR JAYARAMAN AND KEVIN J. DONLY

CHAPTER OUTLINE

Restorative materials used in pediatric dentistry are typically the same as those used in general dentistry. This chapter identifies commonly used materials in pediatric dentistry and provides information that applies specifically to their use. Many materials are available, and in most cases clinical considerations will dictate the choice of the appropriate material. Table 29.1 identifies the most used materials in pediatric restorative dentistry and the relevant clinical considerations. Chapters 30 and 31 discuss the specific clinical restorative techniques associated with these restorative materials.

Bases and Liners

Bases and liners are available to reduce marginal microleakage from the restoration and prevent sensitivity to the underlying tooth structure. Traditionally, preparations of calcium hydroxide, zinc oxide–eugenol, and zinc phosphate were the materials of choice. Currently, glass ionomer cement is a commonly used base material.

Calcium Hydroxide

Calcium hydroxide cements are supplied in a visible light–cured system (Fig. 29.1A) and a two-paste system (Fig. 29.1B). A catalyst paste containing calcium hydroxide, zinc oxide, and zinc stearate in ethylene toluene sulfonamide reacts with a base paste containing calcium tungstate, calcium phosphate, and zinc oxide in glycol salicylate to form an amorphous calcium disalicylate. The alkaline pH (pH 12.5) aids in preventing bacterial invasion. Studies have shown that calcium hydroxide "softens" under amalgam and resin-based composite restorations.[1,2] The results are attributed to hydrolysis of the calcium hydroxide by fluid contamination from dentinal tubules and microleakage. As hydrolysis occurs, occlusal forces cause apical displacement of the restoration, leading to discrepancies and breakdown at the restoration margin. Visible light–cured calcium hydroxide preparations have demonstrated clinical success[3] and may be less susceptible to hydrolysis. When calcium hydroxide is used, a less soluble high-strength base material such as glass ionomer may be placed to overlie the calcium hydroxide.

Zinc Oxide–Eugenol

Zinc oxide–eugenol cement (Fig. 29.2) contains zinc oxide, rosin, and zinc acetate in the powder. The rosin increases fracture resistance, and the zinc acetate is effective in accelerating the reaction rate. The liquid is a preparation of eugenol, which reacts with the powder to form an amorphous chelate of zinc eugenolate. The zinc oxide–eugenol cements are used to provide a sedative effect in deep preparations, but their low compressive strength presents clinical limitations.

To strengthen zinc oxide–eugenol cements, acrylic resin and alumina reinforcers have been added. For example, intermediate restorative material is a polymer-reinforced zinc oxide–eugenol cement. Although these cements are stronger, they remain weaker than the zinc phosphate and glass ionomer cements. When it was evaluated as a base, zinc oxide–eugenol demonstrated significant microleakage in comparison with glass ionomer cement.[4] Because of its sedative effects and years of clinical success, zinc oxide–eugenol remains the material of choice for the pulp chamber filling material after pulpotomies or pulpectomies in the primary dentition. However, reinforced zinc oxide–eugenol cement should not be used for pulpectomies in the primary dentition because it does not resorb well, resulting in remnants of cements in the furcation or periapical areas. Zinc oxide–eugenol cements should be used with caution under resin-based composite restorations because the eugenol can inhibit the polymerization of the resin. A glass ionomer cement base may be placed over zinc oxide–eugenol before the placement of resin-based composite to avoid polymerization.

TABLE 29.1 Commonly Used Biomaterials in Pediatric Dentistry

Materials	Types Available	Composition	Clinical Considerations
Intermediary bases	Calcium hydroxide Zinc oxide–eugenol[a]	Thin pastes of calcium hydroxide or zinc oxide and eugenol suspended in resins	Placed on small areas of cavity preparation deeper than ideal depth Placed on exposed dentin of preparations undergoing acid etching Used for direct pulp capping of permanent teeth Must not be left on enamel of preparations
Amalgam	Lathe-cut Spherical Admixed Unicompositional[a]	Silver (40%–74%) Tin (25%–30%) Copper (2%–30%) Zinc (0%–2%) Mercury (0%–3%)	A high copper (>6%) admixed or unicompositional, precapsulated alloy is recommended for restoration of pit and fissure and interproximal caries in posterior teeth
Stainless steel crowns	Straight sides Precontoured[a] Pretrimmed[a]	Iron (65%–73%) Chromium (17%–20%) Nickel (8%–13%) Manganese, silicon, and carbon (<2%)	Restoration of grossly damaged teeth, usually posterior, must be well trimmed, contoured, polished, and cemented to ensure optimum gingival health
Filled resin-based composite	(Based on filler size) Traditional, 5–30 μm Microfill, 0.04–1 μm[a] Hybrids, 0.04–100 μm[a] (available as auto-cure or visible light–activated)[a]	Dimethacrylate Bisphenol A-glycidyl methacrylate (Bis-GMA) resin or urethane matrix with filler particles of quartz, silicates, or glass	Esthetic restoration of anterior teeth Available for use in class I and II restorations in posterior teeth Microfills provide most polishable surfaces and have excellent esthetics Hybrids demonstrate least shrinkage and wear and have good polish and esthetics Visible light activation provides better polymerization control, better color stability, and less porosity than autopolymerized resins
Cements	Glass ionomer[a] Reinforced zinc oxide and eugenol[a] Zinc oxide–eugenol	Silicate glass containing Ca, Al, F, polycarboxylic acid Zinc oxide reinforced with alumina, polymer, or eugenol Zinc oxide, eugenol	Primary use is cementation of stainless steel crowns or zirconia crowns May be used as a base Glass ionomer may be used as a liner for resins and conservative restorations in primary teeth Reinforced zinc oxide and eugenol most frequently used for obliterating primary pulp chambers after pulpotomy and pulpectomy

[a]Types most frequently used.

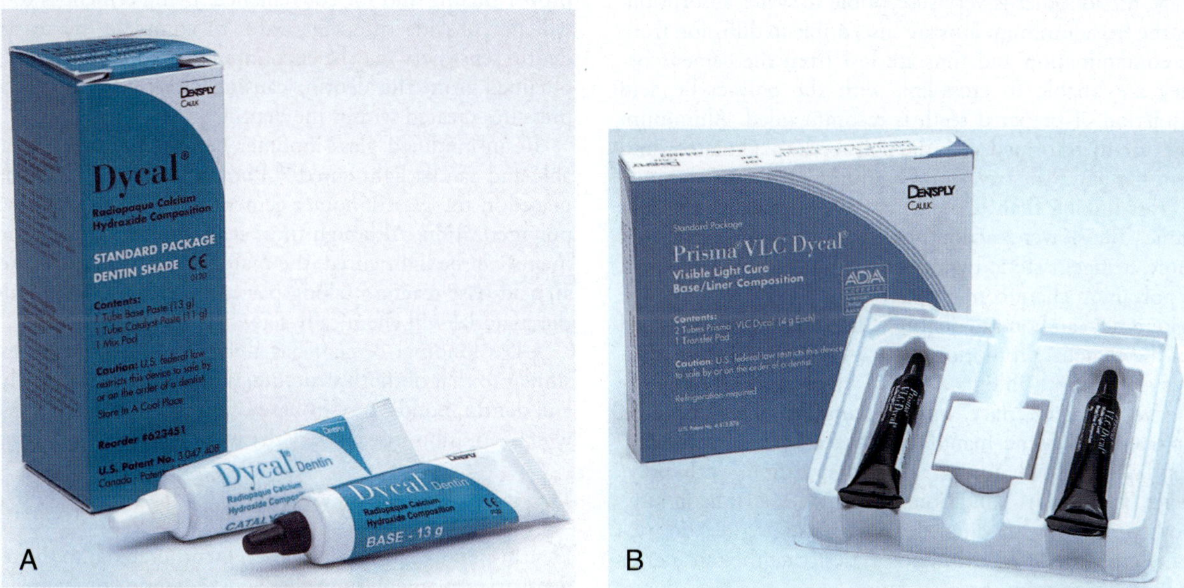

• **Fig. 29.1** Calcium Hydroxide Cements. (A) Two-paste system (Dycal). (B) Visible light–cured system (Prisma VLC Dycal). (Courtesy DENTSPLY Caulk, Milford, DE.)

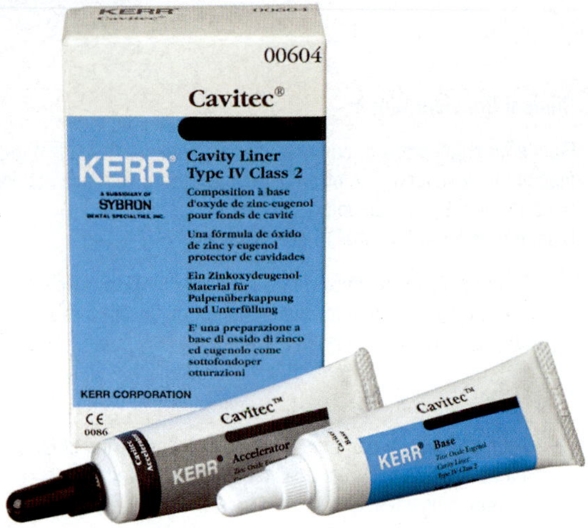

• **Fig. 29.2** Zinc oxide–eugenol cement (Cavitec). (Courtesy Kerr Corporation, Orange, CA.)

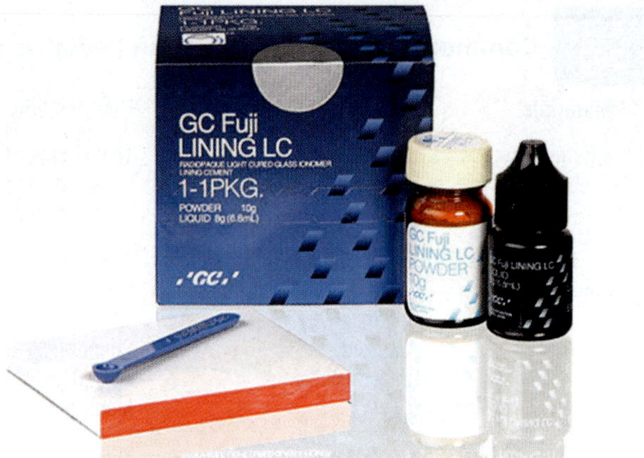

• **Fig. 29.3** Glass ionomer cement (GC Fuji Lining LC). (Courtesy GC America, Alsip, IL.)

Glass Ionomer Cement

Glass ionomer cement (Fig. 29.3) is a commonly used base agent. It creates a physicochemical bond to tooth structure and releases fluoride. Glass ionomer cement consists of calcium aluminosilicate glass particles mixed with polyacrylic acid. The initial reaction stage involves the ionization of polyacrylic acid, which leads to a change in the polymer chains from a coiled to a linear form. The hydrogen ions produced by ionization attack the calcium aluminosilicate glass, which also contains fluoride, and causes the release of metal and fluoride ions. Most of the metal cations (Ca^{2+}, Al^{3+}), divalent or trivalent, respectively, are bound by the ionized polymer to form cross-linked salt bridges. Calcium and aluminum ions bind to polyacrylic acid at the carboxyl groups, and a gel phase is precipitated to form a matrix of the hardening cement. Calcium carboxylates are formed first as a firm gel because of the rapid binding of calcium to the polyacrylic acid chains. This initial set has the property of being able to carve, but at this stage the ionomer is very susceptible to water absorption. Likewise, the free aluminum ions are susceptible to diffusion from moisture contamination and thus are lost from the cement because they are unable to cross-link with the polyacrylic acid chains. Isolation of prepared teeth is recommended. Aluminum salt bridges are then formed with the polyacrylic acid matrix, and the cement hardens. The trivalent aluminum ions ensure a much stronger cross-linking than is possible with the calcium divalent bonds alone. The slower reaction of aluminum ions is attributed to the more stringent steric requirements imposed by a trivalent ion on a polyanion chain configuration.

Glass ionomer can bond to dentin by free hydrophilic carboxyl groups in the cement, promoting surface wetting to form hydrogen bonds at the tooth interface. At the same time, an ionic exchange occurs at the interface, with calcium ions being displaced by phosphate ions. Some manufacturers recommend removing the smear layer, created during cavity preparation, with polyacrylic acid. This tooth "conditioning" provides an uncontaminated tooth surface for bonding. Because the setting reaction requires some moisture, it is critical not to desiccate the tooth after rinsing conditioning from the preparation.

Tartaric acid is added to the glass ionomer cement to accelerate the rate of hardening without decreasing the working time. Itaconic acid may be placed in glass ionomer mixtures to increase the reactivity of the polyacrylic acid to the glass, and polymaleic acid may be added to modify the reaction.

Studies have shown that glass ionomer bases and liners exhibit less marginal microleakage than zinc oxide–eugenol, zinc phosphate, and calcium hydroxide,[4,5] thereby preventing bacterial penetration. Fluoride is released from glass ionomer cement by dissolution and diffusion. Glass ionomer bases and liners have demonstrated the inhibition of secondary caries formation.[6–9] The fluoride released is taken up by both the enamel and dentin adjacent to the material.[10–13] This fluoride aids in creating an inhibition zone that is not susceptible to demineralization, compared with areas adjacent to non–fluoride-releasing materials.[14,15]

Glass ionomer cements are supplied in anhydrous and hydrous forms. Because of the viscosity of the hydrous form, mixing the cement may be difficult. The anhydrous form has a longer shelf life because the polyacrylic acid is dehydrated and placed in the powder. It is critical that glass ionomer be mixed according to the manufacturer's instructions. Glass ionomer cements are available in capsule form, which may help avoid any errors caused by improper mixing and for convenience. If the cement is too thick it will not provide sufficient water to complete the reaction, and dentin sensitivity may be encountered; the necessary water will be obtained from the dentin, causing sensitivity due to hydraulic pressures created within the dentin.

Resin-modified glass ionomer cement preparations are available and can be light cured.[16] Photoinitiated polymers have been placed in the glass ionomer cement formulation to provide light polymerization. Although these resin-modified glass ionomer cements can be light cured, the material sets as a true cement, with an acid-base reaction taking place; therefore, given enough time, the material will chemically set without light curing.

Glass ionomer cement has a coefficient of thermal expansion similar to that of tooth structure; it can protect an underlying base and dentin, bonds to resin-based composite, and releases fluoride, which can inhibit secondary decay.

Dentin-Bonding Agents

Dentin-bonding agents have been incorporated into the restorative dentistry armamentarium. Previously, dentin- or enamel-bonding agents fell into two groups. The first was halophosphorus esters of 2,2-bis[4-(2-hydroxy-3-methacryloyloxypropyloxy)phenyl] propane (Bis-GMA). The second group was categorized as polyurethanes. The polyurethanes are halophosphorus esters of hydroxyethyl methacrylate. Both dentin-bonding agents relied on a phosphate-calcium bond for retention.

Removal of the smear layer was found to increase the effectiveness of the dentin-bonding agents. The newer bonding agents include conditioning or primer components that remove or alter the smear layer over the dentin. This results in the creation of a mechanical bond by the infiltration of monomers into a zone of demineralized dentin, where the monomers polymerize and interlock with the dentin matrix.[17] Most of the contemporary dentin-bonding agents are similar to those previously discussed or are composed of 4-methacryloxyethyl trimellitic anhydride.

Self-etching bonding systems (Fig. 29.4) offer the convenience of etching and bonding simultaneously. Although research demonstrates adequate bonds to dentin and enamel, caution is advised. The products must be used as instructed by the manufacturer, particularly focusing on agitation of the product during placement and the recommended length of application time.[18,19]

Restorative Materials

Amalgam

Traditionally, amalgam was the material of choice for class I and class II restorations. Today amalgam continues to be an effective restorative material.[20,21] A 3-year study of the clinical performance of 260 amalgam restorations (86.4% class II) demonstrated 254 to be successful.[22] It is important to understand the clinical makeup and setting reaction of amalgam to correlate restoration successes and failures with the fundamental properties of the material.

Amalgamation

Dental amalgam consists of an alloy mix of silver, copper, tin, and, in some cases, zinc particles combined with mercury. The alloy particles have either a spherical or comminuted (lathe-cut) configuration. The unreacted alloy particles are termed the *silver-tin (gamma) phase.* These particles are combined with mercury, which acts as a wetting agent of the alloy particles to initiate the setting reaction termed *amalgamation.* The particle surfaces react with mercury to form a cementing matrix, consisting of the gamma 1 and gamma 2 phases. The gamma 1 phase employs the binding of silver and mercury (Ag_2-Hg_3). The gamma 2 phase involves the binding of tin and mercury (Sn_7-Hg). The gamma 2 phase is responsible for early fracture and failure of the comminuted particle amalgam restorations. Tin cannot be eliminated from the alloy because of its importance in the setting reaction and control of dimensional change of amalgam. To avoid the detrimental gamma 2 phase, copper was introduced into the amalgamation reaction. The copper replaced the tin-mercury phase with a copper-tin phase (Cu_6-Sn_5). The copper-tin matrix decreases the corrosion of tin, preventing secondary weakening with subsequent fracture of the restoration.

The amount of mercury needed to complete the amalgamation reaction is contingent on the alloy composition and particle configuration but usually falls between 42% and 54% of the amalgam mix. When mercury exceeds 55%, there is a detrimental reduction in amalgam strength. Spherical alloy particles with the addition of copper require less mercury than comminuted particles to complete the amalgamation process. It is important to point out that once amalgamation occurs, unreacted mercury is not available; the mercury is alloyed with silver, tin, or copper. Zinc is present in some alloy mixes to act as a scavenger for oxygen, which inhibits the formation of copper, silver, or tin oxides, thus weakening the amalgam restoration. Using preencapsulated amalgam (Fig. 29.5) and strictly following the manufacturer's recommendations for trituration and manipulation are critical for achieving restoration success.

Properties

Hardening amalgam may expand or contract depending on the type and manipulation of the material. The American Dental Association[23] requires that there be no more than 20 μm/cm of expansion or contraction after 24 hours.

The compressive strength required by the Council on Dental Materials and Devices[23] for amalgam is 11,600 psi (88 MN/m^2) after 1 hour. Tensile strength is substantially lower; therefore cavity preparation design becomes critical. The preparation should have a design that allows the amalgam to be condensed as a "bulk" of material, avoiding shallow depths and a thin isthmus where fracture may occur. Comminuted and spherical low-copper amalgam demonstrates decreased marginal fracture resistance. This is partially due to the increased creep of these amalgams. Creep is

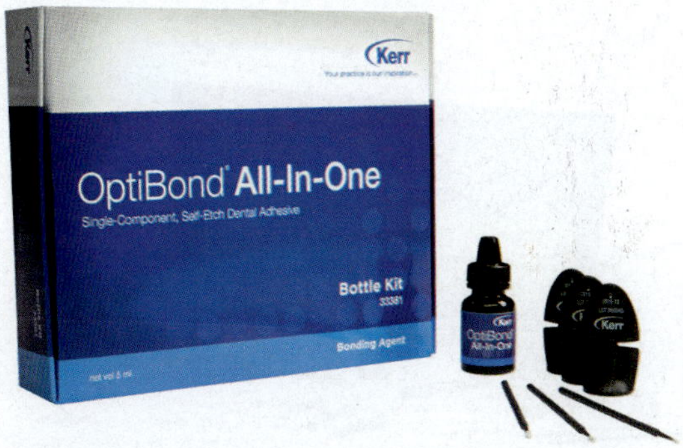

• **Fig. 29.4** Self-etching bonding system (OptiBond All-In-One). (Courtesy Kerr Corporation, Orange, CA.)

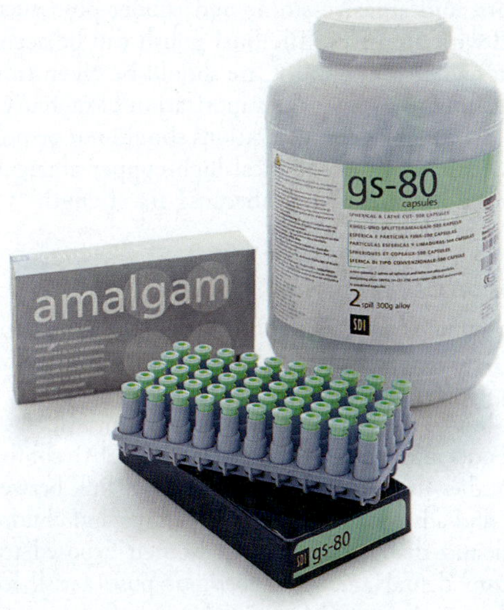

• **Fig. 29.5** Preencapsulated amalgam (GS-80). (Courtesy SDI [North America], Bensenville, IL.)

the dimensional change that occurs when amalgam sustains a load during mastication, a result of the viscoelastic property of amalgam. The American Dental Association requires that an amalgam have a maximum of 5% creep to be certified.

Corrosion, a chemical or electrochemical deterioration of amalgam, occurs at the surface or subsurface. Deterioration may be caused by pitting or scratching secondary to poor condensation, carving, or finishing of amalgam, which allows food or saliva components to attack the chemical matrix. Dissimilar metals in contact with each other can also cause corrosion as a result of galvanic action that encourages the materials to go into the solution. This leads to pitting and food entrapment within the pits, which subsequently causes further corrosion. The gamma 2 phase (tin-mercury) is most susceptible to corrosion; therefore the spherical high-copper amalgams are the least susceptible. Although extensive corrosion can lead to restoration failure, minimal corrosion in conjunction with creep allows open restoration margins to be packed full enough with corrosion byproducts to significantly close these margins.

Condensation

Amalgam should be placed and condensed immediately after trituration, according to the manufacturer's recommendations. Placement of amalgam in small increments is appropriate. Condensation allows force to be applied for material adaptation with a minimum of excess mercury. Use of small condensers with firm pressure on small increments of amalgam minimizes voids within the final restoration. A delay in condensation should be avoided because the initial hardening that occurs after trituration but before condensation may make the effective removal of excessive mercury more difficult. This, in turn, decreases restoration's strength and increases the creep in the material. Moisture contamination should also be controlled because excess moisture causes delayed expansion, particularly in zinc-containing alloys. The use of isolation devices can prevent moisture contamination and isolate the working field effectively.

Finishing and Polishing

Finishing and polishing of the amalgam surface are highly recommended. Small scratches and pits can be removed with finishing burs, and abrasive stones and rubber points can be impregnated with abrasives. The final polish can be accomplished with a tin oxide compound. Care should be taken to use water when polishing to prevent the vaporization of mercury from the amalgam. Most amalgam restorations should not be polished for 24 hours, although the spherical high-copper amalgam can be polished almost immediately because its strength is obtained rapidly.

Concerns on Using Amalgam

Amalgam remains the most controversial dental material in use. Multiple randomized controlled trials and systematic reviews have demonstrated no adverse effect on the nervous system or kidney function, but concerns regarding health risk persist.[24–26] In 2009, the US Food and Drug Administration (FDA) confirmed that clinical studies had not established a causal link between dental amalgam and adverse health effects in adults and children aged 6 and older and that breast milk of women exposed to mercury vapors from dental amalgam does not pose a risk for adverse health effects in infants.[27] Despite these confirmations, the FDA reclassified dental amalgam to a Class II device indicating that it carried some risk. Warning labels were added to disclose the possible harm of mercury vapors and identify mercury content, and its use was contraindicated in persons with a known mercury sensitivity.[28] In 2020, the FDA updated their guidance to avoid the use of amalgam in additional high-risk groups, including pregnant women, women who are planning to become pregnant, nursing women, children (especially those under the age of 6), people with preexisting neurologic conditions, and those with impaired kidney function.[29] Because there was lack of evidence from clinical trials showing harm in these patient populations, the FDA explicitly advised against replacing existing amalgam restorations in good condition.[29]

In addition to health-related fears, environmental concerns have limited the use of amalgam. Amalgam is banned in Norway[30] and Sweden,[31] and it is being phased out in the European Union.[32] The United States and 122 other countries have signed onto the Minamata Convention on Mercury, which seeks to phase out or reduce mercury use in certain products, including dental amalgam.[33]

The combination of parental desires for esthetic restorations, perceived health concerns, and increasing environmental regulation has resulted in a shift from amalgam use to composite or glass ionomer restorations. An analysis of private insurance claims shows use of amalgam in pediatric dentistry has decreased considerably.[34] A recent study conducted in the United States found that the usage of amalgam has declined among the general population from 21.8% in 2017 to 4.1% in 2023.[35] A 2019 survey of members of the American Academy of Pediatric Dentistry (AAPD) found that only 45% of respondents were using amalgam.[36] Regardless, the AAPD best practice on restorative dentistry lists dental amalgam as an option for class I and II restorations in primary and permanent teeth.[37]

Resin-Based Composite

Resin-based composite (Fig. 29.6) has become one of the most widely used contemporary restorative materials over the past 30 years. Currently resin composite is used for sealants and for class I through V restorations in primary and permanent teeth.[38,39] Resin-based composite restorations have been accepted primarily because of their excellent esthetic qualities. Other advantages include relatively low thermal conductivity, preservation of tooth structure in cavity preparation, and advances in the stability of compositional properties of the material.

Conventional resin-based composites were viscous fluid nonvolatile monomers (Bis-GMA) that have filler particles incorporated into the resin. Bowen[40] formulated the Bis-GMA resin by synthesizing a dimethacrylate monomer, the product of the reaction between bisphenol A and glycidyl methacrylate. Many

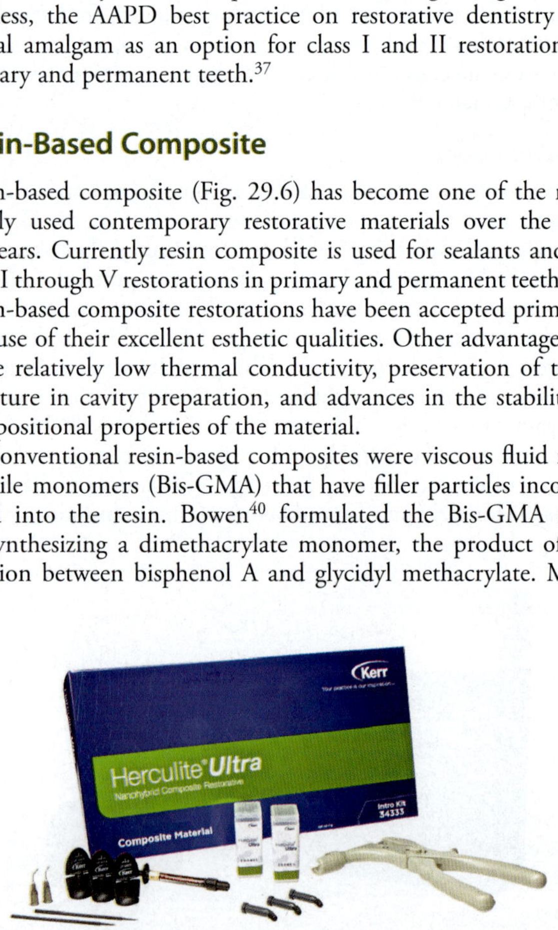

• **Fig. 29.6** Resin-based composite system (Herculite Ultra). (Courtesy Kerr Corporation, Orange, CA.)

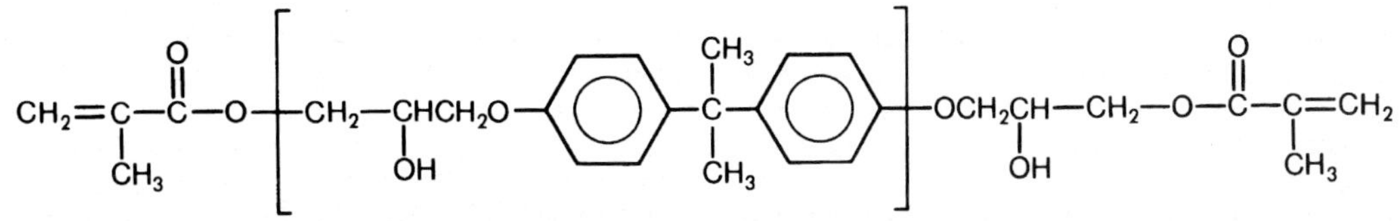

• **Fig. 29.7** Chemical composition of 2,2-bis[4-(2-hydroxy-3-methacryloyloxypropyloxy)phenyl] propane (Bis-GMA).

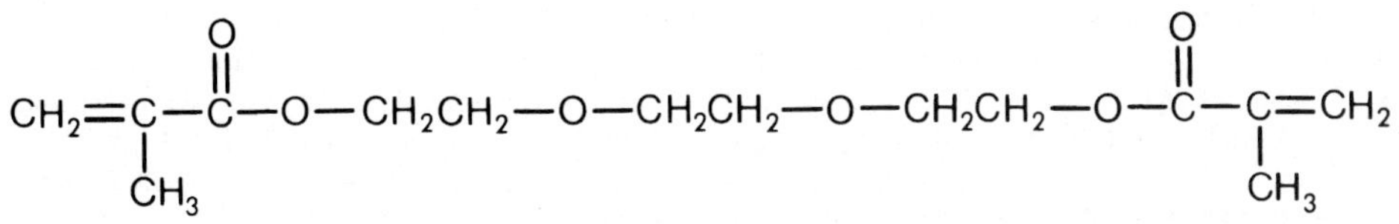

• **Fig. 29.8** Chemical composition of triethylene glycol dimethacrylate (TEGDMA).

contemporary composite restorative materials contain dimethacrylate monomers (Bis-GMA) as the major component of the matrix phase. A relatively low-viscosity monomer (triethylene glycol dimethacrylate [TEGDMA]), which helps produce the desired handling qualities of the material, is an important component of the matrix phase. Fig. 29.7 schematically illustrates the chemical structure of Bis-GMA, and Fig. 29.8 illustrates the chemical structure of TEGDMA.

Incorporated into the monomer matrix are filler particles. A small number of available products contain urethane dimethacrylates rather than the Bis-GMA matrix. Initially, fused quartz and various glasses were incorporated into the Bis-GMA monomer as filler particles, providing a reinforced resin composite. The fillers were coated with a vinyl silane coupling agent, with the silane chemically bonding with the polymer matrix.[41] These particles were usually irregularly shaped to provide mechanical retention in the resin.

Composites available today contain quartz, colloidal silica, borosilicate glasses, and glasses containing barium, strontium, and zinc. Excluding quartz and colloidal silica, these filler particles give the material radiopacity, which is clinically advantageous during radiographic examination. Contemporary posterior resin-based composites contain a high percentage by volume of filler particles. This composition provides wear resistance and more stability.[42] Thermal expansion and polymerization contraction are both reduced by increasing the volume percentage of filler particles. The increased filler content, needed for wear resistance, requires a decrease in matrix resin polymer, therefore allowing for a reduction in the amount of shrinkage that occurs upon polymerization. As the concentration of filler particles increases, the modulus of elasticity increases and tends to minimize shrinkage.[43]

Resin-based composites absorb water, yet hygroscopic expansion is very infrequently sufficient to compensate for polymerization shrinkage.[44,45] Therefore the incremental placement and polymerization of resin-based composite are critical during restorative procedure.[46–49]

Chemically Polymerized Resin-Based Composite

The traditional chemically activated resin-based composites form cross-links during copolymerization of methyl methacrylate and ethylene glycol dimethacrylate. The dimethacrylate monomers polymerize by means of free radical–initiated polymerization to form the organic matrix of a three-dimensional network. This highly viscous monomer can undergo free radical addition polymerization to provide a rigid cross-linked polymer. Usually, the benzoyl peroxide present in one paste acts as the initiator, whereas a tertiary amine (dihydroxyethyl-*p*-toluidine) acts as the catalyst in the other paste.[50]

Visible Light–Polymerized Resin-Based Composite

Today most resin-based composites are visible light–activated materials (see Fig. 29.6). This allows for more controlled, incremental placement of material into a cavity preparation. The visible light–activated composites usually contain a diketone initiator (camphorquinone) and an amine catalyst (dimethylaminoethyl methacrylate). The diketone absorbs light at approximately 470 nm to form an excited state, which, together with the amine, results in ion radicals to initiate free radical polymerization.[51]

DENTAL LIGHT-CURING UNITS

Sharukh S. Khajotia and Fernando L. Esteban Florez

Dental light-curing units are handheld devices that are used for the polymerization of visible light–activated dental materials. The four types of light-curing units that are currently available include quartz-tungsten-halogen (QTH), light-emitting diode (LED), plasma arc curing (PAC), and Argon laser units.

QTH light-curing units are the most widely used, although LED lights are increasingly popular in the United States, and are made of a quartz bulb containing a tungsten filament in a halogen environment. QTH units emit ultraviolet irradiation and visible light (broad-spectrum), which is filtered to limit the wavelength output to between 400 and 500 nm while also minimizing heat. The intensity of light emitted by a QTH bulb ranges from 400 to 1200 mW/cm^2 and can decrease with use. The use of a radiometer is recommended for the routine monitoring of the light intensity, and permitting the built-in fan to cool the QTH bulb is recommended to facilitate optimal function of the unit. These lights deliver lower energy and need a 40-second cure.

LED light-curing units emit light in the blue part of the visible spectrum, typically between 440 and 490 nm, and do not emit heat. Therefore LED units do not require filters. They can be powered by rechargeable batteries because they require low wattage, and they are quieter than QTH units because they do not need a cooling fan. Initial versions of LED units emitted a lower intensity of light, whereas newer versions incorporate multiple LEDs with a variety of ranges of wavelengths to broaden the spectrum of the emitted light and increase the overall intensity in order to adequately polymerize all visible light–activated dental materials. Most manufacturers recommend a 20-second cure with an LED with a minimum irradiance of 800 mW/cm^2, and dentists should check for specific instructions.

PAC light-curing units contain a xenon gas that is ionized to produce plasma. The high-intensity white light emitted is filtered to minimize heat and to limit the output to the violet-blue part of the visible spectrum (400 to 500 nm). Argon laser units emit the highest intensity and emit light at a single wavelength (approximately 490 nm). The higher costs associated with the use and maintenance of the PAC and Argon laser units has limited their widespread use in dentistry.

Visible light–activated dental materials contain an initiator such as camphorquinone (CQ) that absorbs light at the appropriate wavelength (approximately 470 nm for CQ). The free radicals necessary for the initiation of polymerization are generated when the initiator combines with an organic amine such as dimethylaminoethyl methacrylate. The wavelength, intensity, and duration of exposure to light determine the number of photons absorbed by the initiator and therefore impact optimal polymerization. Factors such as light-curing unit intensity, angle of illumination, diameter of the tip of the light source, distance from the light source, and duration of exposure can significantly affect the number of free radicals formed, thereby making this system highly technique sensitive. Initiators other than CQ are also used in visible light–activated materials and are typically activated in the violet part of the spectrum (400 nm). Because they absorb light at different wavelengths than CQ, some curing lights are made with dual- or polywave technology. It is critical that the light-curing unit used emits light at the requisite wavelength for that particular initiator.[52]

Newer light-curing units have higher intensities, typically greater than 1000 mW/cm^2 with an approximate wavelength of 385 to 515 nm, which permit either shorter durations of cure for a given depth of cure or increased depth of cure for a given duration of cure (VALO LED Curing Lights, Ultradent Products Inc, South Jordan, UT). The use of these higher intensity lights can, however, produce higher shrinkage stresses within the restoration. It is important to remember that the type of light-curing unit and curing mode used affect the polymerization kinetics, polymerization shrinkage, and associated stresses, microhardness, depth of cure, degree of conversion, color change, and microleakage in visible light–activated restorations. Lastly, precautions such as protective eyewear and light shields are critical for the safety of the patient and clinic personnel when using dental light-curing units.

In an attempt to reduce polymerization shrinkage, resin molecules longer than Bis-GMA have been placed in resin-based composites. An example would be EMA-6, which can be found in Filtek Z250 (Fig. 29.9; 3M ESPE Dental Products, St. Paul, MN).[53]

Problems that may be associated with light-activated resin-based composites include polymerization toward the light source, sensitivity of composite to ambient light, and variability in the depth of polymerization because of the intensity of light penetration. Polymerization toward the light source may cause the resin-based composite to pull away from the walls of the preparation. Sensitivity of resin-based composite to ambient light may cause initial polymerization before placement of the material into the preparation. Variability in the depth of light penetration, differences in curing light intensity, diameter of the tip of the light source, and time of light exposure can result in variations of polymerization. The benefits of light-activated resin composites include ease of manipulation, control of polymerization, and lack of need for mixing. Since mixing is not required with light-activated composites, it is less likely that air will be incorporated and form voids in the mixture.

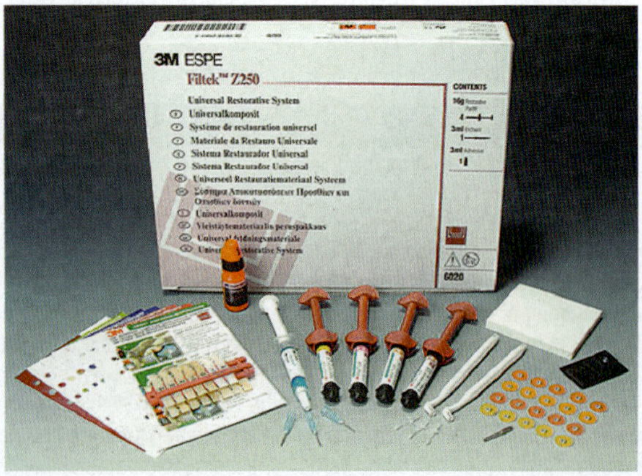

• **Fig. 29.9** Resin-based composite with EMA-6 (Filtek Z250). (Courtesy 3M ESPE Dental Products, St Paul, MN.)

Bulk-Fill Resins

Extensive efforts have been made over the past decade to develop low shrinkage resin-based composites through advances in filler technology and monomer chemistry.[54,55]

Conventionally the maximum incremental thickness of resin-based composite that provided adequate light penetration and polymerization was defined as 2 mm.[56,57] Use of these conventional materials requires a layering technique that is time consuming and has the potential to introduce voids, thus increasing the risk of failure.[58] The risk of failure presents itself clinically by allowing the ingress of bacteria, ultimately leading to secondary caries, pulpal inflammation, necrosis, or postoperative sensitivity.

Recently a new class of resin composite materials, the bulk-fill resin composites, has been introduced. Clinical recommendations suggest that these materials have a greater depth of cure, which allows them to be placed in 4-mm bulk increments and still have adequate polymerization.

This innovative technology is based on changes in monomer chemistry by modifying the Bowen monomer (Bis-GMA: 2,2 bis [4-(2-hydroxy-3-methacryloxypropoxy) phenyl] propane) to create monomers with lower viscosity.[59–62] This new modification is achieved by incorporating hydroxyl-free Bis-GMA aliphatic urethane dimethacrylate or highly branched methacrylates.[63] The outcomes of these changes in monomer and composite organic matrix have been shown to reduce polymerization shrinkage stresses over 70%.[64]

Resin-Based Composite Wear

Initial resin-based composites used for posterior restorations exhibited excessive occlusal wear. Studies have shown that when conventional composites are placed in high stress concentration areas, excessive wear occurs.[65–68] Further investigations pursued factors that might influence the rate of wear, such as the size and hardness of the filler particles, the amount of porosity within the material, and the method of polymerization.[69] It was found that the ceramic filler particles nearly always remained intact. There was no evidence of wear on the particles themselves; they were found to be hard enough to cause wear of the surrounding unfilled resin during mastication until the resin matrix gradually wore away from the particles. Once a critical portion of the filler particle was exposed, it was easily dislodged. Although there seemed to be a correlation between the size of the filler particle and its hardness (larger particles possessing a more critical hardness), substantially larger particles were found to accelerate the wear. Therefore the hardness of particles is not necessarily the most significant factor affecting wear. The ideal material would have particles that have adequate hardness, are distributed within minimal unfilled resin, and have the least abrasion potential during mastication.[70] Thus, more recently, nanoparticles have been introduced as filler particles.

Porosity has been shown to be a major factor in the wear rate of posterior resin-based composites.[69,71] All resin restorations contain a certain degree of porosity and voids. These defects can be minimized by careful placement technique and polishing of the material. Because light-cured composites do not require mixing, they contain fewer voids. Problems of wear appear to be improved with newer composites. Composite resins are vacuum packed to decrease porosity. It is important to note that mixing shades for esthetics may increase the porosity. This problem is created from the incorporation of air during the mixing process. Current posterior resin-based composites show minimal wear. This has been achieved by incorporating a variety of particle sizes into the polymer matrix. The increased filler content decreases the amount of matrix resin polymer. The mechanism of wear is hypothesized to be caused by the loss of the resin matrix. Increasing wear resistance is believed to be possible because the filler particles are closely packed, thereby leaving little unfilled resin exposed.

Marginal Adaptation

The use of resin-based composites for restoring posterior teeth has historically presented the problem of marginal leakage at the resin-tooth interface.[72] This marginal leakage caused teeth with posterior resin-based composite restorations to be more prone to secondary caries than teeth with amalgam restorations. Failure of the composite to bond to the cavity preparation walls and voids in the restorative material have been identified as the causes of inadequate marginal adaptation. This problem has been reduced by (1) using contemporary posterior resin-based composites, which contain a high volume of filler that decreases polymerization shrinkage; (2) using an enamel bevel; (3) using newer dentin-bonding agents and glass ionomer cements; and (4) acid etching the enamel.

Formulations

Enamel-bonding agents

The use of phosphoric acid (35% to 50%) results in an acid-etched surface on enamel that creates an effective mechanical bond with the Bis-GMA enamel-bonding agent. Enamel-bonding agents (Fig. 29.10) are placed over the acid-etched enamel before composite placement. The bonding agents are merely unfilled dimethacrylates and are used because their low viscosity allows easy penetration of the etched enamel surface. The resin matrix of the resin-based composite will then chemically bond to the bonding agent.

Sealants

The use of pit and fissure sealants has been effective in preventing occlusal caries for almost five decades.[73–75] Traditional sealants are hydrophobic and are composed of a Bis-GMA resin structure used in resin-based composites. The Bis-GMA monomer is diluted with low-weight dimethacrylate monomer to make the sealant material a fluid that can easily penetrate the pits and fissures of occlusal surfaces. A new generation of resin-based sealants is formulated with hydrophilic resins that behave favorably in the moist environment (Fig. 29.11). These materials contain no Bis-GMA or bisphenol A derivatives. A recent systematic review found no difference in the retention or caries prevention ability of hydrophilic resin-based sealants compared with conventional sealants resin or glass ionomer sealants at 12-month follow-up; however, future studies are required to investigate long-term outcomes.[76]

Although the use of sealants is an excellent preventive technique, initially there were concerns that caries could occur at sealant margins or where the sealant had partially broken away. The concept of adding fluoride-releasing resins was examined for caries inhibition and found to be effective in vitro.[77] Most sealants currently in use contain fluoride and are light cured. Two component systems that self-polymerize are also available. See Chapter 15 for a discussion of sealant properties.

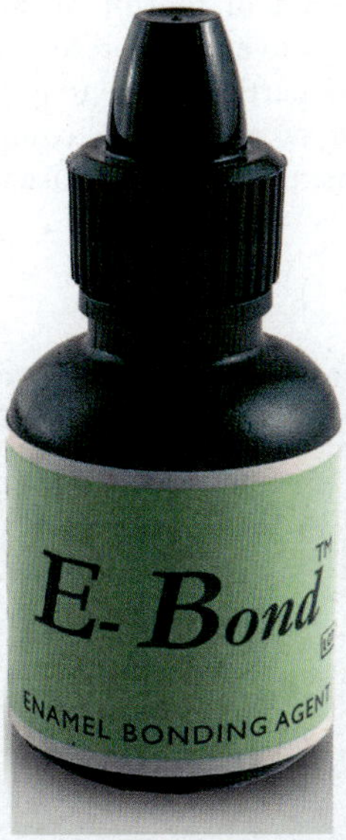

• **Fig. 29.10** Enamel bonding agent (E-Bond). (Courtesy Danville Materials, San Ramon, CA.)

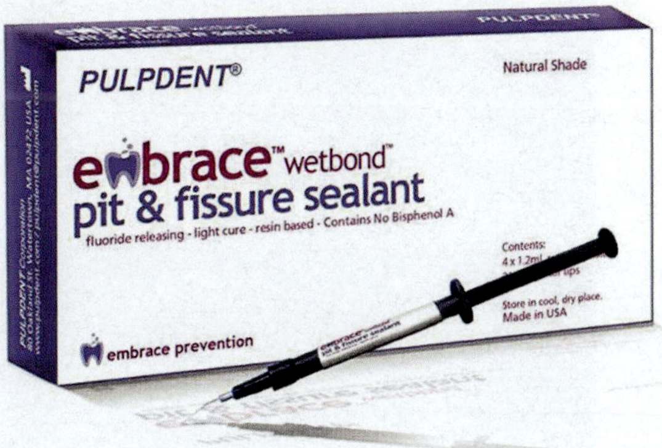

• **Fig. 29.11** Pit and fissure sealant (EMRACE WetBond). (Courtesy Pulpdent Corporation, Watertown, MA.)

Microfilled resin–based composite

Microfilled resin–based composite (Fig. 29.12A) has silane-treated colloidal silica filler particles in a Bis-GMA resin. Traditional microfilled composites contained approximately 50% (by volume) filler particles. Because of the high percentage of resin matrix, the particle configuration, and the small particle size (<1 µm in diameter), this resin composite is easily polished and reaches a high luster. Microfilled composites are recommended for restorations that are highly visible yet encounter minimal stress during mastication. The low percentage of filler results in a decrease in strength and an increase in wear. To compensate for polymerization shrinkage, some of the Bis-GMA resin in the composite is prepolymerized by the manufacturer.

More highly filled (>70% by volume) microfilled resin–based composites are available and can be effectively used in areas where greater wear and stress is anticipated.

Macrofilled resin–based composite

Macrofilled resin–based composite (Fig. 29.12B) has silane-treated filler particles (approximately 80% by volume) in a Bis-GMA resin. The particle sizes are much larger than those found in microfilled systems. Although these particles are larger than those found in the microfilled composites, they are smaller than the conventional resin-based composite particles. The high filler-particle percentage increases wear resistance. Because most of these resin composites are used for posterior restorations, the material is usually radiopaque from the filler type.

Hybrid resin–based composite

Hybrid resin–based composites (Fig. 29.12C) have a combination of small and large particles, representing the size of the particles found in microfilled and macrofilled resin–based composites, respectively. The high percentage of filler particles provides strength and wear resistance, yet the smaller filler particles allow for particles to arrange in close proximity to each other, which can provide minimal polymerization shrinkage and improved ability to polish compared with macrofilled composite. These resin-based composites are considered for restorations that may have stress-bearing areas during mastication but must have a well-polished surface.

Nanofilled resin–based composite

Since the introduction of resin-based composites, the size of filler particles has become smaller. More recently, nanofilled composites (Fig. 29.12D) that contain very small filler particles have been introduced. These resin composites offer the strength of a highly filled resin as well as ability to polish because of the small particles.

Glass Ionomer

Anterior Restorations

Preparations of glass ionomer cements are available in various shades that can be used for anterior restorations.[78,79] The use of glass ionomer for anterior restorations is limited to class III and class V preparations. The low fracture resistance and strength of mechanical bonding to enamel make its use impractical for class IV restorations. Retention of glass ionomer restorations in the

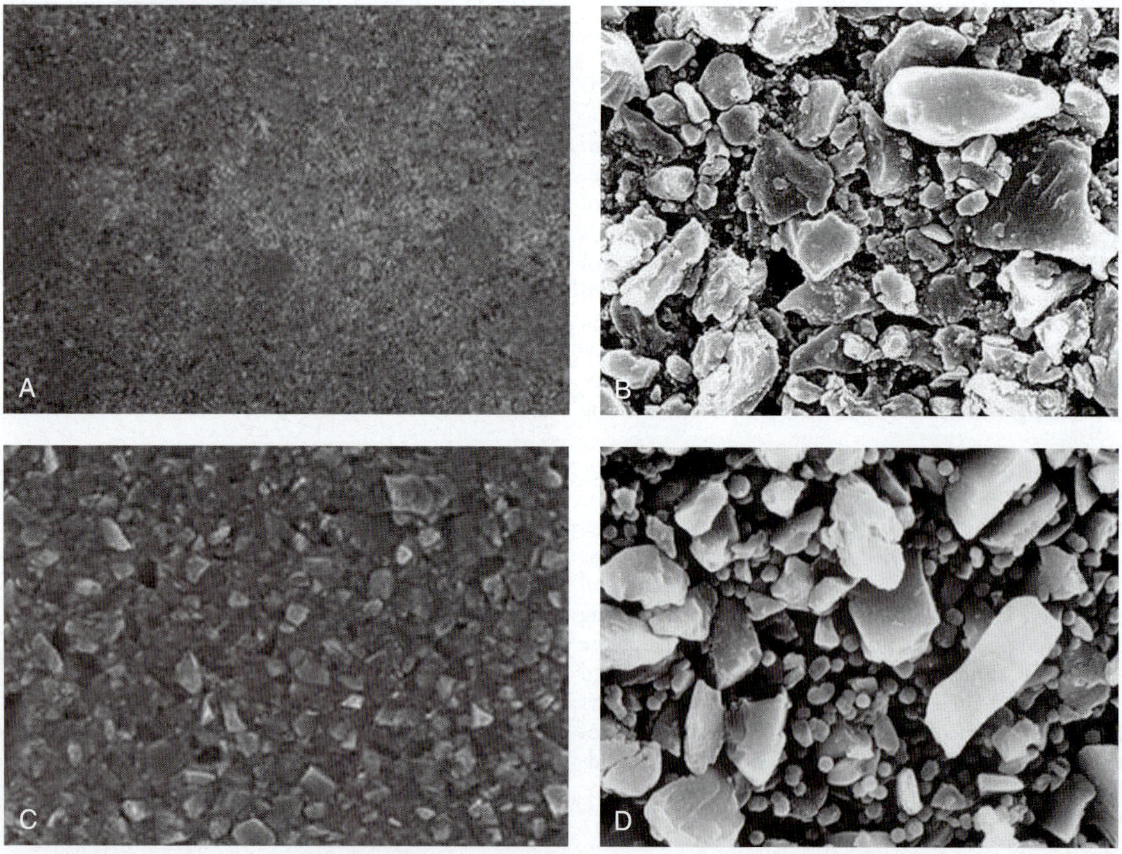

• **Fig. 29.12** (A) Microfill material. (B) Macrofill material. (C) Hybrid material. (D) Nanofill material. (From Freedman G. *Contemporary Esthetic Dentistry*. Mosby; 2012.)

restoration of class V preparations, where the gingival margin is not in enamel, may demonstrate favorable retention when restored with a glass ionomer rather than a resin-based composite. The fluoride release from glass ionomer restorations has been shown to inhibit the development of secondary caries.[77–80]

Posterior Restorations

The major disadvantage of glass ionomer cement as a posterior restorative material is its susceptibility to fracture and wear. Metal particles have been added to glass ionomer cement to increase their strength and wear resistance for posterior restorations. Fracture resistance remains a concern, and critical decisions should be made when using the material for posterior restorations. Investigations have demonstrated the clinical success of resin-modified glass ionomer cement as a posterior restorative material in the primary dentition.[81–85] Again, fluoride release and bonding capabilities are advantages of the glass ionomer cements.

Compomers

Compomers are recommended for use as a pediatric dental restorative material.[86–89] Compomers are a cross between resin-based composite and glass ionomer cement.

The compomers were developed in the hope of bringing the favorable properties of resin-based composite—such as wear resistance, color stability, and ability to polish—to the glass ionomers. An acid-base reaction takes place within the compomer material but is not the primary setting reaction; therefore visible light–polymerization is necessary to complete the setting reaction. Compomers are used with methacrylate primers that bond to enamel, dentin, and the compomer restorative material; therefore, for better retention, it is recommended to etch the tooth structure before placement of the restoration.

Luting Cements

Luting cements are frequently used in pediatric dentistry. Their primary use is for the cementation of stainless steel crowns and orthodontic bands. Zinc oxide–eugenol and glass ionomer are the cements most used. These cements were previously discussed in the section "Bases and Liners." The particles in glass ionomer cement are usually larger than those found in glass ionomer bases. There is less particle surface area available for reaction in the cement; therefore the cement sets more slowly than the base, allowing more working time. The importance of accuracy in the liquid/powder ratio of glass ionomer cement has been discussed. Encapsulated, premeasured cement is available and may be considered for clinical use. Automix syringe tips are available for the resin-modified glass ionomer materials as well.

Bioactive cements have more recently become available in the marketplace. These cements have glass particles incorporated into a resin matrix and have the advantage of bonding to tooth structure. The cements release calcium and fluoride. Manufacturers recommend these cements for cementing stainless steel, porcelain, and zirconia crowns.

The various cements most commonly used in pediatric dentistry and their clinical considerations are presented in Tables 29.1 and 29.2.

Stainless Steel Crowns

Stainless steel is an alloy of iron that is resistant to corrosion because of inclusion of over 10% of chromium. Stainless steel crowns in dentistry are made up of varying compositions of iron, nickel, chromium, and other minor elements.[90] Most of the crowns available in the market are prebelled, precrimped, and prefestooned to be able to adapt to the tooth structure with minimal trimming or contouring. Uncrimped anterior stainless steel crowns are also available. Stainless steel crowns are considered an ideal restorative option for carious or hypomineralized primary and permanent molars. Despite esthetic disadvantage, they are considered for durability, longevity, reliability, efficiency, and cost-effectiveness.

Monolithic Zirconia

Several options are available for restoration of primary anterior teeth.[90] Monolithic zirconia was introduced to dentistry almost two decades ago; more recently, it has been used for complete coverage crowns. The zirconia ceramic crown is very strong in flexural and compressive strength. A highly polished, glossy surface is very favorable to gingival tissue.[91] Monolithic zirconia

TABLE 29.2 Comparison of Dental Cements

Cement	Composition	Working Time	Setting Time	Compressive Strength	Bond Strength to Dentin	Release of Fluoride	Pulpal Response	Removal of Excess
Ideal	—	Medium	Short-medium	Very high	High	Yes	None	Easy
Glass ionomer	Silicate glass containing Ca, Al, F Polycarboxylic acid	Short-medium	Short	High	Medium	Yes	Low	Moderate
Bioactive	—	High	Medium	High	High	Yes	None	Moderate
Zinc oxide and eugenol	Zinc oxide Eugenol	Long	Medium	Low-medium	None	No	None	Easy
Reinforced zinc oxide and eugenol	Zinc oxide reinforced with alumina or polymer eugenol	Long	Medium-long	Low-medium	None	No	None	Easy

Modified from Farah JW, Powers JM. Cements. *Dent Advisor.* 1985;2(1):3.

crowns are now available for the esthetic restoration of primary anterior and posterior teeth.[92] These crowns come with retention grooves in the inner surface of the crown (EZ Crowns, Sprig, Loomis, CA) or without retention grooves (ZR Crowns, NuSmile, Houston, TX). Currently, manufacturers recommend the use of glass ionomer or resin-modified glass ionomer cements for zirconia, including bioactive cements (Bio Cem, NuSmile, Houston, TX; Ceramir, Doxa Dental Inc., Chicago, IL; Activa Bio Active Cement, Pulpdent Corporation, Watertown, MA). An in vitro study has demonstrated that natural teeth opposing zirconia crowns have a more favorable wear than natural teeth opposing porcelain crowns.[93] Although stainless steel crowns had demonstrated superior clinical performance for restoration of primary molars, several studies have found a similar success rate between the stainless steel crown and zirconia crowns.[94,95]

Visit eBooks.Health.Elsevier.com to see full list of references.

30

Restorative Dentistry for the Primary Dentition

TRAVIS NELSON, ELISE W. SARVAS, AND WILLIAM F. WAGGONER

CHAPTER OUTLINE

Pediatric restorative dentistry is a dynamic combination of materials science and technical skill, modified by the behavioral needs of the patient. In recent years there have been many exciting developments in restorative care for children, yet many aspects of primary tooth restoration have not changed for decades (Fig. 30.1). In 1924 G.V. Black outlined several steps for the preparation of carious permanent teeth to receive an amalgam restoration.[1] These steps have been adopted, with slight modification, for the restoration of primary teeth using adhesive materials. In turn, the increased use of adhesive restorative materials and bonding systems has supported a shift to more conservative and esthetic preparations and restorations. Materials such as glass ionomer and resin-based composite convey advantages such as bonding to tooth structure, fluoride release, improved esthetics, reduction of mercury exposure, and conservation of tooth structure. In addition, prefabricated zirconia crowns (ZCs) now offer an esthetic alternative to stainless steel crowns (SSCs). Although few of these esthetic materials have the lengthy track record of older materials, the evidence for their use is constantly improving. Today it is possible to provide durable and esthetic restorations that will satisfy caregivers and children, while lasting the life span of the primary tooth.

Anatomical Considerations of Primary Teeth

Although some primary teeth resemble their permanent successors, they are not miniature permanent teeth. These anatomical differences must be recognized by the operative dentist because they affect restoration choice and preparation design (Table 30.1; Fig. 30.2).

Instrumentation and Caries Removal

Nearly all instrumentation for restorative procedures is carried out with the high-speed handpiece (100,000 to 300,000 rpm, either electric or air turbine) combined with coolant. The coolant may be water spray or air alone. A water spray coolant is often recommended for high-speed instrumentation; however, there is some evidence that air coolant alone may be used without creating irreversible pulpal damage,[2,3] and use of both coolant techniques is taught in many pediatric dental residency programs.[4–6] There are some instances when a water spray coolant is strongly recommended. This is especially true when removing old amalgam restorations or using diamond burs. Regardless of the coolant used, intermittent cutting at intervals of a few seconds with light, brushing strokes should be done to prevent excessive heat generation. Protective masks and eyewear should always be worn when providing restorative treatment.

The low-speed handpiece (500 to 15,000 rpm) is primarily used for caries removal, and occasionally for polishing and finishing procedures. As with high-speed instrumentation, light pressure and brushing strokes should be used when operating the low-speed handpiece. Hand instrumentation is minimal in most primary dentition operative preparations, and it is usually limited to final caries removal.

Although use of a handpiece for caries removal and cavity preparation is by far the most popular and frequently used method, there are at least three other methods for treating carious teeth: air abrasion, laser treatment, and chemomechanical. With these methods, tooth preparations move from the conventional preparations used by G.V. Black to much more conservative, "tooth-saving" preparations used in minimally invasive dentistry.

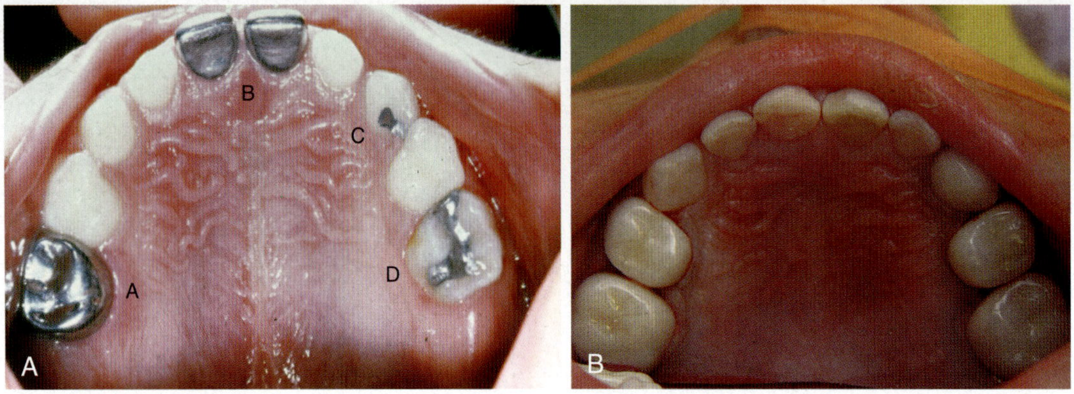

• **Fig. 30.1** (A) Traditionally restored dentition demonstrating: A) Stainless steel crown B) Preveneered steel crowns C) Class III amalgam, and D) Class II amalgam. (B) Primary dentition immediately after restoration with modern esthetic restorations.

TABLE 30.1 Anatomical Differences Between Primary and Permanent Teeth

Anatomical Difference	Clinical Impact
Primary teeth have thinner enamel and dentin thickness than permanent teeth (see Fig. 30.2)	Caries progresses rapidly if not treated
The pulps of primary teeth are larger in relation to crown size, and closer to the outer surface of the tooth, than permanent pulps	Caution must be exercised to avoid iatrogenic pulp exposure
In molars the mesiobuccal pulp horn is the most prominent	Intracoronal restorations are rarely placed on mesial occlusal lesions in primary first molars, due to risk of pulp exposure
Primary molar crowns demonstrate significant cervical constriction	Care must be exercised to avoid overpreparation and loss of the gingival seat of the proximal box in a class II preparation
Primary molars have a more prominent cervical contour than permanent teeth	The buccal bulge of the primary molars is a retentive feature in a stainless steel crown, but it must be removed for a zirconia crown
Enamel rods slope occlusally in the cervical region of the crown in primary teeth	It is not necessary to remove unsupported enamel at the base of the class II box, as is sometimes recommended in permanent tooth preparations
Primary teeth have broad, flat proximal contact areas	Initial caries is more likely to form interproximally in primary molars, whereas pit and fissure lesions predominate in permanent molar
Primary incisors rarely have developmental grooves or mamelons	It is not necessary to develop complex anatomy in primary incisor restorations; full-coverage composite and zirconia crowns have flat facial contours
Primary teeth are whiter in color than their permanent successors	Restorative materials in light shades (e.g., A1, B1) work best for primary teeth
Primary teeth have relatively narrow occlusal surfaces compared with their permanent successors	The size of intracoronal restorations is reduced accordingly

Depending on the type of carious lesions, method of instrumentation, and restorative material to be used, the clinician can opt for a conventional G.V. Black type of cavity preparation or for a more conservative micropreparation. Fig. 30.3 illustrates a continuum of cavity preparation based on size and instrumentation.

Dental lasers have also become popular with some clinicians (Fig. 30.4). Lasers can be used on children for soft tissue surgery, caries prevention, caries diagnosis, biostimulation and pain control, pulp therapy, and cavity preparation.[7] The energy absorbed by the intended tissue is dependent on the wavelength of the laser, meaning specific tissues (e.g., enamel, gingiva) are more readily cut with lasers of specific wavelengths.[8] The various types of dental lasers are named for the active medium that generates photon energy. Carbon dioxide (CO_2), erbium-doped yttrium aluminum garnet (Er:YAG), erbium, chromium-doped: yttrium-scandium-gallium-garnet (Er,Cr:YSGG), diode, and argon are a few of the various laser types available to clinicians.[9] "All-tissue" lasers that can be used for both tooth preparation and soft tissue procedures have become popular with dentists due to their versatility. Among the most common "all-tissue" lasers in use are the isotopic 9.3-micron CO_2 laser (Solea, Convergent Dental, Waltham, MA) and Er,Cr:YSGG lasers (Waterlase, BIOLASE, Foothill Ranch, CA). These devices can be used in restorative dentistry for minimally invasive preparation of pits and fissures, cavity preparation of all classes (I through VI), and treatment of deep dentinal caries. Some advantages of using lasers for cavity preparation include (1) better patient acceptance because they are quiet, (2) no vibration and minimal need for use of anesthetic, (3) minimally invasive

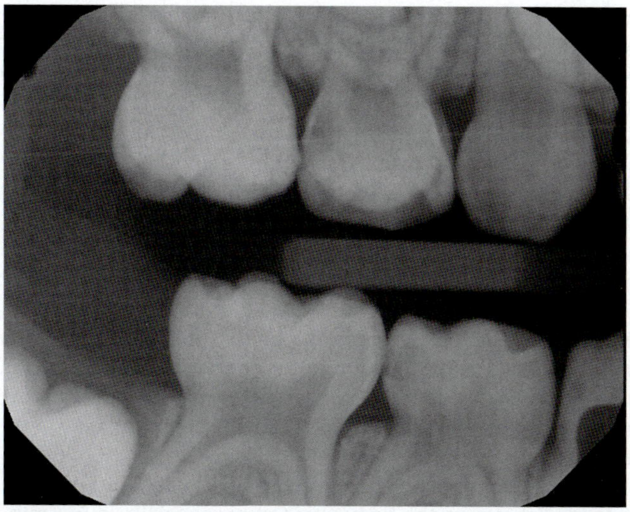

• **Fig. 30.2** Right Bitewing of Primary Dentition. Note the difference in enamel thickness. The enamel of the primary molars is approximately half the thickness of the enamel of the first permanent molars. Also note interproximal caries requiring restoration between the first and second primary molars and the distal of the mandibular primary canine.

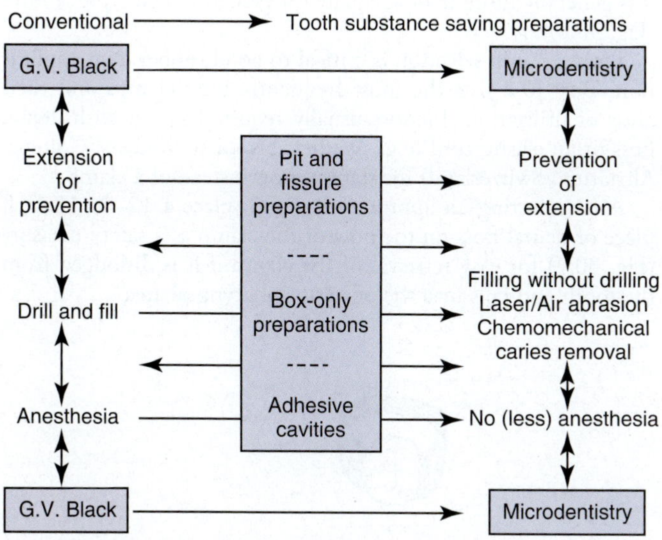

• **Fig. 30.3** Cavity preparation continuum. (Courtesy Dr. Luc Martens, Ghent, Belgium.)

cavity preparation because of the selective absorption of laser light by carious tissue, (4) production of very clean cavity preparations free of a smear layer, (5) minimal thermal increase in the pulp chamber, and (6) the production of cavity preparations with a macroroughened surface that increases surface bonding area for better adhesion of resin-based materials.[10] Some disadvantages include (1) a longer learning curve; (2) significantly higher equipment costs ($30,000 to $150,000 for an all-tissue laser); (3) need for specialized training; and (4) possible need for a traditional handpiece to complete the process, depending on the cavity size and preparation needed.[11] Whenever dental lasers are used, it is important to ensure that patient, staff, and clinician are wearing protective eyewear. Dental lasers also create a plume that contains microflora, gasses, and debris. Therefore it is important to utilize high-speed evacuation during the procedure.[12]

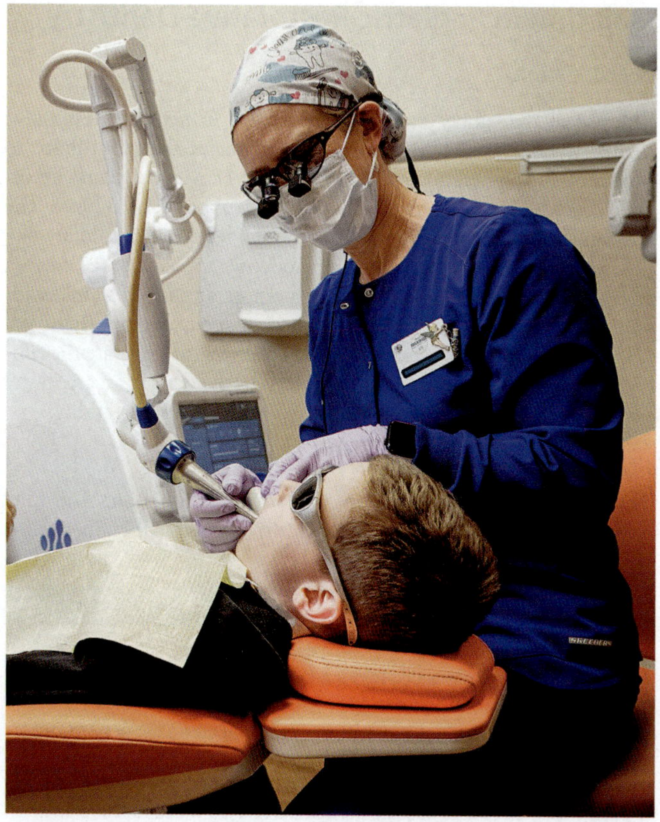

• **Fig. 30.4** Use of laser for operative dentistry. (Courtesy Dr. Jennifer Bryk-Hechko.)

Chemomechanical caries removal is a noninvasive technique that eliminates infected dentin via a chemical agent by means of dissolution.[13] Instead of drilling, a chemical agent such as Carisolv (MediTeam AB, Göteberg, Sweden) or Papacárie (F&A Laboratorio Farmaceutico Ltd., São Paulo, Brazil) is applied to the carious dentin and assisted by hand instruments to remove soft carious material. This method usually does not require anesthesia, preserves sound tooth structure, is nonaerosol generating, and relies on bonded restorative materials for final restoration. Drawbacks to this method include an increase in operator time to remove caries, only certain carious lesions are suitable for its use, a handpiece may still be necessary to gain access to the dentinal or interproximal areas, and data regarding long-term success of the method are limited.[14]

One final aspect to be considered when discussing tooth preparation is the use of magnification during operative procedures. Historically the use of magnification for dental procedures came only with increasing age and failing eyesight, but now the use of magnifying loupes or microscopes is taught from the beginning of dental school training. Loupes are available in a wide range of magnification, but generally 2.5× to 3.5× magnification is recommended for pediatric restorative dentistry. The use of magnification during restorative procedures has several advantages, including an increase in productivity, improvement in outcomes of dental treatment, and greater visual diagnostic abilities.[15] Perhaps most importantly, loupes have been shown to improve posture and assist in prevention of musculoskeletal disorders brought about by poor operator positioning.[16–18]

Isolation in Pediatric Restorative Dentistry

Rubber Dam

The use of the rubber dam is indispensable in pediatric restorative dentistry. Its use conveys numerous advantages that contribute to providing the highest quality of care (Box 30.1). Most pediatric restorative procedures can be completed with the rubber dam in place. The few situations in which it may not be used include the following: (1) in the presence of some fixed orthodontic appliances; (2) when a recently erupted tooth will not retain a clamp; and (3) in a child with an upper respiratory infection, congested nasal passage, or other nasal obstruction. However, even poor nasal breathers may tolerate the rubber dam if a small (2- to 3-cm) hole is cut in the dam in an area away from the operative quadrant to allow for some mouth breathing.

Preparing for Placement of the Rubber Dam

The rubber dam is available in an assortment of colors and may even be scented or flavored. Historically virtually all rubber dams were made of latex; however, the use of latex-free material is now recommended because of concerns regarding latex allergies. A 5 × 5-inch medium-gauge rubber dam is best suited for use in children. The darker the dam, the better the contrast between the teeth and dam. The holes should be punched so that the rubber dam is centered horizontally on the face and the upper lip is covered by the upper border of the dam, but the dam does not cover the nostrils. One method of proper hole placement is seen in Fig. 30.5.

• BOX 30.1 Advantages of Rubber Dam Use

1. Better access and visualization are gained by retracting soft tissues and providing a dark contrasting background to the teeth.
2. Moisture control is superior to other forms of isolation.
3. The safety of the child is improved by preventing aspiration or swallowing of foreign bodies and by protecting the soft tissues.
4. Placement generally results in decreased operating time.
5. Many children tend to become quieter and relaxed with a rubber dam in place. The dam seems to act as a separating barrier so that movements in and out of the oral cavity are perceived by the child as being less invasive than without the dam in place.
6. With a rubber dam in place, a child becomes primarily a nasal breather. This enhances nitrous oxide administration when it has been deemed necessary from a behavioral standpoint.

Punch the smallest number of holes necessary for good isolation of all teeth to be restored. For single class I, V, or VI restorations, only the tooth being restored needs to be isolated. For interproximal lesions, at least one tooth anterior and one tooth posterior to the tooth being restored should be isolated. This allows better access, more ease in placing a matrix, and improved visualization of adjacent marginal ridges for appropriate contouring of the restoration.

When isolating several teeth, instead of punching numerous individual holes in the dam, some clinicians will simply punch two holes approximately one-half inch apart and cut the rubber dam with scissors connecting the two holes. This is called the "slit" or "split" technique and allows for very quick placement of the rubber dam (see Chapter 15, Online Case Study: Rubber Dam Split Dam Technique and Resin Dental Sealant Placement). Moisture control is not as dependable with the slit technique, but it is generally more than adequate for pediatric dental procedures (Fig. 30.6).

Proper clamp selection is critical to good rubber dam application. Box 30.2 lists the most frequently used clamps and their areas of utilization. Incisors usually require ligation with dental floss or an elastic cord (e.g., Wedjet, HySolate Wedjets, Coltene, Altstätten, Switzerland) for stabilization instead of a clamp.[19]

After selecting an appropriate clamp, place a 12- to 18-inch piece of dental floss on the bow of the clamp as a safety measure (Fig. 30.7) for easy retrieval of the clamp if it is dislodged from the tooth and falls into the posterior pharyngeal area.

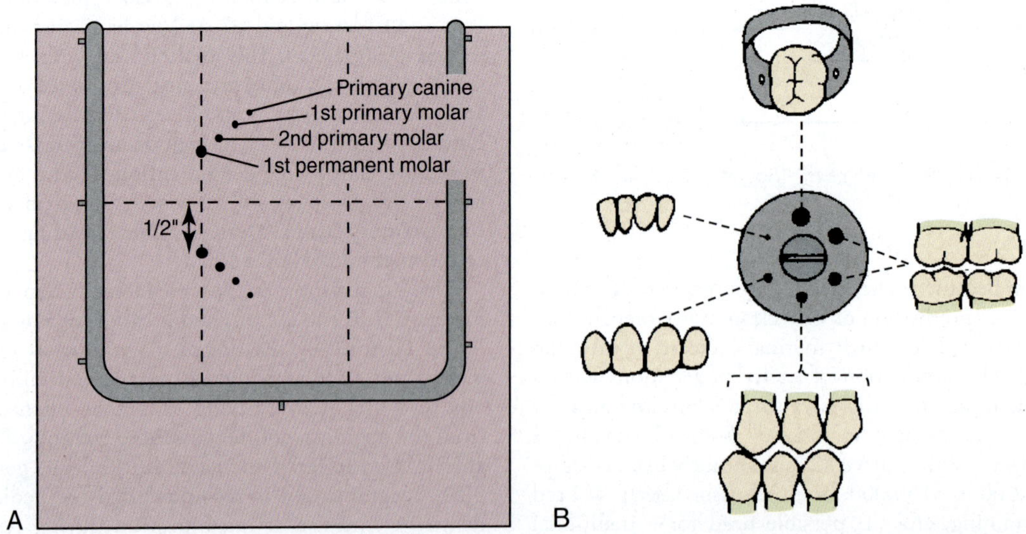

• Fig. 30.5 Preparation of the Rubber Dam. (A) The Young frame is applied to the rubber dam. The upper limit of the frame coincides with the upper edge of the rubber dam material. The dam is divided vertically into thirds, and the area inside the frame is divided in half horizontally. The holes for each tooth are placed as indicated, at a 45-degree angle 3 to 4 mm apart. (B) The rubber dam punch table with corresponding teeth and hole sizes. (B, Modified from The DAE Project. *Instructional Materials for the Dental Health Professions: Rubber Dam.* New York: Teachers College Press, Teachers College, Columbia University; 1982:42.)

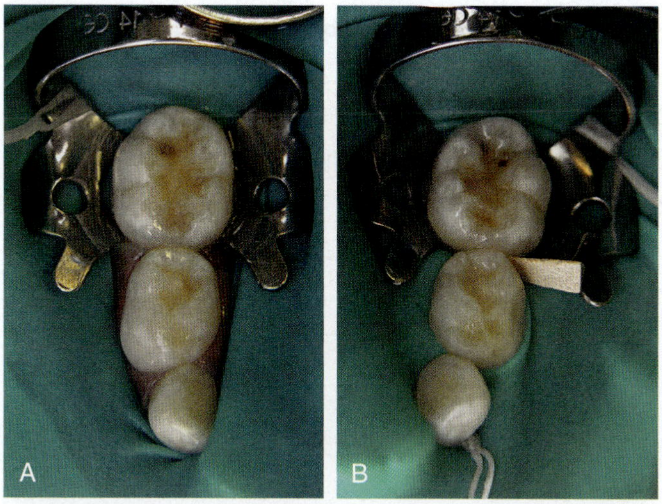

• **Fig. 30.6** (A) Quadrant isolated using slit dam technique. (B) Quadrant isolated with individual tooth holes, prewedge between molars and a floss ligature.

• BOX 30.2 Common Rubber Dam Clamps for Pediatric Restorative Dentistry

Permanent molars: 14, 14A, 8, 8A[a,b,c]
Second primary molars: 26, 27,[c] 3[a,b]
First primary molars/bicuspids/permanent canines: 2, 2A,[a,b] 207, 208[c]
Primary incisors and canines: 0,[a] 00,[b] 209[c]
"A" clamps have jaws angled gingivally to seat below subgingival heights of contour.

[a]Ivory, Heraeus-Kulzer, South Bend, IN.
[b]Hygienic Corp., Akron, OH.
[c]Hu-Friedy Mfg. Co., Chicago, IL.

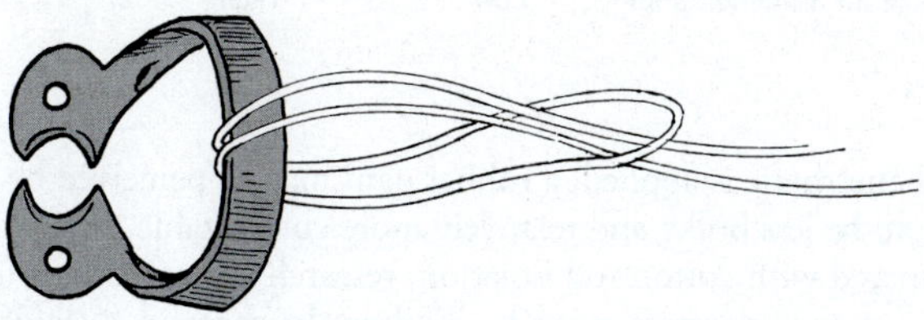

• **Fig. 30.7** A floss safety through the bow of the rubber dam clamp allows for easy retrieval of the clamp, should it become dislodged from the tooth. (Modified from The DAE Project. *Instructional Materials for the Dental Health Professions: Rubber Dam.* Teachers College Press, Teachers College, Columbia University; 1982:66.)

Before trying the clamp on the tooth, floss the contacts through which the rubber dam will be taken. If floss cannot be passed through the contact because of defective restorations or other factors, modification of the contacts or rubber dam will be necessary before placement. Next, using the rubber dam forceps, place the clamp on the tooth, seating it from a lingual to buccal direction. Be certain that the jaws of the clamp are placed below the height of contour and are not impinging on the gingival tissues. After seating the clamp, remove the forceps and place a finger on the buccal and lingual jaws of the clamp and apply gingival pressure to ensure that the clamp is stable and has been seated as far gingivally as possible.

Placement of the Rubber Dam

The punched rubber dam should be lightly stretched onto the rubber dam frame before placement of the clamp. This holds the corners of the dam out of the line of the operator's vision during placement. If the material is stretched too tightly, tension is too great and the clamp may be dislodged when the material is stretched over the bow of the clamp. Next, pull the floss attached to the clamp through the most posterior hole in the dam that has been punched for the clamped tooth. Instruct the child to open the mouth widely and consider placement of a mouth prop. With the index fingers, stretch the most posterior hole of the rubber dam over the bow and wings of the clamp. Sometimes when isolating the most posterior maxillary molars, the bow of the clamp rests very close to the anterior border of the ramus when the mouth is opened wide. This makes slipping the dam material over the bow difficult, but when one simply asks the child to close the mouth slightly, the ramus will move posteriorly and allow the material to slide between the bow and the ramus.

If necessary, adjust the tension of the rubber dam on the frame. Next, stabilize the rubber dam around the most anterior tooth. This may be done by placing a wooden wedge interproximally, by stretching a small piece of elastic cord or rubber dam through the contact, or by ligating with dental floss (see Fig. 30.6). To ligate, place floss (12 to 18 inches) around the crown of the tooth and have the dental assistant hold the floss gingivally on the lingual with a blunt instrument. Draw the floss tightly around the tooth from the buccal and tie a surgical knot below the cervical bulge. Do not cut the ends of the ligature tie because the long ends remind the operator that the ligature is present. After anterior stabilization, all other teeth for which holes have been punched can be isolated. An explorer or similar instrument can be used to invert the rubber dam into the gingival sulcus around each isolated tooth.

Removing the Rubber Dam

To remove the rubber dam when restorative procedures are complete, first rinse away all debris and cut and remove any ligatures used for stabilization. Next, stretch the rubber dam so that the dam's interproximal septa may be cut with a pair of scissors. The clamp, frame, and dam are then removed as a unit with the rubber dam forceps. Inspect the dam and the mouth to see that no small pieces of dam material have been left interproximally. Gently massage the tissue around the previously clamped tooth, rinse, and evacuate the oral cavity.

Alternative Isolation Systems

Today alternative isolation systems are commonly used in pediatric dentistry. These systems incorporate high-volume evacuation, a bite block, and protective barriers for the tongue and cheek. Some systems are made of transparent materials. This increases visibility and allows incorporation of illumination into the mouthpiece (Fig. 30.8). The mouthpieces are constructed of flexible polymer materials that are several millimeters thick but easily adapt to the mouth's contours and provide protection of the soft tissues. These systems reduce moisture and oral humidity to levels similar to a rubber dam. As an added benefit, the design allows the operator to simultaneously work on opposing maxillary and mandibular quadrants. These systems also exhibit continuous evacuation, which may reduce the start/stop time required with the use of high-volume evacuators (HVEs) in four-handed dentistry. A comparison of alternative isolation systems with the rubber dam is found in Table 30.2.

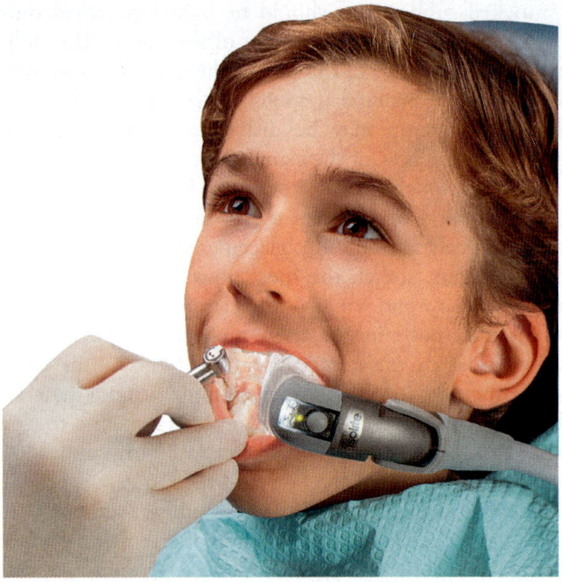

• **Fig. 30.8** Isolite-alternate isolation system. (Courtesy Isolite Systems, Santa Barbara, CA. Used with permission.)

Manufacturers produce mouthpieces in a variety of sizes to accommodate most patients. Two popular systems, Isolite (Isolite Systems, Santa Barbara, CA) and DryShield (DryShield, Fountain Valley, CA), require purchase of specific armamentarium for each dental unit that is equipped. Other systems such as Mr. Thirsty (Zirc, Buffalo, MN) connect directly to existing HVEs. Mouthpieces may be disposable (Isolite, Mr. Thirsty) or autoclavable and reusable (DryShield).

Placement of Alternative Isolation Systems

Step 1: Hold the control head with index finger and thumb. With your other hand, fold the cheek shield onto the tongue retractor. Gently slide the folded mouthpiece into the buccal vestibule on the side to receive treatment. Angle the mouthpiece to allow the lower edge of the tongue retractor to move along the buccal edge of the teeth.

Step 2: Move the bite block onto the occlusal surface of the teeth, just distal to the mandibular cuspid. Instruct the patient to "rest gently" on the bite block to secure.

Step 3: Place the cheek shield into the buccal vestibule. Move the isthmus onto the retromolar pad behind the maxillary tuberosity. Adjust the tongue retractor in the lingual vestibule as needed. Move the bite block distally to provide more vertical working room.

Behavioral Considerations When Using Alternative Isolation Systems

When used properly, both rubber dam and alternative isolation systems can provide good moisture control and protection of oral soft tissues. Although placement of a rubber dam typically requires administration of local anesthetic, alternative isolation systems do not. This may lead users to believe that the alternative system is better tolerated by patients. This observation may be especially true for sealants and other situations in which local anesthetic would not otherwise be used. However, local anesthetic is used for most operative dental procedures. Therefore, when local anesthetic is applied, a rubber dam may be perceived by children to be less bulky and relatively more comfortable. In addition, compared with cotton roll isolation, research indicates that rubber dam use may decrease stress in children. In contrast, a significant percentage of children may feel that the alternative isolation system mouthpiece stretches their mouth and makes them feel as if they are going to gag.[20] Although there has been limited research in this area, in some situations a rubber dam may convey the behavioral advantages of decreased noise, decreased bulk, and enhanced nitrous oxide inhalation through nasal breathing.[21,22]

TABLE 30.2 Contrasting the Rubber Dam With Alternative Isolation Systems

	Rubber Dam	Alternative Isolation Systems (Isolite, Dry-Shield, Mr. Thirsty)
Isolation		
Moisture control	++	+
Reduction of aerosol	+	+
Improves visibility of field	++	+
Continuous evacuation		+
Protection from debris and dropped instruments	++	+
Retracts gingival tissues	+	
Ability to isolate partially erupted teeth	+	++
Saves time	+	++
Illumination		+ (Isolite only)
Behavioral		
Reduces mouth breathing, may increase N_2O inhalation	+	
Reduces talking	++	+
Added noise		–
Challenge in sizing for some children/gagging		–
Local anesthesia required	–	
Implementation		
Cost for disposable supplies	Very low	Moderate
Cost for armamentarium	Low	High

Restoration of Primary Molars

The broad, flat interproximal contact areas and relatively thin enamel of primary molars makes them the most caries-susceptible primary teeth. Although minimally invasive dentistry recognizes that not every caries lesion requires restoration, primary molars serve vital roles in mastication and as maintainers of space for the succedaneous teeth. This has shaped a philosophy of restoring and conserving primary molars, versus extraction.[23]

SSCs, ZCs, adhesive materials such as resin-based composites, glass ionomers, resin-modified glass ionomers (RMGIs), polyacid-modified resin-based composites (compomers), and amalgam are the main materials used in the restoration of primary molars. The following discussion of primary molar restoration has been divided topically based upon the tooth surfaces treated, with specific focus on differences encountered when using a variety of restorative materials.

Amalgam Use in Primary Molars

Favorable handling properties, good longevity, and less technique sensitivity have made amalgam a popular choice for restoration of primary teeth. Although amalgam was historically the material of choice for intracoronal restorations, today it is far less popular than composite resin.[24] This is likely driven by dentist and parent preferences for esthetic restorations and concerns regarding exposure of dentists, patients, and the environment to mercury in amalgam. Today amalgam is banned in several European countries and the US Food and Drug Administration now suggests that children, especially those younger than 6 years of age, are at greater risk for harmful health effects related to amalgam use.[25] For a more detailed discussion of the controversy the reader is referred to Chapter 29. Although many schools no longer teach amalgam as the preferred restorative material for primary teeth, it is included here because it provides the basis of cavity preparation design for intracoronal restorations.

Adhesive Materials in Primary Molars

Compared with amalgam, resin-based composite materials offer the advantages of improved esthetics, elimination of mercury, low thermal conductivity, more conservation of tooth structure, easier reparability, and bonding of the restorative material to the tooth. Disadvantages include an exacting technique, incompatibility with moisture contamination during placement, increased operator time, potential marginal leakage, possible postoperative sensitivity, and a tendency for open contacts. Although it appears that amalgam may continue to offer increased restoration longevity over other alternatives, a number of studies have shown good results for resin-based composite.[26,27] For example, a 5-year longitudinal study showed no statistically significant difference in overall failure rate between composite and amalgam, although composite restorations did require seven times more repairs than amalgam.[28] In recent years the number of clinical trials investigating materials for restoration of primary teeth has grown. A wide variety of products have shown good performance, and it remains up to the clinician to weigh the relative merits of each material.[29,30]

In addition to resin-based composites, polyacid-modified resin-based composites, also known as compomers, RMGIs, and glass ionomers, have all been suggested for use in primary molar restorations. Several clinical studies have evaluated compomer use in primary molars[31–35] and found them to provide useful, predictable restorations. RMGI has also been evaluated in a number of clinical studies.[36–38] Although these restorations demonstrate more color change and occlusal wear than resin-based composites or compomers, they are also more moisture tolerant and release significant amounts of fluoride. This makes them particularly well suited to high caries–risk pediatric populations. Glass ionomer cements have also been used in restoring primary molars but with less satisfactory results than the other adhesive materials.[39,40] Use of glass ionomers for multisurface or large restorations in primary molars, except for teeth with a very limited life span, is generally not recommended.[23,41]

In recent years there has been increasing interest in bioactive restorative materials. The goal of such materials is reducing secondary caries by suppressing bacterial growth and/or improving chemical balance through release of fluoride or calcium phosphate.[42] A number of new products in this category have been released on the market, but more research is still needed to determine their effectiveness.[43] eTable 30.3 describes key differences between amalgam and adhesive restorative materials.

Adhesive Systems for Primary Teeth

Adhesive systems can be classified according to their bonding strategy: total-etch and universal/self-etch systems. Total-etch systems require etching the tooth with phosphoric acid, rinsing, and applying a primer and bonding agent (which may be applied sequentially or as one step), which is then cured. Given that primary dentin has lower mineral content and greater tubule density than permanent dentin, it is susceptible to "overetching" or deeper demineralization, which causes the collapse of collagen fibrils and results in less penetration of resin monomers to form an adequate hybrid layer. Some authors recommend a reduced etching time of primary dentin (e.g., half of the manufacturer's recommended etch time for permanent teeth)[44,45] or application of etchant to the enamel margins of the preparation first and then to dentin.[46]

Universal systems include both "self-etch and rinse" and self-etch with no rinsing step and also include mild pH (pH >2) and strong pH (pH <1) self-etchants.[47] Strong pH systems such as 3M Adper Prompt L-Pop Self-Etch Adhesive (3M, St. Paul, MN) should be avoided for primary dentin to prevent overetching. Mild pH systems such as Scotchbond Universal Adhesive (3M, St. Paul, MN) provide adequate bond strength to primary dentin; however, they have a reduced ability to adequately etch primary enamel. Thus selectively etching enamel and rinsing before adhesive application has been suggested.[48] Weak evidence suggests that a mild, 10-methacryloyloxydecyl dihydrogen phosphate (MDP) monomer-based universal adhesive such as Scotchbond Universal Adhesive may be used in primary teeth.[49] The selective etch and rinse mode is preferred in clinical situations involving a considerable amount of enamel. Clinical data are limited, and further studies are needed to evaluate the long-term bonding performance of universal adhesives in primary teeth.

General Principles for Intracoronal Restoration of Primary Posterior Teeth

Class I Restorations

Amalgam design (available online)

Adhesive Restoration Preparation Design

In large part, class I adhesive restorations follow the same preparation principles as amalgam restorations. However, adhesive materials adhere to noncarious pits and fissures and can be placed successfully in preparations that are more shallow. Therefore the preparation design for adhesive materials is typically more conservative and may incorporate elements of restorative and sealant techniques. This is referred to as a preventive resin restoration (PRR). The steps of preparation and restoration of class I restorations are listed in Box 30.3.

Simonsen and Stallard first described the PRR in 1977.[50] This restoration combines the preventive approach of sealing susceptible pits and fissures with conservative class I cavity preparation of

• BOX 30.3 Steps of Preparation and Restoration of Class I Restorations

1. Administer appropriate anesthesia and place rubber dam/isolation system.
2. Using a no. 330 bur, penetrate the tooth parallel to its long axis in the carious region. Prepare only to the depth required to remove the lesion. **For amalgam:** enter and extend preparation to a depth of 0.5 mm in dentin.
3. Remove carious dentin using a large, round bur or a sharp spoon excavator.
4. Ensure cavity margins are caries-free and refine the final outline form with the no. 330 bur.
5. Rinse and dry the preparation and inspect for caries removal.
6. Place a short bevel (0.5 mm) at the cavosurface margin. This may be accomplished with a tapered diamond bur. *Note:* No bevel should be placed for amalgam, glass ionomer, or RMGI.
7. Place base/liner for pulp protection if indicated.
8. If using a total etch technique, etch the preparation for 10 seconds, ideally applying to enamel margins and then to dentin. Rinse and dry the preparation. If a self-etching adhesive is used, this step is eliminated.
9. Place adhesive in the preparation with a small brush. Gently air dry to disperse a thin layer of adhesive evenly. Polymerize with curing light.
10. With a plastic instrument or a pressure syringe, place the composite in the preparation. **For amalgam:** condense, contour, and carve amalgam according to the manufacturer's instructions. Initial contour is critical for amalgam, as it cannot be immediately adjusted as easily as many adhesive materials. Excess material may lead to heavy occlusion and restoration failure. Inadequate material may reduce restoration strength.
11. Hold the curing light as closely as possible to the composite and polymerize per the manufacturer's instructions. Apply fissure sealant to unrestored surfaces and cure.
12. Remove isolation materials and check occlusion with articulating paper.
13. A round or pear-shaped carbide finishing bur (12–20 flutes) is excellent for adjusting occlusion and finishing the occlusal surface. A lubricated, pointed white stone or rubber finishing point may also be used for polishing.
14. Floss the interproximal areas ensure no excess material remains.
15. Rinse the oral cavity.

RMGI, Resin-modified glass ionomer.

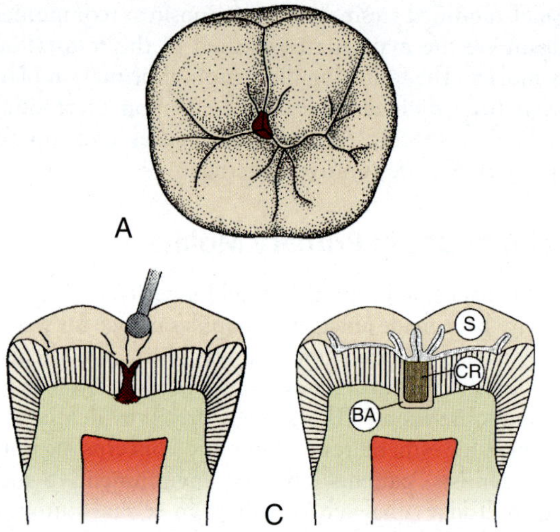

• Fig. 30.10 (A) The occlusal surface of a mandibular second primary molar with a small, discrete area of decay in the central pit. (B) A small round bur is used to conservatively remove the decay. (C) A bonding agent *(BA)* and resin-based composite *(CR)* material are placed in the preparation. Then a sealant *(S)* is applied over all the remaining susceptible pits and fissures.

caries occurring on the same occlusal surface. Instead of the traditional amalgam cavity preparation's "extension for prevention" beyond the area of decay into the adjacent pits and fissures, this technique limits cavity preparation to the discrete areas of decay. This results in a restoration that conserves tooth structure and is both therapeutic and preventive. Although the nomenclature reflects the fact that resin is frequently utilized for the PRR, other adhesive materials (e.g., compomer, glass ionomer, RMGI) may also be used in these restorations.

The PRR is ideally suited for small carious lesions in teeth that would otherwise lose a considerable amount of tooth structure if the extension for prevention treatment were followed.[51] Houpt and colleagues reported 79% retention of PRRs in permanent molars after 9 years and concluded that the PRR was a successful conservative alternative to treatment of minimal occlusal caries.[52] Although long-term retention studies of PRRs in primary teeth are lacking, with retention rates of PRRs and sealants in permanent teeth being very similar, it is not unreasonable to believe that retention rates of PRRs in primary teeth would also be similar to sealant rates.

Teeth that are suitable for PRRs are those that demonstrate small, discrete regions of dentinal caries, often limited to a single pit (Fig. 30.10). As with sealants, the ability to isolate the tooth and keep it dry throughout the procedure is the single most important indication. Amalgam or RMGI, being less sensitive to technique and moisture, is the restorative material of choice if the tooth cannot be kept dry. Many PRRs do not require anesthesia because of the minimal tooth preparation. However, soft tissue anesthesia may be necessary for comfort if placing a rubber dam.

Common Errors With Class I Restorations

Some frequent errors made in class I restorations are (1) preparing the cavity too deep; (2) leaving unsupported enamel; (3) carving the anatomy too deep, leaving insufficient restorative material; (4) undercarving/undercontouring, which leads to subsequent fracture or tooth sensitivity from hyperocclusion; and (5) not including or sealing all susceptible fissures. Note that sealing over restorative materials significantly decreases microleakage[53] and increases the longevity of the restoration.[54,55]

Liners and Bases in Primary Teeth

Evidence suggests that the goal of maintaining tooth vitality is best achieved by reducing pulp exposures. In selective removal, caries may be left over the pulp, with a base/liner applied directly over remaining caries, and the tooth immediately restored.[23] A meta-analysis of indirect pulp cap treatment suggests that glass ionomer, calcium silicate cement, and calcium hydroxide all produced similarly good results regarding maintenance of pulp vitality.[56] However, conventional calcium hydroxide may hydrolyze gradually,[57] leaving a small void underneath the restoration and ultimately weakening it.[58] Therefore when placing a base/liner it is recommended to use RMGI or a resin-based calcium silicate cement product that will ensure dimensional stability over time such as Ultra-Blend plus (Ultradent, South Jordan, UT), Lime-Lite Enhanced (Pulpdent, Watertown, MA), or NeoLINER LC (NuSmile, Houston, TX). Some liner products have lower radiopacity than the restorative materials placed over them.[59] Therefore it is important to avoid using excessively thick liners that could be mistaken for caries in radiographs.

Class II Restorations

General considerations

Preparation of the proximal surface requires additional steps during both preparation and restoration. Placement of an interproximal wedge before and during preparation is highly desirable to achieve a slight separation of teeth and consequently a tighter interproximal contact of the final restoration. The wedge also protects the interproximal gingival tissue during instrumentation and thereby reduces the likelihood of hemorrhage into the proximal box during instrumentation (see Fig. 30.6).

Adhesive Restoration Preparation Design. For resin-based composites, absolute moisture control is a must, making effective use of rubber dam or an alternative isolation system almost mandatory. Unlike amalgam preparations, which have been well defined for years, there is no current consensus about the precise design of a class II adhesive material preparation. A 2001 survey of pediatric dentistry departments in North American dental schools found that 57% of the dental schools teach a conservative "box-only" preparation (with and without retention grooves), whereas 36% use and teach the traditional G.V. Black amalgam preparation.[60] Leinfelder[61] recommended that a class II preparation be primarily restricted to the region of the caries, with little to no occlusal extensions. He also stated that extending the proximal box line angles in "self-cleansing" areas is not necessary and in fact creates a larger restoration that is more prone to occlusal wear. In recent years, bonding agents and adhesive restorative materials have improved dramatically, suggesting that under the right circumstances the slot preparation (Fig. 30.12) may be used effectively.[31,62–64] Although evidence indicates that the slot technique can be successful, experience suggests that a conservative preparation that incorporates mechanical retention such as a small dovetail or a cavosurface margin bevel to increase surface area for bonding should improve retention and overall success of the restoration.[65] Beveling not only increases the surface area to be etched but also removes the aprismatic layer of enamel, which may not etch well and may leave islands of unetched enamel that can act as pathways for bacterial leakage and/or reduce resin bond strength to the enamel.[66] However, it must be noted that placing a bevel in glass ionomer and RMGI restorations may lead to marginal failure, and therefore is not recommended.[23]

In primary teeth, many practitioners limit class II restorations to relatively small two-surface restorations. Three-surface mesial-occlusal-distal (MOD) restorations may be done, but studies have shown that full-coverage crowns are a more durable and predictable restoration for large multiple surface restorations in primary teeth.[67] Messer and Levering[68] reported that SSCs placed in 4-year-old and younger children showed a success rate approximately twice that of class II amalgams, for each year up to 10 years of service. In high caries–risk children treated under general anesthesia, over one-third of those who initially received composite restorations in their molars required retreatment, versus only 8% of those who received SSCs.[69] In the preschool child with large proximal carious lesions, SSCs are preferred to intracoronal restorations because of their durability. Similar-sized lesions in teeth that are within 2 or 3 years of exfoliation may be restored with an amalgam or adhesive material because the anticipated life span is fairly short.[70]

Matrix application

Interproximal restorative matrices aid in restoring normal contour to contact areas and prevent extrusion of restorative materials into gingival tissues. Many types of matrix bands are available for use in pediatric dentistry. Regardless of the type of matrix band used,

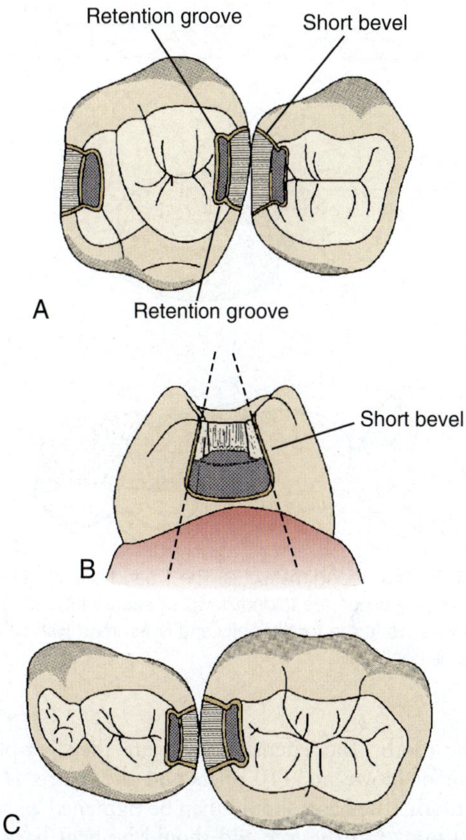

• **Fig. 30.12** Modified Class II Cavity Preparations for Adhesive Restorative Materials. Note the short bevel around the preparations and small retention groves. (A) Maxillary right second and first primary molars (occlusal view). (B) Mandibular second primary molar (proximal view); note occlusal convergence of proximal walls. (C) Mandibular right first and second primary molars (occlusal view).

after it is in place and a wedge firmly inserted, a small ball burnisher can be used to burnish the band against the adjacent tooth in the area of the contact point. This will help provide a tight proximal contact.

1. T band: Allows for multiple matrices, no special equipment is needed.
2. Sectional matrices: Allow for multiple matrix placement, are very easy to use, are not circumferential, must be held in place by a wedge.
3. AutoMatrix (Dentsply Sirona Inc., Charlotte, NC): Allows for multiple matrix placement, is very easy to use, requires special tightening and removal tools.
4. Tofflemire matrix: Used infrequently because it does not fit primary tooth contour well and is difficult to place as multiple matrices. A preassembled, single use, disposable version is available with a narrow band option in the Pro-Matrix system (Young Innovations, Inc. Algonquin, IL).

T bands are available in different sizes, contours, and materials. A straight, narrow, brass T band will work in almost all pediatric restorative procedures.[71] The T-band matrix (Fig. 30.13) is formed by folding the band back on itself in the form of a circle and by folding over the extension wings of the "T" to make an adjustable loop. The band is contoured and positioned onto the tooth with the folded extension wings on the buccal surface. The free end of the band is drawn mesially to pull the band snugly

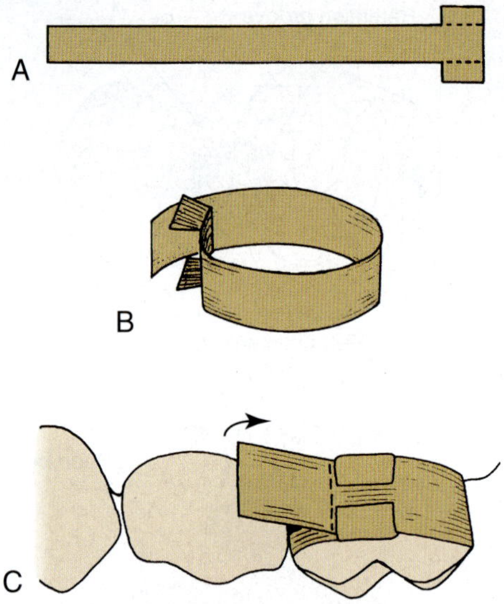

• **Fig. 30.13** (A) The T-band matrix. (B) The T band is formed into a circle, and the extension wings are folded down to secure the band. (C) The T band is adapted to fit the tooth tightly and is trimmed with scissors, and the free end is bent back.

against the tooth. The extension folds are then grasped firmly with a pair of Howe no. 110 pliers and the matrix is removed from the tooth. The band should then be tightened an additional 0.5 to 1.0 mm, and the free end should be bent back over the vertical folds and cut with scissors to a length of 5 to 6 mm. The band is then reseated onto the tooth and wedged. It must fit below the gingival margin of the preparation and must also be at least 1 mm higher than the marginal ridge of the adjacent tooth. The T band is removed by opening the extension wings with an explorer or spoon excavator and allowing the band to open. For cured adhesive restorations the wedge can simply be removed and the matrix lifted from the contact. For amalgam and glass ionomer restorations that have not fully set, scissors are used to cut one end of the band close to the restored proximal surface, the wedge is removed, and the band is then drawn buccally or lingually through the contact.

There are many commercially available sectional matrices. One commonly used in pediatrics is the Strip-T System (Denovo Dental Inc., Baldwin Park, CA). They are stainless steel matrix strips approximately one-half inch long that do not encircle the prepared tooth; instead, they fit only in the prepared proximal area. For small class II preparations, they are very simple to place and use. After placement, they must be firmly wedged to stay in place. They are not recommended for proximal preparations that extend beyond the line angles; a circumferential matrix (or SSC) is more appropriate in that instance.

AutoMatrix is a preformed loop of stainless steel matrix material that is placed on the tooth and tightened with a special tightening tool that comes with the kit (Fig. 30.14). A small pin automatically keeps the tightened matrix tightly bound around the tooth. To remove the matrix, this small pin is clipped (another special tool) and the matrix is easily loosened and removed.

Placement of restorative materials in class II restorations

The steps of preparation and restoration of class II restorations are listed in Box 30.4. The use of adhesive materials is emphasized (with modifications for amalgam described briefly and **available digitally**). If a base or liner is to be used, it should be placed and

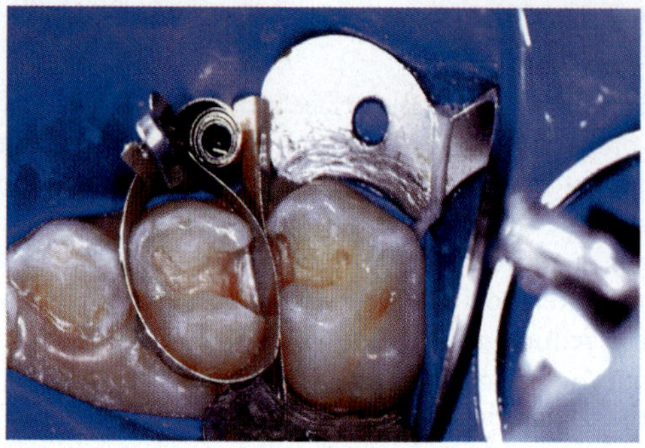

• **Fig. 30.14** A sectional matrix (Strip-T, Denovo) is placed onto a mesio-occlusal preparation of the second primary molar. An AutoMatrix (Dentsply Sirona) is seen placed on the distoocclusal preparation of the first primary molar. The matrix can be tightened to draw the band more closely to the tooth. A wedge secures both in place.

• BOX 30.4 Steps of Preparation and Restoration for Class II Restorations

1. Administer appropriate anesthesia and place rubber dam/isolation system.
2. Place a wooden wedge in the interproximal area being restored.
3. Using a no. 330 bur, prepare the proximal box. Contact should be just broken between the adjacent tooth and the gingival wall such that the wedge is seen. If the gingival wall is made too deep, the cervical constriction of the primary molar will create a very narrow gingival seat. Take care not to damage the adjacent proximal surface.
4. Remove any remaining caries with a sharp spoon excavator or a round bur.
5. Place a short bevel (0.5 mm) at the cavosurface margin. This may be accomplished with a tapered diamond bur. *Note:* No bevel should be placed for amalgam, glass ionomer, or RMGI.
6. Remove the wedge placed at the beginning of the treatment and place a matrix band.
7. While holding the matrix band in place, forcefully reinsert the wedge between the matrix band and the adjacent tooth, beneath the gingival seat of the preparation. The wedge is placed with a pair of Howe pliers or cotton forceps from the widest embrasure. The wedge should hold the band tightly against the tooth but should not push the band into the proximal box.
8. Rinse and dry the preparation and inspect for caries removal.
9. Place base/liner for pulp protection if indicated.
10. If using a total etch technique, etch the preparation for 10 seconds, ideally applying to enamel margins and then to dentin. Rinse and dry the preparation. If a self-etching adhesive is used, this step is eliminated.
11. Place adhesive in the preparation with a small brush. Gently air dry to disperse a thin layer of adhesive evenly. Polymerize with curing light.
12. Place a small increment of flowable composite in the proximal box and cure (incremental fill). Alternatively, leave uncured and proceed directly to next step ("snow-plow" technique).
13. With a plastic instrument or a pressure syringe, place the composite in the preparation.
14. Hold the curing light as closely as possible to the composite and polymerize per the manufacturer's instructions. Apply fissure sealant to unrestored surfaces and cure.
15. Remove the matrix and cure again from buccal and lingual. **For amalgam:** condense, contour, and carve amalgam according to the manufacturer's instructions. Use caution when removing the wedge and the matrix band after placement. Drawing the band in a buccal-lingual direction, as opposed to an occlusal direction, will be less likely to damage the marginal ridge of the newly placed restoration during withdrawal.
16. Remove isolation materials and check the occlusion with articulating paper.
17. Finishing and polishing can be performed immediately after polymerization as described in Box 30.3.
18. When finishing is completed, floss the interproximal areas ensure no excess material remains.

RMGI, Resin-modified glass ionomer.

cured before the etching or adhesive steps. For the total etch technique, the preparation should be etched for 10 seconds with an acid gel, ideally placing it on enamel and then dentin. The etchant should extend well beyond the cavosurface margin to cover any susceptible pits and fissures not included in the preparation. For both total etch and self-etch systems, the application time may be reduced by half of the manufacturer's recommended etch time for permanent teeth.[45] After application of the adhesive, many clinicians place a flowable resin-based composite as a cavity liner. Although not mandatory, it appears that use of a thin (0.5 to 1 mm) flowable liner reduces the voids at the cervical cavosurface margin in class II restorations[72] and may consequently reduce microleakage. The flowable material may be cured before placement of the packable material (incremental fill technique), or packable composite may be applied directly to the uncured flowable liner and the two layers cocured ("snow-plow" technique).[73]

Many resin-based composites and compomers are prepackaged in small ampules that can be injected directly into the preparation. Alternately, a plastic instrument or condenser can be used to pack or condense the composite into the preparation. With conventional restorative composites, no more than 2 mm of composite should be polymerized at one time. This is to allow the curing light to penetrate the full depth of the material. Incremental placement may also reduce polymerization shrinkage, a suspected cause of adhesive failure and postoperative sensitivity. Modern bulk-fill composite materials are more translucent than conventional materials and have decreased polymerization shrinkage. This allows them to be placed in increments of 4 to 5 mm. A large body of research suggests that bulk-fill and conventional composite now exhibit similar clinical performance.[74]

Complete curing or polymerization of the material is very important to the success of the restoration. Undercuring may lead to a weakened restoration prone to failure under masticatory forces. It is important to place the curing light as close as possible to the surface of the resin material during polymerization. When placing the final increment of packable resin, slightly overfill the preparation with material and use a ball burnisher to push the material toward and up over the enamel margins. This will remove excess material and effectively act as a carver. Do not use a cleoid-discoid carver on resin-based composite material. Use the tip of the explorer to carve the marginal ridge away from the matrix band. Remember to always move the instrument from material to tooth, pushing the material toward the margins. If you move instruments from tooth to restoration, you will likely pull material away from the margins, leaving a gap. Place sealant material at margins of restoration and in any unprepared fissures and cure (see Chapter 15 for a discussion of the benefits of sealing restorations). After final cure of the restoration, remove the wedge and matrix band and cure the restoration one more time, directing the light toward the proximal from a buccal or lingual approach. Finishing can begin immediately after polymerization. The occlusal surface is grossly contoured with high-speed carbide finishing burs or fine-finishing diamond burs. Gross contouring of proximal surfaces is accomplished with flame-shaped, high-speed carbide finishing burs and with garnet disks, where accessible. Final finishing can be completed with a white stone or with rubber abrasive points. Fine abrasive disks or strips may also be used for final polishing of accessible proximal margins.

Adjacent or back-to-back class II restorations

Adjacent interproximal lesions are not uncommon in the primary dentition. From the standpoint of time and patient management, it is desirable to restore these lesions simultaneously. After the preparations are completed, matrix bands or segmental matrices are placed on both preparations and a wedge is forcefully inserted between the two bands. Be certain that the placement of the matrices allows a convexity to the proximal surface of both teeth. Sometimes the matrices are positioned such that if the restorative material were placed into the preps, one proximal surface would be vastly overcontoured and the adjacent surface vastly undercontoured. This can be prevented by putting the matrix on one tooth, restoring it completely, and then placing the matrix band on the second tooth and restoring it. However, it is possible to place both matrices and restore simultaneously. With two matrix bands in place, etch and bond both preparations as dictated by the manufacturer's instructions. Next completely fill, contour, and polymerize one of the restorations. To ensure a tight contact between the two restorations, after the first restoration is polymerized, use a small ball burnisher and burnish the matrix band against the newly placed restoration in the area where you want to create the contact point. Then add, contour, and polymerize the material in the second preparation. Remove the wedge and bands; finishing and polishing procedures are identical to single restoration placement.

If amalgam is placed, the technique for placement of adjacent proximal restorations varies slightly. Condensation of the amalgam should be done in small increments, alternately in each preparation, so that the restorations are filled simultaneously. Condensation pressure toward the matrix will help ensure a tight interproximal contact. Carve the marginal ridges to an equal height, and carefully remove the wedge and matrix bands one at a time. Final carving is as described for solitary class II restorations.

Common problems with class II restorations

Class II restorations share many of the errors discussed for class I restorations, with the proximal box being a key area for recurrent decay or restoration loss. Most restorative problems in pediatric dentistry result from not considering the primary tooth's anatomical or morphologic structural characteristics. Marginal failure in the proximal box, often due to excessive flare of the cavosurface margin, is common. Incomplete caries removal or inadequate condensation can also lead to restoration failure.[75,76] Failure of adhesive restorations can also result due to deviation from the manufacturer's recommendations for etchant materials, light cure time, and maximum material depth.

Full Coronal Coverage of Primary Molars

Preformed metal crowns, also referred to as *stainless steel crowns,* were introduced to pediatric dentistry by Humphrey in 1950.[77] Since then, they have become the treatment of choice for primary teeth with large carious lesions or hypoplasia. SSCs are made of a combination of nickel, iron, and chromium. They do not contain mercury or silver (though they are sometimes called "silver crowns"). Although in rare cases hypersensitivity reactions from nickel have been reported for SSCs, as they have been for orthodontic appliances, the release of metal ions is below the normal dietary intake levels.[78] SSCs are generally considered superior to large, multisurface amalgam or adhesive restorations and have a longer clinical life span than two- or three-surface restorations.[68,70,79–81] They are also indicated to create an effective coronal seal and provide stability for weakened dentinal structure in primary teeth that have had vital pulp therapy. The crowns are manufactured in different sizes as a metal shell with some preformed anatomy and are trimmed and contoured as necessary to fit individual teeth.

Precontoured crowns are the most popular, and their use is recommended because their anatomy more closely resembles a natural tooth. These crowns are prebelled, prefestooned, and precontoured. Some trimming and contouring may be necessary but usually is minimal. If trimming of these crowns becomes necessary, the precontour will be lost and the crown will fit more loosely than before trimming. Examples include 3M ESPE Stainless Steel Crowns (Minneapolis, MN); Acero3S crowns (Acero Crowns, Seattle, WA), and NuSmile Stainless Steel Crowns (Houston, TX). **Pretrimmed** crowns have straight, noncontoured sides but are festooned to follow a line parallel to the gingival crest. They require contouring and may require some trimming. These crowns require more time and effort for placement and are no longer widely used. Examples include Unitek stainless steel crowns (3M ESPE, Minneapolis, MN) and Denovo crowns (Denovo Inc., Baldwin Park, CA).

The most common complaint parents have about SSCs is their appearance. Unfortunately, there are no tooth-colored, durable SSCs currently available; however, there are other esthetic full coverage options that have been gaining in popularity since 2010. One such option is a prefabricated ZC for primary teeth (Fig. 30.15). ZCs in adults have been shown to be very esthetic, durable, stain resistant, biocompatible, and retentive,[82] and primary ZCs' clinical performance is similar. A recent systematic review and meta-analysis of primary ZCs concluded that, compared with SSCs, these crowns were associated with better gingival and periodontal health, good retention, high fracture resistance, color stability, high parental acceptance, good marginal adaptation, smooth cosmetic surface, and no recurrent caries.[83,84] Like SSCs, primary ZCs come in six premade sizes and can be prepared, fit, and cemented in a 20- to 30-minute visit. Their indications and placement will be discussed later. Less popular esthetic full coverage posterior alternatives include resin-bonded posterior strip crowns and preveneered molar crowns, which are an SSC with a composite veneer overlay on the buccal and occlusal surfaces (e.g., NuSmile Primary Crowns, Houston, TX; Cheng Crowns, Exton, PA). Because of their infrequent use, they will not be discussed in this chapter. A third type of esthetic crown, introduced in 2022, is made of a high-strength resin polymer (BioFlx, NuSmile Primary Crowns, Houston, TX). It is flexible, metal free, and can be fit and placed like an SSC. Its availability has been limited so little is known about its long-term clinical results. However, a 1-year study comparing it with SSCs indicates that it has potential as an SSC replacement.[85]

SSCs are by far the most frequently used full coverage crown in the primary dentition, but the use of ZCs in both anterior and posterior teeth continues to increase in popularity. The indications for use of both are listed in Box 30.5. The steps of preparation and placement of SSCs and ZCs are listed in Box 30.6 and are shown in Fig. 30.16.

• BOX 30.5 Indications for Use of Full Coverage Primary Molar Crowns

1. Restoration of primary or young permanent teeth with extensive carious lesions. These include primary teeth with extensive decay, large lesions, or multiple surface lesions. First primary molars with mesial interproximal lesions are included in the category because the morphologic appearance that the tooth exhibits results in inadequate support for mesial interproximal restorations.
2. Restoration of hypoplastic primary or permanent teeth.
3. Restoration of primary teeth after pulpotomy or pulpectomy procedures.
4. Restoration of teeth with hereditary anomalies such as dentinogenesis imperfecta or amelogenesis imperfecta.
5. Restorations in disabled individuals or others in whom oral hygiene is extremely poor and failure of other materials is likely.
6. As an abutment for space maintainers or prosthetic appliances (stainless steel crowns only, not zirconia).
7. Strong consideration should be given to the use of full coverage restorations in children who require general anesthesia for dental treatment and demonstrate a high caries risk.

Note: Zirconia crowns are recommended for patients with known metal allergies, or who may require head and neck MRI imaging.

Data from Seale NS, Randall R. The use of stainless steel crowns: a systematic literature review. *Pediatr Dent.* 2015;37(2):147-162.

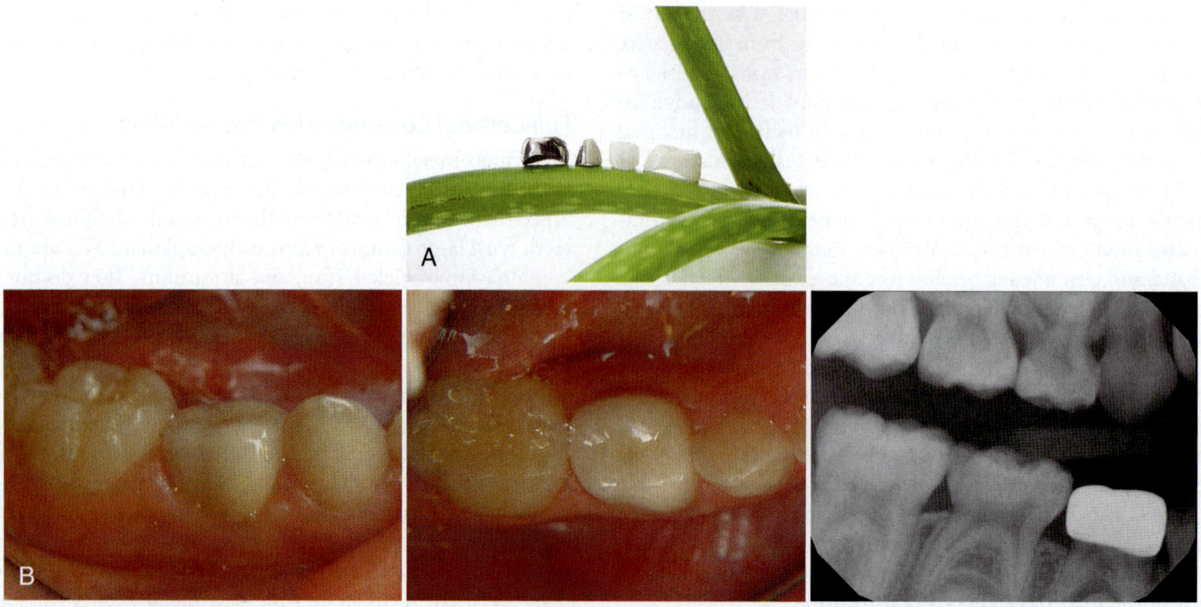

• **Fig. 30.15** (A) Stainless steel, resin face stainless steel, and zirconia crowns. (B) Zirconia crown on first primary molar.

• BOX 30.6 Steps for Preparation and Placement of Stainless Steel Crowns and Zirconia Crowns on Primary Molars

Several different preparation designs have been advocated for stainless steel crowns (SSCs) over the years. Only one such preparation, requiring minimal tooth reduction for SSCs, is discussed here. Necessary adjustments for zirconia crown preparation, fitting, and cementation are noted for each step.

1. Evaluate the preoperative occlusion. Note the dental midline and the cusp-fossa relationship bilaterally.
2. Administer appropriate local anesthesia and place a rubber dam/isolation system. Because gingival tissues all around the tooth may be manipulated during crown placement, it is important to obtain lingual or palatal, as well as buccal or facial anesthesia.
3. Reduction of the occlusal surface is carried out with a no. 169L taper fissure bur or a football diamond. Depth cuts of 1.0 to 1.5 mm can assist with occlusal reduction. Reduce the occlusal surface by 1.5 mm, maintaining the cuspal inclines of the crown (see Fig. 30.16). Establish access to decay with a no. 330 or 169L bur and then remove decay with a large, round bur or with a spoon excavator. *Note: If a zirconia crown is going to be placed, slightly more occlusal reduction (1.5–2 mm) will be necessary.*
4. Proximal reduction is accomplished with the taper fissure bur or thin, tapered diamond. Contact with the adjacent tooth must be broken gingivally and buccolingually, maintaining vertical walls with only a slight convergence in an occlusal direction. Proximal reduction should be approximately 1 mm. The gingival proximal margin should have a feather-edge finish line. Care must be taken not to damage adjacent tooth structure. *Note: For placement of a zirconia crown, proximal reduction should be at least 1.5 mm mesially and distally but also ending in a feather edge.*
5. Round all line angles. For SSCs, buccolingual reduction is often limited to this beveling and is confined to the occlusal one-third of the crown. If problems are later encountered in selecting an appropriate crown size or in fitting a crown over a large mesiobuccal bulge, more reduction of the buccal and lingual tooth structure may become necessary. *Important note: If a zirconia crown is being placed, circumferential reduction including the buccal and lingual surfaces is definitely necessary and all bulges and heights of convexity must be removed, especially on the mesiobuccal. Proximal line angles are rounded. All angles of the preparation should be rounded to remove corners. Avoid an overtapered preparation.*
6. Selection of an SSC crown begins as a trial-and-error procedure. The goal is to place the smallest crown that can be seated on the tooth and to establish preexisting proximal contacts. (*Helpful hint:* Size 4 is a frequently used crown size for molar SSCs.) The selected SSC is tried on the preparation by seating the lingual first and applying pressure in a buccal direction so that the crown slides over the buccal surface into the gingival sulcus. Friction should be felt as the crown slips over the buccal bulge. Some teeth are an "in-between" size, so that one crown size is too small to seat and the next larger size fits very loosely, even after contouring. Further tooth reduction, especially on the buccal and lingual surfaces, may be necessary in these cases to seat the smaller crown. After seating a crown, establish a preliminary occlusal relationship by comparing adjacent marginal ridge heights.

If the crown does not seat to the same level as the adjacent teeth:

- The occlusal reduction may be inadequate
- A gingival proximal ledge may exist
- Contact may not have been broken with the adjacent tooth, preventing a complete seating of the crown.
- The crown may be too long

The crown may be too long. An extensive area of gingival blanching around the crown indicates that the crown is too long or is grossly overcontoured. Some crowns may need to be trimmed slightly for a better fit. Crown and bridge trimming scissors, a heatless stone mounted on the low-speed straight handpiece, and a rubber wheel can be used to neatly trim and smooth an SSC. A properly trimmed crown should extend approximately 1 mm into the gingival sulcus.

The margins of the finished, trimmed steel crown consist of a series of curves or arcs as determined by the marginal gingiva of the tooth being restored. There should be no corners, jagged angles, right angles, or straight lines found on these margins (see Fig. 30.16). *Note: Selection of zirconia crowns is also trial and error; however, when a zirconia crown does not seat completely onto a tooth, the crown cannot be adjusted and more tooth preparation is required until the crown slides over the preparation passively and is completely seated compared with adjacent teeth. If the crown fits very loosely, a smaller crown should be selected. If it does not seat completely, further reduction of the tooth will be necessary. Often the zirconia crown does not seat well because of a gingival ledge on the preparation.* Contour and crimp the SSC to form a tightly fitting crown. Contouring involves bending the gingival one-third of the crown's margins inward to restore anatomical features of the natural crown and to reduce the marginal circumference of the crown, ensuring a good fit. Contouring is accomplished circumferentially with a no. 114 ball-and-socket pliers (see Fig. 30.18A) or with a no. 137 Gordon pliers. Final close adaptation of the crown is achieved by crimping the cervical margin 1 mm circumferentially. The no. 137 pliers may be used for this; special crimping pliers, such as no. 800-417 (3M ESPE; see Fig. 30.18B), are also available. A tight marginal fit aids in (1) mechanical retention of the crown, (2) protection of the cement from exposure to oral fluids, and (3) maintenance of gingival health. After contouring and crimping, firm resistance should be encountered when the crown is seated. After seating the crown, examine the gingival margins with an explorer for areas of poor fit. Observe the gingival tissue for blanching, and examine the proximal contacts. When removing the crown, a spoon excavator can be used to engage the gingival margin and dislodge the crown. A thumb or finger should be kept over the crown during removal so that movement of the crown is controlled. *Note: There is no contouring, crimping, or trimming a zirconia crown.*

7. The rubber dam/isolation system is removed, and special care must be taken when handling the crown in the mouth. A 2 × 2-inch gauze pad should be placed posterior to the tooth being crowned to prevent the crown from dropping into the oropharynx. Place the crown on the tooth, and examine the occlusion bilaterally with the patient in centric occlusion. Look for movement of the crown occlusogingivally with biting pressure, and check for excessive gingival blanching.
8. If the SSC was trimmed, final smoothing and polishing of the crown margin should be performed before cementation to ensure there are no jagged edges.
9. Rinse and dry the SSC inside and out, and prepare to cement it. A glass ionomer or resin-modified glass ionomer cement is preferred for SSCs. The crown is filled approximately two-thirds with cement, with all inner surfaces covered. *Note: Before cementation, the inside of a zirconia crown should be free of contamination. Salivary and hemorrhagic by-products will adhere to the surface of zirconia and cannot be simply washed away. If the crown has been in contact with blood or saliva it is advisable to clean the interior by sandblasting, or use of a decontaminating agent such as Ivoclean (Ivoclar Vivadent, Amherst, NY). This will ensure maximum cement retention. A light-activated resin-modified glass ionomer or bioactive cement is recommended for cementation of zirconia cement. Bleeding is inevitable, due to the subgingival preparation. Achieving excellent hemostasis is imperative to restoration success (see* Fig. 30.26).
10. Dry the tooth with compressed air and seat the SSC completely. Cement should be expressed from all margins. The handle of a mirror or the flat end of a band pusher may be used to ensure complete seating, or the patient may be instructed to bite on a tongue blade. Before the cement sets, have the patient close into centric occlusion and confirm that the occlusion has not been altered. *Note: For zirconia crowns make sure the preparation is free of saliva and blood, and seat the crown gently, tack cure the cement (if light activated), and carefully remove excess cement while keeping the crown stabilized with finger pressure. After cement removal, finish curing the cement from buccal, lingual, and occlusal directions.*
11. Cement must be removed from the gingival sulcus. Excessive glass ionomer cement can be removed immediately with a wet gauze and/or water spray. The interproximal areas can be cleaned by tying a knot in a piece of dental floss and drawing the floss through the interproximal region. A scaler may be needed to remove hardened cement.
12. Rinse the oral cavity well, and reexamine the occlusion and the soft tissues before dismissing the patient. *Note: You cannot adjust the occlusion of an SSC, and it is extremely difficult to adjust a zirconia crown. If the occlusion requires adjustment, consideration should be made to adjusting the tooth opposing the crown.*

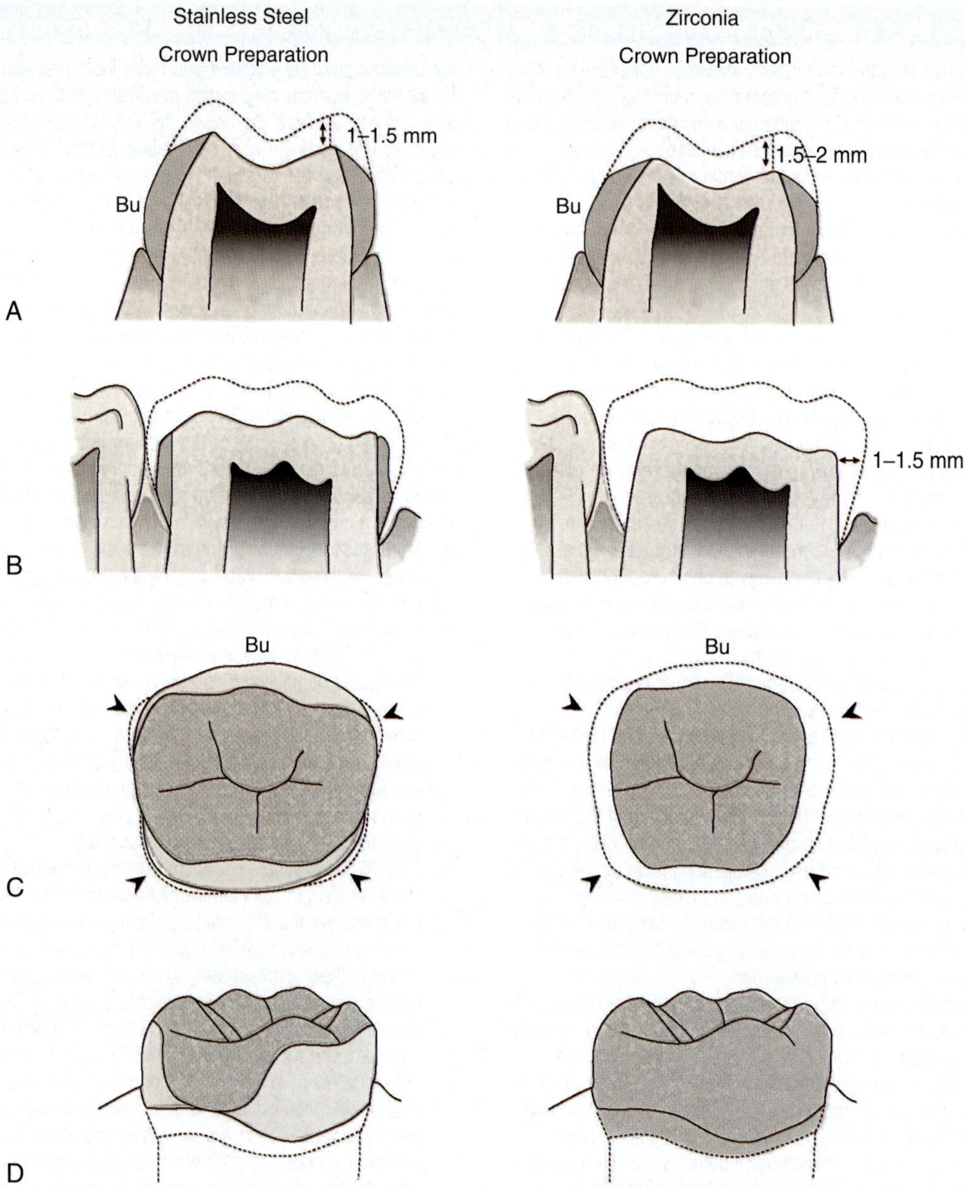

• **Fig. 30.16** Stainless steel crown (SSC) and zirconia crown (ZC) preparation of mandibular second primary molar. (A) Proximal view. Note there is more occlusal reduction for ZCs. (B) Buccal view. Note feather-edge gingival margins on both crown preps but more proximal reduction for zirconia. (C) Occlusal view. Note for SSCs the line angles are just rounded, but circumferential reduction is necessary for the zirconia. (D) Mesiolingual view. For SSCs, lingual and buccal reduction is limited to beveling of the occlusal third, but for zirconia it extends subgingivally to a feather edge. *Bu,* Buccal.

HALL TECHNIQUE OF STAINLESS STEEL CROWN PLACEMENT

N. Sue Seale, DDS, MSD

The Hall technique (HT) of stainless steel crown (SSC) placement is a cost-effective and patient-friendly way to target the biology of dental caries. This minimally invasive technique was first practiced in 1988 by Dr. Norna Hall, a general practitioner in Scotland. It works by entombing caries by fitting an SSC and cementing it over a tooth without local anesthetic, caries removal, or tooth preparation.[1–3] Multiple systematic reviews and randomized clinical trials have concluded that HT is a predictable restorative option with low failure and re-treatment rates compared with traditionally prepared SSCs and other intracoronal restorations.[4–6]

The HT technique is less sensitive than traditional SSC preparation. For placement, the patient should be seated in the dental chair and kept in an upright position because no rubber dam is used and the airway must be protected. No topical or local anesthetic is administered. The clinician chooses the smallest SSC that will seat over the unprepared tooth. It should cover all cusps with a feeling of "spring back," and there should be no attempt to fully seat the crown during try-in. A piece of tape on the occlusal surface may be used to hold the crown for extra security. The chosen SSC is then filled with glass ionomer (GI) cement and seated over the caries-affected tooth, initially using finger pressure and then the patient's own occlusal force if possible. Excess cement is removed, and then pressure is reapplied and the excess cement cleaned again. Then occlusal pressure is maintained by having the child bite on a cotton roll until the cement sets. The high percentage of collagen fibers in the primary periodontal ligament allows for adjustment to the increased occlusal vertical dimension (OVD) over 3 to 4 weeks.[7,8] The superior ability of pediatric masticatory systems to adapt and equilibrate to changes in OVD also may protect against Hall crowns from causing temporomandibular joint dysfunctions (TMDs).

Hall crowns have been shown to be effective for both occlusal and occlusoproximal lesions.[6] Because the HT of SSC placement requires no tooth preparation, occasionally orthodontic separators may be needed in the interproximal areas of the caries-affected tooth to create spacing for easier placement of the crown. The separators may be left in place for several hours or days before the crown appointment.[2,8]

The HT was considered controversial when it was first introduced into the United States due to the initial open bite created and because it does not remove active caries. Studies show the open bite resolved within the first month,[5,8] and entombing caries-affected dentin in teeth parallels the success of a selective caries removal process.[9] Minimally invasive dentistry techniques are successful as long as the seal is maintained and the pulpal status is properly diagnosed pretreatment.[10] To that end, diagnostic radiographs showing the furcation and a thorough clinical history for symptoms are essential when selecting teeth as candidates for the HT.

The HT is indicated in patients who are precooperative, or behaviorally not able to participate in traditional restorative care, yet are not candidates for treatment with sedation or under general anesthesia due to the extent of their individual dental needs, medical complexities, or if using these modalities will be significantly delayed because of available resources. It is also a viable alternative to traditional restorative options when the patient or parent prefers less invasive treatment.[11] The HT of SSC placement can be used similarly to how interim therapeutic restorations (ITRs) have been used in the past, with longer survival time.[12] Permanent molars with enamel hypoplasia and early destruction of the occlusal surfaces can be treated with the HT until the tooth and patient are able to receive a more definitive restoration.

Drawbacks to using HT include parental nonacceptance of the esthetics of an SSC and discomfort in some children during placement.[12,13] Its ease of placement, patient-friendliness, and proven longevity may outweigh these limitations.[14]

References available digitally.

Special considerations for primary crown placement

Placement of Adjacent Crowns. When quadrant dentistry is practiced, it often is necessary to place SSCs or ZCs on adjacent teeth.[65] Tooth preparation and crown selection when placing multiple crowns are similar to that previously described for single crowns. However, there are several additional areas of consideration:

- *Underreduction:* Prepare occlusal reduction of one tooth completely before beginning occlusal reduction of the other tooth. When reduction of two teeth is performed simultaneously, the tendency is to underreduce both.
- *Insufficient proximal reduction:* This is a common problem when adjacent crowns are placed. Contact between adjacent proximal surfaces should be broken, producing an approximately 1.5-mm separation at the gingival level.
- *Order of cementation:* Both crowns should be trimmed, contoured, and prepared for cementation simultaneously. To determine fit, it is generally best to begin placement of the more distal tooth first. The sequence of placement of crowns during cementation should follow the same sequence as when the crowns were placed for fitting. Sometimes crowns that seat quite easily in one placement sequence will seat with great difficulty if the sequence is altered.

Preparing Crowns in Areas of Space Loss. When tooth structure is lost because of caries, adjacent teeth lose proximal contact and drift into space normally occupied by the tooth to be restored. When this happens, the crown required to fit over the buccolingual dimension will be too wide mesiodistally to be placed, and a crown selected to fit the mesiodistal space will be too small in circumference. Placing ZCs in areas of space loss can be extremely challenging and may be a contraindication to their placement because the ZCs cannot be reshaped. The only way to get them to fit in areas of space loss is extensive circumferential tooth reduction. For SSCs, a larger crown, which will fit over the tooth's greatest convexity, is selected and an adjustment is made to reduce mesiodistal width (Fig. 30.17). This adjustment is accomplished by grasping the marginal ridges of the crown with Howe utility pliers and squeezing it, thereby reducing the mesiodistal dimension. Considerable recontouring of proximal, buccal, and lingual walls of the crown with the no. 137 or no. 114 pliers will be necessary (Fig. 30.18). If difficulty in crown placement is still encountered, additional tooth reduction of the buccal and lingual surfaces and selection of another, smaller crown may be necessary. When the area of space loss is in the region of the distal surface of a mandibular first primary molar and difficulty is encountered finding the appropriate size crown because of the space loss, another alternative exists. Select a maxillary first primary molar crown for the opposite side of the mouth and try it on the mandibular tooth. Due to the space loss, often the mandibular tooth preparation resembles a maxillary tooth and may be more suited for placement of the maxillary crown. By selecting the maxillary crown for the opposite side of the mouth, the crown's gingival margin contour in the area of the mesiobuccal cervical bulge fits the mandibular mesiobuccal cervical bulge. If several millimeters of space have been lost, it may be necessary to extract the tooth and place a space maintainer rather than struggling to place a crown on a compromised tooth preparation (Fig. 30.19).

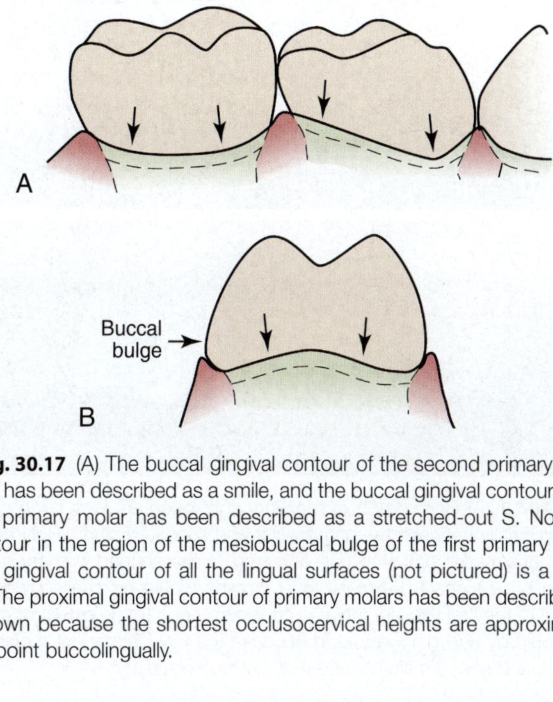

• **Fig. 30.17** (A) The buccal gingival contour of the second primary molar *(left)* has been described as a smile, and the buccal gingival contour of the first primary molar has been described as a stretched-out S. Note the contour in the region of the mesiobuccal bulge of the first primary molar. The gingival contour of all the lingual surfaces (not pictured) is a smile. (B) The proximal gingival contour of primary molars has been described as a frown because the shortest occlusocervical heights are approximately midpoint buccolingually.

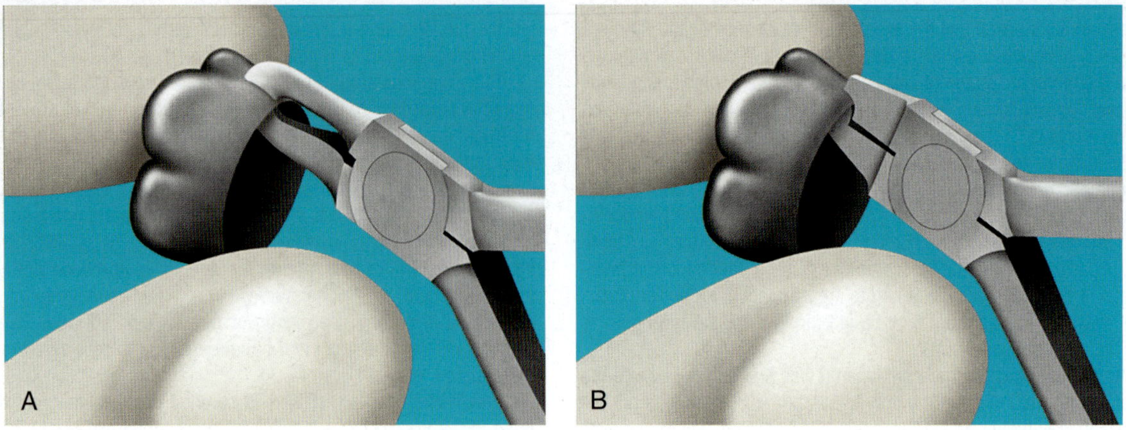

• **Fig. 30.18** (A) Contouring is accomplished with no. 114 pliers. (B) Final crimping is accomplished with no. 800-417 pliers. (Courtesy 3M ESPE, St. Paul, MN.)

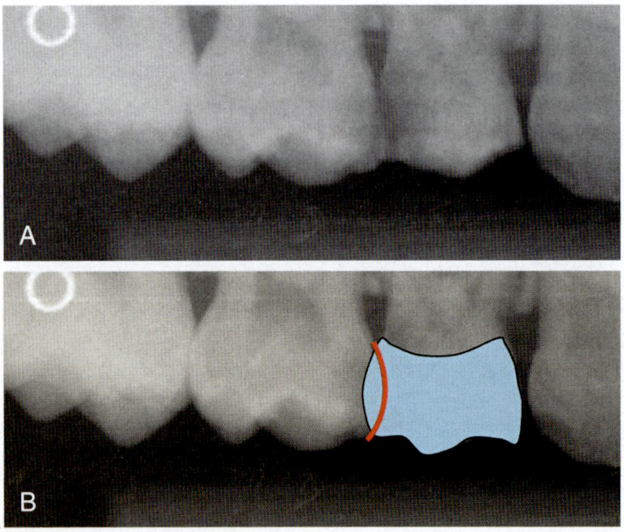

• **Fig. 30.19** (A) Radiograph of maxillary right quadrant with large caries interproximally between the primary first and second molars. (B) Note the space loss/mesial drift that has occurred of the second primary molar. Placing back-to-back stainless steel crowns would be challenging. Extraction of the first primary molar is considered due to the extent of caries (both pulpally and gingivally) and because the first permanent molar has erupted and space maintenance may not be necessary.

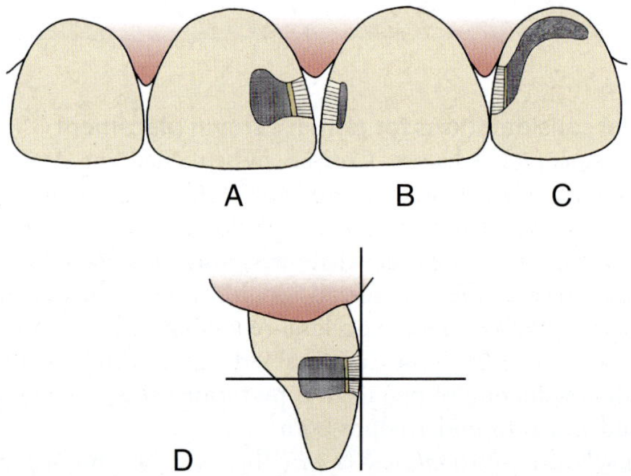

• **Fig. 30.20** Class III cavity preparations (*A, B, C:* labial view). Note that a short bevel is placed on the cavosurface margin of all three preparations. *(A)* Slot preparation with a dovetail (a frequently used class III preparation). The dovetail provides additional retention. *(B)* Slot preparation, used for very small class III carious lesions. *(C)* Modified slot preparation, used when extensive gingival decalcification is evident adjacent to interproximal caries. *(D)* The interproximal box is placed perpendicular to a line tangent to the labial surface.

Restoration of Primary Incisors and Canines

Indications for restoration of primary incisors and canines are generally based on the presence of (1) caries, (2) trauma, or (3) developmental defects of the tooth's hard tissue. In these situations, adhesive materials may be used to restore class III and class V restorations. Class IV restorations may also be done; however, if a great deal of tooth structure has been lost, full coverage with a crown will provide a superior restoration.

Class III Restorations

Class III restorations on primary anterior teeth are very challenging to do well (Fig. 30.20). Caries often extend subgingivally, making good isolation and hemorrhage control difficult. Because of the large size of the pulps of these teeth, the preparations must be kept very small. A simple slot preparation may be used, which merely removes decay and has a short cavosurface bevel.[86] However, in children, especially those with bruxism, experience has revealed that retention of class III restorations solely with acid etching can be inadequate, and additional mechanical retention may be required. Retention can be gained with retentive locks on the facial or lingual surface and by beveling the cavosurface margin to increase the surface area of the enamel etched.[87,88] It has been suggested that preparing the entire facial surface by 0.5 mm and veneering the surface for additional bonding can significantly improve retention of class III restorations.[89]

Restoring the distal surface of primary canines (Fig. 30.21) requires a preparation slightly different from that for incisors. The proximal box is directed at a different angle toward the

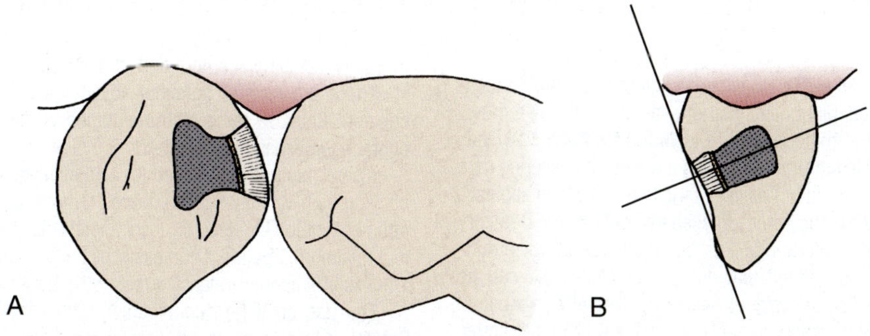

• **Fig. 30.21** Class III Preparation for Primary Canines. (A) The dovetail is usually placed on the lingual surface of maxillary canines and on the labial surface of mandibular canines. A short bevel (not shown) is placed on the cavosurface margin of preparations to be restored with resin-based composite. (B) The proximal box is placed perpendicular to a line tangent to the surface on which the dovetail is placed.

• BOX 30.7 Steps in Preparation and Placement of a Class III Adhesive Restoration

1. Administer appropriate anesthesia and place the rubber dam with ligation of individual teeth.
2. Place a wooden wedge interproximally to protect soft tissues.
3. Prepare the tooth using a no. 330 bur, via facial access. The axial wall is ideally placed 0.5 mm into dentin. The gingival and lingual walls should just break contact with the adjacent tooth, leaving incisal wall to maintain adequate tooth structure.
4. To enhance retention, a dovetail or lock may be placed on the labial or lingual surface (should not extend more than halfway across the labial surface, is kept in the middle third of the tooth, or may extend across the cervical, if there is presence of cervical decalcification).
5. Place a short bevel (0.5 mm) at the cavosurface margin. This may be accomplished with a tapered diamond bur.
6. Remove carious dentin and place base/liner for pulp protection if indicated.
7. Place a plastic or sectional metal matrix. Cut a plastic matrix in half horizontally because they are too wide for primary teeth. The matrix is placed interproximally, and a wedge is reinserted. *Note: A resin strip crown form can be trimmed to cover the preparation only (not the entire crown) to create a custom matrix, which often is easier to use than a matrix strip.*
8. If using a total etch technique, etch the preparation for 10 seconds, ideally applying to enamel margins and then to dentin. Rinse and dry the preparation. If a self-etching adhesive is used, this step is eliminated.
9. Place adhesive in the preparation with a small brush. Gently air dry to disperse a thin layer of adhesive evenly. Polymerize with curing light.
10. With a plastic instrument or a pressure syringe, place the composite in the preparation. Pull the matrix tightly around the cavity preparation with finger pressure and hold until cured.
11. Hold the curing light as closely as possible to the composite and polymerize per the manufacturer's instructions. The light should be directed from both the facial and the lingual surfaces to ensure complete polymerization.
12. Finishing and polishing can be performed immediately after polymerization. The smoothest and most desirable surface of a composite is that which remains after a properly adapted matrix is removed; however, it is difficult to adapt a matrix so accurately that additional adjustment to the margins is unnecessary. Gross finishing or contouring can be performed with fine-grit diamonds or with carbide finishing burs. A flame carbide finishing bur (12–20 flutes) is excellent for finishing the facial and interproximal surfaces. The lingual surface is best finished with a round or pear-shaped carbide finishing bur. A lubricated, pointed white stone may also be used for smoothing. Final interproximal polishing of the restoration is completed with sandpaper strips. These strips will be best used if they are cut into thin strips 2–3 mm in width. Mounted abrasive disks can be used to finish the facial and lingual surfaces.
13. When finishing is completed, remove isolation materials and floss the interproximal areas to check for overhangs and flash.

gingiva. A dovetail may be placed on the facial surface or lingual surface to aid in retention in this high-wear area. The steps in preparation and placement of a class III composite restoration are listed in Box 30.7.

Class V Restorations

Class V restorations are most often needed on the facial surface of canines. To prepare these restorations, access the tooth in the area of caries with a no. 330 bur. Move the bur laterally into sound dentin and enamel, thus establishing the walls of the cavity. The pulpal wall should be convex, parallel to the outer enamel surface. The lateral walls are slightly flared near the proximal surfaces to prevent undermining of the enamel. The final external outline is determined by the extent of caries. Mechanical retention in the preparation can be achieved with a no. 35 inverted cone bur or a no. ½ round bur, creating small undercuts in the gingivoaxial and incisoaxial line angles. For resin-based composites, a short bevel is placed around the entire cavosurface margin. Etching, bonding, material placement, and finishing are like that described for class III adhesive restorations, except that no matrix is used.

ALTERNATIVE RESTORATIVE TREATMENT

Michael J. Kanellis

Atraumatic restorative treatment (ART) is a minimally invasive treatment technique for restoring teeth by means of hand instrumentation for decay removal and fluoride-releasing adhesive materials (glass ionomer) for filling.[1] ART has been promoted by the World Health Organization as a means of delivering care in underdeveloped countries that do not have electricity or access to sophisticated dental equipment.[2] In 2001 the American Academy of Pediatric Dentistry (AAPD) adopted a policy on ART, referring to it as "alternative restorative treatment." The AAPD policy acknowledged that not all dental disease can be treated by "traditional" restorative techniques and recognized ART as a useful and beneficial technique in the treatment and management of dental caries where traditional cavity preparation and placement of traditional dental restorations are not possible. The AAPD further refined their policy and included the technique in a broader discussion of "Interim Therapeutic Restorations" (ITRs).[3] The use of ART in developed countries has led to modifications of the technique that allow for the occasional use of a slow speed handpiece and follow-up care that may include placement of a traditional restoration.

There are several potential advantages to ART when used with young children. Because hand instrumentation is used, the noise and vibration of dental handpieces is eliminated.

Also eliminated is the need for acid etching, water coolant, and the accompanying high-velocity suction. Caries removal using hand instrumentation also often eliminates the need for local anesthesia. Because instrumentation is kept to a minimum, treatment can easily be carried out in the knee-to-knee position. The use of a fluoride-releasing restorative material helps prevent further decay.

The use of ART in combination with silver diamine fluoride, known as SMART (silver modified atraumatic restorative treatment) has been recommended because this combined approach kills bacteria before sealing a cavity with glass ionomer.[4]

References available digitally.

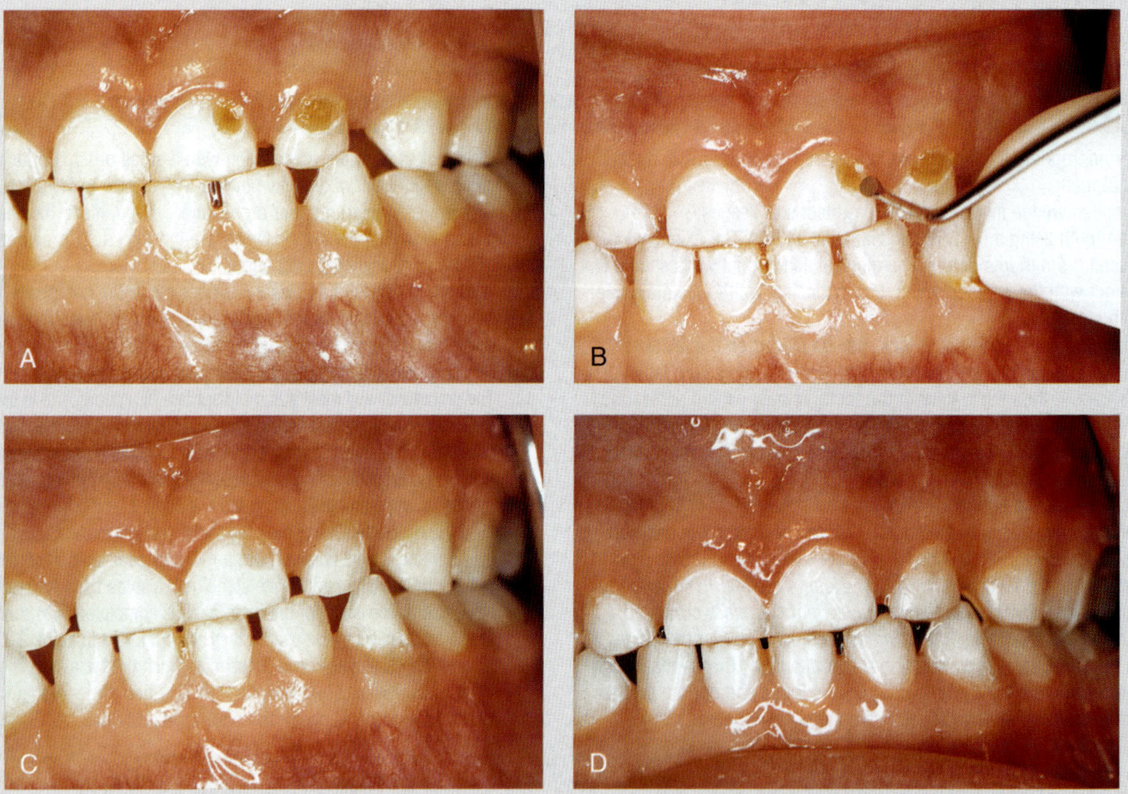

(A) Facial caries evident on incisors and cuspid. (B) Spoon excavator positioned for decay removal. (C) After caries removal with spoon excavator. (D) Teeth restored with glass ionomer restorative material.

Full Coronal Coverage of Incisors

Indications

The indications for full coronal coverage of incisors include the following[90]:

- Large interproximal lesions, or large lesions covering a single surface (e.g., lingual surfaces in early childhood caries)
- Teeth that have received pulp therapy
- Fractures of the incisal edge where an appreciable amount of tooth structure is lost
- Multiple hypoplastic defects or developmental disturbances (e.g., amelogenesis imperfecta, ectodermal dysplasia)
- Discolorations that are esthetically unpleasing
- Teeth with small interproximal lesions that also demonstrate large areas of cervical decalcification (i.e., high caries risk)

It is a challenging task to repair extensively destroyed anterior teeth with restorations that are durable, retentive, and esthetic. There are several methods of providing full coronal coverage to primary incisors, but adhesive resin–based composite crowns (CCs), preveneered SSCs, and preformed ZCs are the most popular (Fig. 30.22). Conventional SSCs and open-face SSCs remain a durable restoration for primary anterior teeth; however, they are often perceived to be esthetically objectionable to parents.[91]

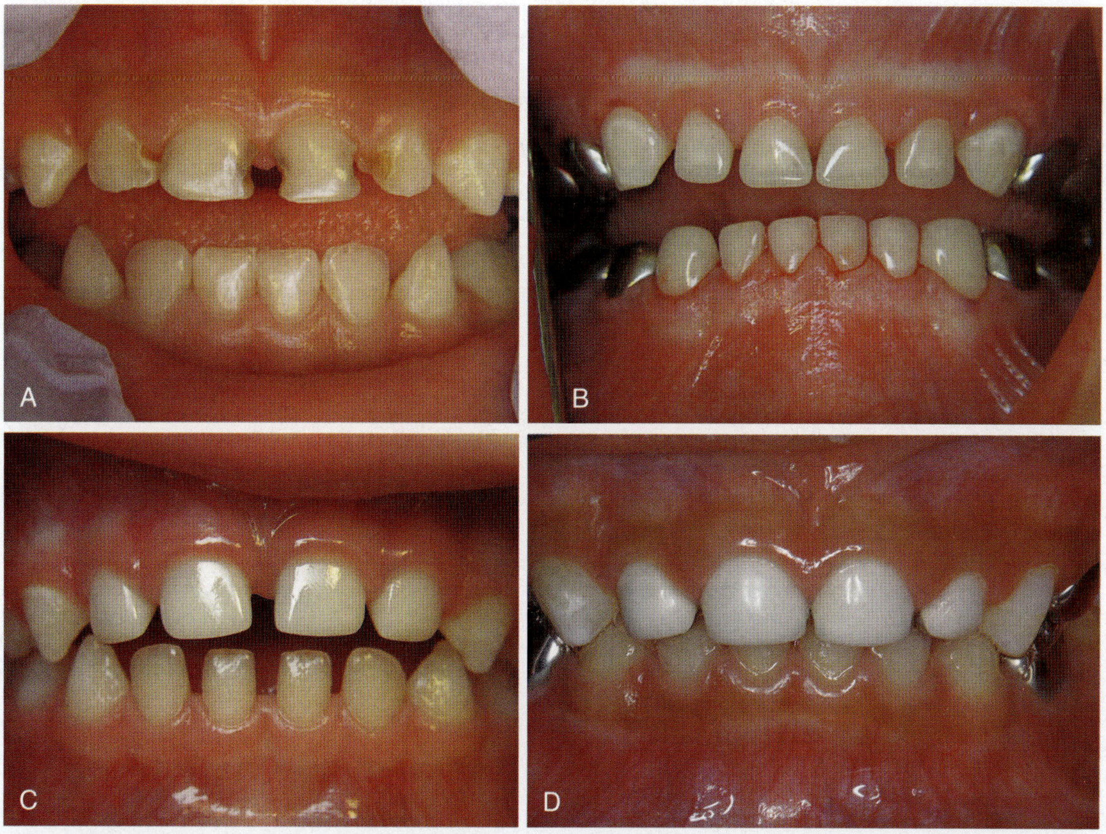

• **Fig. 30.22** Full Coronal Coverage of Primary Incisors. (A) Multiple interproximal carious lesions in primary incisors. The incisors restored with (B). Adhesive resin–based composite crowns (strip crowns). (C) Zirconia primary crowns. (D) Preveneered stainless steel crowns.

The last survey to investigate use of primary anterior crowns was published in 2010, before the introduction of primary ZCs, so we do not have data about current provider preferences.[92] However, anecdotal reports suggest that the use of preveneered and conventional SSCs may be decreasing, with CCs and ZCs on the rise. All have shortcomings (Table 30.4) but may still be used in certain situations.

The adhesive resin–based CC or "strip" crown (i.e., 3M Strip Crown Form [3M ESPE, Minneapolis, MN]) has a long history of clinically satisfactory results with reasonable durability and high parental acceptance.[93,94] Their relative affordability makes them a popular choice to this day. Primary ZCs are the newest anterior pediatric crown type, and several brands are available such as EZCrowns (Sprig Oral Health Technologies, Inc., Loomis, CA), NuSmile ZR (Houston, TX), and Zirconia Kinder Krowns (Kinder Krowns, Eden Prairie, MN). The evidence base for their use has grown over time, with studies suggesting improved retention and durability compared with CCs. Their superior esthetics and improved periodontal health have also made them increasingly popular among parents and clinicians.[95–97] The main concern with the primary ZCs is that the preparation requires significant reduction of the tooth to fit a rigid crown. This may lead to increased incidence in pulp complications that can lead to infection.[98] Traditional SSCs are not frequently used to restore maxillary primary incisors because of the poor esthetics. However, they may be used on severely decayed canines and mandibular incisors, where esthetics are less critical.

The steps for preparation and placement of CCs are listed in Box 30.8 and shown in Fig. 30.23. Because all the anterior crown types have similarities in preparation and placement, noted differences for the preveneered SSCs and ZCs are also listed in Box 30.8.

Preveneered Steel Crowns

Preveneered SSCs for primary incisors and canines (see Fig. 30.22D) provide a one-step esthetic restoration that, unlike CCs or pediatric ZCs, can be placed in the presence of hemorrhage or moisture without affecting the restoration integrity or final esthetic result.[99] They can also be placed on teeth with little remaining tooth structure. Multiple manufacturers make preveneered SSCs: NuSmile, Kinder Krowns, and Cheng Crowns.

Preveneered SSCs have at least three limitations: (1) crimping is limited primarily to the lingual surfaces, but this does not appear to diminish retention because they can be retained as well as crimped anterior SSCs[90]; (2) each crown costs approximately $24 to $32, compared with approximately $6 to $12 for strip crown forms, making an inventory much more costly; and (3) some restorations may develop veneer fractures. If this occurs, replacing the crown, rather than repairing the fracture, will usually provide the fastest, most esthetically pleasing result. One study found fractures or wear of the veneer in approximately 14% of crowns,[100] with canines most likely to be affected. This percentage is slightly less than the incidence of fractures reported with CCs.[94] Parental acceptance for these crowns has been reported to be very high, with more than 90% of parents reporting they were satisfied or very satisfied with their child's preveneered crowns.[101]

TABLE 30.4 Comparison of Full Coverage Techniques for Primary Incisors

Technique	Esthetics	Durability	Time for Placement	Selection Criteria
Resin (strip) crowns[a]	Very good initially; may discolor over time	Retention dependent on amount of tooth structure present and quality of acid etch Can be dislodged fairly easily if traumatized	Time required for optimum isolation, etching, placement, finishing	When esthetics is a great concern Adequate tooth structure remains for etching/bonding Child is not highly prone to trauma Gingival hemorrhage is controllable
Zirconia ceramic crowns[a]	Excellent	Ceramic is very durable, rarely chips or breaks Can be dislodged, especially if prep is excessively tapered or poor cement bond	Like a preveneered crown (prep must fit the crown form)	Adequate tooth structure remains, similar to a strip crown Esthetics of great concern
Preveneered steel crowns	Good	Good; however, facings may occasionally chip or fracture	Comparable to strip crowns; however, must make tooth fit the crown, which adds time	Esthetics is a concern Hemorrhage difficult to control Children with history of bruxism
Steel crowns[b]	Very poor	Very good; a well-crimped, cemented crown is very retentive and wears well	Fastest crown to place	Severely decayed teeth Esthetics of no concern Unable to control gingival hemorrhage Need to place restoration quickly because of inadequate cooperation or time

[a]Restoration of choice esthetically.
[b]Avoid using because of esthetics.

The preparations for preveneered SSCs and ZCs are similar, with some notable differences (see Box 30.8). The operator must keep in mind that the preveneered SSC preparation must be made to fit the crown because the resin-based composite facing is too brittle to permit additional manipulation. Therefore preparation of an incisor for a preveneered SSC is an iterative process. After the preparation is completed, select a crown and try it on the tooth. If the crown does not quite fit, a larger size must be selected or the tooth is further reduced until the crown slides **passively** onto the preparation and the margins are subgingival. Preveneered SSCs should not be forced onto the preparation. They must be fit with only light finger pressure. Too much force during seating can weaken or chip the resin veneer. A passive, sleevelike fit of the crown over the tooth is recommended.[102] Preveneered SSCs do not generally require trimming, and crimping of preveneered SSCs is minimal and limited to the lingual surface only. Preveneered SSCs are best cemented with a glass ionomer cement and may need to be held in place as it sets.

Prefabricated Zirconia Crowns

Prefabricated ZCs for primary incisors and canines provide a highly esthetic restoration (see Fig. 30.22C). Their primary disadvantages include aggressive preparation, a comparably high inventory cost ($20 to $30 per crown), cannot be trimmed or crimped, and cannot be repaired in the mouth. However, it is rare for a ZC to fracture or chip. The most obvious advantages of ZCs are their excellent esthetics, color stability, and durability.[99]

During preparation the operator must keep in mind that the ZC preparation must be made to fit the crown because ZCs will not flex over convexities (Fig. 30.24). Similar to the preveneered SSC preparation, preparation of an incisor for a ZC is an iterative process. Forceful seating can cause the gingival margin of the ZC to break. ZCs cannot be trimmed or crimped, and the occlusion cannot be adjusted easily.

ZCs are best cemented with an RMGI or bioactive cement to maximize retention to the zirconia surface through a chemical bond. It is imperative that hemorrhage and saliva be well controlled before cementing a ZC. Both may interfere with the bond of the RMGI cement to the tooth and/or the zirconia. Zirconia that has been contaminated with blood and/or saliva may lose much of its reactivity to bond well with cements.[103] For this reason, one ZC company (NuSmile ZR Crowns) provides a pink try-in crown that is used for fitting to the prep. After the appropriate size is determined, the try-in crown is exchanged for a noncontaminated white crown of that size, which is not tried on the tooth but is filled with cement and immediately placed on the tooth. The pink try-in crowns may be autoclaved and used multiple times. If a ZC is contaminated by saliva or blood, it should be cleaned internally by either air abrasion (sandblasting) or the use of a cleansing agent specifically for zirconia (Ivoclean, Ivoclar Vivadent, Amherst, NY). Zirconia manufacturers that do not use a try-in crown often place internal retentive grooves inside the crown for added mechanical retention of the cement.

Prosthetic Replacement of Primary Anterior Teeth

Premature loss of maxillary primary incisors because of extensive caries, trauma, or congenital absence may be cause for considering prosthetic tooth replacement for the child.[104] Space maintenance in this region is not generally necessary, and in most instances prosthetic replacement of primary incisors is considered an

• BOX 30.8 Preparation and Placement of Adhesive Resin–Based Composite Crowns With Considerations for Preveneered and Zirconia Crowns

1. Administer appropriate anesthesia.
2. Select the shade of resin-based composite to be used. Then place and ligate the rubber dam. *Note: For zirconia crowns a rubber dam is not typically used.*
3. Select a primary incisor celluloid crown form with a mesiodistal width approximately equal to the tooth to be restored. *Note: For zirconia crowns, estimate the size of crown that best approximates the natural tooth. This reduces the number of crowns that are contaminated during the fitting process.*
4. Reduce the incisal edge by 1.5 mm using a coarse diamond bur.
5. Reduce the interproximal surfaces by 0.5–1.0 mm (see Fig. 30.23). This reduction will allow a crown form to slip over the tooth. The interproximal walls should be parallel.
6. Reduce the facial surface by 1.0 mm and the lingual surface by at least 0.5 mm. Create a feather-edge gingival margin and round all line angles.
7. Remove caries with a large round bur and if pulp therapy is required, complete it now.
8. Place a small undercut on the facial surface in the gingival one-third of the tooth with a no. 330 bur or no. 35 inverted cone. When the resin material polymerizes, engaging the undercut, this serves as a mechanical lock. *Note: This is not required for preveneered or zirconia crowns, but also not contraindicated. However, zirconia crowns must be prepared subgingivally around the full circumference of the tooth to the depth of 1.5–2 mm creating a feather-edge margin (see* Fig. 30.24*). This must be completed after pulp therapy because it will create bleeding.*
9. Trim the selected plastic crown form by cutting away excess material gingivally with crown-and-bridge scissors, and trial fit the crown form. A properly trimmed crown form should fit 1 mm below the gingival crest and should be of comparable height to adjacent teeth. Remember that maxillary lateral incisor crowns are usually 0.5–1.0 mm shorter than those of central incisors. *Note: Preveneered and zirconia crowns are tried on until a crown slides passively over the preparation. If either will not seat passively, more tooth reduction will be necessary until it does seat. Because neither of these crowns flex when being placed onto a preparation, they must not be forced to seat, which could lead to fracture.*
10. After the celluloid crown is adequately trimmed, punch a small hole in the lingual surface with an explorer or a carbide bur to act as a vent for the escape of trapped air as the crown is placed with resin onto the preparation. At this point hemorrhage must be well controlled so it does not interfere with bonding or esthetics. *Note: If the zirconia crown has been contaminated with blood or saliva during try-in, it should be either air abraded internally or cleaned with a zirconia decontaminant (Ivoclean, Ivoclar Vivadent, Amherst, NY).* eFig. 30.26.
11. If a self-etching bonding agent is not used, etch the tooth with acid gel for 10 seconds. Rinse and dry the tooth; then apply an adhesive agent to the entire tooth and polymerize. *Note: This is not required for preveneered or zirconia crowns.*
12. Fill the crown form approximately two-thirds full with a resin-based composite material, and seat onto the tooth. Excess material should flow from the gingival margin and the vent hole. While holding the crown in place, remove the gingival excess with an explorer. *Note: Preveneered crowns are usually cemented with a glass ionomer cement, and zirconia crowns should be cemented with a resin-modified glass ionomer or bioactive cement. A light-activated cement may be used with zirconia crowns. The light will penetrate the zirconia and fix the crown in place with the initial cure.*
13. Polymerize the material. Be certain to direct the curing light from both the facial and lingual directions. *Note: For preveneered and zirconia, allow the cement to set and clean away all excess.*
14. Remove the celluloid form by using a composite finishing bur or a curved scalpel blade to cut the material on the lingual surface and then peel the form from the tooth.
15. Remove the rubber dam and evaluate the occlusion.
16. Little finishing should be required on the facial surface. A flame carbide finishing bur can be used to finish the gingival margin should any irregularities be noted upon tactile examination with an explorer. A round or pear-shaped finishing bur may be used for final contouring of the lingual surface. Abrasive disks are used for final polishing of areas of the crown that require contouring. *Note: For preveneered crowns the proximal-incisal corners may be contoured slightly to give a slightly less "boxy" appearance. Adjustments to zirconia crowns' occlusion or contour are extremely difficult and usually are not attempted.*

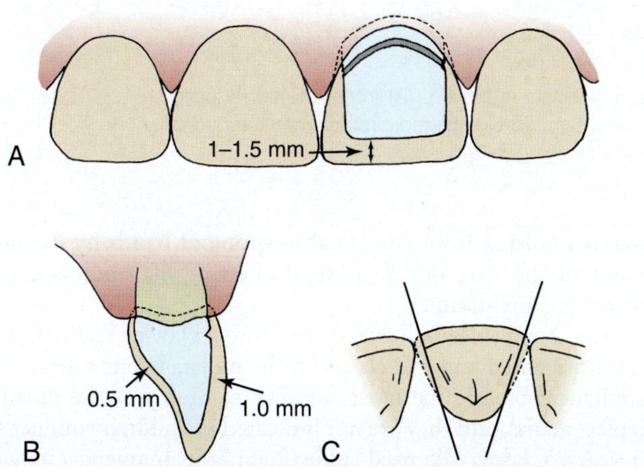

• **Fig. 30.23** Adhesive Resin–Based Composite Crown (Strip) Preparation. (A) Labial view. (B) Proximal view. (C) Incisal view. The proximal slice should be parallel to the natural external contours of the tooth

elective procedure. The most common reason for placement of a prosthetic appliance is parental concern about esthetics.

Lack of compliance in appliance wear and care by the young child are the greatest limitations of, and contraindications for, these appliances. If a young child decides that they do not like the appliance, they will find a way to remove it from their mouth and discard it. Educating parents regarding this fact is essential before the decision to construct an appliance is made.

Prosthetic appliances may be either fixed or removable (Fig. 30.25), and many different designs are used for both. Because of compliance issues, a fixed appliance will almost always be preferred to a removable appliance in young children. When constructing either type, it is best to wait at least 6 to 8 weeks after tooth loss before fabrication. This allows for good healing and gingival shrinkage. However, appliances can be placed the same day the extractions are completed, and the gingival tissue seems to heal and adapt very well around the prosthetic appliance. An anterior deep bite is a contraindication to both fixed and removable appliances.

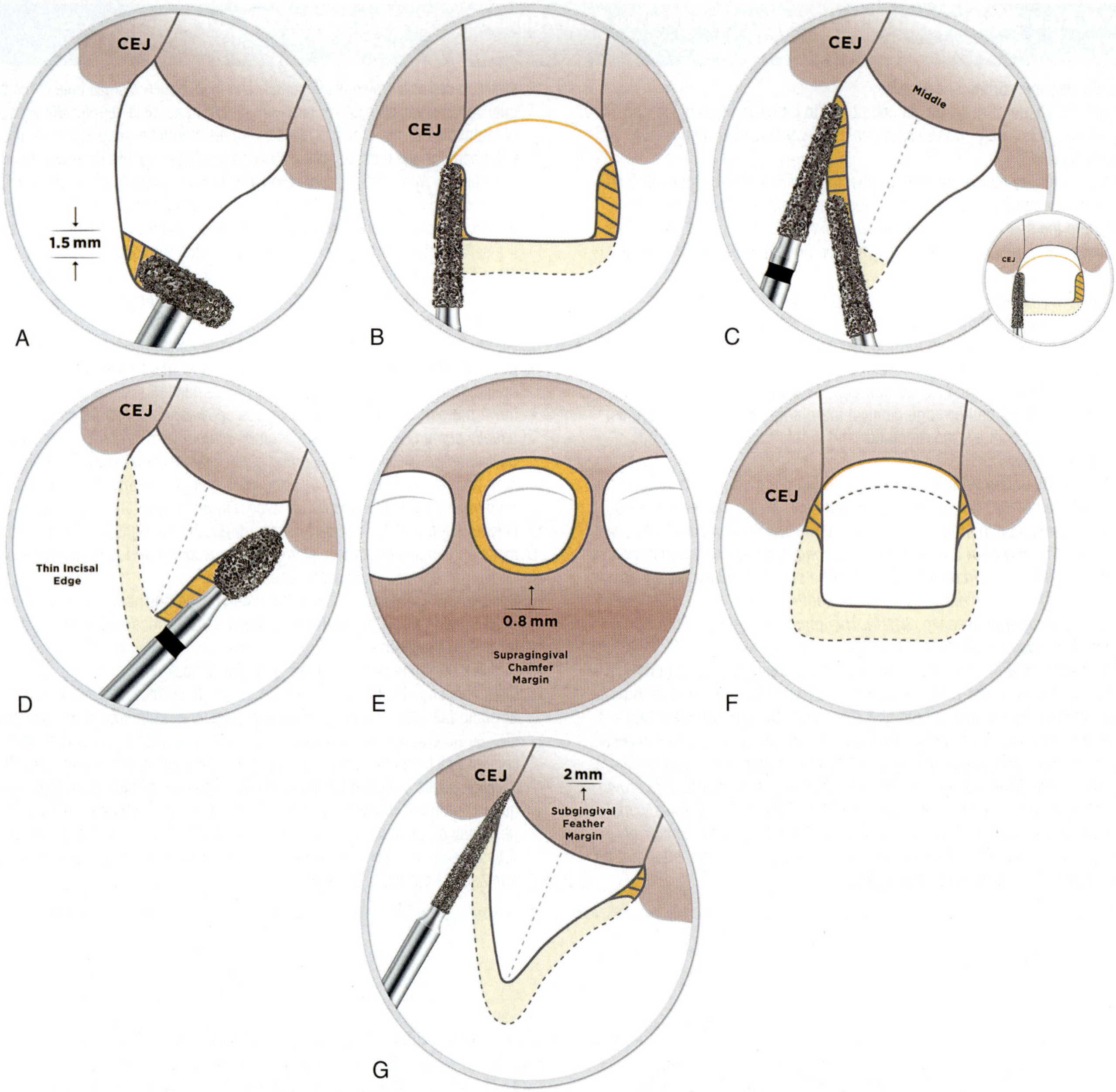

• **Fig. 30.24** Anterior Zirconia Crown Preparation Steps. (A) Incisal reduction. (B) Interproximal reduction. (C) Facial reduction in two planes of space. (D) Cingulum reduction. (E) Completed circumferential reduction. (F) Remaining tooth structure before subgingival reduction. (G) Subgingival reduction.

One fixed appliance design is similar to a Nance space maintainer. It consists of two bands, or preferably steel crowns, connected by a palatal wire to which the replacement teeth are attached. These prosthetic appliances can be fabricated by any laboratory, but they are commercially available through some commercial laboratories such as Space Maintainers Laboratory (SML, Chatworth, CA). This appliance is cemented onto the molars and is not easily removed by the child.[105] The teeth can be made to sit directly on the ridge of the edentulous space (preferred), or acrylic gingiva can be added. Disadvantages of this appliance include (1) possible decalcification around the bands; (2) more difficulty in home cleaning; and (3) bending of the wires with fingers or sticky foods, which may create occlusal interferences and the need for adjustments. Loosening of the bands resulting from continual torquing of bands by the movement of the wire during normal chewing may necessitate frequent recementation.

The removable appliance is similar to a Hawley retainer. It uses circumferential and ball clasps on the molars for retention. These appliances require the most compliance of any of the prosthetic replacements, and they are not indicated in children younger than 3 years. Clasps will need adjustment, the frequency of which depends on the child's handling of the appliances. The greatest advantages of these appliances are that they may be removed for daily cleaning and adjustments can be easily performed by the dentist without having to remove and recement bands.

Visit eBooks.Health.Elsevier.com to see full list of references.

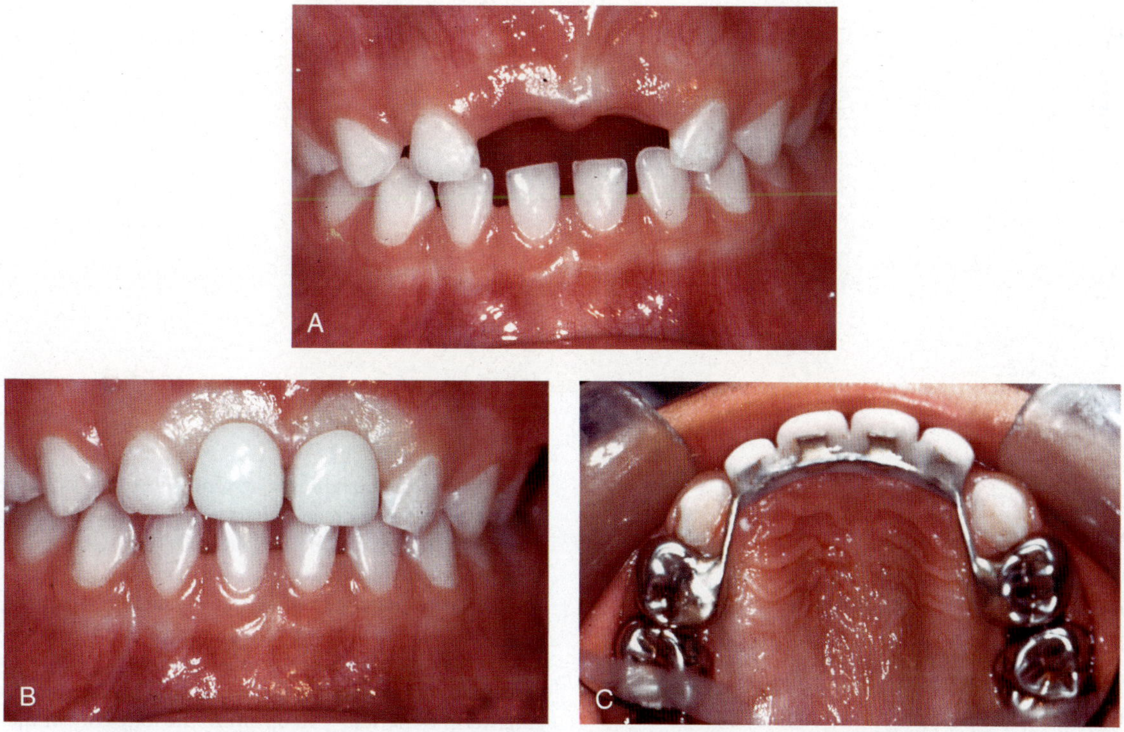

• **Fig. 30.25** Prosthetic Replacement of Primary Anterior Teeth. (A) Edentulous space after extraction of two primary incisors. (B) Fixed prosthetic appliance replacing the two incisors in place. (C) Example of a fixed prosthetic appliance replacing four incisors. *Note:* Stainless steel crowns are used on the first primary molars as abutments. These provide better retention and durability than orthodontic bands.

31 Restorative Dentistry for the Adolescent

DAN BURCH, MARVELLOUS A. AKINLOTAN, AND NINA RAY

CHAPTER OUTLINE

Fundamentals of Material Selection

Material selection plays a crucial role in enhancing dental restorations for adolescents. When choosing a restorative material, it is vital to assess the specific tooth that needs repair, the patient's caries risk, the restoration's location, and the forces it will encounter. Composite resin restorations are a popular choice because they are esthetically pleasing, preserve tooth structure, and contain no mercury. The clinical success of composite resin restoration relies on the adhesive system that provides a durable bond of composite resin to dentin and enamel, effectively sealing restoration margins and minimizing microleakage.[1] To achieve this, a contemporary adhesive system should be used (eFig. 31.1). Contemporary adhesive systems include etch-and-rinse or self-etch systems. Etch-and-rinse adhesive systems, although more technique sensitive, have been shown in laboratory studies to have higher bond strength compared with the self-etch systems.[2] The self-etch systems, in addition to being less technique sensitive, may reduce postoperative sensitivity by leaving behind residue that decrease outward fluid flow from dentin tubules.[3] In vitro data suggest that self-etch systems tend to benefit from selectively etching enamel.[4] There continues to be controversy and limited clinical studies to identify which adhesive system improves the longevity of composite resin restorations, though etch-and-rinse systems seem to provide better long-term esthetics.[3,4] To optimize the longevity of the restoration, the provider should follow the manufacturer's instructions (i.e., some self-etch systems should not be used on uncut enamel) and confirm the adhesive system is compatible with the composite resin. The selection of composite resin restorations can be confusing because a variety of products are available with slightly different physical properties. Essentially there are three types of composite resins that can be used: microfilled, hybrid, and nanofilled. Nanofilled resins have physical properties superior to those of microfills but slightly inferior to hybrids.[5] The mechanical and physical properties of hybrid composite resins are superior to those of microfilled resins because they contain a higher proportion of filler particles. Hybrid resins have traditionally been chosen as a universal restorative material because they can be used in most clinical situations. Microfilled resins are primarily indicated when esthetic restorations are required; because of their particle size, microfilled resins can be polished to an enamel-like luster with more ease and in less time than hybrid resins.

The polymerization of light-activated composite resins is accomplished by using an intense blue light with a peak wavelength of approximately 450 to 470 nm, which corresponds to the absorption peak of camphorquinone (CQ), the most popular photoinitiator.[6] A typical light-curing polymerization unit uses light-emitting diodes (LEDs) to efficiently produce blue light (eFig. 31.2) (see Chapter 29, Dental Light-Curing Units Box for a discussion of curing lights). Light intensity should be regularly monitored with the same measurement device and light guide (eFig. 31.3), and the unit should be repaired or replaced when it no longer meets the manufacturer's specifications.[7]

Eye protection is important when using the curing lights because direct viewing of the light is detrimental to vision.[7] In the absence of protective amber filters, one should avoid looking directly at the light.

Fundamentals of Clinical Technique

Selecting the appropriate shade is a critical initial step in achieving esthetically pleasing dental restorations. Begin by thoroughly cleaning the teeth that need to be matched. Use a rubber prophylaxis cup and flour of pumice to create a clean surface for shade evaluation. Tooth dehydration can significantly alter color perception. Therefore it is crucial to prevent dehydration during shade selection. Dehydrated teeth may appear lighter than their hydrated state. Utilize moistened shade tabs (color guides) to assess the tooth color. Hold the shade tab near the tooth that needs matching. Perform this step under ambient light or indirect sunlight. Avoid using high-intensity operatory lights, as they can distort color perception. Precision and attention to detail during shade selection contribute to achieving a seamless blend with the patient's natural dentition.

Composite resins are available in a range of shades, typically aligned with VITA shade guides (VITA North America, Yorba Linda, CA). However, achieving a perfect color match between composite resins and the VITA guide is rare, and shades can vary across different brands.[8] Recently, the shade range has expanded to accommodate teeth that have undergone whitening or bleaching procedures.

To address shade-matching challenges, some clinicians offer patients a choice between two similar shades. An alternative method involves applying a small amount of composite resin to the tooth surface, polymerizing it, assessing the shade's suitability, and then removing it using a hand instrument. Avoid etching the tooth before this process to ensure uncomplicated removal. Additionally, maintain an uncontaminated field during the insertion of composite resins. The most reliable and cost-effective way to control moisture is using a well-adapted rubber dam. An alternative product is an intraoral vacuum system. Examples are the Isolite (Zyris® Isolite® System, Santa Barbara, CA) and DryShield (Solmetex, Marlborough, MA) systems, which have a flexible plastic mouthpiece that provides retraction of the soft tissues, a bite block, and constant suction. In limited studies, the Isolite system has reduction in spatter and humidity levels similar to a rubber dam (Fig. 31.4).[9,10] Another approach to maintaining a dry field is to use a commercially available lip and cheek retractor (Fig. 31.5). This plastic device, when used with gauze sponges, provides excellent access and good field control.

The use of a base or liner to protect pulp tissue in deep preparations is generally believed to be beneficial. A glass ionomer liner may be used in deep areas of a cavity preparation that is thought to be within 0.5 to 1.0 mm of pulpal tissue (eFig. 31.6). The liner provides chemical adherence to tooth structure and slow release of fluoride.[11]

After adhesive bonding, the photopolymerized composite should be inserted in layers no thicker than recommended by the manufacturer (usually 2 mm), followed by curing the composite according to the manufacturer's instructions (usually 20 seconds minimum with a contemporary curing light; see Chapter 29). Appropriately placed layers and adequate time for light exposure help ensure maximum polymerization and minimize marginal gaps caused by shrinkage. To mimic the translucency of enamel and the opacity of dentin, manufacturers have produced materials with a variety of opacities. These materials should be placed in increments in which the more opaque materials replace dentin, and the more translucent materials replace enamel to produce restorations with similar optical properties to tooth structure.

Plastic or metal instruments are useful for material placement and contouring. Fine sable or camel hair brushes allow the easy contouring and blending of composite resin into the proper form. To prevent composite resin from adhering to the brushes and instruments, they should be lightly touched to the composite resin with a rapid dabbing motion.

After the polymerization process, the contouring and finishing of the restoration is accomplished with carbide finishing burs, ultrafine diamonds, or finishing disks. Fine-pointed burs are

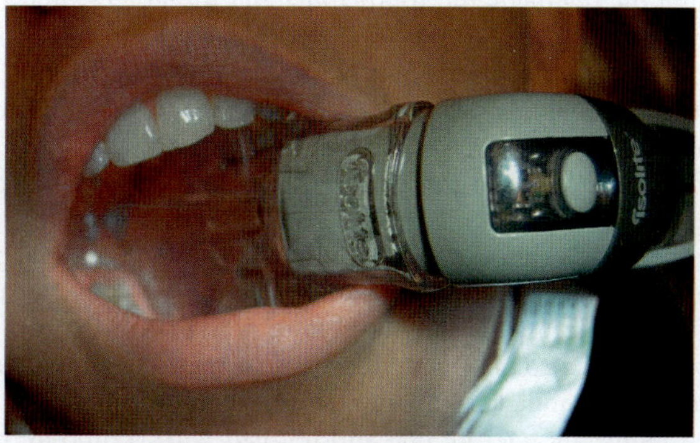

• **Fig. 31.4** Intraoral vacuum system.

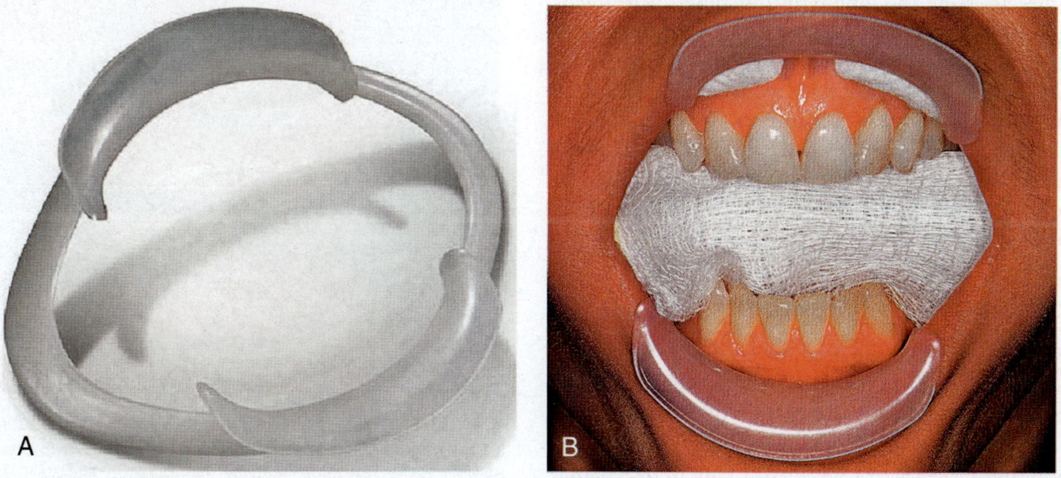

• **Fig. 31.5** (A–B) Isolation of teeth may be enhanced through the use of a lip-retracting device. (A, Courtesy Practicon Dental, Greenville, NC.)

helpful for accessing contour areas that are difficult to reach, such as embrasures. Rounded burs may be used on concave surfaces, and disks may be used on flat or convex surfaces. After contouring and finishing, the restoration should be polished with a series of polishing disks or rubber-abrasive instruments. The final finish and polish of proximal areas are best done with abrasive strips.

Restorations for Fractured Anterior Teeth

Trauma to the front teeth can lead to fractures that involve enamel; enamel and dentin; or enamel, dentin, and pulp. These injuries can raise both pulpal and esthetic concerns and require thorough evaluation through clinical and radiographic assessments (see Chapter 41 for a detailed discussion).

Clinical Technique: Tooth Fragment

If the tooth fragment is available, is relatively intact, and adapts well to the remaining tooth with no encroachment to the biologic width, the fragment can be bonded to the tooth.[12] See Case Study: Management of the Uncomplicated Crown Fracture This technique allows immediate satisfaction by restoring tooth form and function with excellent esthetics and low cost.[13–15] For best results, the fragment should be hydrated. Families should be counseled to place the fragment in saline, Hank's Balanced Solution, or milk while in transit to the dental office. When there is minimal loss of tooth structure, the fragment can be bonded by etching the fragment and tooth and application of a dental adhesive to the fragment and tooth, followed by placement of highly filled flowable composite resin to the fragment and tooth. The fragment is then repositioned and the proximal contacts flossed or a matrix is placed followed by light curing. In this situation the adhesive and flowable composite resin should be light cured together. When there is moderate loss of tooth structure, resin-based composite should be used in lieu of flowable resin and the adhesive should be cured separately. After a direct pulp cap or partial pulpotomy, the internal section of the fragment will need to be modified to allow the best fit. In either scenario, after the fragment is bonded, a shallow double chamber should be prepared along the fracture line and restored with composite resin. This procedure will add strength to the rebonding and minimize the risk for stain at the fracture line (eFig. 31.25B, C).[16,17] Families should be cautioned that the longevity of reattachment is uncertain. Studies assessing the long-term outcomes of reattachment have reported mixed results regarding the survival rates of reattached fragments. One study of 67 patients found similar rates of complications between those with reattachment and those with direct composite restorations.[15] However, another study of 164 patients involving 235 teeth reported a low reattachment survival rate of 42%, leading to higher restorative and biologic failures. In contrast, teeth with direct composite restorations showed a higher survival rate of 65%.[14]

Clinical Technique: Class IV Restoration

Adhesive dentistry has lessened the need for extensive mechanical retentive features in class IV restorations. The primary retentive feature is a beveled enamel cavosurface margin of a minimum of 1.0 to 2.0 mm in length (Fig. 31.7). Beveling allows maximal bond strength and minimizes leakage by exposing the ends of the enamel rods to etching. Because anterior restorations are sometimes subject to strong shearing forces that can be greater than the bond

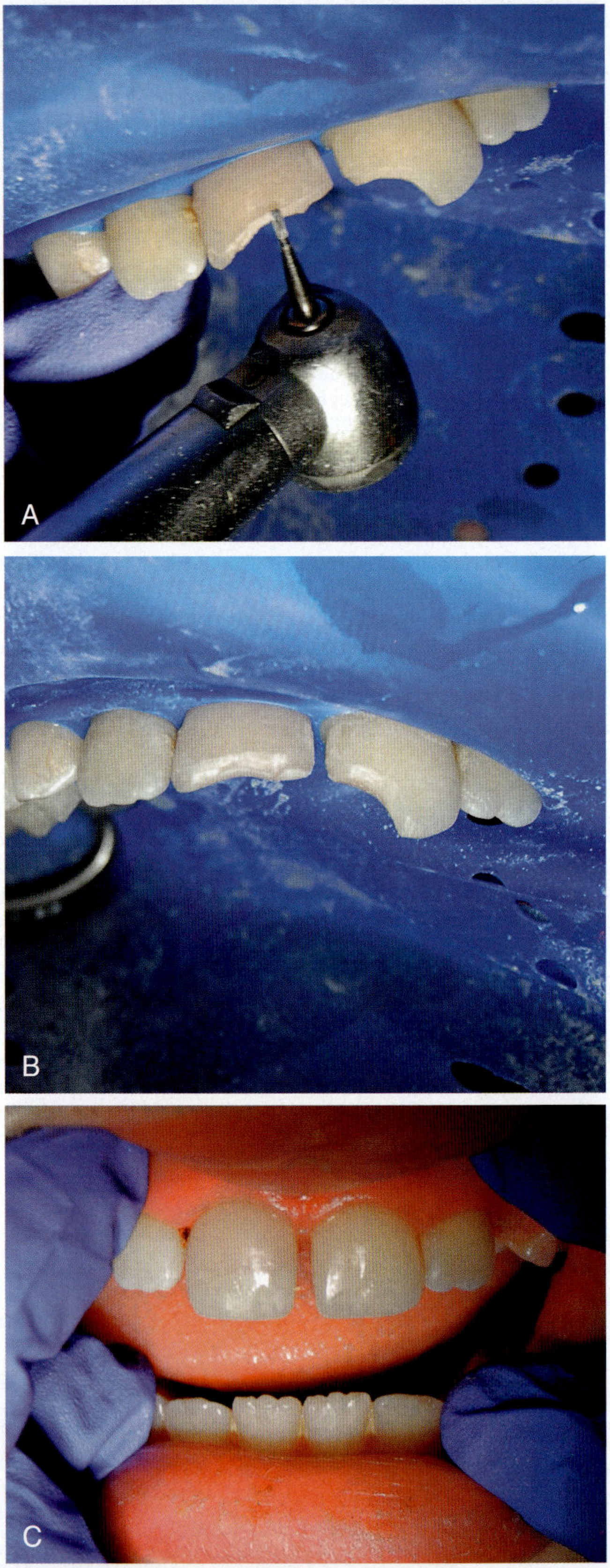

• **Fig. 31.7** (A) The incisal edges of the maxillary incisors were fractured as the result of an accident; a beveled enamel cavosurface margin is placed as a retentive feature. (B) Enamel beveled surfaces of teeth shown in (A). (C) Composite resin restorations of fractured teeth shown in (A) and (B).

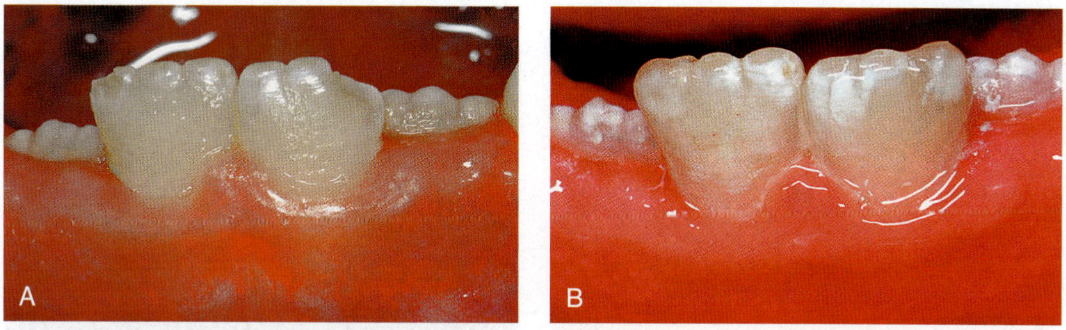

• **Fig. 31.8** (A) The incisal edges of the mandibular incisors were fractured as the result of an accident. (B) Composite resin restorations (Filtek Restorative Material, 3M ESPE) of fractured teeth shown in (A).

strength of the restoration to the tooth, features such as grooves or retentive points may be used to gain additional retentive strength.

After administering anesthesia, followed by isolation, the bevel is prepared with a high-speed rotary instrument. Caries is removed if indicated, and a base or liner may be applied to the exposed dentin. Conditioning of the tooth is achieved in accordance with the adhesive system of choice, with adherence to the manufacturer's directions. A wedged celluloid matrix strip can be used to prevent etching and bonding an adjacent tooth. In addition, anterior matrix systems are available to optimize curvature, anatomical form, and contacts when placing direct composite anterior restorations, such as the Garrison Fusion Anterior Matrix System (Spring Lake, MI) or the Bioclear Matrix system (Bioclear, Tacoma, WA).[18] After placing, finishing, and polishing the restoration, carefully check the restoration for interferences in all excursive movements (Fig. 31.8). Occlusal stresses on the restoration should be minimized.

Some clinicians consider the class IV composite resin restoration an interim restoration for adolescents until a more permanent ceramic crown can be fabricated.[19] However, with modern materials and techniques, the strength and color stability of composite resin class IV restorations are such that they can be considered final restorations that will provide relatively long service.[19] For early adolescents with severely fractured anterior teeth or caries, these restorations can provide years of service, allowing the teeth to mature so that pulpal injury during crown preparation is less likely.

Restoration of Diastemas

Many adolescents consider spaces between anterior teeth (diastemas) unattractive.[20] Historically the only restorative treatment to fill these spaces has been the fabrication of crowns. Improved composite resin materials and acid-etching technology now allow restoration of diastemas with a method that is nondestructive, reversible, and relatively inexpensive. However, patients should be forewarned that fracture and staining are possible drawbacks of composite resin diastema closure and that replacement is likely to be needed after 5 to 10 years.

When an adolescent patient desires diastema closure, careful evaluation and planning are necessary. If the patient is nearing completion of orthodontic therapy but is still undergoing treatment, the restorative dentist may advise the orthodontist about the optimal arrangement of anterior teeth for diastema closure. The orthodontist may then complete active treatment and place the patient into a retention phase before closing the diastema. The use of diagnostic study casts is recommended for evaluation and treatment planning. A diagnostic waxing of the proposed restorative treatment can aid both the patient and the clinician in envisioning the outcome.

Important pretreatment considerations include the size and location of the space or spaces and the size (length and width) and shape of the teeth to be restored. Normally, composite resin is added to the teeth on both sides of the space. For patients who are undergoing orthodontic treatment, one should determine whether the remaining space would best be left in one place, such as the midline between the maxillary central incisors, or distributed over proximal areas throughout the anterior segment. One must also consider the length and width of the teeth to be restored. If the width becomes greater than the length, those teeth appear more squared, leading to an unattractive outcome that may be as displeasing as the original diastema. Because of occlusal patterns and chewing stresses, teeth usually cannot be lengthened with composite resin without creating a high probability of resin fracture. However, light reflections can be used to create the illusion of a longer and narrower tooth when the composite resin is extended to cover most or the entire facial surface. To create the illusion of a narrower tooth, one should form mesial and distal line angles in composite resin that are positioned slightly nearer the middle of the tooth and add definite vertical anatomical highlights (developmental depressions). For some patients the best treatment is partial diastema closure, in which an existing space is made smaller by enlarging the teeth with composite resin but not making the teeth so large that they become esthetically displeasing.

Clinical Technique

After cleaning, shade selection, and isolation, treatment should begin one tooth at a time. The space to be eliminated should be carefully measured via a periodontal probe, calipers, or Boley gauge because after one tooth is restored to eliminate half the space, it is usually difficult to determine how much of the space has actually been restored. The entire labial surface of the tooth should be etched, and bonding agent applied because most of the labial surface will be covered with a thin layer of composite resin to allow a subtle color transition from composite resin to tooth. In addition, covering most of the labial surface allows the use of visual illusions that cause the tooth to look narrower or longer, as described previously.

Composite resin (preferably a resin that is viscous and opaque) should be applied, beginning at the gingival margin of the interproximal area. Using instruments and brushes, one should shape the material to allow a smooth-flowing gingival embrasure without creating an overhanging ledge. The entire proximal surface, as

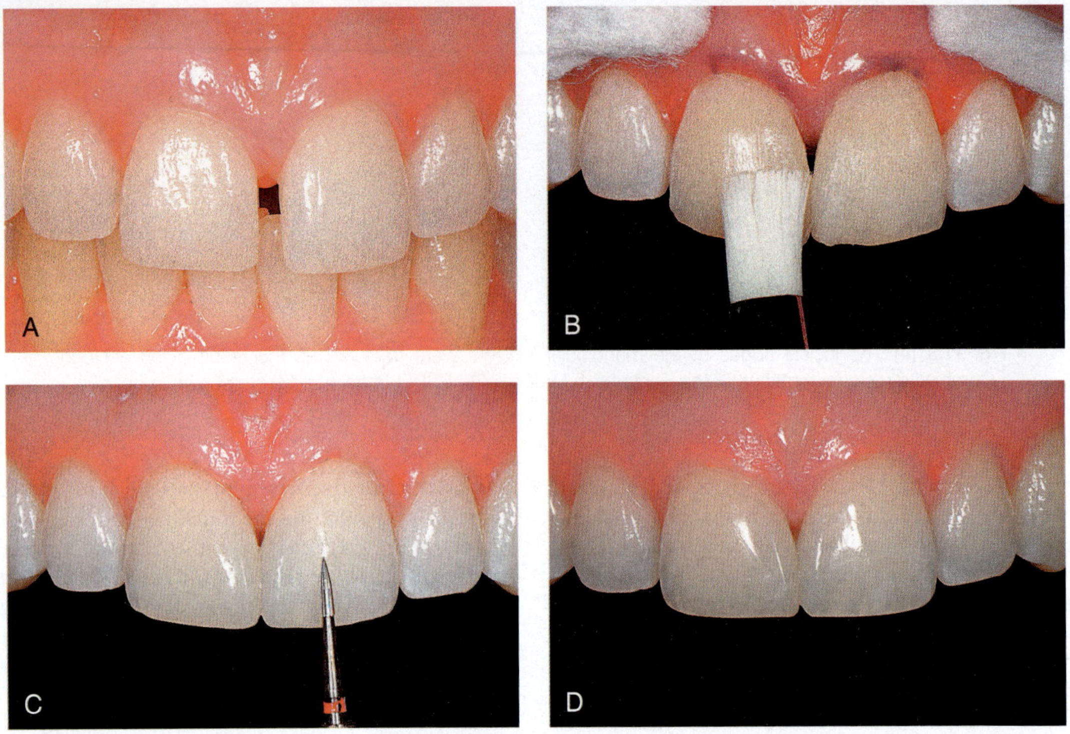

• **Fig. 31.9** (A) Preoperative view of a maxillary midline diastema, which the patient found unattractive. (B) Initial increment of composite resin being contoured with a sable brush before polymerization. (C) Contouring and removing excess composite after buildup of the second tooth. (D) Postoperative view of the completed treatment.

well as the labial surface, can be built up and polymerized at once or incrementally. After this buildup, one should finish the proximal area to the proper contour and polish it. Next, the second tooth is restored similarly. A celluloid matrix and wedge are usually inserted after the gingival increment is polymerized to retain the composite resin and to prevent the restorations from bonding together. Upon completion, the matrix is removed, and contouring and polishing are completed (Fig. 31.9).

Anterior teeth that are unusually small, such as peg lateral incisors, may be restored in the same manner as teeth requiring both mesial and distal diastema closure restorations. Again, careful treatment planning is advised to determine whether the restorations should be done only on the smaller tooth or on both the small and adjacent teeth for maximal cosmetic benefit. Preoperative diagnosis is necessary to determine whether lengthening is feasible. One should forewarn patients that the possibility of fracturing increases as length increases. In situations where fracturing is a concern, a hybrid resin should be used as a substrate and a microfilled resin placed on the surface. This technique increases the strength and esthetic outcome of the restoration.

Restoration of Discolored Teeth

For decades, esthetics has been a crucial aspect of dentistry alongside functionality, but its importance is now greater than ever. Preeruptive tooth discoloration can stem from various causes. The most frequent culprits include trauma, enamel hypoplasia (often due to fluorosis), and childhood antibiotic use. These discolorations range from subtle white or yellow flecks on the enamel surface (referred to as enamel demineralization)[21] to deeper intrinsic bluish-gray hues commonly associated with tetracycline staining.

Vital Bleaching

Vital bleaching techniques are the most conservative because they do not remove tooth structure. They involve the application of peroxide solutions to increase the value (whiteness) of teeth that are unusually dark. Bleaching is often combined with other minimally invasive treatments to conservatively provide maximum results. Peroxide bleaching methods appear to work best on teeth that are mildly discolored, predominantly yellow, and from which the discoloration originates in enamel rather than dentin. The basic methods for vital bleaching are in office power bleaching, custom-fabricated tray bleaching, and over-the-counter bleaching strips.[22]

Power bleaching is an in-office procedure in which a concentrated hydrogen peroxide solution is applied to rubber dam–isolated teeth while heating the teeth, usually with an electric lamp or laser.[23] This method of bleaching may require numerous office visits and often causes temporary tooth sensitivity. Typically, patients who have had this treatment require periodic retreatment to maintain the desired color.

Custom tray or over-the-counter vital bleaching is an at-home treatment. This method of vital bleaching uses a milder peroxide solution (usually 10% carbamide peroxide) that the patient applies and wears outside the dental office, often at night during sleep, for approximately 2 to 3 weeks. At-home bleaching appears to work as well as power bleaching and causes less sensitivity. Concerns were initially raised about the potentially hazardous soft tissue effects of applying peroxide solutions in this manner, but long-term studies of the safety and efficacy of this approach are demonstrating no harmful effects.[24] Vital bleaching also appears to cause limited damage to existing restorations, although these may no longer be a color match after the teeth have been whitened.[25] Over-the-counter bleaching strips can achieve similar whitening effects but take longer to accomplish.[22]

Minimally Invasive Treatments

Discrete hypoplastic white or yellow-brown spots can be improved by the etch-bleach-seal technique, resin infiltration, enamel microabrasion, and/or by making shallow saucer-shaped preparations in enamel to remove the intensely colored tooth structure and then restoring the enamel with composite resin. The etch-bleach-seal technique is the least invasive of all approaches.[26] The "bleach" step of this procedure does not refer to vital bleaching as discussed earlier but refers to the use of sodium hypochlorite. The affected teeth are cleaned with pumice, isolated with a rubber dam, etched with 37% phosphoric acid for 60 seconds, and rinsed. Sodium hypochlorite (5%) is applied and allowed to evaporate. Sodium hypochlorite oxidizes organic material that causes yellow-brown staining. The application process is repeated for 5 to 10 minutes. If improvement is not apparent, the application can continue for 15 to 20 minutes. Some teeth may need to be treated over several appointments. After satisfactory results are achieved, the teeth are sealed with a highly penetrating clear resin or bonding agent.[26]

Resin infiltration (Icon, DMG-America, Englewood, NJ) has also been shown to significantly improve the clinical appearance of white spot lesions (Fig. 31.10) See Case Study: Resin Infiltration.[27] Resin infiltration is discussed in more detail later in this chapter. Microabrasion removes enamel but does not necessitate placement of a restoration. The technique for enamel microabrasion involves application of an acidic abrasive paste by a reduced-speed dental handpiece (Fig. 31.11).[21] Microabrasion is sometimes used in combination with vital bleaching.[28] Limited case reports suggest that a biomimetic peptide (Curodont Repair, vVARDIS, Zug, Switzerland) may be able to improve the appearance of white spot lesions. Future research is needed to verify the effectiveness of this agent on remineralization.[29]

Veneers

Composite resin or porcelain veneers provide a treatment option for patients who have moderate to severe staining of one or more teeth. Patients are most concerned about the appearance of their maxillary teeth as they are more visible in speaking and smiling. In addition, mandibular teeth are often less likely to be successfully veneered because of limited space (insufficient horizontal overlap) and unfavorable forces. For veneer treatment to be successful, the patient must have excellent periodontal health because the placement of veneers will result in contours and margins that require good oral hygiene to maintain gingival health. In addition, patients should be warned that biting on hard objects, such as raw carrots or pencils, may dislodge or break veneers.

Laboratory-Fabricated Veneers

The indirect veneer technique has the advantage of requiring less total chair time because the veneers are fabricated in the laboratory. Excellent esthetically pleasing contours can be achieved with porcelain. Disadvantages include the necessity of two appointments, laboratory expense, and the possibility of creating an excess bulk of restorative material.

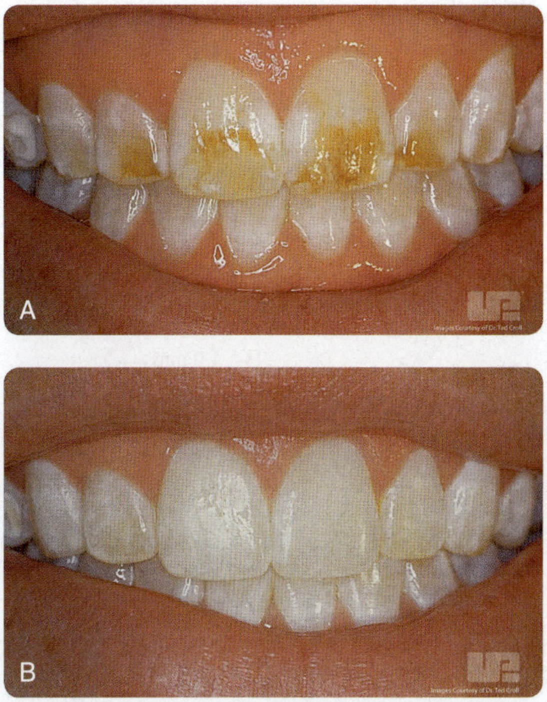

• **Fig. 31.11** (A) Preoperative view of maxillary incisors with white and brown enamel demineralization defects. (B) After enamel microabrasion and home bleaching. (Courtesy Ultradent Products, Inc., South Jordan, UT.)

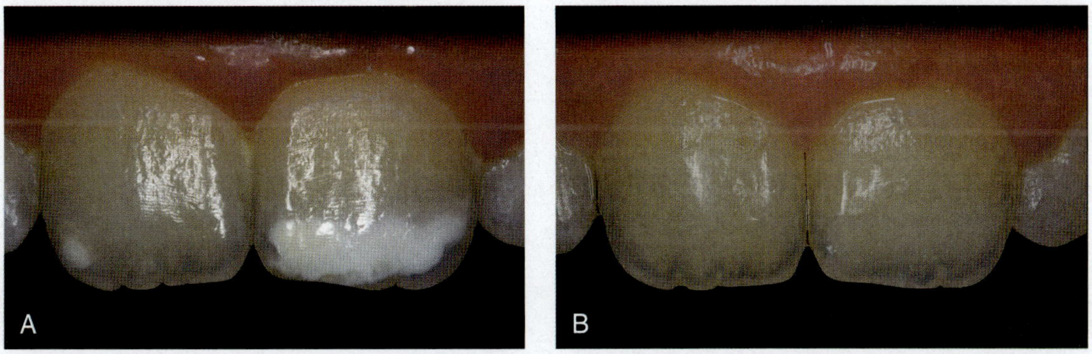

• **Fig. 31.10** (A) Preoperatively the maxillary left central incisor is affected with enamel hypomineralization that presents as a large, white lesion. (B) Postoperatively the esthetics of the tooth is greatly improved after HCl acid etching and resin infiltration. (Courtesy Zafer Cehreli.)

The indirect technique usually requires the removal of some enamel (ideally 0.3 to 0.5 mm, but occasionally more in severely stained teeth) from the facial surface to provide space for the veneer (Fig. 31.12). Tooth preparation is best accomplished with a medium-grit diamond rotary instrument (Fig. 31.13), with the goal of producing a long chamfer finish line throughout the surfaces to be covered. This preparation extends to the proximal surfaces to include the contact areas (Fig. 31.14). Gingivally, the preparation must extend far enough to cover the stained enamel sufficiently to improve the color. For better periodontal health, the finish line should be kept supragingival whenever possible. After the preparation, an accurate impression of the teeth should be made with an elastomeric impression material such as vinyl polysiloxane or polyether.

At the second appointment, one should isolate the teeth and clean them with pumice. After evaluating (using a try-in paste to help hold the veneers in place) and adjusting the veneers, they should be cleaned with the etching gel and silanated according to the manufacturer's recommendations. The preparations should be acid etched individually or in pairs and the veneers bonded in place, beginning with the central incisors. Celluloid matrices help protect adjacent teeth. Photopolymerized or dual-polymerized resins of moderate viscosity are preferred for bonding. Excess resin should be removed from margins with brushes before polymerization. Adequate polymerization time (40 to 60 seconds in each area) should be used because the veneers will shield some light transmission. Finishing and polishing are usually necessary only at the margins and may be done with abrasive strips and rubber cups (Fig. 31.15).

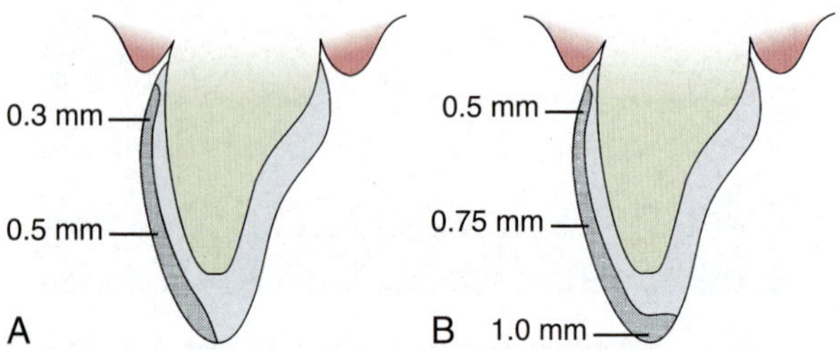

• **Fig. 31.12** Cross-sectional views of a laboratory-processed veneer of ideal thickness without incisal coverage (A) and a veneer of greater thickness with incisal coverage (B).

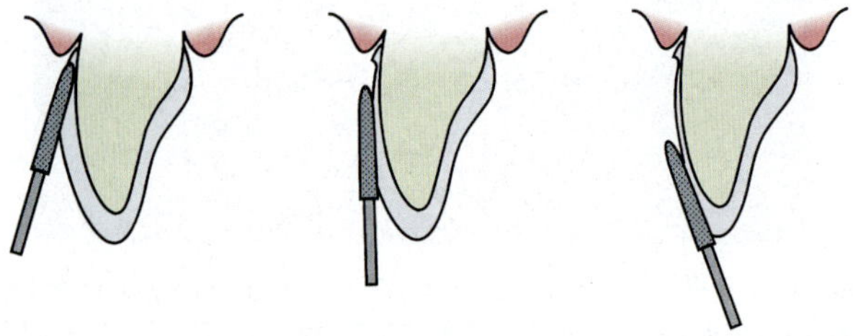

• **Fig. 31.13** Cross-sectional view of the steps in diamond instrument placement needed for preparing the facial surface of a maxillary anterior tooth.

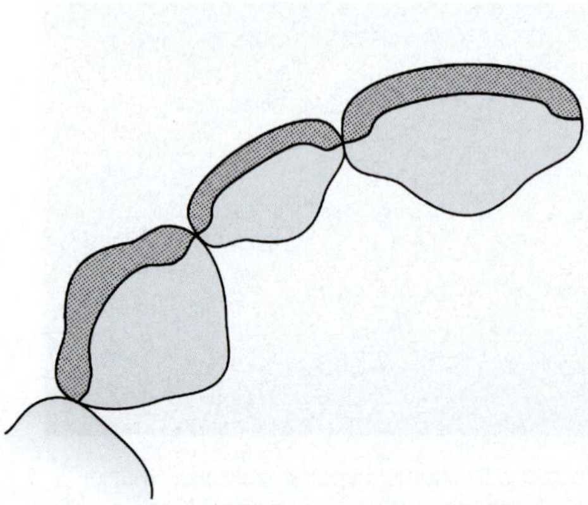

• **Fig. 31.14** Incisal view of veneer preparations.

Direct Veneers

Veneers made of light-polymerized composite resins can be fabricated directly in the mouth. Compared with the indirect type, direct veneers offer the advantages of improved marginal adaptation, placement in one appointment, greater operator control, and no laboratory fee. The disadvantages are that direct veneers require more time, greater skill, and more patience on the part of the clinician. In addition, outcomes are more difficult to predict, and composite resin is more susceptible to staining than porcelain.

The clinical direct technique may be performed with or without any enamel removal. Darkly stained teeth usually require some enamel removal because more composite resin is needed to mask the underlying enamel. The teeth are then pumiced and individually etched, and a bonding agent is applied. Again, celluloid matrices are used between adjacent teeth. Opaquing agents

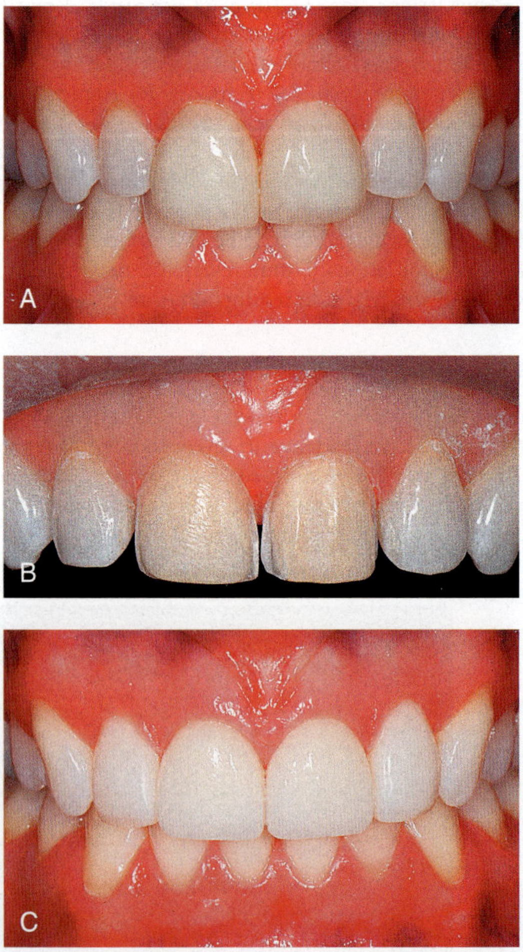

• **Fig. 31.15** (A) Preoperative view of esthetically unpleasing maxillary anterior teeth. (B) Central incisors prepared for porcelain veneers. (C) Porcelain veneers in place.

may then be painted on to cover more intensely stained areas or entire surfaces. For the best appearance, opaquing agents should be used minimally and with care. When dark banding is present, an alternative approach is to remove the band with a round bur and then replace the tooth structure with an opaque hybrid composite resin or resin-modified glass ionomer (RMGI). Next, the composite resin should be applied in a layer 1.0 to 1.5 mm thick and contoured with brushes. The gingival third of the restoration should usually be an opaque yellow shade, and the remaining enamel should be covered with opaque gray or universal composite, overlapping and blending the shades to create a natural-looking, gentle color transition. In many situations a nonopaque shade can be used on the incisal one-fourth to allow a natural, translucent appearance (Fig. 31.16A). After all composite resin has been added to a single tooth and contouring with brushes is complete, the material should be polymerized as recommended by the manufacturer. Finishing and polishing are best done with burs and disks, as described previously.

Strip Crowns

Strip crowns show promising results in anterior restorations but are underused, particularly by general dentists, due to technique sensitivity.[29] Indications include fractured incisors, extensive caries, and hypomineralization, whereas contraindications include insufficient tooth structure, deep bite, and periodontal disease.[30]

Different-sized strip crowns designed for permanent incisors are available and are used to create temporary or intermediate crowns or to serve as a mold to restore a fractured tooth. These strip crowns are made of thin plastic, and dentists can trim them with curved scissors[30] (see Fig. 31.16B–E). Once the crown form is trimmed and adapted to the tooth, the dentist can use a suitable bonding system and any composite materials available in the market. The etching and bonding steps are performed on the tooth, the strip crown is filled with composite, placed on the tooth, and cured. The crown form is "peeled off" and any flash or overhanging composite is polished. Strip crowns are also available for primary teeth (see Chapter 30).

Clinicians have explored modifications to the strip crown technique. In cases where enamel is lacking, such as at the gingival edges, dentists have experimented with dentin replacement using resin-modified glass ionomer cement (RMGIC). By placing a layer of RMGIC to protect exposed dentin before seating the crown form filled with composite resin, they aim to prevent debonding. Another modification involves creating a composite resin short post, known as the "mushroom undercut," by making an undercut in the dentin. This modification enhances the longevity and retention of strip crowns.[30] The strip crown technique, known for its minimally invasive approach, efficiency, cost-effectiveness, and excellent esthetic outcomes, is a preferred choice for managing fractured, carious, or hypomineralized teeth in young patients.[30]

Restorations for Posterior Teeth

Fundamentals of Material Selection

There are numerous materials to select from when restoring the young posterior permanent dentition. In the selection process the dentist should consider the size of the caries/defect, the occlusal forces expected to load on the restoration, the patient's caries risk, the ability to isolate the tooth, and the patient's preference.

Resin Infiltration

Resin infiltration (Icon, DMG-America, Englewood, NJ) is a minimally invasive technique used to restore noncavitated proximal

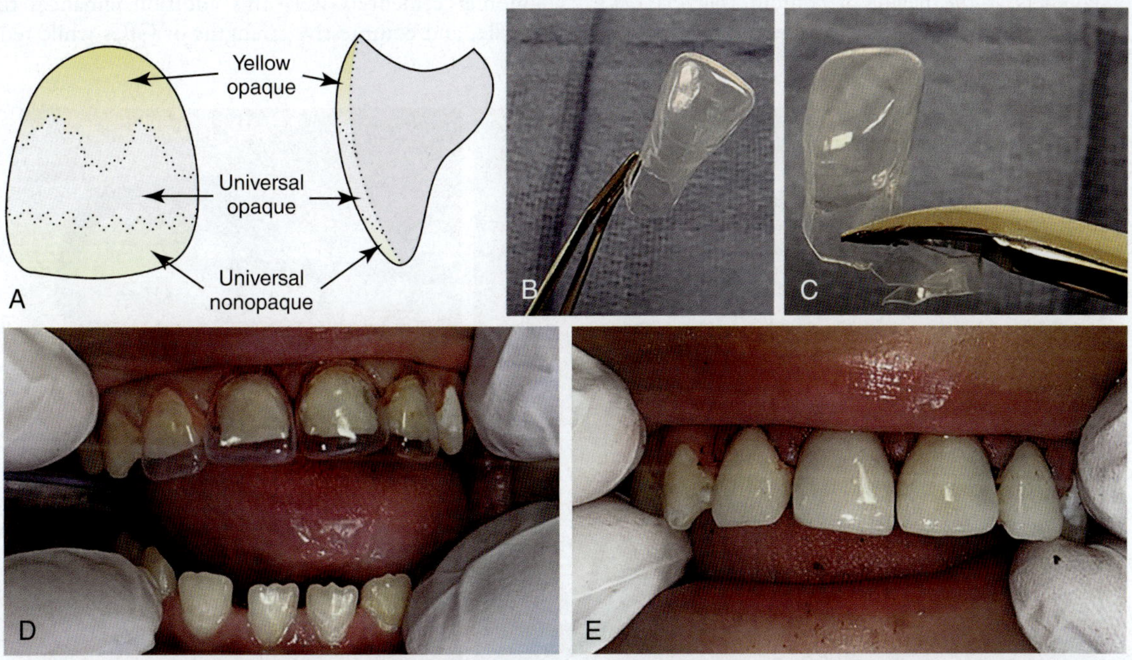

• **Fig. 31.16** (A) The use of overlapping shades of composite resin to create a natural-looking directly placed veneer. (B–E) The use of strip crowns to create a natural-looking directly placed restoration. (Courtesy DENTSPLY Caulk Clear Crown Forms, Milford, DE). (B) Strip crown. (C) Trimming strip crown. (D) Fitting strip crown. (E) Completed restoration.

caries lesions that radiographically extend from the inner enamel to the outer third of dentin[31] (see Fig. 15.19 in Chapter 15). Studies have suggested this technique is more effective at reducing proximal caries progression compared with noninvasive measures such as fluoride varnish and flossing.[32–36]

This technique requires a dry working field and care to protect gingival tissue, such as isolation with a rubber dam. For proximal lesions the teeth must be separated (approximately 50 μm) with a wedge, followed by etching with hydrochloric acid, rinsed for 30 seconds, and then dried to desiccation. The hydrochloric acid removes the hard remineralized outer layer of the lesion, allowing the penetration of the low viscosity resin into the porous enamel. It takes 3 minutes for the resin to penetrate the lesion, excess material is then removed, and the area is light cured from all sides for at least 40 seconds in total. The patient must be followed for caries progression with yearly radiographs; thus preference for this treatment should be for patients who have established a dental home. Because the lesions remain radiolucent in radiographs, patients should be counseled on the importance of notifying other dental providers of the treatment when they leave the practice.

Composite Resin

Composite resin restorations are popular for their esthetics but have drawbacks in the posterior dentition. They have a shorter life span than amalgam,[34,37] are more prone to failure in high-risk patients, and require more precise technique and chair time. However, they preserve tooth structure, and material improvements have been made (see Chapter 29 for a discussion of dental materials). For optimal results, composite resins should be used for appropriately sized restorations, with attention to manufacturer instructions.

Composite resins are sensitive to moisture, and care should be taken to provide adequate isolation. After the preparation is completed, use of a sectional matrix system will provide anatomically correct tight contacts at the height of contour (Fig. 31.17).[35] With the arrival of multiple adhesive systems, care should be taken to confirm that the adhesive system used is appropriate for the clinical situation and the composite is compatible with the adhesive system. The clinician should carefully follow the manufacturer's recommendations for incremental placement, light curing, and polishing the composite of their choice.

Amalgam

Amalgam has been successfully used for restoring teeth for the past 150 years. However, with the demand for esthetically pleasing materials and concern over health-related mercury issues, it has been decreasing in popularity despite evidence that the longevity of amalgam restorations is longer than composite resins.[34] Evidence suggests that there may be no clinically important differences in the safety profile of amalgam compared with composite restorations in neurologic symptoms or immune function.[34]

A disadvantage of amalgam restorations is the required cavity preparation, because it causes greater loss of tooth structure (depending on size of the lesion) compared with composite resin restorations. For large lesions, difficult to isolate areas in nonesthetic zones, and high caries risk patients, amalgam remains an excellent material choice.

Amalgam requires moisture control, but not complete isolation, using a rubber dam or cotton products. It is brittle in thin sections, so the cavity design must provide more bulk. Because it does not bond to the tooth, mechanical retention or undercuts are needed for stability.[36] In addition, to prevent enamel fracture, all unsupported enamel should be removed while retaining a 90-degree cavosurface angle. In addition, to prevent enamel fracture, all unsupported enamel should be removed while retaining a 90-degree cavosurface angle.

Resin-Modified Glass Ionomer

RMGI is created by incorporating resin into traditional glass ionomer cement (GIC). This addition enhances the binding, tensile, and compressive strengths of GICs while reducing their

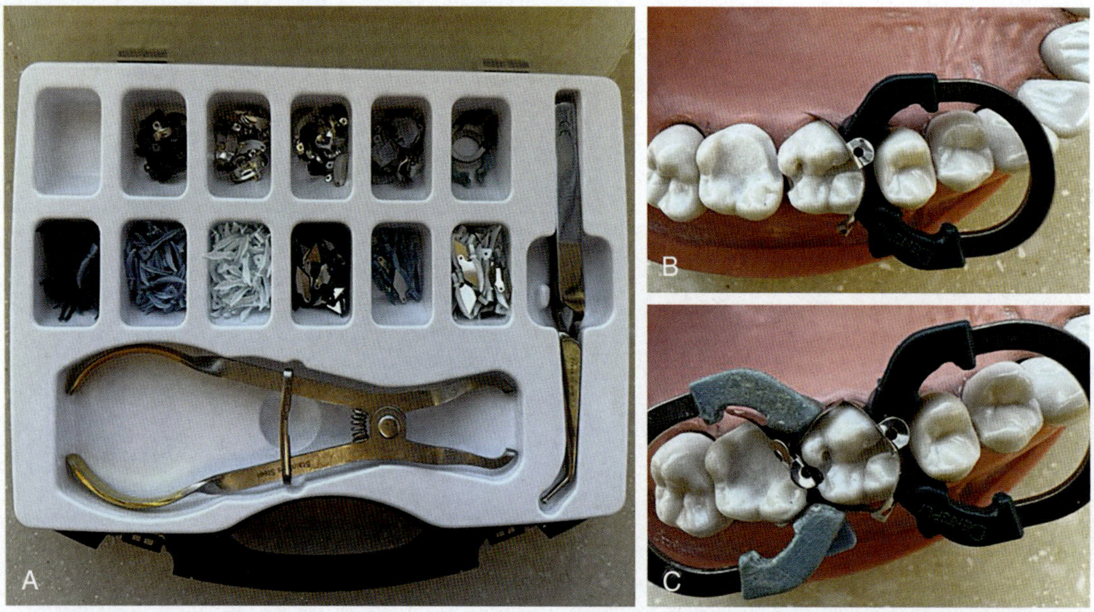

• **Fig. 31.17** (A–C) An example of available sectional matrix systems. (Courtesy DENTSPLY Caulk Palodent Plus Sectional Matrix System, Milford, DE.)

solubility in water, thereby addressing some of the limitations of conventional GIC.[37]

Ionomer-based materials are popular due to their beneficial properties, including chemical adhesion to dental structures, biologic sealing of dentin, biocompatibility, a thermal expansion coefficient similar to that of tooth structure, and anticariogenic effects from fluoride release. However, they also have some drawbacks, such as lower mechanical strength, limited esthetic appeal, and handling difficulties compared with resin composite materials.[38]

There are two main methods of adhesion:

1. Micromechanical interlocking: Glass ionomers are self-etching due to their polyacid component, which results in physical interlocking with the tooth surface.
2. True chemical bonding: RMGI forms ionic bonds between the carboxylate groups on the polyacid molecules and calcium ions in the tooth structure.[39]

Over time, an ion diffusion process occurs between the ions from the cement and the tooth, resulting in strong adhesion and minimal microleakage.[39] RMGI plays a crucial role in preventing caries due to its fluoride release and antibacterial properties. Additionally, RMGI exhibits better flexural strength compared with GICs. However, it is hydrophilic, less soluble, and shows reduced surface crazing.[40,41] Some studies suggest RMGI is comparable to composite in small to medium class II restorations.[42]

Stainless Steel Crowns

Permanent tooth stainless steel crowns (SSCs) may be indicated as an interim restoration for structurally compromised molars for the following conditions: the tooth is partially erupted, orthodontic treatment is indicated to finalize tooth placement in the arch, teeth with severe developmental defects or hypomineralization, and when financial considerations are of concern.[43] There is limited literature reflecting the longevity of permanent SSCs, although one study suggests a success rate of 88% over a 4-year time period.[44]

Significantly more chair time is indicated for the placement of a permanent tooth SSC compared with a primary tooth SSC. The final preparation is similar to that expected for a cast crown but with less tooth reduction. The occlusal reduction is 1.5 to 2 mm; the proximal walls are left in a slightly tapered position with a smooth feather-edge placed just below the level of the free gingival tissue. Unlike primary SSCs, permanent SSCs cannot be left in hyperocclusion and cannot be overextended into the gingival tissues because they are more prone to periodontal issues; hence SSCs for permanent teeth often require trimming. After crimping the SSC, the margins should be thinned and polished to a high shine. A bitewing radiograph is recommended to evaluate the mesial and distal marginal fit before cementation with GIC (Fig. 31.18B).[43]

Enamel Hypomineralization

Enamel hypomineralization is a qualitative enamel defect of unknown origin that affects one or more permanent molars, and frequently the permanent incisors.[45] Globally, the combined prevalence of enamel hypomineralization is estimated to be 14.2%.[46] Enamel defects resulting from molar-incisor hypomineralization (MIH) can vary widely, from mild opacities that have little functional impact to severe posteruptive breakdown (PEB). PEB can develop quickly, leading to sensitivity or pain, increased plaque formation, and caries susceptibility, making cavities challenging to repair. Consequently, this condition is thought to contribute significantly to childhood cavities due to its high prevalence.[46]

Given its common occurrence, enamel hypomineralization should be identified and managed in primary care settings whenever possible. Early detection can result in more effective and less invasive treatment. Generally, the darker the opacity, the softer and more porous the enamel, which increases the risk of substance loss and dentin exposure.[47] Enamel hypomineralization can lead to dental problems that may affect patients' quality of life and pose treatment challenges for dentists.

For anterior teeth presenting with enamel hypomineralization, it is important to note that achieving direct adhesion with composite resin can be challenging. Additionally, hypomineralized teeth often have a normal shape and size, necessitating tooth preparation to create a proper emergence profile and tooth morphology. Consequently, conservative treatments such as tooth whitening and microabrasion should be considered first as less invasive options.

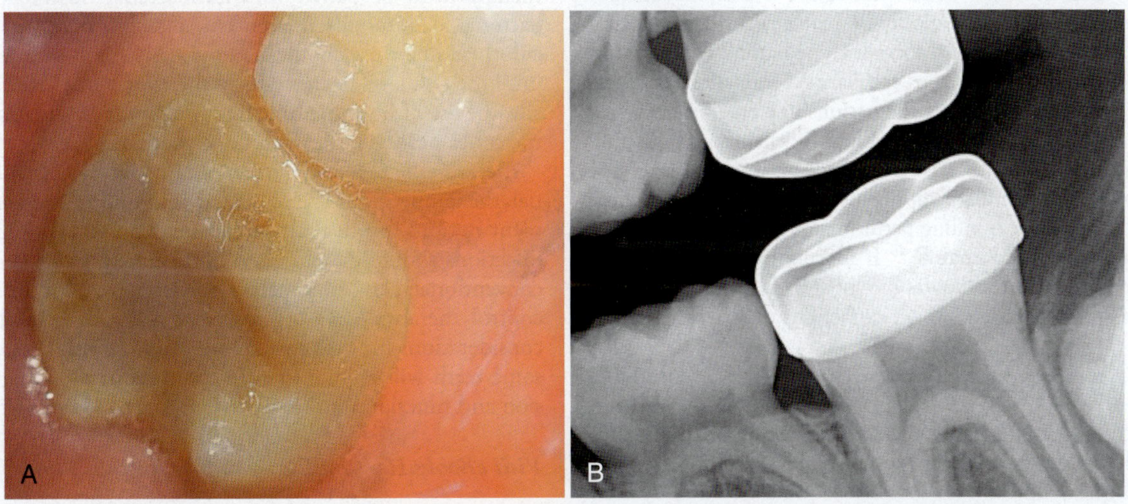

• **Fig. 31.18** (A) Hypoplastic 6-year molar with continued sensitivity despite composite restoration treatment. (B) Bitewing radiograph of stainless-steel crowns before cementation to confirm mesial and distal width of tooth shown in (A).

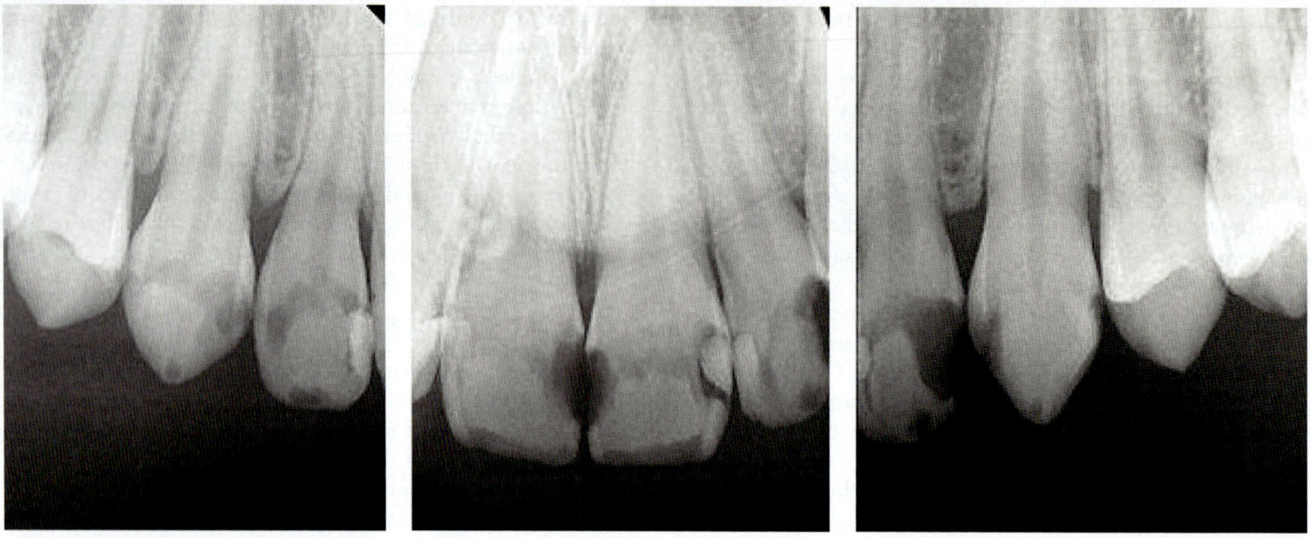

• **Fig. 31.19** Radiographs of a 16-year-old with rampant caries.

Restoring the Hypomineralized Molar

Evaluating the prognosis of affected molar teeth is essential in determining the best treatment. For minimally affected permanent molars with no symptoms or PEB, basic preventive measures like fluoride varnish and fissure sealants are appropriate. If the patient is uncooperative or experiences sensitivity, GIC fissure sealants may be an option. For teeth with hypoplastic defects, such as second molars, restoration with GIC or composite is ideal to minimize the removal of remaining tooth structure (see Fig. 31.18A). When using composite, the margins should be placed on nonaffected enamel because the mechanical bond to affected enamel may fail. When unable to place a resin restoration on unaffected enamel or when unable to obtain ideal restorative conditions (i.e., difficult isolation), a GIC is a reasonable option because the chemical bond will still occur on hard but affected enamel. If the tooth continues to be sensitive or the defect is moderate to severe, a permanent tooth SSC can be used as an interim restoration until a cast crown can be placed (see Fig. 31.18B and see Case: Management of the Hypomineralized Molar).[42] Teeth with severe hypomineralization and a poor prognosis should ideally be managed by a multidisciplinary team, including a specialist pediatric dentist and orthodontist, to evaluate the need for planned extractions if necessary. When considering indirect restorations like onlays or crowns, it is important to assess the amount of healthy enamel, as it directly affects bonding. Using 5% NaOCl, sodium hypochlorite, for enamel deproteinization before applying adhesive has been recommended to improve the bonding performance of resin dental adhesives to hypomineralized enamel.[48] If morphologically acceptable third molars are present radiographically and the long-term prognoses of the affected teeth are poor, extractions may be considered.

Managing Rampant Caries

Rampant caries has been defined as the "suddenly appearing, widespread, rapidly burrowing type of caries, resulting in early involvement of the pulp and affecting those teeth usually regarded as immune to ordinary decay" (Fig. 31.19). The identification of this disease process in the adolescent can be overwhelming for the child, family, and dentist. The underlying etiology of the disease must be identified. Possible etiologies include dietary changes (e.g., habitual intake of sugared drinks or candies), salivary gland dysfunction, systemic conditions, and/or substance abuse. The clinician must determine whether the disease process is rampant caries (as defined previously) or long-term dental neglect. For the adolescent a relationship built on trust with the dentist will be extremely valuable in identifying the etiology of the disease, especially if the disease is associated with drug use.

Although the etiology is being identified and corrected, the progression of the disease should be minimized. Oral health education, diet changes, and high-concentration fluoride products should be introduced, along with considering an antimicrobial rinse. Studies show that relying solely on fluoride and dental restorations in high-risk adults leads to caries progression.[49] Fluoride therapy must be paired with antibacterial treatment to reduce bacterial load, modify the biofilm, and shift the caries balance. A chlorhexidine rinse should be used daily for 1 week each month until the risk level decreases over the course of a year.[49] Additionally, the use of silver diamine fluoride should be discussed to arrest the caries process (at least in nonesthetic zones).

Because the financial burden of rampant caries can be substantial, the family should be presented with multiple restorative treatment options. Teeth that are causing pain and localized areas of infections should be addressed immediately. Resin-modified and conventional glass ionomers are well suited for interim caries control therapy. After urgent needs are met, careful treatment considerations for each sextant are planned with the concept that some teeth will require interim restorations to reestablish occlusion and function until definitive restorations can be placed.

Visit eBooks.Health.Elsevier.com to see full list of references.

32

Pulp Therapy for the Primary Dentition

VINEET DHAR AND MATTHEW K. GENESER

CHAPTER OUTLINE

The primary goal of pulp treatment is to preserve the integrity and health of oral tissues. Early loss of primary teeth can lead to malocclusion and esthetic, phonetic, and functional issues, which may be temporary or permanent. Preserving pulp vitality is essential when possible; however, if not feasible, the pulp can be removed without significantly affecting tooth function.[1,2] This chapter offers a brief overview of the histology of primary pulp, the dentinogenesis process, and factors influencing the dentin-pulp complex's response to stimuli. It also discusses the biologic basis for various pulpal treatment approaches in primary dentition.

Histology

The pulp of a primary tooth is histologically similar to that of a permanent tooth. The dental pulp is a specialized connective tissue of mesenchymal origin surrounded by tubular dentin walls occupying the pulp chamber and the root canal.

The odontoblasts are cells responsible for the synthesis and deposition of the collagen-rich dentin organic matrix, which is further mineralized around the pulp tissue. Therefore dentin and the pulp remain closely associated during tooth development throughout life and are commonly referred to as the *dentin-pulp complex*. The odontoblasts line the periphery of the pulp space and extend their cytoplasmic processes into the dentinal tubules. These cells have several junctions, which allow intercellular communication and help maintain the relative position of one cell to another. Below the odontoblastic layer is the cell-free zone that contains an extensive plexus of unmyelinated nerves and blood capillaries. The large blood vessels and nerves are located in the core of the pulp and are surrounded by loose connective tissue.[2,3] Although this description is correct during active dentinogenesis, it is now accepted that the size of the odontoblasts and the content of their cytoplasmic organelles vary throughout their life cycle and are closely related to their functional activity. The relationship between the size of the odontoblasts and their secretory activity can be demonstrated by differences in their size in the crown and in the root and may express different dentinogenic rates in these two areas of the tooth.[4]

The odontoblasts are highly specialized cells that extend cytoplasmic processes into the dentinal tubules, where they contribute to the main part of the pulp-dentin complex. When this complex is damaged by injury (disease or operative procedures), it reacts to defend the pulp.

The Pulp-Dentin Complex

Dentinogenesis in Healthy State

The inner enamel epithelium and its associated basement membrane have an important role in direct odontoblastic cytodifferentiation. They present bioactive molecules, including growth factors immobilized on the basement membrane that send signals to the cells of the dental papilla, inducing the differentiation of the ectomesenchymal cells into odontoblasts.[3] These cells express specific gene products that will form the highly mineralized extracellular matrix of dentin. Hydroxyapatite forms the main inorganic part of dentin, whereas the organic components consist mostly of type I collagen.[5] During the postmitotic state, the odontoblasts line the formative surface of the matrix and start secreting primary dentin. At the initiation of dentinogenesis, during mantle dentin formation, mineralization is achieved through the mediation of matrix vesicles. Mantle dentin is the first dentin to be formed, has an approximate thickness of 80 to 100 μm, and is almost free of developmental defects.[2]

When mantle dentin formation is completed and the odontoblasts form a tightly packed layer of cells, the matrix of dentin is produced exclusively by the odontoblasts. Although the other cells of the pulp (in the subodontoblastic layer and in the pulp core) support dentinogenesis, they do not have a direct role in primary dentin secretion.[6,7] As the matrix is secreted, the odontoblasts move pulpally, leaving a single cytoplasmic process embedded in a dentinal tubule in the matrix. These tubules, which increase in density near the pulp, confer the property of permeability on the dentin, a feature that has significant clinical importance.[4]

After secretion of the bulk of dentin during primary dentinogenesis, physiologic secondary dentin is secreted at a much slower rate throughout the life of the tooth, leading to a slow reduction in the size of the pulp chamber.[8] The original postmitotic odontoblasts, responsible for primary dentinogenesis, survive for the life of the tooth, unless subjected to injury. These cells remain in a resting stage after primary dentinogenesis, and the physiologic secondary dentin formation represents a basal level of cell activity in the resting tooth stage.[4]

Dentinogenic Response to Injury

In pathologic conditions, such as mild carious lesions or traumatic injuries, the secretory activity of the odontoblasts is stimulated to elaborate tertiary dentin. This will lead to focal secretion of new matrix at the pulp-dentin interface and possibly within the tubules, contributing to the histologic appearance of dentinal sclerosis at the injury site and to a decrease in dentin permeability.[3,9] Thus the formation of tertiary dentin is much faster than the physiologic secondary dentin formation, so this tertiary deposition is regarded as an important defense mechanism of the pulp-dentin complex in response to either pathologic or physiologic insults (attrition).

The nature and quality of the tertiary dentin depend on its tubular structure and influence the dentin permeability of the area. Thus in case of a mild injury, the odontoblasts responsible for the primary odontogenesis can frequently survive the challenge and are stimulated to secrete reactionary dentin beneath the injury site.[10] Because the original odontoblasts are responsible for this matrix secretion, there will be tubular continuity and communication with the primary dentin matrix (Fig. 32.1A).[9] Reactionary dentin might be considered an extension of physiologic dentinogenesis. However, because it is a pathologic response to injury, it should be regarded as distinct from the primary and secondary dentinogenesis. When the injury is severe, the odontoblasts beneath the injury may die; however, if suitable conditions exist in the pulp, a new generation of odontoblast-like cells may differentiate from underlying pulp cells, secreting a reparative dentin matrix. Because this dentin is formed by a new generation of cells, there will be discontinuity in the tubular structure, with a subsequent reduction in permeability (Fig. 32.1B).[11]

A critical question concerns the factors responsible for triggering the stimulation of odontoblastic activity. Although there is still much to learn regarding the molecular control of cell activity in general, and of odontoblastic activity in particular, one family of growth factors, the transforming growth factors (e.g., TGF-β) superfamily, has been reported to have extensive effects on the mesenchymal cells of many connective tissues.[12]

During tooth development, the odontoblasts secrete TGF-β, and some remain sequestrated in the dentin matrix. The sequestrated TGF-β may be released during any process leading to tissue dissolution, like dental caries formation or the use of acid etching, for example. Thus dentin matrix should be considered not as an inert dental hard tissue but rather as a potential tissue store of a cocktail of bioactive molecules (particularly growth factors) waiting to be released, if appropriate tissue conditions prevail.[2,3]

In contrast to reactionary responses, reparative dentinogenesis represents a more complex sequence of biologic processes. The migration and differentiation of pulpal progenitor cells must take place, creating a new generation of odontoblast-like cells, before matrix secretion. A series of stereotypic wound-healing reactions occurs in the pulpal connective tissue, including vascular and cellular inflammatory reactions. In vitro and in vivo experiments on reparative odontogenesis demonstrate that the noninflamed pulp constitutes an appropriate environment where competent pulp cells (potential preodontoblasts) can differentiate into new odontoblast-like cells, forming reparative dentin.[13,14]

Dentin-Pulp Complex Response to Stimuli in Primary Teeth

Although the life span of primary teeth is shorter and the dentin is thinner compared with permanent teeth, the dentin-pulp complex response to dental caries in human primary teeth is similar to that of permanent teeth, including a reduction in the number of the odontoblasts and an increase in the number of inflammatory cells. These are found under the very deep lesions and are less numerous at more distant regions, being almost absent in the radicular apical pulp.[15]

The primary dentition is frequently subjected to stimuli such as trauma or caries with associated pulp inflammation.[16] The same factors affect the dentin-pulp responses in both primary and permanent teeth to external stimuli.

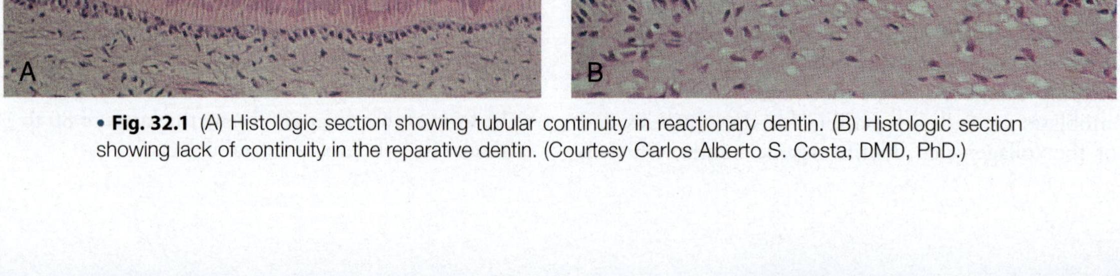

• **Fig. 32.1** (A) Histologic section showing tubular continuity in reactionary dentin. (B) Histologic section showing lack of continuity in the reparative dentin. (Courtesy Carlos Alberto S. Costa, DMD, PhD.)

The inflammatory response of pulp to a stimulus is a continuum, which can be broadly categorized as reversible or irreversible. To accommodate for more biologically driven treatment options, Wolters et al. 2017[17] cclassified pulp inflammation as initial, mild, moderate, and severe pulpitis (Box 32.1). In both initial and mild pulpitis, inflammation is localized to coronal pulp and can be reversed with appropriate vital pulp therapy such as indirect pulp therapy (IPT). Moderate pulpitis is associated with extensive local inflammation confined to coronal pulp and may respond to coronal pulpotomy. Severe pulpitis is suggestive of extensive local inflammation with coronal and possibly radicular involvement, which is likely irreversible.

Deleterious Effects of Microleakage at Restorative Margins

Studies have shown that bacteria and their byproducts play a key role in causing severe pulpal inflammation. This was proven by spontaneous healing of pulp exposures in germ-free animals[18] and by sealing cavity surfaces with zinc oxide–eugenol (ZOE) cement to prevent bacterial contamination.[19] Bacteria in cavities with a remaining dentin thickness (RDT) of less than 0.25 mm cause more severe inflammation than cavities without bacteria.[20] The presence of bacteria always worsens the level of pulpal inflammation, regardless of RDT.[21] In addition, bacteria in class V cavities reduce the number of odontoblasts, especially in deep cavities with an RDT under 0.5 mm. This shows that maintaining an effective seal to protect the pulp from bacterial leakage is crucial for the success of restorative treatments.[22] However, some studies have shown pulpal inflammation in the absence of bacteria,[23] clearly indicating that other factors are also responsible, even if to a lesser extent, for pulp injury after restorative treatment.

The Protective Role of Remaining Dentin Thickness

RDT is an important factor mediating pulpal inflammatory activity, particularly when the RDT is below 0.25 mm.[20] With an RDT below 0.25 mm, a significant decrease in the number of odontoblasts was observed together with minimal reactionary dentin repair.[24] However, when the RDT was above 0.25 mm, the protective tertiary dentin area increased in class V cavity preparations. The RDT significantly modifies the pulpal response: the thicker the RDT, the lower the pulpal inflammatory reaction.[18] The presence of an RDT over 0.5 mm delays the diffusion of noxious materials to the dental pulp and allows the odontoblasts to secrete reactionary dentin, increasing the total distance between the restorative material and the pulp. Any additional decrease in the dentin thickness below 0.5 mm results in a significant reduction in the number of odontoblasts. However, progenitor pulp cells differentiate into odontoblast-like cells, which migrate to the injury site and secrete reparative dentin and may compensate for the reduction in odontoblasts. This reparative dentin decreases the dentin permeability and increases the distance between the restorative material and the pulp, protecting it from noxious products. Thus the RDT appears to provide an important protective barrier against bacterial infiltration, toxins, or any noxious material applied onto the dentin.

Based on the RDT, three situations can be considered:

1. **RDT >0.5 mm** (i.e., initial carious lesions are present and cavity preparation is shallow): A localized reactionary dentin is secreted facing the restoration site, and intratubular mineralization occurs, resulting in pulp protection by significantly decreasing dentin permeability (see Fig. 32.1A).[25,26]
2. **RDT <0.5 mm** (i.e., carious lesion progression indicates a deep cavity preparation): These lesions may lead to partial odontoblast disintegration. Depending on the pulpal inflammatory state, progenitor/stem cells can migrate to the injury site and differentiate to yield a new generation of odontoblast-like cells. These cells are responsible for the deposition of a specific type of tertiary dentin termed *reparative dentin* (see Fig. 32.1B).[27,28]
3. **RDT <0.25 mm**: Deep cavity preparations with RDTs between 0.25 mm and 40 μm lead to poor tertiary dentin repair activity.[20] This results from impaired odontoblast dentin secretory activity caused by cellular injury.[29] Murray et al. demonstrated that the mean number of intact odontoblasts found beneath this kind of cavity preparation was 36% lower than the number found beneath similar preparations with an RDT between 0.5 mm and 0.25 mm. This inability of odontoblasts to provide adequate pulpal repair and pulpal protection after deep cavity cutting has been supported by observations of a persistent inflammatory pulpal response and odontoblast displacement after cavity cutting.[29]

Pulp response to severe inflammation in primary teeth

Primary teeth undergo physiologic root resorption due to programmed osteoclastic activity triggered by localized inflammation and signaling, primarily because of the eruption pressure of permanent teeth. Severe or irreversible inflammation in primary teeth can increase signaling of RANKL (receptor activator of nuclear factor kappa B ligand), which binds to RANK (receptor activator of nuclear factor kappa B) receptors on osteoclast precursors, stimulating their formation and activation and triggering resorptive osteoclastic activities. In addition, elevated proinflammatory cytokines and prostaglandin ED (PGE2) also stimulate osteoclast differentiation and root resorption. The osteoclastic activity is much reduced in permanent teeth, and the mature root structure is often harder to resorb. As a result, primary teeth seem to be programmed to elicit an aggressive immune response to inflammation and therefore are susceptible to premature root resorption.[30,31]

• BOX 32.1 Pulp Inflammation Classification

Initial – heightened but not lengthened response to cold, no sensitivity to percussion, and no spontaneous pain.
Mild – heightened and lengthened response to cold, warmth, and sweet stimuli that can last up to 20 seconds and possible sensitivity to percussion.
Moderate – strong, heightened, and prolonged reaction to cold lasting for minutes, possible sensitivity to percussion, and spontaneous dull pain that is somewhat responsive to pain medication.
Severe – severe, spontaneous pain and clear pain reaction to warmth and cold stimuli and sharp to dull throbbing pain; patients may have trouble sleeping as pain worsens when lying down; tooth is very sensitive to touch and percussion.

Clinical Pulpal Diagnosis

Currently very little or no correlation exists between clinical diagnostic findings and the histopathologic status of the pulp.[32] Among the commonly used pulp sensibility tests, cold pulp testing and electric pulp testing can more accurately diagnose vital teeth compared with the heat pulp testing; however, all three have inherent limitations such as reliance on patients' subjective responses and dentists' interpretations.[33]

Along with sensibility tests, comprehensive medical history, pain characteristics, and thorough extra- and intraoral examinations complemented by selected radiographs will provide the clinician with essential information regarding the pulpal status of a particular tooth or teeth in question. In addition, the source of the discomfort (e.g., trauma or caries, the presence of large, deep, or failed restorations) also plays a critical role in pulpal diagnosis and, subsequently, on the prognosis of the treatment to be provided.

Medical History

When treating a medically compromised child, a more careful approach should be taken.[34] Despite the lack of evidence, for severely immunocompromised patients, the American Academy of Pediatric Dentistry (AAPD) recommends cautious considerations when treating deep carious lesions with close proximity to the pulp. The risk of potential infections, which might be life threatening, drives most clinicians to consider a more radical approach, such as extraction, rather than a more conservative treatment option to preserve the tooth in the arch. In these cases, when pulpally treated teeth are present, close monitoring for signs of pulp degeneration is recommended.[35]

Extra- and Intraoral Examination

The presence of extraoral facial swelling, redness, and/or submandibular lymphadenopathy may indicate the presence of an acute dentoalveolar abscess. In severe situations, facial cellulitis may involve the infraorbital space, resulting in partial/total closure of the eye, limited mouth opening, fever, and malaise. Hospital admission for intravenous antibiotics may be necessary (Fig. 32.2). A careful intraoral and radiographic examination should be conducted to identify teeth with deep cavities or extensive restorations. Diagnosis of pulp necrosis is then reached, and the treatment decision of extraction or root canal therapy is based on the restorability of the tooth, the severity of the infection, assessment of bone loss, lesion proximity to the succedaneous tooth follicle, and patient cooperation.[36]

When examining hard tissues, teeth with questionable diagnoses should be evaluated for abnormal mobility and sensitivity to percussion. The presence of open proximal carious lesions between adjacent teeth creates a space that can serve as a reservoir causing food impaction, providing false-positive response to percussion test (inflammation of interdental papilla rather than acute pulpal inflammation) (Fig. 32.3).

Pain Characteristics

Young children are poor historians; thus parents may be better prepared to report existing symptoms. Stimuli-related responses that cease when the insult is removed (provoked or elicited pain) generally indicate a favorable, reversible status of the pulp that could lead to a more conservative treatment approach such as IPT or pulpotomy. Spontaneous pain refers to complaints of persistent, lingering, or throbbing pain, disturbing sleep and preventing regular activity. This typically indicates an irreversible status of the pulp. Patient symptoms along with clinical examination and radiographic image(s) will lead the clinician to treatment options such as pulpectomy or extraction (Fig. 32.4).

Sensibility Tests

Pulp tests, vitality or sensibility tests, are valuable diagnostic aids in endodontics. Evidence suggests that laser Doppler flowmetry and pulse oximetry are the most accurate diagnostic methods followed by electric pulp testing and cold (thermal) pulp testing.[33] Technologically

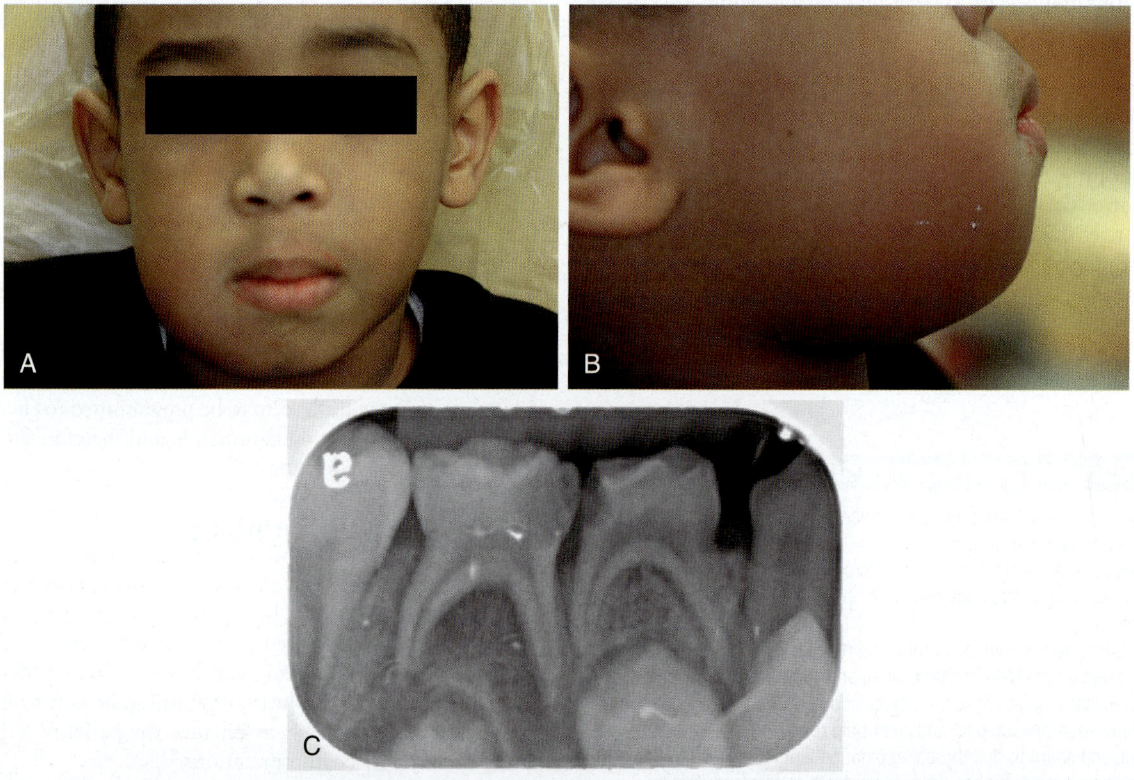

• **Fig. 32.2** (A) Six-year-old male patient with facial swelling caused by deep carious lesion and infection involving tooth #T. (B) Lateral view of same patient, showing redness and extent of cellulitis. (C) Periapical radiograph taken before extraction of the affecting tooth.

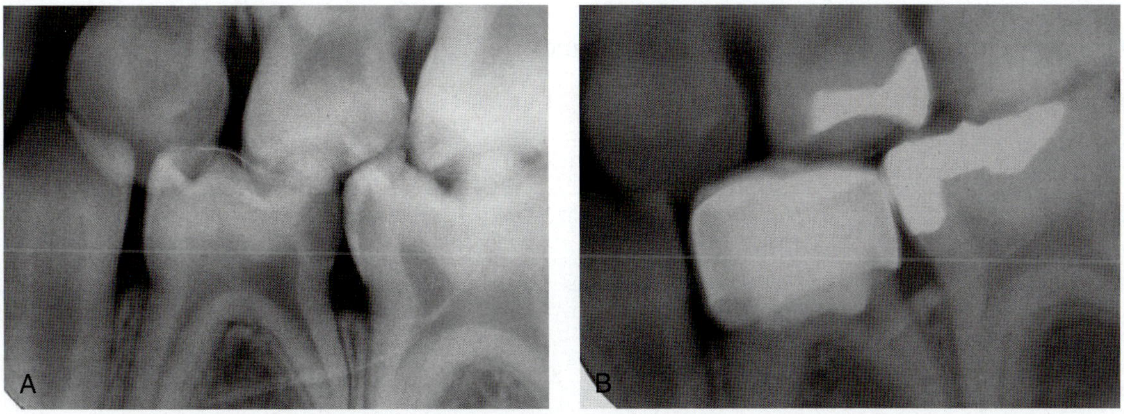

• **Fig. 32.3** (A) Mandibular first and second primary molars with extensive caries and alveolar bone resorption caused by food impaction. The history of spontaneous pain associated with tenderness to percussion may suggest pulp involvement. (B) The same teeth after restoration of the contact point with a stainless steel crown and an amalgam filling. The symptoms disappeared and bone regeneration is evident. (Courtesy Diana Ram, DDS.)

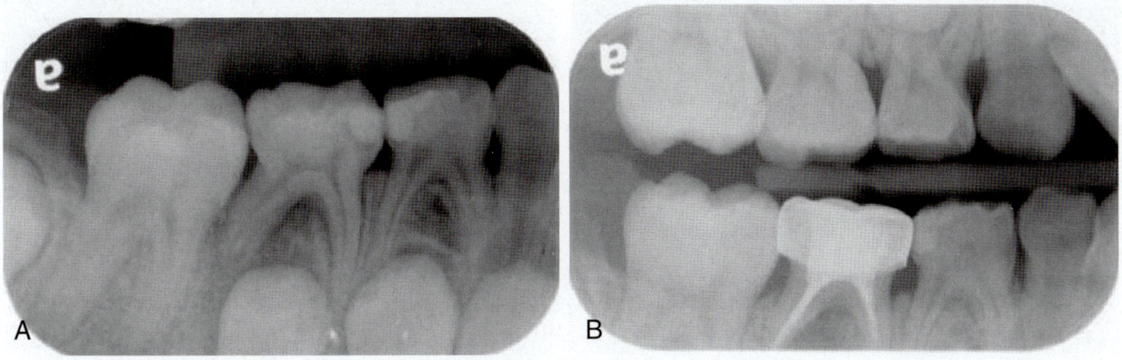

• **Fig. 32.4** (A) Healthy 6-year-old patient with history of spontaneous pain for 2 days pointing to tooth #T. (B) Upon opening, tooth found to be necrotic. Root canal treatment with Vitapex paste performed, followed by a final restoration. (Courtesy Rosa Barnes, DDS.)

advanced tests that detect pulpal blood flow such as laser Doppler flowmetry and pulse oximetry more accurately test the vitality of dental pulp.[33] However, when providing dental care to very young children and/or patients with special healthcare needs, these technologies may require custom-made probes and may lead to unreliable responses due to potential lack of cooperation, signal detection limits, and nonpulpal noise.[3,37] Younger patients may also be more anxious and less reliable because of the subjective nature of the test.[38] To avoid disruptive behavior, when performing percussion and palpation tests in young children, the tip of the finger should be gently used in combination with the tell-show-do technique.[1] The clinician should start the test with a contralateral nonaffected tooth to familiarize the patient with a normal response to the stimuli.

Preoperative Diagnosis of Deep Caries Lesions

Deep caries refers to a carious lesion extending to the inner third of dentin that still has an intact dentin barrier visible on radiographs. Deep caries refers to a carious lesion extending to the inner third of dentin that still has an intact dentin barrier visible on radiographs. When facing deep carious lesions (Fig. 32.3A, 32.10A–B) affecting the primary dentition, limitations exist regarding the determination of the vitality status of the pulp. Percussion and palpation tests, combined with bitewing and selected periapical radiographs, are complementary information that must be obtained. Good quality bitewing radiographs showing the furcation area clearly are essential for an accurate diagnosis. However, in young children in primary and early mixed dentition, especially when using size #0 or #1 films, visibility of the apical third of the primary molar roots and the apical formation of first permanent molars is not always possible. In these situations, a periapical radiograph should be obtained to rule out the presence of internal resorption or periapical involvement.

Integrity and continuity of the lamina dura, together with the presence of trabecular bone in the bifurcation area of primary molars, are indicative signs of a vital pulp. Because of anatomical differences and the superposition of images, clear visualizations of these structures may be difficult to obtain in the maxillary arch.[34] The amount of sound dentin (RDT at least 1 mm) separating the deepest layer of the caries lesion and the pulp horn may also indicate that the pulp is vital.[39]

The texture of the carious lesion can also aid in diagnosis. Soft, friable, grossly denatured dentin is more indicative of a rapidly progressing carious lesion than hard, discolored dentin. Additionally, an open, easily cleansable lesion may be slower progressing than a closed, interproximal lesion that harbors food and debris. Histologic studies show that large interproximal lesions are more likely to have pulpal inflammation than deep occlusal lesions as will be discussed in detail later in this chapter.

A clinical attempt to possibly assess the pulpal diagnosis status of deep caries lesions affecting primary molars using interim

TABLE 32.1 **Diagnostic Principles for Primary Tooth Pulp Diagnosis**

Pulp Diagnosis	Pulpal Status		Pain	Clinical Examination	Radiographic Examination
Reversible	Vital	Inflamed	Asymptomatic or provoked	No furcal/soft tissue involvement, not sensitive to percussion	Deep carious lesion with RDT >1 mm; intact dental lamina
Irreversible			Spontaneous (lingering, throbbing, unprovoked)	No furcal/soft tissue involvement	Deep carious lesion; intact dental lamina
Necrotic	Necrotic	Infected	Spontaneous if periapical tissues involved; may also be asymptomatic for a time	Sensitive to percussion, facial swelling, fistula/sinus tract, mobility	Widened PDL, furcation radiolucency, bone loss, periapical lesion

PDL, Periodontal ligament; *RDT*, remaining dentin thickness.

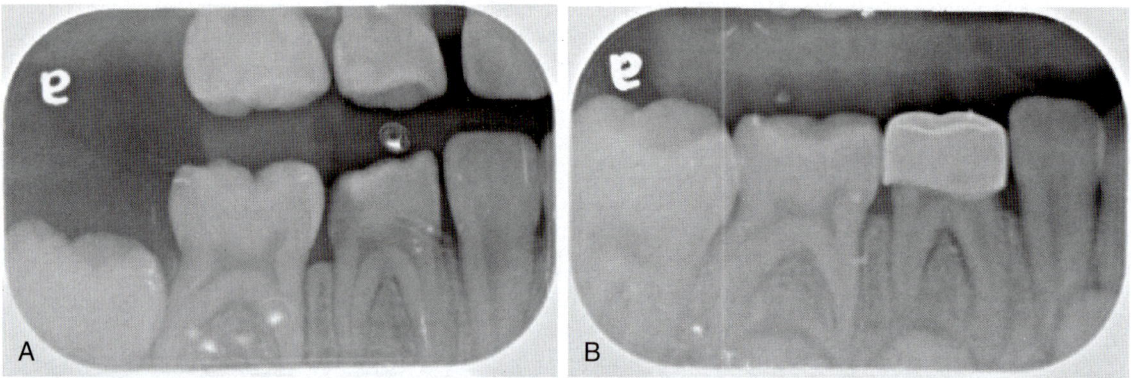

• **Fig. 32.5** (A) Asymptomatic tooth #S selected for indirect pulp treatment. (B) Inadequate stainless steel crown coverage resulted in treatment failure after 1 year. Note enhanced radiolucency in the furcal area of tooth #S. (Courtesy Shawn Hanway, DMD.)

therapeutic restorations has been advocated.[40] Table 32.1 provides a summary of symptoms, clinical signs, and radiographic findings to assist with pulpal diagnoses. For asymptomatic teeth or teeth with reversible pulpal inflammation, to preserve dental structures and avoid further damage to the pulp, conservative approaches such as stepwise excavation and incomplete caries removal should be considered.[41–43] The goal is to prevent bacteria penetration and caries progression from occurring, which could lead to treatment failure (Fig. 32.5). A more detailed explanation is discussed later in the "Vital Pulp Therapy for Normal Pulp/Reversible Pulpitis" section.

Operative Diagnosis

There are instances when a final diagnosis can be achieved only by direct evaluation of the pulp tissue, and a decision about treatment is made accordingly. The bleeding from a direct exposure of the pulp tissue must be assessed; profuse bleeding or purulent exudate indicates irreversible pulpitis or pulpal necrosis. Based on these observations, the treatment plan may be confirmed or changed. For example, if a pulpotomy is planned, the bleeding from the amputation site should be within normal limits (evident in less than 5 minutes with mild cotton pellet pressure). If bleeding persists, a more radical treatment should be undertaken (nonvital pulp therapy or extraction). Excessive bleeding, in the absence of a perforation, is likely an indication that the inflammation has reached the radicular pulp. Conversely, if a pulp polyp is present and bleeding stops normally after coronal pulp amputation, a pulpotomy may be performed instead of a more radical procedure (Fig. 32.6).[44] Direct pulp capping (DPC) of carious exposed primary teeth has shown to have lower success.[45,46]

A schematic diagram for pulpal diagnosis in primary teeth affected by deep carious lesions is presented in Fig. 32.7.

Trauma

Traumatic injuries to the primary dentition can have an impact on the vitality status of the pulp. Discoloration of the crown may indicate internal changes in the pulp canal. Yellow and grayish colors are the most commonly found sequelae of traumatic injuries. Periapical radiographs with clinical examination for sinus tract or gingival swelling will aid in the diagnosis and determination of treatment if needed. (See Chapter 40 for a detailed discussion of sequelae caused by trauma.) Teeth diagnosed with pulp canal obliteration (yellowish discoloration) are vital and should be periodically monitored.

Teeth with light/dark gray discoloration may or may not be necrotic. If asymptomatic with no signs of soft tissue and/or periapical pathology, teeth should be only monitored.[47] The presence of a sinus tract in combination with grayish discoloration of the tooth is a pathognomonic of pulp necrosis (Fig. 32.8).

Correlation Between Histopathologic Status of the Pulp and Deep Caries

Few studies have examined the link between caries depth and pulpal inflammation in primary teeth. Eidelman and Ulmansky analyzed carious, nonrestorable, extracted primary incisors and

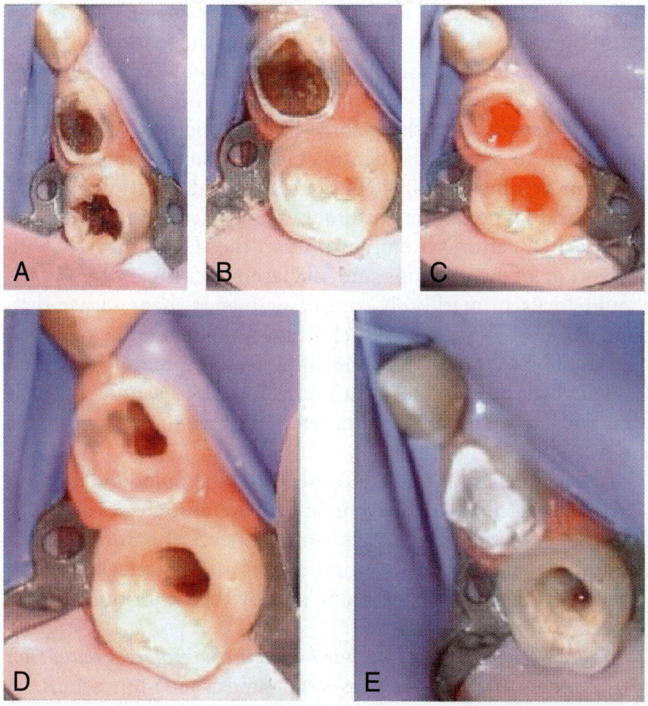

• **Fig. 32.6** (A) First and second primary molars with extensive caries. (B) Pulp exposure after complete caries removal. (C) Extensive bleeding after pulp amputation; the color of the blood is bright red. (D) Bleeding stopped, indicating the tooth is appropriate for a pulpotomy. (E) The pulp stumps are covered with a zinc oxide–eugenol paste. (Courtesy Nathan Rozenfarb, DMD.)

found that when caries removal did not expose the pulp, the pulp was usually normal.[48] This supports the idea that RDT >0.5 mm is important for pulpal health. When pulp was exposed, inflammation was mostly limited to the coronal pulp, making these teeth good candidates for pulpotomy.

Kassa et al.[49] found that deep caries (extending >50% of dentin thickness) caused more inflammation in primary molars with proximal caries than those with occlusal caries. Diagnosing pulp health is crucial for treatment planning but challenging in pulp therapy. Guelmann and colleagues[127] reported a 53% success rate for emergency pulpotomies, attributing early failures (within 3 months) to undiagnosed subclinical inflammation, whereas long-term failures might be associated with microleakage of the restoration. Combining clinical and radiographic data helps improve diagnosis (Table 32.1).

Pulp Treatment Procedures

Different pulp treatment modalities have been recommended for primary teeth. They can be classified into two categories: (1) vital pulp therapy—teeth diagnosed with a normal pulp or reversible pulpitis (pulp protection, IPT, DPC, and pulpotomy), and (2) nonvital pulp therapy—teeth diagnosed with irreversible pulpitis or necrotic pulp (pulpectomy and root filling, and lesion sterilization tissue repair [LSTR]). When the infection cannot be arrested by any of the methods listed, bony support cannot be regained, and the tooth is not restorable, extraction is the treatment of choice (see Fig. 32.7).

Vital Pulp Therapy for Normal Pulp/ Reversible Pulpitis

Terminology

Complete removal of all carious tissue was considered the gold standard 150 years ago.[43] A paradigm shift in carious lesions treatment occurred in the late 1990s with Fusyama[50] suggesting that the superficial layer of grossly denaturated *infected* dentin should be removed, but the underlying layer of partially demineralized caries-*affected* dentin (containing intact, undenaturated collagen fibrils amenable to remineralize) should be preserved during caries excavation.[51,52] These terms are now outdated, particularly the term *infected,* which conveys the idea that dental caries is an infectious or communicable disease that needs to be cured by removing bacteria.[53] Presently, managing a carious lesion includes several options, from the complete, or nonselective, removal of carious tissue, where no visible carious tissue is left before placement of the restoration, to the opposite extreme, where no caries is removed, and noninvasive methods are used to prevent progression of the lesion.[54,55]

A group of cariology experts from 12 countries met in 2015 (the International Caries Consensus Collaboration [ICCC]) to

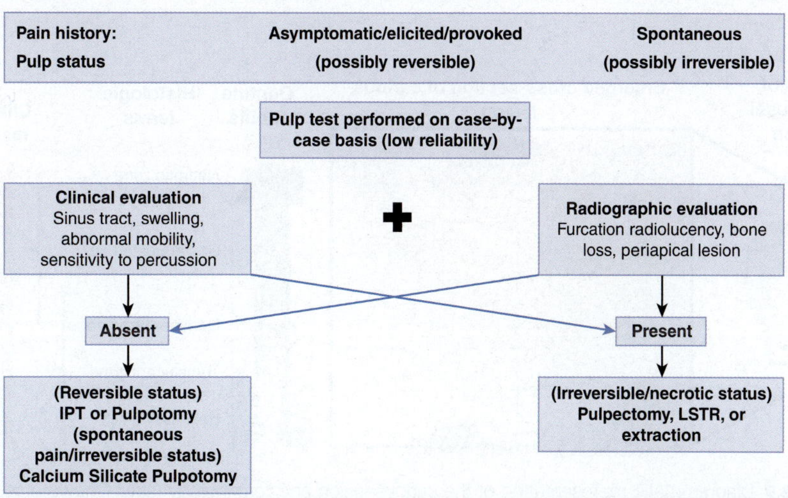

• **Fig. 32.7** Pulpal diagnosis tree for deep carious lesions in primary teeth. *IPT,* Indirect pulp therapy; *LSTR,* lesion sterilization tissue repair.

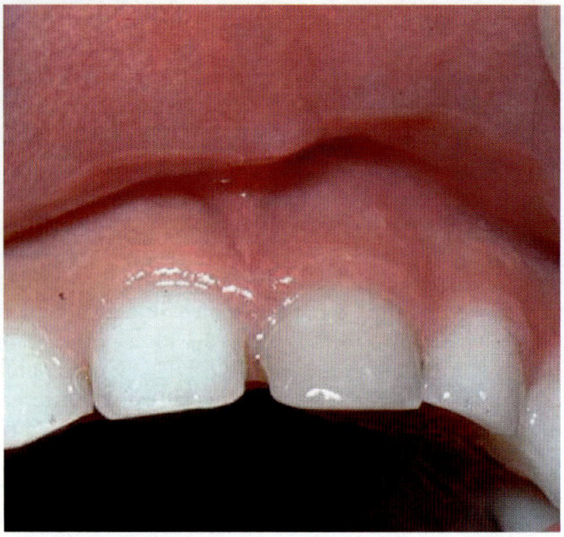

• **Fig. 32.8** Luxation injury affecting tooth #F resulted in grayish discoloration and pulp necrosis with sinus tract.

discuss issues of relevance to cariology researchers, dental educators, and the clinical dentistry community.[43]

In describing the clinical manifestation of caries, these experts agreed that it would be ideal to relate the visual, clinical appearance of the lesion directly to what is taking place histopathologically.[56–58] Although this is not so straightforward, histopathologic investigations of the relationship between the visual appearance of the carious tissue and several parameters such as bacterial invasion, degree of demineralization, and softness of dentin helped develop an understanding of the carious process. As histologic terms are less helpful when communicating with dentists in the clinical setting, and for practical purposes when trying to describe which carious tissue should be removed, the ICCC[43] described the different physical properties associated with the different status of dentin as follows (Fig. 32.9):

Soft dentin will deform when a hard instrument is pressed onto it and can be easily scooped up (e.g., with a sharp excavator), with little force being required.

Leathery dentin does not deform when an instrument is pressed onto it, but it can still be lifted without much force. There might be little difference between *leathery* and *firm* dentin, but leathery is a transition in the spectrum between soft and firm dentin.

Firm dentin is physically resistant to hand excavation, and some pressure needs to be exerted through an instrument to lift it.

Hard dentin: A pushing force needs to be used with a hard instrument to engage the dentin. Only a sharp cutting-edge instrument or a bur will lift it. A scratchy sound or "cri dentinaire" can be heard when a straight probe is taken across the dentin.

As dental caries is a biofilm disease, the ICCC suggests both prevention of new lesions and management of existing lesions should focus primarily on control or management rather than tissue removal. Noncavitated (cleansable) lesions can be managed with biofilm removal (toothbrushing) and/or remineralization. Cavitated (noncleansable) dentin carious lesions cannot be managed by biofilm removal, and remineralization and restorative interventions are indicated.[53]

To remove carious tissue in teeth with vital pulps and without signs of irreversible pulp inflammation, several strategies are available, based on the previously mentioned level of hardness of the remaining dentin.[54] The decision among these strategies will be guided by the depth of the lesion and by the dentition (primary or permanent).

Nonselective removal to hard dentin (complete excavation or complete caries removal) uses the same criteria for carious tissue removal both peripherally and pulpally, and only hard dentin is left. This is considered **overtreatment** and is no longer advocated (ICCC).

Selective removal to firm dentin leaves leathery dentin pulpally, but the cavity margins are left hard/clean after removal. This is the treatment of choice for both dentitions in shallow or moderately cavitated dentinal lesions (radiographically extending less than the pulpal third or quarter of dentin).

Selective removal to soft dentin is recommended in deep cavitated lesions (radiographically extending into the pulpal third or quarter of dentin). Soft carious tissue is left over the pulp to avoid exposure and further injury to the pulp, but peripheral enamel and dentin are prepared to hard dentin to allow a tight seal and a durable restoration. Selective removal to soft dentin reduces the risk of pulp exposure significantly compared with nonselective removal to hard or selective removal to firm dentin.

Stepwise removal is carious tissue removal in two stages. For primary teeth, the second step also adds additional cost, time, and

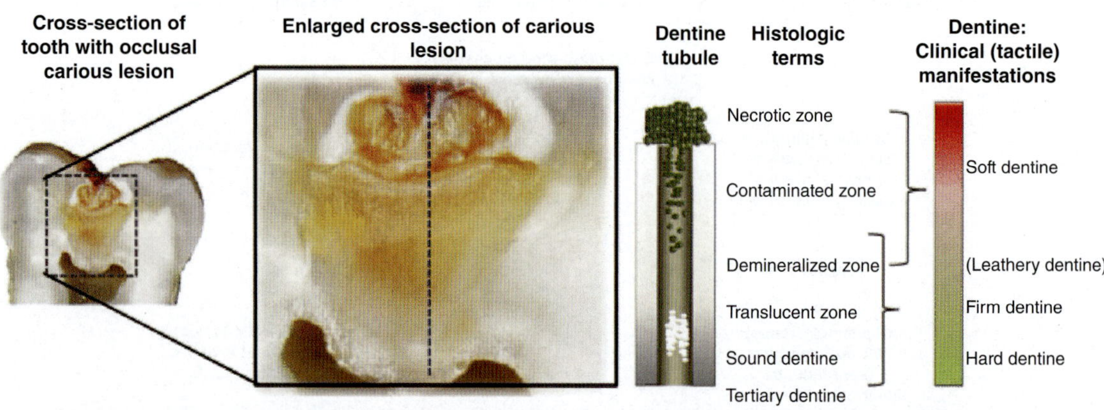

• **Fig. 32.9** Diagrammatic representation of the carious lesion and terminology (after Ogawa et al. 1983). (From Innes NP, Frencken JE, Bjørndal L, et al. Managing carious lesions: consensus recommendations on terminology. *Adv Dent Res*. 201628(2):49-57. doi: 10.1177/0022034516639276)

discomfort for the patient; there is enough evidence that it is not necessary for primary teeth, and selective removal to soft dentin should be carried out.[59]

Protective Base

AAPD guidelines recommend placing a protective base or liner on the pulpal and axial walls to shield the pulp from restorative materials.[35] Dentin is permeable, allowing material movement between the oral cavity and pulp. Previously, pulp inflammation was thought to result from toxic dental materials,[60] but evidence shows it is mainly caused by bacterial invasion.[19,20,61] Marginal leakage and recurrent caries are the leading causes of pulp degeneration under restorations. In deep cavities, thin dentin with large tubules is highly permeable and should be sealed, typically with glass ionomer cement.[62] Modern cavity sealers, including resin cements, glass ionomers, and dentin-bonding agents, enhance bonding and protect the pulp.[62,63] Protective liners or bases should only be placed in deep cavities approaching the pulp (see Chapter 29).

Indirect Pulp Treatment (Selective Removal to Soft Dentin)

IPT is recommended for teeth that have deep carious lesions near the pulp (extending radiographically into the inner third or quarter of the dentin) but have no signs or symptoms of pulp degeneration. IPT is used for deep carious lesions where removing soft dentin may expose the pulp. The deepest carious dentin is left *(selective removal to soft dentin)* and covered with a biocompatible material. Soft dentin over the pulp prevents exposure, and peripheral enamel and dentin are prepared to hard dentin for a secure restorative seal. Complete caries removal from the dentinoenamel junction and cavity walls is essential to prevent microleakage.

IPT results in the deposition of tertiary dentin, increasing the distance between the remaining soft dentin and the pulp, and in the deposition of peritubular (sclerotic) dentin, which decreases dentin permeability. Selective removal to soft dentin reduces the risk of pulp exposure significantly compared with nonselective removal to hard dentin or selective removal to firm dentin (Fig. 32.10).

Clinical experience and a good understanding of the process of caries progression can allow for better control of the "selective caries removal" step. A large round bur (no. 6 or 8) can provide better control in preventing pulp exposure than spoon excavators.[64] The ultimate objective of this treatment is to maintain pulp vitality[65] by (1) arresting the carious process, (2) promoting dentin sclerosis (reducing permeability), (3) stimulating the formation of tertiary dentin, and (4) remineralizing the carious dentin.

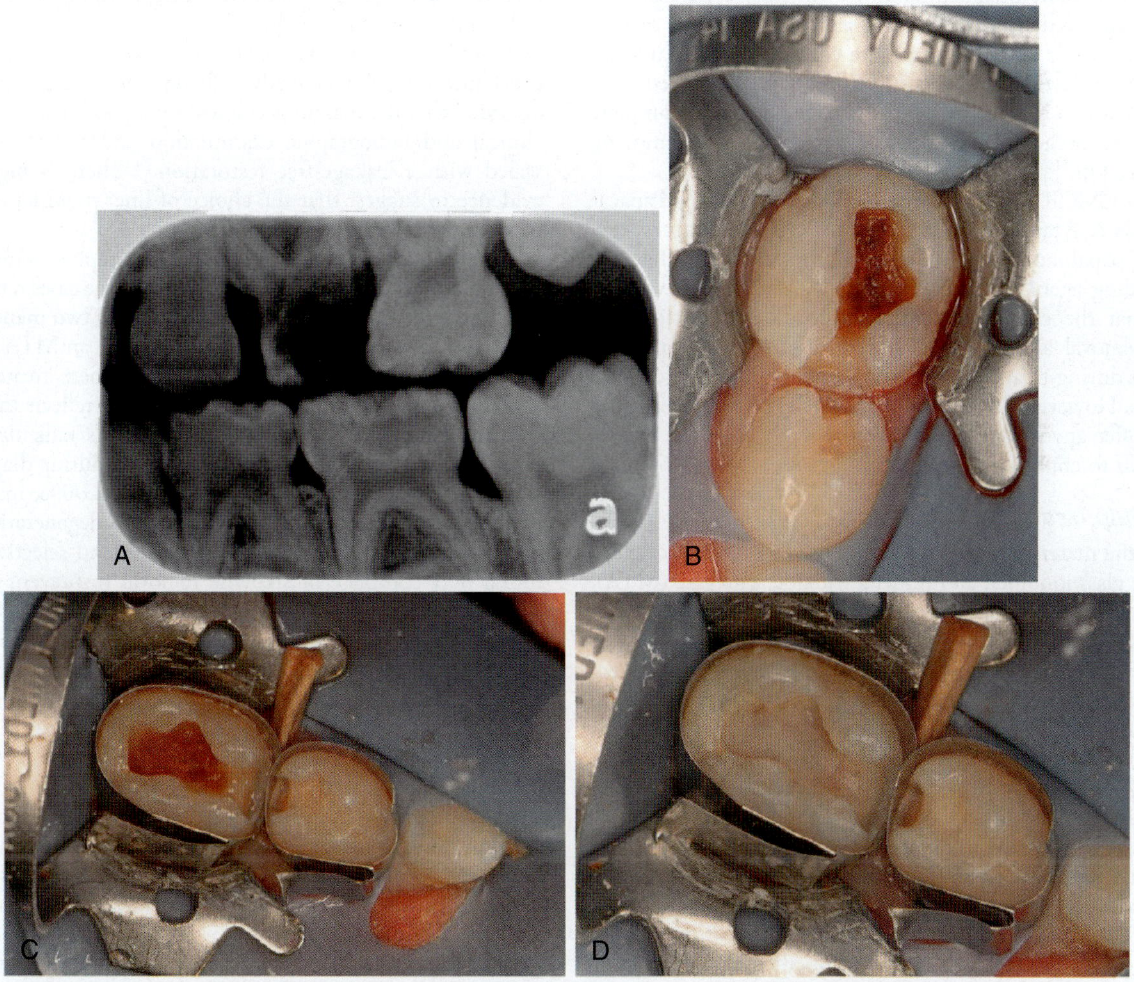

• **Fig. 32.10** (A) Bitewing radiograph showing deep carious lesion affecting asymptomatic tooth #K. (B) Selective caries removal on the pulpal floor (tooth #K) leaving peripheral cavity walls caries free. (C) Cavity preparations ready to be restored. (D) Resin-modified glass ionomer placed on pulpal floor as protective base.

Continued

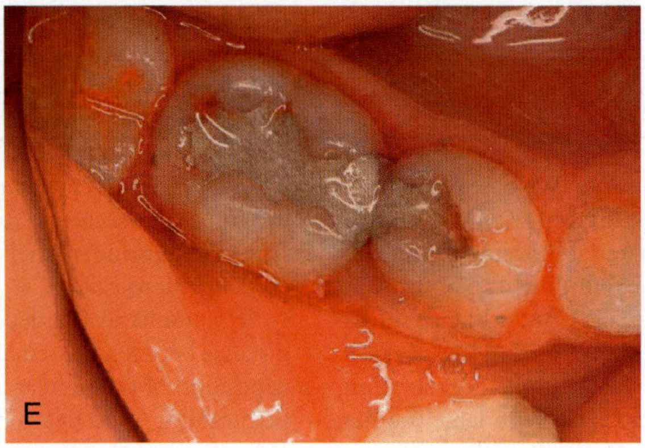

• **Fig. 32.10, cont'd** (E) Final restorations. (Courtesy Ary Kupietzky, DMD, MS.)

Chemomechanical Caries Removal

Several chemomechanical caries removal (CMCR) agents have been developed. CMCR involves chemically softening carious dentin and removing the softened dentin with hand instruments or special burs. One such example is Carisolv (Medi Team Dental, Savedalen, Sweden). A gel made of three amino acids and a low concentration of sodium hypochlorite is rubbed into the carious dentin with specially designed hand instruments. With Carisolv, sound and carious dentin are clinically separated, and only carious dentin is removed, resulting in a more conservative preparation. When a bur is used, healthy tissue is frequently removed. The main drawback to this technique is the time needed to complete the procedure, because it is a much slower process than removing caries with a bur.[66,67]

Another CMCR agent that was developed in Brazil is Papacarie (Fórmula & Ação, São Paulo, SP, Brazil). This product is a gel containing papain, an enzyme similar to human pepsin, that acts as a debriding agent with no harm to healthy tissue. Evidence suggests that the chemomechanical approach is efficacious for bacterial removal and significantly reduces the risk of pain or discomfort during treatment, thereby reducing the need for local anesthetics. However, the technique is more time consuming and does not offer any benefits over selective removal to soft dentin with regards to clinical outcomes.[68,69]

Indirect Pulp Treatment Materials

Presently, the materials most commonly used in IPT are calcium hydroxide, glass ionomer, and mineral trioxide aggregate (MTA). Many historical studies have examined the interaction between tooth tissues and calcium hydroxide, and more recently with MTA. The main soluble component from MTA has been shown to be calcium hydroxide. The clinical response of the tooth to both materials is based on comparable mechanisms involving the dissolution of calcium hydroxide and release of calcium and hydroxyl ions, raising the pH of the environment well above 7.0. Because dentin contains a large store of potentially bioactive molecules, it has been considered that the interaction of a high pH material, such as calcium hydroxide or MTA, may cause the release of some of these molecules. This action is similar to that occurring during the demineralization of dentin during a caries attack, where the pH of the local environment is low.[70]

When resin-modified glass ionomers are placed into a cavity preparation, their initial pH within the first 24 hours is approximately 4.0 to 5.5. Therefore the glass ionomer remineralizes the adjacent dentin, releasing ions and potentially the sequestered bioactive materials as well. The pulpal response to glass ionomer is favorable when a layer of dentin remains between the material and the pulp.

Dentin-bonding agents are recommended for IPT, but concerns remain about their effectiveness.[72] Nakajima et al. found that bond strength to carious dentin is significantly lower than to sound dentin.[73] This raises questions about the bond's integrity and its ability to prevent bacterial invasion and also emphasizes that IPT depends on complete caries removal from the lateral walls and cavosurface margins.

Contrary to previous beliefs, IPT can also be an acceptable procedure for primary teeth with reversible pulp inflammation, provided that the diagnosis is based on a good history and proper clinical and radiographic examination and the tooth has been sealed with a leakage-free restoration.[74] There is high-certainty evidence to suggest that the choice of liner material did not impact the success of IPT after 24 months.[45,46]

A thorough history, clinical, and radiographic examination are essential for accurate diagnosis. However, some cases remain uncertain, affecting prognosis. Fig. 32.11 compares two mandibular first primary molars in the same patient: one with an MTA pulpotomy showing internal root resorption, and its antimere, treated with IPT and composite, appearing normal. This likely reflects the preoperative pulp status, as the pulpotomized tooth's radicular pulp was likely chronically inflamed but undetectable during diagnosis.

IPT success rates in primary teeth exceed 90%, making it the preferred treatment for cases without pulp degeneration. Studies by Ricketts, Dhar, and colleagues recommend selective caries removal over complete or stepwise removal to prevent pulp exposure.[75,76] Research shows IPT is successful,[64,77–80] particularly more than DPC or pulpotomy for deep caries in primary molars.[46,64,77–81] Given its proven success and biologic benefits, we can recommend IPT (selective removal to soft dentin) as the most appropriate treatment for symptom-free primary teeth with deep caries, provided that a proper, leakage-free restoration can be placed.

A recent systematic review and meta-analysis on vital pulp therapy in primary teeth found that IPT and pulpotomy with calcium silicates (MTA and Biodentine, Septodont) had the highest success rates and strongest evidence after 24 months for treating deep caries.[45] In contrast, DPC had lower success rates and weaker supporting evidence.

New experimental strategies use bioactive molecules such as enamel matrix protein (Emdogain [Straumann Canada Limited, Burlington, Ontario]) or TGF-β to stimulate tertiary dentin formation and decrease dentin permeability. However, these are not yet in clinical use.[3]

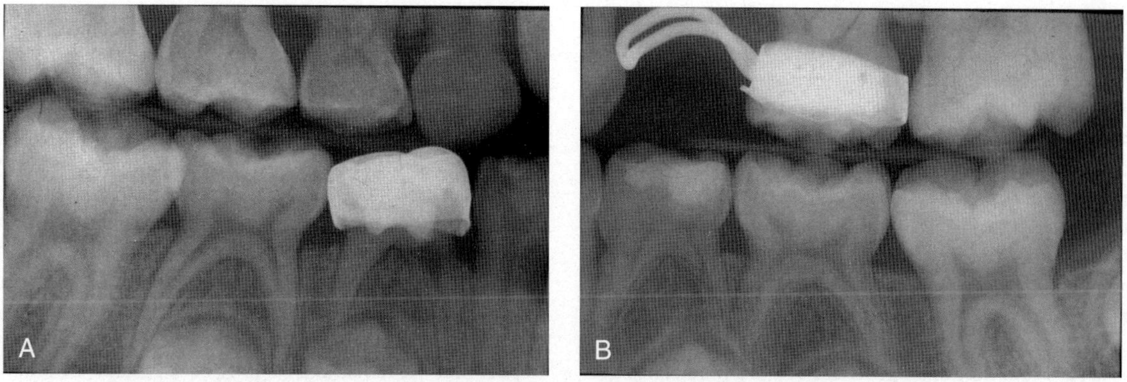

• **Fig. 32.11** Mandibular first primary molars of the same patient 3 years after treatment of deep caries. (A) Tooth #S treated with mineral trioxide aggregate pulpotomy. Internal resorption is evident. (B) Contralateral tooth #L treated conservatively with indirect pulp treatment and a composite restoration. The pulp appears normal.

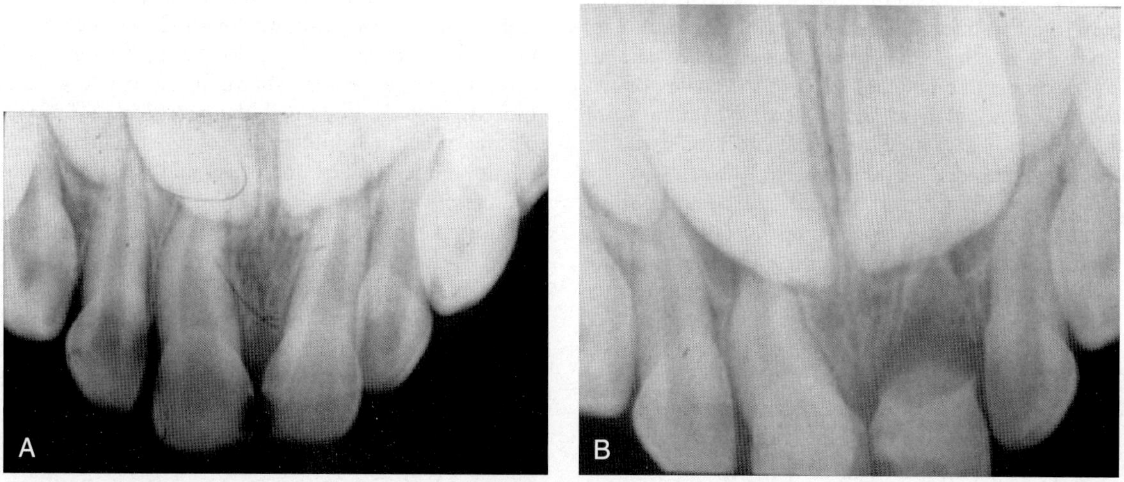

• **Fig. 32.12** (A) Maxillary primary central incisor treated by direct pulp capping with $CaOH_2$ after pinpoint iatrogenic pulp exposure. (B) Extensive internal resorption was evident 6 months later.

Direct Pulp Capping

DPC is performed when healthy pulp is exposed due to trauma or an operative procedure. The tooth must be asymptomatic, with a pinpoint exposure free of contaminants. Calcium hydroxide is placed to stimulate dentin formation and maintain pulp vitality.[2,46] Success is low in primary teeth, with failures leading to internal resorption or acute abscess (Fig. 32.12). Kennedy and Kapala[85] claim that the high cellular content of the primary pulp tissue may be responsible for the increased failure rate of DPC in primary teeth. These authors believe that undifferentiated mesenchymal cells may differentiate into odontoclasts, leading to internal resorption, a principal sign of failure of DPC in primary teeth.

Some advocate for using dentin-bonding agents to provide a seal against bacterial invasion, but results have been inconsistent, with some studies showing poor outcomes.[71,86]

Animal research has shown the good compatibility of mechanically exposed pulps to visible light–activated composite when bacteria are excluded.[18] Araujo and associates[87] reported good clinical and radiographic results in cariously exposed primary teeth 1 year after acid etching and capping with a bonding agent and restoration with a resin-based composite. Based on these reports, Kopel[88] proposed a "revisitation" of the DPC technique in primary teeth. He suggested "gently wiping the dentin floor and the exposed pulp with an antibacterial solution such as chlorhexidine or a fixative such as formocresol or a weak glutaraldehyde solution," replacing calcium hydroxide with dentin-bonding agents. In another publication a year later, Araujo and colleagues[89] examined histologically primary molars with micro-exposures that were successfully treated with a composite acid etch technique and then extracted or exfoliated. These authors observed microabscesses adjacent to the exposure site, and no dentin bridge was formed in any specimen. These results were confirmed by Pameijer and Stanley,[90,91] who concluded that "the belief that any material placed on an exposed pulp will allow bridge formation as long as the cavity is disinfected is a fallacy." In a review on pulp capping with dentin-adhesive systems, Costa and coworkers[92] reported that self-etching adhesive systems led to inflammatory reactions, delay in pulpal healing, and failure of dentin bridging in human pulps capped with bonding agents. They state that vital pulp therapy using acidic agents and adhesive resins seems to be contraindicated.

The effectiveness of TGF-β and bone morphogenetic proteins (BMPs) in inducing reparative dentinogenesis in pulp capping situations in vivo[82–84] provides the basis for development of a possible new generation of biomaterials. Because the specificity of these growth factors to induce reparative processes is not clear, more studies are required to fully explain the kinetics of growth factor release and the sequence of growth factor–induced reparative dentinogenesis.

Guidelines do not recommend DPC for caries-exposed primary teeth,[35,46] but recent trials suggest promising results,[93–95] particularly when materials like MTA, bonding agents, and enamel-derivate protein (Emdogain) with or without prior rinsing of the exposed pulp with saline or an antibacterial solution such as sodium hypochlorite or chlorhexidine, were compared with calcium hydroxide as capping agents. Regardless of the methodology used, very strict inclusion criteria were common to all tested teeth: absence of clinical and radiographic signs and symptoms such as swelling, abnormal mobility, presence of fistula, spontaneous pain, sensitivity to percussion, and furcation involvement. In addition, all exposed pulps had to be limited to 1.0 mm or less. In only one study was rubber dam isolation not used,[95] and bonding agents' techniques were compared with calcium hydroxide as pulp protection. Relative isolation did not interfere with the outcome. A high success rate was only obtained when phosphoric acid and nonrinse conditioners did not directly contact the pulp. Restorations of the treated teeth were performed with amalgam only,[95] amalgam and resin-based materials followed by a sealant coverage,[93] and stainless steel crowns.[94] Coll et al.[45] reported that up to 24 months, "DPC showed lower success rates to IPT and MTA or Biodentine pulpotomies, and the quality of evidence was lower." When long-term results (beyond 24 months) of these procedures are available, more definitive conclusions can be drawn regarding this technique for primary teeth.

Although DPC in primary teeth should still be approached cautiously, it may be viable for exposed pulps in older children, 1 or 2 years before normal exfoliation. In these children, a failure of treatment would not require the use of a space maintainer after extraction, as it would in younger children.

Pulpotomy

Given the evidence supporting IPT, every effort should be made to prevent pulpal exposure when managing deep carious lesions. However, if the pulp is exposed or affected, pulpotomy is the treatment of choice. The AAPD recommends pulpotomy over pulpectomy for vital anterior primary teeth with reversible pulpitis.[46] Pulpotomy is based on the idea that healthy radicular pulp can recover after removing the affected coronal pulp.[1,2] It is contraindicated if there are signs of inflammation beyond the coronal pulp, including swelling, fistula, pathologic mobility, pathologic external or internal root resorption, periapical or interradicular radiolucency, pulp calcifications, or excessive bleeding from the amputated radicular stumps. The ideal dressing should be bactericidal, be safe for the pulp, promote healing, and not interfere with root resorption. Other signs, such as a history of spontaneous or nocturnal pain or tenderness to percussion or palpation, should be interpreted carefully (see Fig. 32.4).

Pulpotomy Agents

Formocresol

A decade ago, the most used pulp dressing material was formocresol (Buckley solution: formaldehyde, cresol, glycerol, and water). Primosch and associates[96] reported in 1997 that the majority of the predoctoral pediatric dental programs in the United States advocated the use of either full-strength formocresol (22.6% of programs) or a one-fifth dilution of formocresol (71.7% of programs) as the preferred pulpotomy medicament for vital primary teeth.

Clinical and radiographic studies have demonstrated that formocresol pulpotomies have success rates ranging from 70% to 97%.[97–100] The use of a one-fifth dilution of formocresol has been advocated by several authors[97,98] because of its reportedly equal effectiveness and potential for less toxicity. This solution is prepared by making a diluent of three parts glycerin and one part water. Four parts of this diluent are then mixed with one part Buckley solution to make the one-fifth dilution.

Although many studies have reported the clinical success of formocresol pulpotomies, an increasing body of literature has questioned the use of formocresol. Rolling and Thylstrup[100] demonstrated that its clinical success rate decreased as follow-up time increased. Furthermore, the histologic response of the primary radicular pulp to formocresol appears to be unfavorable. A classic study claims that, subsequent to formocresol application, fixation occurs in the coronal third of the radicular pulp, chronic inflammation in the middle third, and vital tissue in the apical third.[101] Others report that the remaining pulp tissue is partially or totally necrotic.[102] Several reports have questioned the safety of formocresol,[103,104] and most authorities now agree that formocresol is at least potentially mutagenic, carcinogenic, and toxic when used in high concentrations and under specific conditions in animal studies. However, there are no documented cases of systemic distribution or pathologic tissue changes associated with the use of formocresol in humans.[105] The doses used in animal models far exceed those used in clinical practice; normal clinical doses carry little risk for patients. Indeed, a study examined the presence of formocresol in the plasma of children undergoing oral rehabilitation involving pulp therapy under general anesthesia and showed that formaldehyde and cresol were undetectable above baseline plasma concentration in subjects receiving pulpotomy treatment under general anesthesia.[106] The authors concluded that the levels present were far below those recommended by the US Food and Drug Administration (FDA). It is unlikely that formocresol, when used in the doses typically employed for a vital pulpotomy procedure, poses any risk to children. Nevertheless, amid the controversies and concerns, efforts have increased to find a substitute medicament.

Formocresol is no longer the most commonly taught medicament for pulpotomy. In the United States a 2008 survey detected a trend away from the teaching of 1:5 diluted formocresol, with more using ferric sulfate (FS) for pulpotomy; still, 22% of programs recommended full-strength formocresol.[107] The philosophies and trends on medicaments vary among countries and regions, and even among dental schools, with reported preference for diluted formocresol[108] in Brazilian dental schools, and FS in the United Kingdom and Ireland.[109] Issues regarding the selection of pulpotomy medicaments will be discussed later in this chapter.

Calcium silicate cements

An evidence-based proven alternative to formocresol with reported success rates equal to and even surpassing those of formocresol and all other pulpotomy agents is MTA.[110] MTA was developed by Torabinejad at Loma Linda University in the 1990s, first described in the dental scientific literature by Lee and colleagues[111] in 1993 and approved by the FDA in 1998. It is a mixture of a refined Portland cement, dicalcium silicate, tricalcium silicate, tricalcium aluminate, gypsum, and tetracalcium aluminoferrite; bismuth oxide is also added, making the material radiopaque. Both in vitro and in vivo investigations have shown that MTA has many positive properties such as excellent biocompatibility, an alkaline pH, radiopacity, a high sealing capacity, and the ability to induce the formation of dentin, cement, and bone.[112] A radiograph of two primary molars treated with MTA is presented in Fig. 32.13.

A preliminary study comparing MTA with formocresol, with follow-up periods ranging from 6 to 30 months, found no clinical or radiographic pathologic issues in any MTA-treated teeth. Pulp canal obliteration occurred in 13% of formocresol-treated teeth and 41%

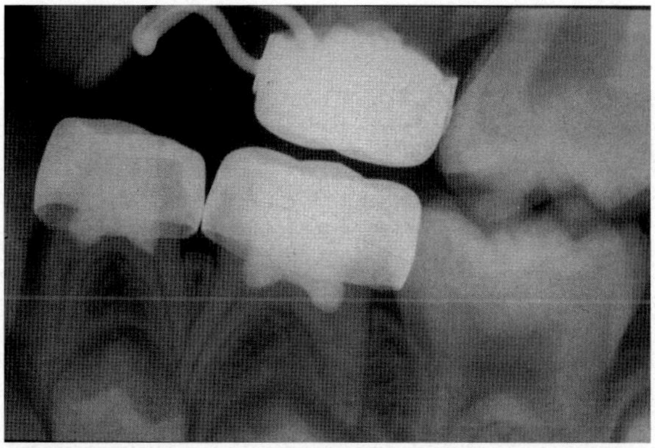

• **Fig. 32.13** Mandibular first and second primary molars 36 months after pulpotomy with mineral trioxide aggregate. Pulp canal obliteration is evident in the distal root of the second molar; both procedures were rated as successful.

of MTA-treated teeth. Internal root resorption, previously observed in FS and diluted formocresol-treated teeth in other studies,[119,121] was not noted in the MTA-treated teeth in this preliminary report.[113]

Longer clinical studies have since been published with high success rates.[114–120] Holan and associates[121] investigated MTA effects in 33 pulpotomized molars during a median follow-up evaluation period of 38.2 months, reporting a success rate of 97%. Farsi and coworkers[122] compared the effect of MTA in 60 pulpotomized molars with those of formocresol followed during 2 years and noted a success rate of 100%.

When MTA was first commercialized, it had a gray coloration; but in 2002 a new white formula was created to improve on the dark color properties exhibited by the gray preparation. White MTA has smaller particles and does not contain tetracalcium aluminoferrite or iron, both of which are found in gray MTA. Cardoso-Silva and colleagues[123] compared the results of gray and white MTA pulpotomies in a sample of 233 primary molars, with a maximum follow-up period of 84 months. The gray MTA had 100% radiographic success, and the white had a 93% success rate. Another interesting finding was that gray MTA showed a significantly higher number of dentine bridge formation than white MTA. MTA is commercially available as ProRoot MTA (DENTSPLY Tulsa Dental Products, Tulsa, OK), MTA-Angelus (Angelus Soluções Odontológicas, Londrina, Brazil), and more recently as Neo-MTA (NuSmile, Houston, TX).

The other most widely recognized calcium silicate cement is Biodentine, which has also been used as a pulpotomy agent with promising results. An 18-month follow-up randomized clinical study found similar results when Biodentine was compared with ProRoot MTA.[124,125]

Based on high quality evidence, Coll et al.[45] reported the 24-month success of MTA pulpotomy to be 94%, followed by Biodentine at 90.4% and formocresol at 86%. Given the higher success of calcium silicates and potential concerns related to formocresol, the recent AAPD guidelines[46] gave a strong recommendation in favor of MTA and Biodentine, and a conditional recommendation for the use of formocresol.

Other pulpotomy medicaments

FS is a hemostatic agent that precipitates proteins in the blood, physically blocking the openings of capillaries, which stops bleeding at the exposure site. It is bacteriostatic and can potentially mask an irreversibly inflamed pulp with its hemostasis activity. There is low certainty data to suggest that FS had significantly lower success rates compared with calcium silicate materials such as MTA, leading to a conditional recommendation against its use.[45,46]

Preliminary studies have investigated the use of 5% sodium hypochlorite (NaOCl) as a primary molar pulpotomy agent. A pilot study by Vargas and colleagues[128] showed promising results after a 12-month period, and a retrospective study[129,130,131] confirmed these findings. Both studies concluded that clinical and radiographic success rates for NaOCl pulpotomies are comparable to FS and formocresol pulpotomies. However, studies with longer follow-up (18 months) were included in a recent systematic review that showed NaOCl pulpotomies to be significantly less successful than formocresol (FC). Thus the current AAPD Clinical Practice Guidelines conditionally recommended against the use of NaOCl.[46]

Nonpharmacotherapeutic approaches to pulpotomy include the treatment of radicular pulp tissue by electrocautery or laser to eliminate residual infectious processes. Although these techniques are currently being used by a number of practitioners, no long-term controlled clinical studies are available to evaluate their success, and studies have shown conflicting results.[132–134]

In summary, the search for alternatives to formocresol as a pulp dressing in primary tooth pulpotomies has revealed MTA and Biodentine as the ideal capping agents in primary tooth pulpotomies.[46,135] Table 32.2 offers a summary of pulpotomy agents.

Pulpotomy Technique

Before local anesthesia administration, a thorough clinical examination should be repeated, including visual examination of the vestibulum, palpation, and percussion of the involved and neighboring teeth. After achieving anesthesia and placing a rubber dam, remove all superficial caries to minimize bacterial contamination before pulpal exposure. Use a no. 330 bur with a high-speed turbine to remove the pulp chamber roof. Amputate the coronal pulp with a sharp excavator or large round bur. This should be done carefully to avoid damaging the pulp or perforating the pulpal floor. Ensure all coronal pulp tissue is removed, as any remaining tissue under dentin ledges can bleed and obscure the condition of the radicular pulp stumps, hindering diagnosis (Fig. 32.14A). The technique is essentially the same for anterior teeth, involving the removal of coronal pulp tissue from the chamber (approximately 2 mm below the free gingival margin) while ensuring that the radicular pulp tissue is not damaged or removed.

After coronal pulp amputation, one or more cotton pellets should be placed over each amputation site, and pressure should be applied for a few minutes. When the cotton pellets are removed, hemostasis should be apparent, although a minor amount of wound bleeding may be evident (see Fig. 32.14B). Excessive bleeding that persists despite cotton pellet pressure may indicate that the inflammation has extended to the radicular pulp. Such signs suggest that the tooth is not a good candidate for pulpotomy, and nonvital pulp therapies/extraction should be considered. No intrapulpal local anesthesia or other hemostatic agent should be used to minimize hemorrhage, because bleeding is a clinical indicator of the health of the radicular pulp. After hemostasis, MTA or Biodentine paste is applied to cover the exposed radicular pulp surface with a margin of not less than 1 mm beyond the pulp dentin interface. A base of either intermediate restorative material (IRM) or resin-modified glass ionomer is placed over the calcium silicate cement. See Case Study: Pulpotomy and Stainless Steel Crown Procedures. The success of an MTA pulpotomy does not seem to be affected by choice of base material.[46]

The formocresol procedure is essentially the same with the medicament placed over the pulp in place of calcium silicate cement. When using formocresol, a cotton pellet moistened with Buckley solution (full concentration or one-fifth solution) is placed over the

TABLE 32.2 **Characteristics of Primary Tooth Pulpotomy Agents**

Agent	AAPD Recommendation as of 2024	Properties	Effect on Pulp	Advantages	Disadvantages
MTA	Strong in favor	Mineral trioxide aggregate cement (refined Portland cement)	Sets hard and seals pulp; stimulates dentin bridging	Biocompatible; excellent sealing properties; antibacterial due to high pH	Cost; stains tooth; difficult handling properties
Biodentine	Strong in favor	Calcium silicate–based cement	Sets hard and seals pulp; stimulates dentin bridging	Biocompatible; excellent sealing properties; antibacterial due to high pH; improved handling properties	Cost
Formocresol	Conditional in favor	Mixture of formaldehyde, cresol, and glycerin; tissue fixative	Fixes the pulp; zone of necrosis	Easy to use; bactericidal	Some concerns for toxicity and carcinogenicity
Ferric sulfate	Conditional against	Hemostatic agent	Causes protein coagulation creating a barrier between the pulp and restorative base	Easy to use; biocompatible	Bacteriostatic; can mask hemorrhagic pulp; lower success rates
Sodium Hypochlorite (NaOCl)	Conditional against	Antimicrobial agent	Disinfects pulpal tissue and can help achieve coagulation/hemostasis	Inexpensive; easy to use	Limited long-term evidence

AAPD, American Academy of Pediatric Dentistry; *MTA*, mineral trioxide aggregate.

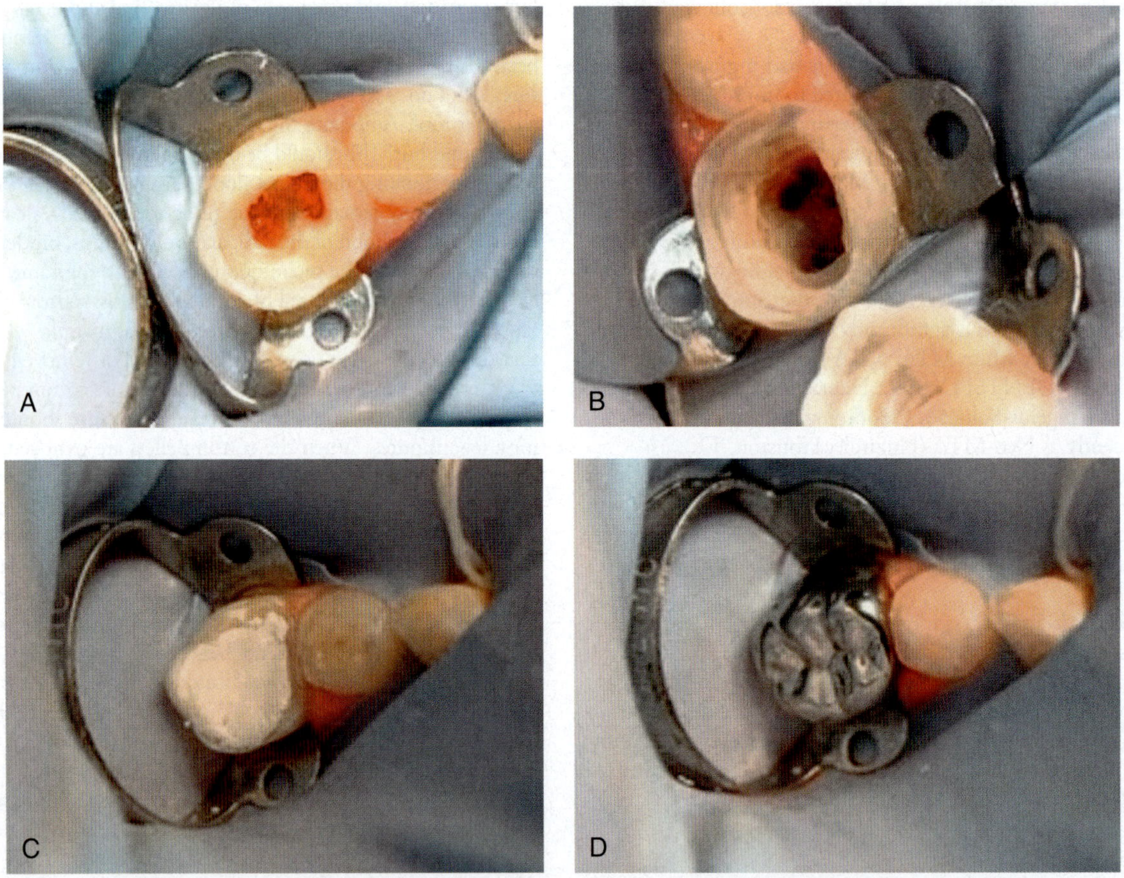

• **Fig. 32.14** Pulpotomy Technique Steps. (A) Pulp chamber after coronal pulp amputation; wide access opening prevents leaving tissue tags. (B) After hemostasis and formocresol application, the tissue at the entrance of the canals shows dark color, a sign of tissue fixation. (C) The pulp stumps are covered by a zinc oxide–eugenol base. (D) The tooth is restored with a stainless steel crown. (Courtesy Nathan Rosenfarb, DDS.)

pulp stumps for 5 minutes. When the pellet is removed, the amputation site should appear dark brown (when a full concentration of formocresol is used) or dark red (when the one-fifth dilution is employed). In both cases, very little or no hemorrhage is present. A base of ZOE (either plain or reinforced) is placed over the amputation site and lightly condensed to cover the pulpal floor. A second layer is then condensed to fill the access opening completely (see Fig. 32.14C).

The final restoration is preferably a stainless steel crown, which should be placed at the same appointment (see Fig. 32.14D). Holan and coworkers[126] observed that pulpotomized primary molars could be successfully restored with one-surface amalgams if their natural exfoliation is expected within 2 years or less. However, if placing the final restoration is not possible, glass ionomer or IRM may be used as an acceptable interim restoration until the stainless steel crown can be placed. The most recent AAPD Clinical Practice Guidelines note that the type of restoration may not influence the success of an MTA pulpotomy, though the recommendation was conditional and based on studies that only offered data for 12 months of follow-up. Although a clinician may choose a restorative material based on clinical expertise, the restoration should be able to restore form and function and be **leakage free**.

In summary, the highest level of success and quality of evidence supports IPT and the pulpotomy techniques of MTA and Biodentine for the treatment of deep caries in primary teeth after 24 months. DPC shows slightly lower success rates compared with IPT and calcium silicate pulpotomies, and the quality of evidence is lower.[46] The comparable success rates for all three vital pulp therapy techniques (IPT, DPC, and pulpotomy) provide more latitude in treatment choices for the practitioner in managing a vital primary tooth with deep caries.

Pulp Therapy for Irreversible Pulpitis or Necrotic Pulp

Vital Pulp Therapy for Irreversible Pulpitis

In cases of extremely deep caries that penetrates the entire radiographic thickness of dentine with no discernable radiographic dentin barrier, the pulp is likely infected and inflamed, regardless of symptoms. Treatment includes non-selective (complete) caries removal, pulp assessment, and calcium silicate full pulpotomy, if hemostasis is possible and there is no necrosis, even when spontaneous pain is present.[136]

Non-vital Pulp Therapy for Irreversible Pulpitis or Necrotic Pulp

In presence of furcation or periradicular involvement or signs of pulp necrosis, non-vital pulp therapies in primary teeth include pulpectomy and lesion sterilization tissue repair (LSTR). The goal of non-vital pulp therapy is to preserve primary teeth, prevent spread of dental infection, and facilitate natural exfoliation of primary tooth. Pulpectomy is a root canal procedure involving complete extirpation of coronal and radicular pulp, followed by debridement, shaping of canals, irrigation, and obturation with a resorbable material. LSTR was developed as a non-instrumentation endodontic procedure in which the necrotic coronal pulp is removed followed by placement of a triple-antibiotic paste in a propylene glycol vehicle to disinfect the root canal systems. Pulpectomy has high success when there is no pre-operative root resorption, while LSTR is preferred for short-term management of non-vital primary teeth with root resorption. The reluctance of some dentists to perform root canal treatments in primary teeth is likely influenced by the behavior guidance challenges that occasionally arise with pediatric patients.

Certain clinical situations may justify nonvital pulp therapy, even with the knowledge that the prognosis may not be ideal. An example of such a case is advanced pulpal involvement of a primary second molar that occurs before the first permanent molar erupts. A premature extraction of the primary second molar without placement of a space maintainer usually results in mesial eruption of the first permanent molar with subsequent loss of space for the second premolar (Fig. 32.15). Although a distal shoe space maintainer is an option, preserving the natural tooth is the preferred treatment. Therefore a pulpectomy or LSTR in a primary second molar is preferable, even if that tooth is only able to be maintained until the first permanent molar has adequately erupted and is followed eventually by extraction of the primary second molar and placement of a space maintainer (Fig. 32.16).

Pulpectomy and Root Filling

Pulpectomy is indicated for teeth with minimal root resorption and irreversible inflammation or necrosis in the radicular pulp. It is contraindicated in teeth with significant root loss, internal or external resorption, or periapical infection involving the succedaneous tooth. Challenges in preparing complex primary root canals and

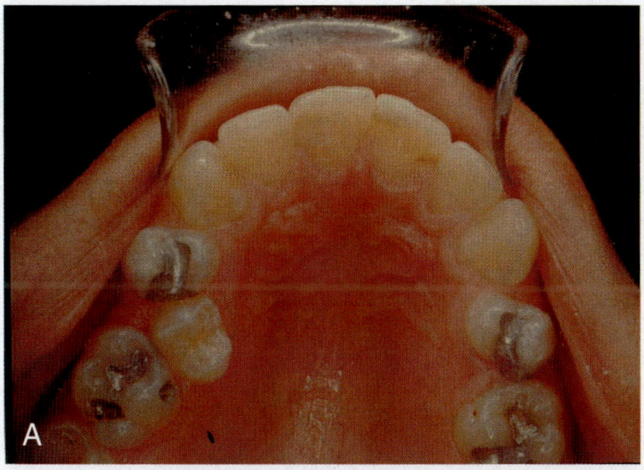

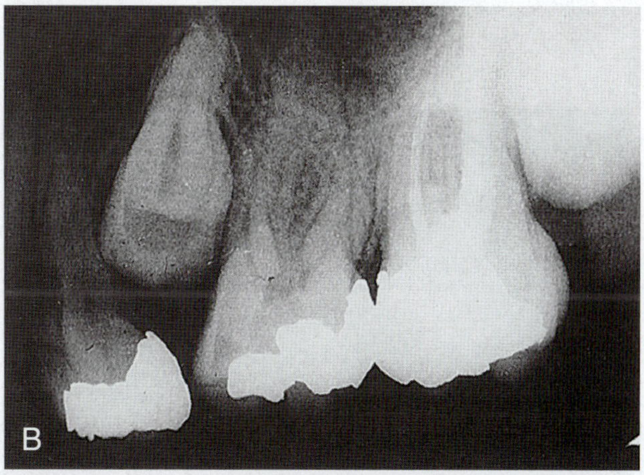

• **Fig. 32.15** (A) Occlusal view of the permanent dentition after bilateral premature extractions of the maxillary primary second molars. The right second bicuspid erupted ectopically, and the left is impacted. (B) Radiograph of the area showing the impacted left premolar. (Courtesy Ilana Brin, DMD.)

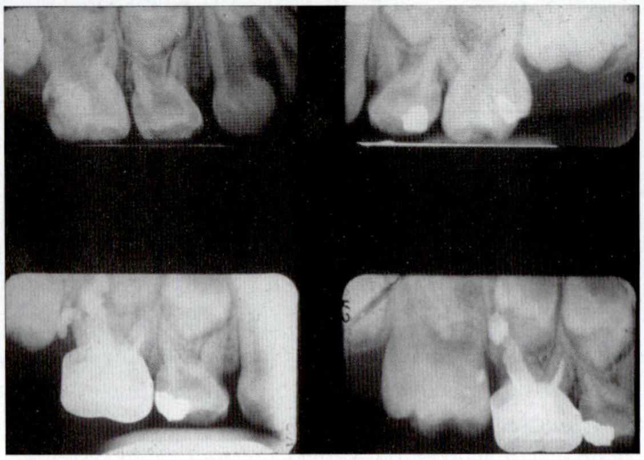

• **Fig. 32.16** Nonvital maxillary second primary molar, treated by pulpectomy with zinc oxide–eugenol (ZOE). *Top left,* Before pulpectomy. *Top right,* Contralateral vital tooth. *Bottom left,* Excess of ZOE in palatal and distobuccal canals. *Bottom right,* Primary tooth successfully retained until eruption of first permanent molar.

concerns about the impact on developing succedaneous teeth may discourage some clinicians. Despite these issues, the success of pulpectomies in primary teeth has led many pediatric dentists to prefer them over extractions and space maintenance in certain cases.

Root canal filling materials

Developmental, anatomical, and physiologic differences between primary and permanent teeth call for differences in the criteria for root canal filling materials. The ideal root canal filling material for primary teeth should resorb at a rate similar to that of the primary root, be harmless to the periapical tissues and to the permanent tooth germ, resorb readily if pressed beyond the apex, be antiseptic, fill the root canals easily, adhere to their walls, not shrink, be easily removed if necessary, be radiopaque, and not discolor the tooth.[137] No material currently meets all of these criteria. Several investigators have evaluated various root filling materials through clinical and radiographic assessments; however, the lack of controls in these studies limits their relevance.[138–144] The filling materials most commonly used for primary pulp canals are ZOE paste, iodoform-based paste, calcium hydroxide, and calcium hydroxide and iodoform in combination.[2]

Zinc oxide–eugenol paste

ZOE is a commonly used filling material for primary teeth in the United States. Camp introduced the endodontic pressure syringe to overcome the problem of underfilling, a relatively common finding when thick mixes of ZOE are employed.[145] However, underfilling is frequently clinically acceptable. Primary teeth frequently present with interradicular radiolucent areas but without periapical lesions, and they sometimes even have some vital pulp at the apex (Fig. 32.17). Conversely, overfilling may cause a mild foreign body reaction, and it has also been associated with increased failure rate compared with underfilling or flush finishing.[146] Success rates with this material varied between 65% and 100%, with an average of 83%, and no significant difference could be observed when ZOE was compared with other calcium hydroxide and/or iodoform pastes.[146–150]

Another disadvantage of ZOE is that it may remain in the alveolar bone for a long time, although it is not certain that this has a clinically significant effect (Fig. 32.18).

Iodoform-based pastes

Several authors have reported the use of Kri paste (Pharmachemie, Zurich, Switzerland), which is a mixture of iodoform, camphor, parachlorophenol, and menthol. It resorbs rapidly and has no undesirable effects on succedaneous teeth when used as a pulp canal medicament in abscessed primary teeth. Further, Kri paste extruded into periapical tissues is rapidly replaced with normal tissue.[146] Sometimes the material is also resorbed inside the root canal (Fig. 32.19).

A paste developed by Maisto has been used clinically for many years, with good results reported.[151,152] This paste has the same components as the Kri paste, with the addition of zinc oxide, thymol, lanolin, and calcium hydroxide.

Although not very popular, calcium hydroxide, in a ready-mixed paste delivered via syringe or in a combination of two pastes (base and catalyst), has also been used as root canal filling in primary teeth. Clinical studies report an average success rate of 88%.[149,150] Vitapex (Neo Dental Chemical Products, Tokyo) or Diapex (Dia-Dent Group International, Burnaby, British Columbia, Canada), as commercialized in North America, include the addition of iodoform and silicone oil to calcium hydroxide, which have been investigated clinically and histologically.[153] This material is easy to apply, resorbs at a slightly faster rate than that of the roots (complete resorption of the excess paste is expected within 2 to 8 weeks[153]), has no toxic effects on the permanent successor, and is radiopaque. For

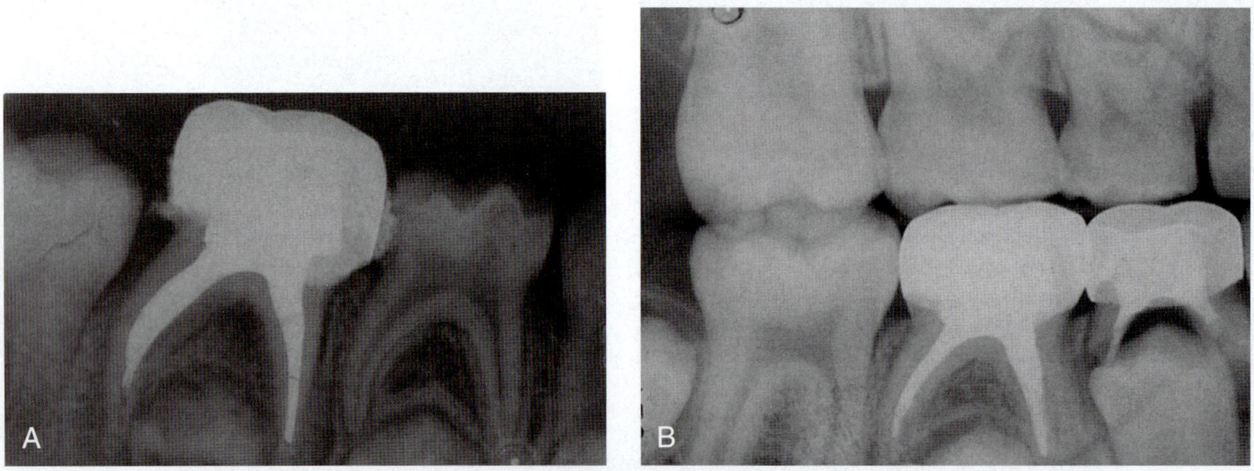

• **Fig. 32.17** (A) Mandibular second primary molar immediately after completion of root canal treatment with Endoflas. Note the interradicular radiolucent area and filling slightly short of the apex on the distal canal. (B) The same tooth 3 years later showing healing of the lesion. (Courtesy Moti Moskovitz, DMD.)

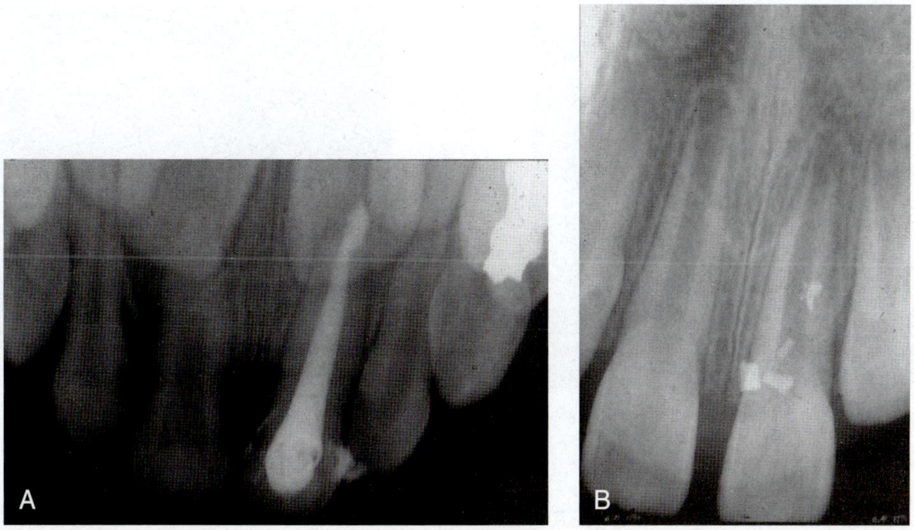

• **Fig. 32.18** (A) Maxillary primary central incisor with excessive zinc oxide–eugenol (ZOE) immediately after pulpectomy. (B) Permanent successor of the root-treated primary tooth showing remnants of ZOE in the alveolar bone. (From Fuks AB, Eidelman E. Pulp therapy in the primary dentition. *Curr Opin Dent*. 1991;1:556-563.)

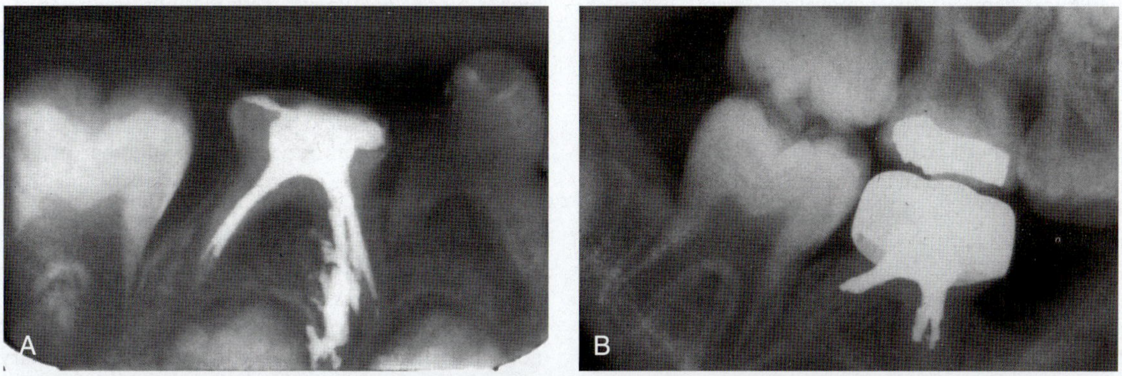

• **Fig. 32.19** (A) Mandibular second primary molar pulpectomy with Kri paste. Note the excess of material immediately after treatment. (B) Nine months after treatment, the material has resorbed considerably and the lamina dura appears normal. (Courtesy Gideon Holan, DMD.)

these reasons, Machida[137] considers the calcium hydroxide–iodoform mixture to be a nearly ideal primary tooth filling material.

Another preparation with similar composition is available in the United States under the trade name Endoflas (Sanlor Laboratories, Cali, Colombia). The results of root canal treatments using Endoflas in a student's clinic reported similar results to those observed with Kri paste.[142] A complete review of filling materials for primary root canals has been published by Kubota and associates.[154] Based on a recent systematic review, AAPD recommends that Endoflas has the highest success, followed by ZOE and then Vitapex.[45]

Pulpectomy Technique

The pulpectomy procedure should be performed as follows: An access opening should be prepared similar to the methods used in a pulpotomy, but the walls may need flaring to facilitate access of the canal openings for broaches and files.[145] Locate each canal orifice and select a properly sized barbed broach. Primary molar roots are curved for succedaneous tooth development, increasing the risk of perforation at the apical portion or coronal one-third of the canal into the furcation.[155] Slightly bending instruments to match canal curvature helps prevent perforations on both outer and inner root surfaces (Fig. 32.20).

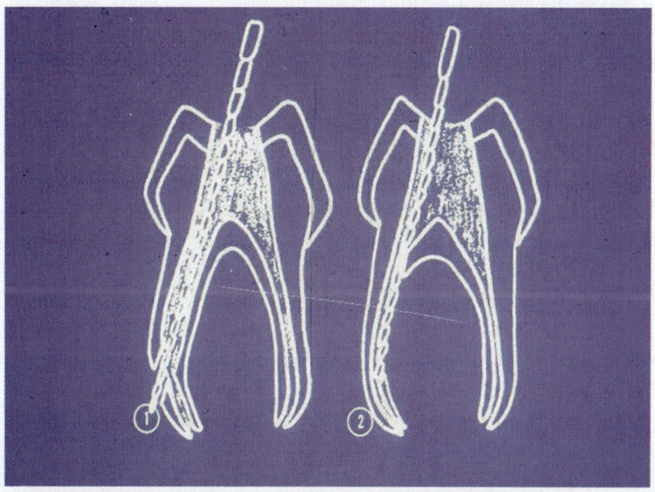

• **Fig. 32.20** Perforations on the convex *(1)* and concave *(2)* aspects of a root of a primary molar caused by injudicious use of root canal instruments.

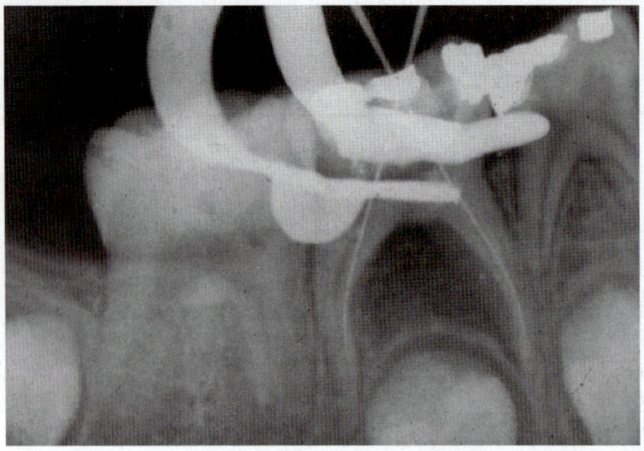

• **Fig. 32.21** Radiographic determination of the length of the canals.

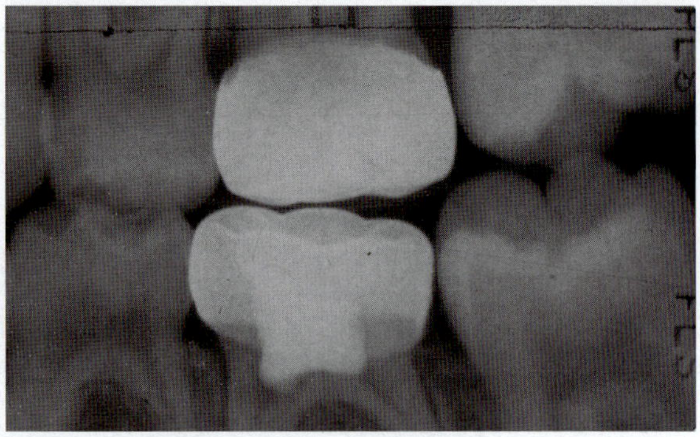

• **Fig. 32.22** Mandibular second primary molar presenting internal root resorption after pulpotomy with ferric sulfate. The area remained unchanged for 30 months.

The broach is used gently to remove as much organic material as possible from each canal. Endodontic files are selected and adjusted to stop 1 or 2 mm short of the radiographic apex of each canal (Fig. 32.21). This is an arbitrary length but is intended to minimize the chance of apical overinstrumentation that may cause periapical damage. The removal of organic debris is the main purpose for filing. A sodium hypochlorite and/or a chlorhexidine solution should be used as an irrigant to aid in removing debris and to ensure optimal decontamination of the canal(s).[143] Because sodium hypochlorite solution may be forced into periapical tissues, it must be used with great caution and minimal irrigation pressure.[156] Sterile saline rinses should follow each chemical irrigant. The canal is dried with appropriately sized paper points. Other methods of canal preparation use nickel-titanium (Ni-Ti) instrumentation,[140,157,158] laser therapy,[159] and ultrasonic instrumentation.[160,161] Advantages of these techniques may include better cleaning and shaping of the canal, promoting a more uniform paste fill. Disadvantages include equipment cost and the learning curve necessary to become proficient with the techniques.

When using ZOE, several filling methods are possible. In larger canals (e.g., primary anterior teeth), coat the canal walls with a thin mixture, then condense a thicker mixture. An endodontic plugger or small amalgam condenser helps compact the paste at the canal orifice. Avoid overfilling. Some primary molar canals may be small and difficult to fill. Commercial pressure syringes have been developed for this purpose. An alternative technique is to use a disposable tuberculin syringe or a local anesthetic syringe, in which the anesthetic capsule is emptied, after which the canal is dried and filled with ZOE paste.

When the root canal is filled with a resorbable paste such as Kri, Maisto, or Endoflas, a Lentulo spiral mounted on a low-speed turbine can be used, facilitating introduction of the material into the canal. When the canal is completely filled (observed by difficulty in introducing more paste), the material is compressed with a cotton pellet. Excessive extruded material is rapidly resorbed (see Fig. 32.19).

Vitapex (Diapex) is prepackaged in a convenient and sterile syringe, and the paste is injected into the canal with disposable plastic needles. This technique is particularly easy to use for primary incisors but less practical for narrow canals of primary molars.[141]

Regardless of the root filling material used, an immediate postoperative periapical radiograph should be taken with two purposes:

1. Evaluate the quality of the fill and consider prescribing antibiotics in cases of excessive overfill.
2. Provide a baseline for assessing and comparing the success of the root canal treatment in follow-up visits.

Overall Success

A recent systematic review reported that pulpectomy showed higher success in primary teeth without preoperative root resorption.[162] Among obturation materials, Endoflas and ZOE were better than iodoform alone. Use of rotary instruments was significantly faster than hand instruments, but it did not influence success. Similarly, method of obturation or root length determination or obturation, type of tooth, number of visits, irrigants, smear layer removal, and timing or type of final restoration did not appear to influence success.[162]

Criteria for Radiographic Success

Traditionally, successful root treatments meant no pathologic resorption with associated bone rarefaction.[138,147] Payne et al. note that clinicians often accept pulp-treated primary teeth with limited radiolucency or pathologic root resorption (Po) if no symptoms occur[163] (Fig. 32.22). Thus clinical outcomes are often reported as higher than radiographic ones because asymptomatic teeth with Po are deemed successful and monitored, provided that parents contact the dentist if problems arise and the patient returns for regular recare visits. This criterion, adopted by many studies including Fuks et al.,[142] sometimes leads to lower overall success rates—for example, in their study the overall success rate was low (69%) because incomplete lesion healing was considered a failure. However, only one tooth was extracted due to pathology and the others were left to follow-up and did not receive subsequent treatment.

Adverse effects of root canal treatment of primary teeth may occur. Disturbances of the development of permanent tooth bud, radicular cysts, and deviation in the eruption of the permanent tooth have been documented.[164] Hence, pulp therapy requires periodic clinical and radiographic assessment of the treated tooth and the supporting structures.

Lesion Sterilization Tissue Repair

LSTR is indicated in primary teeth that show evidence of pulp necrosis. The goal of the "lesion sterilization technique" is to sterilize the lesion, eliminate bacteria, and promote disinfection by placing a mixture of three antibacterial drugs (metronidazole, ciprofloxacin, and minocycline) in a ratio of 1:3:3 with propylene glycol.[165] The concept was developed at the Cariology Research

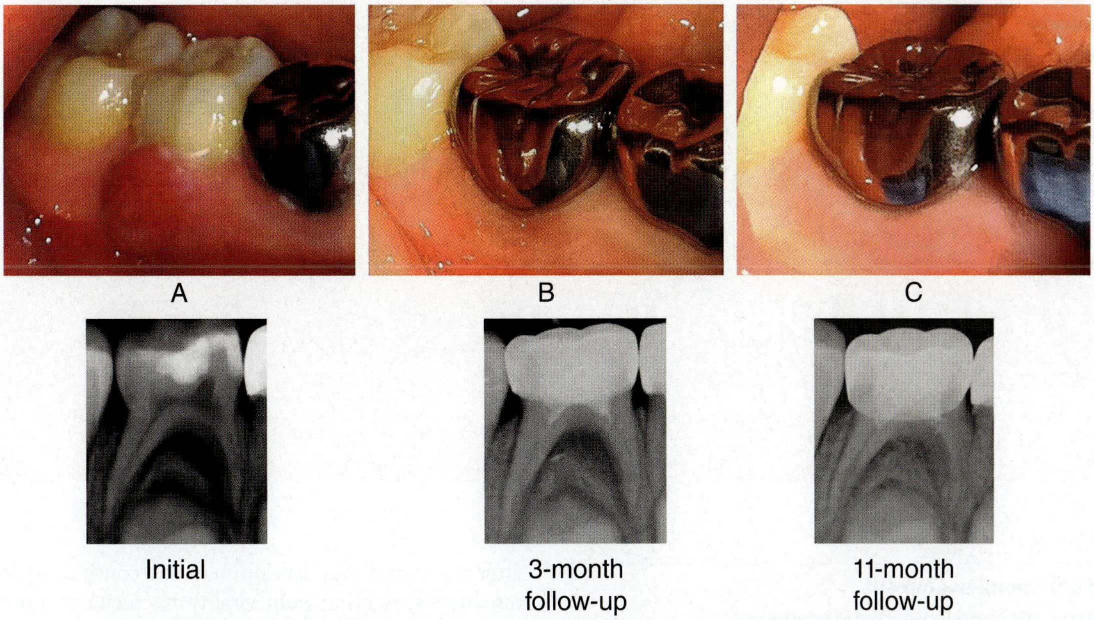

• **Fig. 32.23** (A) Mandibular second primary molar with intraoral abscess and furcal involvement. (B) Three months follow-up after lesion sterilization tissue repair, the tooth is asymptomatic. Note the healing in gingival mucosa and furcation area. (C) Eleven months after treatment, the tooth is asymptomatic, and the gingiva and furcation appear normal. (Courtesy David Burrus, DDS, and Dr. Brian Hodgson, DDS.)

Unit of Niigata University School of Dentistry, Japan.[165] It is contraindicated in teeth with perforated pulp floor, unrestorable teeth, and allergy to any of the antibiotic components.

A recent systematic review[162] reported higher success of LSTR compared with pulpectomy in primary teeth with preoperative root resorption. Therefore it is a viable treatment option to preserve primary teeth with signs and symptoms of pulp necrosis and preoperative root resorption, where pulpectomy is less likely to succeed (Fig. 32.23).

The clinical procedure is very similar to coronal pulpotomy, including obtaining anesthesia, placement of rubber dam for tooth isolation, and access opening to remove coronal (necrotic) pulp. It is suggested to enlarge canal orifices to create medication wells, followed by hemorrhage control with moist cotton pellets and sodium hypochlorite if needed. Once the chamber is dry, the 3-mix paste is placed in the medication well and over the pulpal floor, and the pulp chamber is sealed (for example with glass ionomer) and tooth restored[166] (Fig. 32.24).

The AAPD systematic review noted higher success of LSTR when the 3-mix triple antibiotic paste was altered by replacing minocycline with amoxicillin or clindamycin. This compound is also known as 3Mix alternate. Based on the review, the authors[162] also suggested that instrumenting and/or preparing the root canals did not increase LSTR success. LSTR may be preferred over pulpectomy to preserve nonvital primary teeth with root resorption. However, in absence of long-term studies and occasional case reports of enamel defects[167] and interradicular bone loss[168] related to succedaneous teeth, AAPD's recommendation for use of LSTR was conditional based on 12-month data, and it was advised that the treated tooth should undergo periodic clinical and radiographic evaluation on an annual basis.[162]

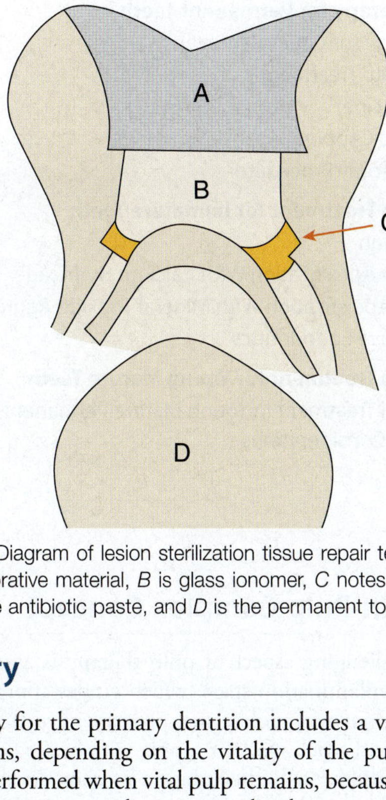

• **Fig. 32.24** Diagram of lesion sterilization tissue repair technique where *A* is the restorative material, *B* is glass ionomer, *C* notes the medication wells for triple antibiotic paste, and *D* is the permanent tooth bud.

Summary

Pulp therapy for the primary dentition includes a variety of treatment options, depending on the vitality of the pulp. Vital pulp therapy is performed when vital pulp remains, because the potential for recovery exists once the irritation has been removed. Nonvital pulp therapies are indicated in teeth showing evidence of chronic, irreversible inflammation or necrosis in the radicular pulp.

Visit eBooks.Health.Elsevier.com to see full list of references.

33

Pulp Therapy for the Young Permanent Dentition

MATTHEW K. GENESER AND VINEET DHAR

CHAPTER OUTLINE

The Dentin-Pulp Complex Concept

The most challenging aspect of pulp therapy is assessing pulpal health or its inflammation stage, which guides appropriate treatment. In children and adolescents, permanent teeth have a more cellular pulp and a rich vascular supply with better healing potential than in adults,[1] and their degree of root development will affect the treatment plan.

Immature permanent teeth (incomplete root development and apical closure) can be present in children from 6 years of age until 3 years after the eruption of the third molars. After apical closure, these teeth are classified as mature teeth. Secondary dentin formation in the pulp chamber and root canal is continuous, beginning after crown and root development and continuing slowly throughout life.[2] Preserving pulp vitality is crucial in young permanent teeth, which have wide root canals. Dentin apposition helps prevent fractures, a common issue in endodontically treated teeth with wide canals.[3] Treatment planning should aim to maintain vitality to support ongoing root development and physiologic dentin apposition. The pulp and the dentin are closely related and are usually looked upon as one unit, the pulp-dentin complex.[4,5] As discussed in Chapter 32, all procedures performed in the dentin will have an effect on the pulp.

Reactions to Caries and Operative Procedures

The molecular and cellular events of primary dentinogenesis are mirrored in dentin-pulp responses to injury. Kuttler[6] proposed the concept of tertiary dentin, which includes a range of responses from the secretion of regular tubular to dysplastic atubular dentin, reflecting reactions to varying stimuli. Tertiary dentin is classified as reactionary (formed by surviving odontoblasts after mild stimuli) or reparative (produced by new odontoblast-like cells after original odontoblast death).[2]

The dentin matrix is considered a reservoir of growth factors and cytokines sequestered during dentinogenesis. During caries progression, these molecules may be released from the dentin degraded by bacterial acids with other components of the extracellular matrix, inducing the formation of reactionary dentin.[6] See Chapter 32, Fig. 32.1. Members of the transforming growth factor (TGF) superfamily, specifically TGF-βs, have received considerable attention in affecting mesenchymal cells and inducing dentin regeneration.

These chemotactants are hypothesized to provide the signals involved in the recruitment, proliferation, and differentiation of the cells to the site of pulp injury to initiate tissue regeneration and dentin bridge formation.

Reparative dentinogenesis encompasses a complex sequence of biologic events involving stem/progenitor cells recruitment and differentiation before matrix secretion at the site of the injury. A few in vivo studies demonstrated that ethylenediamine tetraacetic acid solubilizes dentin matrix components, shows morphogenetic activity, and can induce reparative dentinogenesis.[7]

In addition to the caries process, various factors associated with the method of cavity preparation and restoration can influence the tertiary dentin response. The size of the cavity, the residual dentin thickness (RDT), the etching of the cavity, and the type and method of application of the restorative material have an effect on the type and quality of the tertiary dentin. Several studies have reported that the alterations in the pulp related to the previously mentioned factors are more important than those related to the restorative materials.[8–11] As discussed in Chapter 32, RDT is apparently the most significant factor determining the secretion of reactionary dentin. Maximal reactionary dentin was observed in a study where the RDT in the cavities was between 0.5 and 0.25 mm. Reduced reactionary dentin and reduced odontoblastic survival were observed in teeth with an RDT less than 0.25 mm.[11] In these deep cavities, little more than 50% of the odontoblasts survived, whereas in shallow cavities, odontoblastic survival was about 85% or greater. Despite the cutting of the odontoblastic process, the cells responded by secreting reactionary dentin.

Pulp exposure in young permanent teeth is mainly the consequence of caries or trauma. In carious exposures, the pulp and the dentin are infected, whereas in iatrogenic exposures during operative procedures, only the dentin may be infected; the pulp may sometimes not even be inflamed. In traumatic pulp exposures, the dentin is not infected, and the pulp tissue may remain vital and uninfected if treated soon after the injury.

Clinical Pulpal Diagnosis

Patient History

The medical and dental history should always be carefully documented. The most accurate diagnosis can only come from gathering information from several sources, with thorough clinical and radiographic examinations coupled with an accurate symptom history. The type of pain described by the child, whether it is spontaneous or is precipitated by a stimulus, should be assessed.[12] Sensitivity to pressure may indicate that the pulpal inflammation has extended to the periodontal ligament (PDL). However, this sensitivity may also be the result of a much more innocuous situation such as a sealant placed in excess or a high restoration causing hyperocclusion.[12] Children often report "toothaches" during the eruption of the first permanent molars. In these cases, the dentist should carefully ascertain whether the report is caused by a pericoronitis or by biting on an operculum, rather than by pain resulting from a pulp condition. Food impaction and illness, such as a sinus infection, can also mimic the symptoms of an irreversible pulp condition. In cases of trauma, both patient and caregivers should be asked about the timing and nature of the injury, and whether previous treatment or traumatic incidents have occurred. See Chapter 41.

Clinical Examination

Both extraoral and intraoral examinations are important for the detection of the pulpally involved tooth. Extraoral examination should focus on swelling, local lymphadenopathy, and extraoral sinus tract. Intraoral examination should focus on the tooth suspected as the origin of pain, but all the teeth on the same side should be inspected carefully, because referred pain can occur. The examination includes observation of the soft tissues for redness, swelling, or sinus tract.

Tooth discoloration is also an important finding, especially in traumatized teeth. Examining tissues by palpation and percussion, determining periodontal involvement, and assessing tooth mobility should follow. Special attention should be paid to fractured restorations or those with marginal breakdown, as these may also be indicators of pulp involvement.[13] Additional tests should include thermal and electric pulp test (EPT) of the involved tooth and of an appropriate control tooth. As in primary teeth, sensibility tests, such as thermal and EPT, have limited reliability in young permanent teeth and do not reflect the extent of pulp inflammation.[14,15] Studies concluded that until innervation is completed (after 4 to 5 years in function), the EPT is not a reliable means of determining tooth vitality.[16] Cold test has been found more reliable in immature permanent teeth.[14,15] See Chapter 41 for sensibility tests in traumatized teeth. Reliability of sensibility tests in traumatized teeth, especially in the period adjacent to the traumatic incident, is limited because of possible damage to the pulp innervation system.[17–20]

The presence of extraoral or intraoral sinus tract requires the performance of a tracing radiograph to trace the origin of the infection.[22,24] When the originating tooth is detected, root canal treatment should be performed. Sensitivity to palpation in the vestibule may be indicative of an acute apical pathologic process. Emphasis should be placed on soft tissue swelling or bony expansion in the area, which may indicate the presence of Garré osteomyelitis.[25]

Pain History

The presence of pain, along with the characteristics of the discomfort, have long been used in conjunction with sensibility testing to assign a pulpal diagnosis. These pain findings are very important but may not correlate well to histologic status. Pain to percussion does not indicate the state of pulpal inflammation; rather, it is an indication of inflammation in the PDL. This inflammation is most often a result of pulp inflammation that extended into the PDL or as a sequela of dental trauma.[26] Periodontal probing is part of the intraoral examination and diagnosis, as bone loss is not a consequence of reversible (treatable) or irreversible (untreatable) pulpitis, but rather evidence of pulpal **necrosis.**[24] Diagnosis of reversible pulpitis indicates that the inflammation should resolve and vital pulp therapy (VPT) is a potential treatment option, however, the idea that VPT is only an option for teeth with "reversible pulpitis" is changing, and evidence exists that teeth with irreversible symptoms may also benefit from VPT.[18] Proper treatment depends on the progress of the inflammatory process within the pulp and the degree of root development.

Clinically the difference between reversible and irreversible pulpitis is frequently determined by evaluating the duration and intensity of the pain. Prolonged response to cold stimuli, spontaneous pain, or referred pain will lead to a diagnosis of irreversible pulpitis, but histologic studies suggest that there is no definitive boundary that would make an inflamed pulp unrepairable.[19]

Radiographic Examination

Radiographs should follow a careful clinical examination. Bitewing radiographs are necessary to assess the depth of the caries, the morphology of the pulp chamber, the height of the pulp horns, the integrity and depth of restorations, and the level of bone support. Bitewing views can also demonstrate the presence of a calcified bridge in the pulp chamber, indicating the formation of tertiary dentin by a vital pulp in response to caries or pulp treatment.

On each periapical radiograph, inspection of the PDL continuity should be done to diagnose inflammatory and resorptive lesions. The interpretation of radiographs of young, immature permanent teeth can be difficult because of their normally large and open apex and radiolucent dental papilla. Less experienced dentists treating these teeth should avoid confusing pathologic changes with normal apical anatomy. In a young child, a vertical bitewing with a small size radiograph can be used instead of a periapical radiograph in order to see the periapical area of posterior teeth. Treatment decisions should not be made based on a single radiograph, so an additional radiograph of the antimeres should be taken for comparison. The degree of root development of the affected tooth and the amount of dentin apposition along the canal should be compared with those of the contralateral tooth. It is important to remember that the root canals of permanent teeth are wider in the buccolingual plane than the mesiodistal. Therefore it is difficult to determine the extent of apical closure in a regular radiograph showing only the mesiodistal plane. In the anterior region, radiographs of each central incisor should be obtained separately from a distal angulation to prevent overlapping of the PDL of the central incisor over the lateral incisor. Performing radiography in this manner is mandatory in teeth after traumatic injuries. Lateral external inflammatory root resorption is a common finding in necrotic young teeth after trauma. External replacement root resorption can also be seen after traumatic injuries.[20] (See Chapter 41 for a detailed discussion of trauma sequelae.)

In recent years the use of cone-beam computed tomography (CBCT) in endodontics has significantly increased. CBCT is a technique that produces undistorted three-dimensional digital imaging of the teeth and their surrounding tissues at reduced cost and with less radiation for the patient than traditional scans. The American Association of Endodontics (AAE) and the American Academy of Oral and Maxillofacial Radiology (AAOMR) state that the use of CBCT is justified in cases in which the benefits to the patient outweigh the potential risks of exposure to x-rays, especially in the case of children or young adults. CBCT should only be used when the question for which imaging is required cannot be answered adequately by lower dose conventional dental radiography or alternate imaging modalities.[22]

Direct Pulp Evaluation

In some instances, due to conflicting or illogical symptom and radiographic histories, a definitive diagnosis may be aided by direct visualization of the pulp tissue. The quality (color) and the amount of bleeding from a direct exposure of the pulp tissue can be assessed. A study on primary teeth found that profuse bleeding or deep-purple–colored blood is likely to indicate increased inflammatory mediators and inflammation that extends into the radicular pulp.[23] However, the assessment of blood color is difficult to perform, and the evidence, particularly in permanent teeth, is conflicting. Moreover, the ability to control hemorrhage enables clinical assessment of inflammatory levels and helps identify areas of necrosis.[115] Excessive hemorrhage would indicate that the pulp may have irreversible pulpitis, and the treatment plan may need to be changed. Direct visualization of the pulp may also reveal a dry chamber or purulent exudate within the chamber, which would indicate a level of necrosis that would necessitate nonvital pulp therapy.

Vital Pulp Therapy for Permanent Teeth

Terminology for Caries Removal

Presently, managing a deep carious lesion includes several options, from the complete surgical excision, where no visible carious tissue is left before placement of the restoration, to the opposite extreme, where no caries is removed and noninvasive methods are used to prevent progression of the lesion.[27,28] In describing the clinical manifestation of caries, a group of cariology experts (International Caries Consensus Collaboration [ICCC]) described the different physical properties associated with the different statuses of dentin as follows: *soft dentin, leathery dentin, firm dentin,* and *hard dentin.* (A more complete discussion of the current caries removal terminology can be found in Chapter 32.)

To remove carious tissue in teeth with vital pulps and without signs of irreversible pulp inflammation, several strategies are available, based on the earlier mentioned level of hardness of the remaining dentin.[27] The decision among these strategies will be guided by the depth of the lesion and by the dentition (primary or permanent). *Selective removal to firm dentin* is the preferred treatment for shallow to moderately sized lesions (radiographically extending less than the pulpal third or quarter of dentin), but *nonselective removal to hard dentin* (complete caries removal to hard dentin) is considered overtreatment. For deep cavitated lesions (radiographically extending into the pulpal third or quarter of dentin), *selective removal to soft dentin is recommended.* Soft carious tissue is left over the pulp to avoid exposure, and the walls of the preparation are prepared to hard dentin, to allow a tight seal and a durable restoration. Selective removal to soft dentin significantly reduces the risk of pulp exposure compared with either other caries removal strategy.

An additional option for permanent teeth is *stepwise removal* in which carious tissue is removed in two stages. Soft carious tissue is left over the pulp on the first step, and the tooth is sealed with a provisional restoration that should be durable to last up to 12 months to allow changes in the dentin and pulp to take place. In reentering, after removing the restoration, as the dentin is drier and harder, caries removal is continued. There is some evidence that in such deep lesions the second step might be omitted, as it increases the risk of pulp exposure.[29–32] With evidence showing little progression of caries beneath the sealed restoration and no better outcomes with the second step added, bringing the child back for the second appointment should be carefully considered.

Another form of caries removal that is less frequently used is chemomechanical removal. When a bur is used, healthy tissue is frequently removed along with carious tissue. With this method, sound and carious dentin are clinically separated, and only carious dentin can be removed, resulting in a more conservative preparation. It has also been reported that this method contributes to patient comfort, as it has been said to be painless, requiring less drilling and local anesthesia. The main drawback of this technique is the time needed to complete the procedure, as it has been shown to be much more time consuming than the use of a bur.[33] (See Chapter 32 for a discussion of products.)

Indirect Pulp Treatment

Selective caries removal to soft dentin is more commonly referred to as indirect pulp therapy (IPT). The main objective of IPT is to maintain the vitality of teeth with reversible pulp injury or teeth with deep caries that might otherwise need endodontic therapy if the decay was completely removed.[35] The rationale for this treatment is based on the observation that postmitotic odontoblasts can be induced to upregulate their secretory activities in response to reduced infectious challenge.[39] This results in the deposition of tertiary dentin, which increases the distance between the firm dentin and the pulp, and in the deposition of peritubular (sclerotic) dentin, which results in decreased dentin permeability.

Clinically, IPT is defined as the procedure in which nonmineralizable carious tissue is removed and a thin layer of caries is left at the deepest site of the cavity to prevent pulp exposure.[35] Clinically it is difficult to differentiate between the different layers of carious dentin. As a practical approach, the remaining dentin should feel firm when examined with an explorer. Additionally, it is important to remove the carious tissue completely from the dentinoenamel junction and from the lateral walls of the cavity to achieve optimal interfacial seal between the tooth and the restorative material, thus preventing microleakage. The preferred instrument for caries excavation is a large carbide round bur (No. 6 or 8), because the bur allows better control of the "partial removal caries step" than spoon excavators do.[47] Use of a bur also results in a significant reduction in viable counts of both *Streptococcus mutans* and lactobacilli.[48] Several clinical studies have demonstrated a high percentage of success utilizing this technique.[2,29,31,40] The indication for IPT should be limited to teeth without signs of irreversible pulpitis. In this procedure, the deepest layer of the remaining carious dentin should be covered with a liner. The materials used for these procedures are calcium hydroxide liners, bioactive calcium silicates, and glass ionomer liners, with good results in clinical studies.[30–40]

Until recent years, the dentist's dilemma lay in the assessment of how much caries to leave at the pulpal or axial floor. It was generally believed that the carious tissue that could remain at the base of the cavity preparation was the quantity that, if removed, would result in overt exposure.[41,42] Hence studies suggested that deep carious lesions could be managed by stepwise excavation performed in two visits, which resulted in fewer pulp exposures compared with direct, nonselective, complete excavation. At 1-year follow-up, there was a statistically significant higher success rate with stepwise excavation than with nonselective one-visit treatment.[32,43] At present, there is enough evidence of good clinical and radiographic success without reentering, if the restoration is maintained leakage free.[29,44–46] Both approaches require knowledge of tooth anatomy, clinical experience, and a good understanding of the process of caries progression. Evidence suggests that it would be preferable to leave carious dentin, assuming a clean periphery, rather than being overly aggressive with deep caries removal, running the risk of a pulp exposure that would require additional steps to manage. Finally, leakage-free restoration is essential to IPT success; thus if the tooth is too broken down to allow for a proper intracoronal restoration, placement of a crown should be considered. (Fig. 33.1 demonstrates the IPT technique using a calcium hydroxide liner.)

Protective Liner

The American Academy of Pediatric Dentistry (AAPD)[31] recommends the placement of a protective barrier on the floor of the preparation between the restorative material and the pulp-dentin complex: calcium silicate cements, glass ionomer cements, or calcium hydroxide liners. There is sufficient evidence to show that pulp reaction to dental materials is transitory, and overt inflammation occurs only after bacteria or their byproducts have reached the pulp.[32–34] When bacteria and bacteria-produced irritants have been removed by caries excavation, and a bacteria-tight restoration has been placed, new bacteria are prevented from reaching the deeper portion of the dentin, and the inflamed pulp will have a great opportunity to heal.

Direct Pulp Capping

Direct pulp capping (DPC) may be performed when a small exposure of the pulp is encountered during cavity preparation in teeth with a normal pulp or reversible pulpitis.[35] Direct capping may also be used after a recent clean fracture caused by a traumatic injury. A recent study by Gencerlier et al. found that DPC has favorable outcomes, particularly in permanent molar teeth,[49] and may be underutilized as a treatment modality. The aim of DPC is to maintain pulp vitality by forming a calcified barrier to wall off the exposure, keeping in mind that in teeth affected by caries there is an inflammatory response of the pulp to bacteria or bacterial products.[50–53]

When DPC is indicated, it should be performed immediately after the exposure to prevent contamination of the pulp. Because the extent of the inflammatory process in the pulp cannot be accurately assessed by clinical tests, the diagnosis of reversible (treatable) pulpitis may be sometimes incorrect. In some teeth affected by deep caries, pulp inflammation might have reached the stage of irreversible pulpitis without showing clinical signs.

Pulp Capping Agents

Pulp capping materials should be biocompatible, be nonresorbable, seal well to block bacteria, and promote pulp healing and dentin bridge formation. The bridge should be free of tunnel defects to prevent future bacterial entry.[54]

Mineral trioxide aggregate (MTA) and calcium hydroxide are the most frequently recommended capping materials. The mechanism of action of the two materials in vital pulp treatment are similar, as the main soluble component of MTA is calcium hydroxide.[55] Calcium hydroxide dissolves in an aqueous environment into calcium and hydroxyl ions, creating a high pH in the close environment (~12). This alkaline pH is responsible for the antibacterial activity of these materials.[56] When calcium hydroxide is applied to exposed pulp tissue, its high pH causes a superficial layer of tissue necrosis. This mild irritation stimulates the pulp's natural defense and repair response. In contrast, MTA causes only mild inflammation and necrosis in the underlying pulp, making it less caustic than calcium hydroxide.[57] Calcium ions are released from the capping material, forming inorganic precipitations that have been associated with the mechanism controlling cytologic and functional changes in the interacting pulpal cells.[58]

The high pH and low solubility of calcium hydroxide prolongs its antibacterial effect. However, being water soluble, it might dissolve under leaky restorations and be washed out, leaving an empty space under the filling material. Hard-setting calcium hydroxide cements can induce dentin bridge formation, but they do not provide an effective long-term seal against bacteria or their byproducts.[59,60]

Recent studies suggest that the mechanisms by which calcium hydroxide or MTA stimulate the wound-healing process are related to the solubilizing effect of calcium hydroxide on the dentin matrix component. Growth factors and other bioactive molecules, sequestered within the dentin matrix during dentinogenesis (e.g., TGF-βs), may be released by the action of calcium hydroxide and mediate the changes in cell behavior observed during reparative dentinogenesis.[4,61]

Calcium silicate–based bioactive materials such as MTA present some advantages over calcium hydroxide as the material of choice for DPC. It is a hard-setting, biocompatible material with an antibacterial effect that provides a biologically active substrate for cell attachment. These features make this material effective in preventing microleakage, improving the treatment outcome. As previously mentioned, MTA stimulates reparative dentin formation with

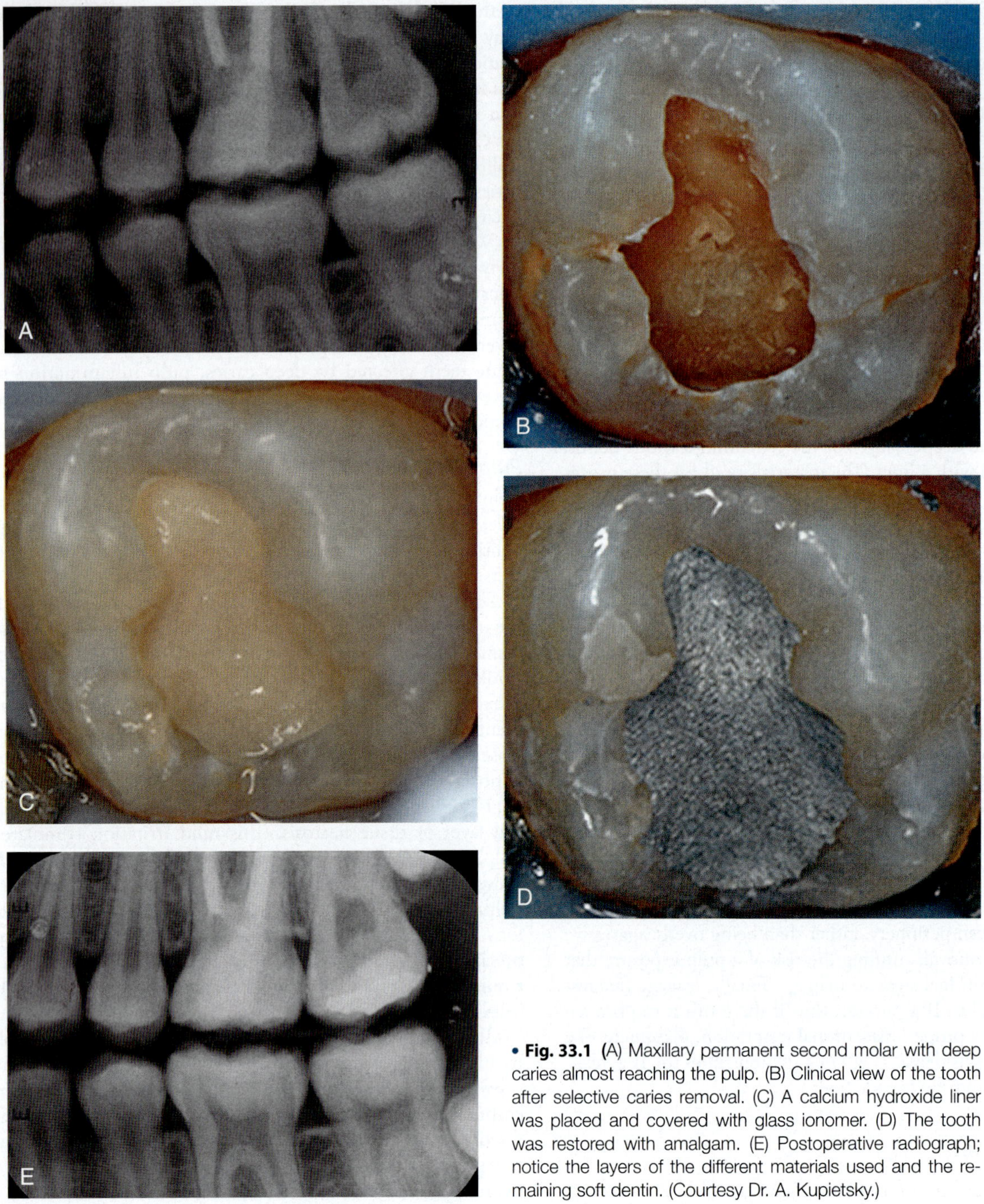

• **Fig. 33.1** (A) Maxillary permanent second molar with deep caries almost reaching the pulp. (B) Clinical view of the tooth after selective caries removal. (C) A calcium hydroxide liner was placed and covered with glass ionomer. (D) The tooth was restored with amalgam. (E) Postoperative radiograph; notice the layers of the different materials used and the remaining soft dentin. (Courtesy Dr. A. Kupietsky.)

negligible pulpal necrosis and minimal inflammatory reaction in the exposed pulp.[57] Tziafas et al. demonstrated that after DPC with MTA in dogs, the underlying pulp tissue was consistently normal, and only at a later stage was some hemorrhage in the pulp core observed. The beginning of a hard tissue barrier was observed after 2 weeks, and reparative dentinogenesis was disclosed after 3 weeks, associated with a firm fibrodentin matrix.[62] It was also demonstrated that, compared with calcium hydroxide, MTA consistently induces the formation of a dentin bridge at a greater rate with a superior structural integrity. Therefore MTA appears to be more effective than calcium hydroxide for maintaining long-term pulp vitality after DPC.[57]

A practice-based, randomized clinical trial evaluated and compared the success of DPC in permanent teeth with MTA or CaOH (calcium hydroxide). The probability of failure at 24 months was 31.5% for CaOH versus 19.7% for MTA (permutation log-rank test, $P = 0.046$). This large randomized clinical trial provided confirmatory evidence for a superior performance with MTA as a DPC agent, compared with CaOH when evaluated in a practice-based research network for up to 2 years.[67]

However, traditional MTA does have drawbacks, one being its propensity for staining tooth material, for both the gray and white versions (Fig. 33.2).[63–66] Therefore the use of traditional MTA in VPT procedures (pulp capping, pulpotomy) is not appropriate in

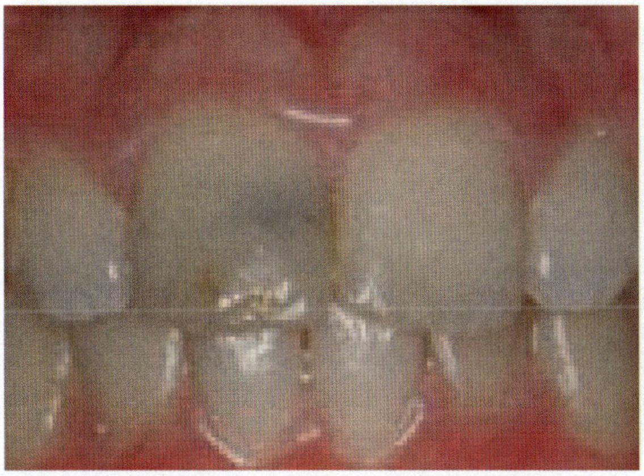

• **Fig. 33.2** Right permanent central incisor 1.5 years after partial pulpotomy using white mineral trioxide aggregate. Notice the gray discoloration of the crown. (Courtesy Dr. E. Nuni.)

the esthetic zone. In anterior teeth, alternatives to MTA (such as calcium hydroxide or Biodentine) should be considered, as these have been shown to have similar outcomes in some studies.[71,72]

Early MTA, derived from Portland cement, has a long history of use in perforation repair and root-end surgery, but the prolonged setting time and difficult handling properties made it difficult to use. Newer calcium silicates are found in capsules or syringes, making them easier to place with faster setting times and are preferred for VPT. Bioceramic materials with similar characteristics to early MTA are Biodentine (Septodont, Saint-Maur-des-Fosses, France), NuSmile NeoMTA (NuSmile, Houston, TX), MTA Angelus (Angelus, Londrina, PR, Brazil), EndoSequence root repair material (Brasseler Savannah, GA), or iRoot BP Plus (Innovative Bioceramix Inc., Vancouver, Canada). New materials continue to be introduced, so the prudent practitioner should carefully evaluate these new products to ensure that evidence of their success is well documented.

Direct Pulp Capping Technique

The tooth should be isolated with a rubber dam and disinfected with sodium hypochlorite (NaOCl). After cavity preparation with high-speed burs under constant water spray and caries removal with slow-speed burs, the cavity should be rinsed with NaOCl (every 3 to 4 minutes), which disinfects the cavity and removes the blood clot, if present, from the pulp exposure site. If the bleeding cannot be controlled within normal bleeding time (up to 10 minutes), it suggests that the pulp inflammation has progressed deeper into the tissue, and the treatment procedure should be modified by shifting to a partial or complete pulpotomy.[68–70] See Chapter 41 for a discussion of the DPC technique for traumatized teeth.

Calcium silicates such as MTA or Biodentine should be prepared according to the manufacturer's instructions and placed directly over the exposed pulp tissue (1.5 to 2 mm thick). The material should then be covered with a glass ionomer liner followed by a permanent restoration.[71] DPC should always be followed by an immediate, definitive, leakage-free restoration, as this leads to higher success rates.[49]

The Pulpotomy Procedure

Immature permanent teeth should be carefully considered for VPT, such as coronal pulpotomy, to allow for continued normal tooth development.[20] Teeth presenting with evidence of irreversible pulpitis (spontaneous pain) have been shown to be successfully treated with pulpotomy, showing that a conservative approach is preferable, particularly in immature permanent teeth.[21] Traditionally, the use of conservative VPT procedures has been more widely accepted for immature permanent teeth, but less so for mature teeth. Material advances, such as the use of MTA and other calcium silicate materials, have allowed for successful use of DPC and coronal pulpotomy procedures in cariously exposed mature permanent teeth, giving another pulpal treatment option.

The pulpotomy procedure involves "cutting into" and removing pulp tissue that has inflammatory or degenerative changes, leaving intact the remaining vital noninflamed tissue, which is covered with a pulp capping agent to promote healing at the amputation site.[69–71] See Case Study: Permanent Molar Pulpotomy. Traditionally, pulpotomy implied the removal of the entire coronal pulp up to the cervical area. Today, the depth of tissue removal is based on clinical judgment: only tissue judged to be inflamed or infected should be removed, because the capping material should be placed on healthy tissue. Although many materials and drugs have been used as capping agents after pulpotomy, the calcium silicate materials (MTA and Biodentine) seem to be the treatment of choice to stimulate dentin bridge formation in young permanent teeth with exposed pulps.[61,67] Aguilar and Linsuwanont reported that partial pulpotomy and full (cervical) pulpotomy provide a more predictable outcome than DPC in teeth with carious exposure.[70]

Partial (Cvek) Pulpotomy Technique

Case Study: Management of Complicated Crown Fractures in Permanent Teeth details the partial pulpotomy technique. The tooth should be isolated with a rubber dam and disinfected with NaOCl solution. In traumatically exposed pulps, only tissue judged to be inflamed should be removed (~2 mm). Cvek[73] has shown that, in exposures resulting from traumatic injuries, pulpal changes are characterized by a proliferative response, with inflammation extending only a few millimeters into the pulp. Care should be taken to remove all the tissue coronal to the amputation site to prevent continuation of bleeding, contamination, and discoloration of the tooth. In teeth with carious exposure, it might be necessary to remove tissue to a greater depth in order to reach noninflamed pulp. Cutting of the tissue with an abrasive high-speed diamond bur with water cooling has been shown to be the least damaging to the underlying tissue.[74] After pulp amputation, the preparation is thoroughly washed with NaOCl or chlorhexidine[75] to disinfect and control hemorrhage. If hemorrhage persists, amputation should be performed at a more apical level.[70] Once hemorrhage has been controlled and the blood clot removed, a dressing of calcium silicate material (MTA or Biodentine) or calcium hydroxide is gently placed over the amputation site. Care should be taken not to push the material into the pulp.[76]

The pulp medicament should be covered with a glass ionomer liner, and a definitive restoration should be placed (Fig. 33.3). If the pulpotomy is successful, a tertiary dentin bridge will be formed; occasionally, obliteration of the pulp may occur. Research has shown that partial pulpotomy after traumatic exposure is successful up to 9 days after pulp exposure, but studies have not shown success rates beyond this time.[77] Treatment soon after the time of exposure is ideal, minimizing pulpal inflammation. Success of this treatment in immature teeth would be continued root development and apexogenesis.

Cervical Pulpotomy

Complete pulpotomy, or cervical pulpotomy, is the surgical removal of the entire coronal pulp. This "traditional" pulpotomy would be

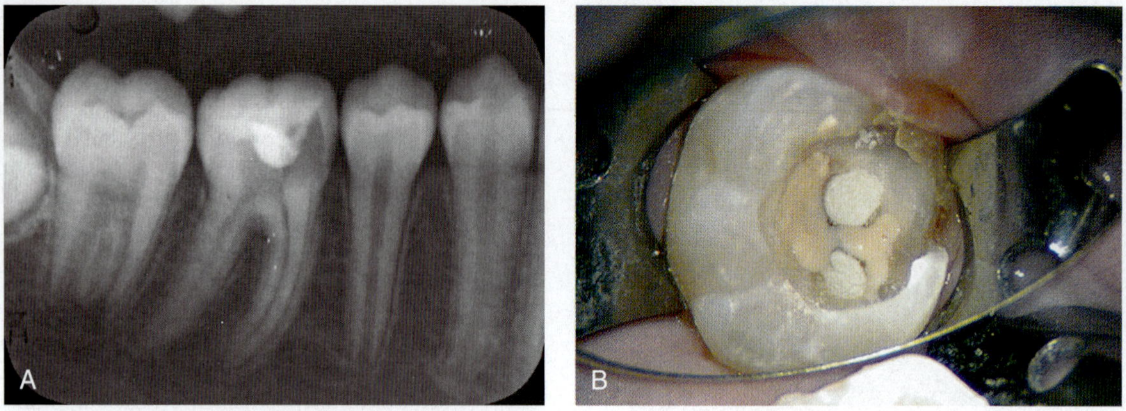

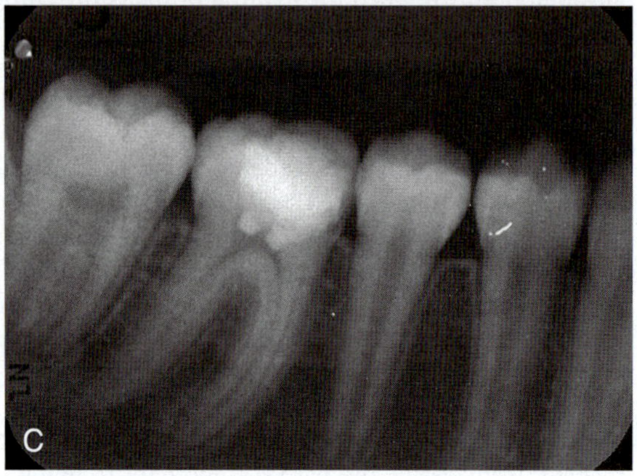

• **Fig. 33.3** Partial Pulpotomy Technique. (A) Mandibular first permanent molar with a broken temporary filling and extensive caries. (B) Clinical view of the tooth showing two amputation sites covered with white mineral trioxide aggregate. (C) The same tooth after 2 months. No symptoms are present, and no pathologic process is evident in the radiograph. It is recommended that the composite temporary filling be replaced by a more definitive restoration (crown) to prevent failure of the treatment caused by microleakage. (Courtesy Dr. E. Nuni.)

considered emergency treatment in a mature permanent tooth with symptoms consistent with irreversible pulpitis, with a follow-up appointment scheduled for a complete root canal treatment.

In immature permanent teeth, however, cervical pulpotomy is performed to allow for apexogenesis and maturation of the root. This procedure is performed in teeth with large carious pulp exposures and has the potential to produce a dentin bridge and complete the formation of the root, with vital noninflamed tissue remaining in the roots. In extreme cases, immature teeth with minimal root formation may be saved by a very deep pulpotomy that can maintain the vitality of the radicular pulp, but these unique situations may require endodontic microscopes and advanced training.

The technique for a routine cervical pulpotomy in immature permanent teeth is similar to that used for primary teeth, and the dressing material should preserve the vitality and function of the pulp. Care should be taken to remove the blood clot before placing the dressing material over the pulp stumps, as its presence may compromise the treatment outcome. It has been demonstrated that leaving the blood clot may result in the formation of dystrophic calcifications and internal resorption. A blood clot may also interfere with dentin bridge formation and serve as a substrate for bacteria in leaky restorations.[78] Calcium silicate materials have been shown to have higher success rates and provide a better long-term seal than traditional calcium hydroxide.[70,79]

Cervical pulpotomy is frequently performed in teeth in which the histopathologic status of the pulp stumps is not clear. Research has shown that teeth with deep caries approximating the pulp and symptoms consistent with irreversible pulpitis may still benefit and see relief of pain from cervical pulpotomy. Taha et al. found that young permanent teeth with irreversible pulpitis could be successfully treated with Biodentine pulpotomy.[79] Initial symptoms of irreversible pulpitis should not be a contraindication to VPT. However, if the symptoms continue and pulpectomy is needed, the MTA or Biodentine may need to be removed using an ultrasonic instrument and an operative microscope.

There is controversy as to the indications for performing root canal treatment after root maturation but before obliteration of the root canal space, which could hinder future root canal treatment. However, prophylactic endodontic treatment is not recommended because of the low percentage of pulp necrosis.[80,81] Hence clinical and radiographic follow-up of these teeth is essential to ensure that pulpal or periapical pathosis is not developing. The roots should show continued normal development and maturogenesis. As with other VPT treatments, placing a definitive restoration as soon as possible is crucial to prevent bacterial leakage and ensure the success of the treatment.[82]

Nonvital Pulp Treatment for Immature Teeth

Apexification

Apexification is a method of treatment for immature permanent teeth in which root growth and development ceased because of partial or complete pulp necrosis. The outcome of this procedure is the inducement of root end closure, but with no canal wall thickening and no continued root lengthening. It can be achieved in two ways: (1) as a long-term procedure using a calcium hydroxide dressing to allow the formation of a biologic hard tissue barrier, or (2) as a short-term (more recent) procedure, creating an artificial apical plug of MTA or other bioceramic material. Apexification is most often performed in traumatized incisors that lost vitality, but it is also used after carious exposures and in teeth with anatomical variations such as dens invaginatus with an immature root. Fig. 33.4 shows an example of a calcium hydroxide apexification for a premolar tooth that ceased root development after partial necrosis.

The apex in immature teeth may present two morphologic variations: divergent with flaring apical foramen (blunderbuss apex) or parallel to convergent. This morphology is difficult to determine because of the two-dimensional image obtained by dental radiographs. In both forms, conventional endodontic treatment cannot be performed, because it is difficult if not impossible to achieve an apical seal that will prevent extrusion of the filling material, thus apexification is necessary. When apexification is carried out successfully in teeth with radiographic signs of rarefying osteitis, healing of the bone will be observed gradually. The tooth should continue to erupt, and the alveolar bone should continue to grow in conjunction with the adjacent teeth. Follow-up is necessary to ensure the absence of adverse posttreatment clinical and radiographic signs.

Long-Term Apexification With Calcium Hydroxide

This mode of treatment requires compliance of both the patient and the parent because of its long duration. Calcium hydroxide apexification is a predictable procedure, and an apical barrier will be formed in 74% to 100% of cases.[83] The most common complication is cervical root fracture because of the thin walls of the cervical part of the tooth, which may fracture easily.[3]

It has been reported that calcium hydroxide significantly increases the risk of root fracture after long-term application (more than 1 month) as a result of structural changes in the dentin. Therefore to reduce this risk in immature teeth, it is advisable to minimize the time needed for apical barrier formation.[84,85]

Apexification is traditionally performed using a calcium hydroxide dressing that disinfects the root canal and induces apical closure. The high pH and low solubility of calcium hydroxide keeps its antimicrobial effect for a long period of time.[86–88]

Calcium hydroxide assists in the debridement of the root canal, because it increases the dissolution of necrotic tissue when used alone or in combination with NaOCl.[89]

The mechanism of action of calcium hydroxide in induction of an apical barrier is still controversial, although it is formed by cells originating from the adjacent connective tissue. The calcified barrier, even when appearing radiographically and clinically complete, is histologically porous and may be composed of cementum, dentin, bone, or osteodentin.[90]

This procedure requires multiple visits and could take a year or more to achieve a complete apical barrier that would allow root canal filling using gutta-percha (GP) and sealer.[91]

It is unclear whether the stage of root development at the beginning of the treatment or the presence of a pretreatment infection affects the time required for barrier formation.[90]

Calcium Hydroxide Apexification Technique

After isolation with rubber dam, coronal access preparation should be wide enough to include the pulp horns to prevent future contamination and discoloration. Gates-Glidden drills can be used in anterior teeth to remove the lingual eminence in the cervical portion of the root canal, facilitating cleaning of all aspects of the canal. The length of the root canal should be determined radiographically with a large GP point, because an electronic apex locator is not reliable in teeth with open apices. Inserting a large paper point to the point of bleeding may also assist in length determination. The working length should be approximately 1 mm short of the radiographic root end. Debridement of the root canal is mainly achieved by irrigations with NaOCl solution. The irrigation should be done without pressure, verifying that the needle is loose inside the root canal and short of the working length. Minimal or no instrumentation is advised to prevent damage to the thin dentin walls. To facilitate disinfection and debris removal from these wide canals, passive ultrasonic irrigation with NaOCl solution is recommended.[92]

A calcium hydroxide dressing in a creamy consistency can then be applied with a Lentulo spiral mounted in a low-speed engine, with specially designed syringes, or with files.

The second visit is scheduled from 2 weeks to 1 month later. The goal in the second visit is to complete the debridement and remove the tissue remnants denatured by the calcium hydroxide dressing that could not be removed mechanically in the first appointment. In addition, the canal should be further disinfected. After disinfection, a thick paste of calcium hydroxide is packed in the root canal to a level apical to the cemento-enamel junction using endodontic pluggers; this will reduce dentin weakening in this fracture-sensitive area.[93] The coronal access should be restored

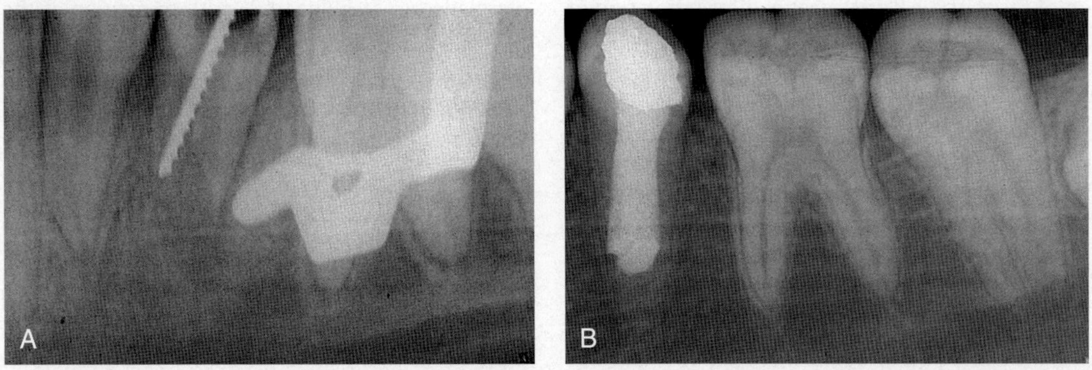

• **Fig. 33.4** (A) Mandibular premolar with incomplete root development caused by partial pulp necrosis. Apexification with calcium hydroxide was instituted. (B) Two years later, apical closure was evident in the radiograph. Root canal treatment was completed using gutta-percha with a root canal sealant. (Courtesy Dr. E. Galon.)

with a filling that will do the following: provide a long-term coronal seal, be easily identifiable if reentry is required, and restore the form, function, and esthetics of the tooth.

The tooth should be monitored clinically and radiographically at 3-month intervals to examine the formation of an apical hard tissue barrier and to confirm the absence of pathology such as root resorption and apical periodontitis. If a calcified barrier is not evident and the calcium hydroxide has been washed out, it should usually be replaced. When a calcified barrier can be seen on the radiograph, the tooth is reopened, and the calcium hydroxide is removed by copious irrigations. The apical area should be gently examined using a GP point and/or through the operative microscope to determine the completeness of the apical barrier. If the barrier is incomplete and the patient feels the touch of the GP point, the apexification procedure is reestablished until a complete barrier is formed. The frequency in which the calcium hydroxide dressing should be replaced is controversial. Some authors support a single application of the material and claim that it is only required to initiate the healing reaction, but others propose to replace the calcium hydroxide only when symptoms develop or if the material appears to have been washed out of the canal when viewed radiographically.[90]

When a completed apical barrier can be traced, the canal is obturated with a permanent root canal filling material (e.g., thermoplasticized GP) and sealer.

Fig. 33.5 shows an immature maxillary central incisor with a necrotic pulp and acute apical abscess treated with calcium hydroxide apexification. The bony lesion healed, and the endodontic treatment was properly completed.

When a calcified barrier is formed coronal to the apex, it should not be perforated in order to fill the tooth to the apical end; the tissue forming the apical barrier should be regarded as healthy tissue, and root canal filling should be placed up to this point.

As noted earlier, immature teeth with thin dentin walls, especially after calcium hydroxide apexification, are at high risk of fracture. The stage of root development seems to be a key factor.[3,85] In order to minimize the risk of fracture, calcium hydroxide should be used for the shortest possible time, after which the root is reinforced, or strengthened, by intracanal placement of a bonded composite resin restoration.[94]

One-Visit Apexification With Mineral Trioxide Aggregate

MTA has been commonly used as an artificial apical barrier in a one-visit apexification procedure. MTA reduces the time needed for completion of the root canal treatment and for restoration of the tooth. The apical barrier is achieved in one visit, and the whole treatment is completed in just a few visits.[95]

MTA characteristics such as low solubility, excellent sealability, biocompatibility, release of calcium hydroxide, high pH, and radiopacity are responsible for its preferable clinical results and popularity as an apical plug material.[96] Other bioceramic materials with similar characteristics can also be utilized, like Biodentine, NuSmile NeoMTA, MTA Angelus, EndoSequence root repair material, or iRoot BP Plus.[67]

The root canal is disinfected during the first visit, similar to the process used in long-term apexification. At the second visit, MTA can be placed in the apical portion of the immature root and will act as an apical plug after setting. It is very difficult to remove the MTA from within the canal after it sets; if retreatment is necessary, apical surgery will most likely be required. Therefore complete debridement and disinfection of the root canal and of the dentin walls are mandatory. This technique has a number of advantages: (1) patient compliance is required but less crucial, (2) cost and clinical time are reduced, (3) the dentin will not lose its physical properties, and (4) it allows for earlier restoration with bonded composite resin within the root canal, thus minimizing the likelihood of root fracture. Disadvantages include the following: (1) may require an operative microscope or referral to an endodontic specialist, and (2) MTA removal after setting is difficult.

Mineral Trioxide Aggregate Apexification Technique

Disinfection of the root canal is achieved as described in the first visit of the long-term apexification. A calcium hydroxide dressing is also indicated to raise the low pH of the inflamed periapical tissue before the MTA placement. Lee et al. have demonstrated that an acidic environment has an adverse effect on the setting and microhardness of MTA.[20,97]

In the second visit, after rubber dam placement, the canal is irrigated and dried. After mixing according to the manufacturer's instructions, a plug of MTA is compacted into the apical 4 to 5 mm of the canal, about 1 mm short of the radiographic apex (Fig. 33.6). Placement of MTA in the apical part is more complicated than the use of calcium hydroxide. The material is introduced into the apical area using special carriers or endodontic pluggers and compacted using hand condensation with indirect ultrasonic activation.[98]

Placement of a resorbable material at the root end (e.g., calcium sulfate; CollaCote, Zimer Dental, Carlsbad, CA) against which the MTA can be compacted has been suggested to keep the MTA within the confines of the canal space but is not required.[99,100]

Proper placement of the material is verified by a radiograph (see Fig. 33.6A). A wet cotton pellet or paper point is placed over the MTA, providing moisture for its setting, and the tooth is sealed with a temporary filling.

After a few days the tooth is reentered, and the hardness of the MTA is examined with an endodontic instrument. In cases where the MTA is not set, its placement should be repeated the same way described. After setting, the root canal filling can be completed using thermoplasticized GP and sealer. The tooth is then permanently restored with a bonded composite resin extending into the canal space in an attempt to strengthen the root.[94] In short roots, the composite resin can be placed in direct contact with the MTA plug (see Fig. 33.6).[20]

Using new-generation bioceramic materials (e.g., Biodentine) can shorten the treatment period even further. The short setting time of this material (~10 minutes) will allow the placement of a permanent root filling and tooth restoration at the same visit of the apical plug placement.[20]

Regenerative Endodontics

Regenerative endodontics is an alternative treatment option for necrotic immature permanent teeth that is based on the observation of spontaneous revascularization that occasionally occurs in immature teeth after traumatic injury.[101–104] The benefit of regenerative endodontics over apexification is that, when successful, root lengthening and apical closure with thickening of the canal walls (maturogenesis) are expected, thus improving the long-term prognosis of the young tooth (Fig. 33.7). A few factors are necessary for a successful endodontic regeneration. These factors include absence of infection within the root canal space, a physical scaffold, stem cells, signaling molecules, and an effective coronal seal.[105,106]

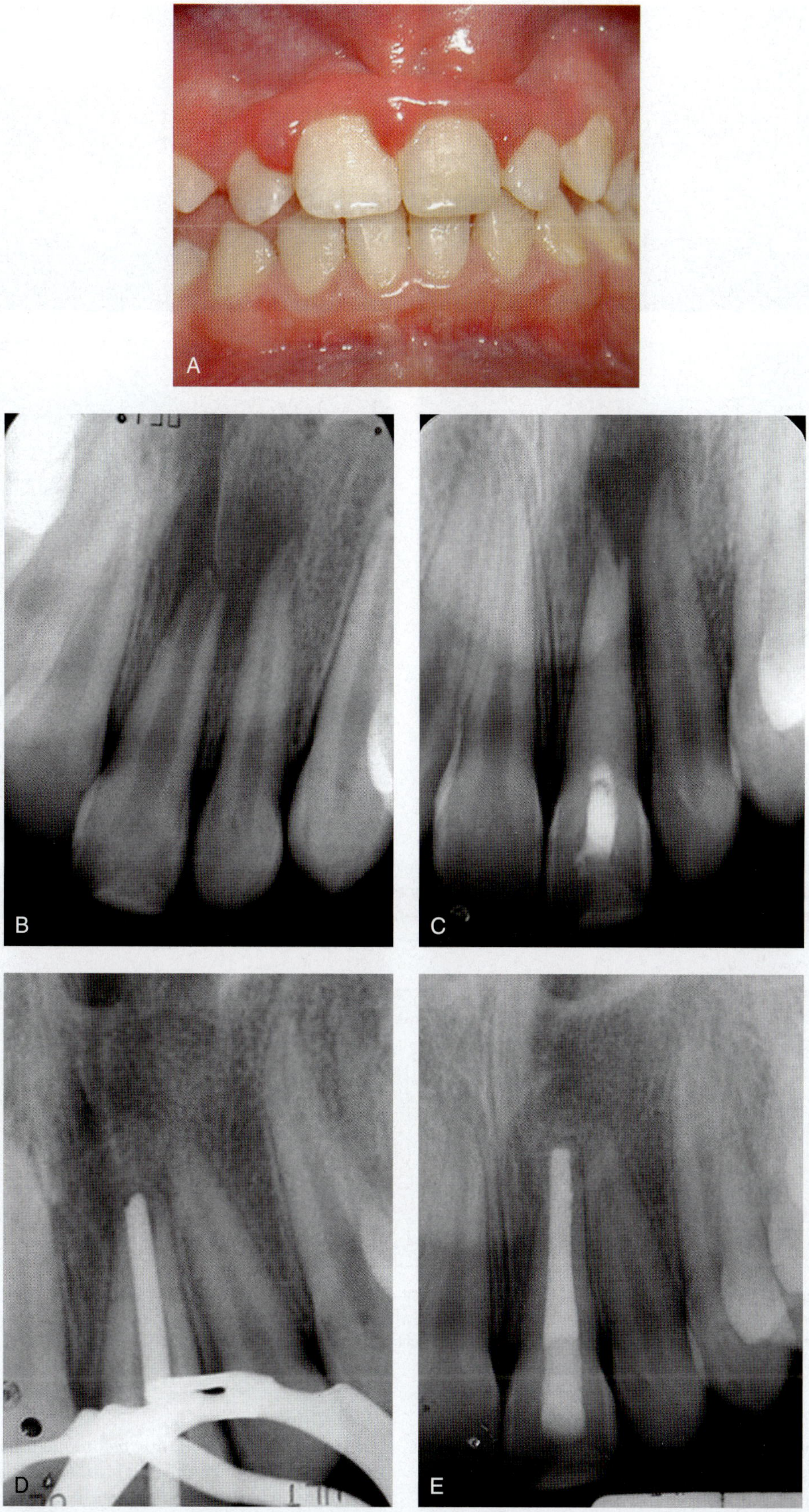

• **Fig. 33.5** **(A)** Clinical photograph of a traumatized left central incisor with an acute apical abscess (notice the vestibular swelling). **(B)** Radiograph of the same tooth showing an incompletely formed root, an open apex, and periapical bone destruction. **(C)** Radiograph of the tooth filled with a calcium hydroxide paste to achieve apexification. **(D)** Radiograph showing the completeness of the apical barrier checked with a gutta-percha point. **(E)** The tooth after root canal filling with gutta-percha and sealer. (Courtesy Dr. Z. Elazary.)

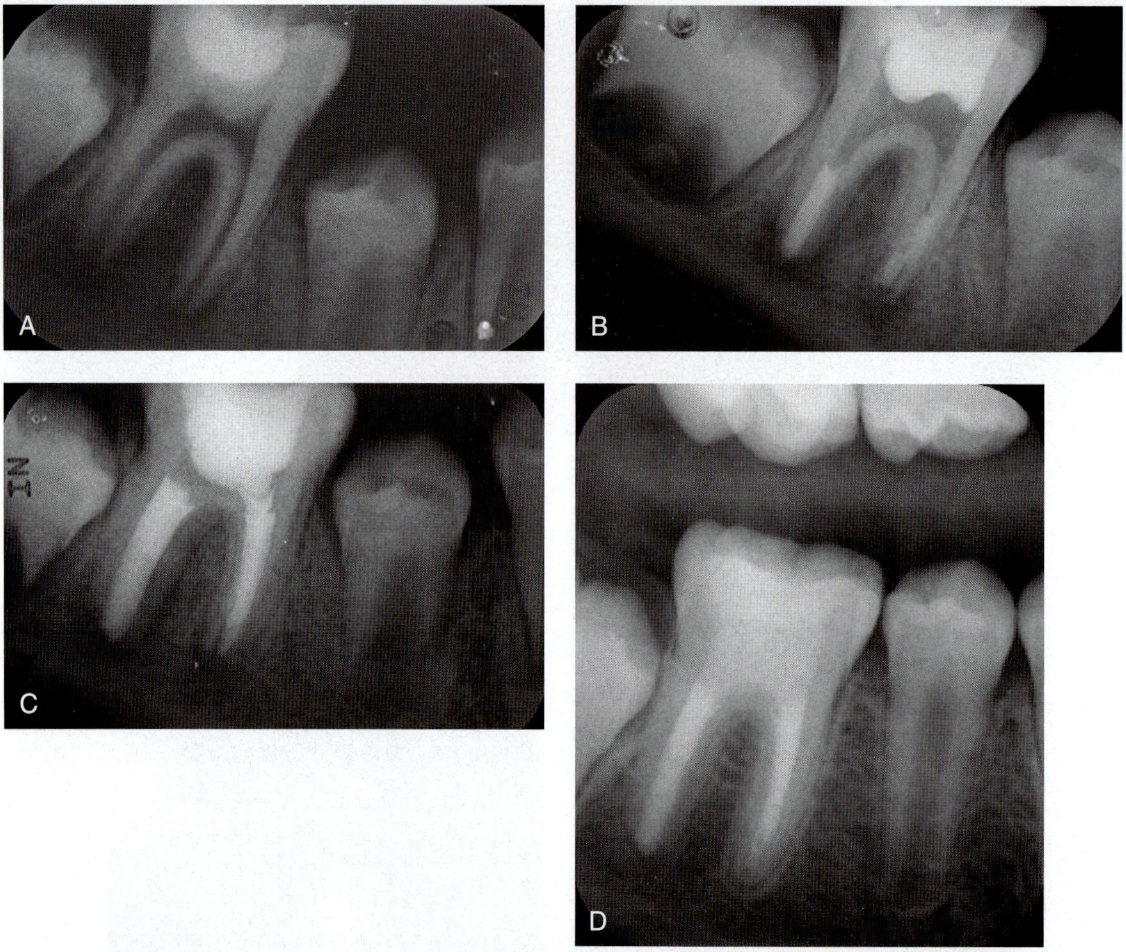

• **Fig. 33.6** (A) Immature mandibular molar with periapical pathologic radiolucent areas. (B) Apical plugs with mineral trioxide aggregate (MTA). (C) Warm gutta-percha filling over the hardened MTA plugs. (D) Successful follow-up after 15 months showing healing of the periapical lesions. (Courtesy Dr. E. Nuni.)

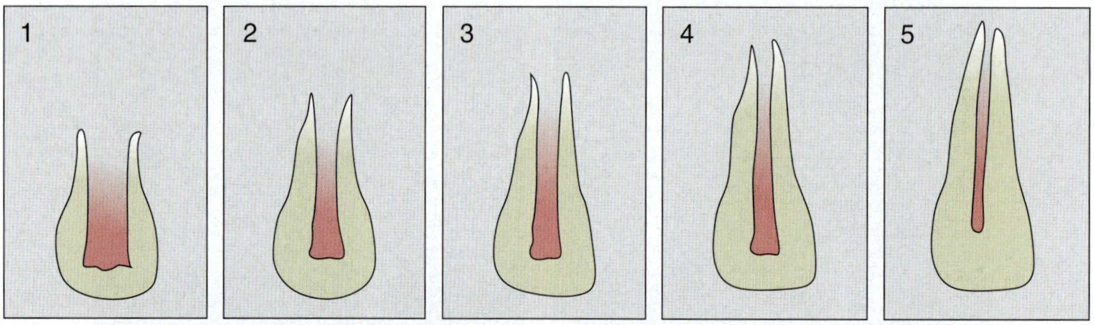

• **Fig. 33.7** Examples of Stages of Root Development of Teeth. Teeth with root maturation stages 1 through 3 are candidates for regenerative techniques. A root with maturation stage 4 is a candidate for either regenerative procedures or mineral trioxide aggregate apexification.

The nature of the hard and soft tissue formed as a result of revascularization is not clear. Radiographic evidence of changes in root length and wall thickness does not necessarily indicate a regeneration of functional pulp tissue and the formation of new dentin and cementum. Histologic studies in dogs and humans suggest that in some cases these radiographic changes may be a result of deposition of cementum-like and bonelike tissues, meaning an ingrowth of PDL tissue instead of pulp tissue.[20,106–110]

Technique

The regenerative endodontic technique usually requires at least two treatment visits.[116] In the first visit, under rubber dam isolation, the root canal is disinfected using irrigation solutions (like 1.5% NaOCl) that are then rinsed with saline to minimize cytotoxicity to the stem cells in the apical tissue. An intracanal dressing of calcium hydroxide or low concentration of triple antibiotic paste is placed and sealed with a temporary restorative material for 1 to 4 weeks.

At the second appointment, under rubber dam isolation, the remaining paste is removed with copious irrigation. The canal is dried and bleeding is introduced into the canal space through the apical foramen to create a scaffold on which a new tissue will grow and repopulate the canal space. Alternatives such as platelet-rich plasma, platelet-rich fibrin, or autologous fibrin matrix can also be used. Bleeding is stopped 3 to 4 mm below the access preparation to allow for restorative material. Application of MTA or bioceramics and a good coronal seal is the last step of the treatment (see Chapter 41, Fig. 41.10).[111]

Advances in the field of material sciences, stem cell biology, and dental tissue engineering have raised the possibility of using biology-based treatment strategies to regenerate functional dental tissues. In the short-term future, regeneration of an individual tooth structure is a more realistic approach than a regeneration of an entire tooth.[112]

Nonvital Pulp Treatment for Young Mature Teeth

Root Canal Treatment in Young Mature Permanent Teeth: Special Considerations

Root canal treatment in mature teeth of children and adolescents is similar to that performed in adults. However, because of their wider canals and thinner dentinal walls in comparison with those of adult patients, special precautions may be needed, as described in this section.

Access

The coronal access should be wide enough to include the pulp horns to prevent future contamination and discoloration. During opening of the access cavity, care should be taken to remove only a minimal amount of dentin in the canal orifices. Removing too much dentin will weaken anterior teeth and may cause perforation in molars.

Instrumentation

The length of the root canal should be determined carefully using radiographs; an electronic apex locator or paper points can also be used. Though the root canals are larger, they may be curved, so instrumentation should be done with precurved instruments in anticurvature filing motions. The use of crown-down procedures and nickel titanium rotary instruments will ease the preparation of the root canal.

Irrigation

Irrigation during root canal treatment should be done only after making sure that the rubber dam is placed properly and that leakage of fluids into the mouth cannot occur accidentally. The needle of the irrigation syringe is placed loosely in the root canal to avoid pushing the irrigation solution beyond the apex. NaOCl is used in various concentrations (0.5% to 5.25%) as the preferred irrigation solution.[113]

Intracanal Dressing

In teeth with infected root canals, the emphasis is on disinfection and removal of tissue remnants. Because effective mechanical preparation of wide canal walls is difficult, it is recommended that treatment be done in two sessions, with placement of an antiseptic dressing between visits. Calcium hydroxide paste is the preferred dressing material because it dissolves tissue remnants.[89]

The placement of the dressing material can be accomplished using a Lentulo spiral shorter than the length of the root canal, specially designed syringes, or files.

Isthmus

The isthmus is a thin communication between two or more root canals in the same root that contains pulp tissue. Any root containing two canals or more has a high incidence of isthmi.[114]

An isthmus is formed when a root projection cannot close itself, and it will be larger in children where root formation is not fully complete. These weblike connections between root canals are part of the root canal system. They can function as a reservoir for bacteria and therefore should be cleaned and obturated during root canal treatment.[114]

Obturation

The apical foramen in young teeth is large, and adaptation of a master cone should be done carefully to avoid extrusion of filling materials that can easily occur during obturation. Lateral condensation requires more accessory GP points; initial points should be placed such that they will not block access to the canal. Filling with warm GP or using warm condensation techniques should be done cautiously to avoid overfilling.

In some cases, fabrication of a customized master cone is favorable. A GP point is fitted several millimeters short of the apex; the apical 2 to 3 mm are softened (with a solvent or a heat source) and tamped gradually into place. The completed customized cone represents an impression of the apical portion of the canal preventing extrusion of filling material during obturation.[20]

Visit eBooks.Health.Elsevier.com to see full list of references.

34

Pediatric Oral Surgery: Principles and Techniques

DAVID M. AVENETTI

CHAPTER OUTLINE

Introduction to Pediatric Oral Surgery: Principles and Practices

Pediatric oral surgery encompasses a wide range of procedures, such as extractions, management of infections and trauma, and more complex procedures, such as biopsies and frenectomies.[1] These procedures require understanding children's anatomy while considering the need for behavior guidance and interdisciplinary collaboration.

Scope of Pediatric Oral Surgery

Standard pediatric oral surgery procedures necessitate careful planning and utilizing age-appropriate techniques. Pediatric extractions are frequently performed due to advanced caries, orthodontic treatment needs, or traumatic injuries.[2] Extractions must be performed with appropriate techniques to minimize trauma and promote healing without disrupting ongoing dental development. Children's developing teeth and bone density require careful approaches to preserve the underlying permanent teeth and ensure proper skeletal development. Managing odontogenic infections, including abscesses and cellulitis, is important to prevent the spread of infection and its effects on systemic health. Infection management in children is especially critical, as untreated infections can lead to more severe complications affecting both oral and general health.[3]

Due to their active lifestyles, children are at considerable risk for traumatic dental injuries, which can include facial fractures, injury to teeth and supporting structures, or soft tissue damage.[4,5] Effective management may involve repositioning and splinting damaged teeth, particularly preserving developmental structures. Unlike adults, children's growth and the development of their permanent dentition must be considered when providing treatment (see Chapters 40 and 41 for a detailed discussion of trauma).

Pediatric oral surgery also includes more complex procedures like biopsies, management of impacted teeth, frenectomies, and, in rare cases, implants or autotransplantation. These specialized interventions require understanding pediatric anatomy and growth patterns to minimize invasiveness and protect developing teeth and surrounding structures. Although these procedures may be beyond the scope of many dentists, understanding the indications for these procedures is imperative as part of comprehensive dental care and proper case selection.

Preoperative Assessment

The preoperative assessment is key to comprehensively understanding the patient's needs. Assessment includes a thorough medical and dental history evaluation, comprehensive examination, risk assessment, and knowledge of the child's behavioral and psychological needs. Proper informed consent and effective communication with both the child and their caregivers help build trust and ensure a positive surgical experience.

Medical and Dental History

A comprehensive medical history is a fundamental component of the preoperative assessment, especially when systemic conditions, allergies, and medication interactions can complicate or increase the risk associated with surgical interventions[6] (see Chapter 35, Fig. 35.2 for a sample medical history). In addition to standard medical questions, dentists should consider conditions that might increase surgical risk, such as bleeding disorders, cardiovascular conditions, respiratory conditions, neuromuscular disorders, or immunodeficiencies. Understanding the patient's past and current medications can help avoid adverse events during and after surgery.

When a child's medical condition poses an increased risk for potential complications, it is necessary to obtain consultations from appropriate medical professionals. This approach ensures a complete understanding of any precautions that may be needed. The dental history must also be reviewed, which may include previous dental treatment and the patient's tolerance to dental care.

Risk Assessment

Risk assessment in pediatric patients must consider the patient's age, developmental level, and any underlying medical conditions. Children with specific medical histories, such as asthma, epilepsy, or bleeding disorders, may present higher risks during surgery. The dentist must anticipate potential emergencies and be prepared to handle them. Familiarity with pediatric emergency protocols and training in managing complications is essential, as unexpected reactions may arise during procedures (see Chapter 35).

Physical Examination

The physical examination includes both extraoral and intraoral assessments. Extraoral evaluation should consist of a soft tissue examination of the head and neck, noting any asymmetry, lymphadenopathy, soft tissue injuries, and range of motion of the temporomandibular joint. Intraorally, the dentist should carefully examine the teeth, gums, soft tissues, and any potential sites for surgery. The dentist should also consider the need for future space maintenance after extractions of primary teeth. Failure to provide timely space maintenance can lead to issues like the mesial migration of permanent teeth, which may complicate future orthodontic alignment.

Radiographic Assessment

Preoperative radiographs are essential to establish diagnoses of the tooth (restorability) and surrounding tissues (furcal and periapical areas; see Chapter 17 for a discussion of radiographic techniques and Chapters 40 and 41 for a discussion of appropriate radiographs for traumatized teeth). Additionally, radiographic imaging often includes two or more periapical radiographs of the same area to assess the buccal, lingual, facial, or palatal relationships of impacted or supernumerary teeth. A three-dimensional (3D) radiograph may be necessary in specific cases, such as identifying supernumerary or impacted teeth adjacent to cleft sites. Three-dimensional imaging has increasing applications in pediatric dentistry and can be a useful tool with proper case selection.[7]

Behavioral and Psychological Considerations

Understanding and addressing behavioral and psychological aspects are fundamental in pediatric oral surgery. Dental anxiety, fear of the unknown, and potential behavioral issues are common in children. Using age-appropriate language and positive framing can make the experience less daunting for the child and encourage cooperation. Techniques such as tell-show-do, distraction, positive reinforcement, and, if needed, premedication or moderate sedation can make the experience more manageable for young patients.[8] When sedating pediatric patients, strict adherence to sedation monitoring guidelines is necessary to ensure safe delivery of care[9] (see Chapters 26 and 27 for detailed discussions of nonpharmacologic and pharmacologic behavior guidance techniques).

Parental concerns also play a role in a child's comfort. Engaging caregivers in the process and addressing their questions can provide reassurance, which in turn helps calm the child (see Chapter 26 Case Study: Prepared Parents, Prepared Children, Positive Coping). Building rapport and explaining each step of the procedure can foster a trusting environment conducive to cooperation.

Informed Consent and Patient/Parent Education

In pediatric cases, obtaining informed consent involves clear, understandable communication with the patient and their parents or guardians. Dentists must ensure that caregivers understand the planned procedure and potential risks, benefits, and alternatives. The informed consent process should also involve educating caregivers about postoperative expectations, such as pain management, activity restrictions, and signs of possible complications. Effective communication requires using simple, nontechnical language and visual aids when appropriate to ensure the family fully comprehends the procedure (see Chapter 26 for a detailed discussion of informed consent).

Extractions in Pediatric Patients

Performing extractions on children requires a modified approach due to anatomical differences, the smaller size of the oral cavity, and considerations related to the developing dentition. The approach includes proper preoperative assessment, choice of suitable instrumentation, proper technique, and careful management of the child's comfort and anxiety.

Indications for Extraction

The need for extraction in pediatric patients can arise from various conditions. Unlike in adult dentistry, extractions may be recommended earlier in children to prevent adverse effects on dental development. Some common indications include caries, trauma, crowding/orthodontic needs, infection, and developmental anomalies, which are described in Box 34.1.

Armamentarium for Pediatric Extractions

The instruments used in pediatric extractions are often distinct from those used in adults. Pediatric instruments are smaller, allowing for easier placement in a child's smaller oral cavity. Smaller instruments are more easily concealed within the operator's hand, which can reduce the child's anxiety by restricting their view of the instruments. Instruments such as the no. 150S and no. 151S forceps are widely used in pediatric extractions and feature smaller working ends (beaks) that align more closely with the morphology of primary teeth,[10] reducing the risk of damage to surrounding tissue or underlying permanent tooth buds (Fig. 34.1). eTable 34.1 lists the recommended surgical armamentarium for pediatric procedures. The use of cow horn mandibular forceps, common in adult dentistry, is contraindicated in primary teeth due to the risk of injury to developing premolars (Fig. 34.2). Careful use of elevators adjacent to restorations, such as stainless steel crowns, is necessary to prevent dislodgement. Restorations near erupting single-rooted teeth may become dislodged with minimal force, warranting caution.

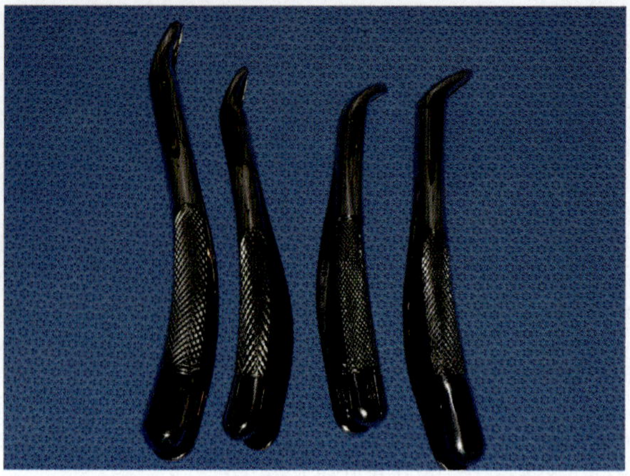

• **Fig. 34.1** Extraction Forceps. Left to right, no. 150, no. 150S, no. 151S, and no. 151. The smaller size of the "S" forceps is appreciated.

• BOX 34.1 Common Indications and Treatment Considerations for Tooth Extractions

1. **Caries:** When caries severely compromises structural integrity or extend into the pulp and cannot be treated with restorations and/or pulpotomy, extraction may be necessary to prevent infection or abscess formation.
2. **Trauma:** Injuries such as root fractures, luxations, or avulsions often lead to the extraction of teeth, especially primary teeth, if the trauma compromises the integrity of the tooth or poses risks to the underlying permanent teeth.
3. **Crowding and orthodontic needs:** When teeth crowd the dental arch or contribute to malocclusion, extraction of primary teeth and/or permanent premolars may be recommended to provide space for properly aligned permanent teeth.
4. **Infection:** Odontogenic infections often require extraction to prevent the spread of infection and avoid systemic complications. In immunocompromised and medically compromised children, this is particularly important to mitigate health risks.
5. **Developmental anomalies:** Supernumerary teeth or teeth severely affected by molar incisor hypomineralization and caries may necessitate extractions.

Techniques for Extraction

The extraction technique in pediatric patients parallels adults in principle but incorporates adjustments for young patients' unique anatomy and psychological needs. A common approach is to show the child a curette or other benign instrument and explain the procedure using age-appropriate language, such as describing the feeling of pressure and a tooth "dancing out." Profound anesthesia is essential, as the sensation of pain can make it challenging to regain a child's confidence, and advanced behavior guidance techniques may be required. See Chapter 28 for a discussion of local anesthetic techniques.

General Technique Considerations

Before an extraction, the dentist should explain the surgical procedure and the expected postoperative recovery course. This allows parents to make special postoperative arrangements, such as the need for a soft diet or childcare support.

Positioning is critical to ensure the child is comfortable and safe while reducing the risk of swallowing or aspirating objects. Several factors make it possible for the child patient to aspirate or swallow foreign objects during dental treatment.[11] These include (1) the common practice of treating the child patient in a reclined position, (2) poor visibility because of the smaller oral cavity and the proportionately larger tongue of the child, and (3) the increased likelihood of unexpected movements by the child. The child should be positioned with the upper jaw at a maximum 45-degree angle relative to the floor and with a gauze screen or rubber dam to protect the posterior airway (Fig. 34.3).

The dentist should be located where he can easily control the instrumentation, have good visual access to the surgical site, and control the child's head. The fingers of the dentist's nondominant hand are then placed in the patient's mouth on either side of the tooth being extracted. The role of the nondominant hand is to help control the patient's head; to support the jaw being treated; to help retract the cheek, lips, and tongue from the surgical field; and to palpate the alveolar process and adjacent teeth during the extraction (see Fig. 34.3). See Case Study: Extraction of Primary Molar and eVideo 34.1.

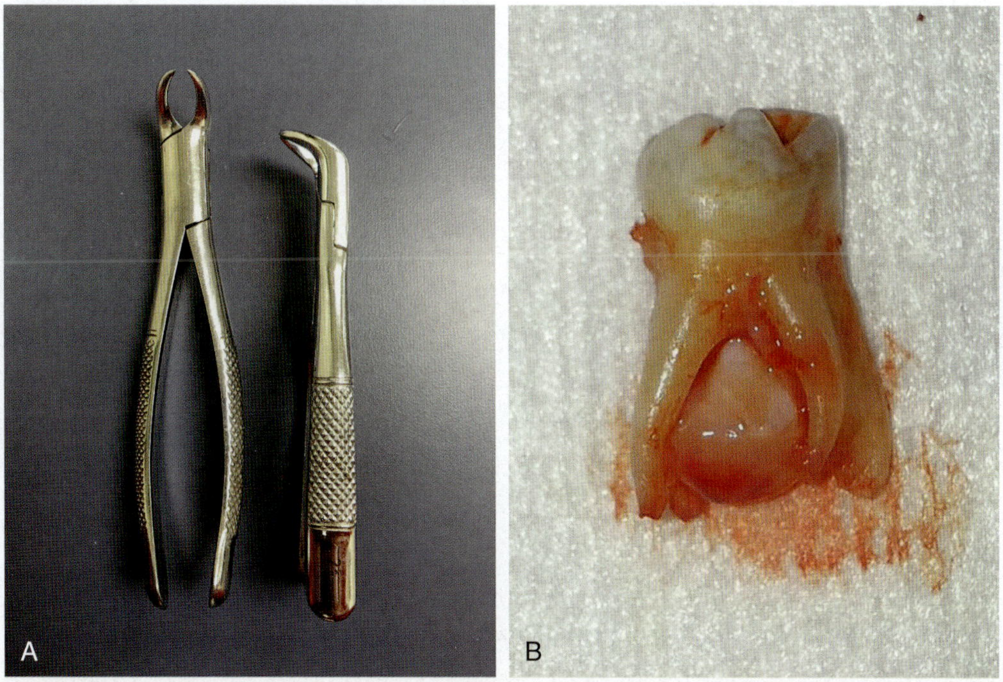

• **Fig. 34.2** (A–B) The use of cow horn mandibular forceps is contraindicated for primary teeth due to the potential for injury to the developing premolars. (B, Courtesy Gabriel Dominici.)

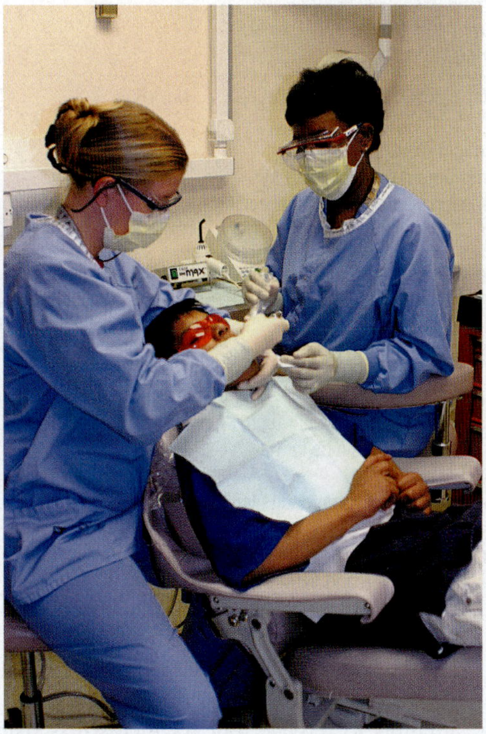

• **Fig. 34.3** To help prevent aspiration of extracted teeth, the child is positioned so that the upper jaw is at a 45-degree angle to the floor.

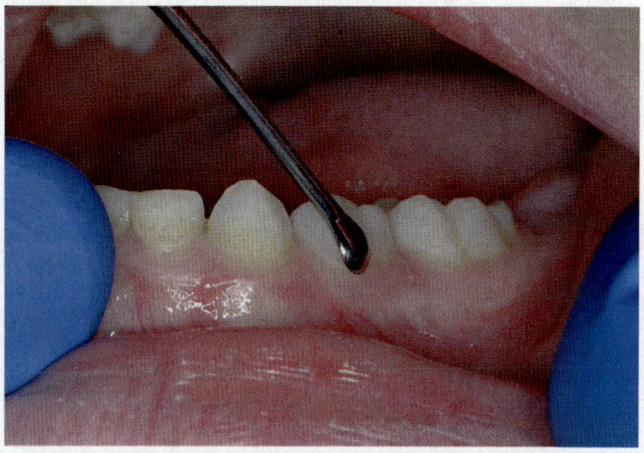

• **Fig. 34.4** A periosteal elevator is used to separate the epithelial attachment of the tooth before extraction.

Extraction Procedure

Profound local anesthesia is required. Using a dental curette or periosteal elevator, the dentist separates the epithelial attachment of the tooth to be extracted (Fig. 34.4). This step minimizes trauma to surrounding tissue and is especially important for multirooted teeth. Appropriate elevators are used to luxate the tooth, noting that the force is created by placing the elevator between the bone and tooth being extracted, not by elevating against adjacent teeth (Fig. 34.5). Care is taken to avoid damaging adjacent or underlying teeth, especially in primary teeth with thin roots and less dense supporting bone. The extraction is then performed via the proper forceps technique (Fig. 34.6). A description of the surgical technique for each type of tooth is seen in Table 34.2. Ensuring adequate luxation, especially for severely decayed teeth, can facilitate easier forceps delivery and minimize the possibility of tooth fracture. Careful and coordinated movements by both the dominant and nondominant hands reduce the risk of complications (Figs. 34.7 and 34.8).

The surgical site is evaluated visually after the tooth is removed from its socket. If granulation tissue is present, it should be gently removed with a surgical curette; however, aggressive manipulation of a curette in a primary tooth socket is contraindicated due to the

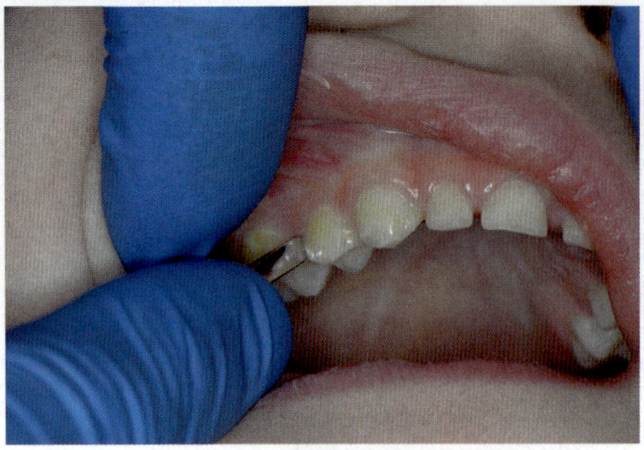

• **Fig. 34.5** A no. 301 straight elevator is used to luxate the tooth. Extreme care is taken to prevent accidental luxation of adjacent teeth.

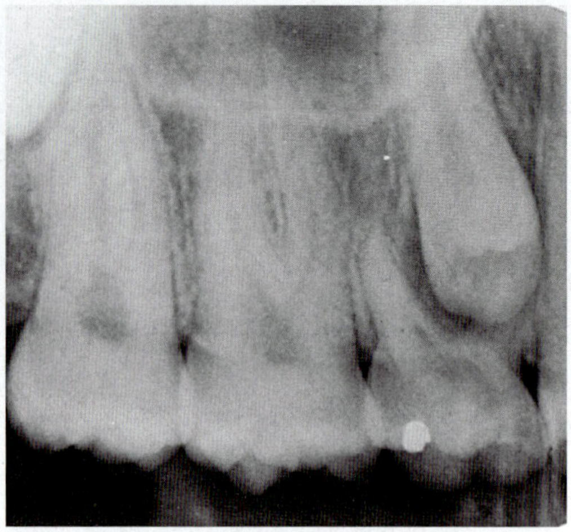

• **Fig. 34.6** Primary molars with roots encircling the developing premolar may have to be sectioned to prevent accidental extraction of the premolar.

TABLE 34.2 Recommendations for Extraction Technique by Primary Tooth Type

Primary Tooth Type	Recommendation for Technique	Forceps
Maxillary anterior teeth *(central incisors, lateral incisors, canines)*	Adequate local anesthesia should include infiltration of the maxillary anterior vestibule and the incisive papilla (nasopalatine block) for lingual anesthesia. Release the epithelial attachment, then luxate with a no. 301 straight elevator. Use anterior forceps along the long axis of the tooth, positioning the beaks apical to the cementoenamel junction. Apply slight rotary and vertical movements (apical thrust, twist, and pull). If roots show resorption, take care to avoid fracturing the roots.	No. 1
Maxillary molars	Ensure adequate anesthesia with maxillary infiltration and palatal injection or greater palatine block. Release the epithelial attachment, then luxate with a no. 301 straight elevator. Use maxillary universal forceps for extraction, initiating palatal movement first, followed by alternating buccal and palatal motions. Apply slow, continuous force to expand the alveolar bone and extract without fracture.	No. 150S
Mandibular anterior teeth *(incisors, canines, premolars)*	Ensure adequate anesthesia with mandibular infiltration and lingual injection or inferior alveolar nerve block (IANB) supplemented by infiltration. Use rotational movements to extract single-rooted teeth. Avoid force on adjacent teeth to prevent their luxation or dislodgement. This can be particularly challenging when crowding is present.	Variable forceps are available designed with small beaks for mandibular anterior teeth (i.e., No. 44)
Mandibular molars	Adequate anesthesia through an IANB, with potential additional long buccal block. Infiltration with articaine infiltration shows promising evidence for primary tooth extractions in the mandible in lieu of IANB. Support the mandible with the nonextraction hand to prevent injury to the temporomandibular joints. After luxation with a no. 301 straight elevator, use alternating buccal and palatal motions to extract the tooth. Apply slow, continuous force to expand the alveolar bone and extract without fracture.	No. 151S

potential for damage to the succeeding tooth bud. The operator should palpate the facial and palatal or buccal and lingual aspects of the surgical site to feel for any bone irregularities or alveolar expansion. Digital pressure should be sufficient to return the alveolus to its presurgical configuration if gross expansion has occurred.

Managing Fractured Primary Tooth Roots

In some cases, root fractures can occur, particularly in primary molars with divergent roots or in teeth undermined by caries. Aggressive attempts to retrieve root fragments may damage the succedaneous tooth. If the root tip is small or deeply situated, leaving it in place for natural resorption by the erupting permanent tooth is often preferable as normal physiologic resorption should occur.[12] However, extracting the root tip becomes particularly important in cases of active infection, such as cellulitis. Larger root fragments may be removed with minimal manipulation if they are readily accessible, and instruments such as root tip picks can assist. Intraoperative radiographs can help identify residual root fragments and decide if they should be left or retrieved

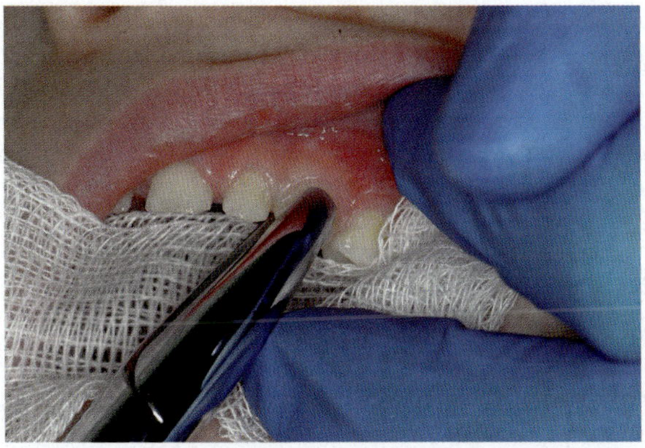

• **Fig. 34.7** Rotational movements and buccolingual motions are used to extract primary incisors. The dentist's nondominant hand helps control the child's head, supports the jaw being treated, retracts adjacent soft tissues, and palpates the alveolar process and adjacent teeth during extraction. Also note the gauze screen in the oral cavity to aid in preventing aspiration or swallowing of extracted teeth.

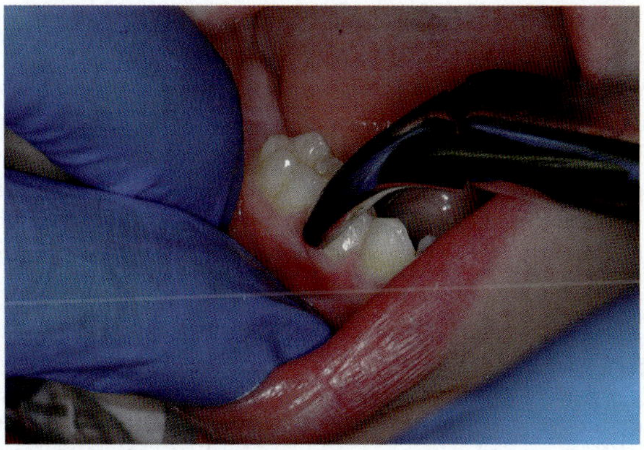

• **Fig. 34.8** The nonextraction hand supports the mandible during extraction of mandibular molars.

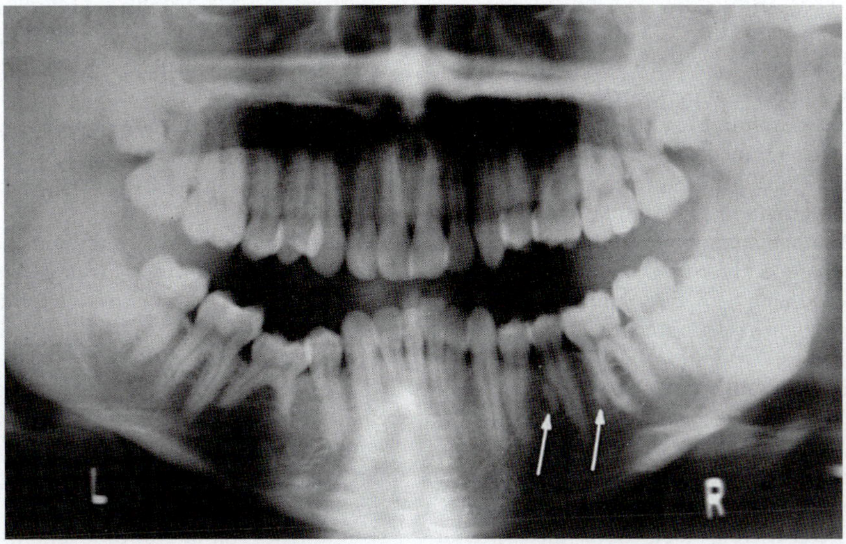

• **Fig. 34.9** In this patient, unresorbed primary root tips *(arrows)* did not impede eruption of the succeeding premolar. Also note that in the area of congenitally missing #29, the primary molar roots of tooth #T are not being resorbed and the occlusal surface of this tooth is well below the occlusal plane (i.e. Tooth #T is infraoccluded).

(Fig. 34.9). When fragments are intentionally left to resorb, documentation and parent notification are essential redundant to beginning of sentence.[13]

Sectioning Teeth and Use of a Surgical Handpiece in Extractions

Sectioning teeth may be appropriate when the tooth cannot be extracted as a single unit due to factors such as multirooted teeth, extensive caries, impacted or ankylosed teeth, and in cases of limited access[14] (Figs. 34.6 and 34.10). When roots diverge significantly or are curved, sectioning allows for the removal of individual roots without excessive force, minimizing trauma to surrounding structures. Teeth with significant structural compromise due to caries may fracture under extraction force so that sectioning can facilitate controlled removal. Sectioning helps isolate parts of an ankylosed tooth for easier removal when the tooth is embedded deeply or fused to the bone.[14] In cases where access

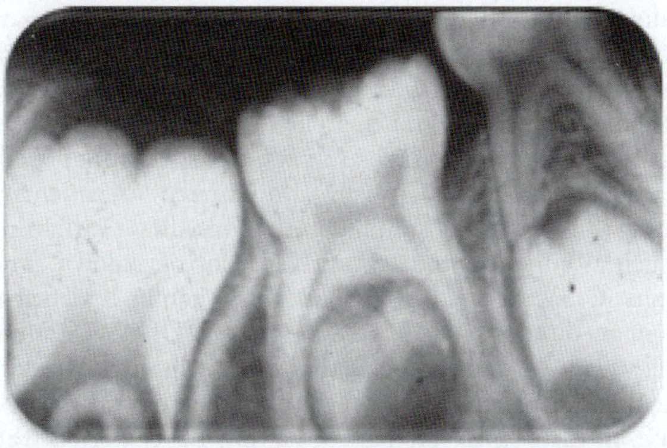

• **Fig. 34.10** For the ankylosed primary second molar, the crown should be sectioned with a fissure bur in a buccolingual direction down the midline of the tooth so that the detached portions of the crown and roots can be elevated separately.

is restricted (e.g., third molars or posterior teeth), sectioning reduces the need for excessive manipulation.

A surgical handpiece should be used to avoid the risk of air emphysema from traditional air-driven handpieces.[15] Using a surgical handpiece to section teeth can reduce the force required for extraction, preserving surrounding tissues and minimizing postoperative complications. Removing the overlying bone with a surgical handpiece exposes the tooth for easier extraction in impacted or partially erupted teeth.

Postoperative Care

Postoperative care in pediatric extractions can help minimize complications and promote effective healing. Detailed instructions for bleeding control, pain management, and dietary adjustments should be provided to both the child and their caregiver, ideally before the procedures begin[16] (see "Postoperative Care and Follow-Up in Pediatric Oral Surgery is correct (section is on page 434" later in this chapter).

Management of Bleeding

Local Measures

In surgical procedures, bleeding is controlled through both local and systemic measures. Local bleeding control interventions at the extraction site assist with minimizing blood loss. Direct pressure is one of the most effective methods, achieved by having the patient bite down on the gauze placed directly over the surgical site. This encourages clot formation and compresses blood vessels to reduce bleeding. Another common technique is suturing, which stabilizes tissues, reduces the risk of continuous bleeding, and helps retain the blood clot. However, suturing over an infected site is not recommended (see "Suturing in Pediatric Oral Surgery" later in this chapter).[17] Additionally, hemostatic agents, such as Gelfoam (Pfizer, New York, NY), Surgicel (Johnson & Johnson MedTech, Arlington, TX), collagen-based products, and topical thrombin, can be applied to the site to promote clotting, especially in cases where pressure alone is insufficient.[18] Last, vasoconstrictors found in local anesthetics such as epinephrine can help control bleeding by constricting blood vessels, thereby reducing blood flow and enhancing clot stability. These local measures provide options to manage bleeding during most surgical procedures effectively.

Systemic Measures

Bleeding can also be managed through systemic measures when indicated. Appropriate medical consultations are required for patients who may experience anticipated bleeding, and therapies are often coordinated with hematologists or other specialized physicians.[19] Systemic drugs, such as tranexamic acid, work by stabilizing blood clots and are usually administered to patients with bleeding disorders or those at high risk of bleeding. Antifibrinolytics, such as aminocaproic acid, prevent clot breakdown, whereas vitamin K may be used in patients with vitamin K deficiencies. Certain medications, such as desmopressin (DDAVP), stimulate the release of von Willebrand factor, which helps improve clotting, particularly in patients with mild hemophilia or von Willebrand disease. In cases where the patient has low platelet levels (thrombocytopenia), a platelet transfusion may be administered to promote clotting. Platelets are critical in hemostasis, serving as the primary mediators of initial plug formation at sites of vascular injury. For patients with known bleeding disorders like hemophilia, replacing specific clotting factors (e.g., factor VIII or IX) before surgery ensures the blood can clot normally. Given that surgical procedures are likely to produce more bleeding than traditional periodontal or restorative procedures, providers must be prepared to prevent and manage bleeding using a variety of local and/or systemic measures when indicated.

Third Molar Extractions: Current Philosophies, Indications, and Timing

Current Treatment Philosophies

The approach to third molar (wisdom tooth) extractions is increasingly patient specific, balancing preventive care with the risks of surgery. The debate whether to extract prophylactically or to monitor asymptomatic third molars is ongoing. The American Association of Oral and Maxillofacial Surgeons offers the following position statement: "Predicated on the best evidence-based data, third molar teeth associated with disease or at high risk of developing disease should be surgically managed. Active clinical and radiographic surveillance is indicated in the absence of disease or significant risk of disease."[20] Potential problems associated with impacted third molars are risk of pain and/or infection, damage to neighboring teeth, caries, periodontal disease, and pathology associated with tooth follicles (e.g., cysts, tumors).

Indications for Extraction

When third molars have sufficient space to erupt and are not associated with any symptoms or pathology, extraction may not be necessary. Third molar extraction is indicated when the tooth poses a risk for acute pain or infection, pericoronitis, caries that cannot be restored, an associated cyst or other pathology, or periodontal disease. Prophylactic removal of asymptomatic third molars is also indicated when there is insufficient space to accommodate the erupting tooth,[21] to facilitate orthodontic treatment (e.g., a third molar impeding eruption of a second molar), or when the tooth is likely to be nonfunctional. Systematic reviews indicated that there is no higher risk of crowding among patients who retained third molars compared with those who had third molars removed. Crowding increased in both groups without any significant difference, so preventing crowding is not an indication for third molar removal.[22,23] Prophylactic removal of partially erupted mesially angulated third molars has positively affected oral health-related quality of life.[24] In cases where a patient has hypodontia or tooth loss in one or more quadrants, third molars may be strategically saved as a tooth replacement option; for example, in cases of molar incisor hypomineralization (MIH) where first permanent molars are extracted to allow drifting of the second permanent molars and increased space available for third molar eruption. For this reason, careful consideration of the entire dentition is necessary before extracting one or more third molars.[25]

Timing of Extraction

According to the American Association of Oral and Maxillofacial Surgeons, the most appropriate time to extract third molars is between 16 and 25 years of age,[20,21] which may facilitate faster healing with fewer complications. Waiting until after 25 may be more challenging due to completely formed roots on third molars, denser bone, and a higher chance of delayed healing.[26,27]

Risks of Extraction

Some more common risks of extraction include pain, swelling, and postoperative bleeding. Less common risks include nerve injury that can lead to temporary or permanent paresthesia, infection (such as alveolar osteitis), fracture of the mandible, or risks associated with anesthesia.[28–30] Dry socket and bisphosphonate-related osteonecrosis of the jaw (BRONJ) primarily affect adults. Still, they must be considered in adolescents who demonstrate risk factors for these conditions, such as those who take bisphosphonates or smoke. Careful planning, conservative techniques, and thorough patient education minimize these risks. Early intervention for high-risk teeth and monitoring of asymptomatic cases ensures optimal long-term outcomes.

Odontogenic Infections in Pediatric Patients

Odontogenic infections, originating in the teeth or their supporting structures, are relatively common in children and adolescents. These infections are often initiated by untreated caries, trauma, or other dental conditions that allow bacteria to invade the pulp, leading to an inflammatory response. Periodontal abscesses are less common in children than adults. Although many pediatric odontogenic infections are localized and can be effectively managed in-office, certain cases can escalate, spreading beyond the dentition and causing potentially serious health complications.[31]

Types and Causes of Odontogenic Infections

A periapical abscess develops when caries or trauma allows bacteria to penetrate the pulp and spread to the periapical tissues, causing pain, localized swelling, and potentially purulent discharge in the affected area. Periapical abscesses may also affect surrounding tissue and bone, leading to potential damage to developing permanent teeth if left untreated (i.e., localized enamel hypoplasia/Turner tooth).

Cellulitis is a diffuse, spreading bacterial infection of the soft tissues that can occur when an odontogenic infection is not promptly treated. This infection is more concerning than a localized abscess, as it involves multiple anatomical spaces and can spread rapidly.[32] Because of the developmental nature of pediatric bones and soft tissues, the infection can invade the fascial spaces and spread to deep spaces, presenting a higher risk to systemic health.[31–33] Understanding how infection involving particular spaces may be associated with specific signs/symptoms can help clinicians assess acuity and potential sources of infection (Table 34.3). The progression of odontogenic infections can be more rapid in children due to lesser bone density, necessitating early and effective intervention. Although uncommon, serious complications can occur when the infection spreads beyond the dentition, such as cavernous sinus thrombosis, a brain abscess, airway obstruction, sepsis, or mediastinal spread. Managing cellulitis can be challenging because it has a wide variability of clinical presentation due to the involvement of multiple anatomical structures, polymicrobial etiology, and differing disease progression.

Diagnosis and Clinical Signs

Recognizing the signs and symptoms that suggest a severe infection is critical for determining the appropriate treatment approach. Classic signs of infection include the following:

1. *Redness, swelling, and pain:* These are the hallmarks of an abscess or cellulitis, indicating an inflammatory response in the infected area. Facial asymmetry, infraorbital swelling, or swelling extending near or below the inferior border of the mandible indicate more serious odontogenic infections (Fig. 34.11).
2. *Systemic temperature increase:* A fever greater than 101°F (38.3°C) can signal that the infection has spread beyond the local site and may involve deeper tissues.
3. *Difficulty swallowing or breathing:* In advanced cases of cellulitis, swelling may interfere with normal breathing and swallowing (dysphagia), which requires urgent medical attention.
4. *Voice changes, fatigue, and nausea:* These symptoms, along with excessive sweating and dehydration (often due to reluctance to eat or drink), are indications of a more severe systemic infection requiring immediate intervention.

When systemic symptoms such as elevated body temperature, difficulty swallowing, or visible spread of the infection appear, urgent evaluation and potential hospitalization may be needed.

Treatment Approaches

Managing odontogenic infections in children focuses on prompt and effective removal of the infection source (i.e., endodontic therapy or extraction) and prevention of further spread. Treatment combines surgical and pharmacologic approaches based on infection severity, patient cooperation, and medical status. Social factors also play a role (i.e., If extraction is delayed or swelling worsens, how likely is the family to obtain timely care, given possible social and economic constraints?).

Minor Infections

A pulpectomy (removal of the infected pulp), lesion sterilization/tissue repair (see Chapter 32), or extraction of the infected tooth can be effective for localized abscesses without systemic involvement. These procedures eliminate the source of infection and allow the affected tissues to begin healing. Removing the infected tooth is often preferred if the integrity of the tooth is compromised or if there is a high risk of reinfection. Oral antibiotics are not indicated if the dental infection is contained within the pulpal tissue or the immediate surrounding tissue.[34] Antibiotic therapy is indicated in cases of systemic infection[34,35] (see "Antibiotics and Other Medications" later in this chapter for a discussion of antibiotic therapy).

Serious Infections

Assessment

For more severe infections, incision and drainage (I&D), along with treating the offending tooth, are often required. I&D involves making a small incision to release pus and reduce pressure in the affected area, draining the infection and facilitating faster recovery.[36] I&D is particularly important for cases where the infection has spread to deeper fascial spaces. The procedure may not always produce purulent discharge, but it can shift the local environment from a more gram-negative anaerobic series of bacteria to aerobic gram-positive bacteria, which leads to a more favorable microbiology that is more susceptible to antibiotics.[36]

When systemic symptoms are present, concurrent inpatient treatment with intravenous (IV) antibiotics may be necessary. Hospital-based treatment is not only more effective in controlling rapidly spreading infections but also reduces the likelihood of serious complications while allowing close monitoring of the patient's disposition.[37,38] Research indicates that immediate

TABLE 34.3 Summary of Head and Neck Spaces, Borders, and Infection Risks

Space	Borders	Odontogenic Infection Risk
Buccal space	• Lateral: Skin of cheek • Medial: Buccinator muscle • Superior: Zygomatic arch • Inferior: Mandible	Infections from maxillary or mandibular molars, particularly premolars and first molars
Sublingual space	• Superior: Oral mucosa of the floor of the mouth • Inferior: Mylohyoid muscle • Lateral: Mandible	Infections from mandibular premolars or molars with roots above the mylohyoid
Submandibular space	• Superior: Mylohyoid muscle • Inferior: Hyoid bone • Lateral: Mandible • Medial: Digastric muscle	Infections from mandibular molars with roots extending below the mylohyoid
Submental space	• Superior: Mylohyoid muscle • Inferior: Skin of the chin • Lateral: Anterior belly of digastric muscle	Infections from mandibular anterior teeth, particularly incisors
Parapharyngeal space	• Medial: Pharynx • Lateral: Medial pterygoid muscle • Posterior: Carotid sheath • Anterior: Pterygoid fascia	Infections from mandibular molars or infections spreading from submandibular or sublingual spaces
Pterygomandibular space	• Medial: Medial pterygoid muscle • Lateral: Mandibular ramus • Superior: Lateral pterygoid muscle	Infections from mandibular molars, often associated with inferior alveolar nerve block complications
Canine (infraorbital) space	• Superior: Orbital floor • Inferior: Buccinator muscle • Lateral: Levator anguli oris • Medial: Nasal cavity	Infections from maxillary canines or first premolars
Masseteric space	• Lateral: Masseter muscle • Medial: Lateral surface of the mandible • Superior: Zygomatic arch	Infections from mandibular molars, especially third molars
Lateral pharyngeal space	• Medial: Pharyngeal wall • Lateral: Medial pterygoid muscle • Superior: Skull base • Inferior: Hyoid bone	Infections spreading from submandibular, sublingual, or retropharyngeal spaces
Retropharyngeal space	• Anterior: Pharyngeal constrictors • Posterior: Prevertebral fascia • Lateral: Carotid sheath	Infections spreading from parapharyngeal space or severe odontogenic infections
Ludwig angina	• Involves submandibular, sublingual, and submental spaces	Severe bilateral infections of mandibular molars spreading to multiple spaces, causing airway compromise

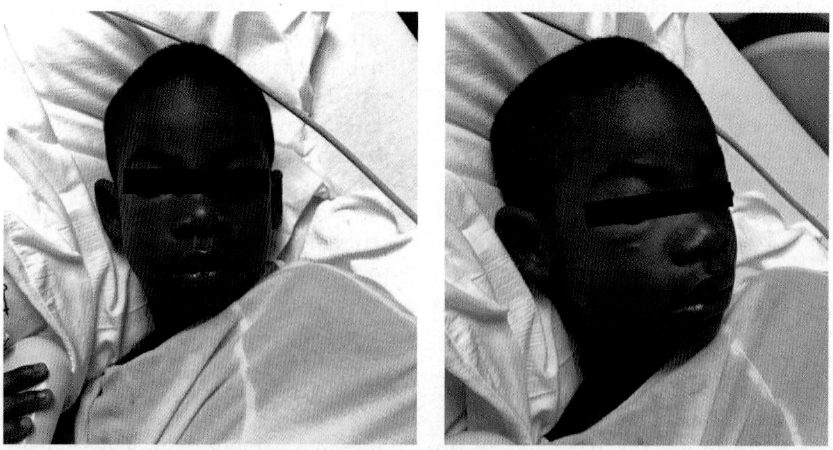

• **Fig. 34.11** A child with right facial cellulitis and swelling due to an abscessed tooth.

treatment of the causative tooth, coupled with IV antibiotics, is significantly more cost-effective and results in shorter hospital stays than treating with antibiotics alone.[38] Situations in which hospital admission may be necessary include swellings that may spread to high-risk areas (i.e., involving the inferior orbit of the eye or extending to the inferior border of the mandible), high fever with malaise, trismus or difficulty swallowing, or respiratory distress.[39]

If not treated promptly, odontogenic infections can lead to serious complications. Potential complications of untreated or inadequately treated odontogenic infections include orbital cellulitis, cavernous sinus thrombosis, brain abscess or meningitis, temporary blindness, airway obstruction, sepsis, and mediastinal spread of infection.[37] Infection spread to the cavernous sinus can result in a blood clot, causing vision changes, headache, and neurologic deficits.[40] This rare, but life-threatening, complication requires urgent intervention. Brain abscesses require intensive medical and sometimes surgical treatment. Severe cellulitis can obstruct the airway, and in extreme cases, the infection can cause sepsis or spread to the mediastinum, requiring emergency surgery and intensive care.[41]

Incision and drainage technique

After confirming the need for I&D, the surgical site may be cleansed with an antiseptic solution such as chlorhexidine gluconate. Profound local anesthesia is required, but anesthesia should not be injected directly into the pus accumulation. In young or anxious children, sedation may be used to ensure cooperation and reduce distress. A small, controlled incision (i.e., with a no. 15 blade) is made over the most fluctuant part of the abscess, often in the buccal mucosa or soft tissue surrounding the infected area. The incision should be deep enough to reach the abscess cavity without causing excessive tissue damage.[42] Intraoral incisions are generally preferred for esthetic reasons and to avoid scarring. The cut is kept small to minimize trauma but wide enough to allow thorough drainage of purulent material.[32,36]

Once the incision is made, gentle pressure is applied to the area to encourage complete drainage of pus from the abscess cavity. The clinician may use a blunt instrument, such as a hemostat, to carefully break up any loculations or fibrous septa within the abscess to ensure all pockets of infection are drained. This step is essential to prevent recurrence and enable the antibiotic treatment to be more effective. After draining the pus, the abscess cavity is flushed with a sterile saline solution or chlorhexidine to remove any remaining debris and bacteria. This irrigation step helps reduce the bacterial load and supports faster healing. In some cases, especially for large or multilocular abscesses, a small rubber drain or gauze strip may be placed in the incision to prevent premature closure and encourage continued drainage. The drain is typically secured in place and left for 24 to 48 hours, after which it can be removed during a follow-up visit.

After the procedure, caregivers are provided with instructions on maintaining oral hygiene, monitoring for signs of recurrence, and managing discomfort with age-appropriate pain relievers. Antibiotic therapy is continued as prescribed to support infection control. Patients and caregivers are advised to watch for signs of complications, such as fever, swelling, or prolonged pain, and to return for follow-up visits to assess healing and drain removal (if indicated). Facial swellings not responding to initial antibiotic therapy should be reevaluated and additional or alternative antibiotics may be recommended, and other sources of infection should be considered. Follow-up appointments are also an opportunity to address any underlying risk factors, such as poor oral hygiene or dietary habits, to reduce the likelihood of future infections and identify other treatment needs.

Trauma Management in Pediatric Patients

Diagnosis and assessment of traumatic dental injuries is discussed in detail in Chapters 40 and 41 with a focus on teeth and supporting structure. This section will consider surgical interventions, soft tissue injuries, and facial fractures associated with traumatic injuries.

Patients who present with facial trauma may also have acute life-threatening injuries such as chest or abdominal trauma or more significant head or neck injury. The dentist must ensure that there is no loss of consciousness or any other serious injuries before addressing the facial injuries. Initial care should be directed to a medical assessment, including pain control, hemorrhage control, patient reassurance, wound cleansing if possible, and tetanus prophylaxis when indicated.[43,44] Care should be taken to account for all teeth. In cases of avulsion or crown fractures, in which teeth cannot be accounted for, chest or abdominal radiographs may be needed to locate swallowed or aspirated teeth, whereas soft tissue radiographs may be indicated to rule out crown fragments embedded through, for instance, a lip laceration. Soft tissue injuries of the face or oral cavity are summarized in Table 34.4 along with their treatment approaches. When there is tissue damage that involves a break of the skin, great care must be taken to be certain that no foreign objects are left hidden within the wound (eFig. 34.12).

Surgical Interventions

Soft tissue injuries with lacerations are typically managed with primary closure. Small lacerations may heal well without sutures, but larger or deeper wounds often require layered suturing to ensure proper healing and reduce scarring.[45,46] Small lacerations of the wet portion of the lips, gingivae, alveolar mucosa, or tongue usually heal very well, even if left unsutured. A resorbable suture is commonly used intraorally, especially in children, because silk sutures have the disadvantage of needing removal. Large lacerations should be closed, regardless of their location, and multilayer wound closure may be indicated for very deep lacerations or for lacerations that extend from the face into the oral cavity (through-and-through lacerations).[46] Principles of a layered closure include a watertight mucosal closure, followed by closure of the muscular, facial, subcutaneous, and skin layers, as necessary. Facial lacerations are always reapproximated first at significant anatomical structures, such as the vermilion border, columella of the nose, or eyebrows.[45] Malalignment of these structures produces a noticeable cosmetic defect. It is generally advisable to refer to an oral surgeon or a plastic surgeon if the laceration crosses the vermilion border of the lip.

In cases of severely intruded teeth, gentle surgical repositioning may be necessary in accordance with the Dental Traumatology Guidelines for the Permanent Dentition. For surgical repositioning, local anesthesia is administered. Forceps are placed as apically as possible, and the tooth is loosened with both rotational and buccolingual movements. Elevation before repositioning may be necessary. Once the proper tooth position is established, the bone should be compressed to minimize the periodontal ligament space by applying finger pressure both labially and lingually. When access is challenging, a soft tissue releasing incision may be necessary

TABLE 34.4 Soft Tissue Oral Injuries: Types, Definitions, and Management

Type of Injury	Definition	Management
Abrasion	Superficial injury involving the scraping away of the epithelial layer of soft tissue	• Clean the area with saline or chlorhexidine • Apply an antibiotic ointment to prevent infection • Cover with a protective dressing if needed
Contusion	Bruising of the soft tissues without a break in the skin, caused by blunt trauma	• Apply cold compresses to reduce swelling • Monitor for signs of underlying bone or tooth injury • Provide analgesics if necessary
Laceration	A tear in the soft tissue, varying in depth and severity, often caused by sharp objects or trauma	• Irrigate with sterile saline to remove debris • Suture deeper or extensive wounds • Consider antibiotics and tetanus prophylaxis
Puncture wound	A deep injury caused by a sharp or pointed object penetrating the soft tissue	• Clean thoroughly with saline • Avoid suturing deep puncture wounds to allow drainage • Consider antibiotic prophylaxis • Monitor for signs of infection
Avulsion of soft tissue	Complete tearing away of a section of soft tissue from its attachment	• Control bleeding with pressure • Reattach tissue if possible using sutures • Ensure a clean wound area • Consider antibiotics and tetanus prophylaxis
Burn	Injury caused by exposure to heat, chemicals, or electrical sources affecting oral tissues	• Rinse with cool water for heat burns • Neutralize and flush chemical burns immediately • Apply a soothing agent (e.g., Orabase) and manage pain • Refer for severe cases
Soft tissue foreign body	Insertion of an object or debris into soft tissues	• Remove the foreign body carefully using local anesthesia and appropriate instruments • Irrigate with saline • Administer antibiotics if the wound is contaminated • Monitor healing

to access the tooth. Clean the affected area with saline or chlorhexidine and suture gingival lacerations if necessary. Teeth should be splinted until the periodontal ligament reattaches and the tooth has adequate bone support. The tooth is stabilized using a flexible splint, and splinting times vary depending on the severity of the trauma (see Chapter 41).

Management of Facial Fractures

Facial fractures in children are relatively uncommon compared with adults, accounting for approximately 5% to 15% of all facial trauma cases.[43] The lower incidence is primarily attributed to anatomical factors such as greater cranial-to-facial ratio, increased elasticity of facial bones, and protective fat pads. The most common etiologies include falls, sports-related injuries, motor vehicle accidents, and interpersonal violence, with age influencing the mechanism—falls predominate in younger children, whereas sports and motor vehicle accidents are more common in adolescents.

The mandible is the most frequently fractured facial bone in children, followed by the nasal bones, zygomatic complex, and orbital rim.[47,48] The pattern of injury varies by age, with younger children exhibiting fewer complete fractures due to the elasticity of developing bones. Management of pediatric facial fractures aims to restore function, prevent growth disturbances, and minimize psychological impact. Signs and symptoms of mandibular, maxillary, and facial fractures are shown in Box 34.2. Nondisplaced fractures are often managed conservatively with observation and a soft diet, whereas displaced or complex fractures may require closed or open reduction with fixation.[44] Techniques are modified to accommodate developing dentition and growth centers, with a preference for resorbable fixation materials when possible. Early intervention by a multidisciplinary team, including pediatric dentists, oral surgeons, and plastic surgeons, is essential

• BOX 34.2 Signs and Symptoms of Facial Fractures

Maxillary or Midface Fractures

- Altered occlusion
- Numbness in the infraorbital nerve distribution
- Double vision
- Periorbital ecchymosis (bruising)
- Facial asymmetry or edema
- Subcutaneous emphysema (skin cracking upon palpation)
- Nasal hemorrhage
- Ecchymosis of the palatal or buccal mucosa
- Mobility or crepitus upon manipulation of the maxilla

Mandibular Fractures

- Numbness in the mental or inferior alveolar nerve distribution
- Altered occlusion
- Periauricular pain
- Ecchymosis or abrasion of the chin
- Facial asymmetry or edema
- Ecchymosis of the floor of the mouth or buccal mucosa
- Mandibular hemorrhage
- Mandibular deviation on opening or limited opening
- Mobility or crepitus upon manipulation of the mandible

for optimal outcomes. Immobilization, pain control, and antibiotics for open fractures are essential steps. An oral maxillofacial surgeon ideally manages definitive treatment to ensure proper alignment and support normal facial growth.

Long-Term Follow-Up and Monitoring

Follow-up care is important to monitor healing, assess complications, and address any long-term sequelae. Monitoring of tooth necrosis and other sequelae via clinical and radiograph examination is discussed in Chapters 40 and 41. For facial lacerations, monitoring is necessary to assess for any scarring or cosmetic effects. If scarring is pronounced, a referral to a plastic surgeon may be recommended.

Pharmacomanagement in Pediatric Oral Surgery

Effective pharmacomanagement is important in pediatric oral surgery to ensure patient comfort, manage pain, and to manage the risk of infection or existing infection. Children have unique pharmacologic needs due to their developing physiology, varied responses to medications, and potential sensitivities to certain drugs.

Pain Management

Pain management in pediatric oral surgery is essential for minimizing discomfort and ensuring a positive treatment experience, as poorly managed pain can result in heightened anxiety or reluctance to seek future dental care. Although analgesics can be given in response to pain, administration of analgesics before local anesthesia wears off, and on a regular dosing schedule (instead of waiting until pain is experienced) preemptively manages pain.[49]

Intraoperative Pain Management

Local anesthetics are discussed in detail in Chapter 28; however, the important surgical principle is that adequate local anesthesia is necessary to achieve desirable outcomes. Although lidocaine with epinephrine can be effective for most procedures, even in the presence of swelling, articaine shows strong penetration through bone and may be beneficial for infiltration and/or supplemental injections when anesthesia may be difficult to achieve.[50] Articaine is lipophilic and can diffuse more easily in areas of swelling where pH may be lower. Unless patients have a contraindication to using epinephrine, local anesthetics with epinephrine extend the effectiveness time. Nitrous oxide is often beneficial for children undergoing extraction or surgical procedures for its analgesic properties as a supplement to local anesthesia. Placement of a nasal hood can be challenging for children who have incurred dental or facial trauma.

Nonpharmacologic approaches are also beneficial in pediatric pain management. Distraction (toys, screen time, stories), comforting touch, controlled breathing, relaxation techniques, and cognitive coping strategies are all effective approaches to multimodal pain management in children.[51] These techniques are discussed in Chapter 26.

Postoperative Pain Management

Ibuprofen and acetaminophen are standard over-the-counter (OTC) medications for managing postoperative pain in children. Ibuprofen is often preferred for its antiinflammatory properties, which help reduce both pain and swelling after procedures. Acetaminophen is an alternative for children who cannot tolerate nonsteroidal antiinflammatory medications. Combination therapy of ibuprofen and acetaminophen, administered in alternating doses, can offer enhanced pain control without the need for stronger prescription medications.[52] Pediatric dosing is discussed in detail in Chapter 28. A dose of acetaminophen or ibuprofen should be taken before the local anesthetic wears off to ensure there is a bridging of pain management. To supplement OTC medications, cold items such as ice packs to the face (applied to the face in 15-minute intervals or as long as tolerated) and popsicles can assist with managing pain and reducing swelling.

Prescription Analgesics

In cases of severe pain, such as after complex surgical procedures, additional pain control may be necessary. Counseling the parent that some pain is normal after a surgical procedure can help set realistic expectations, as some parents may assume their child should experience no discomfort. Anticipatory guidance should be provided because pain and swelling can peak around 48 hours after a procedure.

In general, opioids are not recommended due to the risk of adverse reactions from hyperresponders or hyporesponders and the potential for dependency.[53,54] The use of codeine and its alternatives, oxycodone, hydrocodone, morphine, and tramadol, for children as an analgesic is not recommended by the American Academy of Pediatrics. Chapter 27 discusses opioid analgesics in detail. Opioids are reserved as rescue medications for severe "breakthrough" pain. In this scenario, a patient is using an OTC analgesic on an appropriate schedule (i.e., every 6 hours); is attempting adjunct, nonpharmacologic approaches; and is still experiencing severe pain (pain score of 7 to 10). A patient may be prescribed a few doses of an opioid such as hydrocodone (0.2 mg/kg/dose up to 5 mg per dose) or oxycodone (0.1 to 0.2 mg/kg per dose up to 5 mg per dose).[55] Prescriptions should not exceed 50 morphine milligram equivalents per day or have a longer duration than 3 days.[55] Patients requesting pain management at the end of opioid therapy should be reevaluated.

Sedation and General Anesthesia

Sedation and general anesthesia (GA) play an important role in pediatric oral surgery, especially for young or highly anxious children who may not tolerate procedures under local anesthesia alone. Safety protocols and guidelines are essential to use these methods effectively and responsibly. Sedation is discussed in detail in Chapter 29. IV sedation is generally reserved for older children and adolescents undergoing complex or lengthy procedures. This method is usually used to provide a deeper and more controlled sedative effect, but it requires specialized training and equipment.[9] Due to the higher risks associated with IV sedation, it should be conducted in a facility equipped to handle potential complications, with readily available resuscitation equipment and trained personnel.

GA is indicated for extensive surgical procedures, cases involving children with significant behavioral challenges, or those with special healthcare needs. GA provides complete unconsciousness, ensuring the child remains still throughout the surgery. GA should only be administered in a hospital, specialized surgical center, or well-equipped office-based anesthesia suite by a licensed anesthesiologist. Before GA, a preoperative evaluation assesses the child's health status, including any history of respiratory issues or allergies. Postoperative recovery is closely monitored to ensure safe discharge.

Antibiotics and Other Medications

Antibiotics are not routinely used in pediatric oral surgery but may be indicated in certain cases to prevent or manage infection. The pharmacology and types of antibiotics are discussed in Chapter 18. Facial lacerations and puncture wounds may require topical and/or oral antibiotic agents. Intraoral puncture wounds and lacerations that appear to have been contaminated by extrinsic bacteria, debris (e.g., dirt, soil, gravel), foreign body, open fractures, and joint injury have an increased risk of infection and should be managed by systemic antibiotics.

Prophylactic antibiotics may be prescribed for children with systemic conditions before extraction or procedures involving significant tissue manipulation, such as cyanotic cardiac conditions. Additionally, prophylactic antibiotics may be warranted for children at elevated risk of infection, such as immunocompromised patients. The same prophylaxis regimens as those used for infective endocarditis prophylaxis are appropriate in immunocompromised patients (see Chapter 18 for a discussion of antibiotic prophylaxis for infective endocarditis, noting the trend away from using clindamycin as an alternative to amoxicillin).

For infections that can be managed in the clinical or outpatient setting, oral penicillin or amoxicillin is generally the empirical first choice.[56] Amoxicillin is favored due to its broad spectrum and convenient dosing schedule. As described by the American Academy of Pediatric Dentistry (AAPD) guideline on the use of antibiotic therapy for pediatric patients, the usual dosing for children $<$40 kg in weight is 20 to 40 mg/kg/day in divided doses every 8 hours (maximum single dose 500 mg), and for children $>$40 kg it is 250 to 500 mg every 8 hours. In cases of penicillin allergy, clarithromycin and azithromycin are recommended as alternatives. Azithromycin is dosed 10 to 12 mg/kg on day 1, single dose (maximum 500 mg), followed by 5 to 6 mg/kg once daily for the remainder of treatment (2 to 5 days). A loading dose increases the plasma concentration of the antibiotic more quickly to effectively manage an infection. Clindamycin is still considered a suitable alternative for patients with penicillin allergies; however, its use is declining due to gastrointestinal side effects, including the risk of *Clostridioides difficile* colitis. When additional coverage for gram-negative bacteria is needed, clindamycin, metronidazole (with penicillin/amoxicillin), or a regimen of amoxicillin clavulanate potassium may offer broader microbial coverage.[56]

For aggressive infections, patients may be treated with IV antibiotics in a hospital setting. Ampicillin/sulbactam, clindamycin, or a combination of penicillin with metronidazole are commonly used in hospitalized pediatric patients. Patients may be discharged with a prescription for a course of oral antibiotics after the initial infection is managed by IV antibiotics. In specific cases, adjunct medications such as antiinflammatory agents, corticosteroids, or topical anesthetics may be used to manage pain, swelling, or inflammation. For example, corticosteroids are occasionally prescribed postoperatively to minimize severe swelling, especially in cases involving extensive tissue manipulation. Prednisone, methylprednisolone, or dexamethasone can be given over a short course to control inflammation. Dexamethasone can be given as 4 mg orally as a loading dose, then 2 to 4 mg every 12 hours for 1 to 2 days in children 2 to 6 years old, or 4 to 8 mg orally as a loading dose, then 4 mg every 12 hours for 1 to 2 days in children 6 to 12 years old.[57] These are administered infrequently, at low doses, and for a short duration to avoid side effects such as adrenal insufficiency.

Special Procedures in Pediatric Oral Surgery

Various specialized oral surgery procedures may address unique conditions affecting children. These include soft tissue biopsies, management of impacted teeth, frenectomies for restrictive frenula, implants in limited cases, and autotransplantation as an alternative to implants in growing children. Each procedure requires thorough consideration of the child's developmental stage, specific anatomy, and potential outcomes. Pediatric patients are still developing, and some conditions may resolve or lessen with age. For example, in cases of ankyloglossia (tongue-tie), the tongue's movement and function may improve with natural growth, sometimes reducing the need for surgery. Determining the best age for a procedure can prevent complications. For instance, performing a frenectomy too early may lead to reattachment, whereas waiting may enable better outcomes with a single surgery. See Chapter 48 for a discussion of tethered oral tissues.

Biopsy and Pathology

Biopsies aid in diagnosing oral lesions and conditions that may range from benign growths to more serious pathology. Biopsies are typically indicated when a lesion or abnormality does not resolve with conservative management or when there is concern that the lesion may represent a more serious pathology. Common indications for biopsy in pediatric dentistry include persistent swellings or growths, nonhealing ulcers, pigmented lesions (especially with noticeable change), and vascular lesions, which may or may not have radiographic changes.[58,59]

In general, lesions that persist beyond 2 weeks without a clear diagnosis or fail to respond to initial treatments may need a biopsy for accurate diagnosis. Chronic ulcers that do not resolve on their own may indicate underlying autoimmune or infectious processes or even malignancy. Unusual color changes, such as dark or bluish lesions, may warrant a biopsy to rule out malignancy or vascular malformations. These lesions are monitored closely, especially if they change in size, shape, or color over time. Vascular lesions can present unique risks, as they can bleed significantly during surgical procedures. Chapter 19 offers a more detailed discussion of oral pathologic lesions. Proper evaluation with palpation, auscultation for a bruit, and possibly a needle aspiration can help determine the best approach and should be done by skilled providers in the appropriate environment.

Types of Biopsies

The two main types of biopsies performed in pediatric dentistry are excisional and incisional biopsies. An excisional biopsy involves the complete removal of a small lesion, typically less than 0.5 cm in diameter. Excisional biopsies are ideal for lesions that are well-contained and likely benign.[58] They serve both diagnostic and therapeutic purposes, as the entire abnormal tissue is removed. An incisional biopsy is used for larger lesions where removing the entire lesion may not be feasible or necessary for diagnosis. Instead, a representative section of the lesion is excised, allowing for diagnostic analysis. This approach is beneficial when the lesion is extensive or suspected to be malignant.

After the biopsy is taken, proper handling of specimens is essential to ensure accurate diagnostic outcomes. The tissue sample should be immediately placed in a formalin solution to preserve cellular structure and transported to a pathology laboratory for analysis. Care should also be taken to avoid contamination and drying of the sample. For pediatric patients, using resorbable sutures for wound closure is typically preferred to avoid a follow-up visit for suture removal.

Suturing in Pediatric Oral Surgery

Suture Types and Materials

Selecting the appropriate suture type is essential for promoting healing and minimizing stress for young patients. Although the term "resorbable" is commonly used in clinical practice, manufacturers broadly categorize them into absorbable based on the body's enzymatic degradation of the material and nonabsorbable types (nylon or silk) when this degradation process does not occur. Absorbable sutures, such as plain gut, chromic gut, and synthetic materials like polyglactin with a reverse cutting needle are typically preferred in pediatric patients.[60] These sutures naturally dissolve over time, eliminating the need for removal, which can reduce follow-up visits and alleviate anxiety in children. For soft tissue closures and cases where sutures are in hard-to-access areas, absorbable sutures are especially useful. A size 3-0 (or "000") is a common suture size with a ½ or ¾ reverse cutting needle shape. Common suture materials are presented in Table 34.5.

Technique

Interrupted sutures using 3-0 absorbable suture material with a reverse cutting needle are commonly used in pediatric oral surgery due to their versatility, ease of placement, and the ability to adjust each suture independently.[61] Before placing sutures to close a wound or incision, tissue edges must be well approximated and free of tension as sutures placed under tension are likely to fall out or tear through tissue.[62] Using needle drivers (with a crosshatch pattern made for holding the needle securely), insert the needle perpendicular to tissue surface on the buccal or lingual surface about 2 to 3 mm from the wound edge to avoid tearing the tissue (Fig. 34.13). Traditional hemostats can be used if needle drivers are not available. Pass the needle through the tissue on the subcutaneous side, bringing it out on the opposite side of the wound.[61] Once the suture is in place, tie a secure knot with a gentle pull, ensuring the wound edges are approximated without excessive tension. The knot should lie on one side of the wound and not over the wound edges. Carefully trim any excess suture material, leaving a short tail to prevent irritation. Throughout the procedure, avoid excessive force on the needle or suture material to minimize tissue trauma. Pediatric tissues are delicate, so maintaining a gentle technique promotes smoother healing and reduces postoperative discomfort. Using small, resorbable sutures and gentle handling contributes to a better recovery experience for young patients. Additional sutures may be placed and are usually 3 to 4 mm apart.

Management of Impacted Teeth

Impacted teeth, particularly maxillary canines, are a common concern in pediatric dentistry because they have a high rate of ectopic eruption.[63] Timely diagnosis and intervention are critical for preserving proper alignment and reducing the need for more complex treatments in the future[64] (see Chapter 25 for a detailed discussion of diagnostic approaches and extraction recommendations for the primary canine). For teeth that cannot be redirected and remain impacted, cone beam computed tomography (CBCT) offers 3D imaging, which provides highly detailed information on the impacted tooth's position in relation to other structures.

Surgical Management of Impacted Canines

If the impacted tooth has favorable positioning (e.g., the tooth is not inverted or laying horizontal) and incomplete root development, passive eruption can often be achieved by exposing the crown and allowing natural forces to facilitate eruption.[65] In some cases, only a minor incision of soft tissue is needed to expose the tooth, whereas in some case removal of bone is also necessary.

In cases where the crown of the permanent canine overlaps the lateral incisor root by more than 50%, the chance of normal eruption diminishes. Thus in cases where active (facilitated) eruption is necessary, the crown of the tooth is surgically exposed and an orthodontic bracket or chain is attached to gradually bring the tooth into proper alignment.[66,67] This technique is beneficial when the tooth is in a challenging position or when root development is complete. Ensuring adequate space for the impacted tooth to erupt is essential for eruption. Orthodontic appliances or

TABLE 34.5 Characteristics of Common Suture Materials

Suture Material	Type	Resorbable	Time Until Resorption	Characteristics
Plain gut	Natural	Yes	7–10 days	Fast-absorbing, made from animal collagen; low tensile strength, often used for mucosal closures
Chromic gut	Natural	Yes	10–21 days	Treated with chromic salts to slow absorption; moderate tensile strength; used in oral mucosa and soft tissue
Polyglycolic acid	Synthetic	Yes	28–30 days	Absorbable braided suture; maintains strength longer than gut; often used in soft tissue closure
Polyglactin (Vicryl)	Synthetic	Yes	56–70 days	Braided, resorbable; good handling and knot security; common for internal sutures
Silk	Natural	No[a]	N/A	Nonresorbable braided suture; good handling, but higher risk of infection in some areas; used in skin and mucosal closures

[a]Other nonresorbable sutures include nylon, polypropylene, and polyester, which have high tensile strength and minimal tissue reaction.

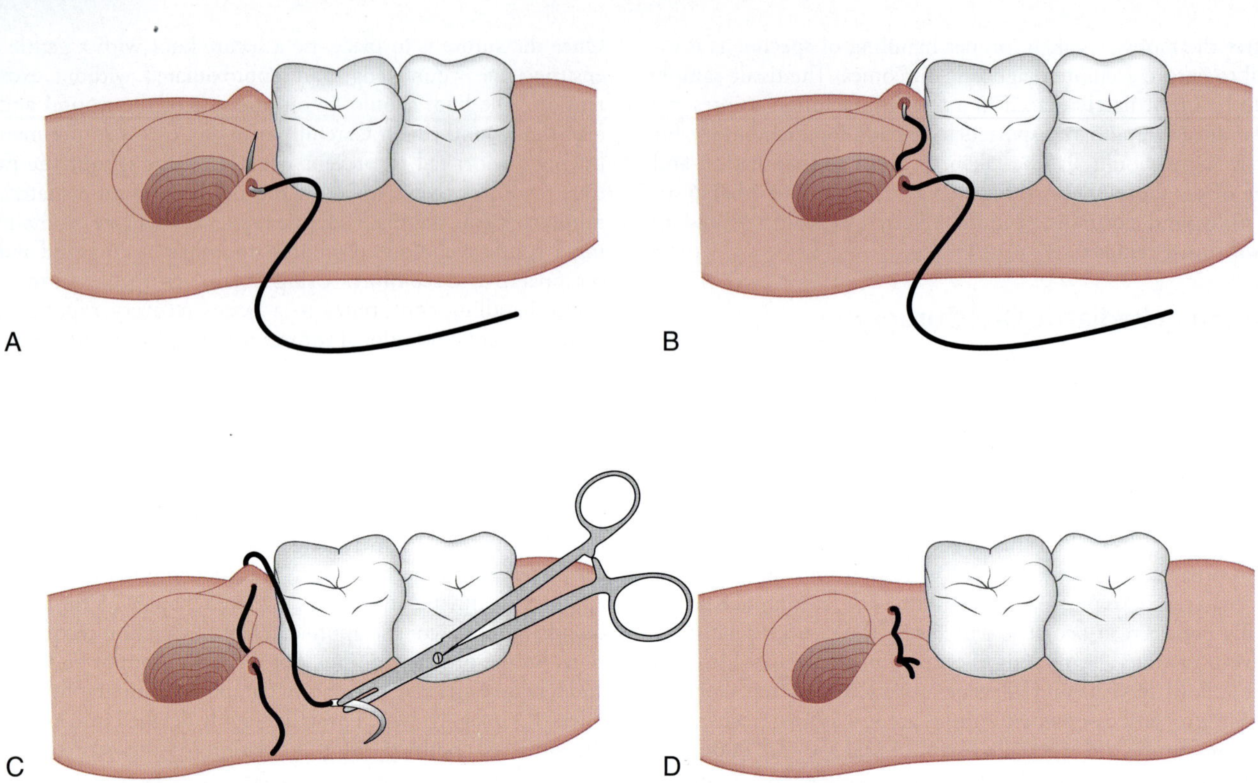

• **Fig. 34.13** Interrupted Suturing. (A) Needle passes through buccal papilla on the "outside" of the wound. (B) Needle passes through lingual papilla on the "inside" of the wound. (C) Suture is pulled through to shorten tail. (D) Knot is tied, often with a surgeon's knot.

other appliances can be used to create space, allowing the tooth to erupt into the arch without interference.[67] Care must be taken to avoid disturbing the cementum or root structure of the impacted tooth, as trauma can increase the risk of ankylosis, which would prevent proper eruption.

Surgical Management of Mesiodens and Supernumerary Teeth

Supernumerary teeth occur most commonly in the anterior maxilla and are referred to as mesiodens when positioned near the midline. The prevalence of supernumerary teeth ranges from 0.5% to 3.8%; conical mesiodens are the most frequent type in pediatric patients.[68] They can occur singly, in pairs, or in higher numbers.[69] Early identification is essential, as supernumerary teeth can disrupt normal tooth eruption, cause malocclusion, and lead to crowding, delayed eruption, or resorption of adjacent teeth.[70] They can be diagnosed through clinical examination and confirmed with radiographs, typically a maxillary occlusal, panoramic or, if necessary, a CBCT scan to better assess the exact position and orientation of the extra tooth.

In cases when a mesiodens is not inverted and erupts on its own, it can simply be extracted when the crown is sufficiently erupted. In cases where the mesiodens does not erupt but is impeding eruption of incisors, a more complex surgical approach is necessary.[71] The timing for the removal of supernumerary teeth depends on the child's age, the tooth's position (buccal, midalveolar, or palatal), and its effect on surrounding structures. The extraction should be delayed until the root of the successor is one-half to two-thirds developed, with removal before the root formation of adjacent permanent teeth to minimize the risk of misalignment or delayed eruption.[71,72] Maxillary central incisor root completion is usually 9 to 10 years of age, and maxillary lateral incisors is 10 years, on average, so referrals and treatment should precede this by 1 to 2 years. In some cases, if the mesiodens does not cause immediate issues or affect surrounding teeth, a clinician may delay extraction until later in the mixed dentition stage.[71,72] An example would be a mesiodens that does not erupt but is located palatal to maxillary incisors and does not obstruct the normal eruption of the incisors.

The standard surgical technique involves creating a small flap incision over the affected area to expose the supernumerary tooth. The flap must provide adequate visibility while preserving gingival tissue. After flap elevation, careful use of a dental handpiece allows for minimal bone removal around the supernumerary tooth, enabling safe extraction with limited trauma. Elevators are used to luxate the tooth gently, and, if the root is malformed or if the tooth is fused with another, the tooth may be sectioned for easier removal. During the procedure, it is necessary to avoid disturbing the roots of adjacent permanent teeth, especially in cases where the supernumerary tooth is near the developing dentition. If the successor has eruption potential (an open apex), then the soft tissue can be closed, and the tooth can be monitored for continued root development and eruption. If the successor has minimal eruption potential (i.e., a fully formed root with a closed apex), then the "expose and bond" to assist with active eruption can occur at the same time the surgical extraction is completed.[73,74] This must be coordinated with the orthodontist if appliances are needed to create space or facilitate eruption.

Potential Complications and Postoperative Care

Complications of supernumerary tooth extraction include swelling, minor bleeding, and potential infection. Rarely, there may be injury to adjacent tooth buds, particularly in younger patients. Postoperative care includes pain management with age-appropriate analgesics and guidelines for a soft diet for a few days to reduce trauma at the surgical site (see "Postoperative Care and Follow-Up in Pediatric Surgery" later in this chapter).

Follow-up appointments allow providers to monitor healing and assess the eruption pattern of the surrounding permanent teeth, as the removal of supernumerary teeth can positively affect the alignment and spacing of the dentition. Regular radiographic monitoring may also be recommended to detect any residual effects on the developing teeth. Early diagnosis, careful timing, and a minimally invasive approach can significantly reduce the effect of supernumerary teeth on the child's developing dentition.

Implants in Pediatric Patients

Dental implants are generally avoided in growing pediatric patients due to the need for complete skeletal growth for long-term stability.[75] However, in select cases, implants may be considered for older adolescents who are close to skeletal maturity and have lost teeth due to trauma or congenital absence.[75] In some conditions, such as ectodermal dysplasia, early implants may be recommended to assist with the retention and stability of prostheses but are not generally placed for individual tooth replacement.[76]

Timing is a key consideration when considering implants for pediatric patients. Placement before skeletal maturity is generally avoided, as the implant can become misaligned as the surrounding bone continues to grow, leading to noticeable defects.[77] Growth is generally complete around age 18, with a tendency for females to cease growth slightly before 18, whereas males may cease growth slightly later. Everyone follows a different growth trajectory and should therefore be assessed individually. Growth can be determined by general anthropometrics (i.e., height), hand-wrist films or other long bones in the body, cervical vertebral maturation, or serial cephalometric radiographs.

Growth is particularly problematic in the maxillary anterior region, where vertical bone growth is significant during adolescence.[77,78] Implant placement in younger patients may also involve bone grafting if alveolar bone volume is inadequate. In such cases, careful long-term monitoring and follow-up are essential to evaluate osseointegration and ensure proper alignment with adjacent teeth. The potential for future implant placement is a key consideration when evaluating all possible treatment options, such as retained primary second molars with missing successor premolars or anterior teeth extracted due to trauma. The sequential treatment plan must facilitate the option for future implant placement.

Autotransplantation

Autotransplantation involves relocating a tooth from one site in the mouth to another within the same individual. An appropriate donor tooth must be identified as an initial step in the treatment planning process. It is a viable option for addressing congenitally missing teeth in one arch when combined with arch length discrepancies or clinical signs of tooth crowding in the opposite arch.[79] It is also suitable for replacing teeth with poor endodontic or restorative prognosis and managing cases of cleft lip and palate or developmental dental anomalies and is a valuable option for growing patients who need a replacement tooth but are not suitable candidates for implants due to their ongoing growth.[80] It can also be used in cases of impacted canines to move a tooth from an undesirable location to its ideal location. Unlike implants, which osseointegrate and impede alveolar development, autotransplanted teeth have vital periodontium and are compatible with the eruption process of adjacent teeth and ongoing bone growth of the maxillary or mandibular arch.[81] The recipient site determines what is a suitable donor tooth. In the maxillary anterior region, the donor tooth is often a single rooted premolar with an open root apex (approximately two-thirds developed), which has the capacity to maintain vascularity or revascularize and continue root development in its new location.[82–84] Third molars can replace missing first or second molars.[84] Autotransplantation is a specialized procedure presented in this chapter as a consideration for treatment planning. The procedure itself is usually completed by providers with advanced training (see Chapter 46 for further discussion).

Surgical Management of Ankylosed Teeth

Ankylosed teeth, characterized by fusion of the tooth's root to the alveolar bone, pose significant challenges for extraction due to the absence of a periodontal ligament.[85] Ankylosis is confirmed through clinical signs (e.g., lack of mobility, infraocclusion, and a dull sound when tapping with the handle of an intraoral mirror) and radiographic evidence (e.g., loss of periodontal ligament space). Ankylosis is generally described as mild, moderate, or severe. The teeth most often affected are traumatized permanent incisors and primary second molars. Teeth with mild ankylosis usually exfoliate without intervention when a successor premolar is present, so monitoring is usually sufficient as supraeruption of opposing teeth and tipping of adjacent teeth do not usually occur (see Fig. 34.10).[86] In the presence of moderate ankylosis where a distinct vertical defect is present (noted with an occlusal step and mesial tipping of the distal tooth), space maintenance may be necessary.[87] Other efforts to reduce supraeruption of the opposing tooth and tipping of adjacent teeth can include composite resin buildups or stainless steel crown placement.[88–90] Chapter 24 offers a discussion of treatment options for an ankylosed primary molar.

In cases of severe ankylosis, surgical intervention should be completed before the primary tooth becomes completely submerged.[88,89] When the determination to extract an ankylosed tooth is made, surgical management typically involves careful treatment planning and technique. When multiple teeth are affected or the ankylosis is moderate to severe, referral to an oral surgeon may be more appropriate, whereas isolated extractions of mildly ankylosed teeth may be more predictable (see previous discussion of sectioning ankylosed teeth).

Complications in Pediatric Oral Surgery

Pediatric oral surgery, while generally safe, carries inherent risks due to the anatomical, physiologic, and developmental differences between children and adults. Complications can range from minor issues like delayed healing to more serious concerns, such as nerve damage or anesthesia-related complications, which are described in Table 34.6.

Prevention and Risk Mitigation

Preventing complications in pediatric oral surgery requires a multifaceted approach beginning with a thorough preoperative assessment. As discussed previously, a comprehensive medical and

TABLE 34.6 Surgical Complications and Their Management

Problem	Description	Management
Anesthesia-related complications	Children may experience respiratory depression, allergic reactions, or postanesthetic nausea and vomiting due to differences in metabolism and sensitivity to anesthetics. Respiratory arrest is rare.	Supportive care such as oxygen therapy, careful monitoring in a controlled environment, and administration of antiemetics (e.g., ondansetron) for nausea. Immediate medical attention for allergic reactions. Document reactions for future reference.
Aspiration of tooth	Proper patient positioning and pharyngeal protection (eg, rubber dam, Isolite, or throat screen) are essential to prevent aspiration if a tooth dislodges from forceps due to operator error or patient movement.	If a tooth cannot be retrieved and aspiration is suspected, immediate medical referral for chest imaging is warranted.
Delayed healing	Delayed healing can result from poor postoperative care, underlying medical conditions, or infection, affecting the child's ability to eat, speak, and maintain oral hygiene.	Advise a soft diet, gentle brushing, and age-appropriate antimicrobial mouth rinses. Follow-up evaluations are necessary to rule out underlying conditions or infection. Consider additional interventions like chlorhexidine rinses.
Hemorrhage	Prolonged bleeding may occur, especially with extensive soft tissue manipulation or undiagnosed bleeding disorders. Pediatric patients generally have better hemostasis, but complications can arise.	Apply pressure with gauze, use local hemostatic agents (e.g., Gelfoam or Surgicel), and potentially suture the site to promote clot formation. If bleeding persists, caregivers should contact the dentist or oral surgeon for possible medical/systemic intervention.
Infection	Postoperative infections can lead to localized swelling, pain, and fever. Children are more vulnerable due to developing immune systems and potentially less thorough hygiene habits.	Administer appropriate antibiotics (e.g., amoxicillin or azithromycin for penicillin-allergic patients). Severe infections may require surgical drainage of abscesses. Irrigate the affected areas and recommend antiseptic rinses.
Nerve damage	Rare nerve damage may occur during procedures involving the mandibular canal, mental nerve, or inferior alveolar nerve, leading to temporary or permanent sensory loss or paresthesia.	Immediate reevaluation if nerve damage is suspected. Conservative treatment focusing on monitoring sensory return. If damage persists, refer to a specialist. Corticosteroids may be considered to reduce inflammation and aid recovery.
Soft tissue trauma	Due to the small oral cavity and developing dentition, there is a risk of damaging adjacent tissues during surgery, causing swelling, bruising, and discomfort.	Apply soothing topical agents, recommend a soft diet, and use ice packs to minimize swelling and bruising. Monitor for signs of infection, as trauma can increase the risk of secondary infections.
Unusual pain or swelling	Some swelling and discomfort are normal, but caregivers should be alert to severe or worsening symptoms, which can indicate complications.	Antiinflammatories, antipyretics, and cold compresses can help with mild to moderate pain and swelling. Swelling that interferes with breathing or swallowing requires immediate medical intervention.

dental history with attention to the need for prophylactic antibiotics should be obtained, and radiographic evaluations can reveal anatomical details that may complicate surgery.

Risk management also involves proper communication and consent. Parents and older pediatric patients should be instructed on appropriate postoperative care and the need for follow-up appointments. Effective management of complications requires prompt intervention and a clear understanding of pediatric care protocols. When unanticipated events occur, they should be noted and discussed with the family. Table 34.6 outlines strategies to manage surgical complications.

Postoperative Care and Follow-Up in Pediatric Oral Surgery

The AAPD offers the resource "Postoperative Instructions for Extractions/Oral Surgery," which aims to minimize complications and promote healing.[16] The following are key postoperative instructions for patients who have had oral surgery.

Bleeding control: Gauze should be placed at the extraction site, with the child instructed to bite down gently for approximately 15 minutes. In younger or sedated children, an intraoral gauze pack extending out of the mouth prevents accidental swallowing.

Diet: Following surgery, children should consume soft, cool foods that are easy to chew and will not irritate the surgical site (i.e., yogurt, applesauce, scrambled eggs, and smoothies). Hot, spicy, or acidic foods should be avoided. Parents may also be advised to avoid foods with small particles, such as rice, which may lodge in the surgical site. The use of straws should be discouraged to prevent dislodging the blood clot.

Activity restrictions: Children should rest after surgery and avoid strenuous activities (i.e., running/jumping) for the first 24 to 48 hours to reduce the risk of bleeding and swelling. Parents should monitor their child's activity level and discourage behaviors such as touching or disturbing the surgical area.

Pain management: Pediatric doses of analgesics, such as ibuprofen or acetaminophen, are recommended (see Chapter 28 for a discussion of pain management). Nonpharmacologic measures like cold compresses can also reduce swelling and pain. For more involved surgeries, see previous discussion of pain management.

Oral hygiene: Parents should encourage gentle brushing, avoiding the area around the surgical site for the first few days. In some

• BOX 34.3 Postoperative Healing Timeline for Extraction Sites

- **Day 1–2:** Blood clot forms, site appears red with slight swelling; mild discomfort or minor bleeding may occur.
- **Day 3–4:** Clot stabilizes, and initial granulation tissue begins forming; site may appear less red.
- **Week 1:** Granulation tissue proliferates, covering the socket; swelling and discomfort significantly reduce.
- **Weeks 2–3:** Granulation tissue matures, and early epithelialization occurs; site appears pink and smoother.
- **Weeks 4–6:** Bone remodeling begins under the soft tissue; socket is fully covered with epithelium and may feel firm.
- **Months 3–6:** Significant bone healing; complete bone fill may take longer in larger defects.

cases, rinsing with a mild saltwater solution or an antiseptic rinse can help keep the area clean without disturbing the healing tissue. Maintaining hygiene reduces oral bacteria and promotes healing.

Follow-up care: A follow-up appointment allows the dentist to monitor healing, detect any late-developing complications, and ensure that growth and development remain on track. In cases of trauma, follow-up is essential for evaluating pulpal and periodontal ligament status. Parents should be informed about the warning signs of complications and seek prompt follow-up care if these symptoms occur Table 34.6. Understanding what healing should look like in the days, weeks, and months after extractions can help the practitioner identify normal versus abnormal healing as shown in Box 34.3.

Future Directions in Pediatric Oral Surgery

The field of pediatric oral surgery is advancing rapidly, driven by new technologies, evolving research, and a focus on improved patient outcomes. Technologic advancements are revolutionizing pediatric oral surgery, particularly through tools like 3D imaging, laser surgery, and conservative surgical techniques.

3D Imaging

Traditional two-dimensional x-rays can only provide limited information on the complex anatomy of a child's developing oral structures. In contrast, 3D imaging, such as CBCT, offers detailed, multidimensional views that enhance diagnostic accuracy and surgical planning. CBCT allows clinicians to assess impacted teeth, root structures, and bone density with precision, reducing surgical risks and improving outcomes. This technology also facilitates virtual treatment planning, enabling surgeons to simulate procedures and anticipate challenges before entering the operating room.

Laser Surgery

Laser technology is making pediatric oral surgery less invasive and more precise. Lasers minimize bleeding and swelling, reduce the need for sutures, and often allow for a faster recovery with less postoperative discomfort. Laser techniques are especially beneficial for soft tissue procedures, such as frenectomies and biopsies. For example, diode and CO_2 lasers can remove soft tissue lesions or treat ankyloglossia (tongue-tie) with minimal pain and faster healing. Laser surgery is also associated with a reduced risk of infection and scarring, making it an appealing option for young patients and their caregivers.

Research and Clinical Trials

Ongoing research and clinical trials are shaping the future of pediatric oral surgery, focusing on safety, efficacy, and long-term outcomes.

Regenerative techniques: Researchers are exploring the potential for regenerative treatments to repair or replace damaged tissues. Stem cell research and tissue engineering are promising avenues that could eventually allow tooth structures, bone, or soft tissue regeneration. Such advancements could drastically reduce the need for more invasive surgical procedures, particularly in cases of trauma or congenital disabilities where growth and development are still ongoing.

Pain management: Pain management remains a critical area of research as practitioners seek safer and more effective ways to manage postoperative discomfort in children. Studies are examining alternative analgesic methods, including nerve blocks, long-acting local anesthetics, and nonopioid medications, to provide effective pain relief with minimal side effects. Research on nonpharmacologic approaches, such as cold therapy, acupuncture, and psychological techniques, also holds promise for pediatric patients who may benefit from a combination of methods for comprehensive pain management.

Infection control and antibiotic stewardship: Pediatric oral surgery often involves prophylactic antibiotics to prevent postoperative infections. However, with rising concerns about antibiotic resistance, clinical trials are exploring optimal antibiotic use, alternative infection control methods, and wound care innovations that reduce the need for antibiotics. For instance, studies on antimicrobial mouth rinses, local antibiotic gels, and low-dose systemic antibiotics are being conducted to ensure effective infection control while minimizing antibiotic overuse.

Conclusion

Mastering pediatric oral surgery includes applying key principles, preoperative assessments, proper technique for extractions, and understanding the management of infections. A structured approach with careful technique and communication ensures success and supports recovery. Collaboration with families and healthcare professionals improves outcomes. Staying updated on new techniques and research helps maintain high standards of care and positive experiences for pediatric patients.

Visit eBooks.Health.Elsevier.com to see full list of references.

PART 4

Special Considerations

35 Medical Emergencies

MATTHEW R. COOKE AND R. JOHN BREWER

CHAPTER OUTLINE

Medical Emergencies in the Pediatric Dental Office

Medical emergencies occur within the practice of pediatric dentistry.[1] A medical emergency is defined as a sudden, unexpected deviation from the normally expected pattern (normal physiology). Emergencies can occur with anyone: the patient, parent/guardian, or other individuals who accompany the patient, the dentist, or the staff.[1]

Morbidity

All types of medical emergencies occur. Some are seen more frequently (allergic reactions, asthma, cardiac arrest, diabetes mellitus, hyperventilation, seizures, and syncope) and will be discussed later in the chapter. Acute events result in morbidity, a diseased state, disability, or poor health due to any cause.[2]

Mortality

Emergencies in the pediatric dental office may threaten the patient's life. However, only on rare occasions is death the outcome. Objectives in medical emergency training include management of morbidity to prevent mortality.[1]

"Swiss Cheese Model" of Accident Causation

Medical emergencies are the result of system failure.[3] Every step in a process has the potential for failure. The ideal system is similar to sliced Swiss cheese. This model is often referred to as the "Swiss cheese model" of accident causation.[3] The holes represent opportunities for failure, and each slice serves as a "defensive layer" in the process. An error may allow a problem to pass through a hole in one layer, but in the next layer the holes are in different places, allowing the issue to be identified. Each layer serves as a defense against additional errors that impact the total outcome (Fig. 35.1A).[3] Catastrophic errors occur when the holes align for each step in the process, allowing all defenses to be defeated (see Fig. 35.1B).[3]

The Swiss cheese model includes both active and latent failures or "sins of commission and sins of omission." Active failures are the unsafe acts that can directly cause an accident. Latent failures refer to not acting when indicated to prevent or manage a situation. Both types of failure contribute to catastrophic outcomes. The Swiss cheese model is respected and considered useful, but it may not explain all medical emergencies in the pediatric dental office.[4]

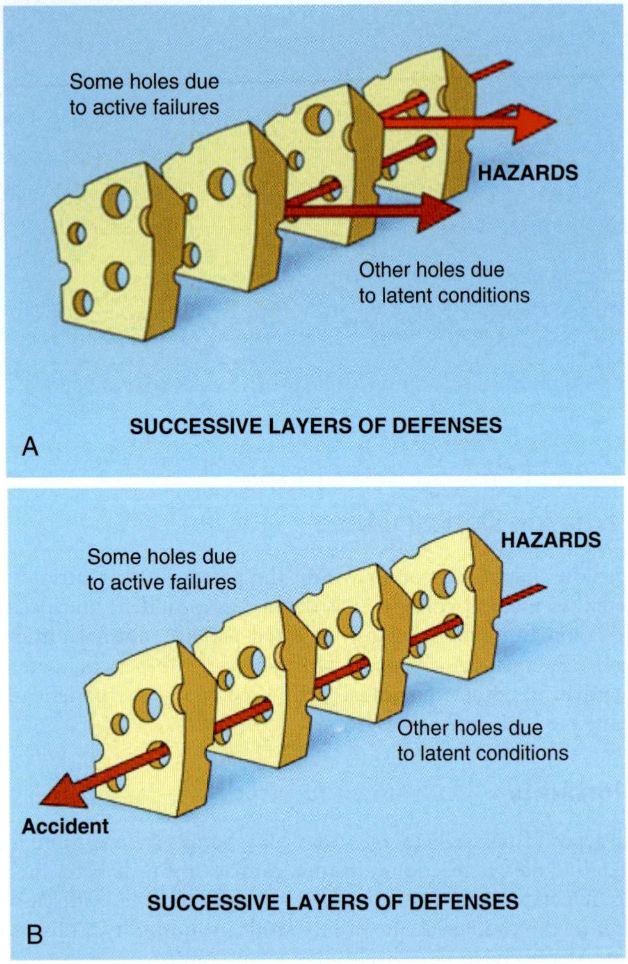

• **Fig. 35.1** (A–B) Swiss cheese illustration. (From Reason J. *Human Error.* Cambridge University Press; 1990.)

Fear, anxiety, and pain are often associated with the surgical specialty of pediatric dentistry. Acute stress reactions result in surges of endogenous catecholamines.[1] The physiologic response may be conducive to the development of a medical emergency.[5] Add highly vasoactive drugs, such as local anesthetics and vasoconstrictors, used for almost all pediatric dental procedures, and the probability for a medical emergency increases.[1] Other drugs, such as antibiotics, sedatives, and analgesics, also carry the potential for producing acute, life-threatening reactions from toxicity or allergy.[1]

Recognition and action are key steps. Because pediatric dentists are not routinely managing medical emergencies, there may be uneasiness when expected to handle a crisis in the dental office. However, what may be an emergency to one provider may be a normal occurrence to another.[6] Responsibilities of the pediatric dentist include prevention, preparation, basic life support (BLS), basic emergency medicine procedures, and procurement of help.[7] Patients may require transfer by Emergency Medical Services (EMS) personnel to an appropriate medical facility for definitive diagnosis and treatment. Upon recognition of a medical emergency, the pediatric dentist should attempt to stabilize the patient.

Prevention of Medical Emergencies

Undoubtedly, preventing the occurrence of medical emergencies is most desired.[1] Studies show that a complete system evaluation of all dental patients can prevent approximately 90% of life-threatening situations.[8–10] The remaining 10% will occur despite the best preventive efforts.[9] Knowledge of acute and chronic conditions allows for medical optimization and risk reduction, thus decreasing the probability of a medical emergency.[1,9] Completing a pretreatment assessment or evaluation is essential and is accomplished with a complete medical history and physical examination. A medical consultation should be considered, when indicated.[1]

History and Physical Examination

Knowledge of existing medical conditions, which predispose the patient, will prevent the vast majority of emergency situations.[1,8,9] Assessment of the patient's psychological outlook to dental treatment should also be included. The medical history is generally obtained via a written questionnaire, which is completed by the patient or parent.[11,12] Many standardized forms are available, but they may require modification for pediatric dental practice. These forms should include questions pertaining to any present or past medical conditions, allergies or adverse drug reactions, hospitalizations, surgeries, and medications (Fig. 35.2). Questions regarding dental concerns as well as past dental treatment are frequently included (see Chapter 10). The dentist should review this form, note positive findings, and conduct a brief interview with the patient to clarify and expand on the questionnaire. Clarifications and further explanations of positive findings should also be written by the dentist in the record, documenting that these questions were thoroughly addressed.[12] An example of this would be if a parent notes "asthma" on the medical history form. Asthma is the second most prevalent chronic condition in pediatric patients and it has multiple forms (mild, intermittent through severe, persistent). It is the responsibility of the pediatric dentist to obtain more information than the mere fact that the patient currently has or has had asthma in the past. The dentist should further document the frequency and severity of the asthma attacks, what causes them, how they are managed, and whether past episodes were ever so severe that treatment was emergently needed in the hospital or emergency room. Also, it is prudent to determine when the last attack occurred, and finally whether the patient is breathing easily today. Based on the assessment of these documented clarifications, the dentist may feel comfortable providing the needed dental treatment at that appointment or may decide to postpone treatment until the patient is medically optimized by his or her physician.[12]

The physical examination should include baseline vital signs (blood pressure, pulse rate and rhythm, respiratory rate and character See Chapter 7, Table 7.2 for normal vital signs by age), a thorough head and neck examination, and observation of general appearance (gait, mental status, skin tone and color, etc.).[12] Further physical evaluation should be dictated by the dentist's training, expertise, and plan.[12,13]

A complete history and physical examination will give the pediatric dentist insight into preexisting conditions that potentially may lead to a medical emergency.[1,12] Conditions involving the cardiac, pulmonary, and endocrine systems are of greatest concern. Patients with a history of seizures also warrant special consideration. Knowledge allows the development of treatment protocols that decrease the likelihood of a serious medical event. These protocols may involve prophylaxis for infective endocarditis, proper timing of appointments, or the use of sedation/anesthesia for stress-induced condtions.[1,13–15]

MEDICAL HISTORY

Child's Full Name ________________________________ Date of Birth ______/______/______

Child's Physician/Pediatrician ________________ Child's Pediatrician's Telephone:________________

Pediatrician's Address: ____

Medications or Treatments

1. Is your child up to date on immunizations? ☐ No ☐ Yes
2. Is your child currently taking any medication (prescription, over-the-counter medicines, or inhalers)? ☐ No ☐ Yes
3. Has your child ever received radiation or chemotherapy or is it planned? ☐ No ☐ Yes

If yes to any of the above, please explain: ________________________________

Allergies

1. Is your child allergic to any medication? ☐ No ☐ Yes
2. Is your child allergic to latex? ☐ No ☐ Yes
3. Any other allergies such as skin, food, etc.? ☐ No ☐ Yes

If yes to any of the above, please explain: ________________________________

Please indicate if your child has or has a history of any of the following:

Growth and Development:

☐ Birth complications/premature ☐ Physical growth ☐ Delayed growth ☐ Intellectual disabilities
☐ Behavioral problems/disorders ☐ Learning disabilities ☐ Communication difficulties ☐ None of these

If yes to any of the above, please explain: ________________________________

Central Nervous System:

☐ Cerebral palsy ☐ Epilepsy (seizures)/convulsions ☐ Fainting ☐ Autism spectrum disorder
☐ Speech, hearing, vision problems ☐ Hydrocephaly ☐ None of these

If yes to any of the above, please explain: ________________________________

Heart Problems:

☐ Congenital heart disease ☐ Heart murmur ☐ Heart damage from rheumatic fever
☐ High blood pressure ☐ Any other heart problems ☐ None of these

If yes to any of the above, please explain: ________________________________

Blood:

☐ Blood transfusion ☐ Anemia ☐ Sickle cell disease/trait ☐ Cancer
☐ Bruise easily ☐ Frequent nosebleeds ☐ Bleed excessively from small cuts ☐ None of these
☐ Other blood disorder

If yes to any of the above, please explain: ________________________________

Breathing:

☐ Asthma ☐ Shortness of breath ☐ Difficulty in breathing
☐ Pneumonia ☐ Cystic fibrosis ☐ Any other breathing problem ☐ None of these
☐ Snoring ☐ Obstructive sleep disorder

If yes to any of the above, please explain: ________________________________

• **Fig. 35.2** Sample medical history questionnaire.

Continued

Digestive system:
☐ Stomach/intestinal problems ☐ Hepatitis ☐ Jaundice or liver problems ☐ Other
☐ Eating disorders/problems ☐ Unexplained weight loss ☐ Reflux/GERD ☐ None of these
If yes to any of the above, please explain: ______

Reproductive/Urinary system:
☐ Bladder/kidney problem ☐ Is the patient pregnant or possibly pregnant? ☐ None of these
If yes to any of the above, please explain: ______

Glands:
☐ Diabetes ☐ Thyroid disorders ☐ Gland problems ☐ None of these
If yes to any of the above, please explain: ______

Skin:
☐ Skin problems ☐ Rash/hives, eczema ☐ Cold sores or canker sores ☐ None of these
If yes to any of the above, please explain: ______

Arms/Legs:
☐ Limitations of arms or legs ☐ Arthritis ☐ Joint bleeding ☐ None of these
☐ Joint replacement ☐ Muscular dystrophy ☐ Muscle weakness
If yes to any of the above, please explain: ______

Hospitalizations

Has your child been hospitalized? ☐ No ☐ Yes
If yes, please list hospital, date, and reason: ______

Please check any of the illnesses that your child has now, has recently been exposed to, or has had in the past:

☐ HIV/AIDS ☐ Tuberculosis (TB)
☐ Scarlet fever ☐ Methicillin resistant staphylococcus aureus (MRSA)
☐ Substance abuse, alcoholism, drug addiction
☐ Upper respiratory infection, common cold, sinus infection, or tonsillitis
☐ Sexually Transmitted disease (genital herpes, gonorrhea, syphilis, other)

Is your child presently being seen by a physician? ☐ No ☐ Yes
If yes, for what reason:
______

Is there any other significant medical history pertaining to this child or his/her family that the dentist should be told?
☐ No ☐ Yes
If yes, describe: ______

______ ______ ______
Signature (Parent or guardian) Relationship to child Date

• **Fig. 35.2, cont'd**

Medical Consultation

Consultation with the physician of a medically compromised patient is highly advised before treatment.[1,12] The outdated concept of obtaining "medical clearance" from a medical consultant before initiation of a dental procedure has now been superseded by requesting the consultant's statement that "the patient is in optimal condition for the planned procedure."[1,12] The information obtained should help the dentist develop the safest treatment plan for the mutual patient.

Patient Monitoring

Monitoring is continuous observation of physiologic parameters over time.[13] The dentist and/or trained staff member should always be monitoring/observing the patient.[12–24] The level of monitoring necessary to safely treat a pediatric dental patient depends on the procedure to be provided, the patient's underlying medical condition, and the management technique used.[1,13,23,24]

When changes are detected, an intervention can be implemented, preventing potentially dangerous situations.

Monitor/observe the general appearance of the patient, including the level of consciousness, level of comfort, muscle tone, color of the skin and mucosa, and respiratory pattern. For the majority of healthy patients being treated with local anesthesia alone or with minimal sedation as defined by the American Dental Association, this is all the monitoring that is necessary.[23] The patient should never be left alone once drugs (local anesthetics or sedative agents) are administered.[21,22,24,25]

Moderate sedation requires a time-based record including blood pressure, pulse, and pulse oximetry. Waveform capnography is strongly recommended.[13] A precordial stethoscope should also be used (Fig. 35.3).[13] Electrocardiography monitoring should be considered, though at this time it is not a requirement for

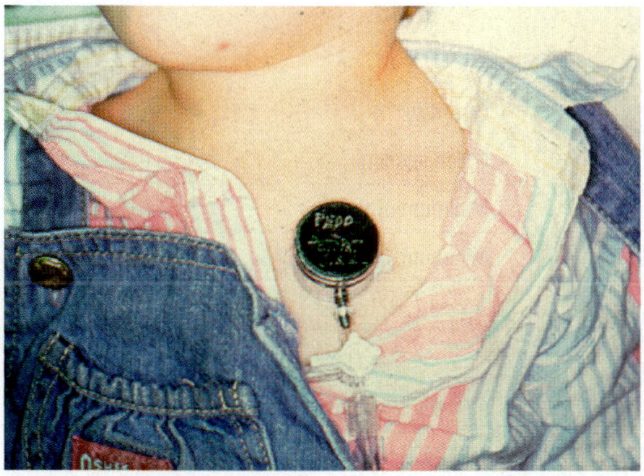

• **Fig. 35.3** Use of a precordial stethoscope.

moderate sedation in children under 12 years of age.[13] These measures are particularly important for patients with whom continual verbal contact is difficult or undesirable[13] (see Chapter 27 for a detailed discussion of monitoring during sedation). Deep sedation and general anesthesia require advanced monitoring, as the patient is unconscious.[21,22] (*Note:* These services should only be provided by practitioners who are properly trained.) Presedation and discharge vital signs, including pulse rate, respiratory rate, and blood pressure, should always be obtained unless prevented by the lack of patient cooperation.[13] Patients should return to baseline before discharge.[13,21,22]

Preparing for Office Emergencies

All dentists and staff members must master basic life support (BLS) at the healthcare provider (HCP) level of training[1,26] and should also receive additional medical emergency training, which includes simulated medical emergency scenarios. Advanced Cardiac Life Support (ACLS) and Pediatric Advanced Life Support (PALS) are required if providing office-based sedation.[13,21,27,28] The reader is referred to the American Heart Association's publications on emergency cardiovascular care. Additionally, using cognitive aids like the Stanford Emergency Manual[29] or ADSA's "10 Minutes Saves a Life!"[30] may be invaluable in guiding teams through complex emergencies.

Personal Preparation

Although dentists cannot be expected to manage every medical emergency, they can anticipate the most likely high-risk situations in their practice.[1,31] Emergency situations that might logically occur as a direct result of medications or techniques must be anticipated and well understood.[1] Examples include local anesthetic toxicity reactions and respiratory depression secondary to sedation.[31] The dentist must be prepared to quickly carry out an action plan to manage the situation.[31,32] Personal preparation for the dentist should include, at a minimum, a working knowledge of the signs, symptoms, course, and therapy for common treatable conditions.[31,32]

Staff Preparation

The office should have an emergency plan in place. Each team member should know what is expected in an emergency.[1,32–37] Responsibilities of the team include dentist and staff providing patient care, staff to phone 911, staff for documentation, staff for assisting other patients and family members, and staff to direct EMS to the patient.

A team approach to medical emergencies will provide for organized management of emergency situations.[1,32] Closed-loop communication is essential in these scenarios, ensuring that instructions are clearly understood, and tasks are accurately completed. Regularly scheduled mock medical emergency drills will keep the team protocol running smoothly and reduce panic in an actual emergency.[32,33]

Backup Medical Assistance

The dentist and staff should be prepared to manage medical emergencies until EMS arrives, which may take 20 to 40 minutes, even in cases of cardiac arrest.[1,25,27] Dentists and staff should not rely on nearby physicians; it is their responsibility to manage the emergency until EMS arrives.[1,32,33,36] Paramedics should be requested over basic emergency medical technicians when feasible.[1]

Office Preparation: Emergency Equipment

Table 35.1 details recommended emergency equipment for the pediatric dental office. Emergency equipment for pediatric patients must be appropriately sized (infant through adolescent) and available[1,13,31,33] (Fig. 35.4).

Oxygen is the primary emergency drug in the dental office.[33] It requires specialized equipment for administration. An oxygen source capable of delivering greater than 90% oxygen at flows of 10 L/min for a minimum of 1 hour is ideal. This means that an "E" cylinder is the minimum size required. Pediatric dental patients rarely suffer myocardial infarction or cardiac arrest as the initiating medical event.[28] Drug-induced respiratory depression and loss of a patent airway during unconsciousness are much more likely to occur.[13,38,39] Hypoxemia (low oxygen content in the arterial blood) will be the final common pathway to morbidity and mortality in the majority of severe pediatric medical emergency situations.[28,38,39] Therefore establishment and maintenance of a proper airway and respiratory function is paramount.[13,33]

Adequate oxygenation is easily ensured by the administration of supplemental oxygen.[28] If the patient is adequately breathing spontaneously, oxygen may be delivered by way of a face mask, nasal mask, or nasal cannula prongs.[28] A nonrebreather face mask should be available, as this delivers the highest concentration of oxygen to the spontaneously breathing patient for the most serious medical emergencies.[28] However, should the patient cease breathing during an emergency situation, positive pressure ventilation will be necessary.[28] Although mouth-to-mouth ventilation, or preferably mouth-to-mask ventilation, is possible, this delivers only about 17% oxygen from the rescuer's lungs and is not ideal, but certainly better than no ventilation in a patient who is not breathing.[33] A positive-pressure oxygen delivery system (bag-valve-mask device) that can be connected to a high-flow oxygen source is considered essential equipment to deliver oxygen to the apneic patient (Fig. 35.5).[13,28,33] The bag-valve-mask device, face masks, and oxygen cylinder should all be together in one central location in the office.[1,13,33]

A high-volume suction device is another piece of equipment that is considered essential for the management of medical emergencies.[1,13,28] Emergency situations, especially those involving an obtunded patient, often induce vomiting.[40,41] The aspiration of vomitus can be disastrous, leading to pneumonia and death.[40–44]

TABLE 35.1 Emergency Equipment

Equipment	Description	Quantity
Suction and suction tips	High-volume suction system	Office suction
	Large-diameter round-ended suction tip (Yankauer suction)	Minimum of 2
Oxygen delivery system	Positive pressure via bag valve mask device (Ambu bag)	Minimum 1 infant, 1 child, 1 small adult, 1 large adult
	Nasal cannulas basic oxygen mask	
	Nonrebreather oxygen masks	
Airways	Oral and nasal (with appropriate sizes)	1 of each size
Patient monitor	Stethoscope, pulse oximeter, glucometer	1 of each
	Blood pressure cuffs (pediatric and adult)	
Automatic external defibrillator	Pediatric and adult pads available	1 of each
Syringes for drug administration	Disposable syringes and 18-g needle	4 3-mL syringes

If performing office-based sedation it is advised to have the following emergency equipment:

- Advanced airways
  - [a]i-gel/LMA adult and pediatric (with hands-on medical emergency training)
- Cardiac monitor
- Capnography
- IV/IO equipment
- Mucosal atomization devices
- Nebulizer masks

[a]i-gel (Intersurgical Ltd, Wokingham, Berkshire, UK).
IO, Intraosseous; *IV,* intravenous; *LMA,* laryngeal mask airway.

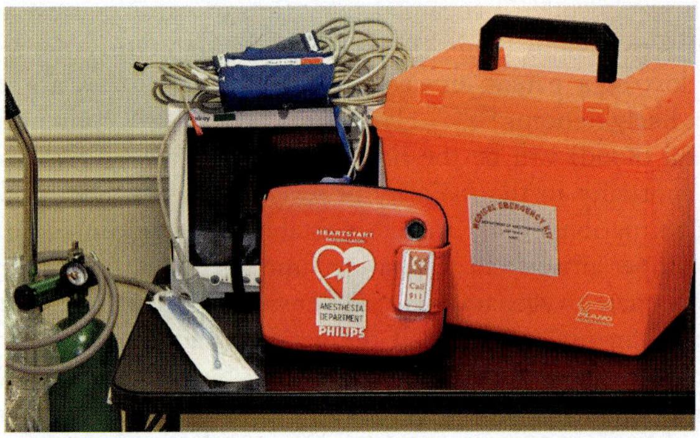

• **Fig. 35.4** Recommended emergency equipment for the pediatric dental office.

This can usually be minimized or prevented by proper patient positioning and suctioning.[41] Most dental offices contain high-volume suction equipment for restorative dentistry purposes. A Yankauer type of suction configured and connected to the high-volume evacuation dental suction unit is recommended for suctioning the mouth and pharynx (Fig. 35.6).

Other emergency items that may be needed include syringes and needles for drug administration, oropharyngeal and nasopharyngeal airways, basic monitoring devices that are appropriately sized, and automated external defibrillators (AEDs) capable of electrical therapy delivery for both children and adults.[1,33] For pediatric dentists who provide office-based sedation, the armamentarium for establishing intravenous (IV) access and advanced airway equipment (i-gel [Intersurgical Ltd, Wokingham, Berkshire, UK]/laryngeal mask airway [LMA], endotracheal tubes) should be available.[13,21]

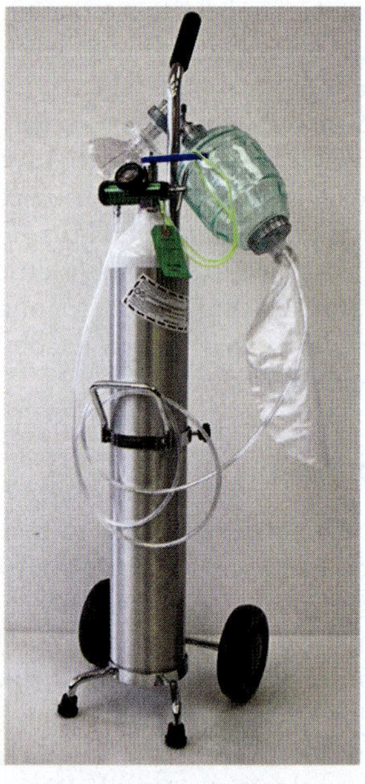

• **Fig. 35.5** Bag-valve-mask apparatus to deliver positive pressure ventilation to a nonbreathing patient.

Emergency Drugs

Medical emergencies do not always require rescue drugs.[1,31] Emergency drugs should be administered when there is a clear indication that the agent is needed.[33] There are 10 basic drugs (Table 35.2) that a pediatric dentist should have in their emergency kit (Fig. 35.7).[1,23,27,28,31–33] Pediatric dentists who

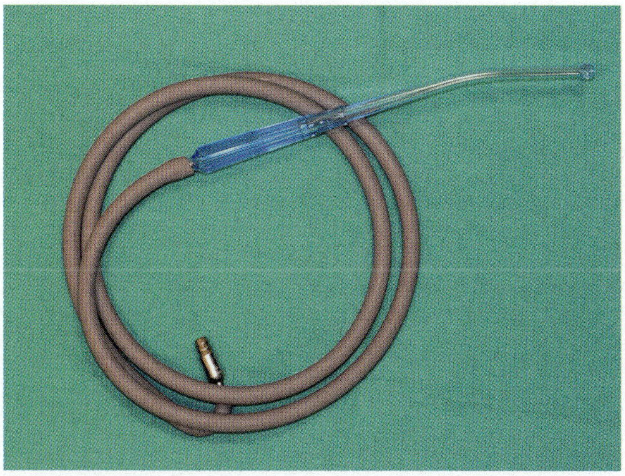

• **Fig. 35.6** A Yankauer type of suction tip enables effective suctioning without damaging surrounding tissue.

provide office-based sedation are required to have additional drugs available.[13,20,21]

Pediatric dentists should assemble their own drug kit instead of purchasing a commercial one,[33,45–47] as these kits are often expensive and not tailored to individual needs[1,33] (eFig. 35.8). Relying on a commercial kit can create a false sense of security. Emergency drugs and equipment should be stored in a single, accessible location known to the entire dental team.[1,32,33]

The pediatric dentist is responsible for knowing what drugs are available, along with indications, contraindications, dosages, and side effects.[28,33,45–47] When an emergency occurs, this may be difficult to remember; therefore it is advised to have a set of emergency drug cards as a reference.[28,47,48] It is also important to know the expiration date of rescue drugs and keep them current.[1,32,33]

Various state regulations may require specific drugs not listed in Table 35.2. The list contains only superficial information and must be expanded upon as needed.

TABLE 35.2 Emergency Drugs

Albuterol	
Indications	Treatment of bronchospasm in either asthma attack or allergic reaction
Action	B_2-adrenergic receptor agonist, which causes bronchodilation
How supplied	Metered-dose inhaler and premixed 2.5 mg/3 mL nebulized solution
Amount to keep in office	1 inhaler and 3 premixed albuterol for nebulized treatments
Dosage	2 puffs; ideally should have a spacer; may repeat as needed 2.5 mg/3 mL premixed via O_2 powered nebulizer; may repeat as needed
Side effect	Tachycardia, anxiety, shakiness in arms, hands, legs, feet
Aspirin	
Indications	Suspected acute coronary syndrome or myocardial infarction
Action	Antiplatelet agent; inhibits thromboxane synthesis
How supplied	Chewable tablet (81 mg preferable)
Amount to keep in office	1 bottle baby aspirin (81 mg)
Dosage	(4) 81 mg chewable
Side effects	Dyspepsia (initially)
Diphenhydramine	
Indications	Allergic reactions of slower onset, or less severity than anaphylaxis; adjunct drug with epinephrine in severe allergic reactions
Action	Histamine (H_1) receptor antagonist that blocks the response of the H_1 receptor to histamine
How supplied	50 mg/mL vial and oral tabs 25 mg/tab
Amount to keep in office	(3) 50 mg vials and (1) box of 25 mg tablets
Dosage	1 mg/kg IM/IV; max 50 mg
Side effects	Dry mouth, sedation
Epinephrine	
Indications	Anaphylaxis, severe persistent asthma, bronchospasm
Action	Sympathomimetic that stimulates both α- and β-adrenergic receptors, increasing heart rate and blood pressure, relaxing bronchial smooth muscle, and inhibiting histamine's action (antagonism of the physiologic effects of histamine)
How supplied	1:1000 (1 mg/mL) ampule, autoinjector 0.3 mg/mL (EpiPen) and 0.15 mg autoinjector (EpiPen Jr)
Amount to keep in office	(1) EpiPen Adult, 0.3 mg; (1) EpiPen Jr, 0.15 mg (2) 1:1000 ampules, 1 mg

Continued

TABLE 35.2 Emergency Drugs—cont'd

Dosage	Adult: 0.3 mL (0.3 mg)
	Pediatric: IM pediatric dose 0.01 mg/kg up to a maximum of 0.3 mg/dose
Side effects	Sinus tachycardia, supraventricular tachycardia and ventricular tachycardia, hypertension, chest pain, anxiety, and headache
Glucose (Oral)	
Indications	Treatment of very low blood sugar (hypoglycemia), most often in people with diabetes mellitus
Action	Will raise blood sugar if patient is able to swallow
How supplied	37.5 g tube
Amount to keep in office	(4) 37.5 g tubes
Dosage	Swallow 37.5 g; may repeat as necessary
Side effects	N/A
Midazolam (Versed)	
Indications	Anticonvulsant for management of status epilepticus (recurrent of sustained seizures >2 min) or seizures from local anesthetic overdose
Action	Anticonvulsant; enhances GABA-A receptor activity
How supplied	5 mg/mL in 1-, 2-, 5-, 10-mL vials
Amount to keep in office	1 mg/mL and 5 mg/mL in 10-mL vial; (1) vial each is suggested
Dosage	IV/IM/IN: Adult 2 mg (max dose 10 mg); pediatric dose IN 0.2 mg/kg; supplemental doses may be considered if seizures have not resolved within 5–10 min
Side effects	Sedation; respiratory depression or arrest
Naloxone	
Indications	Blocks or reverses the effects of opioid medication, including depressed respiratory effort or loss of consciousness. Naloxone is used to treat a narcotic overdose in an emergency situation
Action	Opioid antagonist
How supplied	0.4-mg/mL vials; 0.4-mg/mL multidose vials; 2-mg prefilled syringe
Amount to keep in office	(5) 0.4 mg/mL vials or (1) 0.4 mg/mL multidose vial
Dosage	Adult dose 0.4–2 mg every 3–5 min; max dose: 10 mg
	IV/IM/IN: Pediatric dose 0.01–0.1 mg/kg every 3–5 min as needed based on response; max dose: 10 mg
Side effects	Abrupt reversal of opioid effects in persons who are physically dependent on opioids may precipitate an acute withdrawal syndrome, which may include aches, fever, sweating, runny nose, sneezing, weakness, shivering or trembling, nervousness, restlessness or irritability, diarrhea, nausea or vomiting, abdominal cramps, increased blood pressure, and tachycardia; flash pulmonary edema potential for resedation
Nitroglycerin	
Indications	Chest pain as a result of angina or myocardial infarction
Action	Nitrates cause reduction in left and right ventricular preload through peripheral arterial and venous dilation (predominantly venous)
How supplied	Tablets 0.4 mg or spray 0.4 mg metered dose
Amount to keep in office	1 bottle
Dosage	0.4 mg sublingual every 3–5 min until pain is resolved Administer only if the blood pressure is above 100 systolic and the heart rate is between 60 and 100 beats/min
Side effects	Headache, facial flushing, hypotension
Oxygen	
Indications	Any medical emergency where the patient is having respiratory distress and hypoxemia
Action	Increased concentrations of oxygen will increase the amount of oxygen dissolved in the blood, relieving the symptoms caused by low oxygen levels in tissues
How supplied	Cylinders

TABLE 35.2 Emergency Drugs—cont'd

Amount to keep in office	Minimum (1) E cylinder with adjustable regulator 0–15 L
Dosage	If pulse oximetry is <94%, medium to high concentration, 8–15 L/min via basic or rebreather mask. If pulse oximetry is >94%, low concentration is all that is necessary, 2–4 L via nasal cannula
Side effects	Increased myocardial ischemia/damage when given in high concentrations, when pulse oximetry is >94%
Flumazenil (Romazicon)	
Indications	Indicated to reverse oversedation and respiratory depression Required if sedating with benzodiazepines
Action	Benzodiazepine antagonist
How supplied	0.1 mg/mL, 5 mL, and 10 mL multidose vials[a]
Amount to keep in office	(1) 0.1 mg/5 mL multidose vial
Dosage	Adult dose: 0.2 mg IN/IM repeat every minute; max dose is 1 mg
	Pediatric dose: 0.01 mg/kg IN/IM with a maximum dose of 0.2 mg as initial dose; may repeat up to max dose of 1 mg
Side effects	May induce seizure activity; potential for resedation

[a]Not FDA approved.
FDA, US Food and Drug Administration; *GABA*, γ-aminobutyric acid; *IM*, intramuscular; *IN*, intranasal; *IV*, intravenous.

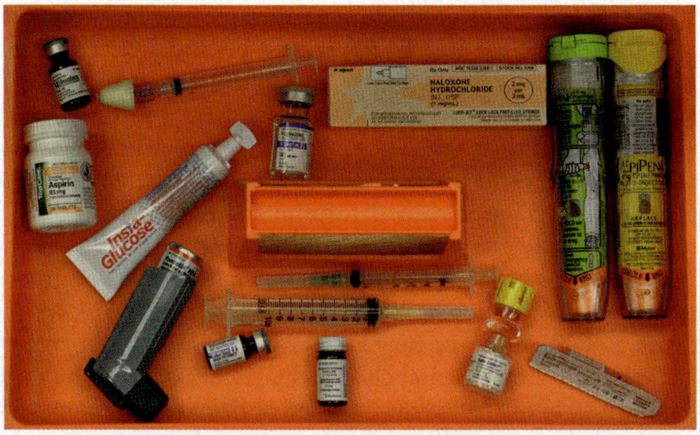

• **Fig. 35.7** Emergency drugs.

Aspirin

Although this drug is unlikely to be needed by the pediatric patient, he or she is brought to the dental office by adults who may require emergency medical management.

Epinephrine

Epinephrine is the treatment of choice for life-threatening emergencies including anaphylactic reactions and severe asthmatic attacks unresponsive to albuterol.[1,33,49] It is also an early ACLS drug for cardiac arrest.[27] If a pediatric dentist is administering drugs to patients, including local anesthetics, epinephrine must be available in case of allergy.[1,33]

Glucose

Simple sugar, as opposed to complex carbohydrates, should be available for ingestion in cases of suspected hypoglycemic shock.[33] Examples of simple sugar include sugar packets emptied into coffee, nondiet soda, or dissolving candies such as Life Savers.[33] IV dextrose can be given by those competent in establishing IV access.

Other optional medications

The pediatric dentist may consider having available a respiratory stimulant, such as ammonia inhalant crushable capsules.[31,47] Commonly, these drugs are found in dental offices taped to cabinets in the operatory to help arouse a patient with unconsciousness secondary to suspected syncope.[1] Other medications to consider in the emergency kit include a corticosteroid, such as methylprednisolone (Solu-Medrol) or hydrocortisone (Solu-Cortef) for acute adrenal insufficiency.[1,50,51] These may also serve as an adjunct to allergy management.[49]

Other agents for cardiovascular urgencies or emergencies could be included. Drugs used in the treatment of hypotension, hypertension, tachycardia, and bradycardia should be available for use by pediatric dentists with advanced training (ACLS and PALS) and who are well versed in their use.[25,27]

One other consideration is intralipid.[24] Lipid emulsion therapy is an effective treatment for systemic toxicity resulting from local anesthesia overdose.[16,24,52] This condition occurs when local anesthetics, such as lidocaine, are absorbed into the bloodstream at toxic levels, potentially causing serious cardiac and neurologic complications, including seizures, arrhythmias, and cardiac arrest. Lipid emulsion therapy involves the IV administration of a lipid-rich solution, which acts as a "lipid sink" to sequester lipophilic anesthetic molecules from target tissues, thereby reducing their plasma concentration and mitigating toxic effects.[53] This therapy has been shown to improve cardiac function and reverse neurologic symptoms rapidly, making it a critical intervention in cases of local anesthetic systemic toxicity. Prompt recognition and treatment with lipid emulsion can significantly enhance patient outcomes and reduce the risk of severe complications.[24,52]

Management of Medical Emergencies in the Dental Office

Medical emergencies should be approached systematically[31,33] following basic principles (Box 35.1).[1,31,33] Management should be

• BOX 35.1 Steps for Management of Medical Emergencies

The five basic steps include (the CABs):
- (P)—Position
- (C)—Circulation
- (A)—Airway
- (B)—Breathing
- (D)—Definitive treatment

For all emergencies:
1. Discontinue dental treatment.
2. Call for assistance/someone to bring oxygen and emergency kit.
3. Position patient to ensure open and unobstructed airway.
4. Monitor vital signs.
5. Be prepared to support respiration, support circulation, provide cardiopulmonary resuscitation, and call for emergency medical services.

consistent, even if a definitive diagnosis is not clear, improving efficiency and reducing anxiety for the dental team.[31–33]

Position

Patients who are unconscious or have a decreased level of consciousness should be placed supine.[32] This will minimize the work of the heart, increase return of pooled blood from the extremities, and increase vital blood flow to the brain. If the patient is awake, the patient can be placed in a position of comfort (sitting position or semireclined).[32]

Circulation ("C")

The first assessment step is to determine whether the patient has a pulse.[27,28,48] The carotid pulse is the easiest and most accurate in the adult and child patient (Fig. 35.9).[32] The carotid artery lies just under the sternocleidomastoid muscle in the neck. Do not palpate both carotid arteries simultaneously as pressure on the baroreceptors of the carotid sinuses may precipitate reflex bradycardia.[27] When assessing the infant, the brachial pulse should be palpated.[28,48]

While assessing pulse, evaluate chest movement.[28,48] If there is good rise and fall of the chest and a pulse, the patient likely has circulation. If the patient has no chest movement or a very slow, gasping type of breathing (agonal breathing), then assume there is no circulation.[27,28,48] Begin chest compressions immediately (Box 35.2).[48] EMS should simultaneously be activated. Allow full recoil of the chest after each compression; do not lean on the chest after each compression.[48] Compressions should be fast and deep.[48]

Airway ("A")

If the supply of oxygen to the lungs is interrupted, rapid deterioration will occur, resulting in brain cell damage, cardiac arrest, and death.[1,28,32] After determining the patient has a pulse, assess for an adequate airway.[27,28,48] The upper airway may be obstructed by progressive swelling, trauma, a foreign body, or other factors.[54,55]

The most common cause of airway obstruction is the tongue.[56] When a patient becomes obtunded or unconscious, the musculature supporting the mandible and tongue will become relaxed. This allows the base of the tongue to fall against the posterior pharyngeal tissues creating an obstruction. Children with enlarged tonsils are particularly vulnerable to this type of airway obstruction.[57] Tilting the head back (head-tilt maneuver or cervical extension; Fig. 35.10) and thrusting the jaw forward (chin-lift or jaw-thrust maneuver) will help open the obstructed airway.[32] Oral or nasal airway devices are also useful in keeping the tongue forward in the unconscious or deeply obtunded patient.[27,28] These devices should not be used in conscious patients because they tend to induce gagging and vomiting.[28]

If the airway is obstructed by a foreign body, such as a cotton roll or dental device, management depends on the patient's condition.[26,32] If the patient is conscious and can cough or vocalize, allow him or her to expel the object with his or her own efforts.[26] If after a short period of time this is clearly ineffective, or if the patient uses the universal choking sign of placing the hands around the neck, the initial step should be to deliver abdominal thrusts (Heimlich maneuver).[26,58–61] Sitting or standing behind the patient, place one fist below the xiphoid process over the mid to upper abdomen; clench it with the other hand and pull up and back forcefully.[26,58] This maneuver pushes the diaphragm up and produces a sustained forceful increase in intrathoracic pressure, expelling air through the larynx and hopefully dislodging the obstruction.[26,58] Abdominal thrusts should be performed in rapid succession until successful or loss of consciousness.

The abdominal thrust may be modified for the patient who is lying down (as in the dental chair). The rescuer delivers the thrust with the heel of the hand from the side or front of the patient. The abdominal thrust should not be performed in infants less than 1-year-old because of their relatively large abdominal organs (especially the liver), which could be damaged.[26] In these cases, a chest thrust maneuver should be delivered. Use the heel of the hand positioned over the midsternum, similar to the position of chest compressions during cardiopulmonary resuscitation (CPR).[26]

If the object is not expelled, consciousness will be lost. EMS should be activated as soon as possible. Begin CPR or BLS, chest compressions, and head-tilt-chin-lift maneuver.[26,28] If a foreign body is visible, remove it, but do not perform blind finger sweeps because they may push obstructing objects farther into the pharynx

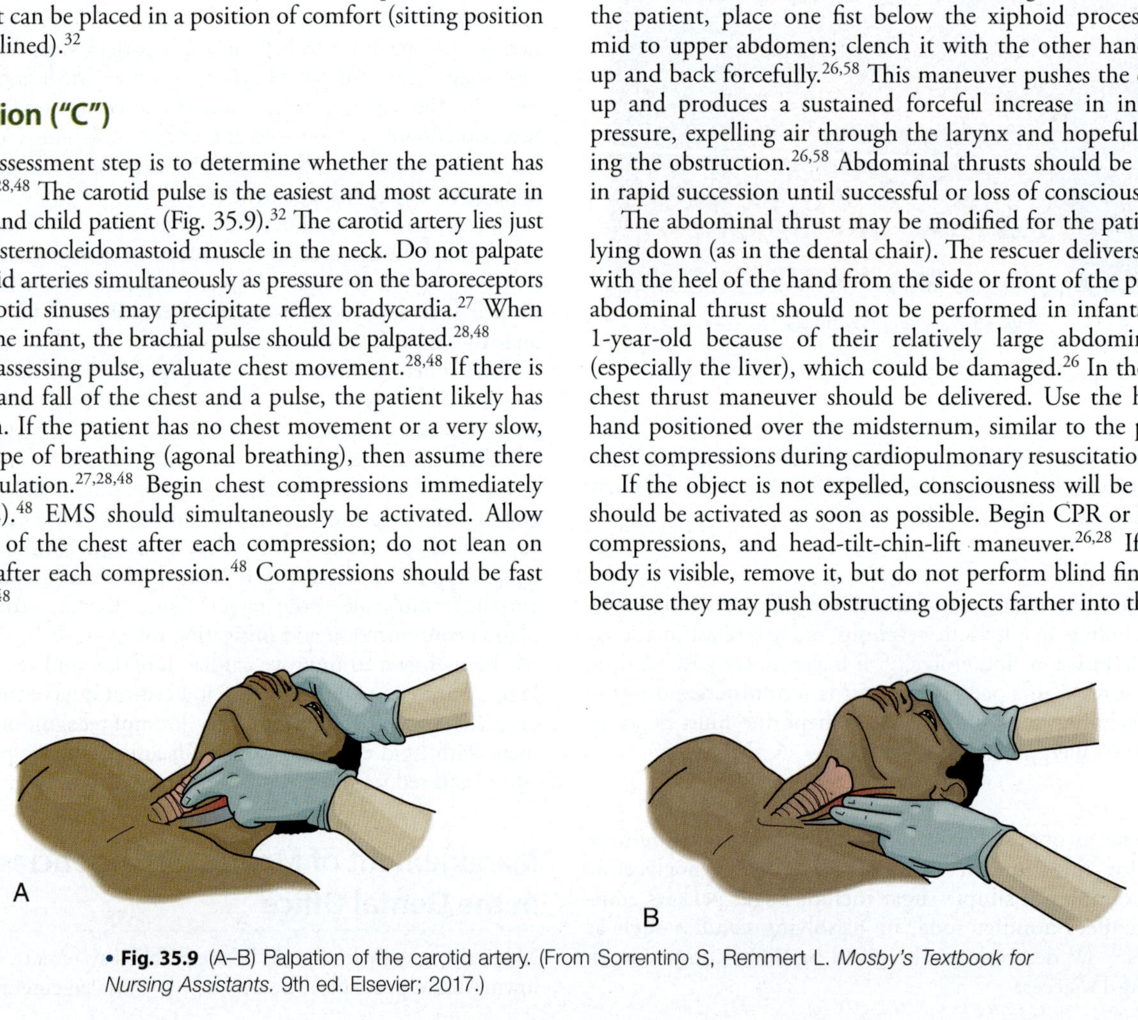

• **Fig. 35.9** (A–B) Palpation of the carotid artery. (From Sorrentino S, Remmert L. *Mosby's Textbook for Nursing Assistants.* 9th ed. Elsevier; 2017.)

• BOX 35.2 Compressions

The compression rate is 100–120 per minute. Compressions are done in the lower half of the sternum, midnipple line. The compression depth is as follows:

Adult (puberty and above): 2"–2.4" in depth
Child (age 1 to prepuberty): 2" in depth
Infant (discharge from hospital to age 1): 1½ in depth

The compression to ventilation ratio is

30:2 single rescuer
30:2 two rescuer adult
15:2 two rescuer, infant and pediatric cardiopulmonary resuscitation

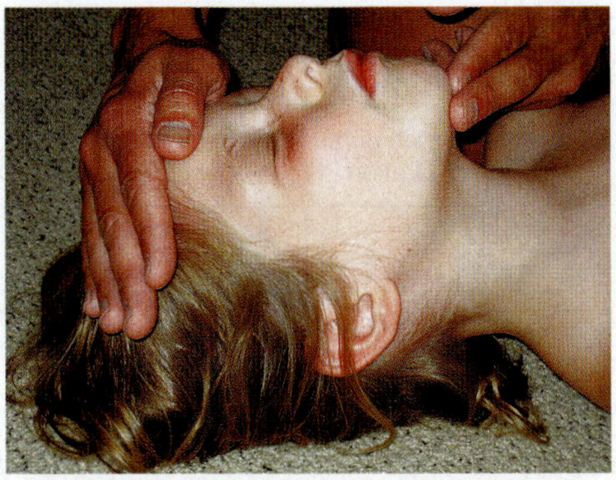

• **Fig. 35.10** Head-tilt/chin-lift maneuver. (From Malamed SF. *Medical Emergencies in the Dental Office.* 7th ed. Elsevier; 2015.)

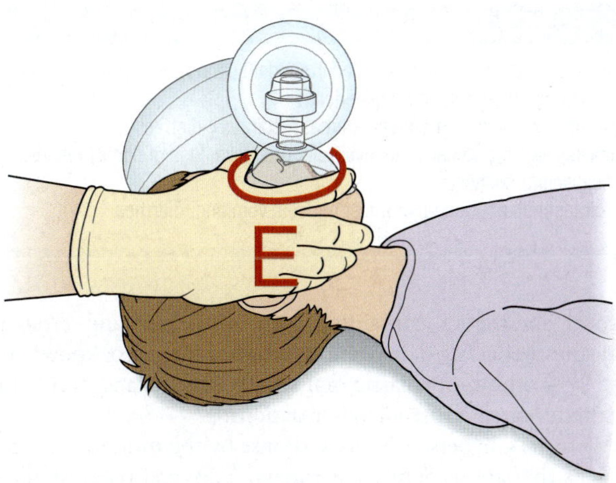

• **Fig. 35.11** Hand position ("C and E") for bag valve mask for ventilation.

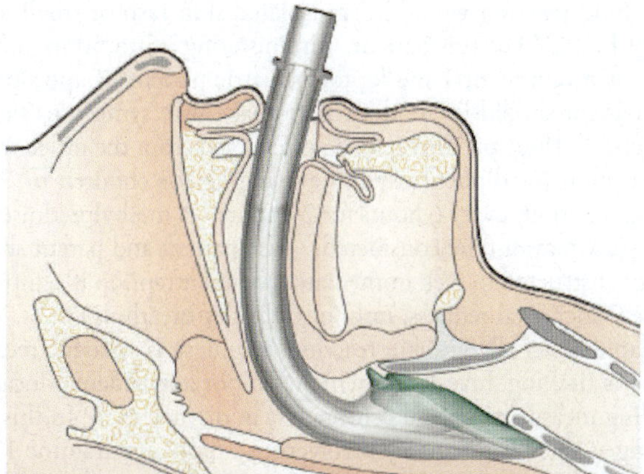

• **Fig. 35.12** The i-gel single-use supraglottic airway device. (Courtesy Intersurgical Inc., East Syracuse, NY.)

and may damage the oropharynx.[26] Attempt to give two breaths and continue with cycles of chest compressions and ventilations.[26,28] There should be only very brief intermittent evaluations of the upper airway to determine whether the foreign body has been dislodged or could be seen and removed. If ventilations are difficult because of the obstruction, reattempt head-tilt/jaw-thrust and consider an oral or nasal airway.[26,28] Caution should be used when placing an airway so as not to distalize the foreign object, worsening the obstruction.[62] Dentists with training may perform laryngoscopy, endotracheal intubation, transtracheal jet ventilation, or cricothyroidotomy, if skilled in these techniques.[33]

Breathing ("B")

Once the airway is managed, rise and fall of the chest should be observed.[1] If there is no rise and fall of the chest, or breathing appears to be inadequate, then ventilating the patient is necessary.[26] In the office setting, ventilation is best achieved by using an appropriately sized bag valve mask.[26,62,63] A bag-valve-mask system, such as an Ambu bag (Ballerup, Denmark), is considered essential emergency equipment for every dental office.[33] The bag valve mask may require two people to operate correctly.[28] One rescuer seals the mask, making the letter "C" and "E" with their fingers and the other squeezes the bag to ventilate (Fig. 35.11). The bag valve mask should be connected to an oxygen source (E tank at minimum) at 15 L/min to ensure 100% oxygen delivery.[28] Bag-mask ventilation is the most critical emergency management skill to master.[63,64]

If there is a palpable pulse (≥60 beats/min) but there is inadequate breathing, give rescue breaths at a rate of 12 to 20 breaths/min (1 breath every 3 to 5 seconds) until spontaneous breathing resumes.[26] Reassess the pulse every 2 minutes.[26]

Ventilate with 100% oxygen. Do not hyperventilate, as outcomes are worse when patients are hyperventilated.[27,28,65,66] If unable to properly ventilate using a bag valve mask, an oral or nasal airway should be inserted.[28] Consider an advanced technique when unsuccessful with the oral or nasal airway.[28,33] For the novice intubator, an effective advanced technique may be the i-gel LMA (Intersurgical Ltd, Wokingham, Berkshire, UK) (Fig. 35.12).[33,67,68]

Definitive Therapy ("D")

The "D" represents definitive therapy.[1,32] Once circulation, airway, and breathing are managed, treatment options, including drug administration, should be considered[32,69] based on risk versus benefit.[1] If the cause is clear or related to treatment, definitive therapy may be necessary.[28,32,69]

Common Medical Emergencies

Allergic Reactions

The primary agents employed in pediatric dentistry that provoke allergic reactions are penicillins and latex.[69,70] Sulfite antioxidants

• BOX 35.3 Severe Systemic Allergic Reactions

A severe reaction most likely will occur suddenly and manifest in all systems:
Skin: flushing, urticarial, and angioedema
Respiratory: wheezing, laryngeal edema, respiratory distress
Cardiovascular: hypotension, tachycardia, dizziness, loss of consciousness, cardiovascular collapse
Gastrointestinal: abdominal cramps, nausea, vomiting, diarrhea

in local anesthetics containing vasoconstrictors and ester-type local anesthetics used in topical products are also known triggers.[71,72] Common pediatric oral sedative agents and amide local anesthetics rarely cause allergic reactions.[1,72]

Allergy is a hypersensitivity response by the immune system to antigens that are recognized as foreign.[73] Several types of allergic reactions may occur.[74] They range from mild to severe and treatment varies depending on the type of reaction.[74–76] The type I, immediate, or anaphylaxis reaction is of most concern.[1,75,76]

A mild reaction would be an isolated skin rash or small number of hives.[75] For this patient, administering 25 to 50 mg of oral diphenhydramine or 1 mg/kg for pediatric patients is appropriate. The patient should be monitored to make sure symptoms do not worsen.[1,31] These patients may be discharged from the office with a prescription for diphenhydramine 1 mg/kg for children or 25 to 50 mg for adults every 6 hours for 24 hours.[1] A methylprednisolone dose pack may also be considered.[77] The patient and parent should also be instructed to seek immediate medical attention if symptoms worsen (increased redness, rash, or difficulty breathing).[1]

Rapid-onset allergic skin reactions manifest as systemic redness, urticaria (itching, hives), erythema (rash), or angioedema (localized swelling measuring several centimeters in diameter).[1,75] In this case as long as there is no airway involvement, diphenhydramine 1 mg/kg up to 50 mg should be administered intramuscularly (IM).[69] Activate EMS if recovery is not immediate.[1] Recognize that this moderate reaction may rapidly progress to a severe/anaphylactic reaction, which a true life-threatening emergency (Box 35.3).[78]

As a general rule, the more rapid the onset and the more intense the symptoms, the more severe the generalized reaction will become.[1,78] Edema that involves the face and neck may rapidly progress to airway obstruction and death.[78] Respiratory symptoms follow skin reactions in generalized anaphylaxis.[1,78] Constriction of bronchial smooth muscle causes respiratory distress. The principal recognizable sign is wheezing, a distinctive breathing sound associated with bronchoconstriction and similar to an asthmatic attack.[78] As the obstruction worsens, the patient has increasing difficulty exchanging adequate volumes of air.[78]

Cardiovascular involvement, which could lead to life-threatening hypotension, occurs in 45% of patients.[49,78] Hypotension is produced by the vasodilating effects of histamine and other mediators of the response. Reflex tachycardia, arrhythmias, and eventually cardiac arrest may follow. The management of a severe, immediate reaction is discussed later.[49,78]

Management

Terminate the suspected agent, begin BLS protocol (circulation, airway, breathing [CAB]), activate EMS, and administer 0.3 mg of epinephrine IM for an adult or 0.15 mg for the pediatric patient (EpiPen and EpiPen Jr, respectively)[1,49,79] (Fig. 35.13). Epinephrine at the dose of 0.01 mg/kg to a maximum initial dose of 0.3 mg must be administered to reverse the deleterious effects of histamine (bronchoconstriction and vasodilation).[1,49,79]

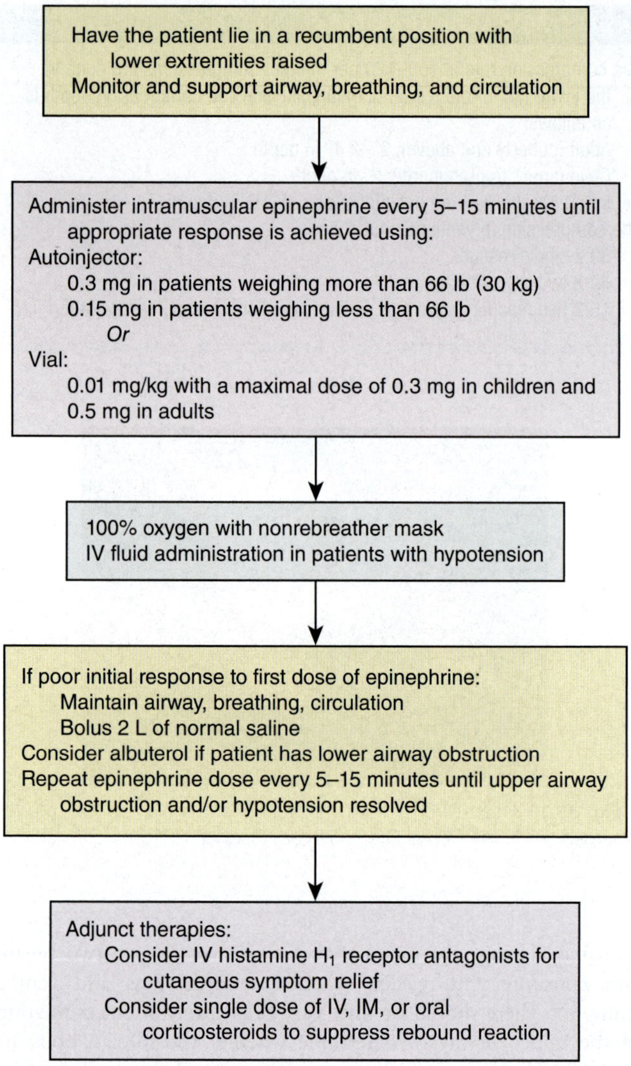

• Fig. 35.13 Management of anaphylaxis in the outpatient setting. *IM,* Intramuscular; *IV,* intravenous. (Data from Lieberman P, Kemp SF, Oppenheimer J, et al. The diagnosis and management of anaphylaxis: an updated practice parameter. *J Allergy Clin Immunol*. 2005;115 [3 suppl 2]:S483–S523.)

Administration may need to be repeated every 5 to 15 minutes if symptoms recur and EMS is not yet on the scene.[49] Oxygen therapy, two puffs of the albuterol inhaler, and diphenhydramine may also be administered. The patient who suffers from severe anaphylaxis must be transported to the hospital for additional treatment with antihistamines and corticosteroids.[49]

Asthma (Acute Bronchospasm)

Asthma is a common medical emergency that may occur in the dental office.[1,31,69] It is estimated that approximately 17 million Americans suffer from asthma.[79] This results in approximately 2 million visits to the emergency department each year and approximately 5000 to 6000 deaths per year.[1,79]

Asthma is an inflammatory airway disorder causing intermittent airflow obstruction.[80,81] Patients have heightened airway sensitivity, increased muscle contraction, and excessive secretions. Bronchospasm and wheezing result from smooth muscle constriction,[1,82] while thick secretions and edema block small airways, each leading to airway compromise.

Signs and symptoms of an acute asthma attack include chest congestion, cough, wheezing, dyspnea, use of accessory muscles, anxiety, restlessness, apprehension, tachypnea, tachycardia, increase in blood pressure, diaphoresis, confusion, nasal flaring, and cyanosis.[1]

The primary type of asthma in children is allergic or extrinsic asthma, which is mediated by immunoglobulin (IgE) antibodies.[1,82] This asthma attack is triggered by specific allergens such as pollens, dust, and molds.[82,83] The process may produce various signs and symptoms from mild wheezing and coughing to severe dyspnea, cyanosis, and even death.[81–83]

Acute attacks of extrinsic asthma usually occur with diminishing frequency as the child ages and may disappear in later life.[1] In adults, the primary type of asthma is intrinsic asthma. With intrinsic asthma, attacks may be precipitated by infections, cold weather, exercise, and stress.[84,85] Some overlap may occur in the types of asthma.

A thorough history should be documented in the record as previously described (see "History and Physical Examination").

Efforts should be made to avoid precipitating factors, and patients should be instructed to continue their medications before the appointment.[1] Patients should bring their albuterol inhaler, as it is the primary rescue inhaler.[31,69] In cases of wheezing or respiratory distress, the patient should be seated upright and administer two puffs of albuterol.[1] If the inhaler is unavailable, the dentist should provide one from the office emergency kit. In most cases, albuterol inhalation will effectively abort the asthmatic attack.[1] If this fails to reverse the bronchospasm, oxygen should be administered. This may likely be status asthmaticus, a true medical emergency.[31,81,86] If the dentist believes the attack may be life-threatening, 0.01 mg/kg (maximal initial dose, 0.3 mg) of epinephrine (1:1000) should be injected IM and EMS activated.[31] Epinephrine should be beneficial within a few minutes in most cases. Early administration of a corticosteroid IM may also be helpful in severe attacks, although the onset is rather slow.[77]

Management

Terminate the dental procedure. Reassure the patient and place him or her in a position of comfort. Assess CABs and administer two puffs of albuterol inhaler or 2.5 mg albuterol/3 mL nebulized solution via an oxygen-powered nebulizer mask at 6 L/min. If the patient is unresponsive to treatment, activate EMS. Reassess CABs, deliver oxygen in high concentration, and consider administering epinephrine 0.3 mg (1:1000) IM for an adult or 0.15 mg (1:1000) for a child (EpiPen and EpiPen Jr).[1,31,87]

Cardiac Symptoms (Acute Coronary Syndrome)

Pediatric dentists will not see many patients with acute coronary syndrome (ACS). However, parents and grandparents who accompany the patient may develop these symptoms.[1] The chief complaint is usually chest pain, typically described as tightness or pressure in the chest. The severity can range from minimal to a severe crushing type of discomfort. Pain may radiate to the neck, back, jaw, and/or down one or both arms. Associated symptoms include dyspnea, nausea, vomiting, and diaphoresis.[27,88] The patient may also experience profound weakness.[27]

Management

Place the patient in a position of comfort and perform physical assessment with vital signs. Activate EMS and administer aspirin (81 mg × 4 chewable) and nitroglycerin 0.4 mg (if the heart rate is between 60 and 100 and BP is >100 systolic). Administer oxygen at 4 L/min if the pulse oximeter is less than 90%. Repeat nitroglycerin as needed every 5 minutes (up to three times) as long as heart rate and blood pressure remain stable.[88]

Cardiac Arrest

The American Heart Association reports 326,200 cases of out-of-hospital nontraumatic sudden cardiac arrest annually, with 9 of 10 victims dying.[89,90] This event can occur anywhere, including the dental office, and affects people of all ages, including infants.[1] Common causes include thrombosis, cardiomyopathy, and prolonged QT interval,[1,90] and predisposing conditions may go undetected. Medications, such as attention-deficit/hyperactivity disorder (ADHD) drugs, antidepressants, and antibiotics, can contribute.[91] Warning signs include dizziness after exertion, unexplained loss of consciousness, or a family history of sudden death under age 50.[91–96] Timely recognition and management are crucial in cases of cardiac arrest.[1,27,28]

Management

Assess the circulation by checking for a pulse while looking for adequate chest rise and fall. Activate EMS and obtain the AED with the emergency kit and oxygen. Begin chest compressions at a rate of 100 to 120 a minute, with good recoil at the appropriate depth, as described earlier in this chapter, until the AED arrives. Once the AED arrives, turn it on, and follow the voice prompts.[27,28] If a shock is advised and delivered and the patient does not recover, immediately, resume chest compressions and ventilations at the appropriate intervals. If an advanced airway is placed (LMA, i-gel), compressions become continuous, and the ventilations are given at a rate of 1 breath every 6 seconds for adults and 1 breath every 2 to 3 seconds for pediatric patients. The AED will analyze every 2 minutes. Continue BLS until EMS arrives or the patient has a return of spontaneous circulation.[27,28] The AED is indicated for everyone including infants. Pediatric electrode pads should be used for children under 55 lb (25 kg).[28]

Diabetic Emergencies

Diabetes mellitus involves insulin production and/or resistance,[97] leading to impaired carbohydrate, fat, and protein metabolism, and untreated results in hyperglycemia.[98] Chronic hyperglycemia causes vascular damage and affects the cardiovascular system, nerves, kidneys, and other organs.[1,97] Type 1 diabetes, common in children,[99] results from loss of pancreatic β-cell function and requires daily insulin injections.[1,98] Emergencies in children can stem from hypoglycemia or hyperglycemia.[1] Prolonged low insulin levels cause high blood glucose, leading cells to break down fat and protein for energy, producing ketones and causing diabetic ketoacidosis (DKA).[98] DKA develops over several days, not suddenly, and typically does not present as an acute emergency in the dental office though the condition can lead to coma or death.[1] If a diabetic patient appears unwell or has acetone-scented breath, they should seek medical attention immediately.[1,98]

If a diabetic patient, who appears well, has a sudden deterioration in cognition or loss of consciousness in the dental office, the condition is more likely to be due to acute hypoglycemia or insulin shock.[1,69,98] The usual scenario involves a patient who has taken his or her morning insulin and has forgotten to eat a meal or has ingested inadequate carbohydrates.[1]

Exercise and stress may also increase carbohydrate utilization and lower blood glucose concentrations.[100,101]

Glucose and oxygen are the primary metabolic sources for brain cells.[98] As serum glucose levels decrease, symptoms appear.[101] The sympathetic nervous system will attempt to raise blood glucose levels, resulting in tachycardia, hypertension, anxiety, and sweating.[97,98] If not corrected, the patient will develop slurred speech, ataxia, and eventually loss of consciousness.[1] Seizures may also occur.

Most diabetic patients are well attuned to this phenomenon and carry a carbohydrate source to be ingested in this event.[101,102] However, if carbohydrate is not ingested and the blood glucose concentration continues to decrease, cerebral function will deteriorate. Alterations in mood, strange activity, and inappropriate responses to questions may be early clinical indicators.[97,98] Patients in this condition may be confused with those having excessive alcohol ingestion.[1]

Recommend patients continue with their daily regimen and eat their normal diet.[1] This should prevent hypoglycemia (<80 mg/dL blood glucose). The exception to this rule is when patients are instructed to have nothing by mouth (NPO) before sedation or general anesthesia.[102,103]

Management

Place the patient in a position of comfort and assess (CABs) the patient. Obtain a blood glucose (if possible) and provide definitive care.[1] Management of hypoglycemia involves the administration of glucose.[101,102] The oral route is used if the patient is conscious and is experiencing early symptoms. Oral glucose tabs 37.5 g can be administered and repeated as necessary. Sugar dissolved in juice or a sugar-containing soft drink may also be used. Simple sugars are more rapidly absorbed than complex carbohydrates. Should the patient become unconscious, BLS should be initiated.[104] Definitive care requires IV access and 50% dextrose IV. This will rapidly bring a return to consciousness. Administering glucose orally is unadvisable if the patient is significantly obtunded or unconscious, as aspiration or airway obstruction may occur. Glucagon may also be considered.

Hyperventilation Syndrome

Hyperventilation syndrome is a maladaptive anxiety reaction that primarily occurs in apprehensive patients who attempt to hide their anxiety.[105] The syndrome is often triggered by an anxiety-provoking event such as local anesthetic adminstration.[1] The patient is usually unaware of the fact that he or she is breathing rapidly. Respiratory rates increase (25 to 30 breaths/min) with an increase in tidal volume. Increased ventilation causes a marked reduction in the blood carbon dioxide.[105,106] The decrease in the arterial partial pressure of carbon dioxide ($PaCO_2$), referred to as hypocarbia, causes a physiologic vasoconstriction of the arteries supplying the brain. The result of the decreased blood flow leaves the patient feeling dizzy and light-headed, which further enhances the anxiety, worsening the condition in a vicious cycle.[1] Other symptoms that may occur include numbness and tingling of the extremities and perioral area, muscle twitching and cramping, seizures, and loss of consciousness.[105–107]

Management

Management of hyperventilation involves early recognition.[1] Reassurance, patient rapport, and calmly coaching the patient to breathe slowly may be sufficient to stop the process.[1] Oxygen administration will worsen the syndrome.[106] If the cycle cannot be broken, steps should be taken to increase the $PaCO_2$.[1] This can be accomplished simply by having the patient rebreathe exhaled CO_2-containing air. Raising $PaCO_2$ should reverse the process. Extended periods of rebreathing are not recommended, as hypoxia should be avoided.[1] Sedation or general anesthesia for future treatment may be appropriate.

Seizures

Seizures are clinical manifestations of paroxysmal excessive neuronal brain activity.[1] Uncontrolled electrical discharge within the central nervous system (CNS) results in sensory or motor activity, altered visceral function, abnormal motor movements, changes in mental acuity, and unconsciousness.[1]

There are various types of seizures. Generalized (tonic-clonic) seizures may be life-threatening.[1] Generalized seizures are manifested in four phases: prodromal, aura, convulsive (ictal), and postictal. The prodromal phase consists of subtle changes that occur over minutes to hours. It is usually not clinically evident to the practitioner or the patient. The aura is a neurologic experience that the patient goes through immediately before the seizure. It is specifically related to the trigger areas of the brain in which the seizure activity begins. It may consist of a taste, a smell, a hallucination, motor activity, or other symptoms. A given patient's aura is often the same for all seizures. As the CNS discharge becomes generalized, the ictal phase begins.[108]

Consciousness is lost, the patient falls to the floor, and tonic, rigid skeletal muscle contraction occurs. Clonic movements begin, producing rapid jerking of the extremities and trunk. Breathing may be labored during this period, and patients may injure themselves. This tonic-clonic phase usually lasts 1 to 3 minutes.[108–110] As the clonic phase ends, the muscles relax and movement stops. A significant degree of CNS depression is usually present during this postictal phase.[108] Caution must be exercised in the postictal phase as there may be respiratory depression. Often, the patient has amnesia from the prodromal phase throughout the entire seizure.[1]

Management

Management of a seizure consists of clearing the area, gentle immobilization (stabilization), and positioning of the patient to prevent self-injury.[1,111,112] Postictal management is critical as this is when the patient is likely to become obtunded or hypoglycemic.[111] Ensure adequate ventilation (airway management) and provide supportive care, as indicated. Consider a blood glucose level to rule out hypoglycemia if the patient is unarousable.[1,111]

Single seizures do not require drug therapy because they usually are self-limiting. Should the ictal phase last longer than 5 minutes or if seizures continue to develop with little time between them, a condition called *status epilepticus* has developed.[108,109] This may be a life-threatening medical emergency because the uncontrolled muscle activity can result in hyperthermia, hypoglycemia, increased oxygen consumption, tachycardia, hypertension, impaired ventilation, and cardiac arrhythmias.[109,110] IV administration of an benzodiazepine anticonvulsant (diazepam, lorazepam, or midazolam) should be administered.[31,113] In the pediatric dental office, where IV access may not be available, the condition may be managed with IM midazolam, 0.2 mg/kg to a maximum of 10 mg or intranasal midazolam 0.2 mg/kg up to 1 to 2 mg.[114–116] Airway management postadministration is essential as benzodiazepines can cause respiratory depression. EMS should be activated for transport to the hospital.[114]

Syncope

Syncope is the most common medical emergency in the dental office.[117,118] While less common in young children, it is very prevalent among teenagers and young adults.[1] Factors that predispose patients to syncope include, but are not limited to, anxiety, pain, and stress.[1,119]

Vasodepressor syncope, or the simple faint, is the most common type of syncope and cause for loss of consciousness in the dental office.[1] This maladaptive stress reaction activates the fight-or-flight response of the sympathetic nervous system. Endogenous epinephrine and norepinephrine are released into the circulation, resulting in a large increase in blood flow to the muscles of the body. If the muscles are contracting, as would be the case if the individual were running, normal blood flow is maintained. However, in the dental chair, little or no muscle contraction is occurring, thus the blood pools in the muscles, effectively decreasing the relative blood volume available to the central circulation and therefore the brain. The heart rate initially increases in an attempt to maintain the blood pressure, but as ventricular filling decreases because of poor venous return, reflex mechanisms slow the heart rate to improve filling of the ventricles. Thus a patient who is anxious with initial hypertension and tachycardia develops hypotension and bradycardia. Cerebral perfusion is then compromised, causing loss of consciousness or fainting. Early in the process, as blood flow to the brain decreases, the patient feels dizzy or light-headed. This phase of the condition is called *presyncope,* and the patient may lose normal skin color in the face and lips. Presyncope usually begins rapidly.[1]

If presyncope is recognized in a susceptible patient and managed quickly, loss of consciousness may be prevented. Management consists of positioning the patient supine, lowering the head, and raising the legs above the heart to augment blood flow to the brain by gravity. Cardiac output will be increased and adequate cerebral perfusion will be restored. Administration of oxygen is appropriate in any emergency involving a decrease in brain perfusion.

If the process of syncope continues, the sympathetic nervous system will fatigue, and the parasympathetic nervous system will suddenly become dominant. This vagal response results in a sudden, severe decrease in heart rate and blood pressure. Blood flow to the brain is compromised, and consciousness is lost. However, if the patient is quickly placed in the supine position with legs elevated, loss of consciousness from syncope will likely resolve. Although consciousness may be regained fairly quickly, recovery of heart rate and blood pressure may be quite slow. If loss of consciousness does not return in less than 1 minute, it is not syncope. All syncope cannot be assumed to be vasovagal; however, treatment is essentially the same.[1,119]

Management[1,31,69]

Position the patient supine, with legs slightly elevated, and administer oxygen. Airway, breathing, and circulation should be monitored and supported as needed.[1] Tight and constrictive clothing should be loosened and vital signs monitored. Ammonia inhalants may stimulate and be beneficial.[31]

If recovery of consciousness is delayed beyond 5 minutes or is incomplete after 15 to 20 minutes, medical assistance should be sought.[1,69] Drug therapy is usually not indicated with syncope unless the heart rate or blood pressure remains dangerously depressed after positioning. In such a case, epinephrine could increase heart rate and improve cardiac output.[27]

After a syncopal episode, the patient may be discharged after a period of watchful waiting and return of vital signs to acceptable levels. The risk of repeat syncope is, however, greater for some time after the episode.[119] The patient should not operate a vehicle and should arrange for alternative transportation if needed.

Sedation-Related Emergencies

Procedural sedation in pediatric patients carries significant risks, which can be minimized but not entirely eliminated through careful preprocedure assessments of the patient's medical history and conditions.[12,13] These assessments help predict how the sedation process might interact with the patient's health.[13]

Candidates for Sedation in Pediatric Dentistry

Most pediatric patients are suitable candidates for minimal to moderate sedation in a pediatric dental setting.[6,12,13] However, selecting a child for in-office sedation requires the pediatric dentist to consider the patient's American Society of Anesthesiologists (ASA) status, develop a detailed sedation plan, and prepare for potential emergencies.[6,13] See Chapter 27 for a a detailed discussion of patient selection for sedation.

The American Academy of Pediatric Dentistry (AAPD) and the American Academy of Pediatrics (AAP) have collaborated on a joint document titled "Guidelines for Monitoring and Management of Pediatric Patients Before, During, and After Sedation for Diagnostic and Therapeutic Procedures."[13] This document provides comprehensive guidelines to ensure the safe sedation of pediatric dental patients, covering all aspects of care from presedation evaluation to postsedation monitoring and management.[13]

Pediatric patients have specific physiologic differences that make them more vulnerable during sedation.[6,13] They have a lower physiologic reserve and higher oxygen consumption rates compared with adults. The unique physiologic and anatomical characteristics of pediatric patients necessitate careful dose calculation, constant monitoring, and readiness to manage emergencies.[6,13,120]

Rescue Skills for Deeper Levels of Sedation

Studies indicate that children often pass from the intended level of sedation to a deeper, unintended level.[13,121,122] Therefore the ability to rescue a patient from a deeper level of sedation is essential. Practitioners must be equipped to rescue from one level deeper than the intended sedation[13–15,22,23]:

- Minimal sedation requires skills to rescue from moderate sedation.
- Moderate sedation requires skills to rescue from deep sedation.
- Deep sedation requires skills to rescue from general anesthesia.

Practitioners should have the necessary skills and equipment to manage various sedation levels.

Airway Management and Perioperative Respiratory Adverse Events

A significant portion of adverse outcomes in pediatric sedation and anesthesia is related to airway management failures, rather than primary cardiac events..[38,39] If the airway is compromised, it can quickly lead to hypoxia, bradycardia, and potentially cardiac arrest. To maintain a patent airway, the following steps are crucial[6,13]:

1. Proper positioning of the head with neck extension
2. Performing a jaw thrust and/or chin lift
3. Inserting a nasal or oral airway
4. Providing positive pressure ventilation with a bag valve mask
5. Inserting a supraglottic device (i-gel) if needed

Perioperative respiratory adverse events (PRAEs) are significant complications that can occur during the perioperative period, which encompasses the time immediately before, during, and after surgery.[6,123] As previously stated, these events are particularly concerning in pediatric patients, where airway management failures can lead to serious morbidity or even mortality. Therefore developing and implementing effective airway management strategies tailored to the unique needs of pediatric patients is of utmost importance.[6,13,123] Recent upper respiratory infections, asthma, and exposure to secondhand smoke, including vaping and marijuana, can increase the risk of reactive airway issues for several weeks.[6,124] Awareness of these factors can help anticipate and manage potential PRAEs.[124]

The following is a list of some common PRAEs and detailed strategies for managing specific airway-related complications.[6,13,123]

Laryngospasm

Laryngospasm is a reflexive closure of the vocal cords that can obstruct the airway. It is a common perioperative complication in children, requiring prompt intervention to prevent serious outcomes. The management steps include the following[125]:

1. **Suction the airway:** Clear any secretions or debris to reduce irritation and obstruction.
2. **Perform a jaw thrust:** This maneuver helps open the airway by lifting the tongue and epiglottis away from the posterior pharyngeal wall.
3. **Provide positive pressure ventilation:** Use a bag valve mask to deliver positive pressure ventilation, which can help overcome the spasm.
4. **Administer IM succinylcholine:** If necessary, give 3 mg/kg of IM succinylcholine to relax the vocal cords. Be prepared to manage potential bradycardia with atropine at 0.02 mg/kg IM.

Bronchospasm

Bronchospasm[126] involves the constriction of the bronchial smooth muscle, leading to wheezing and difficulty breathing. It is often triggered by underlying reactive airway disease or irritants. The management steps include the following:

1. **Administer albuterol:** Use 2.5 mg of albuterol mixed with 3 cc normal saline via a nebulizer mask with oxygen at 6 L/min or administer two to four puffs of an albuterol inhaler.
2. **Use albuterol with metered-dose inhaler (MDI) adapter/bag valve mask:** If the patient is obtunded, use an albuterol inhaler with an MDI adapter and bag valve mask for effective delivery.
3. **Administer IM epinephrine:** For severe bronchospasm, administer IM epinephrine (0.15 mg for patients <60 lb, 0.3 mg for patients >60 lb) to reduce airway inflammation and open the airways.

Airway Obstruction, Hypoxia, and Apnea

Rapid intervention is crucial in cases of airway obstruction, hypoxia, and apnea. The management steps include the following[13,31,126]:

1. **Provide oxygen:** If pulse oximetry is <90% with a respiratory rate >12 breaths/min deliver 15 L of oxygen via a rebreather mask.
2. **Assist ventilation:** If pulse oximetry is <90% and the respiratory rate is <10 to 12 breaths/min, assist ventilation with a bag valve mask at one breath every 3 seconds.
3. **Reposition the airway:** Perform a jaw thrust and/or chin lift.
4. **Insert an airway:** Nasal trumpet or oral airway.
5. **Administer reversal agents:** Use reversal agents if necessary, such as Narcan (0.01 mg/kg) for opioid reversal and flumazenil (0.01 mg/kg) for benzodiazepine reversal.
6. **Insert supraglottic device (LMA)**
7. **Tracheal intubation**
8. **Surgical airway**

Emesis

Aspiration of gastric contents is a serious risk during anesthesia. Managing emesis[126] effectively can prevent aspiration and related complications. The management steps include the following:

1. **Position the patient:** Place the patient in the Trendelenburg position (head down at least 15 degrees) and roll them onto their side to reduce the risk of aspiration.
2. **Clear vomitus:** Use large-bore suction to clear vomitus from the airway.
3. **Provide oxygen:** Titrate oxygen to maintain pulse oximetry >90%.
4. **Assist ventilation:** If necessary, assist ventilation to ensure adequate oxygenation and ventilation.

Foreign Body Airway Obstruction

Foreign body aspiration[126] can quickly lead to complete airway obstruction. Prompt and decisive action is required to resolve the obstruction. The management steps include the following:

1. **Perform abdominal thrusts:** Continue until the object is cleared or the patient becomes unconscious.
2. **Begin chest compressions:** If necessary, perform up to 30 chest compressions to dislodge the object.
3. **Visualize and suction:** Attempt to visualize the object, suction if needed, and ventilate the patient, repeating the steps as necessary

Maintaining Competency

Competency in emergency airway management is crucial and is best maintained through frequent simulation and team training.[6,13,127] Understanding and following emergency airway management algorithms are fundamental for safe sedation practices and successful patient rescue.

Knowledge of Sedative Agents

Practitioners must have an in-depth understanding of the sedative agents they intend to use, including their potential complications (see Chapter 27 for a discussion of sedative agents).[6,13] Numerous reviews and handbooks are available for reference on sedating pediatric patients. Specific situations, such as the delivery of general anesthesia and monitored anesthesia care by anesthesiologists or other practitioners, are beyond the scope of this chapter.

Recommendations

Managing medical emergencies in a pediatric dental office requires not only technical skills but also a well-structured cognitive approach. This chapter outlines a systematic cognitive framework to effectively handle various emergencies in pediatric dentistry. The authors recommend the following:

- Be prepared by further expanding on this material.
- **Utilize decision-making algorithms:**
  - **Emergency protocols:** Follow established protocols for specific emergencies, ensuring a step-by-step approach.
  - **Critical thinking:** Apply clinical judgment to adapt protocols to the specific situation.
- Understand drug-related emergencies that may result from pharmacologic agents being utilized in daily practice.

Visit eBooks.Health.Elsevier.com to see full list of references.

36 Children With Disabilities

JESSICA WEBB

CHAPTER OUTLINE

Overview of Disability

Disability

A *disability* is a physical or cognitive impairment that limits a person's ability to take part in activities and participate.[2] Activities are the tasks of daily life such as hygiene, self-care, and managing a household.[2] Participation refers to life pursuits and interactions with others such as school, work, social engagement, and community involvement.[2]

Conditions causing disability may be present at birth (e.g., Down syndrome), may appear during childhood (e.g., autism spectrum disorder [ASD]), may be acquired later in life (e.g., brain or spinal cord injury), or they may be secondary to a chronic health condition (e.g., visual impairment or limb loss secondary to diabetes).[2]

Developmental Disability

Developmental disabilities are a broad category of conditions that begin during the developmental period and may be physical, cognitive, or behavioral.[3] Developmental disabilities affect daily functioning and typically continue throughout a person's lifetime.[3]

Intellectual Disability

Intellectual disability (ID) is defined by "significant limitations in both intellectual functioning and adaptive behavior that originates before the age of 22."[4] Intellectual functioning refers to one's ability to learn, reason, and problem solve.[4] Adaptive behavior includes conceptual skills, such as the ability to understand money and time; social skills, such as being able to understand and follow laws and avoid being victimized; and practical skills, such as navigating healthcare and transportation systems.[4] ID occurs in approximately 1% to 3% of the population.[5]

Physical Disability

Physical disability arises from a condition that limits "physical functioning, mobility, dexterity, or stamina."[6] These conditions may be static, such as a physical disability from cerebral palsy (CP), or progressive such as muscular dystrophy.[2]

Sensory Disability

Sensory disabilities result from impairments to any of the senses, such as vision, hearing, smell, taste, touch, and/or spatial awareness.[7]

Most commonly, sensory disabilities refer to visual impairments, which include low vision and blindness, deaf and hard of hearing, or both.[7] Sensory processing differences are not caused by impairments to the senses.[8,9] Instead, they result from the way in which sensory stimuli are processed.[8,9] This is discussed further in the section "Sensory-Adapted Dental Environment."

Chronic Health Conditions

Chronic health conditions are "conditions persisting over a period of time that require health care and/or limit activities of daily living."[10] They include conditions such as allergies/anaphylaxis, asthma, dental caries, obesity, seizure disorders, diabetes, and mental health conditions.[10]

Medically Complex

Children with medical complexity (CMC) are children who "have multiple significant chronic health problems that affect multiple organ systems and result in functional limitations, high healthcare need or utilization, and often the need for or use of medical technology."[11]

Children With Disabilities

Children with disabilities, like all children, are a heterogenous population. They may have a disability due to a syndrome such as a child with Down syndrome having an ID (see Chapter 37), secondary to medical complexity such as pediatric malignancy (see Chapter 39), or they may have a disability such as a developmental disability that is not related to a syndrome or medical complexity.[2] Similarly, disabilities can co-occur with syndromes, chronic health conditions, and medical complexity that are unrelated, or children may have multiple disabilities such as an ID and a sensory impairment.[12]

Biopsychosocial Model of Disability

There are many models that help conceptualize disability. The model that healthcare providers are most commonly trained in, implicitly or explicitly, is the *medical model* of disability.[13] The challenge with this model is that it medicalizes disability, informs attitudes in healthcare and society that those with disabilities are less than, and overlooks the lived experience of disability.[13] The *social model,* in contrast, recognizes that people have impairments but holds that what makes a condition disabling are the societal attitudes and lack of inclusion.[13]

The model that is widely accepted is the *biopsychosocial model.*[13,14] This model aims to capture that disability is dynamic and composed of not only the health condition(s) the person has, but aspects of their unique situation, ability to engage in activities, and ability to participate meaningfully, which influences the experience of their disability Fig. 36.1.[13,14] Although this model is a bit cumbersome to use for individual patients in a clinical setting, conceptually it reveals how disability is a complex phenomenon and a given condition cannot be generalized from person to person. What it means to have a disability is different for each individual; for example, two children may have the same diagnosis of CP or ASD, but the way in which they experience disability is unique to each of them. As clinicians, it is important to be knowledgeable about the health conditions of patients and to have a solid clinical foundation, but to use that as a starting point for understanding patients rather than assuming it is comprehensive.

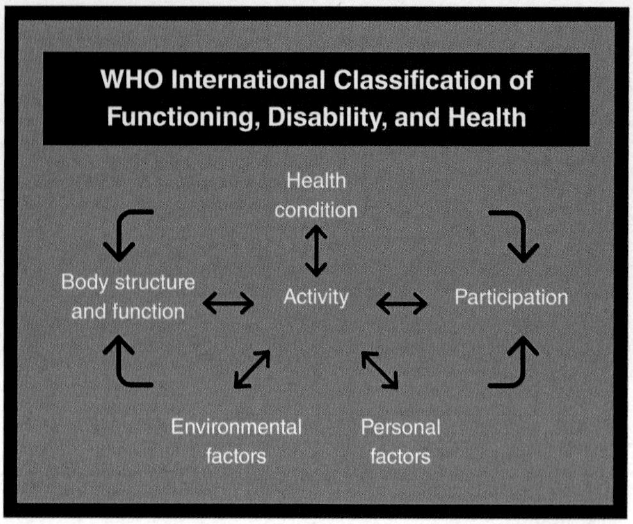

• **Fig. 36.1** WHO international classification of functioning, disability, and health.

Neurodiversity

Neurodiversity recognizes that neurologic functioning and processing exists on a spectrum and holds that variation is a part of human diversity to be accepted and embraced.[15] It maintains that neurodivergence, such as in those with intellectual disabilities or ASD, is not problematic, but instead values the perspective of those who are neurodivergent and celebrates neurologic diversity.[15]

Children With Disabilities in the Dental Setting

Approximately 17% of children have a developmental disability, and any dentist caring for children will undoubtedly have the opportunity to work with this patient population.[16] Common developmental disabilities include ID, ASD, CP, and Down syndrome (discussed in Chapter 37).

Assessment

Caring for children with disabilities begins with a comprehensive patient assessment, just as it does with any patient. It is essential to ensure a complete, accurate, and current history that includes medical diagnoses, medications, surgical history, hospitalizations, allergies, sensory sensitivities, behavioral considerations, and safety concerns as part of the medical, dental, social histories, and chief complaint collected and updated at each visit for all patients.[17] It may be necessary to request records from other providers, such as the primary care provider, specialty providers, and therapists, as well as consult, coordinate care, and communicate with those providers.[17]

The assessment should also involve understanding the patient's ability to communicate and cooperate.[17] This information may initially be collected before the visit in writing/electronically or verbally by staff. This allows for appropriate scheduling and planning, for needed records to be requested, and for communication without the child present, especially if the child's behavior is such that detailed or lengthy conversations are difficult or if such discussions increase the child's anxiety about healthcare visits. However, the parent interview should be reviewed and discussed between the dentist and parent before examination or treatment. Often it can be helpful to have an introductory visit where the dentist can conduct the parent interview, assess cooperation and communication, and introduce the child to the dental office without the expectation of examination to desensitize them to the new environment.[17]

Common Developmental Disabilities

ID is often combined with developmental disability as intellectual and developmental disabilities (IDDs) to capture individuals who have an ID and other disabilities.[18]

ASD occurs in approximately 1 in 36 children and occurs in boys almost four times as often as it does in girls.[19] There is no test such as a genetic or blood test to detect ASD; it is diagnosed based on clinical criteria.[20] The etiology of ASD is not well understood, but it is multifactorial.[20] Risk factors for ASD include having a sibling with ASD, fragile X syndrome, complications during birth, and older parents.[20] ASD is characterized by deficits in social communication, restricted and repetitive behavior or interests, and symptoms presenting in the developmental period that have a clinically significant impairment and are not better explained by another diagnosis such as ID.[21] Historically, Asperger syndrome and pervasive developmental disorder were distinct diagnoses, but in the current criteria these have been included under the umbrella of ASD.[21] Predictors for cooperation for children with ASD in the dental setting include ability to read, age, toilet training status, expressive language, and concurrent diagnoses.[22] When cooperation is limited and protective stabilization is considered, this technique was more acceptable to parents whose children with ASD had been treated with the use of protective stabilization previously.[23] The dental implications of having ASD may include behavioral or sensory challenges to home hygiene and preventive care or treatment in the dental setting, restrictive diets, and habits with oral implications such as bruxism, pica, or self-injurious behavior.[24]

CP is a condition caused by abnormalities that occur during fetal or infant brain development.[25] It results in motor dysfunction and often includes ID, seizure disorders, speech and language disorders, musculoskeletal conditions, behavioral challenges, gastrointestinal conditions, and feeding difficulties sometimes resulting in gastrostomy tube (G-tube) use.[25] People with CP often have contractures, necessitating consideration for positioning in the dental setting and may contraindicate the use of protective stabilization.[26,27] Dentally, people with CP are more likely to have malocclusion, specifically class II malocclusion and anterior open bite, bruxism, sialorrhea, mouth breathing, delayed tooth eruption, and retention of food in the mouth due to the inability to effectively clear the oral cavity.[28–30]

Risk of Social Isolation

Often, children with disabilities are reduced to their diagnoses and much of their time is dedicated to healthcare and therapeutic appointments rather than engaged in other aspects of childhood. Belonging is a fundamental human need, and a lack of social interaction leads to social isolation and loneliness.[31] Children with IDD in particular often have limited opportunities to make and maintain developmentally appropriate peer friendships.[32] They are often excluded and are at greater risk of loneliness.[31] Loneliness has negative effects on mental health, behavior, and social emotional development, and those effects often carry over into adulthood.[31] A key component to meaningful friendship is reciprocity, which is often missing in the relationships of children with disabilities whose relationships can predominantly consist of family, healthcare providers, and therapists.[32] Although we want dentists to have positive relationships with their patients with disabilities, dentists can do more to improve the health of their patients with disabilities by being aware of the social isolation for which these patients are at high risk.

Parents

Parents who have children with disabilities may face a variety of stressors. These include *intellectual stressors* in understanding the diagnosis, its scope, and the implications.[27] They may also encounter *instrumental stressors,* such as financial challenges in caring for their child, navigating insurance and the healthcare system, and managing additional tasks that may be needed.[27] Families may have *emotional stressors* around the diagnosis and care of their child.[27] Factors such as emotional stress, exhaustion, and disagreements between parents about the care of the child may lead to parental depression.[27] Extended family, such as grandparents, may experience denial or negative emotions around the diagnosis of a child with a disability, which may make the family feel even more isolated, or they may be an additional source of support and caregiving.[27] Parent networks where parents are able to learn and receive support have been shown to be very effective.[27,33]

Siblings

Siblings of children with disabilities have unique experiences and needs as well. Some children may worry, feel guilty, exhibit behaviors to get attention similar to their sibling, or take on extra responsibility to relieve their overburdened parents.[27] Often siblings of children with disabilities demonstrate increased maturity, responsibility, tolerance for differences, closeness to family, self-confidence, and independence.[27]

Implications for Dentists

Although it is beyond the scope of the dentist to identify and manage all the social support and resources for children with disabilities and their families, dentists can play an important role in connecting them with support and resources. Dentists are uniquely positioned to share resources and facilitate connections as they typically see patients and families every 6 months and see the siblings and the child with the disability. This is a frequency and level of interaction with the family that many other healthcare providers do not have.

Awareness of the benefits of social and recreational activities for children with disabilities, the instrumental needs families may have, and the potential need for information and support for families allows the dentist to recognize need and/or opportunities when interacting with families to share resources.

Beyond being aware of the potential needs for children with disabilities and their families, dentists can familiarize themselves with local resources for social, recreational, and support programs, such as local chapters of national support organizations like Parent to Parent for parent support; Sibshops for sibling support; local chapters of diagnosis-specific groups such as the National Down Syndrome Society; and inclusive social, leisure, and recreational activities (e.g., The Best Buddies program, therapeutic horseback riding programs through the Professional Association of Therapeutic

Horsemanship, and inclusive activities such as Special Olympics or Outdoors for All, Girl Scouts, or inclusive summer camps).[34–42]

Dentists can also share government assistance programs, mental health resources, translation services, training and employment resources, and afterschool and recreational programs to facilitate connecting families to needed resources. This includes the resource of dialing "211," a nationwide program that aims to minimize the difficulties with navigating convoluted governmental and community agencies by connecting individuals and families directly to resources for food, housing, clothing, and utility assistance, healthcare and mental health resources, and childcare services. Exploring city, county, and state governmental websites to learn about programs and resources such as parks and recreation programs or department of health resources; asking interdisciplinary colleagues such as pediatricians, social workers, and mental health providers; and learning about local community programs are all ways to familiarize oneself with local resources.[43] Ideally, dental offices can display or provide contact information for resources to share with families when appropriate. Dentists can also ensure that the community events they host or participate in are inclusive to children with disabilities.

Ableism

Ableism is the belief, which may be conscious or unconscious, that those with disabilities are less than.[44] There are a variety of ways that ableism is perpetuated both in society, generally, and healthcare, specifically, such as lack of physical access for those with limited mobility, disparaging remarks about those with intellectual disabilities, and representations of people with disabilities in the media that reinforce stereotypes. In healthcare, ableism has been apparent in people with intellectual disabilities being denied procedures such as organ transplants, presuming that symptoms are related to the disability rather than addressing them, and assumptions about the quality of life of people with disabilities.[45–49] Everyone has unconscious bias; the goal is to be aware of it and work to mitigate it.[45] A useful tool can be the Implicit Association Test by Harvard's Project Implicit: the disability-specific assessment is available at https://implicit.harvard.edu/implicit/takeatest.html.[50]

Ableism in Language

The language used by healthcare professionals must balance being clinically accurate, respectful of patients and their families, and inclusive of the disability community broadly. Words can be reflective of historical biases as well as influence beliefs; this underscores the importance of using words that do not reinforce negative and antiquated notions of disability. Word choices rooted in ableism should be avoided with the goal of utilizing terminology that reflects a neutral attitude about disability. This includes avoiding outdated terminology, euphemistic language, stereotypes, words with negative connotations, and using disability as an insult.[51]

Terms such as "mental retardation" and "handicapped" are outdated and have been replaced with "intellectual disability" and "disabled," respectively. Rather than using "normal" or "able-bodied," use "nondisabled."[52]

Euphemistic terms such as "differently abled," "handicapable," and "special needs" should be avoided as they are considered patronizing.[52] Clinicians will observe that the term "special needs" is ubiquitous in the healthcare setting and literature, particularly in pediatrics, but should note the move away from this terminology and aim to replace it with "disabilities."[52] Furthermore, as previously discussed, people with disabilities are a heterogenous group and terms like "special needs" do not provide meaningful accuracy or adequate specificity in the clinical setting. Although often well-intentioned, comments such as calling those with disabilities "inspirational" or "brave" reinforce the stereotype that living with a disability is a somehow diminished life and to simply endure it or to parent and love a child with a disability is heroic.[52] People with disabilities may do things that are inspirational or brave, so these comments should be reserved for actions that warrant their use instead of characterizing their existence as remarkable.[52]

Common phrases such as "wheelchair bound" or "confined to a wheelchair" should be replaced with simply stating that the person "uses a wheelchair."[51] This eliminates the negative connotation of being "bound" or "confined." Additionally, it is more accurate, using a wheelchair facilitates mobility rather than being an object of "confinement." Furthermore, some individuals who utilize wheelchairs for mobility may be able to stand or walk to an extent and it is important to avoid language that reinforces stereotypes. Discussing the diagnoses of patients is another area where negative connotations and stereotypes often arise. Terms like "suffers from" or "afflicted with" ought to be replaced with simply stating that the patient "has a diagnosis of ___." The aim is to use accurate and neutral language when discussing disability.[51] It is not appropriate to use disability as an insult or descriptor of something negative. Although this may seem obvious, there are commonly used terms that are rooted in disability such as "retarded," "crippled," and "spastic" that are often used out of habit and without awareness of their etiology or the impact they have on people with disabilities.[52]

Changing language requires effort, being open to feedback, and continued learning to stay contemporary, as language is ever-evolving. As healthcare providers, it is important to use appropriate and clinically accurate language to engage with colleagues; to model appropriate language to dental teams, patients, and society more broadly; and to use language that makes patients and families feel welcome and included in our practices. A helpful resource to stay contemporary is the National Center on Disability and Journalism style guide.[51]

Person-First and Identity-First Language

Person-first language aims to counter the practice of referring to people with disabilities as their diagnosis such as "a Downs child" and instead put the person first by saying "a child with Down syndrome."[51–53] The goal of person-first language is to recognize a patient's personhood over their diagnosis. Typically, person-first language is the default unless the patient prefers identity-first language, and it is more commonly used in pediatrics. There are some disability communities that may generally favor person-first language, for example, the Down syndrome community.[54]

Identity-first language aims to capture the idea that many disabled people view their disability as a part of their identity, and take pride in it and in the community to which they belong.[51–53] They may view that person-first language reinforces the notion that disability is wrong or stigmatizing by trying to separate their disability from their identity, and they may choose to have their disability come first such as identifying as "disabled," "Deaf," or "autistic."[51–53,55] Identity-first language is more commonly used with adults and in the Deaf and autistic communities.[51,52,55]

Barriers to Care

Individuals with disabilities face barriers when attempting to access healthcare. Some of them are broad and systemic, and some are challenges to providing care in the clinical setting.

Systemic Barriers to Care

Systemic barriers to people with disabilities accessing healthcare include physical access to healthcare facilities or devices such as a panoramic radiograph machines, communication barriers, and inadequate access to transportation.[17,56–58] Financial barriers are common due to lack of insurance coverage, high out-of-pocket costs, and high deductibles.[17,56–58] Often there is a lack of awareness of the need for dental care, or even if there is awareness of the need, there may be competing or higher priority healthcare or therapeutic needs for people with disabilities.[17,56,58] There can also be challenges with finding providers who are adequately trained and prepared to care for patients with disabilities.[58] As is the case in society more broadly, individuals with disabilities also face ableism and implicit bias when accessing healthcare.[57,58]

Clinical Barriers to Care

Once healthcare is accessed by people with disabilities, there may be barriers to providing care in the clinical setting. People with disabilities may have atypical presentations of symptoms and/or difficulty communicating symptoms.[58] For example, a child with an ID may have dental pain that presents as a change in behavior. This exacerbates the difficulty in accessing care in that problems may go unrecognized and untreated until they are severe and/or urgent. There can be a lack of useful diagnostic systems, such as ability to capture radiographs or compete pulp testing, on a patient who is unable to cooperate. There may also be a lack of continuity of care for people with disabilities. This may be due to turnover in home caregivers so there are no caregivers who know the patient well. This also may be due to high turnover in healthcare providers, such as for patients who receive care in university or hospital settings, which are often safety nets for this population, but have a high turnover of trainees.[58]

Barriers to Evidence-Based Dentistry

A significant barrier to providing quality care to patients with disabilities, specifically those with ID, is a lack of evidence to inform clinical care, behavior guidance, and decision-making. Most studies involving people with IDD in the dental literature were observational or epidemiologic yielding a dearth of interventional studies and randomized control trials, and a consequent lack of higher level evidence.[59]

The lack of research including people with IDD cannot adequately be addressed without historical context. Historically, people with IDs have had research abuses committed against them when they have been used as research subjects to yield data that are beneficial to the general population, for example, the Willowbrook and Vipeholm studies.[60–63] In these studies, people with IDD were intentionally given diseases so they could be used as subjects in research to benefit nondisabled populations. This is distinct from the thoughtful inclusion of people with IDD as research participants to benefit people with IDD by improving the ability to receive evidence-based healthcare that is tailored to their unique needs. Although there have been significant improvements in ethical research and elimination of abuses, there has not been adequate inclusion of people with IDD in meaningful research for the benefit of people with IDD.[64] There are barriers that can make it challenging to include this patient population in research such as difficulty having ideal clinical conditions that are helpful for quality research, lack of adequate cooperation, challenges with long-term follow-up, difficulty complying with research protocols, challenges to the informed consent process, and difficulty with identifying representative samples of people with IDD (often convenience samples are used that may not adequately represent people with IDD).[64] This leaves clinicians with a lack of robust evidence to inform clinical care and best practices for diagnosis, treatment, and prevention for people with IDD.

Oral Health of Children With Disabilities

Oral Hygiene

Children with disabilities often have significantly greater plaque, poorer oral hygiene, and poorer gingival health.[65–69] This may be due to physical disabilities limiting dexterity, behavioral challenges making home hygiene difficult, comorbid conditions or malocclusions resulting in mouth breathing, or lack of ability to effectively clear the oral cavity due to neuromuscular limitations.

Caries Risk

Studies are inconsistent if the caries rate of those with IDD is comparable or different than those without disabilities, but studies do tend to show that those with IDD do have more untreated caries, have more missing teeth due to caries, and have fewer restored teeth.[67,68]

Children with disabilities are a heterogeneous group and caries risk is multifactorial with biologic, environmental, socioeconomic, and behavioral factors.[70] Caries risk should be determined individually based on each child and a preventive plan should be tailored to their unique needs.[17,70] Specifically, for children with disabilities, consuming greater than four sugar-sweetened beverages per week was associated with caries.[71]

Caries risk factors to consider in children with disabilities include sugary medications or medications placed in fermentable carbohydrates to make them more palatable, sensory sensitivities leading to preferences for soft foods or avoidance of home hygiene, use of fermentable carbohydrates for behavioral rewards, fermentable carbohydrates to promote weight gain, avoidance of fluoridated toothpaste due to inability to expectorate excess, reduced salivary flow due to medications or health conditions, inability to adequately clear the oral cavity after eating, enamel defects, and behavioral challenges to oral hygiene and preventive dental visits.[17,70,72,73]

Oral Hygiene and Caries Prevention Strategies

Toothbrushing and the use of fluoridated toothpaste have been shown to be effective caries prevention strategies in children with IDD.[17,65,66,69,74] Studies are inconsistent regarding whether power toothbrushes are more effective than manual toothbrushes in people with IDD; this variability may be due to sensory sensitivities and/or behavioral challenges.[74] Toothbrush selection depends on what works for each individual patient and their unique needs.[17]

Given the best evidence currently available, the strategies with demonstrated efficacy for children with IDD are toothbrushing, the use of fluoridated toothpaste, limiting sugar-sweetened beverages, and individualized caries risk assessment and preventive strategies based on individual caries risk factors.[17,65,66,69–71,73,74]

Trauma Risk and Management

Children with disabilities are at a greater risk for traumatic dental injuries.[17,75] This is due to a variety of factors such as motor skill and coordination challenges increasing risk of falls, seizure disorders, visual impairment increasing fall risk, excess overjet, lip incompetence, bruxism, increased risk of abuse, nonnutritive habits, and self-injurious behavior.[17,75] Comprehensive dental care for children with disabilities ought to include anticipatory guidance regarding traumatic dental injuries.[17] When managing traumatic dental injuries in children with disabilities, relevant factors to consider include co-occurring medical conditions, immunocompromise, allergies, medications, ability to cooperate, habits, and self-injurious behavior.[76,77]

Behavior Guidance

Behavior guidance, both nonpharmacologic and pharmacologic, are discussed in depth in Chapters 26 and 27. There are potential additional challenges to cooperation for children with disabilities due to difficulties with communication, intellectual and/or developmental disabilities, anxiety in the healthcare setting, oral aversion, sensory sensitivities, and/or fatigue from many healthcare visits and procedures.[17] There are also additional considerations for standard nonpharmacologic and pharmacologic behavior guidance for children with disabilities.[17]

Nonpharmacologic behavior guidance techniques demonstrated to be effective in patients with IDD are reinforcement, modeling, desensitization, distraction, relaxation, communication strategies, and adaptation of the clinical environment.[78] Specifically, audiovisual distraction, sensory-adapted dental environments (SADEs), and picture exchange communication system (PECS) Fig. 36.2.[79]

Pharmacologic behavior guidance may be indicated more commonly for children with IDD, chronic health conditions, and/or medical complexity. This may be due to dental needs exceeding the child's ability to cooperate, dental fear due to extensive interactions with healthcare and/or procedures, the need for modification of treatment with premedication, preoperative admission or additional postoperative monitoring, and/or the need to complete dental treatment in one visit due to medical complexity.[17] Children with IDD, chronic health conditions, medical complexities, and/or at high risk for airway compromise may have contraindications to procedural sedation or general anesthesia in the office setting, and may need to be treated in a hospital setting.[17,80,81] For example, patients who are hypertonic or hypotonic, or have craniofacial anomalies such as a hypoplastic midface, retrognathic mandible, or potential atlantoaxial instability have more challenging airways to maintain.[81]

Best Practices

Often the approach when working with children with disabilities is to take existing best practices in dentistry and attempt to modify them for children with disabilities. Given the lack of robust evidence to inform the care of this patient population discussed previously, this is an appropriate strategy and can be very effective; however, it can often be inadequate. In addition to utilizing evidenced-based dentistry and oral health best practices for our patients with disabilities, it is effective to also utilize best practices in the field of disability and apply them to dentistry.

Strengths-Based Approach

Utilizing a strengths-based approach is a useful practice with any patient or family and is considered a best practice when working with patients with disabilities and their families.[82] A *strengths-based approach* focuses on understanding the strengths and areas of competence for a patient or family and then working to support and leverage those strengths and competencies.[83] This contrasts with a *deficit-based approach,* which focuses on limitations. An additional advantage of this approach is that it can be employed by the entire dental team who can be taught and encouraged to seek out areas of strength and competence and to build and encourage from there.

Universal Design

Universal design is the practice of "designing all products, buildings and exterior spaces to be useable by all people to the greatest extent possible."[84] Universal design recognizes that the impact of a disability is not just the disability of itself, but the way in which products, buildings, and spaces exacerbate the disabling effects of a condition by not being designed with physical or social inclusivity in mind.[84] This concept aims to make design modifications to maximize the universal usability of products, structures, and spaces by people with a range of abilities and to do so without needing modifications or segregation.[84] An example of this is curb cuts that facilitate access for those who use wheelchairs, allow for greater ease when pushing a stroller, provide critical information to those with visual impairments using mobility canes, and allow for people to wheel a suitcase or cart up a curb. Ideally, universal design should be incorporated from the time of idea conception so that it is integrated into the design rather than needing to modify it after the fact to be inclusive.[84] Universal design includes accessibility, but is a distinct concept. Accessibility focuses on access to the physical environment, predominantly for those who use wheelchairs, such as ramps, elevators, and wider doorways. Although accessibility is necessary and a move in the right direction, it does not include a diversity of users; it focuses on buildings and is less thoughtful about products, and it tends to promote separateness with different entrances and seating areas, which does allow physical access but may result in social segregation. For example, a movie theater may be accessible with ramps, automatic doors, and designated wheelchair seating, but if a teenager that uses a wheelchair wants to go to the movie with friends she may be excluded from sitting with the group, so the physical access is inadequate to make the prototypical high school experience of going to the movies with a group of friends inclusive, even though it is accessible. Table 36.1 shows how universal design can be incorporated into the dental setting.

Patient- and Family-Centered Care

Patient- and family-centered care is rooted in the value of partnership between clinicians and families, which is broadly defined.[86] The evolution to patient- and family-centered care from simply family-centered care, aims to capture the importance of including the patient in the process in a developmentally appropriate manner.[86] This partnership based approach honors that; families know the child with a disability best, the day-to-day interactions

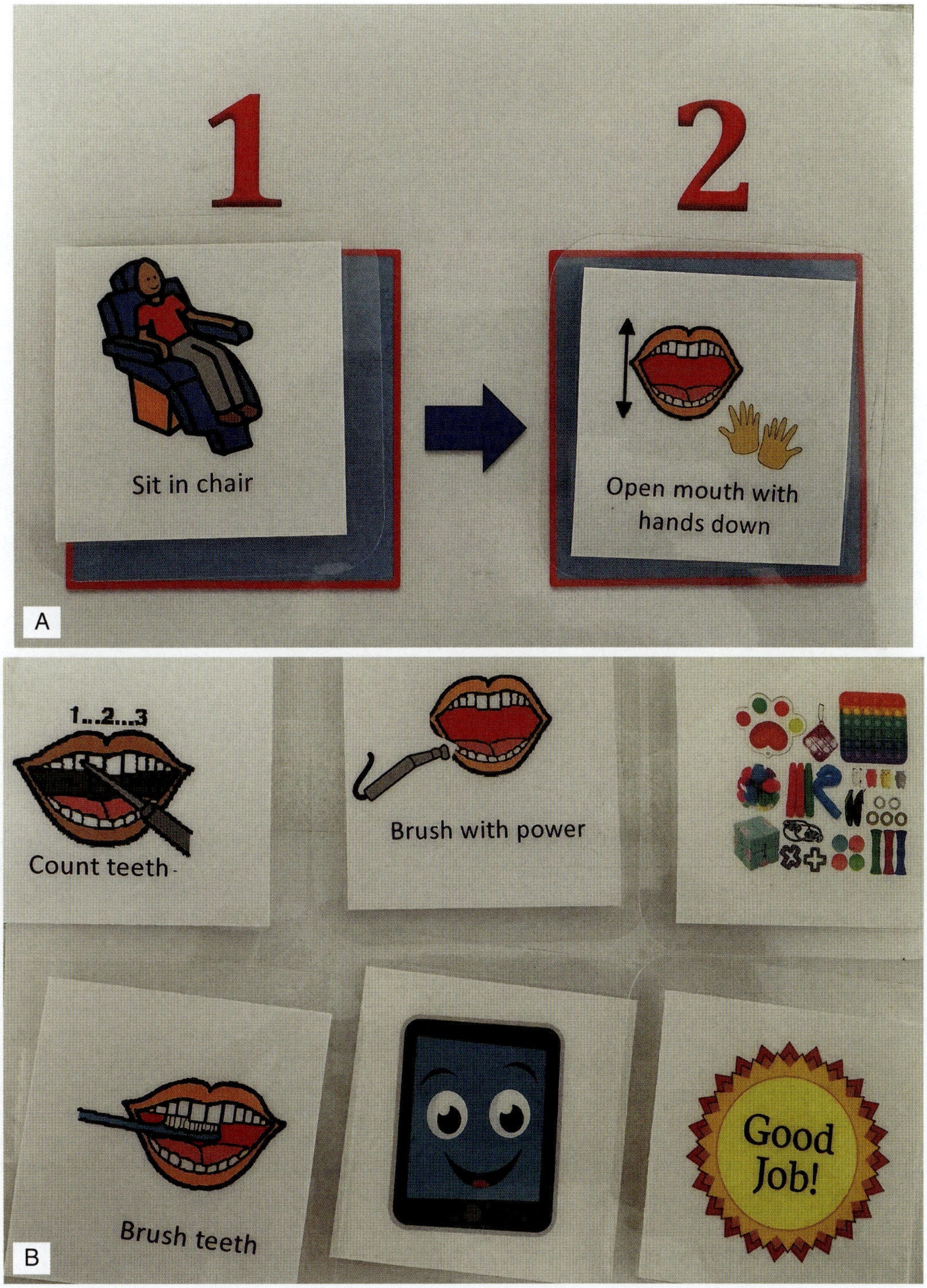

• **Fig. 36.2** (A–C) Example of picture exchange communication (PECS).

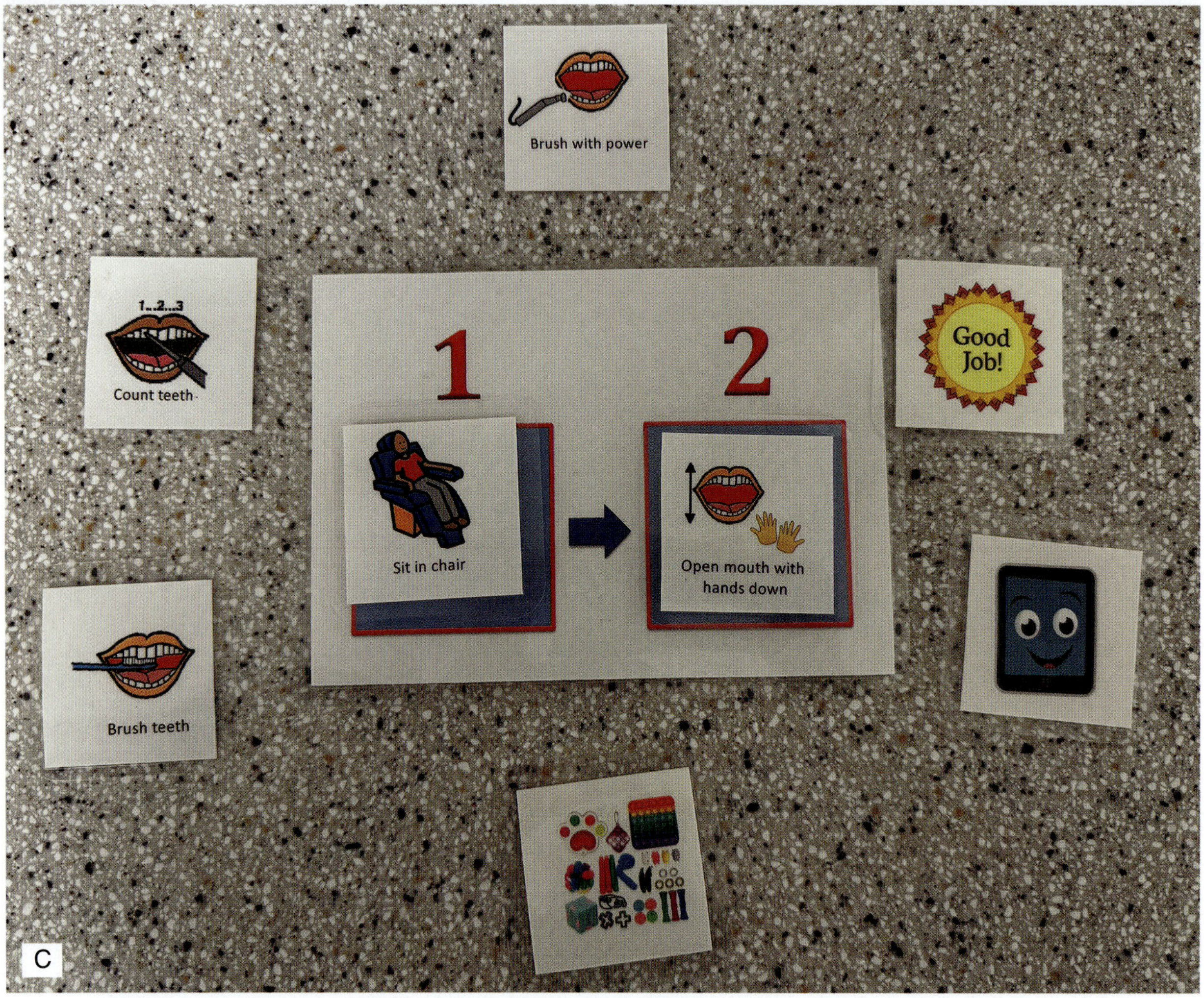

• **Fig. 36.2, cont'd**

TABLE 36.1 Universal Design in the Dental Setting

Physical access	• Ramps instead of curbs/steps • Lever door handles instead of knobs • Grab bars • Seat level counters • Keep walkways and ramps decluttered and free of tripping hazards • Accessible family restrooms
Written materials	• Large print for printed materials • Ability to adjust font size for electronic materials • Alt text for images • High contrast between text and background • Offer an auditory option • Enable keyboard navigation
Auditory information	• Closed captioning • Transcripts
Sensory modifications	• Dimmable lights • Adjustable volume • Minimize scents and fragrances

From DisabilityEtiquette.pdf. https://www.unitedspinal.org/pdf/DisabilityEtiquette.pdf. Accessed April 3, 2024.

and interventions are more meaningful to health and wellbeing than periodic visits to health care providers, for an intervention to be effective inclusion of the family is critical, well-supported families are able to better care for children, and providers change over the child's life but the family members are more constant.[86] The core tenants of patient- and family-centered care include listening and respect; flexibility; sharing complete, honest, and unbiased information; providing and/or ensuring support; collaboration; and recognizing and building upon strengths.[86] Patient- and family-centered care has been shown to improve outcomes, overall satisfaction with healthcare experiences, resource utilization, and decrease healthcare costs.[47]

Sensory-Adapted Dental Environment

Sensory processing is the neural system interpreting sensory input from the body and the environment.[8,9] Types of sensory input include proprioceptive, vestibular, olfactory, gustatory, visual, auditory, and tactile sensory domains.[8,9] *Sensory processing differences* are common in children with developmental disabilities.[87] There is a diagnosis of *sensory processing disorder,* but this diagnosis is out of the scope of practice for a dentist to make, and it is distinct from sensory processing differences that are associated with having a developmental disability.[8] Sensory processing differences occur in between 40% and 80% of children with neurodevelopmental disabilities and between 3% and 11% of adults with neurodevelopmental disabilities compared with 2.8% to 6.5% of the neurotypical population.[87,88] Given that sensory processing differences are more common in children with neurodevelopmental disabilities than adults with neurodevelopmental disabilities, they are likely a function of developmental immaturity and diminish with maturation.[89] Often there is greater awareness of sensory processing differences in children with ASD; however, the occurrence of sensory processing differences in children with ASD is comparable to children with neurodevelopmental disabilities more broadly, and ought to be considered for all children with neurodevelopmental disabilities, not just ASD.[89] With that said, children with ASD have demonstrated more severe sensory processing differences and more significant responses.[89]

Children with sensory processing differences may be *hyperresponsive* to sensory input, which yields a sensory avoidant response or negative reaction to sensory stimuli, or they may be *hyporesponsive* to sensory input, which results in sensory-seeking behaviors or strong sensory preferences.[8,9,89] Sensory hyperresponsivity and sensory hyporesponsivity can coexist in the same child; they may be sensitive to light and sound and seek tactile stimulation.[9] Sensory processing differences can lead to difficulty with emotional regulation and subsequent behavioral challenges.[8] This is particularly relevant in the dental setting both because behavior is a variable in the ability to provide dental examination and treatment, and because the dental environment with its bright lights, high-pitched noises, strong smells, laying in a reclined position, strange tastes, gritty and sticky textures, and moving chairs is rife with sensory stimulation in all sensory domains.

Sensory adaptation of the environment is an evidence-based intervention that has been shown to reduce pain, increase concentration, decrease maladaptive behaviors, offer a pleasant experience, provide relaxation, and provide sensory input for people with neurodevelopmental disabilities, and it has been modified specifically for the dental setting Fig. 36.3.[90–95] SADE has been shown to increase relaxation and cooperation in all children, but it was more significant for children with neurodevelopmental disabilities compared with neurotypical children.[79,93–95]

Consider all sensory domains when creating a sensory adapted dental environment (Table 36.2). There are a variety of factors to consider when selecting sensory equipment for the dental setting.

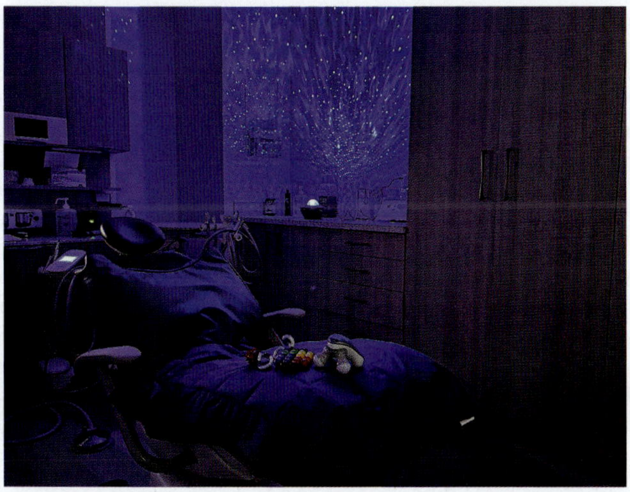

• **Fig. 36.3** Image of a sensory-adapted dental environment.

TABLE 36.2 Elements of a Sensory-Adapted Dental Environment

Sensory Domain	Intervention
Visual	• Light projector • Bubble tube • Rope lights • Sunglasses • Turning off overhead lights and using only the dental light and/or headlamp
Auditory	• Auditory stimulation that is pleasant, but not upregulating such as nature sounds or classical music • Noise-canceling headphones (may impede communication with the dental team)
Tactile	• Tactile balls that are textured or filled with materials such as sand • Pop its • Bubbles
Olfactory	• Scented and unscented hoods for nitrous oxide to accommodate both those with hyperresponsiveness and hyporesponsiveness to olfactory input • Scented nitrous oxide hood can be utilized with only oxygen if nitrous oxide is not indicated • Washcloth with essential oils
Gustatory	• Flavored and unflavored options when possible
Vestibular	• Vibrating pillow or mat • Handheld massagers • Lowering and reclining the chair before having the patient sit/lay in it as moving furniture can be disconcerting to patients with sensory sensitivities
Proprioceptive	• Pad for the dental chair such as the Specialized Care Company Stay N Place chair liner • Beanbag chairs • Placing a lead vest on the patient • Weighted blankets

Safety is, of course, of significant importance. Choking hazards should be avoided and the dentist should be aware of patient allergies, as they may affect materials selected or modifications used, such as essential oils. Equipment must be durable and cleansable between patients for infection control purposes. Single-use options may be considered when feasible, such as small individual bottles of bubbles that can be given to the family after the appointment rather than a large bottle that is reused with multiple patients. Another option is to use the patient's own sensory items when possible, such as having the family bring the patient's own noise-canceling headphones, tactile sensory equipment, or weighted blanket. When selecting sensory equipment for the dental setting, consider sourcing items from occupational therapy suppliers as those items are designed for sensory interventions in therapeutic settings and are more durable and cleansable for use by multiple patients in a clinical setting.

Communication

Children with disabilities may have limitations to their receptive and/or expressive language and some may not use speech at all.[17]

Communication and language disabilities do not mean there is an ID.[17] Additionally, communication is much broader than language. It can be helpful to engage the parent or caregiver as a resource to better understand how the patient best communicates in both receiving information and expressing needs and preferences. It is important to always speak directly to the patient even if the patient has limitations in receptive or expressive language.[81] A significant portion of communication is nonverbal and speaking to the patient allows for eye contact, tone, and facial expressions even if there is a lack of communication via speech.[81] Discussions about the patient with the family/caregivers should be inclusive of the patient to the extent possible.[81]

Helpful strategies include positioning oneself at eye level to patients, giving patients time to acclimate to the presence of the dentist instead of charging at the patient and initiating the examination, and employing calm nonverbal communication. Offering the patient choices when possible is a useful strategy, such as if they wish for the dental chair to go up first or back first or if they would like their top teeth brushed first or their bottom teeth. This accomplishes two important aims: it gives the patient a sense of control, which can mitigate dental anxiety, and when the patient asserts their preference and it is honored, it builds trust and rapport with the dental team member. Patients may utilize augmentative and alternative communication (AAC), so dentists should familiarize themselves with these and discuss preferred communication strategies with the patient and family.[81]

Some children with ASD may use echolalia in their speech communication. *Echolalia* is repeating the speech of others, it can be speech from either other people or heard on media such as radio, television, movies, online videos, or computer games.[96] Echolalia may be immediate or delayed.[96] Historically, echolalia, while speech, was dismissed as not communication, but is now recognized as meaningful and functional communication.[96] Echolalia can be a way for patients to communicate their anxiety and a method to self-regulate. It can also be a way to engage with patients and build rapport in a way that feels safe and comfortable to them. A diagnostic criterion of ASD is having repetitive and restrictive interests, often providing children with ASD an opportunity to discuss these interests can make them feel more comfortable and build rapport with the dentist.[21] Additionally, these interests can be leveraged with nonpharmacologic behavior guidance techniques. For example, for a child interested in trains, the prophy angle or slow-speed handpiece may bounce like a train, or the high-speed handpiece may whistle like a train whistle. Some people with ASD find eye contact difficult, sometimes even described as painful, and sometimes described as limiting their ability to take in information from their other senses when they are forcing it. Therefore eye contact should not be pushed for in individuals with ASD and is not considered reflective of attention or listening.

Social Stories

Social stories are visual representations of social or novel situations that help prepare a child for a dental visit.[97,98] They are predominantly used for children with ASD, but may be useful for other children with intellectual or developmental disabilities, and are geared toward specific targeted skills, such as going to the dentist.[97,99]

Although meta-analyses indicate that generalizability is difficult, they may be helpful for many children.[98–100,101] Advantages of social stories include that they are low cost and simple to make, so there is little downside to offering or attempting them as an option.[97,99]

A social story includes photos of the environment and the different phases of the process with captions about what to expect or what should be done Fig. 36.4.[97,98] The parent or caregiver can review the social story before the appointment to help prepare the patient.[99] The images can be illustrations or photographs depending on what is better suited for the child.[97–99] They can be generic dental social stories or specific to the practice the child is visiting. Photos of the dentist and staff with faces visible, followed by photos of the dental team in personal protective equipment such as masks, gloves, and gowns, is a useful strategy.[97] Social stories may be printed for the child to review or may be shown to the child digitally on a smartphone or tablet.[97]

Desensitization

Desensitization is the process of utilizing gradual stimulus exposure to teach dental skills.[81,102] It is essentially practicing going to the dentist for children who benefit from more repetition to learn skills or overcome anxieties in the dental environment.[81,102] It allows for the modification of behaviors to facilitate dental treatment.[81,102] When anxiety-provoking situations or environments are avoided, anxiety increases.[81,102] When there are successive, controlled exposures to anxiety-provoking stimuli that are reinforced with pleasant experiences, anxiety can be reduced.[81,102] Desensitization benefits from the natural maturation in children and this can have a synergistic effect with desensitization visits.[81] Desensitization can be individualized to each patient depending on their specific anxieties, strengths, motivations, and schedule.[81]

There are a variety of relevant factors when considering desensitization as an approach. Oral health status is a critical factor to consider. If the child has active disease or acute dental disease, that should be addressed before beginning desensitization rather than taking the time that desensitization requires while the disease is not being addressed and/or progressing.[81] Desensitization should be developmentally appropriate, and the pacing and steps should be tailored to the child's capabilities.[81] Additionally, be aware of the child's expressive and receptive communication to ensure communication relevant for desensitization is feasible.[81] Ensure discussions with the parents/caregivers take into account their preferences, scheduling constraints, and geographical considerations as well as the dentist setting realistic expectations for desensitization.[81] For example, due to the regular visits required for desensitization, families traveling a significant distance may not be good candidates, and desensitization may not be as productive if it is done when the child is fatigued such as after school or after therapeutic appointments. Desensitization is a gradual process, and ideally, visits should end on a positive note. Communicating this process clearly to parents will help ensure the family and the dentist are aligned on what desensitization visits will look like, as they are typically quick, progress may not be noticeable at any individual visit, and the goal is to make it a pleasurable experience and have the visit end well, rather than trying to do more because the patient is doing well. Desensitization requires time and effort on the part of the family and the dental team.[81] During the planning process, ask about what is motivating and rewarding to the child, so that there is a plan for reinforcement at the end of the desensitization visits.[81] Regarding the dental team, although desensitization requires frequent visits, they are usually brief, require minimal setup, and some of them may be done by trained staff depending on the child's behavior and needs.

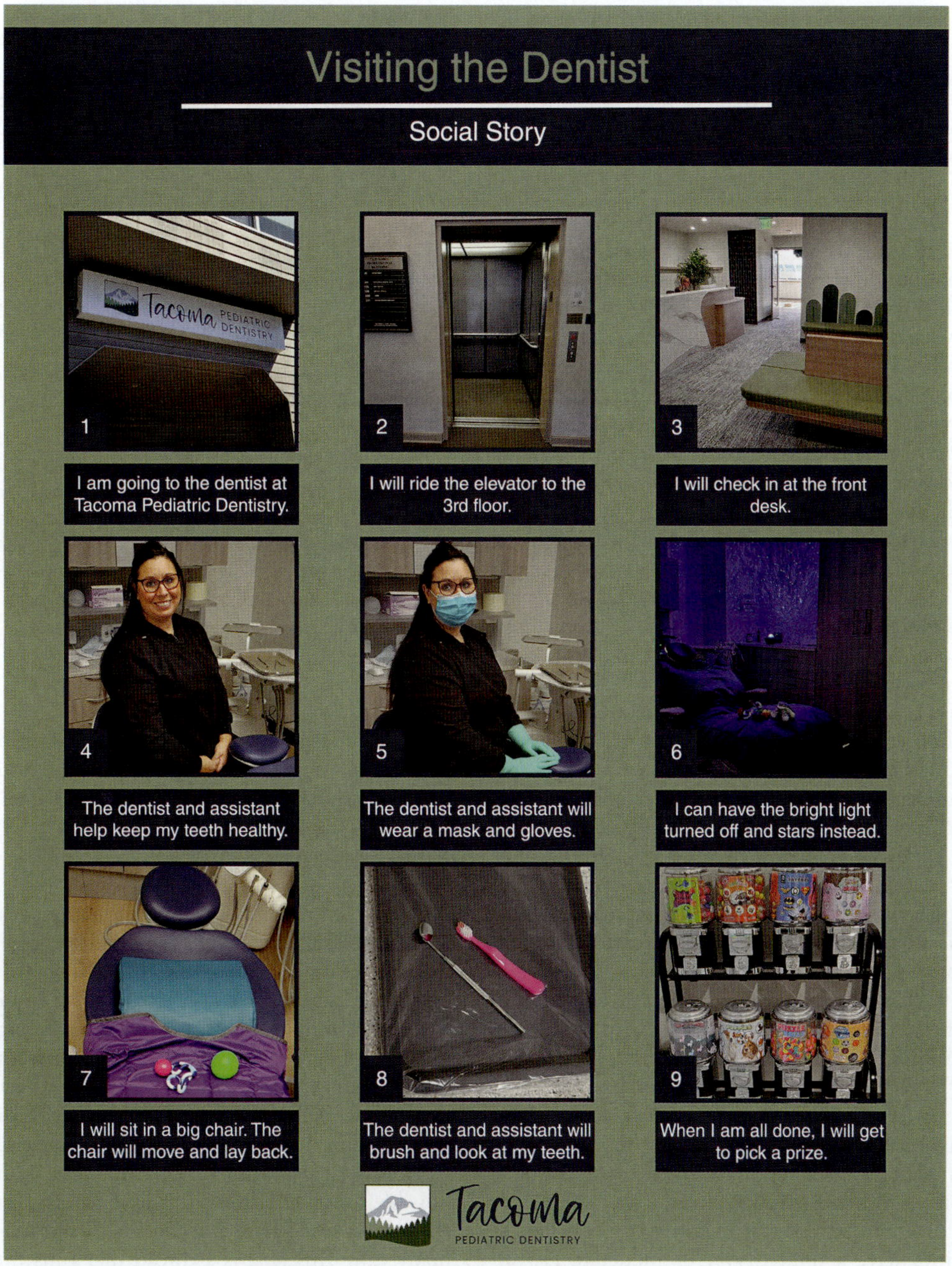
Visiting the Dentist
Social Story
1
I am going to the dentist at Tacoma Pediatric Dentistry.
2
I will ride the elevator to the 3rd floor.
3
I will check in at the front desk.
4
The dentist and assistant help keep my teeth healthy.
5
The dentist and assistant will wear a mask and gloves.
6
I can have the bright light turned off and stars instead.
7
I will sit in a big chair. The chair will move and lay back.
8
The dentist and assistant will brush and look at my teeth.
9
When I am all done, I will get to pick a prize.
Tacoma
PEDIATRIC DENTISTRY

• **Fig. 36.4** Example of a dental visit social story.

The skills that the dentist starts with will depend on the existing skills and what the priority is for the dentist and the parent/caregiver. From there, start with an existing skill in the dental environment or a similar environment. The goal is to then build on that skill by leveraging it into another skill or increasing the duration of the skill, for example, shifting a toothbrush prophylaxis to a mirror-only examination. At the next visit, it may be a good idea to start with the original skill, then shift to the new skill, so that the dentist is starting from a place of comfort and competence before practicing the new skill. The next goal may be increasing the duration, such as transitioning from the child simply allowing the mirror to enter the oral cavity to gradually building the tolerance for a complete intraoral examination with a mirror.

There should be one priority for the visit, either a new skill leveraged from an existing skill or increasing the duration of an existing skill. Having multiple goals for one visit often results in no or minimal progress toward any of them. This does sometimes make visits seem brief and repetitive to the parent and/or the dentist, but it is exactly that repetition that mitigates the anxiety of the child.

To the extent possible, try to keep as much as is feasible consistent for desensitization visits, such as the room, assistant, dentist, and routine. Consider providing the parent/caregiver with a plastic dental mirror so that families can practice at home, especially if they can do it in the same order such as brushing and then using the mirror at home so that routine can be replicated in the office during desensitization visits. Gloves are a choking hazard and suffocation risk so use caution in providing them to families for practice. If the child struggles with a new skill or increased duration, if possible, shift to a skill they are likely to be successful with, so that the visit can end on that success. After the success, ending desensitization visits with a reinforcer is an effective strategy. Reinforcers can be those typically used by the practice such as stickers, toys, etc., or can be customized by the family to the child's unique interests and motivators.

Transition

Improvements in healthcare have led to the increased life expectancy of those with disabilities.[103] This means that more children with disabilities will survive until adulthood, and that adulthood is longer for those with disabilities than it was in the past.[103] Historically, it was common for pediatric dentists to continue to see patients with disabilities into adulthood.[103] However, the longer life span of those with disabilities means an increased need for lifelong oral healthcare that is often better provided by general practitioners and other dental specialists.[103] Additionally, with more adults with disabilities, the pediatric dental workforce cannot possibly begin to care for all of the adults with disabilities while continuing to meet the needs of pediatric patients.[103]

Transition is a key component of facilitating oral healthcare throughout the life span of people with disabilities.[103] Transition is the developmentally appropriate process of transferring from pediatric to adult care, services, and resources.[27,103] This occurs across many settings and services for families including educational, financial, housing, recreational, support services, and healthcare.[27,103,104] This can be a challenging and stressful time for the family due to the volume and magnitude of change, and because often there are less resources for adults with disabilities than for children, there is often a feeling of falling off a resource and support cliff.[104] Pediatric dentists can best facilitate transition and support families by discussing and preparing for transition well in advance so that it is an expected and facilitated experience rather than a sudden surprise Table 36.3.[103,105,106]

The significant barrier to transition is often access to general dentists who are knowledgeable and comfortable with caring for people with disabilities, medical complexity, and/or chronic health conditions.[103,105,107,108] Supporting additional training for the hands-on care of this patient population in dental schools, advocating for adult dental benefits, and supporting enhanced reimbursement for patients with disabilities and medical complexities are critical to address this gap on a systems level.[103,105,107,108]

It is important to note that the vast majority of people with intellectual disabilities have a mild (85%) or moderate (10%) ID.[5] Only 4% have severe ID and about 1% having profound ID.[5] Generally, those with mild to moderate ID can be seen in the traditional dental setting and are able to cooperate for examination, preventive care, and the majority of treatment. Those with IDD and those with chronic medical conditions or medical complexity can largely be treated in the office setting with accommodation and modification.[103]

TABLE 36.3 Strategies for Transition[103,105,106,108–112]

Transition Practices	Transition Resources
Forge relationships with general practitioners	Special Care Dentistry Association directory
Advocating for adult dental benefits and for general dentists to have hospital privileges	Dental school and hospital-based clinics and training programs
Discuss transition with families in early adolescence to foster time for processing and planning	County and state oral health resources and programs
Provide care summaries to facilitate transition	Got Transition resources
Offer continued communication, support, and consultation to general dental colleagues throughout the transition process and beyond	Participate in Special Olympics Special Smiles and connect colleagues for hands-on opportunities to work with individuals with developmental disabilities

Conclusions

Going to the dentist is a life skill, and an adult with a disability who can allow for a dental examination, and possibly even treatment, is going to be more likely to be able to access care. Dentists caring for children are always balancing immediate dental needs with developing children's ability to feel comfortable in the dental setting, cooperate for examination and treatment, and ability to access lifelong oral healthcare; it is no different for children with disabilities. When caring for children with disabilities, consideration should be given to fostering the development of skills that will allow for participating in dental care. Although it may not be possible for all children with disabilities to grow into adults who are able to cooperate for care in the traditional dental setting, many can. This goal is a thread that runs throughout treatment and care planning so that the oral health of patients is addressed not only in the present moment, but throughout their lives.

Visit eBooks.Health.Elsevier.com to see full list of references.

37 Congenital Genetic Disorders and Syndromes

REBECCA L. SLAYTON AND ERIN EALBA BUMANN

CHAPTER OUTLINE

Practicing dentists are confronted daily with conditions that are either primarily genetic or have a significant genetic contribution in their etiologies. Common conditions such as tooth agenesis are now known, in many cases, to be caused by specific genetic mutations. Many syndromes involve craniofacial structures and have associated dental anomalies. Frequently other major malformations are present in addition to the craniofacial anomalies. Advances in the Human Genome Project have led to the discovery of the genetic basis of many of these disorders that include craniofacial and dental anomalies as part of the spectrum of the disease. Understanding the disease at this level permits the practitioner to provide a more precise diagnosis of the disease, a more appropriate treatment, and a more accurate prognosis of the outcomes of care.

Dental practitioners are aware of the environmental and behavioral risk factors that contribute to poor oral health. Patients and their parents are routinely counseled about the risks involved with cigarette smoking, smokeless tobacco, alcohol, poor oral hygiene, sweetened beverages, a diet high in carbohydrates, and traumatic injuries to the head and mouth. The two most common dental diseases—dental caries and periodontal disease—are complex and have both environmental and genetic components. As information about the genetic makeup of individuals increases, there will be additional genetic susceptibility or resistance factors identified that will influence the severity of oral diseases. Once these factors are identified, there will be tests that can be performed well before the occurrence of disease. This will permit practitioners to educate patients about the importance of their behaviors and to tailor their preventive strategies more specifically for each patient. Some of these will be in-office tests, whereas others will require the use of an outside laboratory. The application of appropriate tests and ultimately the interpretation of the test results and the management of the oral disease will be the responsibility of the dentist. Therefore practicing dentists must understand the basis of the test, how it is performed, and how the results are interpreted. Understanding the basis for many of the genetic tests available today requires an understanding of basic genetic concepts as well as the current technologies that are available for testing.

Basic Genetic Concepts

A person's genome is made up of the DNA in all 46 chromosomes in the nucleus of each cell of the body. Each cell has 23 pairs of chromosomes. One chromosome of each pair is inherited from each parent. Two of the chromosomes are called sex chromosomes (X and Y), whereas the remaining chromosomes (numbered

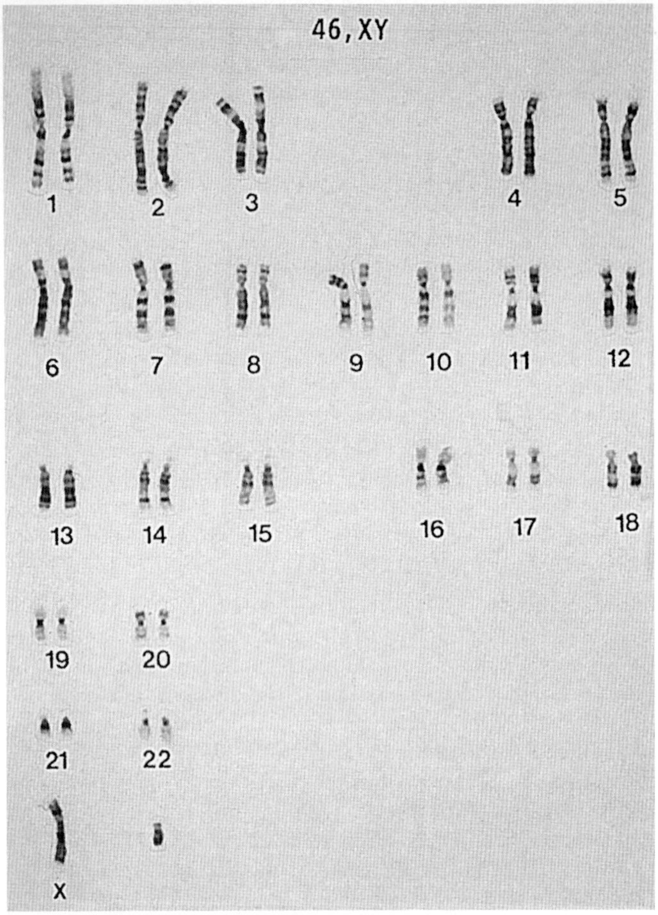

• **Fig. 37.1** Karyotype of a normal male.

1 through 22) are called autosomes. Males have one X and one Y chromosome; females have two X chromosomes. In each cell of a female, one of the X chromosomes is randomly inactivated. This is an important determinant of the severity of X-linked genetic disorders, as discussed later. The technique used to look at all the chromosomes in a cell and to determine the sex of a fetus from amniotic fluid is called karyotyping (Fig. 37.1). This technique also identifies major chromosomal anomalies such as trisomy (an extra chromosome), translocations of one part of a chromosome to another, or large chromosomal deletions.

Each chromosome is made up of a double-stranded DNA helix composed of a series of four nucleotides and a sugar-phosphate base. Each of the four nucleotides (adenine, thymine, cytosine, and guanine) is paired with a specific complementary nucleotide to form the double helix. Adenine always pairs with thymine, and cytosine always pairs with guanine. The ability of a single strand of DNA to bind to a complementary strand of DNA or RNA forms the basis of many of the diagnostic tests performed today.

Genes are sequences of DNA that are transcribed into messenger RNA and then translated into proteins. Each chromosome contains thousands of genes, and the entire human genome is estimated to have approximately 20,000 protein-coding genes. The exquisite control of gene expression is essential for the proper growth, development, and functioning of an organism.

Although each cell contains the same DNA and therefore the same genes, only a small percentage of those genes are active or expressed, depending on the time of development and the type of cell. Cells in the epidermis need some different proteins than cells in the developing tooth or in the kidney, and each cell type has a complex regulatory process to ensure that the right genes are expressed and translated into the necessary proteins at the proper time.

Molecular Basis of Disease

Traditionally, genetic diseases have been thought of in terms of Mendelian inheritance patterns. This means that a mutation present in a gene transmitted to a child from one or both parents results in the child either having the disease or being a carrier of the disease. As we have learned more about genetics, additional mechanisms of inheritance have been identified that make it more challenging to predict both the occurrence and the severity of disease. It is not uncommon for a genetic disease to be the result of a new or "de novo" mutation. In this case there would be no history of the disorder on either side of the family. Recently it has been found that advanced paternal age is associated with craniosynostosis syndromes such as Apert and Crouzon syndromes.[1,2] Other types of non-Mendelian inheritance patterns include imprinting, DNA triplet repeat expansion, mitochondrial DNA defects, and complex disorders in which multiple genes may be involved and in which sequence changes increase or decrease a person's susceptibility to disease.

Inheritance Patterns

Autosomal Dominant

In autosomal dominant inheritance, the transmission is vertical from parent to child. An affected parent has a 50% chance of passing along the defective gene to a child of either sex. Autosomal dominant inheritance may occur in the family initially as a new mutation or may have been present in the family for multiple generations. Nonsyndromic dentinogenesis imperfecta can be an example of an autosomal dominant disorder. The gene for type II dentinogenesis imperfecta has been identified (dentin sialophosphoprotein; *DSPP*) and is located on chromosome 4. Incomplete or reduced penetrance, which primarily occurs in autosomal dominant disorders, can occur when an individual carrying the mutation may not clinically exhibit the disease but still be capable of transmitting the mutation to their children.

Autosomal Recessive

An autosomal recessive disorder manifests only when an individual has two copies of the mutant gene. Most frequently each parent has one copy of the defective gene and is a carrier, and there is a 25% chance that both mutant genes will be passed on to their offspring. Male and female offspring will be equally likely to be affected. Fifty percent of the time the offspring will get one copy of the mutant gene from one parent and will be carriers, and 25% of the time the offspring will get two normal copies of the gene. Although autosomal recessive disorders are relatively uncommon, the carrier status in certain populations can be significant. For example, 1 in 25 people of northern European descent are carriers of mutations in the cystic fibrosis transmembrane regulator gene (CFTR), which causes cystic fibrosis.[3] Genetic diseases more common among people of Asian and African descent are β-thalassemia and sickle cell anemia, respectively.[4,5]

X-Linked

Mutations in genes located on the X chromosome result in X-linked genetic disorders. Because females have two X chromosomes and one is randomly inactivated in each cell, they are carriers and do not normally manifest the disorder. Males, on the other hand, have only one X chromosome, which is inherited from their mothers. A son has a 50% chance of inheriting the defective gene from his mother and manifesting the disease. A daughter also has a 50% chance of inheriting the defective gene from her mother but will then be a carrier. X-linked disorders often appear to skip a generation because an affected male will only pass the mutation in his X chromosome to his daughter, and she will serve as a carrier to the next generation. Disorders with X-linked inheritance include hemophilia A, X-linked hypohidrotic ectodermal dysplasia, fragile X syndrome, and X-linked amelogenesis imperfecta. Occasionally, as a result of nonrandom X inactivation, females may have mild symptoms of an X-linked disorder.

Chromosomal Anomalies

In the previous examples, defects in one or both copies of a gene are responsible for the occurrence of a genetic disorder. Some disorders result from defects in chromosomes that result in extra copies of one or more genes, entire deletions of one or more genes, or translocation of one part of a chromosome with another. Generally chromosomal anomalies result in multiple physical defects as well as mental and developmental delay. Down syndrome is the result of a trisomy (three copies) of all or part of chromosome 21. The duplicated part of the chromosome leads to an extra copy of all the genes on that part of the chromosome. The dosage of gene products in each cell is highly regulated. Extra copies of genes lead to excess gene products that interfere with the necessary balance in the cell. Extra or missing chromosomal material frequently results in miscarriages and/or multiple birth defects.

Multifactorial Inheritance

Most common diseases of adulthood (such as diabetes, hypertension, and manic depression) as well as most congenital malformations (cleft lip/palate and neural tube defects) can be the result of multiple genes and gene-environment interactions. This is also true for the most common dental diseases (periodontal disease and dental caries). Multifactorial traits are thought to result from the interaction between multiple genes with multiple environmental factors. The most convincing evidence for this type of inheritance comes from twin studies. If a trait is multifactorial with a significant genetic component, monozygotic (identical) twins will both have the disease significantly more frequently than dizygotic (fraternal) twins. This has been demonstrated in multiple studies for dental caries among twins raised apart and provides strong evidence that there is a genetic component to dental caries susceptibility.[6,7] More recently, researchers have completed a genome-wide association study designed to identify genetic loci associated with the susceptibility or resistance to dental caries.[8] These include *MMP10, MMP14,* and *MMP16*[9]; enamel matrix genes[10]; *MPPED2* and *ACTN2*[11]; and the region near the gene *PKD2.*[12]

Nontraditional Inheritance

Other types of inheritance patterns that do not fit the traditional Mendelian patterns and have been identified are imprinting and triplet repeat expansion. Imprinted genes are turned off by methylation of the gene. This process controls the level of expression of a particular gene in the offspring. Depending on whether the imprinted gene is inherited from the mother or father determines whether the child has a particular disease. In some cases, if the imprinted gene is inherited from the father, the child has one disease, but if the same imprinted gene is inherited from the mother, the child has a different disease. Two disorders that exemplify this are Prader-Willi syndrome and Angelman syndrome. If the child inherits the imprinted gene region from their father, they have Prader-Willi syndrome, and if inherited from their mother, it is manifested as Angelman syndrome.[13]

DNA triplet repeat expansion is a phenomenon where strings of repeated nucleotides increase in number. For example, within a particular gene, there may be 200 copies of the trinucleotide repeat "TAG." Smaller numbers of repeats are often referred to as a premutation, but when the repeats are expanded in an offspring, they may cause the gene to be inactivated (often by methylation). Diseases caused by this type of defect include Huntington chorea and fragile X syndrome.

Epigenetic mechanisms affect the expression of genes and can be caused by environmental chemicals, developmental processes, drugs, or aging. These changes are not the result of DNA sequence alterations but rather are caused by factors such as DNA methylation and histone acetylation. These modifications activate and deactivate parts of the genome at specific times and in specific cells. Epigenetic tags react to environmental stimuli such as diet, toxins, and physical activity. Because these tags can be maintained over multiple generations, offspring may be influenced by epigenetic changes that occurred in grandparents or great grandparents and may not have been manifested in the parents. Although the term *epigenetics* was coined in 1942, its relevance to inheritance of disease susceptibility has attracted substantial attention in recent years. There is evidence to suggest that epigenetics plays a part in autism,[14] cancer,[15] suicidal ideation,[16] and periodontal disease.[17] Future studies on the epigenome are likely to lead to new approaches to risk assessment and the treatment of complex disorders.

Dentist as Dysmorphologist

The word *dysmorphic* describes faulty development of the shape or form of an organism. Facial features in a child are frequently referred to as dysmorphic when they vary from what is considered normal. Features such as the spacing between the eyes, the position and shape of the ears, and the relative proportions of the maxilla and mandible are either within the range of normal or vary enough to be considered dysmorphic. Many genetic syndromes result in dysmorphic facial features that frequently help to diagnose the syndrome. For example, children with Down syndrome have inner epicanthal folds, upslanting palpebral fissures, and maxillary hypoplasia. This causes unrelated children with Down syndrome to have a similar appearance to each other.

There are four basic mechanisms that result in structural defects during development. The first is malformation, the second is deformation due to mechanical forces, the third is disruption where there is a breakdown of tissues that were previously normal, and the fourth is dysplasia or a failure of normal organization of cells into tissues. It is not uncommon for humans to have at least one "minor" difference. This includes things such as hair whorls, inner epicanthal folds, aberrant positioning of oral frenula, or preauricular pits. Although the occurrence of single differences such as these is relatively common and often presents as a familial trait, there are a number of studies that have demonstrated that a child who has three minor differences has a much greater chance of having a major anomaly such as a defect in brain or heart development.[18–20] This illustrates why it is important for healthcare professionals to be careful observers of their patients and to be familiar with the facial features that are considered to be normal or abnormal.

In general, the children seen in a dental practice fit into one of three categories. They may be normally developed, they may have been diagnosed with a developmental anomaly (either physical or mental), or they may have a developmental anomaly that has not been diagnosed. Pediatric dentists and general dentists are in the unique position of seeing their patients regularly. This contrasts with the typical physician who may only see patients when they are ill or less regularly. This frequent interaction between dentists and their patients gives the dentist the opportunity to observe a child's growth and development and to note changes that are not within the range of normal. As healthcare professionals, it is incumbent on all dentists to recognize disease in their patients and to make the appropriate referrals for definitive diagnosis and treatment.

Dentists are trained to observe and examine the mouth, face, and other craniofacial structures. Coincidentally, many inherited diseases in humans involve malformations of the craniofacial region. Accurate diagnosis of developmental anomalies and their related disorders relies on the ability of the clinician to recognize and differentiate between normal and dysmorphic physical characteristics. According to the text *Smith's Recognizable Patterns of Human Malformation,* 12 of the 26 categories of malformations used for diagnostic purposes involve features of the head or neck.[21] Several are limited to oral structures, such as hypodontia, microdontia, micrognathia, and cleft lip/palate. In addition, understanding the full spectrum of malformations associated with certain syndromes is essential for the safe and effective treatment of patients with these disorders.

Because dentists concentrate their diagnostic expertise on the face and mouth, they may be more likely to observe anomalies that are suggestive of major developmental malformations. Dentists who can recognize potential genetic disorders can also provide a valuable service to their patients by offering appropriate referral to a medical geneticist or a genetic counselor.

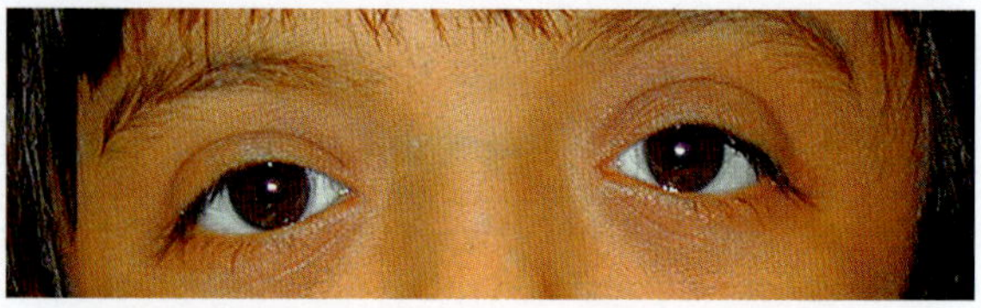

• **Fig. 37.2** Hypertelorism.

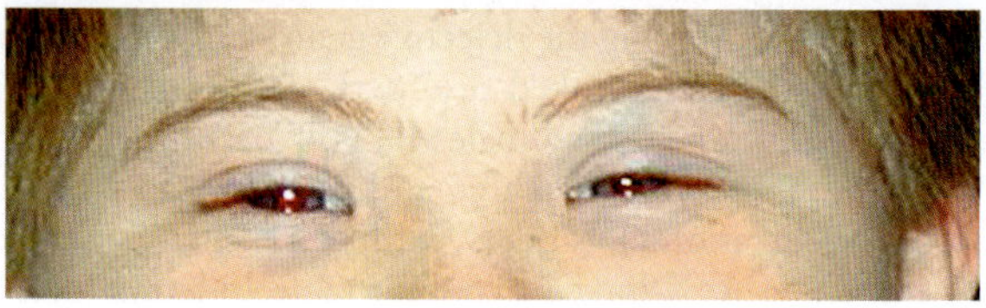

• **Fig. 37.3** Inner epicanthal fold.

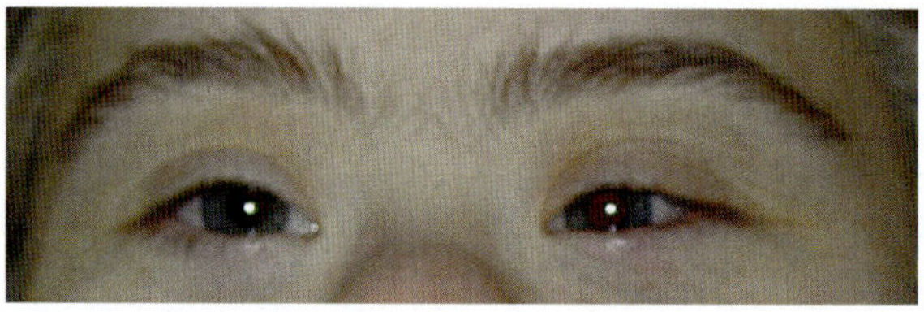

• **Fig. 37.4** Upslanting palpebral fissures.

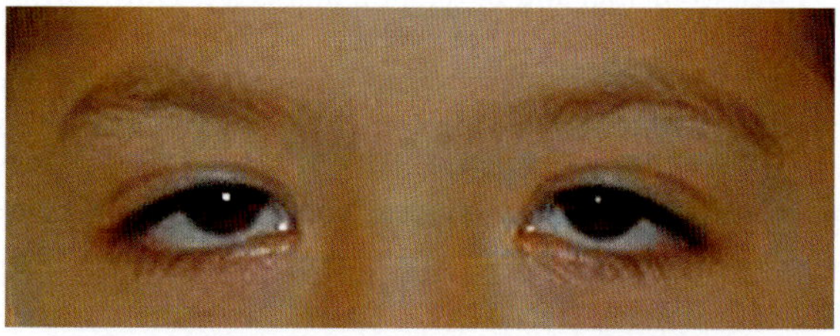

• **Fig. 37.5** Downslanting palpebral fissures.

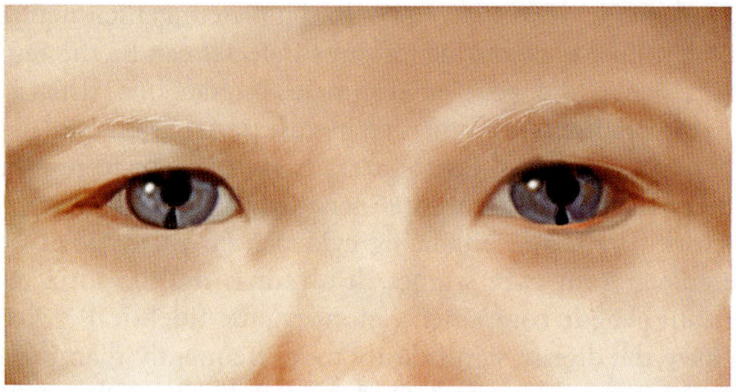

• **Fig. 37.6** Coloboma of the iris. (From Kaban LB, Troulis MJ. *Pediatric Oral and Maxillofacial Surgery*. Saunders; 2004.)

Ocular Anomalies

Minor anomalies that affect the eyes and ocular region include abnormal orbital size and position, widely spaced eyes (hypertelorism) (Fig. 37.2), inner epicanthal folds (Fig. 37.3), slanting of the palpebral fissures (upward or downward; Figs. 37.4 and 37.5), a fused eyebrow (synophrys), blue sclera, and coloboma of the iris ("cat eye"; Fig. 37.6).

Auricular Anomalies

There are several minor anomalies that affect the outer ear (auricle) and the preauricular region. These include preauricular tags or pits (Fig. 37.7), low-set and malformed ears (Fig. 37.8), protruding ears, and slanted ears.

Anomalies of the Mouth and Oral Region

Anomalies in this region include lower lip pits (Fig. 37.9), bifid uvula, clefts, asymmetries, tongue abnormalities, abnormally shaped jaws, and prominent or full lips. Attached or short frenum, as seen with ankyloglossia ("tongue-tie"), or low attached maxillary labial frenum is also a fairly common anomaly in the oral region. A full description in this region is critical to proper care. One example is that many clinicians typically lump numerous forms of cleft lip and cleft palate into a couple of subsets, but the full breadth of description such as unilateral or bilateral cleft lip and/or the range of cleft uvula to full palate shows the complexity and variation of a disease.

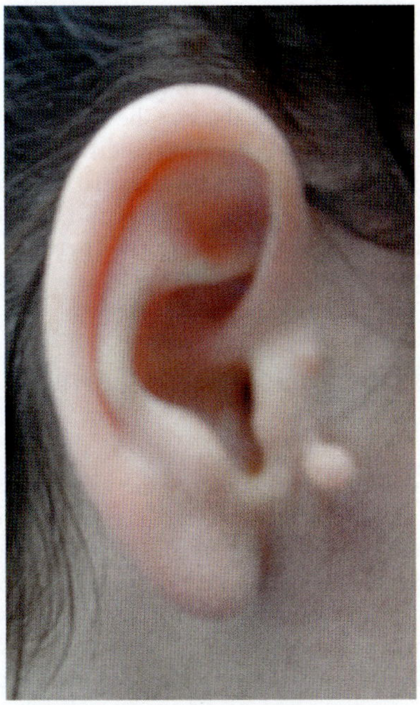

• **Fig. 37.7** Ear tag.

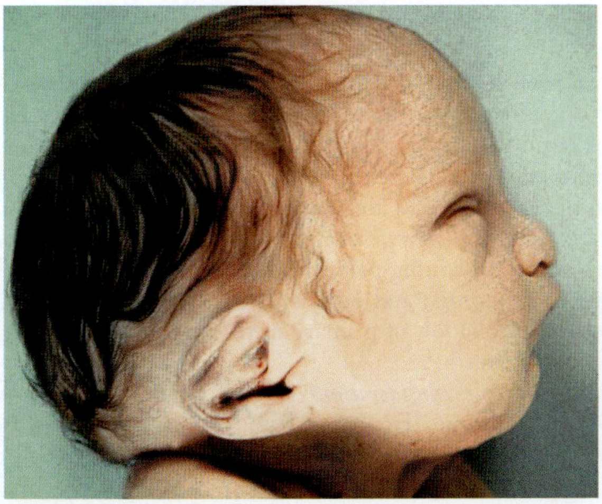

• **Fig. 37.8** Low-set malformed ears. (From Gilbert-Barness E, Kapur RP, Oligny LL, et al. *Potter's Pathology of the Fetus, Infant and Child.* 2nd ed. Mosby; 2007.)

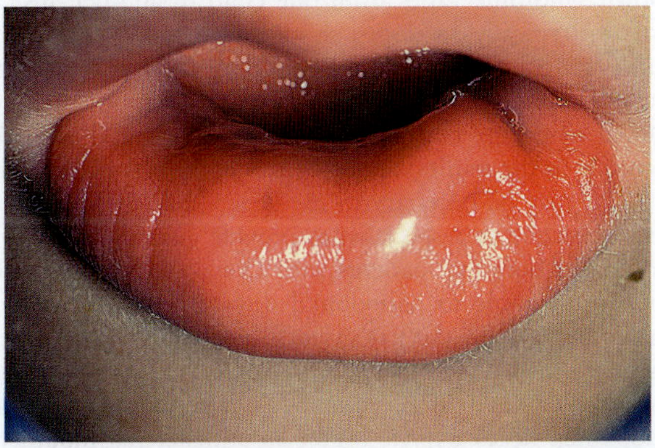

• **Fig. 37.9** Lower lip pits.

Dental Anomalies

Anomalies of tooth development are relatively common and may occur as an isolated finding or in association with other minor and major anomalies or as part of a syndrome. Dental anomalies are discussed in detail in Chapter 20.

Along with managing the oral health of patients, a dentist's first responsibility is to recognize disease, whether it is in the mouth or in another part of the body. An additional responsibility is to know what to do when anomalies are identified in a patient. We are fortunate to be in an era where there is a wealth of information at our fingertips. With access to a computer and the Internet, both healthcare practitioners and the lay public can find information about a specific disorder in minutes. There are several extremely valuable and reliable resources on the Internet, including databases of published research articles, databases for inherited or rare diseases, and websites dedicated to information about specific syndromes (Box 37.1). For those without access to the Internet, there are a variety of valuable and frequently updated textbooks that provide information about syndromes that involve craniofacial anomalies.[21,22]

Why is it important for dentists to pay attention to potential developmental problems with their child patients, and what should dentists do if a developmental anomaly or syndrome is suspected? First, the dentist is responsible for the patient's overall health, not just the health of the mouth or teeth. Patients rely on healthcare providers to diagnose problems and inform them of those problems so that they can obtain appropriate and timely treatment. Second, there are many syndromes with features that influence how a dentist provides care for patients. For example, many children with Noonan syndrome have a congenital heart defect that may require the use of prophylactic antibiotics before dental treatment. Patients with Down syndrome frequently have congenital cardiac anomalies and, in addition, are at higher risk for periodontal disease as adults. Both syndromes require that a dentist modify the way he or she provides treatment to such patients.

When an anomaly is suspected but not diagnosed, the dentist should know how to gather the appropriate background information

• BOX 37.1 Sources of Genetic Information

National Center for Biotechnology Information: https://www.ncbi.nlm.nih.gov/
Online Mendelian Inheritance in Man: https://www.omim.org/
National Human Genome Research Institute: www.genome.gov/
Genetic Education for Health Professionals: www.ashg.org/education/Health_Professionals.shtml
Genetic Alliance: geneticalliance.org/
National Organization for Rare Disorders: www.rarediseases.org/
National Foundation for Ectodermal Dysplasias: www.nfed.org/
National Society of Genetic Counselors: www.nsgc.org/
American Society of Human Genetics: www.ashg.org/
March of Dimes: www.marchofdimes.com/
FACES: The National Craniofacial Association: www.faces-cranio.org/
American Cleft Palate-Craniofacial Association: www.acpa-cpf.org/

from the parent and, if necessary, refer the patient to a medical geneticist for further evaluation. Most teaching hospitals have a department of medical genetics that a child could be referred to for evaluation. In some areas, there are also outreach clinics where medical geneticists and genetic counselors travel to smaller towns to evaluate patients. Availability of genetic counselors in a particular area (in the United States) can be determined from the website of the National Society of Genetic Counselors (http://www.nsgc.org/page/find-a-gc-search). The database can be searched by entering a ZIP code and the number of miles a patient is able or willing to travel for care. Alternatively, practitioner name, practice type, or location can be used as search queries. As with any referral, it is important to send a letter or email to the physician or genetic counselor explaining why you are sending the patient for evaluation.

When discussing potential developmental anomalies with parents, it is important to be very sensitive to their concerns and to avoid causing undue alarm. Depending on the circumstances, it may be best to observe the child at multiple appointments (assuming that there are treatment needs) and to get to know the family better before broaching the subject. On the other hand, when there are obvious concerns and a timely diagnosis is indicated, an immediate referral should be made. One group of disorders that a dentist is likely to be the first to diagnose is the ectodermal dysplasia syndromes. Frequently parents become concerned when their 2- or 3-year-old child does not have any visible teeth or has conically shaped teeth. This should be recognizable to a dentist who sees children as a developmental anomaly that warrants further investigation. At this age, children frequently have sparse hair, but the combination of hypodontia, sparse hair, and dry skin should lead a dentist to refer this child to determine whether he or she has a form of ectodermal dysplasia. Similarly, if a child who is 10 or 12 years old has not lost any primary teeth, a dentist should investigate further to determine the reason why the teeth have not exfoliated. In children with cleidocranial dysplasia, Gardner syndrome, and trichorhinophalangeal syndrome, multiple supernumerary teeth may be present that block the eruption of the permanent teeth; but there is also a genetic defect that keeps teeth from erupting even after the supernumerary teeth are removed.

Because the genetic defects that cause many dominantly inherited syndromes can occur as new mutations, the child may be the first person in the family to experience the disorder. It is always important to ask about family history of disease, but absence of disease in the family does not preclude the occurrence of disease in the child.

When the child has been diagnosed with a particular disorder, frequently the disorder is rare enough that a dentist may not be familiar with it. In this case it is important to gather as much information about the characteristics of the disorder before treating the child. Again, one of the most useful resources for this is the Internet. The database known as Online Mendelian Inheritance in Man (OMIM; www.ncbi.nlm.nih.gov/omim) is maintained and updated regularly by Johns Hopkins University. The database can be searched by entering the name of the syndrome or by entering clinical characteristics of the syndrome, such as hypodontia and sparse hair. After searching for a particular term, the database will give a list of disorders that include that term within the text of the description of the disorder. In addition, there are references that are linked to the National Library of Medicine database of published literature (PubMed; see Box 37.1), so that abstracts of articles about the disorder can be easily accessed or downloaded. This is a free database that is available to anyone with an Internet connection and is also how information was gathered for the charts supporting the following section of this chapter. Information about syndromes is also available via the National Organization for Rare Disorders (NORD; www.rarediseases.org/). This site also has a large database of rare diseases. To view full reports of a disease you must be registered. Two reports per day are available at no charge to registered users. There is currently no charge for registration.

Syndromes/Disorders With Craniofacial Anomalies

It is not possible in a single chapter to discuss every syndrome that includes malformations involving the face or mouth. The following section focuses on a subset of disorders that are either more commonly seen in the dental office or have such dramatic dental and oral manifestations that all dentists should be aware of them. It is recommended that every dental office has access to information about genetic disorders via both the Internet and one or more textbooks.

Down Syndrome

Inheritance pattern: Chromosomal, sporadic.

Gene(s): Trisomy 21.

General manifestations: Hypotonia; cardiac anomaly in about 40% of cases; increased risk for atlantoaxial instability; increased risk for seizures, gastroesophageal reflux, and sleep apnea; intellectual disability; and increased risk for leukemia (acute lymphocytic leukemia [ALL] and acute myeloid leukemia [AML]).

Craniofacial/dental manifestations: Brachycephaly; inner epicanthal folds; upslanting palpebral fissures; low-set, small, folded ears; microdontia; and increased risk for periodontal disease, delayed exfoliation of primary teeth, and delayed eruption of permanent teeth.[21]

Dental treatment considerations: When treating children with Down syndrome (Fig. 37.10), the primary concerns are to determine the need for subacute bacterial endocarditis prophylaxis and the child's ability to cooperate. If a child has had surgery to repair a congenital heart defect, he or she may or may not need subacute bacterial endocarditis prophylaxis, depending on when the surgery was performed and on the presence of any residual defect. This should be confirmed with the parent or the child's cardiologist. The behavior of children with Down syndrome varies from one child to another, just as it does for typically developed children. It is inappropriate to assume in advance that such a child will be uncooperative for dental treatment. Yet some children and young adults with Down syndrome may be very uncooperative and difficult to examine in the traditional dental setting. When behavior is an issue, it may be necessary to use general anesthesia and/or to refer the child to a specialist to provide quality care. It is important to note that patients with Down syndrome are much more susceptible to periodontal disease. The dentist should make this clear to the parent and should stress early development of good oral hygiene habits including thorough, supervised daily toothbrushing with a fluoridated toothpaste; flossing; and, when necessary, the use of an antibacterial mouth rinse such as 0.12% chlorhexidine.

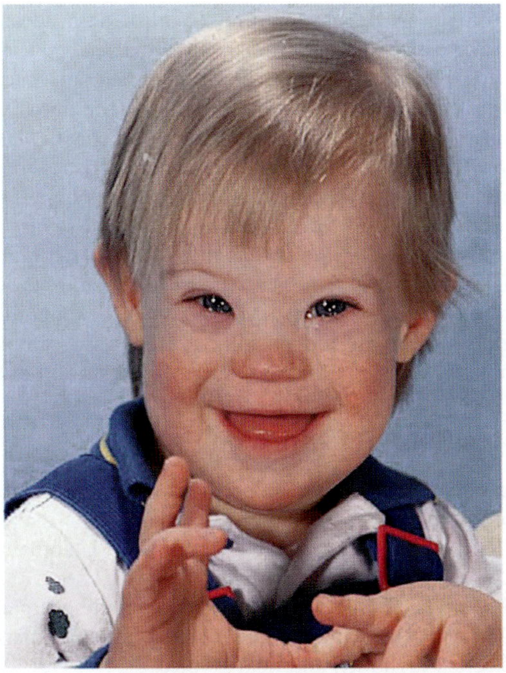

• **Fig. 37.10** Typical facies of a child with Down syndrome, including flat nasal bridge, epicanthal folds, and upslanting palpebral fissures. (From Zitelli BJ, Davis HW. *Atlas of Pediatric Physical Diagnosis.* 5th ed. Mosby; 2007.)

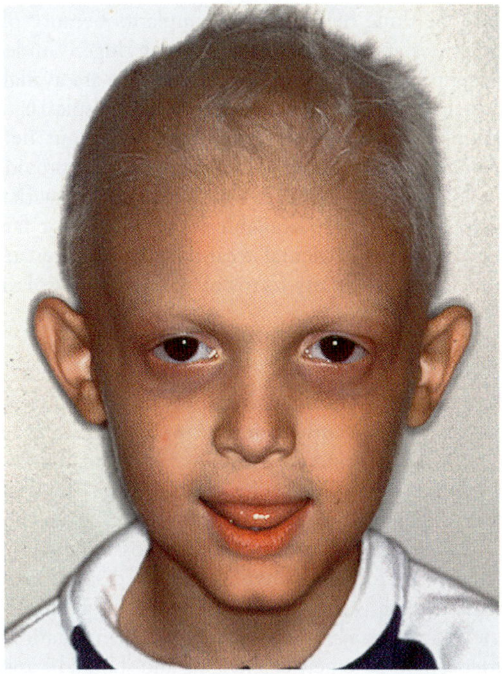

• **Fig. 37.11** A child with ectodermal dysplasia showing sparse hair. (From Proffit WR, Fields HW, Sarver DM. *Contemporary Orthodontics.* 5th ed. Mosby; 2013.)

Ectodermal Dysplasia

Inheritance pattern: X-linked recessive, autosomal dominant, and autosomal recessive.

Gene(s): See Table 37.1.

General manifestations: Sparse hair, dry skin, absence of sweat glands, normal mental status, eyes sensitive to light, may overheat easily,[21,23] and dysplastic and slow-growing nails.[21,23]

Craniofacial/dental manifestations: Full lips, small nose; hypodontia, conical or malformed teeth, deficient alveolar ridge, and relatively flat palate.

Dental treatment considerations: There are more than 150 forms of the ectodermal dysplasia syndrome that affect one or more of the tissues derived from the ectoderm (Figs. 37.11 and 37.12). Although the best known condition is the X-linked hypohidrotic form, there are also autosomal dominant and autosomal recessive forms with symptoms that range from mild with hypodontia only to a more severe form with many structures affected, in addition to a cleft lip and palate and anomalies of the fingers (ectrodactyly–ectodermal dysplasia–clefting syndrome caused by mutations in *TP63*). Children with hypohidrotic ectodermal dysplasia frequently lack most primary and permanent teeth. This leads to underdevelopment of the alveolar ridges and makes the fabrication of dentures more challenging.

When ectodermal dysplasia is inherited as an X-linked or autosomal dominant disorder, parents are usually familiar with the disorder because other family members may have been affected. However, the disorder may also be caused by a new mutation or inherited as an autosomal recessive trait. When this happens, the family may be completely unaware of the manifestations of this disorder. It is not uncommon for the dentist to be the first person to recognize ectodermal dysplasia in a child. Parents become concerned when their child has few if any erupted teeth by 2 to 3 years of age and often seek a dentist's advice. At this age, it is usually possible to assess the developing teeth using maxillary and mandibular occlusal radiographs. These will establish whether the dental development is delayed, if the primary teeth are missing, or if there is some other process that is interfering with tooth eruption. If primary teeth are not present, the child should be referred to a medical geneticist and/or genetic counselor for a thorough evaluation.

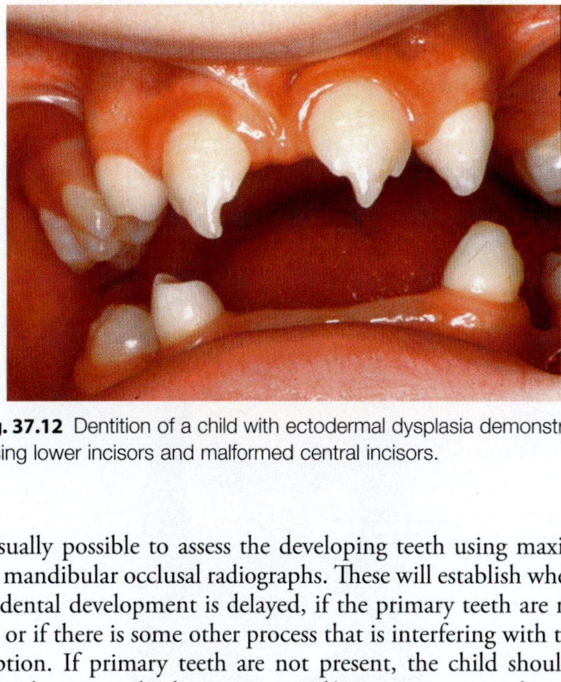

• **Fig. 37.12** Dentition of a child with ectodermal dysplasia demonstrating missing lower incisors and malformed central incisors.

Dentists can provide a great service to children with ectodermal dysplasia by fabricating dentures at a young age and by educating the family about future treatment options. Dentures can be fabricated for young children as soon as they are cooperative enough to tolerate impressions. Because of their tendency to overheat, the use of protective stabilization for extended lengths of time in a very young child is contraindicated. As these children grow and mature, other options become available to them including implants and implant-retained dentures. Frequently bone grafts must be done before placing implants because of the reduced thickness and height of the alveolar ridge. Guidelines for the treatment of these patients at various ages are available from the National Foundation for the Ectodermal Dysplasias (NFED). Information is available online from NFED about dental care (https://nfed.org/learn/library/). This organization provides information and support to families who have children with ectodermal dysplasia. Grants are available from NFED for families to help defray the cost of dental treatment and for researchers to better understand the many forms of ectodermal dysplasia.

Cleidocranial Dysplasia

Inheritance pattern: Autosomal dominant or new mutation.

Gene(s): Runt-related transcription factor 2 (*RUNX2*),[24] msh homeobox 2 *(MSX2),* and core-binding factor, β-subunit *(CBFB).*

General manifestations: Moderate short stature, normal intelligence, and partial to complete absence of clavicles.

Craniofacial/dental manifestations: Frontal bossing, brachycephaly, late closure of fontanels, hypertelorism, delayed eruption of permanent teeth; supernumerary teeth, and impacted teeth.

Dental treatment considerations: The dental manifestations of this disorder can be extremely challenging and should be approached by a multidisciplinary team including a pediatric dentist, oral surgeon, orthodontist, and prosthodontist (Fig. 37.13). The pediatric dentist often serves as the case manager who brings the team together and facilitates communication among the other specialists and the patient's family. Children with cleidocranial dysplasia may have as many as 60 supernumerary teeth or as few as one. Surgical removal of these extra teeth must be done with the appropriate timing and frequently involves multiple surgeries during childhood and adolescence. Once the supernumerary teeth have been removed, orthodontic forces are usually required to bring the permanent teeth into position. The timing of orthodontic treatment is crucial because appropriate anchorage must be established in advance, and often the first permanent molars are impacted.

It is possible that the delayed eruption of permanent teeth (and delayed exfoliation of primary teeth) will be the initial sign that something is abnormal in the child's development. Because this is a relatively rare disorder and its general characteristics are not life-threatening, it may go undetected by the child's physician. Again, this is an opportunity for dentists to provide a service to their patients by recognizing the potential for a genetic condition and referring the child to a medical geneticist for a definitive diagnosis. Evaluation of a child with retained primary teeth should include a panoramic radiograph and possibly a cone-beam computed tomography scan for enhanced localization and position of teeth.[25]

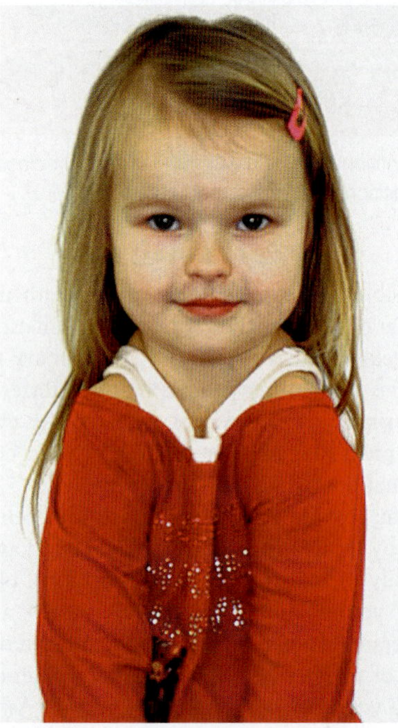

• **Fig. 37.13** A child with cleidocranial dysplasia. (From Cobourne MT, DiBiase AT. *Handbook of Orthodontics*. Mosby; 2010.)

Williams-Beuren Syndrome

Inheritance pattern: Autosomal dominant or new mutation; can be chromosome 7q11.23 deletion syndrome.[26]

Gene(s): 7q11.23 region, elastin *(ELN),* LIM domain kinase 1 *(LIMK1),* and replication factor C *(RFC2).*[27]

General manifestations: Cardiovascular anomalies (supravalvular aortic stenosis), infantile hypercalcemia, outgoing personality, intellectual disability, and hoarse voice.

Craniofacial/dental manifestations: Stellate pattern in the iris,[28] hypodontia, enamel hypoplasia, prominent lips, and wide mouth.

Dental treatment considerations: Children and adults with Williams-Beuren syndrome can provide both fun and a challenge to your practice (Fig. 37.14). Their charming, friendly personality endears them to everyone. However, their hypersensitivity to sound and easy distractibility can make it necessary to spend extra time and patience during dental treatment. Because of the frequent cardiovascular anomalies associated with this disorder, it is essential to determine whether there is a need for subacute bacterial endocarditis prophylaxis before dental treatment. If the parent is unsure about this, the dentist should contact the child's cardiologist and document the physician's advice in the patient's record.

Fragile X Syndrome

Inheritance pattern: X-linked.

Gene(s): Fragile X mental retardation-1 *(FMR1).*[29,30]

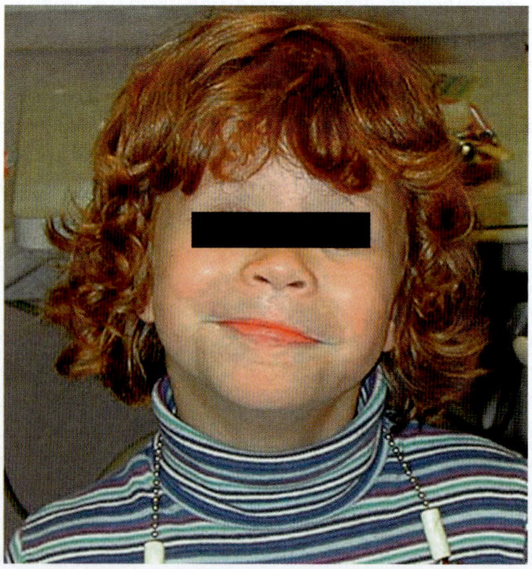

• **Fig. 37.14** Facies of a child with Williams-Beuren syndrome.

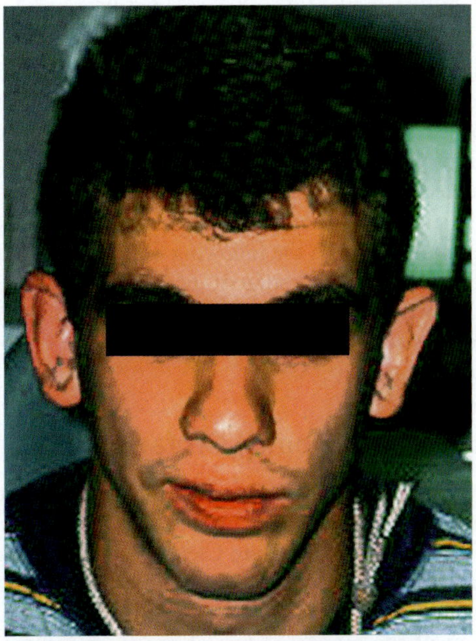

• **Fig. 37.15** A young man with fragile X syndrome.

General manifestations: Intellectual disability, autism in 60%, and macroorchidism.[21]

Craniofacial/dental manifestations: Macrocephaly, prognathism, and large ears.

Dental treatment considerations: Fragile X syndrome is documented as the cause of intellectual disability in almost 6% of males with intellectual disability (Fig. 37.15). In the dental clinic, treatment issues primarily center around the child's behavior and ability to tolerate dental procedures. This is further complicated in children who also have autism. As is true for many persons with special needs, their oral health is the responsibility of a parent or other care provider. For this reason, it is important for the dentist to provide the caregiver with the information and tools required to assess and maintain good oral hygiene and healthy dietary practices for these children.

Osteogenesis Imperfecta

Inheritance pattern: Autosomal dominant, autosomal recessive, or sporadic.

Gene(s): See Table 37.2.

General manifestations: Mild to severe bone fragility, short stature; normal intelligence, hearing impairment in adulthood, hyperextensible joints, and deformity of limbs.

Craniofacial/dental manifestations: Triangular facies, blue sclera, occasional dentinogenesis imperfecta, and delayed eruption of teeth.

Dental treatment considerations: Osteogenesis imperfecta is a heterogeneous disorder resulting from both quantitative and qualitative defects in type I collagen. Even though genes in type I collagen have been identified, many of the newly identified genes are noncollagenous in nature. Symptoms range from mild to severely deforming to lethal.[31] Osteogenesis imperfecta type I is a mild form and may go undiagnosed until the child's first bone fracture. In some cases, parents of children with an undiagnosed mild form of osteogenesis imperfecta have been accused of child abuse when an unreported previous fracture is detected radiographically. It is important for a physician to rule out osteogenesis imperfecta when questions of previous fractures are being evaluated. Osteogenesis imperfecta type II is lethal at birth or shortly thereafter. Osteogenesis imperfecta type III is a severe form where children have extreme bone fragility and by early childhood may have had as many as 30 fractures. They are frequently not ambulatory and have a history of surgeries that includes placement of rods in their legs and spine. Osteogenesis imperfecta type IV is intermediate in severity between type III and type I. These children have moderate short stature, bone fragility, and significant bone deformity. Dentinogenesis imperfecta can be present in children with osteogenesis imperfecta types I–V or VII (Fig. 37.16). Dental treatment for patients with osteogenesis imperfecta should be approached with great care and with guidance from the parent to determine what the child can tolerate. Active or passive immobilization of patients with osteogenesis imperfecta is not recommended. If behavior at a young age makes treatment in the traditional dental setting infeasible, other options such as general anesthesia should be considered. When a child with dentinogenesis imperfecta presents in a dental office, especially when there is no history of this disorder in the family, the dentist should consider the possibility that the child also has osteogenesis imperfecta. A referral to a medical geneticist for evaluation is appropriate if there is any doubt about the diagnosis.

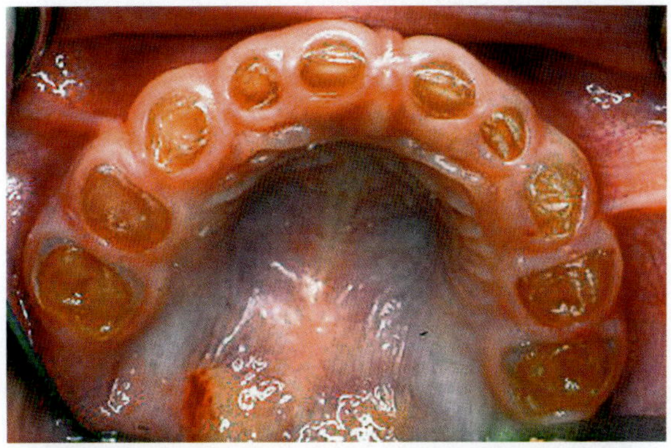

• **Fig. 37.16** Dentinogenesis imperfecta in the primary dentition.

Treacher Collins Syndrome

Inheritance pattern: Autosomal dominant, autosomal recessive, or sporadic.

Gene(s): Treacher Collins–Franceschetti syndrome 1 *(TCOF1)*[32] and polymerase I, RNA, subunit B, C, and D (POLR1B, POLR1C, and POLR1D).

General manifestations: Normal intelligence, conductive hearing loss, pharyngeal hypoplasia, and occasional congenital heart defect.

Craniofacial/dental manifestations: Downslanting palpebral fissures, lower eyelid coloboma, malar hypoplasia, mandibular hypoplasia, malformation of external ear, and cleft palate or submucous cleft.

Dental treatment considerations: The severe micrognathia in some patients with Treacher Collins syndrome contributes to dental crowding and may make intubation difficult if treatment under general anesthesia is required (Fig. 37.17 and 37.18). Frequently orthognathic surgery is required during childhood or adolescence. Dental practitioners should consult with the child's physician to confirm the absence of other medical

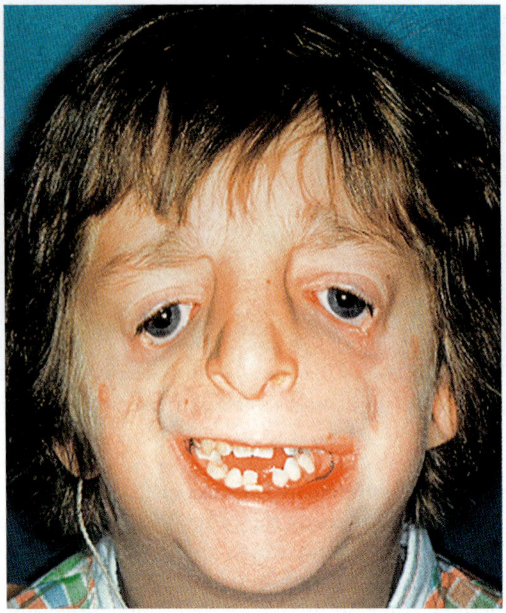

• **Fig. 37.17** Facies of a child with Treacher Collins syndrome. (From Nanci A. Ten Cate's Oral Histology: Development, Structure, and Function. 8th ed. Mosby; 2013.)

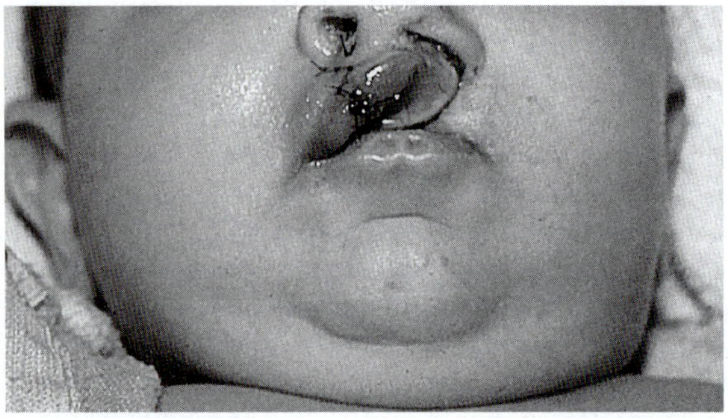

• **Fig. 37.18** Cleft lip/palate in a child with van der Woude syndrome.

conditions such as congenital heart defects that might dictate modifications in how dental treatment is delivered.

Van der Woude Syndrome

Inheritance pattern: Autosomal dominant or sporadic.

Gene(s): Interferon regulatory factor 6 *(IRF6),*[33] Grainyhead-like 3 *(GRHL3).*[34]

General manifestations: Normal intelligence and good general health.

Craniofacial/dental manifestations: Lower lip pits, cleft lip/palate, cleft uvula, hypodontia, and occasional ankyloglossia.

Dental treatment considerations: Cleft lip and/or palate may occur as a solitary finding or as part of a syndrome. It is estimated that approximately 70% of children with van der Woude syndrome have mutations in the gene *IRF6.*[33] Recently mutations in the gene *GRHL3* were found to lead to almost identical orofacial clefting phenotypes as seen in *VWS1* and has since been designated as *VWS2.* Children with van der Woude syndrome may have lower lip pits alone or in combination with cleft lip and/or cleft palate. Because the symptoms are limited and affected individuals have normal intelligence, this disorder could be confused with nonsyndromic cleft lip/palate. It is important that children with cleft lip/palate or with lip pits only be seen and evaluated by a craniofacial anomalies team to determine the cause and heritability of their disorder. In addition, this type of team approach is important for providing coordinated, timely treatment of children with cleft lip/palate. Many hospitals have cleft lip/palate or craniofacial teams that include specialists from the following disciplines: plastic surgery, craniofacial and/or oral surgery, pediatric medicine, pediatric dentistry, orthodontics, speech pathology, audiology, prosthodontics, social work, and medical genetics (see Chapter 38 for more information).

Isolated (Nonsyndromic) Orofacial Clefts

Inheritance pattern: Autosomal dominant or non-Mendelian inheritance pattern with gene-environment interactions.

Craniofacial/dental manifestations: Cleft lip and/or palate.

Dental treatment considerations: Orofacial clefting, a group of anatomical birth defects where there is a gap or break in normal structures of the mouth, is one of the most common human developmental disorders, affecting 1 in every 600 newborns worldwide. The prevalence is high in East Asian and Native American (3.6 per 1000 births) populations and low in African-ancestry populations (0.3 per 1000 births). Cleft lip and/or palate are nonsyndromic or isolated ~70% of the time, whereas the other ~30% are syndromic. There are more than 400 syndromes with cleft lip and/or palate as part of the phenotype. The etiology of orofacial clefting is complex and heterogeneous, with both genetic and environmental influences. Isolated cleft lip/palate has been reported to be associated with mutations in a number of genes. Environmental factors include environmental toxins and consumption of phenytoin, retinoic acid derivatives, alcohol, and folate antagonist drugs during pregnancy. Isolated cleft lip with or without cleft palate and cleft palate only are two different entities. Cleft lip with or without cleft palate are more common in male patients but cleft palate alone is more common in female patients. Orofacial clefting exhibits phenotypic variability in terms of severity and the orofacial structures that are affected. The microforms of cleft lip with or without cleft palate include small defects of lip and/or alveolar arch, scarlike ridges above the lip, and defects of the superior orbicularis oris muscle, which can be visualized only by ultrasonography.[35] The microforms of cleft palate consist of bifid uvula and submucous palatal clefts. The ability to detect the microforms is crucial in identifying the carriers of the mutations.

Hypophosphatasia

Inheritance pattern: Autosomal dominant, autosomal recessive, or sporadic.

Gene(s): Alkaline phosphatase *(ALPL).*[36]

General manifestations: Normal or short stature, bone fragility, and bowed lower extremities.

Craniofacial/dental manifestations: Premature loss of teeth (most commonly primary incisors) due to lack of cementum, and craniosynostosis.

Dental treatment considerations: There are four forms of hypophosphatasia ranging from mild to lethal. The milder form that presents in childhood after 6 months of age results in premature loss of primary teeth and craniosynostosis. All types demonstrate decreased levels of serum alkaline phosphatase. Although this is a relatively rare disorder, dentists should be aware of its existence so that an appropriate referral can be made. Frequently the first sign of this disorder is the premature loss of a mandibular primary incisor without a history of trauma. The exfoliated tooth typically has no root resorption, and histologic analysis will show a lack of cementum. In the mild form of this disorder, the dental manifestations may be the only symptoms. A systematic review of enzyme replacement therapy using asfotase alfa found this to be an effective treatment for infants, children, and adults with hypophosphatasia.[37]

Apert Syndrome

Inheritance pattern: Autosomal dominant with complete penetrance. Most cases are sporadic. The majority of sporadic cases are associated with older paternal age.

Gene(s): Fibroblast growth factor 2 *(FGFR2)*.[38]

General manifestations: Intellectual disability, ocular proptosis, hypertelorism, strabismus, symmetrical syndactyly of hands and feet, and moderate to severe acne during adolescence.

Craniofacial/dental manifestations: Acrobrachycephaly as a result of craniosynostosis, especially of coronal sutures; flat occiput; wide midline calvarial defect extending from glabella to posterior fontanel; midface underdevelopment leading to relative mandibular prognathism and severely crowded teeth; highly arched palate with lateral palatal swellings; depressed nasal bridge; and cleft soft palate or bifid uvula.

Dental treatment considerations: Most of these patients require orthodontic treatment with orthognathic surgery to move the maxilla forward; even with intellectual disability, most patients cooperate well enough in the dental office to tolerate orthodontic treatment.

Crouzon Syndrome

Inheritance pattern: Autosomal dominant with variable expression. Many sporadic cases are associated with older paternal age.

Gene(s): Fibroblast growth factor receptor 2 *(FGFR2)*[39] and fibroblast growth factor receptor 3 *(FGFR3)*.

General manifestations: Intellectually normal, conductive hearing loss, cervical spine anomalies, and calcification of stylohyoid ligaments.

Craniofacial/dental manifestations: Craniosynostosis; increased digital markings on skull radiographs; hypertelorism; exotropia; ocular proptosis secondary to shallow orbits is a consistent feature resulting in exposure conjunctivitis and keratitis; and underdeveloped maxilla leading to crowding of maxillary teeth, ectopic eruption of the maxillary first permanent molars, and posterior crossbite; lateral palatal swellings.

Dental treatment considerations: Most of these patients require orthodontic treatment with orthognathic surgery to move the maxilla forward; patients with Crouzon syndrome usually cooperate well in the dental office.

Genetic Testing

Many genetic tests available today are used to diagnose specific inherited disorders such as cystic fibrosis, Huntington disease, or fragile X syndrome. These tests are typically ordered and interpreted by medical geneticists or genetic counselors. Genetic tests for inherited disorders involve screening for specific mutations or chromosomal disruptions. A second category of genetic tests screen for genetic risk factors for various disorders that have a genetic component. This includes disorders such as familial breast cancer and Alzheimer disease. Testing positive for one of these risk factors does not guarantee that one will get the disease, but it does indicate that an individual is at increased risk of developing the disease. This information allows one to make changes in their life to decrease additional risk factors for that disease.

In recent years DNA sequencing technologies have advanced significantly, allowing whole-genome sequencing for an individual using a saliva sample at the cost of less than $1000. Other technologies that have improved the ability to detect disease-causing mutations include whole-exome sequencing and microarray-based comparative genomic hybridization (CGH).[40]

Identification of genetic risk factors for dental caries and for periodontal disease is the goal of dental researchers. It is conceivable that, in the near future, in-office genetic tests will be available to predict the caries risk or periodontal disease risk of an individual patient. Using the results of these tests, the dentist will be able to develop a targeted prevention plan to minimize the severity of disease for that individual.

Ethical, Legal, and Social Implications of the Human Genome Project

In the past, patients have not been denied dental insurance because of preexisting dental disease, and a thorough dental examination is not usually required for a patient to qualify for dental benefits. The result is that dentists may not be aware of the potential for discrimination to which some patients are susceptible because of their health history. Genetic testing that identifies a person's risk for disease before he or she has any manifestations of the disease introduces a new level of information about an individual's health and insurability that has not been available in the past. In many cases, the ethical, legal, and social implications of the information learned from the Human Genome Project are still being evaluated.

Visit eBooks.Health.Elsevier.com to see full list of references.

38

Cleft Lip and Palate

MATTHEW K. GENESER AND VEERASATHPURUSH ALLAREDDY

CHAPTER OUTLINE

Orofacial clefts are one of the most common head and neck birth defects worldwide, affecting children of all socioeconomic and cultural backgrounds. The overall prevalence rate is roughly 1 in 700 live births, but there is much variation depending on geographical location.[1] In the United States, it is estimated that nearly 1 in 1000 babies are born with an orofacial cleft.[2] Clefts may involve the lip, alveolus, and palate in various combinations. Half of all orofacial clefts involve both the palate and the lip. Clefts that are isolated to the palate are less common.[2]

Children born with an orofacial cleft often have complex medical and dental conditions, necessitating the need for care from healthcare teams involving multiple specialists.[3] Common conditions that occur in children with orofacial clefts are hearing difficulty, speech and language disorders, middle ear abnormalities, psychosocial issues, and dental abnormalities. Pediatric dentists serve an important function on these multidisciplinary teams, as they will not only provide a dental home, but will also often coordinate the many aspects of treatment.[4]

Cleft Lip and Palate Team

Typically, a cleft lip and palate team is composed of members drawn from multiple specialties, as shown in Table 38.1, each of whom plays a pivotal role in the overall care for patients with cleft lip and palate. Key procedures and interventions take place throughout childhood, as shown in Fig. 38.1, although the exact sequence and timing will vary depending on the characteristics of the child's cleft and the philosophy of the cleft lip and palate team members.

Anatomy

The palate is divided into a primary and a secondary palate at the incisive foramen. The primary palate extends anteriorly from the incisive foramen and includes the premaxilla, lip, nasal tip, and columella, as shown in Fig. 38.2. The secondary palate extends posteriorly from the incisive foramen and includes the hard and soft palates as well as the uvula.

Classification of Cleft Lip and Palate

The cleft lip and palate has a long history of varied and sometimes conflicting classification systems.[5] In 1931, Veau grouped palatal clefts into four forms based on anatomical position: clefts of the soft palate, clefts up to the incisive foramen, clefts extending through the alveolus unilaterally, and clefts extending through the alveolus bilaterally.[6] Veau's system is still used today, but other systems exist and debate continues regarding how to best classify clefts. Regardless of the system utilized, understanding the anatomy of the oral cavity is the basis for understanding the classification system as shown in Fig. 38.3.

Cleft lip is classified as being complete or incomplete based on the extent of the cleft as well as unilateral or bilateral depending on whether it affects one or both sides. An incomplete cleft of the lip does not involve the complete thickness of the lip but has a band of tissue intact across the cleft. Conversely, a complete cleft of the lip involves the entire vertical thickness of the lip and is more often associated with a cleft of the alveolus.

Cleft palate is defined in a similar fashion, as either complete or incomplete as well as unilateral or bilateral, as shown in Fig. 38.4. A complete cleft of the palate involves both the primary and secondary palates as well as the alveolus. There is also the less common possibility of an isolated cleft palate,[7] which usually involves the secondary palate, posterior to the incisive foramen. This occurs in 1 in 1500 live births in the United States.[2]

A less severe form of cleft palate is a submucous cleft, which is a deformity in which there is a defective muscle union across the soft palate but the oral mucosa is intact. Classically, this presents as a bifid uvula, an absent posterior nasal spine, and a transparent band of mucosa at the midline of the palate called the zona pellucida. A submucous cleft often goes undiagnosed until the toddler years, and one of the first signs is hypernasal speech.[8] This abnormal speech pattern is a result of a velopharyngeal dysfunction, which occurs in roughly half of patients with submucous cleft palate.[9]

TABLE 38.1 Members of a Typical Cleft Lip and Palate Team

Member	Role
Plastic surgeon	Early surgical interventions, including lip adhesion and/or primary lip repair as well as esthetic surgical procedures throughout growth to minimize scarring and improve facial features
Pediatric otolaryngologist	Early surgical interventions, including lip adhesion and/or primary lip repair, palate repair, velopharyngeal surgery, and other possible surgical interventions such as ear tubes
Oral and maxillofacial surgeon	Depending on training, may play a role in surgical repair of lip and palate Commonly involved in extractions, bone grafting procedures, and distraction osteogenesis
Geneticist	Counsels families on the risk of having future children with CLP Determines whether clefting is a part of a syndrome or an isolated event
Pediatric dentist	Provides a dental home for children with CLP or other craniofacial abnormalities May play a role in presurgical molding techniques (e.g., NAM) Prevention of dental disease in high-risk populations as well as restorations and interceptive orthodontics
Orthodontist	May play a role in presurgical molding techniques (e.g., NAM or Latham) Early treatment for alignment and expansion of constricted dental arches and comprehensive orthodontic treatment
Prosthodontist	Restores dentition to full function and esthetics in adolescence and adulthood
Audiologist	Follows milestones for normal hearing and work with otolaryngologist to determine whether ear tubes are needed
Speech pathologist	Follows milestones for speech development Works with local speech therapists to devise a program that will maximize speech development Input is important when the decision has to be made regarding velopharyngeal surgery
Nurse	Provides support and counseling for families Coordinates many aspects of medical care Works with families to develop a program for feeding, particularly early in life
Psychologist	Assesses child's mental and emotional well-being throughout life Helps child adjust to stages of life and offers assistance and support when needed
Social worker	Provides support and assistance to families, helping overcome barriers, allowing the best possible care to be delivered to the child Financial assistance, transportation, local arrangements, and school programs are a few examples

Makeup of group and roles will vary depending on a number of factors including geographical location, hospital policies, and available specialists.
CLP, Cleft lip and palate; *NAM*, nasoalveolar molding.

Causes of Cleft Lip and Palate

Clefts of the lip and palate may result from isolated mutations, syndromes (as shown in Box 38.1), environmental factors, teratogen exposure (including alcohol and tobacco), or a combination of all four. Genetics plays a strong role in the development of orofacial clefts, both syndromic and nonsyndromic, but it is known that genetics is not the sole determinant of whether or not a child will develop a cleft.

During normal development, the facial prominences appear at the end of the fourth embryonic week. These prominences are derived from the neural crest and consist of maxillary prominences laterally as well as a frontonasal prominence. Nasal placodes, located on either side of the frontonasal prominence, appear during the fifth embryonic week, eventually forming the nasal pits, which are bordered by the lateral and medial nasal prominences. The fusion of the medial nasal prominences forms the nasal tip, columella, and philtrum as well as a portion of the upper lip. The fusion of the maxillary prominences forms the remainder of the upper lip. These fusion events take place during the seventh embryonic week.

The palate begins to form during the fifth embryonic week, continuing through the twelfth embryonic week. The primary palate is formed when the medial nasal prominences fuse, only at a deeper level. The secondary palate begins to form soon after the primary palate is fused, around the seventh embryonic week. This results from fusion of the lateral palatine shelves, beginning at the incisive foramen in the eighth week and ending at the uvula in the twelfth embryonic week.

• BOX 38.1 Common Syndromes and Abnormalities Associated With Cleft Lip and Palate

Apert syndrome
Beckwith-Wiedemann syndrome
CHARGE syndrome
DiGeorge syndrome
Goldenhar syndrome
Kabuki syndrome
Klippel Feil syndrome
Pierre Robin sequence
Stickler syndrome
Treacher Collins syndrome
Van der Woude syndrome
Velocardiofacial syndrome

Challenges and Anomalies Associated With Cleft Lip and Palate

Children with cleft lip and palate may suffer from a number of other complications and conditions. A common presentation

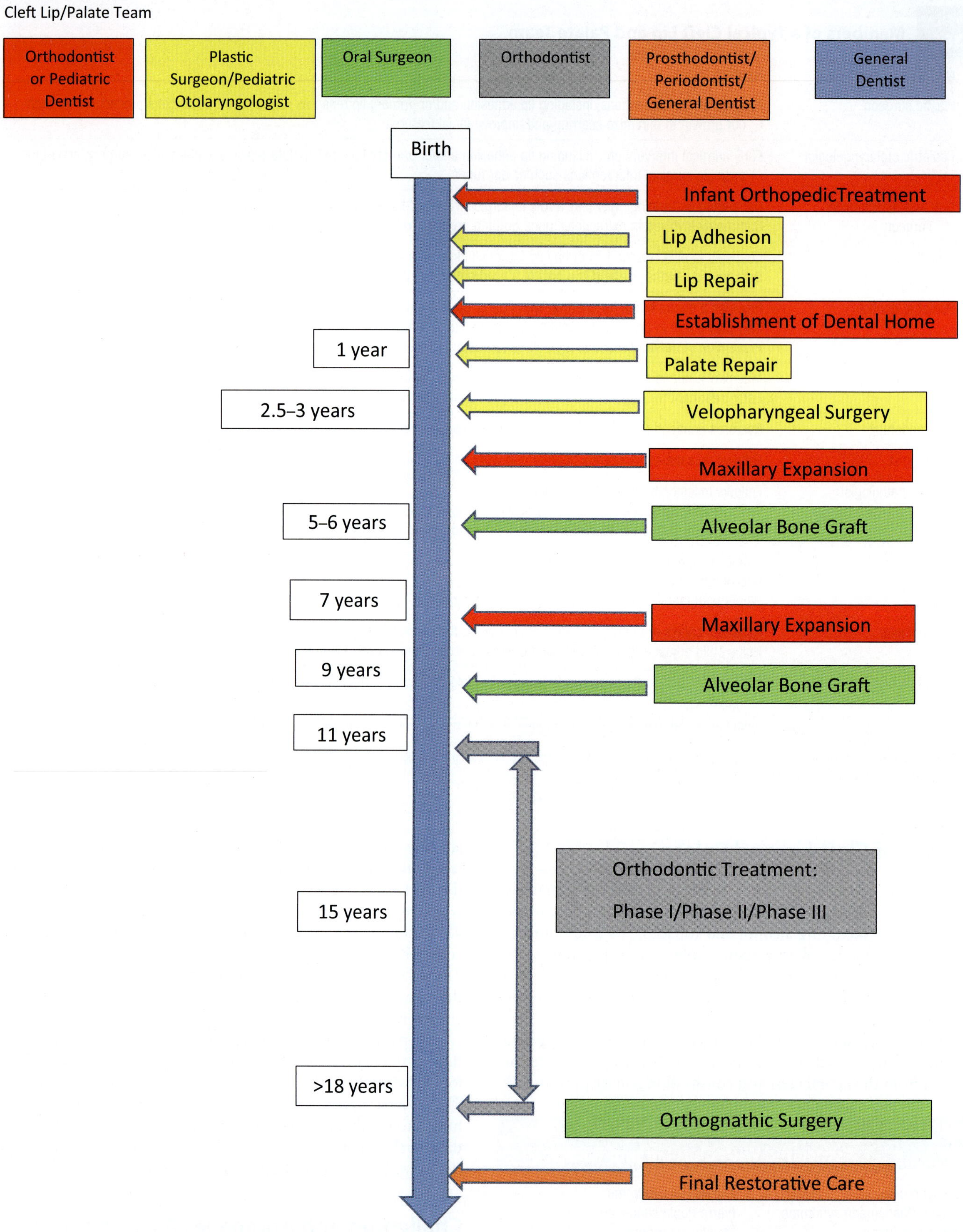

• **Fig. 38.1** Timeline of common treatments and surgical interventions for children with cleft lip and palate.

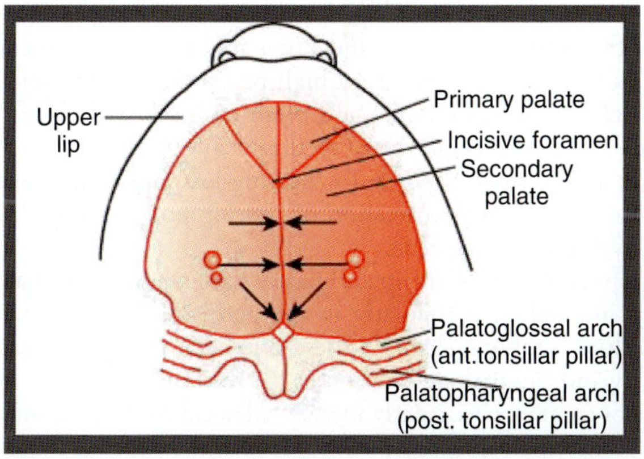

• **Fig. 38.2** Primary and secondary palate divided by the incisive papilla. *Ant.*, Anterior; *post.*, posterior. (From Holzman R. Airway management. In: Davis P, Cladis F, eds. *Anesthesia for Infants and Children.* Elsevier; 2017: 349-369.)

for patients with cleft lip and palate is the concurrent presence of micrognathia and glossoptosis. Together, this triad is commonly referred to as Pierre Robin sequence, as shown in Fig. 38.5, named after Dr. Pierre Robin who described this in the 1920s.[10] This sequence occurs in a number of syndromes and a major concern for these children is airway obstruction due to the malposition of the tongue. It has become common for children with Pierre Robin sequence to have mandibular distraction osteogenesis at a very young age to prevent upper airway obstruction.[11]

Children with cleft lip alone usually have little difficulty feeding and can often nurse or bottle-feed normally. Children with a cleft palate often struggle to feed due to the limited or absent ability of the infant to create suction and suck to feed.[12] To help families navigate these feeding challenges, nursing professionals will demonstrate unique bottles and feeding methods to determine what works best for each child and family, as shown in Fig. 38.6.

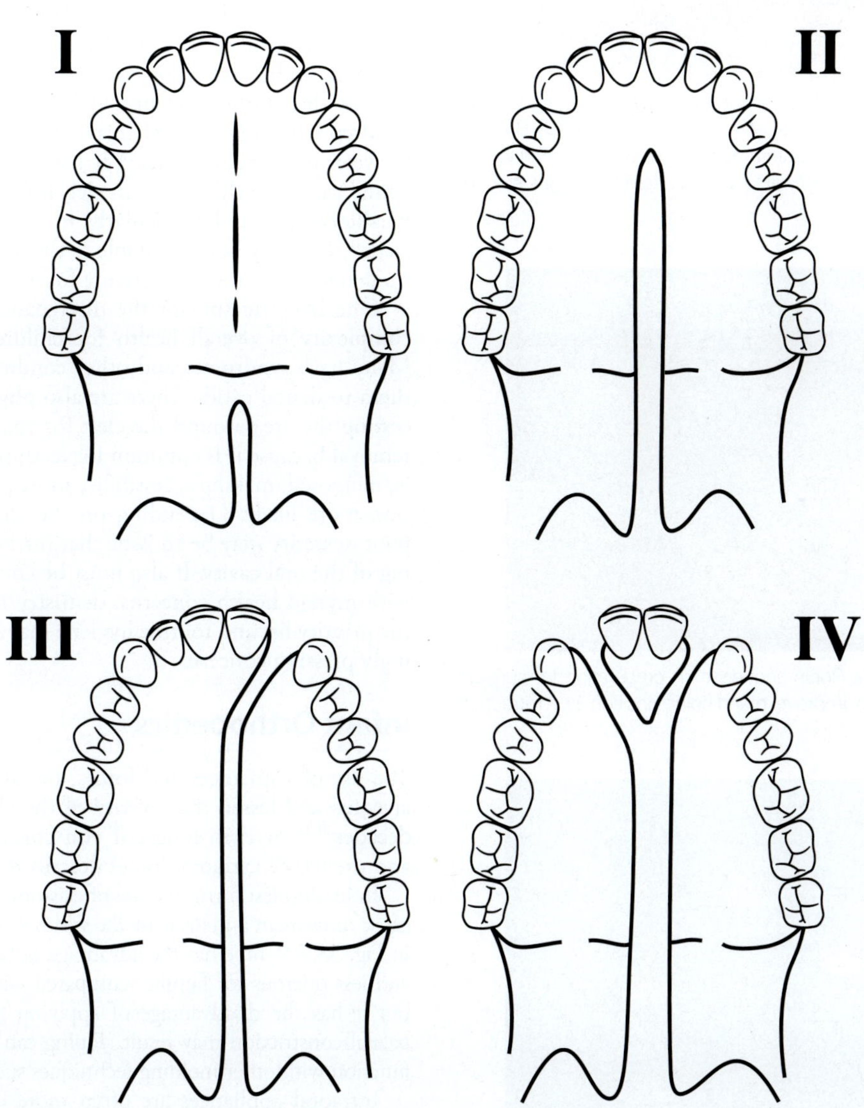

• **Fig. 38.3** Classification of cleft palate. *I*, Incomplete cleft of secondary palate. *II*, Complete cleft of the secondary palate. *III*, Unilateral complete cleft of primary and secondary palate. *IV*, Bilateral complete cleft of the primary and secondary palate. (Courtesy Monica Byrne.)

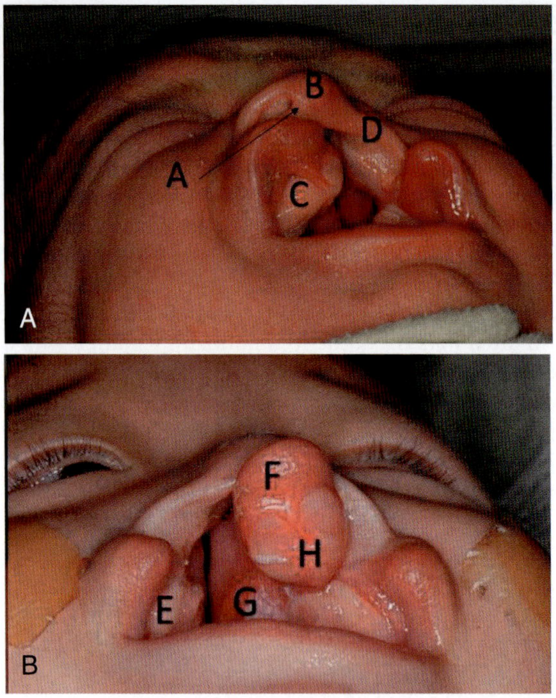

• **Fig. 38.4** (A) Unilateral complete cleft lip and palate. *A,* Columella; *B,* Nasal tip; *C,* Greater segment of alveolus; *D,* Alar rim. (B) Bilateral complete cleft lip and palate. *E,* Lateral shelf of alveolus; *F,* Prolabium; *G,* Vomer; *H,* Premaxilla. Note erupting primary tooth on right side of premaxilla.

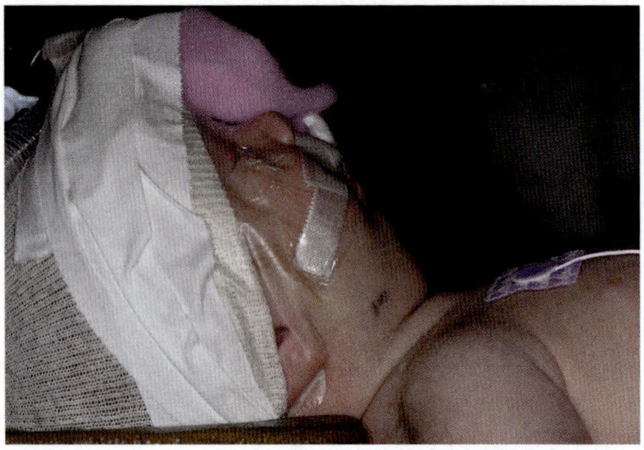

• **Fig. 38.5** Child with Pierre Robin sequence (in preparation for surgical placement of distractors to improve mandibular position by distraction osteogenesis).

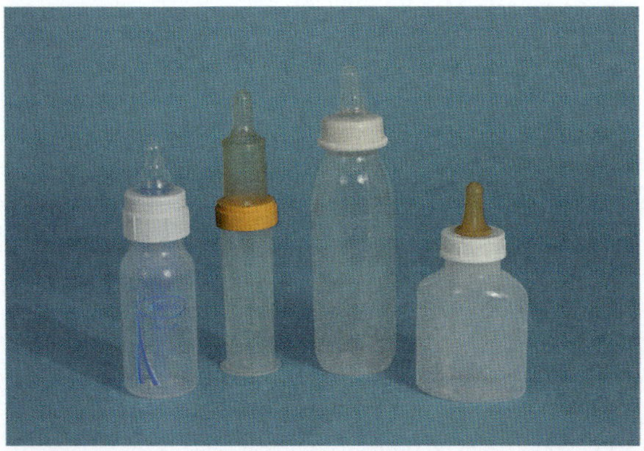

• **Fig. 38.6** Bottles commonly used for children with cleft lip and palate.

Another common challenge for children with cleft lip and palate is frequent otitis media and other middle ear abnormalities. Studies have shown that a very high percentage of children with cleft palate require ear tubes and often multiple sets of ear tubes during childhood as a result of recurrent infections.[13] It is important to screen these children for hearing loss and intervene early because delays in the correction of hearing problems can hinder the development of speech.

Individuals with cleft lip and palate have a higher incidence of dental anomalies, particularly in the permanent dentition, than individuals without clefts.[14] These anomalies vary in degree of severity and can include rotation of the teeth near the cleft, hypoplasia of enamel, particularly in teeth adjacent to the cleft, missing teeth, and supernumerary teeth.

Hypodontia, or missing teeth, occurs more commonly in patients with cleft lip and palate and it occurs more frequently in the permanent dentition compared with the primary dentition. The tooth most likely to be missing is the lateral incisor with the prevalence being higher on the side with the cleft.[15] The prevalence of missing lateral incisors increases as the extent of clefting increases, from cleft lip alone to cleft palate alone to cleft lip and palate.[15]

One question that has proven to be difficult to answer is, "Do children with orofacial clefts have higher rates of dental caries?" Research in this area is contradictory, with numerous studies from around the world showing significantly higher caries rates for children with clefts,[16,17] whereas other studies show no difference between these populations.[18] It has been shown that the rate of dental caries for children with cleft lip and palate is greater in the maxillary arch and particularly in those teeth adjacent to the cleft.[16] This may be attributable to the hypoplasia and other structural anomalies more commonly found in these teeth.[19]

One likely reason for the discrepancies in caries rates is the complexity of overall health for children with orofacial clefts. Many have syndromes and other conditions that can predispose them to dental caries. There are also physical challenges with accessing the area around the cleft for routine hygiene and plaque removal because it is common for teeth in and around the cleft to be malposed, making accessibility more difficult and plaque retention more likely. Depending on the child's physical challenges, poor dexterity may be an issue that further complicates the cleaning of the oral cavity. It also must be considered that for children with myriad health concerns, dentistry may not rank as high on the priority list and routine hygiene may suffer due to more seemingly pressing concerns.

Infant Orthopedics

The use of appliances and forces, in various forms, to mold the alveolus and lessen the severity of the cleft has been around for decades[20,21] or even longer if you consider Hoffman's head cap and the use of extraoral forces described in the late 1600s.[22]

In its simplest form, the use of elastomeric tape to apply force can cause movement and decrease the width of the alveolar cleft, as shown in Fig. 38.7.[23] Tape has the advantage of being relatively inexpensive and less onerous for families compared with other molding devices, but it has the disadvantage of applying forces indiscriminately, so palatal constriction may result. Taping can be done alone or in conjunction with other molding techniques such as intraoral appliances.

Intraoral appliances are often more cumbersome to use, but they do maintain the palatal width, as force can be applied in smaller areas and with greater precision. Recently these intraoral appliances have gained acceptance on many craniofacial teams

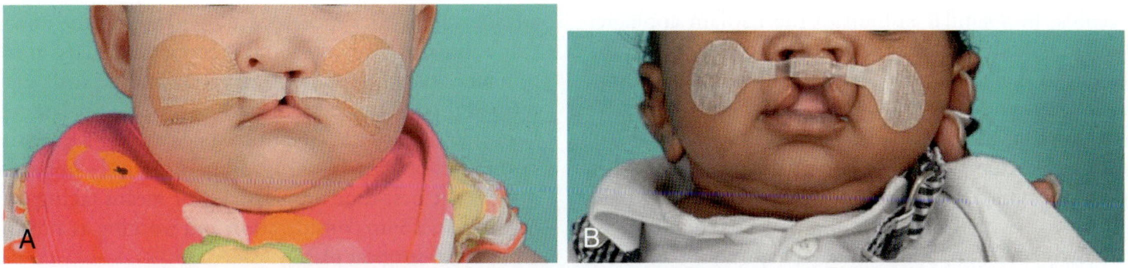

• **Fig. 38.7** Elastomeric Taping. (A) Child with a unilateral cleft. (B) Child with a bilateral cleft.

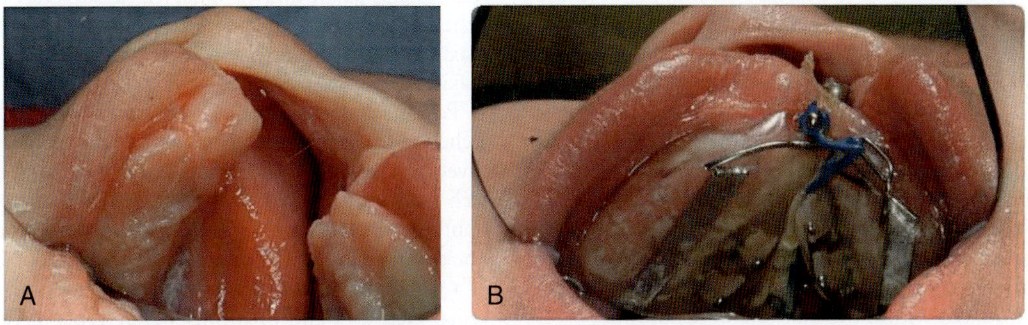

• **Fig. 38.8** (A–B) Latham appliance.

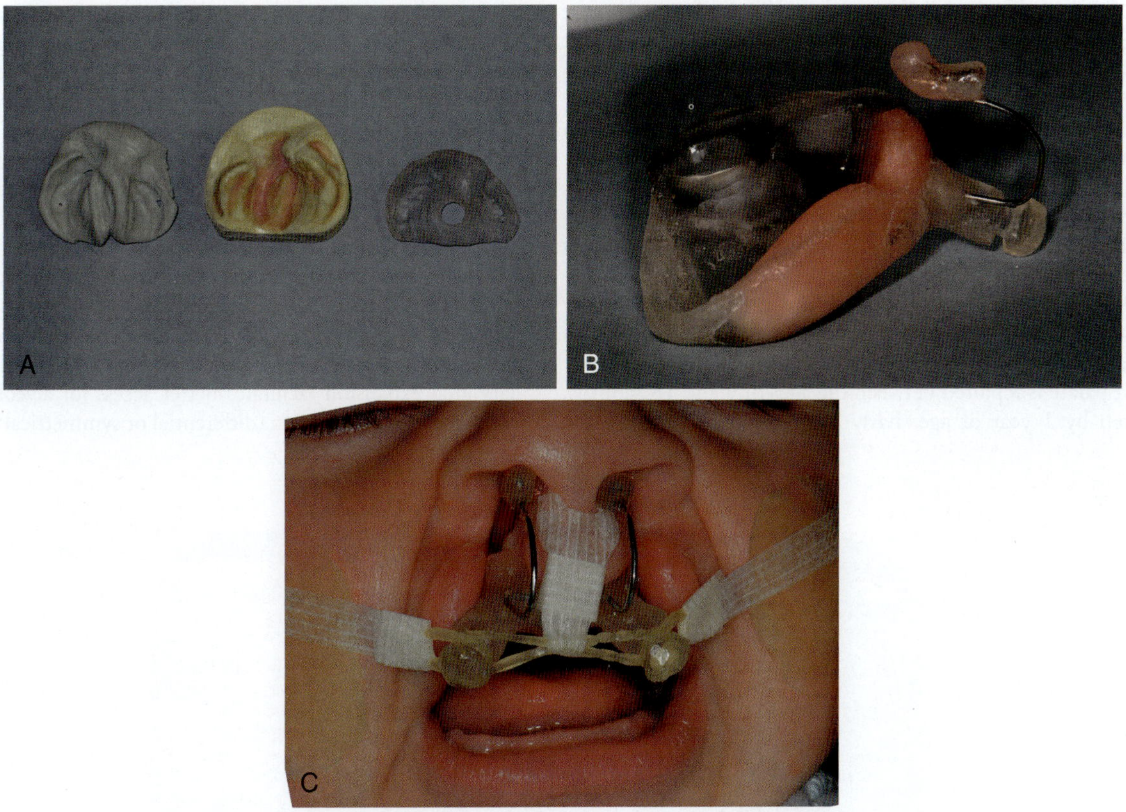

• **Fig. 38.9** Nasoalveolar Molding (NAM) Appliance. (A) Fabrication of NAM appliance. (B) NAM appliance. (C) NAM and taping for presurgical orthopedics.

worldwide and are a hot topic of research. The Latham appliance shown in Fig. 38.8 is an appliance that is surgically placed into a young child's mouth and retained to the palate with a screw.[24] The Latham appliance is adjusted regularly to reduce the cleft size. The advantage of this appliance is that compliance is not required, but the disadvantage is increased surgical interventions in a very young child, both at the time of insertion and at the time of removal.

One less invasive method, pioneered by Dr. Barry Grayson and his team at New York University, is nasoalveolar molding (NAM), as shown in Fig. 38.9.[25] This method uses an acrylic plate to mold the bony alveolus, in a similar fashion to the Latham appliance and early appliances like the Hotz plate, but it is removable and uses a nasal stent to shape the cartilage of the nose, in an attempt to improve symmetry and decrease the need for future invasive surgical correction that may cause scarring and hinder growth.

The NAM appliance is worn throughout the day and held in place by tape to the child's cheeks. Changes are made to the plate incrementally by the dental professional, and over time the bony segments are slowly moved to a more favorable position, lessening the amount of surgical correction that is needed to bring the lip segments together while simplifying the surgical approach for the nose. NAM has even been shown to decrease the number of future surgical interventions that are typically performed for esthetics.[26]

An Overview of the Timeline of Interventions

Many procedures are required for children born with cleft lip and palate, as outlined in Fig. 38.1. The earliest intervention is often infant orthopedic treatment (see previous section). The goal of infant orthopedic treatment is to enhance the surgical repair of lip and nose by establishing a proper skeletal base.[27–29] A wide variety of approaches are used, with one of the most popular being NAM, which is initiated within the first few weeks of life.[30]

A cleft lip is repaired between 3 and 6 months of age after infant orthopedic treatment. A few craniofacial centers may elect to perform another surgery called a nasolabial (lip) adhesion before repairing the cleft lip, although this has largely fallen out of favor in the United States. The nasolabial (lip) adhesion procedure is purported to reduce the extent of undermining and minimize labial tension at the time of lip repair.[31] Any surgical intervention in a young child has to be considered carefully, and traditionally cleft repair surgeries have been subject to the "rule of 10s." This rule states that a child must be 10 pounds in weight, have a hemoglobin value greater than 10 g/dL, and be older than 10 weeks of age before the surgical intervention.[32] This rule is not an absolute, but one must certainly consider the risk of taking a very young baby under general anesthesia when planning care, and this is one reason that nasolabial (lip) adhesion has fallen out of favor.

A cleft palate is repaired between the ages of 9 and 18 months, most often by 1 year of age. Early repair of the palate has the advantage of better speech development, but the downside is that scar tissue can form and inhibit proper maxillary growth, leading to malocclusion (typically class III malocclusions and skeletal pattern) and poor facial esthetics. Conversely, if palate repair is done late, after 18 months, the opposite is true and growth may occur normally but speech will likely be negatively impacted.[33] Determining the best time for palate repair means taking these competing priorities into consideration and working as a team to develop an optimal surgical plan.

If speech development is suboptimal, a velopharyngeal surgery may be performed between 2.5 and 3 years of age.[34] Repair of the cleft lip and palate and velopharyngeal surgeries are performed by either a plastic surgeon, pediatric otolaryngologist, or an oral and maxillofacial surgeon with advanced training in pediatric craniomaxillofacial surgery.

Patients with clefts of the alveolus often have collapsed maxillary arches and require alveolar bone grafting, as shown in Fig. 38.10. Alveolar bone grafting enables the surgeon to obtain maxillary arch continuity, provide support for the dentition to erupt, and stabilize the maxillary arch before any orthodontic treatment.[35–41] The timing of alveolar bone grafting is dependent on the presence of a viable maxillary permanent lateral incisor adjacent to the alveolar cleft area and proximity of the roots of central incisors to the alveolar cleft.[35–41] If a viable permanent lateral incisor is present or if the root of the developing maxillary central incisor is too close to the alveolar cleft, alveolar bone grafting is recommended by 5 to 7 years of age. A number of craniofacial centers elect to perform the alveolar bone grafting at a later time, closer to eruption of the maxillary permanent canines. The most frequently used donor site for alveolar bone grafting is the iliac crest because of ease of access and abundance of bone.[27,40] Alternative donor sites include the mandibular symphysis, rib, cranial bones, and tibia. A few craniofacial centers also use bone morphogenetic protein (BMP).[27,40] This alveolar bone grafting procedure is usually performed by an oral and maxillofacial surgeon.

It is recommended that maxillary arch expansion be performed before alveolar bone grafting to establish proper arch form and to address transverse discrepancies, as shown in Fig. 38.11.[27,34] Maxillary arch expansion facilitates better access for alveolar bone graft sites. Maxillary expansion (differential or symmetrical) is performed

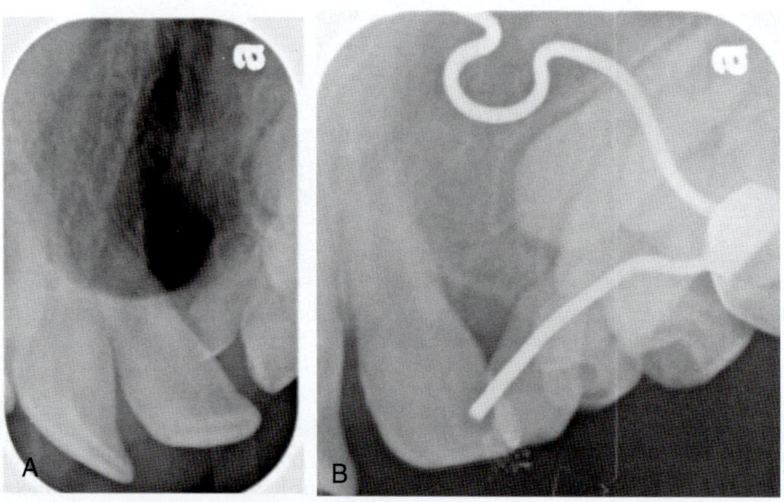

• **Fig. 38.10** Bone Grafting. (A) Alveolar defect in a patient with complete cleft lip and palate. (B) Alveolar defect repaired with an alveolar bone grafting procedure.

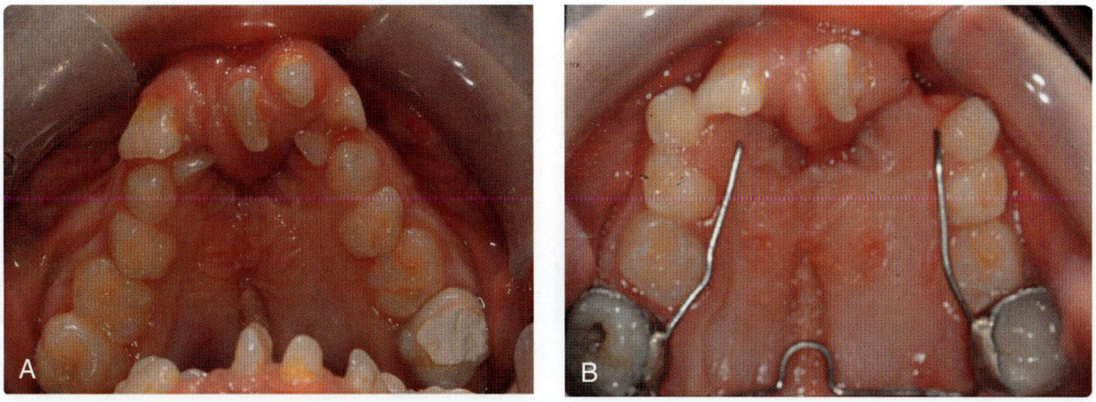

• **Fig. 38.11** (A–B) Maxillary arch in a patient with bilateral complete cleft lip and palate. (Note the collapsed anterior segment of the maxillary arch before expansion.)

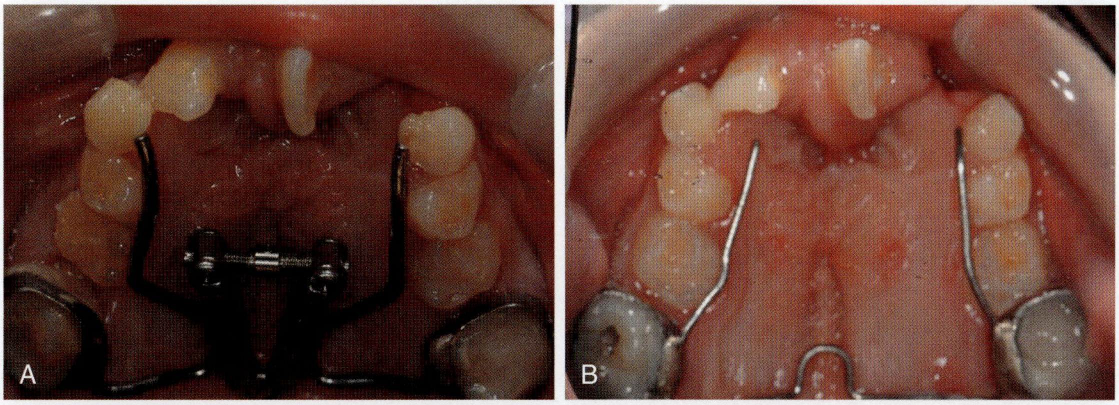

• **Fig. 38.12** Palatal Expansion. (A) Differential expansion with a fan-shaped expander was needed to address the collapsed maxillary arch. (B) Retain expansion with a transpalatal arch appliance.

either by the pediatric dentist or by an orthodontist on the cleft lip and palate team and appliances vary, as shown in Fig. 38.12.

After alveolar bone grafting, the patient is typically followed periodically by the cleft lip and palate team. It is recommended to obtain radiographs of the grafted area 3 to 6 months after the procedure to assess if there is sufficient bone in the grafted area. The eruption pattern of the permanent dentition is closely observed and if indicated, a limited phase of orthodontic treatment (often in the maxillary arch only) is completed during the mixed dentition phase. It is important to keep in mind that teeth can be orthodontically moved into the grafted areas. This will also ensure that the alveolar bone grafts will be successful. For alveolar bone grafts to be successful in the long term, they should be placed under some mechanical stress. This stress can be placed by either permanent teeth erupting through the grafts or by orthodontically moving teeth into the grafted areas. Teeth should never be moved into areas where the alveolar bone graft has failed as this leads to a high risk of devitalizing teeth. The goals of limited maxillary arch orthodontic treatment are to align and level the maxillary arch, correct crossbites, create space for facilitating eruption of permanent teeth, and treat impacted or ectopically erupting teeth, as shown in Fig. 38.13.

During the early teenage years, if it is determined that the amount of anteroposterior skeletal discrepancy is too large, then maxillary distraction osteogenesis is indicated.[42,43] This procedure is performed by an oral and maxillofacial surgeon after eruption of all permanent teeth into the arch. The orthodontist aligns and levels the maxillary arch and prepares the patient to undergo the maxillary distraction osteogenesis procedure. Until a few years ago, maxillary distraction was accomplished by a rigid external distractor (RED) appliance, as shown in Fig. 38.14. Internal distractors, as shown in Fig. 38.15, are being increasingly used by oral and maxillofacial surgeons in place of the more cumbersome extraoral appliances.[43,44]

The patient is followed during the teenage years, and the orthodontist determines the timing of a comprehensive phase of orthodontic treatment. If there are no significant skeletal discrepancies to address, the orthodontic treatment can be initiated after eruption of all permanent teeth. If large skeletal discrepancies exist, it is recommended that a comprehensive phase of orthodontic treatment in conjunction with an orthognathic surgery be initiated after completion of growth.

Role of the Dentist

Children born with cleft lip and palate face a long and difficult road through the healthcare system. They will have many interventions by myriad providers. One must consider the

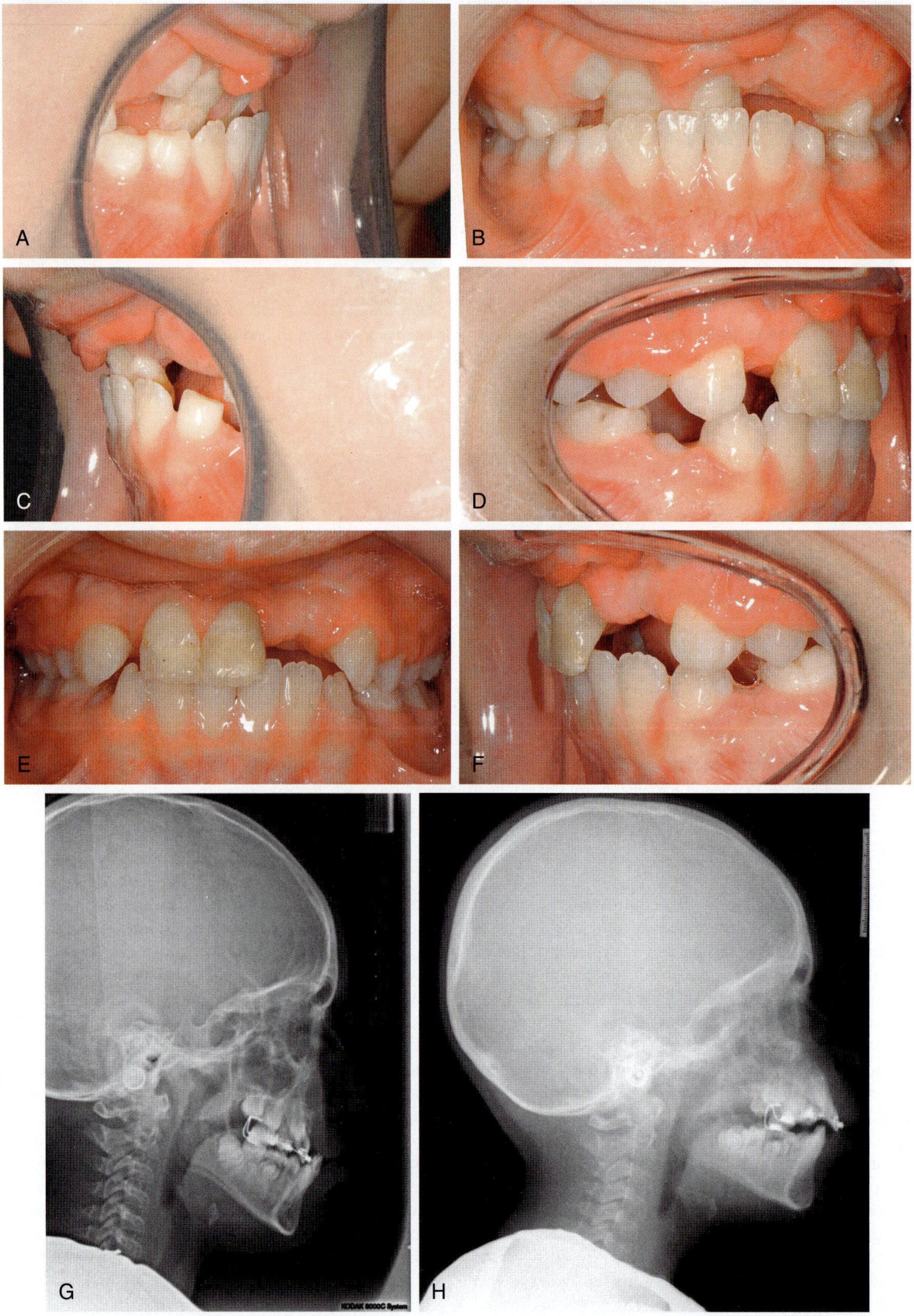

• **Fig. 38.13** Orthodontic Treatment. (A–C) Pretreatment photographs. (D–F) Posttreatment photographs. (G) Pretreatment cephalometric film. (H) Posttreatment cephalometric film.

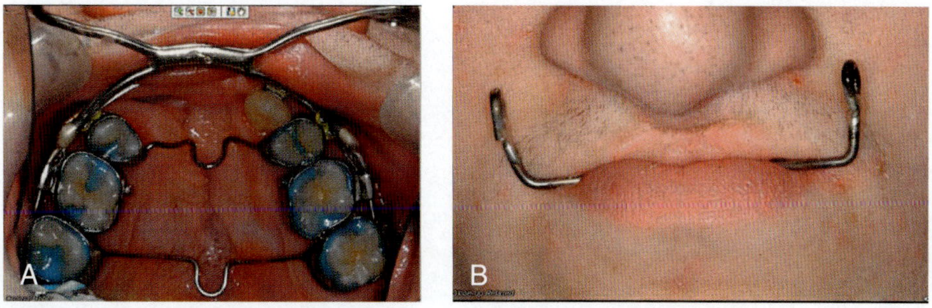

• **Fig. 38.14** (A–B) Setup for a rigid external distractor appliance.

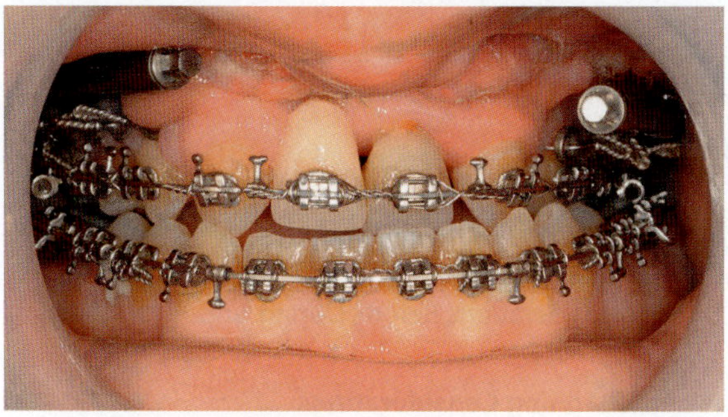

• **Fig. 38.15** Internal distractors.

impact this will have on the physical, mental, and emotional well-being of the child and work closely with other members of the healthcare team to provide the most comprehensive care possible. Even if a dentist is not an active member of a cleft lip and palate team, he or she must have the knowledge to refer to the proper provider at the proper time. A pediatric dentist has a unique opportunity to work with these children and their families from infancy into young adulthood and play a key role in the promotion of optimal oral health as well as ensuring that the family is able to properly navigate the complexities of the healthcare environment.

Visit eBooks.Health.Elsevier.com to see full list of references.

39

Dental and Oral Considerations for Inherited and Acquired Diseases

EVELINA KRATUNOVA, CATHERINE HONG, AND MARCIO A. DA FONSECA

CHAPTER OUTLINE

Inherited Coagulation Disorders

Hemophilia

Hemophilia encompasses a group of inherited coagulation disorders characterized by defective or deficient clotting factors leading to impaired hemostasis.[1] Hemophilia A (factor VIII deficiency) and hemophilia B (factor IX deficiency) have an X-linked recessive pattern.[1,2] Hemophilia A is more common and more severe, with a prevalence of 1 in 5000 male live births compared with 1 in 30,000 for hemophilia B.[1,3] The disorder manifests through varying symptoms of bleeding based on clotting factor activity levels: severe (<1% of normal levels), moderate (1% to 5%), and mild (6% to 40%).[1] Severe hemophilia typically presents with spontaneous or minor trauma-induced bleeding, whereas mild forms might not be noticeable until the patient undergoes a significant hemostatic challenge, such as surgery or trauma.[1–3] Although severe hemophilia predominantly affects males due to its X-linked inheritance, there have been rare instances in females and mild symptoms reported in female carriers.[2] Common sites of bleeding are the oral mucosa, soft tissues, brain, and joints. Late complications include neurologic issues and joint deformities from repetitive bleeding.[1–3] Diagnosis includes a thorough review of the patient's and family's bleeding history, assessment of factor activity level, and genetic testing.[1] The condition should be suspected when a male patient presents with unusual bleeding with normal platelet count, bleeding time, thrombin time, and prothrombin time, but a prolonged activated partial thromboplastin time.[1–3]

Treatment strategies involve both prophylactic and on-demand intravenous administration of clotting factors, primarily factor VIII or IX, through plasma-derived, recombinant, or modified concentrates.[1–3] For mild hemophilia A, desmopressin acetate (1-deamino-8-d-arginine vasopressin [DDAVP]) can be used to stimulate the release of factor VIII, achieving peak levels within an hour. The presence of inhibitors in 20% to 30% in hemophilia A and 5% of hemophilia B complicates treatment, necessitating bypassing agents or immune modulation to manage bleeding.[1,2]

Von Willebrand Disease

Von Willebrand disease (VWD) is the most prevalent inherited bleeding disorder, affecting approximately 1% of the population with no sex predilection.[4] It impairs hemostasis due to either a deficiency or dysfunction of von Willebrand factor (VWF), an important element for blood clot formation and for carrying factor VIII. A partial quantitative deficiency of VWF accounts for 75% to 85% of cases.[4]

Dental Considerations for Patients With Inherited Coagulation Disorders

Dental management for patients with bleeding disorders requires coordination with the patient's hematologist. The necessity and type of coagulation factor replacement are determined by the hemostatic diagnosis, bleeding diathesis severity, and the nature of the dental procedure.[5] Options for systemic replacement therapy vary and may include presurgical testing, such as desmopressin trials or screening for inhibitors.[2]

Antifibrinolytic agents, such as aminocaproic acid and tranexamic acid, are used to prevent clot dissolution postoperatively by inhibiting plasminogen's activation to plasmin. These agents reduce fibrinolytic activity in oral mucosa and saliva and serve as adjuncts to systemic factor replacement therapies addressing underlying coagulation issues.[2,5] When possible, local infiltration is preferred to nerve blocks to minimize hematoma risk. Sedation or general anesthesia may be considered to limit injections into sensitive areas. Endodontic treatment may be considered to avoid extractions in high-risk patients. Surgical approaches should allow for easy management of bleeding, avoiding flaps to reduce bleeding areas, and ensuring primary surgical closure.[5]

Adjunctive hemostatic agents, such as oxidized regenerated cellulose, gelatin matrix, and microfibrillar collagen can be used to enhance clot stability and prevent postoperative bleeding.[5] Electrocautery and suturing are options, albeit with caution, to avoid additional bleeding risks or tissue damage. Pressure application is a key technique for achieving hemostasis. Firm pressure should be applied for at least 30 to 60 minutes without interruption to prevent continued bleeding. Techniques for managing postoperative bleeding include reapplying pressure packs, using hemostatic agents in the sockets, and reinjecting with local anesthetic containing epinephrine, although care must be taken due to potential for rebound vasodilation. Other measures include the removal of exophytic clots to allow proper pressure application, use of astringents like the "tea-bag trick" for its tannic acid, and advising patients to limit physical activities. Acetaminophen is preferred over nonsteroidal antiinflammatory drugs (NSAIDs) for pain management due to its efficacy in relieving pain without increasing the risk of bleeding.[2,5]

Anemia

Anemia is characterized by a reduction in red blood cell (RBC) mass or blood hemoglobin (HGB) concentration, typically arising from decreased RBC production, increased RBC loss, premature RBC destruction (hemolysis), or a combination of these mechanisms.[6,7] Diagnosis is made when hematocrit (HCT) or HGB fall at or below the 2.5th percentile for a person's age, and sex.[6] The etiology includes immune hemolytic disease, infection, hereditary disorders, and iron deficiency, either due to diet or blood loss in older children.[7] Patient assessment includes a detailed history of symptoms, family history of anemias or hemoglobinopathy, and a thorough physical examination. Laboratory testing comprises complete blood count with RBC indices and a peripheral blood smear.[6,7]

Hemolytic anemia results from the premature destruction of RBCs. RBC abnormalities, such as inherited hemoglobinopathies and enzyme deficiencies, result in intrinsic hemolytic anemia, whereas extrinsic forms are caused by external factors like autoimmune diseases, systemic conditions, medications, and toxins that damage RBCs.[6,7] Conditions like hemolytic uremic syndrome, thrombotic thrombocytopenic purpura, and disseminated intravascular coagulation can also lead to hemolytic anemia. Furthermore, mechanical damage to RBCs, such as that caused by artificial heart valves, can contribute to hemolytic anemia.[6,7] The pathophysiology, clinical manifestations, and treatment approaches for anemia depend on the underlying cause, highlighting the importance of a comprehensive diagnostic evaluation to guide appropriate management strategies.

Dental Considerations for Patients With Anemia

A thorough preoperative assessment is essential, including a detailed medical history and a consultation with the patient's physician. Employing atraumatic techniques and local hemostatic measures to minimize bleeding is important because anemic patients have a reduced capacity to tolerate blood loss.[7,8] An increased susceptibility to infections in some anemic patients necessitates aseptic techniques and, where advised, the use of prophylactic antibiotics. For procedures with potential for respiratory compromise, oxygen saturation levels should be monitored, and supplemental oxygen should be available, especially in those with severe anemia. Dental professionals should address potential nutritional deficiencies related to anemia, such as iron, vitamin B_{12}, or folate deficiencies, by educating patients on the importance of a balanced diet and referral to a nutritionist. Effective pain and stress management, comprehensive postoperative care instructions for monitoring complications, regular follow-ups, and coordination with the healthcare team are all vital components to dental care.[8]

Sickle Cell Disorders

The HGB molecule, a tetramer that is soluble and does not polymerize, plays an essential role in RBC function.[9] Normal RBCs contain three types of HGB: A, which is composed of two α and two β globin chains and comprises 96% to 98% of the total HGB; A2, made up of two α and two δ chains, accounting for 1.5% to 3.2% of the total HGB; and fetal HGB, consisting of two α and two γ chains, making up 0.5% to 0.8%. Newborns' blood consists predominantly of fetal HGB (60% to 80%), which reduces to 10% to 20% within the first 3 to 6 months of life.[9]

A point mutation in the β globin gene leads to the production of sickle hemoglobin (HGBS), a defective hemoglobin tetramer consisting of two α and two βS globin chains.[10] When deoxygenated, HGBS becomes poorly soluble causing the RBCs to sickle. These sickle-shaped erythrocytes are rigid, leading to hemolysis, vascular dysfunction, and chronic endothelial damage.[10] The life span of these cells is 12 to 17 days compared with the normal 120 days.[10] These are among the most common inherited blood disorders, primarily affecting individuals from tropical and subtropical regions or with ancestry from areas such as Africa, the Middle East, the Mediterranean, India, the Caribbean, and South America. The incidence varies by region, from 0.3% to 22%.[10,11]

Sickle cell trait (SCT) is a generally asymptomatic carrier state where one allele of the β globin gene carries the HGBS mutation and the other allele is normal. SCT is associated with a reduced risk of severe malaria and hospitalization in areas endemic for *Plasmodium falciparum* malaria.[11] Sickle cell disease (SCD) refers to cases with one βS globin mutation plus a second β globin gene mutation, manifesting clinically with anemia and laboratory evidence of sickling.[10,11] SCD typically becomes apparent in the first 6 months of life as fetal HGB is replaced by HGBS. Clinical manifestations include anemia, vasculopathy, and painful sickle cell crises. The chronic manifestations of SCD result from chronic organ ischemia and infarction, with the compromised immune system predisposing individuals to chronic bone problems. Acute chest syndrome is a leading cause of death and hospitalization among patients with SCD.[10] Treatment for SCD includes supportive care measures such as folic acid supplementation, daily antibiotic prophylaxis for children, and management of vaso-occlusive pain episodes with adequate hydration and pain control.[11] Hydroxyurea and L-glutamine may also be used for symptomatic cases.[10,11] Hematopoietic stem cell transplantation (HSCT) can be curative. In December 2023, SCD became the first disease ever approved by the US Food and Drug Administration (FDA) to be treated with gene editing for children over 12 years of age. Conventional gene therapy is also available.

Dental Considerations for Patients With Sickle Cell Disorders

A comprehensive medical history should be obtained, including the specific type of SCD, the current treatment regimen, and any complications, including previous episodes of sickle cell crises.[12] Patients with SCD may have a different response to pain due to their condition and previous painful experiences.[11,12] Effective pain management strategies should be employed, as stress can trigger sickle cell crises. Stress reduction techniques should be utilized in the dental office and sedation methods, such as nitrous oxide or sedatives, should be considered for anxious patients to minimize the risk of inducing a crisis.[12]

An increased risk of infections in patients with SCD requires strict aseptic technique and prophylactic antibiotics may be recommended by the patient's physician before invasive dental procedures.[12] Hypoxia and dehydration during dental procedures can precipitate sickle cell crises.[10] Nitrous oxide is typically safe for these patients.[12,13] For lengthy procedures, vital signs should be monitored, and supplemental oxygen may be considered. Atraumatic extraction techniques and local measures to control bleeding should be used due to the altered blood clotting dynamics in SCD patients. Consultation with the patient's hematologist should be sought about the need for any preoperative or postoperative hematologic interventions. Elective dental procedures should be scheduled during periods when the patient is stable and free from recent episodes of sickle cell crises.[12]

Glucose-6-Phosphate Dehydrogenase Deficiency

Glucose-6-phosphate dehydrogenase (G6PD) deficiency is the most common inherited RBC enzymatic defect, affecting approximately 400 million people worldwide.[14] It results from a genetic defect in the G6PD enzyme within RBCs that protects erythrocytes from oxidative damage.[15] Exposure to oxidants leads to the depletion of reduced glutathione, causing RBCs to become rigid and nondeformable making them susceptible to destruction by macrophages in the marrow, spleen, and liver. Intravascular hemolysis can also occur, leading to hemoglobinemia and hemoglobinuria.[14,15] This condition is inherited in an X-linked pattern, where heterozygous females are typically unaffected carriers, and homozygous or heterozygous females with skewed lyonization may present with hemolytic anemia.[15]

G6PD deficiency is historically categorized into class I (severe enzyme deficiency [<10% of normal] associated with chronic hemolytic anemia), class II (severe enzyme deficiency but with only intermittent hemolysis upon exposure to oxidant stress), and class III (moderate enzyme deficiency [10% to 60% of normal] with intermittent hemolysis). Manifestations include neonatal jaundice and episodic or chronic Heinz body hemolytic anemia, with acute episodes usually triggered by certain oxidant medications (e.g., dapsone, methylene blue, rasburicase, primaquine, tafenoquine), chemicals (e.g., henna or naphthalene), foods (e.g., fava beans), or infections. There is also an increased susceptibility to infection in some very severe variants and a possible protective effect against malaria.[14,15] Diagnostic testing for G6PD deficiency involves screening tests measuring units of G6PD enzyme activity per gram of HGB. Management of the condition depends on the severity of the deficiency and the clinical manifestations with an emphasis on avoiding known triggers and managing symptoms as they occur.[15]

Dental Considerations for Patients With G6PD Deficiency

A comprehensive medical history should include past hemolysis episodes, current medications, and known triggers. Drugs that can cause oxidative stress, including certain local anesthetics, analgesics, and antibiotics, should be avoided due to their potential to trigger hemolysis.[15,16] Hemolytic episodes can also be triggered by stress and pain; therefore the use of appropriate anesthetics and sedation methods for effective pain management and stress reduction should be employed to minimize this risk.[15] Infections trigger hemolysis necessitating the use of strict aseptic techniques. Prophylactic antibiotics may be considered, after consultation with the patient's physician, to prevent infections without inducing hemolysis.[15,16] Vigilance for acute hemolysis signs, such as sudden pallor, jaundice, dark urine, and back pain during or after dental procedures, is crucial. Immediate medical attention is required if hemolysis is suspected. Consultation with the patient's physician is essential before and after administering medications for dental procedures to ensure their safety in individuals with G6PD deficiency.[15,16]

Gastroenterology

Gastroesophageal Reflux Disease

Gastroesophageal reflux, characterized by regurgitation, is common in infants and usually resolves by 18 months of age.[17] Gastroesophageal reflux disease (GERD) is a reflux with pathologic complications. Symptoms include recurrent regurgitation persisting beyond 2 years, refusal of solid foods, frequent heartburn, dysphagia, asthma not responding to standard treatment, recurrent pneumonia, and chronic hoarseness or stridor.[17] Diagnosis relies on history and physical examination, barium contrast radiography to rule out anatomical abnormalities, and endoscopy with histology. Endoscopic evaluation is central for identifying esophagitis caused by GERD, and eosinophilic esophagitis should be considered as a differential diagnosis. The management of GERD is customized for each individual and may encompass antacids or histamine type 2 receptor antagonists for symptom relief; lifestyle adjustments like weight management for overweight individuals, elevating the head during sleep (in older children) and avoiding foods that exacerbate symptoms; prokinetic agents to improve gastric emptying; and, in certain instances, antireflux surgery, such as fundoplication.[17]

Dental Considerations for Patients With Gastroesophageal Reflux Disease

Patients with GERD should be assessed for signs of acid erosion of the teeth such as tooth sensitivity and enamel loss. Fluoride treatments are recommended to remineralize enamel, and dental sealants are indicated to protect teeth from acid exposure.[18] Teeth should not be brushed immediately after acid reflux episodes to avoid further enamel erosion; instead, rinsing the mouth with water or a fluoride mouth rinse to neutralize the acid and waiting at least 30 minutes before brushing are recommended. Practices that increase saliva production, such as chewing sugar-free gum, are encouraged to help neutralize acid in the mouth.[18] Restorative options for significant enamel erosion include composite restorations, crowns, or veneers. Regular dental checkups and cleanings are encouraged to monitor the progression of enamel erosion and manage any developing dental issues promptly.[18] Referral to a gastroenterologist for assessment and potential treatment should be made if signs of GERD are observed.

Celiac Disease

Celiac disease (CD) is a genetic sensitivity to dietary gluten and related proteins, leading to immune-mediated inflammation in the small intestinal mucosa, affecting 0.5% to 1% of the population.[19] Gluten, found in wheat, barley, and rye, triggers this condition. Adopting a gluten-free diet typically results in morphologic improvement of the small intestinal mucosa within weeks to months, but symptoms and mucosal damage can recur if gluten is reintroduced. The prevalence of CD is notably higher among individuals with Down syndrome, type 1 diabetes mellitus (T1DM), selective IgA deficiency, autoimmune thyroid disease, and Turner and Williams syndromes.[19,20] Symptoms include malabsorption (manifesting as diarrhea, steatorrhea, and weight loss), nutrient deficiencies, and histologic changes like villous atrophy, which are observable on small intestinal biopsy.[20] Nongastrointestinal manifestations may include dermatitis herpetiformis, delayed growth and pubertal development, neurologic disorders, behavioral symptoms, arthritis, dental enamel defects, liver disease, and an association with hyposplenism. Silent CD refers to cases with mild or minimal symptoms but positive celiac serologies.[19,20] Diagnosis is confirmed through serologic tests, endoscopy, and biopsy. Treatment primarily involves a strict gluten-free diet with compliance essential for successful management.[20]

Dental Considerations for Patients With Celiac Disease

Patients with CD often exhibit dental enamel defects that may affect the esthetics and structure of the teeth. It can lead to delayed dental development, including late eruption of teeth, and delayed growth and pubertal development, which may affect orthodontic planning and treatment.[21] Individuals with CD may experience a higher incidence of aphthous ulcers, which can cause significant discomfort and may affect oral intake and nutrition.[20] CD can be associated with reduced saliva production, causing xerostomia, which increases the risk of dental caries, oral infections such as candidiasis, and discomfort. Malabsorption can lead to deficiencies in essential vitamins and minerals, such as calcium, vitamin D, and iron, affecting oral health and healing leading to an increased risk of periodontal disease and delayed wound healing. Patients with CD require regular dental checkups to monitor for enamel defects, caries, and other oral health issues.[21]

Inflammatory Bowel Disease

Inflammatory bowel disease (IBD) encompasses two distinct disorders: ulcerative colitis (UC) and Crohn disease (CrD).[22] The etiology and pathogenesis of IBD are not fully understood. Symptoms include abdominal tenderness or pain, oral ulcers, or perianal disease, and laboratory findings such as anemia, hypoalbuminemia, and elevated inflammation markers, can be present. Extraintestinal manifestations may involve the skin, joints, liver, eyes, and bones, with growth failure and pubertal delay more common in CrD.[22] IBD has a peak incidence between 15 and 30 years of age, with 20% of CrD and 12% of UC cases occurring before age 20. Diagnosis is confirmed through clinical examination, laboratory tests, imaging, and biopsy.[22–25]

Crohn Disease

CrD is an immune-mediated inflammatory disease that can affect any part of the intestinal tract, most commonly the ileum, ileum and cecum, or the ileum and entire colon, leading to transmural inflammation.[25] About 30% of patients may experience gastritis and upper intestinal tract inflammation. The incidence of CrD is roughly 5 to 10 new cases per 100,000 individuals annually, with 20% to 25% of these cases occurring in children under 18 years of age.[23] The disease's etiology and pathophysiology, influenced by genetic and environmental factors, involve potentially gene mutations that can trigger an inflammatory response to intraluminal antigens.[23]

Symptoms include intestinal manifestations (abdominal pain, weight loss, diarrhea, and hematochezia) and extraintestinal manifestations affecting the skin, eyes, joints, and hepatobiliary and respiratory systems. Up to 40% of children with CrD may develop oral lesions such as mucogingivitis, and aphthous-like ulcers.[23,24] Growth failure affects about 30% of children and adolescents, with significant perianal disease also being common.[23] Treatment requires assessing and monitoring disease location and activity, utilizing MRI, endoscopy, and colonoscopy with biopsies for a treat-to-target approach. Therapeutic options vary with disease severity and may include glucocorticoids, aminosalicylates, immunomodulators (azathioprine, 6-MP, methotrexate), anti-tumor necrosis factor (TNF) drugs, or combination therapy. For oral lesions, topical corticosteroids, and for lip lesions, a 0.1% triamcinolone application may be beneficial. Comprehensive healthcare monitoring encompasses growth, nutritional status, infection risk, psychological issues, and cancer surveillance.[22,23]

Ulcerative Colitis

UC is an immune-mediated inflammatory disease targeting the mucosal layer of the colon and rectum, often presenting in adolescence and early adulthood, though it can occur earlier.[22] Its clinical presentation ranges from mild to moderate UC, marked by diarrhea (often bloody), weakness, anemia, abdominal pain, and weight loss, to acute severe UC, which involves severe abdominal pain, hematochezia, tenesmus, fever, leukocytosis, and hypoalbuminemia. Treatment approaches for UC and CrD share similar goals but differ, particularly regarding 5-aminosalicylic acid use (more central in UC) and the role of surgery.[24]

Dental Considerations for Patients With Inflammatory Bowel Disease

Patients with UC and CrD may present with various oral manifestations, including mucogingivitis, aphthous ulcers, swelling, fissures, specific oral Crohn lesions, tissue tags, labial, intraoral or gingival swelling, and cobblestoning of the oral mucosa. These signs can be among the first indicators of the disease or its exacerbation and require dental professionals to be adept at recognizing them for early diagnosis and management.[22–25]

IBD can lead to deficiencies in essential nutrients such as zinc; vitamins B, C, D, and K; calcium; iron; and protein. These deficiencies can manifest as glossitis, purpura, acrodermatitis enteropathica, hair loss, and brittle nails, and can contribute to periodontal disease. Medications for CD and IBD, including glucocorticoids and immunomodulators, can have side effects such as increased risk of oral candidiasis and delayed wound healing. Modifications in dental treatments may be required due to the patient's weakened immune system, medication side effects, or the need for specific management like antibiotic prophylaxis in certain cases to prevent infections.[24,25] Regular dental checkups are vital for early detection and management of oral health issues associated with IBD.

Diabetes Mellitus

T1DM is characterized by insulin deficiency due to the destruction of pancreatic beta cells. It is one of the most prevalent chronic diseases in childhood, accounting for about 85% of all diabetes cases in individuals under 20 years old worldwide.[26] Its incidence varies globally with two age peaks for presentation at 5 to 9 years and 10 to 14 years.[26] Genetic susceptibility and environmental factors play a role in its onset. Classic symptoms include polyuria, polydipsia, weight loss, lethargy, and often diabetic ketoacidosis, particularly in children under 6 years of age. Early diagnosis is crucial, with fasting plasma glucose levels ≥126 mg/dL or symptomatic hyperglycemia with plasma glucose ≥200 mg/dL being diagnostic criteria, alongside an oral glucose tolerance test.[26,27] Insulin therapy, tailored to individual and family needs, is essential for managing T1DM, with various preparations and delivery systems available, including rapid, short, intermediate, and long-acting insulins. Intensive insulin therapy, using multiple daily injections or an insulin pump, alongside regular blood glucose monitoring, is vital for optimal glycemic control. Psychological support for patients and their families is also important to address the increased risk of depression and anxiety, which can affect glycemic control.[28]

Type 2 diabetes mellitus, marked by hyperglycemia, insulin resistance, and relative insulin secretion impairment, has seen rising incidence in younger populations over the past 20 years, linked to increased childhood obesity. Management focuses on maintaining glycemic control and treating comorbidities, highlighting the need for comprehensive care in managing pediatric diabetes.[26]

Dental Considerations for Patients With Diabetes Mellitus

Children with diabetes are more susceptible to periodontal disease and consider saying opportunistic oral infections, such as candidiasis. Due to xerostomia and potentially higher sugar levels in saliva, diabetic children may also have an increased risk of dental caries. Diabetes can impair healing, making postsurgical care critical, thus extra caution and monitoring after dental procedures are necessary to prevent complications. For children experiencing frequent hyperglycemia or associated gastroesophageal reflux, there is an increased risk of dental erosion.[26–29]

Appointments should be scheduled at times when blood glucose levels are typically better controlled, often in the morning, and the child should eat to prevent hypoglycemia. For extensive treatment plans, shorter, more frequent dental appointments are suggested to reduce stress and fatigue.[29] Preventive care should be emphasized, including the application of fluoride varnish and dental sealants, to protect against caries. Before any invasive procedure, good glycemic control should be ensured to reduce the risk of postoperative infection and improve healing. When there is compromised glycemic control or needed procedures with a high risk of infection, antibiotic prophylaxis may be indicated in consultation with the child's physician. Techniques to minimize stress during dental visits should be employed, as stress can affect blood glucose levels. Clear postoperative instructions should be provided to caregivers, focusing on the signs of infection or delayed healing and the importance of maintaining glycemic control. Measures to increase saliva flow and hydration should be encouraged to combat xerostomia.[26–29]

Epilepsy

Epilepsy is a prevalent neurologic disorder globally affecting over 65 million individuals across various age groups, with a higher incidence observed in children under 1 year and adults over 50 years.[30] It is defined by the tendency to experience unprovoked epileptic seizures, which are manifestations of abnormal, excessive, or synchronous neuronal activity in the brain. This condition not only implicates the neurobiologic aspects of seizures but also encompasses significant cognitive, psychological, and social consequences, emphasizing the broad impact of epilepsy beyond its neurologic basis.[30,31]

Contemporary classification and understanding of epilepsy and seizures categorizes seizures based on their onset as either focal or generalized. Focal seizures originate from a specific area of the brain and may occur with preserved consciousness ("focal aware seizures") or impaired consciousness ("focal impaired awareness seizures"). They can manifest through various symptoms, including automatisms and behavior arrest, and sometimes progress to affect both hemispheres, leading to "focal to bilateral tonic-clonic seizures." Generalized seizures involve both sides of the brain from the onset and include types such as myoclonic, absence, atonic, tonic, clonic and tonic-clonic seizures, each with distinct characteristics.[30]

Epilepsy syndromes are defined clusters of features that include specific seizure types, electroencephalogram (EEG) findings, and sometimes genetic etiologies, providing a framework for targeted management and prognosis. Refined epilepsy classification has enhanced the accuracy of diagnosis and treatment approaches, reflecting the diverse manifestations of this condition.[31]

The etiology of epilepsy is multifactorial, with structural, genetic, infectious, metabolic, and immune factors contributing to its development. Despite comprehensive evaluations, the cause remains unknown in many cases. Epilepsy imposes a significant burden, with a lifetime risk of approximately 3.9% and a higher prevalence in males. The long-term prognosis varies, and challenges exist, including increased mortality rates, the risk of sudden unexpected death in epilepsy, and associated neuropsychosocial comorbidities.[30,31]

The diagnosis of epilepsy is based on the occurrence of at least one unprovoked seizure and the likelihood of future seizures, assessed through clinical examination, patient history, EEG, and neuroimaging. EEG plays an important role in determining the seizure type and location, whereas MRI is preferred for identifying structural causes of seizures. Despite advancements, approximately 30% of patients have drug-resistant epilepsy, characterized by the failure of two or more antiepileptic drugs (AEDs) to control seizures effectively.[30,31] Treatment strategies aim to stop seizures or reduce seizure frequency with minimal side effects, utilizing a range of AEDs classified as narrow-spectrum (for specific seizure types) or broad-spectrum (for a wide range of seizures). Newer AEDs generally present fewer side effects compared with older ones. Beyond medication, treatment may involve ketogenic diets, surgery, or neuromodulation techniques such as vagus nerve stimulation (VNS) devices, tailored to the individual's specific condition and type of epilepsy syndrome.[30]

Dental Considerations in Patients With Epilepsy

Understanding the type of seizures, their control level, and medication compliance are essential. Dental professionals should take precautions to minimize the risk of aspiration of loose teeth, poorly retained dental appliances, and crowns during a seizure.[32] Phenytoin can cause gingival overgrowth, which may worsen with poor oral hygiene. Regular dental cleanings and strict oral hygiene at home are important to decrease this side effect. Patients are prone to dental trauma during seizures, thus mouthguards may be recommended for those with frequent seizures.[30–32] Dental lights could potentially trigger seizures in some patients, especially those with specific epilepsy syndromes, such as juvenile myoclonic epilepsy and epilepsy with eyelid myoclonia (Jeavon syndrome). Sunglasses or lighting adjustments during dental treatment can minimize this risk. Many AEDs can cause dry mouth, increasing the risk for dental caries and oral discomfort. Mood changes associated with some AEDs also necessitate a supportive and understanding approach during dental visits.[30–32]

There is no contraindication to the use of local anesthetics with vasoconstrictors in patients with epilepsy. For patients with a VNS device, caution should be exercised to avoid damaging the generator during dental procedures, particularly with the use of electrocautery. The device may need to be turned off by the neurologist for procedures using ultrasonic or electric devices, such as electrocautery. Patients with seizures may have a ventriculoperitoneal (VP) shunt to manage hydrocephalus. Careful manipulation of the head and neck is necessary to avoid disconnection, breakage, or migration of the shunt. Antibiotic prophylaxis before invasive dental procedures is not necessary for patients with a VP shunt. Dental offices should be prepared to handle a seizure emergency, with staff trained in seizure first aid and protocols in place for managing such events safely (see Chapter 35).[32]

Asthma

Asthma is a chronic respiratory condition characterized by airway inflammation, which leads to bronchoconstriction, edema, and increased mucus production. It manifests through episodic attacks of wheezing, chest tightness, shortness of breath, and coughing.[33] Asthma is the most common chronic respiratory condition in childhood worldwide, affecting approximately 14% of children and young people. This condition affects physical activities, school attendance, and quality of life. Its etiology is multifaceted involving a complex interplay of genetic predisposition, environmental exposures, and immunologic factors.[33,34]

Genetically, children with a family history of asthma or atopic diseases are at a higher risk of developing asthma. Environmental allergens, such as dust mites, pet dander, pollen, mold, and tobacco smoke, are significant triggers. Respiratory infections in early childhood, especially viral, contribute to the development and exacerbation of asthma. Children with asthma often have a heightened sensitivity to specific allergens, leading to an overactive immune response that causes airway inflammation and hyperresponsiveness.[33]

Asthma can be classified based on severity, control, and underlying pathophysiologic mechanisms. Severity is categorized into intermittent, mild persistent, moderate persistent, and severe persistent, and it is determined by the frequency of symptoms, nighttime awakenings, and lung function. Control-based classification divides asthma into well-controlled, partly controlled, and uncontrolled, based on symptom frequency, impact on daily activities, and rescue medication use. Pathophysiologic classifications include allergic (eosinophilic) asthma, nonallergic asthma, exercise-induced bronchoconstriction, and occupational asthma, highlighting the diverse triggers and inflammatory patterns.[33,34] The diagnosis relies on a combination of clinical history, physical examination, and lung function tests, such as spirometry, which may be challenging in younger children. Therefore diagnosis often also considers the presence of common triggers, response to asthma medications, and the pattern of symptoms.[33]

Management aims to control symptoms, reduce the frequency and severity of exacerbations, and minimize the need for emergency care. Identifying and minimizing exposure to known allergens and irritants can reduce asthma symptoms and the need for medications. Pharmacologic treatment includes long-term control medications and quick-relief (rescue) inhalers. Inhaled corticosteroids (ICS) are part of asthma maintenance therapy and are effective in reducing airway inflammation. Long-acting β-agonists, leukotriene receptor antagonists, and in some cases, theophylline is added for additional control. Short-acting β-agonists are used as rescue therapy for acute symptoms. For severe, treatment-resistant asthma, biologic therapies targeting specific components of the immune response (e.g., anti-IgE, anti-IL5, anti-IL4R) offer personalized treatment options to reduce exacerbations and improve lung function.[33,34] Effective asthma management includes regular follow-ups to monitor control and adjust treatment as needed.

Dental Considerations in Patients With Asthma

Asthma increases the risk of dental caries due to mouth breathing, xerostomia from medication, enamel defects, use of sucrose-rich medications, and acidic environments from dry powder inhalers. Inhalers often contain lactose to mask bitterness and asthmatics may drink more sodas and juices to relieve dry mouth, raising caries risk further. Acidic medications and GERD can cause dental erosion. Additionally, long-term use of ICS and oral dryness may result in oral fungal infections. Patients must rinse their mouths with water or fluoride mouthwashes postmedication use and maintain optimal oral hygiene practices.[35] A comprehensive understanding of asthma, including a detailed history such as the frequency of exacerbations in the past year, limitations in daily activities, sleep disturbances, medication usage, adherence to therapy, and existing comorbidities, is important. Patients should bring their inhaler to dental appointments.[35]

In children with severe asthma, fluoride varnishes containing colophony should be avoided due to potential sensitivity reactions. The patient's physician should be consulted before the use of nitrous oxide inhalation or passive immobilization as these are relative contraindications in severely asthmatic children. Consults regarding the need for supplemental corticosteroids are indicated for patients on long-term ICS therapy to decrease the risk of adrenal crisis during dental procedures. The use of rubber dam isolation during dental treatments can minimize exposure to aerosols, tooth dust, and dental material residues, reducing the likelihood of an asthma attack.[35]

Cystic Fibrosis

Cystic fibrosis (CF) is an autosomal recessive genetic disorder characterized by mutations in the CF transmembrane conductance regulator (CFTR) gene and occurs in all races and ethnicities, though it is most common in people of Northern European ancestry. The CFTR gene is essential for the transport of chloride and bicarbonate ions across epithelial cells. Mutations result in the production of thick, sticky mucus that blocks various organs, including the lungs and pancreas. CF is diagnosed through elevated sweat chloride levels and the presence of two disease-causing mutations.[36] Treatment has advanced significantly, focusing on CFTR modulators (ivacaftor) and combination therapies (lumacaftor-ivacaftor and tezacaftor-ivacaftor), which correct protein processing and improve function for those with the common phe508del mutation. Despite the high costs and varying patient responses, these treatments have improved lung function, nutritional status, and quality of life, underscoring the importance of early diagnosis and personalized management strategies.[36] CF can affect nutritional and growth patterns often leading to CF-related diabetes and infertility as well as severe respiratory and digestive system complications. Treatment regimens typically include mucus thinners, airway clearance techniques, antibiotics, and pancreatic enzyme supplements, with lung transplantation considered for advanced disease stages.[36] The median survival age of affected patients is 47.4 years in the United States.[36] Active treatment and comprehensive management, including nutritional support, routine vaccinations, and psychological counseling, are critical for improving quality of life and extending survival.[36]

Dental Considerations in Patients With Cystic Fibrosis

Dental management in patients with CF presents unique challenges due to the disease's systemic effects and treatment complications. Oral manifestations may include enamel defects (hypomineralization/hypoplasia) from long-term antibiotic use and systemic infections, associated with tooth hypersensitivity and esthetic concerns.[37] The combination of medication-induced xerostomia, mouth breathing, a high-calorie diet, consumption of sugary drinks to mask medication bitterness, and use of inhalers containing lactose can also contribute to a higher risk of dental caries.[36,37] Patients with CF also have a higher risk for oral *Candida,* linked to impaired salivary gland function, inhalation antibiotic, and steroid therapy. Addressing vitamin deficiencies, liver disease, and CF-related bone disease is critical, necessitating the monitoring for prolonged postoperative bleeding due to vitamin K deficiency and potential osteonecrosis from therapy.[37]

Caution with NSAIDs and antibiotics is advised due to increased allergic reaction rates in CF patients and acetaminophen is usually preferred for pain management. Dental treatment settings must minimize patient-to-patient contact to prevent cross-contamination with *Pseudomonas aeruginosa* and employ thorough cross-infection control.[36,37] Special precautions during dental procedures, including the use of a rubber dam, are essential to reduce aspiration and respiratory distress risks. Sedation strategies and nitrous oxide use require careful evaluation and physician consultation to ensure patient safety. Regular dental checkups are essential for early detection and management of caries, gingivitis, periodontal disease, and enamel defects common in CF.[37] Coordination among dental professionals, pulmonologists, and other healthcare providers is vital, ensuring integrated dental care plans that complement the broader medical management of CF.[37]

Congenital Heart Disease

Congenital heart defects (CHDs) are structural abnormalities of the heart or intrathoracic great vessels that occur during fetal life, making it the most common birth defect.[38,39] The worldwide prevalence of CHD from 2010 to 2017 was estimated at 9.4 per 1000 live births, representing a significant increase from previous years, especially for mild CHD, such as ventricular septal defect (VSD), atrial septal defect (ASD), and patent ductus arteriosus (PDA).[40] Their cause includes both genetic and environmental factors, such as maternal consumption of ethanol, ingestion of certain medications during pregnancy, poorly controlled maternal diabetes, and viral infections during pregnancy.[38,39] Genetic syndromes associated with CHD include trisomy 13, 18 and 21; Turner syndrome; CHARGE syndrome; Williams syndrome; and 22q11.2 deletion syndrome.[38] Prenatal ultrasound can diagnose CHD but fetal echocardiography is the principal diagnostic mean.[39,41] Advances in medical and surgical treatment have led to an improvement in survival. Heart transplantation is indicated for patients with end-stage heart failure, cardiomyopathies, and for those cannot have corrective or palliative surgical procedures.[42] However, there is limited availability and acceptability of heart transplantation in children.

Children with CHD have risk factors for neurodevelopmental delays, particularly those with cyanotic heart conditions and single ventricle.[38,43] Higher rates of attention deficit hyperactivity disorder, autism spectrum disorder, anxiety, depression, aggression, and deficient adaptive functioning are seen in this population.[38,43]

CHD can be noncyanotic and cyanotic ("critical CHD"), which can be divided into right heart obstructive lesions, left heart obstructive lesions, and mixing lesions. Acyanotic lesions include ASD, PDA, and VSD; the latter is the most common heart defect in children. Cyanotic right heart obstructive lesions (e.g., pulmonary atresia, tricuspid atresia, and tetralogy of Fallot) lead to decreased pulmonary flow.[39] Left heart obstructive lesions cause decreased systemic flow and include hypoplastic left heart syndrome and coarctation of the aorta. In mixing lesions, there is a mixing of pulmonary and systemic blood flow, as seen in transposition of the great arteries and truncus arteriosus.[39]

Pediatric Infective Endocarditis

Increased survival rates of children with CHD have led to more cases of infective endocarditis (IE), a complex disease that is difficult to diagnose and manage.[44] Although rare in children, its incidence is increasing, and it can lead to significant morbidity and mortality. IE can also affect individuals with a normal heart structure, such as in those who are immunocompromised and have indwelling catheters.[44] *Streptococcus viridans* and *Staphylococcus aureus* are the most common causative organisms.[44] Prolonged intravenous antibiotic therapy (minimum 4 weeks, often 6 to 8 weeks) should start as early as possible and surgical intervention may be necessary in children at high risk for life-threatening complications (e.g., heart failure).[44] In general, pediatric IE has a good prognosis with low risk of recurrence after surgical management.

The 2021 update to the American Heart Association guidelines emphasizes the importance of good oral health and regular dental checkups to prevent IE.[45] Antibiotic prophylaxis is recommended only for patients at highest risk of IE who are undergoing invasive dental procedures. The most common antibiotic regimen prescribed is oral amoxicillin 50 mg/kg (maximum 2 g) taken 30 to 60 minutes before the procedure. Clindamycin is no longer recommended for patients allergic to penicillin due to its more frequent and severe reactions than other antibiotics. Instead, penicillin-allergic patients can be prescribed azithromycin, clarithromycin, or doxycycline.[45]

Pediatric Cancer

Cancer is the second most common cause of death in children aged 1 to 14 years after accidents, and the fourth most common cause among adolescents (aged 15 to 19 years) in the United States.[46] In 2022, the most common cancers in children were leukemias, myeloproliferative, and myelodysplastic diseases followed by central nervous system (CNS) tumors and lymphomas.[46] In adolescents, the most common cancer was CNS tumors.[46] Although the overall cancer incidence rate in children and adolescents has increased, pediatric cancer research has steadily made progress and the 5-year survival rate for all pediatric cancers has surpassed 80%.[46–48]

The treatment approaches in pediatric oncology are radiation therapy (RT), chemotherapy (CT), HSCT, and, more recently, immunotherapy and targeted therapies. It is beneficial for pediatric dentists to possess some knowledge about the mechanistic nuances inherent in the various antineoplastic therapies to better appreciate the rationale and objectives for dental clearance and to prevent/manage the type of oral complications encountered with these treatments.

RT uses ionizing radiation to kill cancer cells through the generation of free radicals. The extent of destruction depends on RT doses and the radiosensitivity of the tissue/structure in the exposed field (i.e., higher radiosensitivity → higher damage). Bone marrow, eye, and lymphatic tissues are highly radiosensitive, whereas bone, connective tissue, and muscle are the least radiosensitive. RT is associated with a lifelong risk of osteoradionecrosis of the jaw (ORNJ) with doses ≥60 Gy to the head and neck region. Other significant effects of head and neck RT are permanent salivary gland hypofunction and trismus[49–51] predisposing patients to very high risk for rapidly progressing dental decay.[52]

The main mechanism of cytotoxic CT is the inhibition of cell proliferation and growth. Most agents do not differentiate between cancer and healthy tissues; thus rapidly dividing healthy tissues (hair follicles, skin, oral mucosa, and the bone marrow) are affected. Cytotoxic CT regimens are broadly classified into myeloablative and nonmyeloablative regimens.[53] High-dose myeloablative CT is typically indicated for hematologic malignancies and results in a significant fall in the leukocyte, erythrocyte, and platelet counts, starting within 5 to 7 days after regimen administration (Table 39.1). The nadir occurs between 10 and 14 days and is followed by count recovery in 3 to 4 weeks. Nonmyeloablative regimens are reduced in intensity and do not completely suppress the bone marrow, resulting in a less drastic decline in patient's blood counts. Such regimens are used in the maintenance phase for the treatment of hematologic malignancies or as adjuvant treatment for a variety of solid organ malignancies. Depending on the intensity of the CT regimen received, patients will experience varying risks for oral mucositis development, opportunistic infections, and bleeding. A typical CT regimen/schedule for acute lymphoblastic leukemia (ALL) can be broadly grouped in four treatment phases.

1. *Remission induction* aims to reduce disease burden and achieve complete remission. This phase generally lasts 28 days and involves the use of a myeloablative regimen typically consisting of glucocorticoids, vincristine, asparaginase, and occasionally anthracycline.

TABLE 39.1 Normal Blood Count Reference Values

Blood Component	Normal Values
Hemoglobin (g/dL)	Males: 13.5–17.5; females: 12.3–15.3
Hematocrit (%)	Males: 41.5–50.4; females: 35.9–44.6
White blood cell count	4,000–10,000/mL
Platelet count	150,000–450,000/mm^3
Differential	**Normal Values**
Neutrophils (polymorphonuclear leukocytes)	Segmented: 56 Bands: 3
Lymphocytes	34
Monocytes	4
Eosinophils	2.7
Basophils	0.3

Data from McPherson RA, Pincus MR, eds. *Henry's Clinical Diagnosis and Management by Laboratory Methods.* 21st ed. Saunders; 2007:1404-1418.

2. *Consolidation/late intensification* aims to minimize the development of drug cross-resistance through intensified treatment to kill remaining leukemic cells.
3. *Maintenance/continuation therapy* aims to suppress leukemic growth through continued administration of lower intensity CT, usually consisting of daily 6-mercaptopurine, weekly methotrexate, and periodic intrathecal therapy. The optimal duration of maintenance therapy has not been established, but the average is 2 to 3 years.
4. *CNS treatment* is used to eliminate cancer cells within the CNS, which is a sanctuary for leukemic infiltrates due to the inability of systemically administered chemotherapeutic drugs to cross the blood-brain barrier. It is incorporated into all phases of ALL therapy and involves an intrathecal injection of a single agent (usually methotrexate) or a combination of chemotherapeutic agents with high-dose systemic CT. The use of cranial irradiation is increasingly limited to only patients with the highest risk of CNS relapse because of the higher adverse effects including neurocognitive deficits, endocrine issues, growth impairment, and secondary CNS tumors.[54]

Hematopoietic Stem Cell Transplantation

HSCT is the intravenous infusion of hematopoietic stem cells to replace and restore blood cell production in patients whose bone marrow or immune system is defective, such as in hematologic disorders, congenital immunodeficiencies, lipidoses, and inborn errors of metabolism.[55] The stem cells can be obtained from the bone marrow in the iliac crest and other bones, peripheral blood, and from the placenta or umbilical cord blood. Autologous HSCT is where the transplanted cells are the patient's own stem cells. Syngeneic HSCT is where the donor is the identical twin. Allogeneic HSCT is where the transplanted cells are derived from a related (preferred) or an unrelated donor. In the latter type, there is a risk of graft-versus-host disease (GVHD), which is a major cause of toxicity and mortality in HSCT recipients. The likelihood of GVHD is influenced by the degree of human leukocyte antigen (HLA) matching. The HLA system is located on the short arm of chromosome 6 and the goal is to type/match the donor's HLA class I and II antigens as closely as possible to those of the recipient. If a suitable HLA-matched donor is not identified, other alternatives are mismatched unrelated donor (less than 9 of 10 HLA alleles), umbilical cord blood donor, and haploidentical donor.[55]

HSCT can be divided into five phases: (1) conditioning, (2) stem cell infusion, (3) neutropenic phase, (4) engraftment phase, and (5) postengraftment phase. Conditioning commences a few days before the stem cell infusion and can be myeloablative, which causes complete bone marrow aplasia, or reduced intensity conditioning, which is less toxic. The latter regimen is used for children who are unable to tolerate myeloablative conditioning due to significant comorbidities. The stem cell infusion itself is a relatively straightforward process associated with minimal toxicity in most cases. As a consequence of the conditioning therapy, the patient has minimal or no functional immune system in the neutropenic phase, which lasts approximately 2 to 4 weeks, during which susceptibility to infections is very high. The engraftment phase is usually evident between days 20 and 30, sometimes earlier, by increased peripheral leukocyte and platelet counts. The last postengraftment phase can last for months to years and requires monitoring for acute and chronic transplant-related adverse effects. This is particularly pertinent in children as the conditioning regimen and other aspects of HSCT can impair growth and development as well as increase the risk of secondary malignancies (e.g., oral squamous cell carcinoma, posttransplant lymphoproliferative disease).[55,56]

Specific to allogeneic HSCT is the development of acute (within 100 days of HSCT) or chronic (>100 days after HSCT) oral GVHD. The oral presentations of acute GVHD include erythema, erosions, ulcers, and lichenoid lesions. In the absence of cutaneous manifestations, making a definitive diagnosis of acute oral GVHD is challenging because of the nonspecific oral presentations and the difficulty to differentiate it from CT-induced oral mucositis. The classical presentation of chronic oral GVHD is lacy or reticulated white plaques on the tongue, buccal mucosa, lips, and/or palate. Mucoceles may also be present in the palate and are thought to arise from minor salivary gland inflammation. Oral GVHD can be managed with topical moderate to high–potency corticosteroids.[57] Due to the increased risk of squamous cell carcinoma in patients with chronic oral GVHD, such patients should be reviewed at close intervals to detect signs of early oral cancer development.[58]

Immunotherapy and Targeted Therapy

With an increased understanding about the unique biologic characteristics of childhood cancers and the recent availability of immunotherapy and targeted therapies, clinical research has shifted focus to incorporate these agents into conventional cancer treatment regimens. This transition is further fueled by the well-documented detrimental late effects of RT and CT in pediatric oncology. The basis of cancer immunotherapy is to harness the patient's immune system to recognize and eradicate cancer cells. The main types of immunotherapy are chimeric antigen receptor (CAR) T-cell therapy, checkpoint inhibitors, monoclonal antibodies, cytokine therapy, cancer vaccines, and oncolytic virus therapy. Particularly noteworthy is the remarkable success witnessed with CAR T-cell therapy for pediatric B-cell ALL.[59] Of significance to pediatric dentistry is the association of such agents with oral toxicities to include aphthous-like ulcers (e.g., mammalian target of rapamycin inhibitors), lichenoid lesions, geographical tongue (e.g., bevacizumab), gingival hyperplasia (e.g., vemurafenib), and oral hyperpigmentation (e.g., imatinib).[60]

Oral Complications From Cancer Therapy

Several antineoplastic treatment modalities are associated with extensive oral cavity morbidity (Box 39.1). This can compromise the delivery of cancer treatment (e.g., delay or reduction in intensity), which negatively affects survival rate, increase treatment costs, and diminishes the quality of life. The common oral complications associated with RT, CT, and HSCT are oral mucositis, oral pain, opportunistic infections, salivary gland dysfunction, and taste disturbances.[57,61,62]

Among these complications, oral mucositis (Fig. 39.1) is reported to be the most painful and debilitating, occurring in almost all children receiving high-dose head and neck RT and 40% of children who receive CT/HSCT. The CT agents most associated with oral mucositis are cytarabine, doxorubicin, etoposide, melphalan, fluorouracil, and methotrexate. In severely immunosuppressed patients, oral mucositis is a risk for systemic infection as the disrupted mucosa barrier can serve as a portal of entry for bacteria to enter the bloodstream.[63,64] Basic oral care protocols (i.e., atraumatic cleansing of the oral tissues, toothbrushing,

• BOX 39.1 Oral and Craniofacial Complications of Cancer Therapy

Acute Complications From Chemotherapy, Head and Neck Radiotherapy, and Hematopoietic Stem Cell Transplantation

Acute oral graft-versus-host disease
Dysphagia
Gingival bleeding
Mucositis
Oral facial pain (due to oral mucositis, peripheral neuropathy, vinca alkaloid agents)
Opportunistic bacterial, fungal and viral infections
Salivary gland dysfunction (i.e., changes in quantity and/or quality of saliva)
Sialadenitis (radiation only)
Taste changes
Xerostomia

Long-Term Complications From Head and Neck Radiotherapy

Opportunistic fungal and bacterial infections
Mucosal fibrosis
Muscular fibrosis
Radiation caries
Risk of osteoradionecrosis of the jaw
Risk of secondary head and neck malignancies
Salivary gland hypofunction
  Trismus
  Xerostomia
Dental and craniofacial developmental abnormalities (also with chemotherapy)

Long-Term Complications of Allogeneic Hematopoietic Stem Cell Transplantation

Chronic oral graft-versus-host disease
Risks of squamous cell carcinoma and posttransplant lymphoproliferative disease
Dental and craniofacial developmental abnormalities

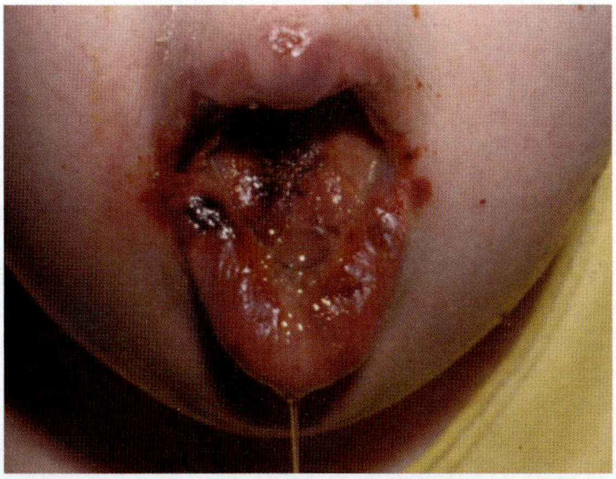

• **Fig. 39.1** Moderate mucositis caused by chemotherapy in a 5-year-old patient.

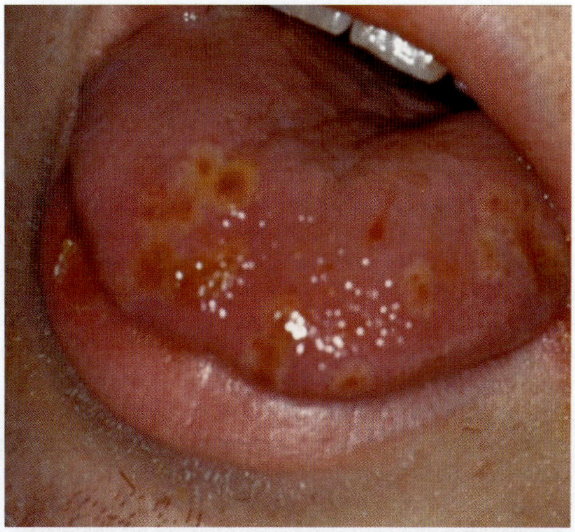

• **Fig. 39.2** Herpetic lesions on the tongue and lip of an immunosuppressed patient.

lubricating the lips and oral mucosa surfaces, and use of bland mouth rinses such as saline) are appropriate despite the absence of high evidence studies.[65] Extrapolation of available evidence from the adult literature suggests the benefits of benzydamine mouthwash, cryotherapy, and intraoral photobiomodulation therapy (with low-level laser therapy) for oral mucositis management.[65] Patient-controlled analgesia is helpful in relieving pain associated with oral mucositis.[66]

A common opportunistic viral infection in immunocompromised patients is recurrent herpes simplex virus (HSV) infection. As such, most institutions routinely prescribed antiviral prophylaxis before HSCT for HSV-seropositive patients. HSV ulcerations (Fig. 39.2) in immunosuppressed patients often appear atypical and can involve any intraoral site, including nonkeratinized areas. A swab of the base of the lesion can be performed and sent to the laboratory for confirmation, preferably via molecular technique due to the quicker turnaround time (within 24 to 48 hours). Oral candidiasis is another common opportunistic infection in this population. There is sound evidence to support the benefits of partially and completely absorbed antifungal agents (e.g., clotrimazole) in the prevention and treatment of oral candidiasis, while agents that are not absorbed through the gastrointestinal tract (e.g., nystatin) are ineffective for prevention and treatment in the immunosuppressed population.[67]

Salivary gland dysfunction is usually transient for children undergoing CT and is managed symptomatically. In contrast, head and neck RT doses as low as 20 Gy can cause permanent salivary gland hypofunction, which is associated with rapidly progressing dental caries if stringent preventive oral care measures are not instituted.[51]

A late effect of cancer treatment unique to children is the impact on growth and development.[68] Children under 5 years of age who undergo myeloablative CT and multimodality regimens and/or HSCT are at greater risk for dental disturbances such as tooth agenesis, complete or partial arrest of root development with thin tapered roots, early apical closure globular, conical crowns, dentin and enamel opacities and defects, microdontia, enlarged pulp chambers, taurodontism, and abnormal occlusion (Fig. 39.3).[68,69] Craniofacial abnormalities, specifically the retardation of the vertical growth of the condyles and mandibular growth, have also been reported.[70,71]

Dental Considerations Before, During, and After Cancer Treatment

For patients undergoing high-dose head and neck RT, the goals are to eradicate local risk factors to minimize ORNJ risk and to

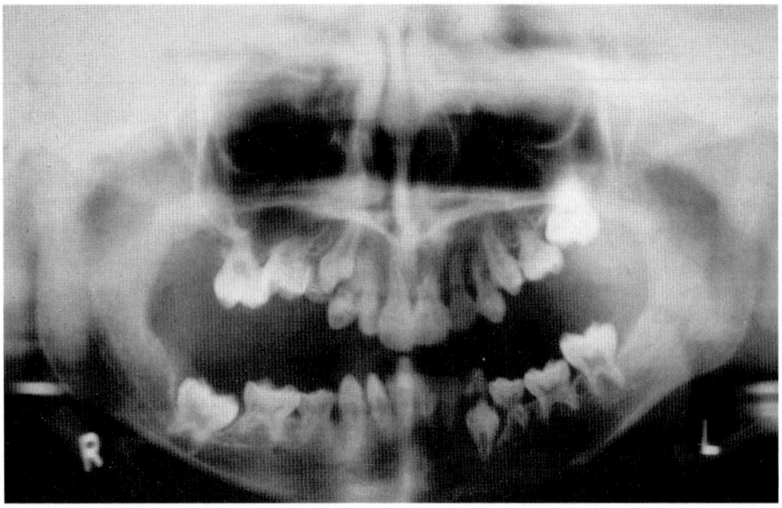

• **Fig. 39.3** Long-term effects on dental development in a 14-year-old boy conditioned with chemotherapy and total body irradiation before a hematopoietic stem cell transplant at age 13 months of age.

provide anticipatory preventive oral care strategies.[72,73] In patients undergoing CT and HSCT, the objective of dental clearance is to prevent and minimize the occurrence of opportunistic infections as well as the potential for systemic spread of local infections during cancer treatment. The two major differences between patients who only receive CT and those who undergo HSCT include the following: (1) in HSCT, there are no cycles of CT with periods of rest in between when the blood counts return to normal and (2) the prolonged immunosuppression after HSCT, with most immune functions only fully restored at approximately a year after HSCT if chronic GVHD or other complications are not present. The implication is the stronger justification to eradicate all disease and complete all dental treatment before HSCT.[72,73]

Before cancer treatment, provision of child and patient education regarding the acute and chronic side effects of the various antineoplastic treatment modalities may likely motivate patients to be more compliant with the recommended oral care protocols.[65,72,73]

Treatment Planning Considerations

The patient's medical history must include information about the underlying disease, time of diagnosis, past and upcoming antineoplastic treatment modality (including dates), treatment-associated complications, infections (both oral/local and systemic), current immune and hematologic status, medications, allergies, and hospitalizations.[72,73] Many patients receiving CT are given a central line, which is an indwelling catheter inserted into the right atrium of the heart, useful for obtaining blood samples and administering chemotherapeutic agents. Presently, there is no scientific evidence for antibiotic prophylaxis before invasive dental procedures for patients who have a central line, even though it may be common practice in some institutions. Knowledge of the patient's oral healthcare habits and regularity of visiting the dentist are helpful to assess awareness, and likelihood to comply with oral care recommendations.[72,73]

A consideration pertinent in patients undergoing cancer treatment is the status of the immune and hematologic systems. Some patients may be at risk for prolonged bleeding caused by the disease itself (e.g., leukemias) and/or from the antineoplastic treatment modality (i.e., CT induced). In the absence of other comorbidities, clinically significant bleeding is unlikely to occur with platelet counts greater than 20,000/mm^3. The thresholds for platelet levels whereby elective dental procedures can be performed varies between guidelines; generally elective dental procedures can be performed when the platelet count is greater than 50,000/mm^3, with attention paid to measures for controlling prolonged bleeding.[74] Other preprocedure coagulation tests (e.g., prothrombin time, activated partial thromboplastin time) may be warranted for patients with liver dysfunction or underlying coagulopathies. Neutrophils are the body's first line of defense; therefore the risk and extent of infection are inversely related to their levels. When the absolute neutrophil count (ANC) is less than 1000/mm^3 (or 500/mm^3 in some institutions), elective dental care should be deferred because the risks for procedure-related infections and bacteremia increase greatly.[72,73] In cases of emergency dental care, the physician must be consulted before any invasive dental procedure is initiated.

All patients should undergo a thorough head, neck, and oral cavity examination with radiographs where indicated before initiation of cancer treatment.[72,73] Some patients may complain of oral paresthesia's caused by leukemic infiltration of the peripheral nerves, whereas others may report dental pain mimicking irreversible pulpitis in the absence of a dental/periodontal infection. This can be a side effect of vincristine and vinblastine, two commonly used vinca alkaloid chemotherapeutic agents.[72,73,75] In this case, the patient should avoid triggers that exacerbate the discomfort, and analgesics can be prescribed for pain control. The pain usually resolves within a few days or weeks after cessation of the causative agent.

All dental pathology should be ideally eliminated before initiation of cancer treatment.[72,73] However, in situations when there is limited time, oral/dental pathology that are at high risk for causing complications during cancer therapy and procedures that require adequate time for healing should be prioritized. Eradication of acute and chronic infections, management of symptomatic teeth, extractions, and removal of sources of irritation are prioritized over restorative or endodontic treatment of asymptomatic carious teeth, and replacement of faulty restorations.[72,73,76,77] Temporary restorations can be placed, and nonacute dental treatment can be delayed until the patient's health is stabilized. When there is sufficient time before cancer treatment, dental scaling and prophylaxis should be performed, defective restorations should be repaired, and teeth with sharp edges should be polished. Extraction of primary teeth with pulp infections is indicated to minimize the risks for local and systemic complications of failed pulp therapy during immunosuppression periods.

Clinically and radiographically sound pulp-treated teeth should present no threats.[72,73,77] Endodontic treatment of asymptomatic permanent teeth with periapical involvement can be delayed if the patient is neutropenic. During immunosuppression, the classic signs of infections (e.g., swelling and purulent exudate) may not be present, resulting in a higher chance of a missed diagnosis.[78] Thus radiographs are vital to determine the presence of periapical or bifurcation pathologic processes in patients who complain of oral/dental pain but with no signs of dental infection. Symptomatic nonvital permanent teeth should ideally receive root canal therapy (or extraction if deemed more appropriate) at least 1 week before initiation of cancer therapy.[72,73,77] If root canal therapy or extraction are not possible due to medical reasons (e.g., severely neutropenic or thrombocytopenic), pharmacologic management with antimicrobials and analgesics or a pulpectomy can be performed first. Definitive treatment such as completion of root canal therapy or extraction (with the exception of a patient undergoing high-dose head and neck radiation) can be scheduled at a later time when the patient's medical condition permits.

Partially erupted molars can become a source of infection because of pericoronitis. If the dentist deems it to be a potential risk, the overlying gingival tissue should be excised. Loose primary teeth can be left to exfoliate naturally. To minimize bacteremia, the patient should be counseled to avoid playing with them. If the patient cannot comply with this recommendation or is greatly bothered by the discomfort, the loose tooth should be removed. Impacted teeth, root tips, partially erupted third molars, teeth with periodontal pockets greater than 6 mm, teeth with acute infections, and nonrestorable teeth should be ideally removed 2 weeks before cancer therapy to allow for adequate healing.[72,73,77]

For extractions, local measures to control bleeding, such as pressure packs, sutures, gelatin sponges, topical thrombin, or microfibrillar collagen, should be readily available and instituted if deemed necessary.[72,73,77] Surgical procedures must be as atraumatic as possible, with no sharp bony edges remaining and satisfactory closure of the wounds. Other than the patient's immune status, the need for antibiotic coverage to prevent systemic bacteremia during the extraction (preprocedure antibiotic prophylaxis) or postextraction local site infection (postoperative antibiotic course usually for 1 week) is influenced by the procedure's complexity and the presence of the infection at the procedure site.[72,73,77]

Fixed orthodontic appliances and space maintainers should be removed if the patient has poor oral hygiene and/or the treatment regimen carries a risk for the development of moderate to severe mucositis. Appliances can harbor food debris, compromise oral hygiene, and serve as mechanical irritants, increasing the risk for secondary infections. Removable appliances and retainers that fit well can be worn if tolerated by the patient who exhibits good oral care.[72,73,77]

During Active Cancer Treatment

In this phase, the pediatric dentist's main roles are to assist the primary team with the management of odontogenic/periodontal pain and infection, and acute or chronic oral complications that arise from the antineoplastic treatment modalities to maintain and optimize oral functions. This may include, but is not limited to, ruling out dental infections as potential causes of fever and septicemia, diagnosing oral pathology, and administering topical agents for pain management (e.g., bland mouth rinses, sucking on ice chips). Elective dental treatment is avoided in this phase. For an acute dental infection, antibiotic therapy (usually intravenous) and analgesics are preferred over surgical intervention.[79] If the infection progresses (e.g., airway compromise) despite pharmacologic management, the pediatric dentist should discuss the plan for surgical management in liaison with the medical oncology team.

After Cancer Treatment

For patients in the maintenance phase of the CT and those who are 1-year post-HSCT with favorable prognosis, it is likely that their hematologic status is close to normal. Dental procedures can be performed routinely, but it is prudent to verify the blood counts before an invasive procedure. For patients who had received head and neck RT doses ≥60 Gy, consultation with the patient's medical doctor regarding the benefit of hyperbaric oxygen therapy before extraction of permanent teeth is warranted due to the risk of ORNJ.[80] Orthodontic treatment may start or resume after completion of cancer therapy and after at least a 2-year disease-free survival.[81] By this time, the risk of relapse is decreased, and the patient is no longer on immunosuppressive drugs. However, the clinician must assess for dental developmental disturbances caused by the cancer therapy, especially in children who received treatment before the age of 5 years (see Fig. 39.3).[68,69,71] Dahllof et al. described the following strategies for provision of orthodontic care for patients with dental sequelae: (1) use appliances that minimize the risk of root resorption, (2) use lighter forces, (3) have shorter treatment duration, (4) choose the simplest method for the treatment needs, and (5) do not treat the lower jaw.[82] For patients with persistent and profound impairment of immune function (e.g., in cases of chronic GHVD), regular dental examinations with radiographs can be performed but elective dental work, including prophylaxis, should be avoided.[57] If a dental emergency arises, the patient's physician must be consulted before treatment is instituted.

Oral Hygiene, Diet, and Caries Prevention Throughout Cancer Treatment

Regardless of the child's hematologic status, routine oral hygiene remains an important best practice to decrease oral complications during cancer therapy.[65,83] Thrombocytopenia should not be the sole determinant of oral hygiene as patients are able to brush without bleeding at widely different platelet counts.[72,73] There is some evidence that patients who perform intensive oral care have a reduced risk of developing moderate to severe oral mucositis.[84] A regular soft toothbrush or an electric brush used at least twice daily is the most efficient means to reduce dental biofilm.[72,73] Sponges, foam brushes, and super soft brushes cannot provide effective mechanical cleansing and should be used only in cases of severe oral mucositis when the patient cannot tolerate a regular brush. Brushes should be air-dried between uses, and a toothpaste without heavy flavoring agents should be considered because such agents can irritate the tissues.[72,73] Patients who have poor oral hygiene or periodontal disease can rinse with aqueous chlorhexidine rinse until the gingival health has been restored. When oral mucositis is present, rinses containing alcohol and flavoring agents should be avoided because they can dehydrate and irritate the mucosa.[72,73] Periodontal infection is a major concern because colonizing organisms can cause bacteremia. The child with cancer may be at high risk for dental caries because of dietary issues, treatment-induced xerostomia or salivary gland hypofunction, and sucrose-rich pediatric medications. Fluoride supplements, varnish, silver diamine fluoride, and neutral rinses or gels are indicated for patients at risk for caries.

Visit eBooks.Health.Elsevier.com to see full list of references.

40

Introduction to Dental Trauma: Managing Traumatic Injuries in the Primary Dentition

GIDEON HOLAN AND DENNIS J. MCTIGUE

CHAPTER OUTLINE

An injury to the teeth of a young child can have serious and long-term consequences, leading to their discoloration, malformation, or possible loss. The emotional impact of such an injury can be far reaching. It is therefore important that the dentist treating children is:

1. Experienced in guiding the behavior of young children in order to minimize their fear and anxiety of treatment.
2. Knowledgeable in the techniques for managing traumatic injuries.
3. Readily available during and after office hours to provide treatment.

If any of these conditions cannot be met, the child suffering a dental injury should immediately be referred to a specialist.

The purpose of this chapter is to provide a straightforward approach to managing dental injuries in the primary dentition. Techniques for diagnosis, treatment, and follow-up care are described. Fundamental issues covered in this chapter—such as the classification of injuries, history, examination, and pathologic sequelae of trauma—pertain to both the primary and permanent dentitions. Chapter 41 will focus on the management of injuries to young permanent teeth and will refer to this chapter for the information just noted. The principles gleaned from both chapters should enable the dentist to manage the great majority of dental injuries encountered in children.

Etiology and Epidemiology of Trauma in the Primary Dentition

The most frequently injured teeth in the primary dentition are the maxillary incisors. Primary molars are rarely injured, and when injury occurs, it is usually caused by indirect trauma (e.g., blows to the underside of the chin, causing the mandible to close forcefully against the maxilla).[1] Primary incisors tend to be luxated more than permanent teeth. This is because of the spongy nature of the bone in young children[2] and to the lower root/crown ratio in comparison with that of permanent teeth. It has been reported that injuries occurring while a child is using a pacifier tend to be tooth displacement rather than fractures.[3]

Although reports of injuries in preschool children presenting for dental treatment show that the majority of children suffer from luxation injuries,[4,5] epidemiologic studies in the community show that crown fractures (mainly enamel fractures) are the most common injuries to the primary teeth.[6–9] It has also been found that the incidence of an injury is higher among children who have already experienced a previous traumatic crown fracture.[10] These injuries, however, may result in only minor inconveniences that do not motivate parents to seek professional dental advice.

By the age of 5 years, one out of three children have experienced traumatic dental injuries.[11] The peak age of injuries to the primary teeth is 2 to 4 years when children are developing mobility skills.[12] Children with protruding incisors, as in developing class II malocclusions, are two to three times more likely to suffer dental trauma than children with normal incisal overjets.[13–17]

Another major cause of dental injuries in young children is automobile accidents. Unrestrained children who are seated or standing often hit the dashboard or windshield when the car is stopped suddenly. All states now have laws mandating the use of child restraints in automobiles, and it is hoped that universal adoption of these laws will decrease the incidence of such trauma to children.[18]

Children with chronic seizure disorders experience an increased incidence of dental trauma. Frequently, these high-risk children wear protective headgear, and the fabrication of custom mouthguards for them is indicated as well (see Chapter 42).

Another serious cause of dental injuries to young children is child abuse. Often overlooked by the dental profession, up to 50% of abused children suffer injuries to the head and neck. Cardinal signs of abuse are injuries in various stages of healing, tears of labial frena, repeated injuries, and injuries whose clinical presentation is not consistent with the history reported by the parent.[6] Battered children frequently lie to protect their parents or out of fear of retaliation. Dentists are required by law to report cases of suspected child abuse (see Chapter 43 for more specific details).

Classification of Injuries to Teeth

Tooth fractures may involve the crown, root, or both (Figs. 40.1–40.3; see also Figs. 41.1–41.3). Fractures of the crown may be limited to the enamel, may involve the dentin, or may include the pulp. Injury to the pulp is the most complicated and demanding to manage. Fractures involving only enamel or enamel and dentin are termed "uncomplicated"; "complicated" fractures include the pulp.[11]

As just mentioned, luxation (displacement) injuries are the most common types of injuries to primary teeth that are treated in the dental office. These injuries damage supporting structures of the teeth, which include the periodontal ligament (PDL) and the alveolar bone (see Fig. 40.1). The PDL is the physiologic "hammock" that supports the tooth in its socket. Maintaining its vitality is the primary objective in the management of all luxation injuries. Several types of luxation injury occur.[11]

1. Concussion: The tooth is not mobile and is not displaced. The PDL absorbs the injury and is inflamed, which leaves the tooth tender to biting pressure and percussion.
2. Subluxation: The tooth is loosened but is not displaced from its socket.
3. Intrusion: The tooth is driven into its socket. This compresses the PDL and commonly causes a crushing fracture of the alveolar socket (Fig. 40.4 and see Fig. 41.15).
4. Extrusion: This is a central dislocation of the tooth from its socket (Fig. 40.5 and see Fig. 41.16A). The PDL is usually torn in this injury.
5. Lateral luxation: The tooth is displaced in a labial, lingual, or lateral direction. The PDL is torn, and contusion or fracture of the supporting alveolar bone occurs (Fig. 40.6 and see Fig. 41.16B).
6. Avulsion: The tooth is completely displaced from the alveolus. The PDL is severed, and fractures of the alveolus may occur (Fig. 40.7 and see Fig. 41.17).

History

Obtaining an adequate medical and dental history is essential to proper diagnosis and treatment. The medical history should already be on record if the child suffering an injury is brought to their regular dentist. Frequently, however, a parent will take an injured child to the closest dentist or to one known to treat children. Thus with the confusion of a young, injured child entering the office for possibly the first time and disrupting the day's schedule, the potential to forget to gather important historical informa-

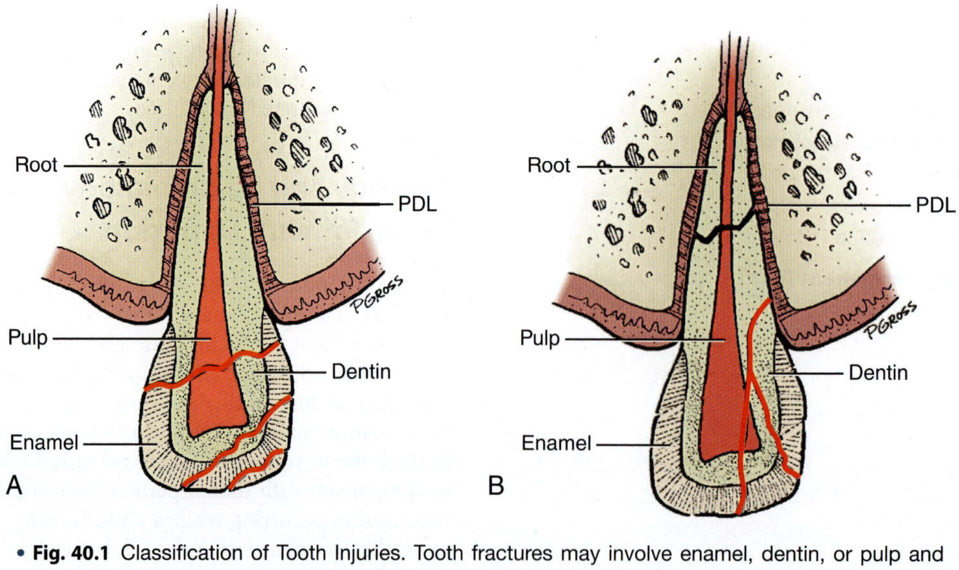

• **Fig. 40.1** Classification of Tooth Injuries. Tooth fractures may involve enamel, dentin, or pulp and may occur in the crown (A) or the root (B).

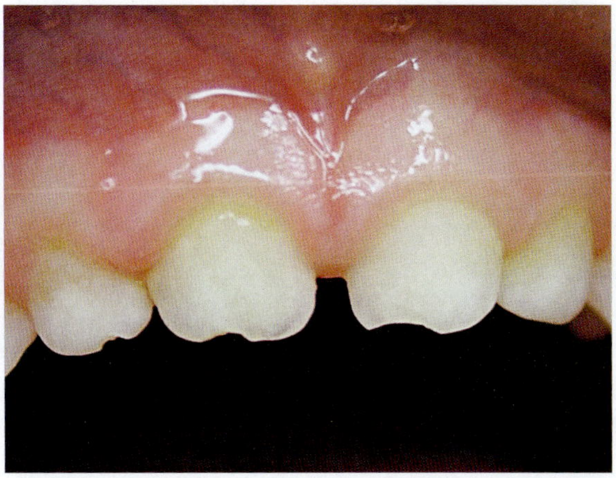

• **Fig. 40.2** Fracture of enamel and dentin in both maxillary primary central incisors.

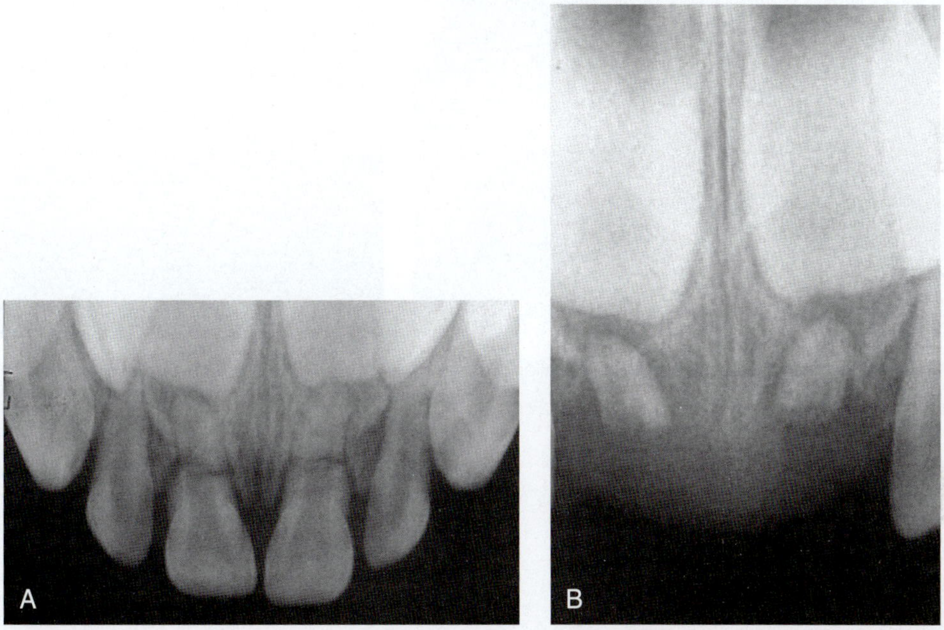

• **Fig. 40.3** (A) Root fracture of both maxillary primary central incisors. (B) Apical fragments of the root fractured maxillary primary central incisors after extraction of the coronal fragments.

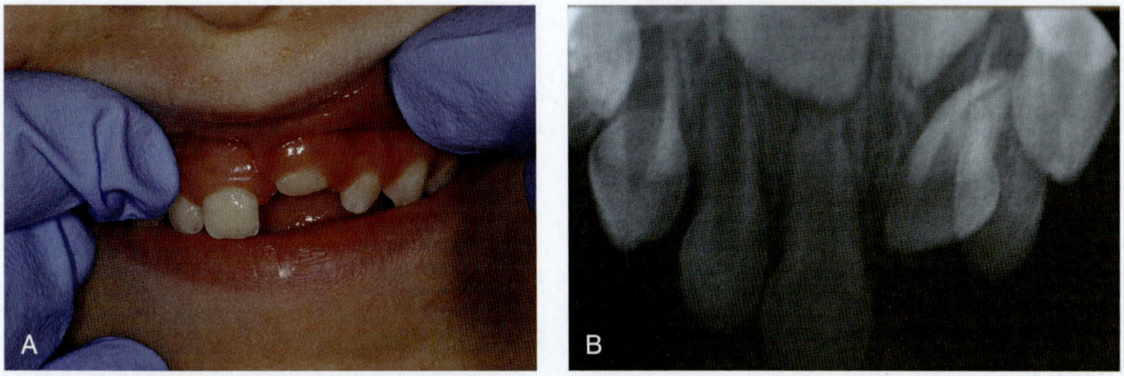

• **Fig. 40.4** (A) Intruded maxillary left primary central incisor. (B) Periapical radiograph showing the left maxillary primary central incisor after intrusion. The shortened and more opaque image of the intruded tooth, compared with that of the right central incisor, indicates that the root has been pushed labially and away from the underlying permanent tooth. (From McTigue DJ. Managing injuries to the primary dentition. *Dent Clin North Am.* 2009;53[4]:627-638.)

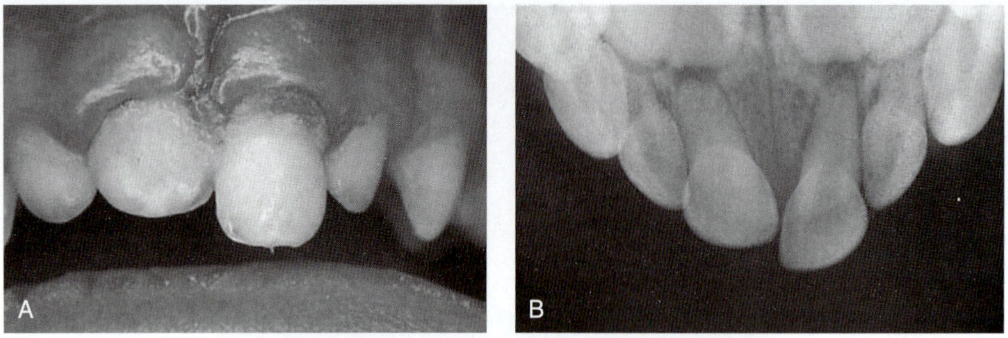

• **Fig. 40.5** Extrusion of the Left Maxillary Primary Central Incisor. (A) Clinical view. (B) Radiographic view. Notice the pulp canal obliteration in the right maxillary primary central incisor, which resulted from a previous injury.

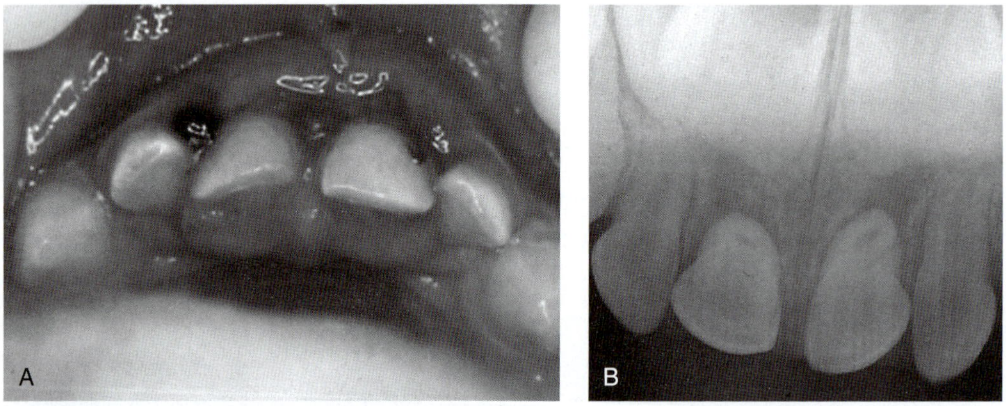

• **Fig. 40.6** Lingual Luxation of Both Maxillary Primary Central Incisors. (A) Clinical view. (B) Radiographic view.

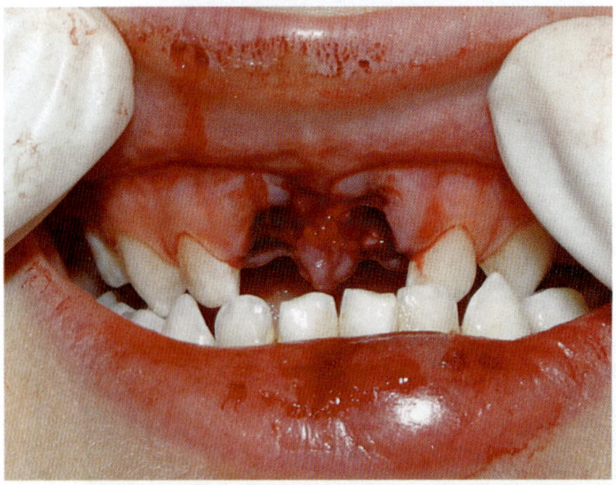

• **Fig. 40.7** Avulsion of maxillary right and left primary central incisors.

tion is great. The use of a trauma assessment form to help record data and organize the management of care is highly recommended (Fig. 40.8).

Medical History

Routine data on the patient's general health should be obtained. Historical information particularly relevant to the dental injury includes the following:

1. Cardiac disease, which may necessitate prophylaxis against infectious endocarditis
2. Bleeding disorders
3. Allergies to medications
4. Seizure disorders
5. Medications
6. Status of tetanus prophylaxis

The issue of tetanus protection is particularly important when a child has suffered a dirty wound (e.g., an avulsion), a deep laceration, or an intrusion injury in which soil is embedded in the tissues. Wounds containing necrotic tissue, dirt, and foreign material should be cleaned and debrided as an essential part of tetanus prophylaxis. Children acquire active immunity through a series of five injections of adsorbed tetanus toxoid, usually completed by the age of 4 to 6 years. These are normally administered as part of the diphtheria-tetanus-pertussis vaccinations. Children should then receive a booster of tetanus toxoid at 11 to 12 years of age and again 5 years later.[19] An increasing number of reports have indicated that children in the United States are not receiving their childhood immunizations appropriately. If there is any question about the adequacy of a child's tetanus protection, the child's physician should immediately be consulted.

History of the Dental Injury

Three important questions are asked in gathering the dental history: *when, where,* and *how* did the accident occur? The time elapsed since the injury occurred is a major factor in determining the type of treatment to be provided. The dentist should also determine whether the tooth had been injured previously or whether the injury had first been treated elsewhere.

SCHOOL of DENTISTRY
DEPARTMENT of PEDIATRIC DENTISTRY

Child's Name ______________ Student ______________
Age ______ Sex ______ Race ______ Faculty ______________
Place of Injury ______________ Chart No. ______ Date ______
Date of Injury ______________
Time of Injury ______________
Time Elapsed Since Injury ______________

HISTORY
Chief Complaint ______________ Previous Trauma ______________
Past Medical History ______________
Past Dental History ______________
How Injury Occurred ______________
Tetanus Protection: ☐ No Yes ☐ Date of Last Booster ______________

EXTRAORAL ASSESSMENT

CNS Status
☐ Unconsciousness ☐ Amnesia
☐ Unequal Pupil Size ☐ Headache
☐ Fixed Pupil ☐ Nausea
☐ CSF from Ears ☐ Disorientation
☐ CSF from Nose ☐ Loss of Smell
☐ Nystagmus ☐ Seizure
☐ Vertigo
Describe ______________

Hard Tissue
☐ Cranial Fracture ☐ Zygoma Fracture
☐ Mandibular Fracture ☐ Infection
☐ Maxillary Fracture
Describe ______________

Soft Tissue
☐ Laceration ☐ Abrasion
☐ Contusions ☐ Infection
☐ Swelling ☐ Embedded Material
Describe ______________

INTRAORAL ASSESSMENT

Hard Tissue
☐ Alveolar Fracture ☐ Palatal Fracture
Describe ______________

Soft Tissue
☐ Lips ☐ Frenum
☐ Buccal Mucosa ☐ Tongue
☐ Gingiva ☐ Palate
Describe ______________

Dental Occlusion
Molar ______ Cuspid ______
Overjet ______ mm Overbite ______ %
Open Bite ______ Crossbite ______
Classification Deviation Induced by Trauma ______
Describe ______________

RADIOGRAPHS
☐ Periapical ☐ Occlusal
☐ Lateral Anterior ☐ Panorex
Other ______________
Pathology ______________

• **Fig. 40.8** Trauma assessment form. *CNS,* Central nervous system; *CSF,* cerebrospinal fluid; *PDL,* periodontal ligament.

Continued

DENTAL FINDINGS

Fracture **Class I** **Class II** **Class III** **Class IV**

Draw Injury

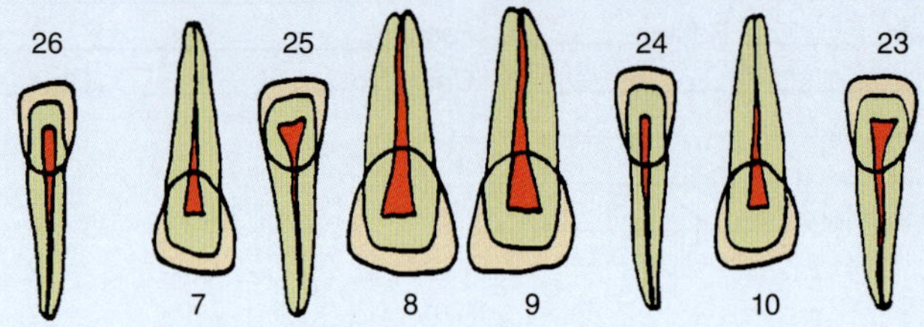

Involved Teeth ______________________

Tooth Response — Pulp and PDL

Tooth No.				
Exposure				
Hemorrhage				
Heat				
Cold				
Contamination				
Percussion				
Mobility				
Vitalometer				

Displacement

☐ Intrusion ☐ Subluxation
☐ Extrusion ☐ Lateral Luxation
☐ Avulsion

Color

☐ Normal ☐ Dark ☐ Light

SUMMARY AND DIAGNOSIS

Crown ______________________

Pulp ______________________

Root ______________________

Periapical Tissue ______________________

Alveolar Process ______________________

Root Displacement ______________________

Restoration ______________________

Fragments ______________________

TREATMENT

Soft Tissues ______________________

Pulp ______________________

Restoration ______________________

Splinting ______________________

Medication ______________________

Recall Follow-up

☐ 2 weeks ☐ 3 weeks ☐ 6 weeks
☐ 3 months ☐ 6 months

Other ______________________

• **Fig. 40.8, cont'd** Tooth figures represent primary teeth; Numbers above/below each tooth represent permanent, succedaneous tooth.

Where the injury occurred sheds light on its severity. Did the toddler slip and hit the coffee table in the living room, or did she fall off her parent's bicycle in the park? This information can help determine the need for tetanus prophylaxis as well as signal a need to rule out more serious injury to the child.

How the accident occurred obviously provides the dentist with the most information regarding severity. Displaced or fractured teeth may be the most obvious sign of injury in a child who has sustained head trauma, so a dentist may be the first health professional to examine the child. Clinical markers for potential intracranial injury include vomiting, loss of consciousness, severe mechanism of injury (i.e., motor vehicle crash or fall from high distance), severe or worsening headache, amnesia, and nonfrontal scalp hematoma. Children under the age of 2 with any of these signs are at increased risk of closed head injury. Positive findings indicate immediate medical consultation.[20]

As previously discussed, the possibility of child abuse can also be ruled out through a careful dental history. Any history of previous dental injuries should also be determined because their sequelae may complicate diagnosis of the current injury.

Directing attention to the specific teeth involved, the dentist should ask the child if there is spontaneous pain from any teeth. Positive findings here may indicate pulp inflammation that is caused by a fractured crown or injuries to the supporting structures, such as the extravasation of blood into the PDL. Does the child experience a thermal change with sweet or sour foods? If so, dentin or pulp may be exposed. Are the teeth tender to the touch or tender while chewing? Does the child note a change in occlusion? These findings may indicate a luxation injury or an alveolar fracture.

Oral Health Quality of Life

"Does impaired dental esthetics after traumatic injuries to the primary dentition affect the child's quality of life?" This question was investigated, and contradictory findings were presented. One study found that 4- to 5-year-olds have negative social perceptions and self-perceptions regarding altered dental esthetics,[21] but other publications reported that the oral health-related quality of life of the children and their families was not influenced by traumatic dental injuries.[22,23]

Clinical Examination

Once the medical and dental histories are complete, the dentist is ready to begin the clinical examination. It is very tempting to focus immediately on a fractured or displaced tooth and thus miss other important injuries. A disciplined approach to a complete clinical examination should be followed in diagnosing every traumatic injury.

Extraoral Examination

A complete examination should rule out injuries to the child's facial bones. The facial skeleton should be palpated to determine discontinuities of facial bones.[24] Extraoral wounds and bruises should be recorded. The temporomandibular joints should be palpated, and any swelling, clicking, or crepitus should be noted. Mandibular function in all excursive movements should be checked. Any stiffness or pain in the child's neck necessitates immediate referral to a physician to rule out cervical spine injury.

Intraoral Examination

All soft tissues should be examined and any injuries recorded. The presence of foreign matter in lacerations of the lips and cheeks, such as tooth fragments or soil, should be identified. Removal at the initial appointment will eliminate chronic infection and disfiguring fibrosis.

The occlusion should be checked to identify possible occlusal disturbances that may result from oral luxation of the maxillary incisors.

Each tooth in the mouth should be examined for fracture, pulp exposure, and dislocation. In some crown fractures, only a very thin layer of dentin remains over the pulp, so that the pulp's outline can be seen as a pink tinge on the dentin. The dentist should be very careful not to perforate this dentin with an instrument.

Displacement of teeth should be recorded, as well as horizontal and vertical tooth mobility. Increased mobility of an injured primary tooth is an indication of damage to the PDL unless the tooth is near natural exfoliation. Reaction to palpation and percussion of teeth is recorded. Percussion sensitivity is a good indicator of PDL inflammation.

Pulpal vitality testing is not routinely performed in the primary dentition. This is because the testing requires a relaxed and cooperative patient who can report reactions objectively, and some young children lack the ability to do so.

Radiographic Examination

Indications for Radiographs

Radiographs are an important part of the diagnosis and management of dental injuries. They allow the clinician to detect root fractures, extent of root development, size of pulp chambers, periapical radiolucencies, extent and type of root resorption, degree of tooth displacement, position of unerupted teeth, relationship between the injured primary teeth and their permanent successors, jaw fractures, and the presence of tooth fragments and other foreign bodies in soft tissues. Although some radiographs will show negative findings at the initial appointment, they are nonetheless important as baseline documentation. Subsequent radiographic evidence can thus be compared with the initial films.

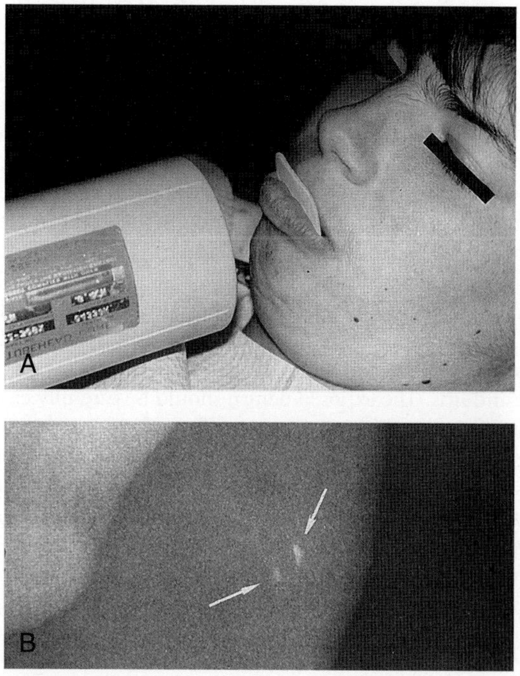

• **Fig. 40.9** (A) Positioning film to detect the presence of tooth fragments in the lip. (B) Radiograph demonstrating tooth fragments in lip *(arrows)*.

Radiographic Techniques

There is no "standard series" of radiographs for dental injuries. All films taken should clearly show the apical areas of traumatized teeth (see Fig. 40.15).

To determine the presence of foreign bodies such as tooth fragments in the lips or tongue, one-fourth of the normal exposure time is used. The film is placed beneath the tissue to be examined, and the radiograph is exposed (Fig. 40.9).

Timing of Follow-Up Radiographs

As noted previously, many pathologic changes are not immediately apparent in radiographs. After approximately 3 weeks, periapical radiolucencies that are caused by pulpal necrosis can usually be detected. In addition, inflammatory root resorption may be evident at this time. After approximately 6 to 7 weeks, replacement resorption, or ankylosis, may be seen. Thus there is adequate rationale to obtain postoperative radiographs at 1 month after the injury. In the absence of any clinical signs or symptoms—such as the development of swelling, fistula, mobility, tooth discoloration, or pain—additional films are not indicated until 6 months after the injury. If changes are to appear radiographically, they usually do so by this time.

Clinical Photography

Photographs are recommended to document the initial injury as well as healing responses. The almost universal availability of cell phone cameras also makes it practical for parents/caregivers to forward providers good images of injuries, thus facilitating triage and treatment planning.[25]

Emergency Care

Injuries to the Hard Dental Tissues

Clinical pathways outlining treatment options for all primary tooth injuries are located at the end of the chapter in eFigs. 40.28–40.31.

Cracks and Fractures of the Enamel and Dentin Without Pulp Exposure

Enamel cracks and small fractures are common findings in primary teeth (see Fig. 40.2). It is believed that even fractures exposing dentin in primary teeth have no deleterious effect on the pulp and need not be covered.[25] In the case of larger fractures, treatment is often indicated to restore esthetics. Various methods have been suggested to restore the fractured crown, including the use of strip crowns, preformed esthetic crowns, and open-faced steel crowns (see Chapter 30).

If it is decided to avoid crown restoration, possibly owing to the child's age and/or behavior, sharp edges at the fracture line can be smoothed with abrasive disks to prevent irritation to the tongue and lips. The exposed dentin should be carefully examined to ensure that there is no exposure of the pulp. If tooth fracture is associated with a wounded lip, then a radiograph of the lip should be obtained to rule out the presence of tooth fragments trapped in the soft tissue (see Fig. 40.9). Late complications, such as coronal discoloration (see later), usually are attributed not to the fractured crown but to overlooked minor displacement of the tooth and obstruction of blood supply to the pulp.

Fractures of the Enamel and Dentin With Pulp Exposure

Deep fracture of the crown may be associated with exposure of the pulp, usually at the pulp horn. If the pulp horn is exposed at its incisal edge, it may not bleed and therefore may go unnoticed. A red point of blood can be seen if the pulp is exposed at a deeper level. If not treated immediately, a widely exposed pulp may proliferate, resulting in a pulp polyp.[26]

Several treatment options are available for crown fracture with pulp exposure in primary teeth, including pulpotomy, pulpectomy, and extraction.[27] The vitality of the tissue and the time elapsed since the injury dictate the treatment of choice. If the pulp tissue is vital, a cervical pulpotomy can be performed (see Chapter 32). Ram and Holan suggest that a partial pulpotomy technique is indicated to preserve pulp vitality in a young primary tooth with a wide-open apex and thin root dentin walls.[28]

Pulp exposure is sometimes overlooked or neglected, and no treatment is rendered. The unavoidable outcome is a necrotic and infected pulp with consequent swelling or fistula. If massive external inflammatory root resorption is detected or if the follicle of the underlying permanent tooth bud is involved in the inflammatory process, the tooth must be extracted as soon as possible. Leaving such teeth untreated increases the risk of damage to the permanent incisor. If there is no evidence of inflammatory external root resorption, some clinicians attempt to save these teeth with complete pulpectomies. The principle of this treatment is complete removal of the necrotic pulp, filling the pulp canal with a resorbable paste, and providing esthetic restoration of the crown. (For further details, see Chapter 32.)

Permanent incisors succeeding infected and root-treated primary incisors may show mild enamel defects that could be attributed to both the inflammatory process and over instrumentation during the endodontic procedure.[29]

Crown-Root Fractures

Fractures involving both the crown and the root of primary teeth are rare. The teeth in this type of injury are split into two or more fragments, with one main fragment remaining firm and the other fragment becoming loose because of injury to its periodontal fibers (Fig. 40.10). The two fragments should be separated to determine whether the pulp has been exposed. The loose fragment should be removed, allowing inspection of the main fragment's exposed dentin. Pulpotomy is the suggested treatment for such exposures, with subsequent esthetic reconstruction of the crown. If the fracture goes deep into the alveolus, creating a periodontal pocket in the space previously occupied by the loose fragment, both fragments should be extracted.

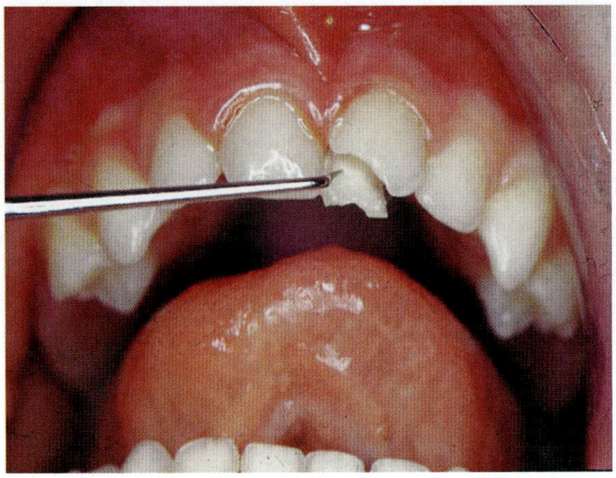

• **Fig. 40.10** Clinical view of a left maxillary primary central incisor with crown-root fracture. The palatal fragment is mobile and attached by gingival fibers only.

Root Fractures

Root fractures are also rare in primary teeth.[30,31] Both fragments may remain close to each other, with the tooth presenting slight mobility and sensitivity to percussion (see Fig. 40.3). If the coronal fragment is pushed away from the apical part of the root, it frequently assumes a lingual inclination that may interfere with the occlusion unless the child has an open bite. In this case the coronal fragment should be extracted. Attempts to remove the apical fragment should be avoided, as such action may harm the developing permanent successor. These apical fragments usually resorb as part of the physiologic process of tooth replacement.[30] If no disturbance to the child's occlusion exists, the tooth may be left untreated and the parents provided with instruction for thorough oral hygiene and soft diet for a limited time (see "Information and Instructions for Parents," later in this chapter). The PDL attached to the mobile coronal fragment may recover, with decrease in tooth mobility and sensitivity to percussion. Unlike permanent teeth, there is no intention to cause repair of the fracture with calcified tissue in root-fractured primary teeth; thus immobilization of the tooth, though reported in the literature as a treatment option,[33] is unnecessary. Splinting the tooth is recommended only to alleviate sensitivity during routine function.

Injuries to the Chin

An injury to the chin may produce a sudden forceful closure of the mandibular teeth with their maxillary opponents. As a result, a wide range of injuries may affect molar teeth.[32] These include minor enamel fractures, fractures with dentin exposure that may imitate a carious lesion on the radiograph, crown-root fractures with or without pulp exposure,[33] and injuries to the PDL.[34] In addition, fracture of the mandible may occur mainly in the symphysis, mental, and subcondylar areas (Fig. 40.11).[35] These injuries have also been correlated with cervical spine fractures.[36]

The exposed dentin in fractured posterior teeth increases the risk of pulp irritation and may become carious. It can therefore be covered by a composite resin if the area of exposure is small. If the fracture is large or extends below the gum line, a stainless steel

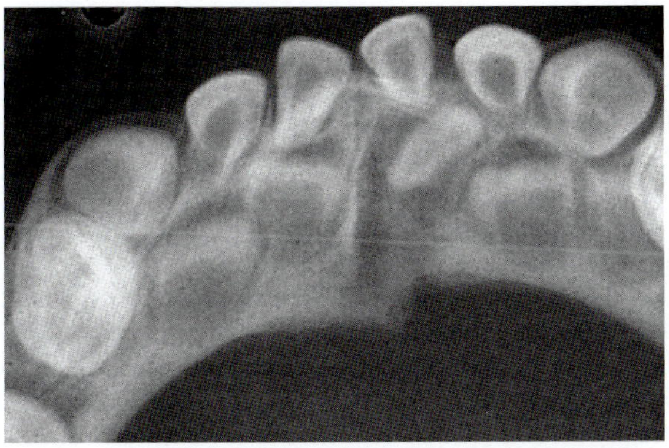

• **Fig. 40.11** Fracture of the mandible in a baby as a result of trauma to the chin.

or zirconia crown are preferable. When the pulp is exposed and the crown restorable, pulpotomy and crown (stainless steel or zirconia) is the treatment of choice. Otherwise, the tooth must be extracted and space maintenance considered.

Injuries to the Supporting Tissues

Concussion and Subluxation

Teeth suffering concussion injuries are sensitive to percussion without any additional sign. Subluxated teeth also present with increased mobility and widening of the periodontal space. If the teeth are examined shortly after the injury, signs of bleeding from the gingival crevice can be seen (Fig. 40.12). Concussion and subluxation are mild injuries that often go unnoticed. Parents, if questioned, may recall the injury when a late complication develops, such as tooth discoloration (see "Coronal Discoloration").[37]

Usually, no treatment is required except for a soft diet for a limited time and thorough oral hygiene to prevent contamination of the damaged PDL (see "Information and Instructions for Parents").

Intrusion

Intrusion is one of the most complicated injuries to the primary incisors. Clinically, the tooth may disappear completely into the surrounding tissues, or the incisal part may remain visible with its clinical crown shorter than that of an adjacent nontraumatized tooth. After intrusion, the PDL is compressed and the root surface is tightly pressed against the alveolar bone, resulting in reduced mobility. Percussion of an intruded tooth produces a metallic sound and does not provoke pain. Bleeding from the gingival sulcus is visible shortly after the injury. A swollen upper lip due to edema and/or hemorrhage can often be seen.

The root of the primary incisor is normally close to the labial surface of the permanent tooth. If the root of the primary tooth is pushed against the crown of the permanent incisor, it may severely damage the developing tooth bud. Immediate removal of the primary tooth may relieve the pressure and minimize the damage.[38] It is therefore extremely important to determine as soon as possible after the injury if the root of the primary tooth contacts the permanent tooth or has been pushed labially and away from the labial surface of the permanent successor. Fortunately, the root apex of maxillary primary incisors has a labial curvature, leading the root away from the permanent tooth in more than 80% of cases.[39]

Several clinical and radiographic signs support the diagnosis of labial alignment of the root:

- Palatal inclination of the crown
- Hemorrhage and hard swelling palpated in the vestibule due to fracture of the labial bone plate by the root of the primary tooth
- A shortened and more opaque image of an intruded incisor compared with an adjacent nondisplaced tooth (see Fig. 40.4B)
- Proper alignment of the permanent successor as seen on a periapical radiograph

Absence of such signs should alert the operator to suspect palatal displacement of the primary tooth root with subsequent displacement of the permanent tooth.

Some authors suggest the use of lateral extraoral radiographs, although a study has shown that this technique does not contribute to assessment of the relation between the root of the intruded tooth and the labial surface of the permanent tooth. In addition, it is only beneficial in children younger than 20 months.[40]

Intruded incisors that do not risk the permanent teeth can be left to spontaneously reerupt. Reeruption begins within 2 to 3 weeks but can be delayed for more than 6 months. In many cases the teeth do not erupt back to their original position but into a rotated alignment (see Fig. 40.23). An estimate of reeruption can be made by measuring the distance between the incisal edge of a partially intruded tooth and a tongue depressor placed between fully erupted teeth on either side of the intruded tooth (Fig. 40.13). Repeated measurements at recall visits allow estimation of the rate of reeruption. It should be emphasized that increase of the clinical crown (the distance between the incisal edge and the gingival margins) is not an indication of reeruption. Decrease in the size of edematous gums may erroneously be viewed as reeruption. Surgical reposition and splinting of the intruded primary incisor has also been suggested as a treatment option.[41–43]

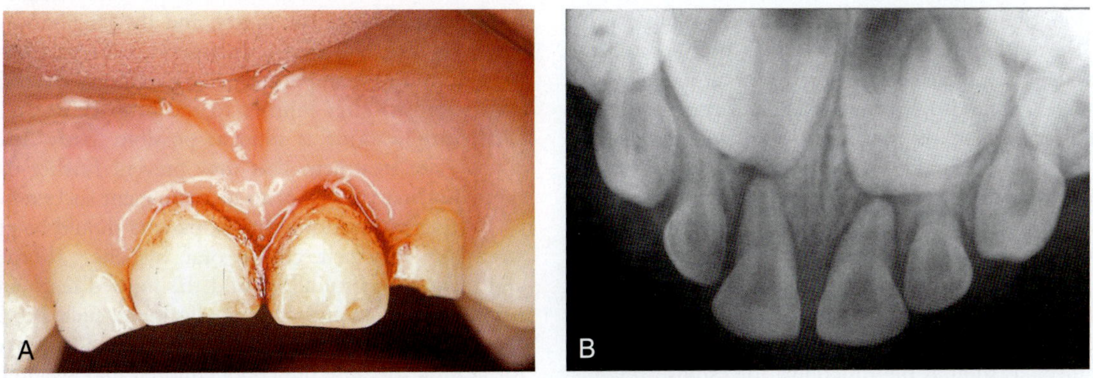

• **Fig. 40.12** (A) Clinical view of subluxation of the left maxillary primary central incisor and slight extrusion of the adjacent central incisor. (B) Radiograph of both teeth showing widening of the periodontal ligament.

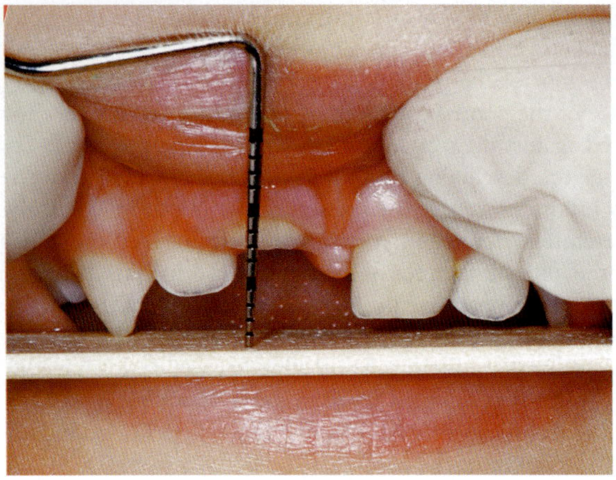

• **Fig. 40.13** Measuring the positions of intruded maxillary right primary incisors relative to their antimeres using a tongue depressor.

Extrusion

An extruded tooth is clinically elongated relative to adjacent unaffected teeth. The tooth presents increased mobility and sensitivity to percussion. Bleeding from the gingival sulcus can be seen shortly after the injury. A periapical radiograph of an extruded tooth will show widening of the PDL, especially around the apex (see Fig. 40.5). The more the tooth moves out of the alveolar socket, the higher the chances of disruption of the blood supply and development of pulp necrosis. Extrusions resemble lingual luxation in many features; thus the approach to both types of injuries should be similar (see "Lingual Luxation").

Lingual Luxation

In the case of lingual luxations, the crown moves in a palatal direction while the apex is pushed labially. It is sometimes difficult to distinguish between lingual luxation and intrusion. The palatal inclination of the crown may interfere with the occlusion unless the child has an open bite. The tooth presents with increased mobility and sensitivity to percussion. Signs of bleeding may be evident around the tooth (see Fig. 40.6A). The upper lip is often swollen, with signs of hemorrhage due to fracture of the labial bone plate by the tooth apex. A periapical radiograph will show a radiolucent gap between the apex and the alveolar bone (see Fig. 40.6B). The luxated tooth presents a shortened and more opaque image compared with an adjacent unaffected tooth.

Many clinicians recommend extraction of severely luxated primary teeth because they may potentially damage the succeeding permanent incisor. Some parents insist that everything be done to save anterior primary teeth, and if the child is seen shortly after the injury and before the formation of a coagulum, the tooth can be repositioned. The tooth must then be splinted for 7 to 14 days, and root canal treatment is indicated because rupture of the blood supply to the pulp is expected in cases of severe luxation.[29] The cost-benefit ratio of retaining these teeth, the potential need for advanced behavior management techniques, and the potential for injury to the succeeding permanent teeth must be explained to the parents.

In the case of open bite without occlusal interference, the functional forces of the tongue may push the crown into a labial position. Occlusal interferences can sometimes be eliminated by creating an intentional open bite by adding composite "buttons" to the occlusal surface of the maxillary or mandibular first molars. These are removed as soon as the functional forces push the lingually luxated tooth into its original position. This technique is indicated when the luxated teeth are seen after the formation of a blood clot in the alveolus several hours after the injury. Extraction of the luxated teeth is indicated in the case of severe fracture of the labial bone plate.

Parents should be provided with strict instructions for good oral hygiene to prevent migration of microorganisms between the root and the gums with subsequent infection of the PDL (see "Information and Instructions for Parents").

Avulsion

Avulsion of a primary incisor is a common outcome of dental trauma in young children (see Fig. 40.7). The high crown-root ratio of primary incisors and the resilience of the bone are contributing factors. In about 75% of cases involving avulsion of a primary incisor, the developing permanent successor is damaged.[44] Most articles, textbooks, and guidelines recommend that avulsed primary incisors should not be replanted because the permanent tooth may be damaged during insertion of the root back to its socket and because of the risk of aspiration.[45,46] Case reports suggest shortening of the root by 2 to 3 mm before replantation to prevent such damage.[47] If a child arrives at the dental office with a tooth that has been avulsed and replanted by his or her parents, the parents should be apprised of the risks and costs versus benefits of keeping that tooth. A splint and root canal treatment with a resorbable paste will be required in the attempt to save the tooth until its natural exfoliation and to prevent inflammatory resorption of the root.

Avulsed primary teeth should be accounted for to rule out potential aspiration. If the tooth cannot be found, the child should be referred for further evaluation by a pediatrician.[48]

Information and Instructions for Parents

Teledentistry in Case of Traumatic Injury to the Primary Teeth

This section intends to advise dentists how to guide concerned parents whose child had recently experienced a traumatic injury to the primary teeth. The main limitations of teledentistry are the inability to get an unmediated impression of the injury outcomes, and the impossibility to take and evaluate an x-ray. Therefore teledentistry is not a substitute for a dental visit. However, based on description and images of the affected tissues provided by parents or caregivers, the dentist can determine the urgency and timing of a clinical visit and suggest immediate and simple actions that can prevent infection, alleviate pain, and create favorable conditions that may later help in the healing process.

Information and Instructions Provided at the Emergency Visit

Parents should be informed about possible complications of the injury, prognosis of the injury, and the likelihood of damage to the permanent successors. Instructions for parents are aimed at preventing late complications (e.g., infection of the PDL and pulp necrosis) after injuries to the primary teeth and detecting such complications as soon as possible. Early detection allows appropriate treatment that may prevent further damage to the injured primary tooth or to its permanent successor.

In cases of luxation injuries, parents should be given strict instructions for their child's oral hygiene. Thorough cleaning and plaque removal all around the injured teeth are imperative. Application of an antiseptic medicament, such as 0.2% chlorhexidine gluconate, to the injured gingivae can improve the chances for healing. Because preschool children may swallow the solution while rinsing, cotton-tipped applicators soaked with the solution should be used to gently apply the antiseptic to the gingival crevices of the injured teeth. This should be repeated several times a day, especially after meals, for 7 days. At this time the gingival fibers are expected to be healed.

The child should be placed on a soft diet for several days to prevent intense forces on the tooth and to allow its stabilization. Antibiotics are only indicated in cases with severe damage to the oral soft tissues, which could lead to secondary infection.

The timing of follow-up examinations is based on the type of injury sustained. Pathologic sequelae such as pulpal necrosis and inflammatory root resorption can frequently be detected radiographically in 1 month. Parents should be instructed to bring the child in earlier if they suspect any deterioration in the condition of the injured teeth, such as redness, swelling, or the appearance of a fistula in the gums above the injured tooth and, in case of discoloration, increased mobility or sensitivity of the tooth.

Pathologic Sequelae of Trauma to the Teeth

Complications after traumatic injuries to primary teeth may appear shortly after the injury (e.g., infection of the PDL or dark discoloration of the crown) or after several months (e.g., yellow discoloration of the crown and external root resorption). It is currently not possible to accurately identify the histopathologic condition of a dental pulp based on clinical symptoms. The following terms describe a spectrum of clinical signs and symptoms that accompany inflammation and degeneration of the pulp and/or PDL.

Reversible Pulpitis

The pulp's initial response to trauma is pulpitis. Capillaries in the tooth become congested, a condition that can be clinically apparent upon transillumination of the crown with a bright light. Teeth with reversible pulpitis may be tender to percussion if the PDL is inflamed (e.g., after a luxation injury). Pulpitis may be totally reversible if the condition causing it is addressed, or it may progress to an irreversible state with necrosis of the pulp.

Infection of the Periodontal Ligament

Infection of the PDL becomes possible when detachment of the gingival fibers from the tooth in a luxation injury allows invasion of microorganisms from the oral cavity along the root to infect the PDL. Loss of alveolar bone support can be seen on a periapical radiograph (Fig. 40.14). This diminishes the healing potential of the supporting tissues. Subsequently, increased tooth mobility accompanied by exudation of pus from the gingival crevice will require extraction of the injured tooth. Parents should be informed about the risk of infection and provided with appropriate instructions to minimize such risk.

Irreversible Pulpitis

Irreversible pulpitis may be acute or chronic, and it may be partial or total. Acute, irreversible pulpitis after a dental injury can be painful if the exudate accompanying the pulpal inflammation cannot vent. Most frequently in children, however, inflammatory exudates are quickly vented and the pulpitis progresses to a chronic, painless condition.

Pulp Necrosis and Infection

Two main mechanisms can explain how the pulp of injured primary teeth becomes necrotic: (1) infection of the pulp in cases of untreated crown fracture with pulp exposure and (2) interrupted blood supply to the pulp through the apex in cases of luxation injury leading to ischemia. Not all luxation injuries result in a necrotic pulp. Surprisingly, intruded primary teeth, unlike permanent teeth, maintain the vitality of their pulp.[39] Though untreated teeth with exposed pulps are expected to develop swelling or fistulas, injured teeth with avascular necrosis may remain asymptomatic both clinically and radiographically.[49] Loss of pulp vitality due to a traumatic injury at an early stage of root development results in the arrest of dentin apposition and cessation of root development (Fig. 40.15).

Periapical radiolucencies indicative of a granuloma or cyst are frequently evident radiographically in necrotic anterior teeth (Fig. 40.16A). In addition, a parulis is often clinically evident at the level of the involved tooth's root apex (see Fig. 40.16B). Controversy exists regarding the most appropriate treatment of

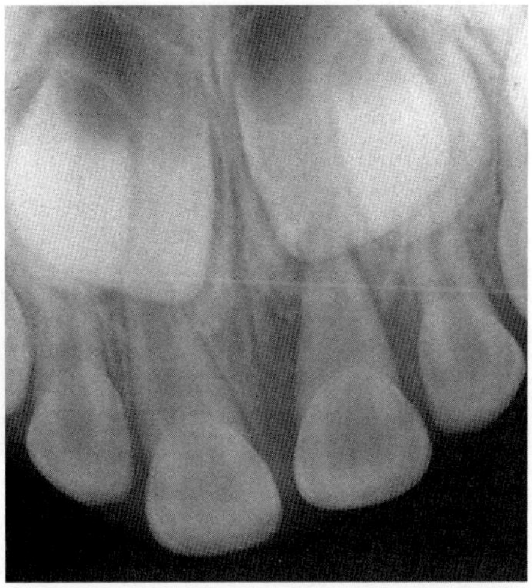

• **Fig. 40.14** Infection of the Periodontal Ligament. This radiograph shows the left maxillary primary central incisor after injury to the supporting tissues. Infection of the attachment apparatus resulted in loss of alveolar bone at the medial aspect of the root.

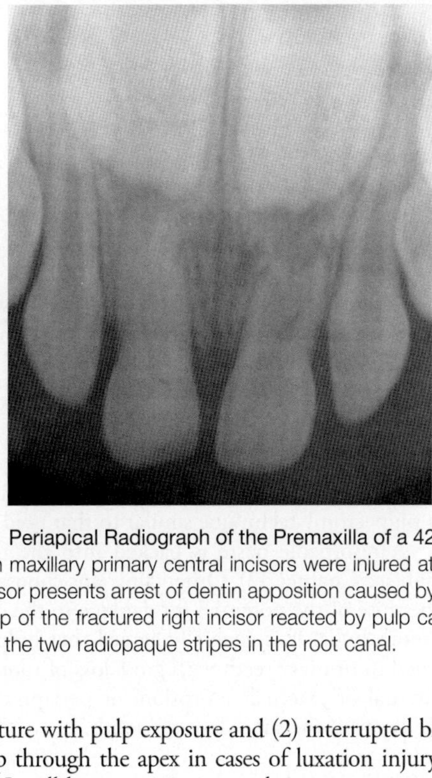

• **Fig. 40.15** Periapical Radiograph of the Premaxilla of a 42-Month-Old Child. Both maxillary primary central incisors were injured at 18 months. The left incisor presents arrest of dentin apposition caused by pulp necrosis. The pulp of the fractured right incisor reacted by pulp canal obliteration. Notice the two radiopaque stripes in the root canal.

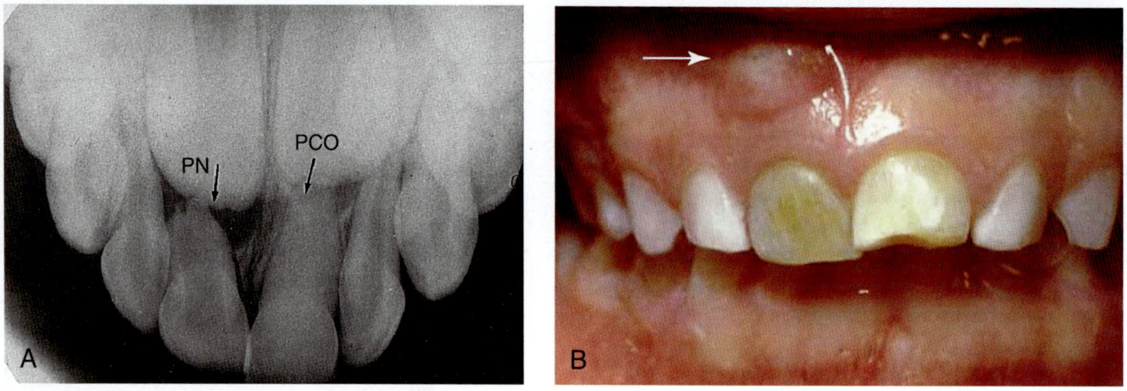

• **Fig. 40.16** (A) Pulp canal obliteration *(PCO)* in the patient's left primary central incisor and pulp necrosis *(PN)* in the right primary central incisor. (B) In the same patient, a parulis is present at the apical level of the necrotic right central incisor *(arrow)*.

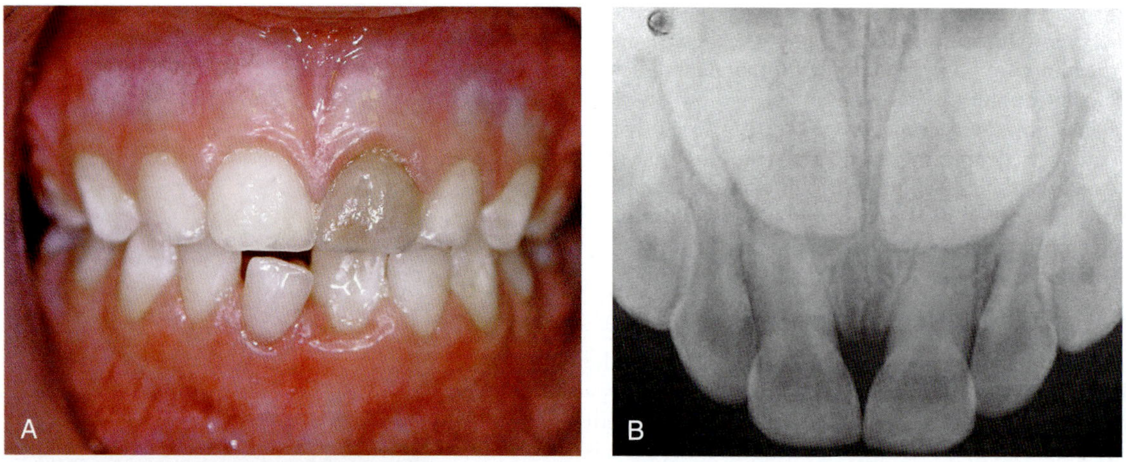

• **Fig. 40.17** (A) Left maxillary primary central incisor 1 year after color change because of trauma. This clinical view shows no pathologic signs except dark discoloration. (B) Periapical radiograph showing no pathology associated with the injury.

primary anterior teeth with necrotic pulps. Some clinicians treat them with a pulpectomy technique similar to that used in permanent teeth.[50] A resorbable paste is packed into the thoroughly cleansed canal (see Chapter 32). Other clinicians choose to extract these teeth because of the potential for damage to the developing permanent tooth buds. It is generally agreed that pulpectomy is contraindicated in primary teeth with gross loss of root structure, advanced internal or external resorption, or periapical infection involving the crypt of the succedaneous tooth.

Coronal Discoloration

As a result of trauma, the capillaries in the pulp occasionally hemorrhage, leaving blood pigments deposited in the dentinal tubules. In mild cases, the blood is resorbed and very little discoloration occurs, or that which is present becomes lighter in several weeks. In more severe cases, the discoloration persists for the life of the tooth (Fig. 40.17).

From a diagnostic standpoint, discoloration of primary teeth does not necessarily mean that the tooth is nonvital, particularly when the discoloration occurs 1 or 2 days after the injury. Dark discoloration that persists for weeks or months after the injury is more indicative of a necrotic pulp.[49,51] Nevertheless, in the primary dentition of a healthy child, color change alone does not indicate a need for pulp therapy or extraction of the tooth. Additional signs and symptoms of infection—such as periapical radiographic radiolucency, mobility, swelling, fistula, or pain—must be evident before further treatment is indicated.

Crown discoloration is the external expression of changes in the pulp-dentin complex that become visible through the almost transparent enamel. Crown discoloration of primary incisors is a common posttraumatic finding and is often the only evidence of trauma to the tooth. Discoloration of a primary tooth can be noticed earlier and seen better if viewed from the palatal aspect by transillumination than by direct observation of its labial aspect. The variety of colors is traditionally divided into three main groups: pink-red, yellow, and dark (gray-brown-black).

Pink discoloration that is observed shortly after the injury may represent intrapulpal hemorrhage. Rupture of blood vessels in the pulp as a result of the injury allows extravasation of red blood cells into the surrounding pulpal tissue, resulting in a reddish hue of the crown that becomes visible shortly after the injury.

A reddish hue noticed long after the injury is usually caused by internal resorption in the pulp chamber. In both cases follow-up is the only treatment option. Although the hemorrhage eventually dissolves and disappears, the resorption process continues and results in early loss of the crown. The apical part of the root can be left untouched, awaiting its spontaneous resorption. It can be removed, if necessary, but care must be taken not to damage the permanent successor.

Yellow discoloration of primary incisors can be seen when the dentin is thick and the pulp chamber narrower than usual (see Fig. 40.16). This condition is termed pulp canal obliteration (PCO). It has been shown that PCO can be seen on radiographs without the corresponding yellow discoloration of the crown.[52] Although PCO is a pathologic process, it has no known deleterious effects and therefore does not necessitate any treatment except follow-up. (See further discussion later.)

Dark discoloration of primary teeth is the most controversial posttraumatic complication in terms of the significance of the change in tooth color. The term "dark" refers to a variety of shades, including black, gray, brown, and intermediate hues.

When the pulp becomes necrotic or when pulpal hemorrhage occurs, red blood cells lyse and release hemoglobin. Hemoglobin and its derivatives, such as hematin molecules that contain iron ions, invade the dentin tubules and stain the tooth dark.[53,54] If the pulp remains vital and eliminates the pigments, the dark discoloration may fade, with subsequent restoration of the original color.[55] If the pulp loses its vitality and cannot eliminate the iron-containing molecules, the tooth may remain discolored.

If dark discolored primary incisors present additional signs such as swelling, fistula, or a periapical radiolucent defect, the diagnosis of pulp necrosis is easy. Controversy exists when the dark coronal discoloration is the only evidence of trauma to the tooth (see Fig. 40.17A). It has been found that over 70% of untreated dark discolored primary incisors remained without radiographic or clinical pathology.[56] Furthermore, asymptomatic primary incisors with persistent dark discoloration of the crown after trauma contain a necrotic or partially necrotic pulp.[39] It is not yet clear why some teeth acquire different hues of dark discoloration. An attempt to investigate the variations in the dark colors failed to show a correlation between the various shades and the condition of the pulp.[57] A study evaluating the effect of root canal treatment compared with follow-up only of asymptomatic dark discolored primary incisors showed that there is no difference in the fate of the primary incisors and the eruption pattern and appearance of the permanent successors.[58] It is therefore important to note that in the primary dentition of a healthy child, color change alone does not indicate a need for pulp therapy or extraction of the tooth.

Rapidly Progressing Root Resorption

Rapidly progressing root resorption (previously referred to as "inflammatory" resorption) can occur either on the external root surface or internally in the pulp chamber or canal (Fig. 40.18, see also Fig 41.13). It occurs subsequent to luxation injuries and is related to a necrotic pulp and an inflamed PDL.[59] It can progress very rapidly, destroying a tooth within months. Clinicians who choose to treat a patient with this condition when it occurs in the primary dentition use a resorbable paste of calcium hydroxide, iodoform or zinc oxide, and eugenol as an endodontic filling material. The operator should be aware of the possibility that the zinc oxide eugenol paste may not be completely resorbed with the root of the primary incisor and remain permanently in the surrounding tissue.[60]

Internal Resorption

The predentin, an unmineralized layer of organic material, covers the inner aspect of the dentin and protects it against access of odontoclasts. When the pulp becomes inflamed, as in cases of traumatic injury, the odontoblastic layer may lose its integrity and expose the dentin to odontoclastic activity, which is then seen on radiographs as radiolucent expansion of the pulp space. Eventually this process reaches the outer surface of the root, causing root perforation. If the coronal dentin is completely resorbed, the red color of the resorbing tissue becomes visible through the enamel. If internal resorption is detected early enough, it can be treated by removing the affected pulp, cleaning, rinsing, and filling the root canal with a resorbable paste.

External Resorption

The cementoblast layer and the precementum serve as a shield, protecting the root from involvement in the perpetual remodeling process of the surrounding bone. In nontraumatized primary teeth, external root resorption is part of the physiologic process of replacing the primary dentition with permanent teeth. In primary incisors sustaining traumatic injuries, external root resorption may appear as an accelerated unfavorable pathologic reaction. A variety of patterns of pathologic external root resorption can be seen in primary incisors after traumatic injury.

Rapidly progressing external root resorption, as in permanent teeth, is a rapid process characterized clinically by increased mobility of the tooth, sensitivity to percussion, a dull sound produced by percussion, and often a fistula or swelling in the gums above the tooth. Radiographically the PDL space is widened, and the root surface is irregular (Fig. 40.18). This condition may develop within a few weeks of the injury. Removal of the necrotic and probably infected pulp may stop the rapid phase of the resorption process; however, because of the unfavorable preexisting conditions, the benefit of root canal filling in saving the tooth is questionable. Traumatized primary incisors with rapidly progressing external root resorption and evidence of infection should therefore be extracted. It has been shown that root canal treatment in traumatized and infected primary incisors is highly correlated with enamel defects in the permanent teeth.[61]

External surface root resorption is characterized by gradual elimination of the root dentin with preservation of the PDL. The resorption process affects the apex of the root only, which becomes rounded, and progresses until natural exfoliation or traumatic avulsion occurs (Fig. 40.19). As the resorption progresses, bone replaces the space previously occupied by the root and separates the primary tooth and its permanent successor. Sometimes an intermediate stage exists in which osteoclasts attack the root along its apical half, leaving the coronal half unaffected. This type of external root resorption has been termed "atypical external root resorption."[56,62,63] The apical half is finally completely resorbed, leaving a shortened root with a rounded apex. The clinical appearance imitates that of natural but early exfoliation.

Root resorption associated with expansion of the permanent tooth follicle can be seen mainly, but not exclusively, in traumatized incisors with dark coronal discoloration (Fig. 40.20A). The follicle of the permanent tooth expands gradually and often does not become visible until close to the normal shedding age, even if the teeth were injured at an early age. Expansion of the follicle of the permanent tooth is rarely expressed clinically, and dark coronal discoloration is the only reason to suspect it.[64]

Occasionally, the hard expansion of the labial bone above the injured primary incisors can be observed or, better, palpated (see Fig. 40.20B). Usually, the primary tooth sheds normally and is followed by normal eruption of the permanent teeth.[56]

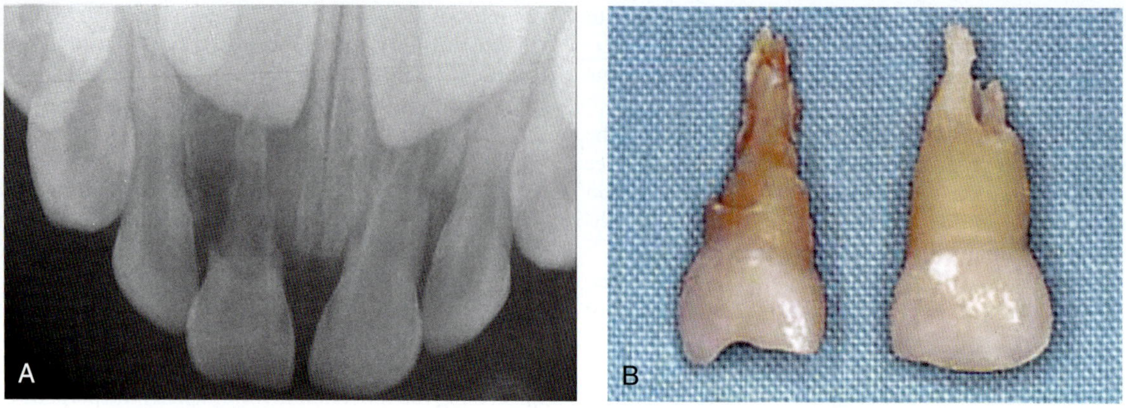

• **Fig. 40.18** (A) Periapical radiograph of the maxillary primary central incisors showing external inflammatory root resorption as a result of traumatic injury several months earlier. (B) The affected teeth after extraction. Notice the irregularity of the resorbed root surface.

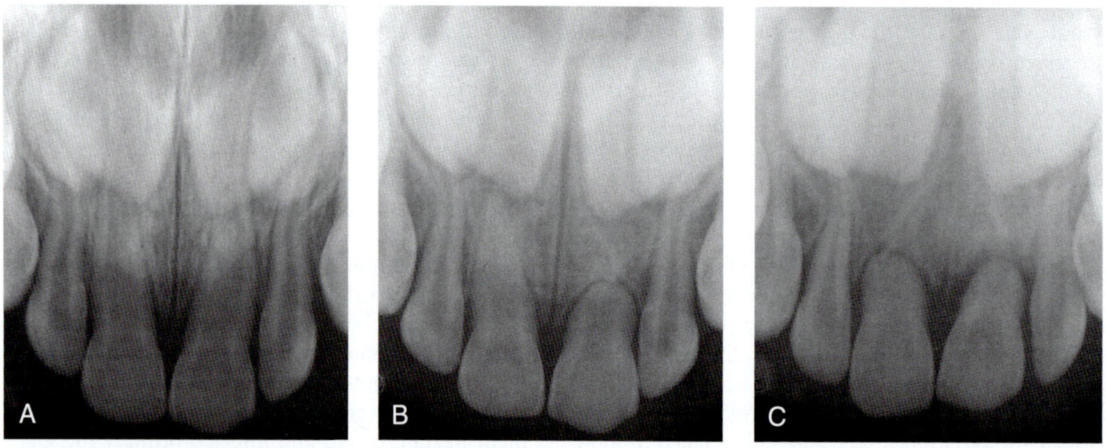

• **Fig. 40.19** Periapical Radiograph of Maxillary Primary Central Incisors With External Surface Root Resorption. (A) Shortly after the injury. (B) Twelve months after the injury. (C) Twenty-seven months after the injury.

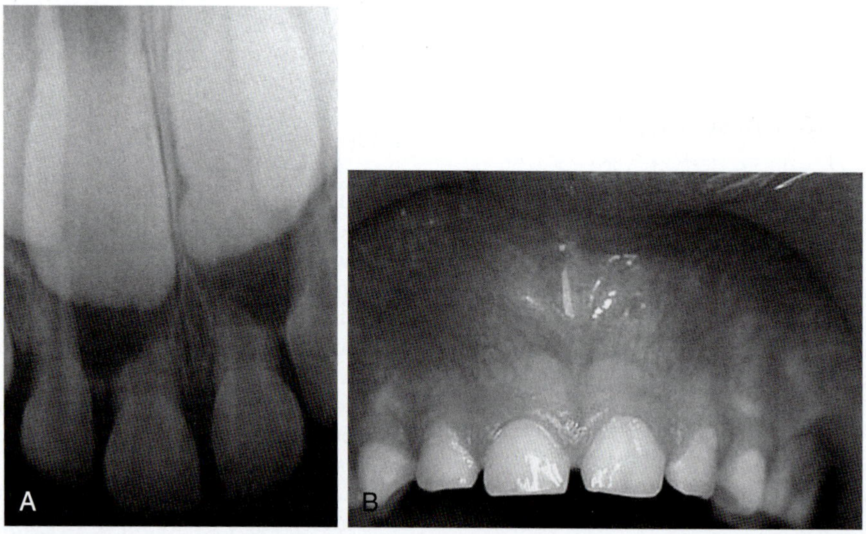

• **Fig. 40.20** (A) External root resorption associated with expansion of the follicle of the developing permanent tooth. (B) Clinical view that shows no pathologic signs except a hard expansion of the bone in the vestibule above the tooth.

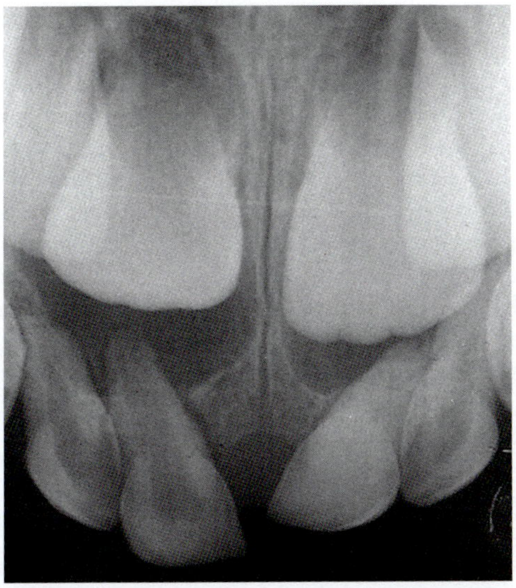

• **Fig. 40.21** Radiograph showing an infected expansion of the follicle of the permanent incisors with deflection of the right maxillary permanent central incisor from its normal alignment.

Occasionally, a dilated follicle becomes infected or the permanent tooth is deflected from its normal alignment (Fig. 40.21). Immediate extraction of the primary incisors is mandatory in these cases.

Replacement External Root Resorption

Replacement external root resorption, also known as ankylosis, results after irreversible injury to the PDL. Alveolar bone directly contacts and fuses with the root surface.[59] As the alveolar bone undergoes normal physiologic osteoclastic and osteoblastic activity, the root is resorbed and replaced with bone. Ankylosis occurs more often in intruded primary teeth, and they eventually become infraoccluded (Fig. 40.22).[39] Ankylosed primary teeth should be extracted if they cause a delay in or an ectopic eruption of a developing permanent tooth.

Pulp Canal Obliteration

PCO is the result of intensified activity of the odontoblasts that results in accelerated dentin apposition. Gradually, the pulp space narrows to a state in which it cannot be seen on a radiograph (see Figs. 40.5B, 40.15, 40.16A, and 40.22). PCO is a common finding in primary incisors after traumatic injuries and is often associated with yellow coronal discoloration.[65,66] As yet, however, the exact mode by which the impact to the tooth affects the odontoblasts is obscure. Although scientifically defined as a pathologic process, clinically it is not regarded as having deleterious effects. Ninety percent of primary teeth that have undergone PCO resorb normally[67]; therefore treatment in the primary dentition is usually not indicated.

Complications After Intrusion

Approximately two-thirds of intruded primary incisors reerupt and survive without any complications more than 3 years after the injury.[39] In most cases, however, the teeth do not return to their original position but reerupt into a rotated alignment (Fig. 40.23). If the child still uses a pacifier, it may occupy the space of the crown of the intruded tooth and prevent its reeruption back to the occlusal level. Intruded primary teeth may fail to reerupt if the root has been pushed out of the alveolar bone into the surrounding soft tissues (Fig. 40.24). These teeth should be extracted. Another reason for failure of intruded incisors to reerupt is damage to the PDL during the injury that results in ankylosis. It is not yet clear whether intervention is needed to remove the ankylosed tooth or if the root can be resorbed spontaneously with subsequent exfoliation of the tooth.

Periodontal breakdown due to infection is the main reason for loss of primary incisors after intrusion.[39] This can be prevented by

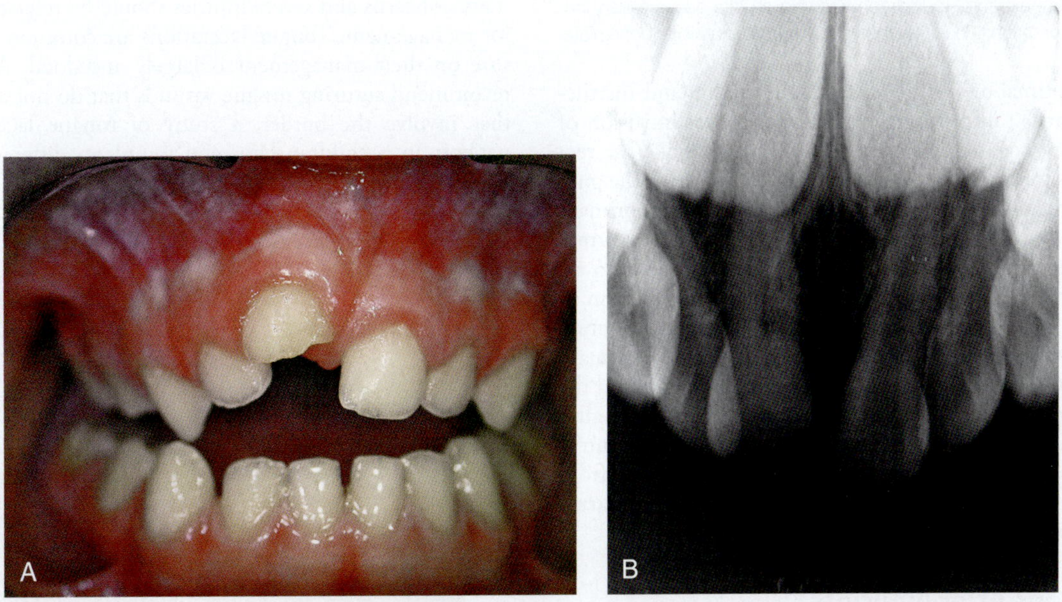

• **Fig. 40.22** (A) Clinical view showing infraposition of the maxillary right primary central incisor after an intrusion injury many months earlier. (B) Radiograph demonstrating ankylosis and pulp canal obliteration of the intruded primary incisor.

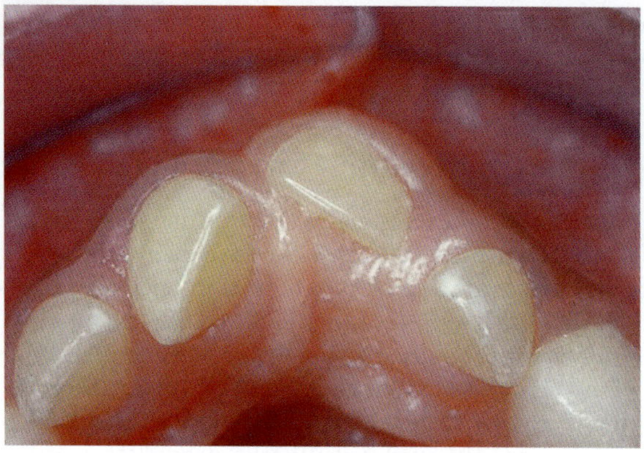

• **Fig. 40.23** Clinical View of the Maxillary Primary Incisors. Both central incisors were completely intruded and reerupted several weeks after the injury but into a rotated alignment. The teeth are clinically asymptomatic.

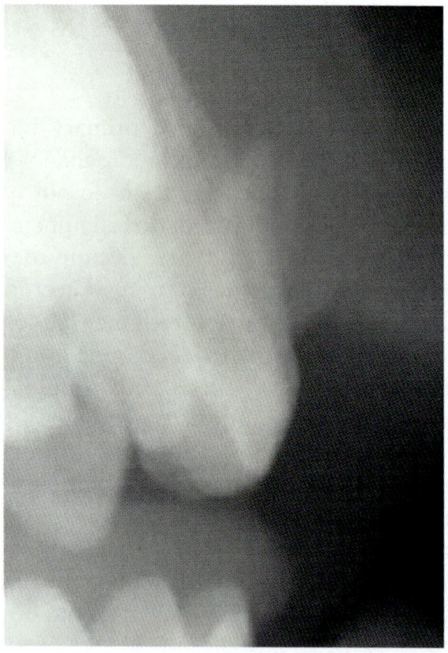

• **Fig. 40.24** Lateral extraoral radiograph showing an intruded maxillary primary central incisor that has been pushed out of the labial alveolar bone plate.

maintaining optimal oral hygiene (see "Information and Instructions for Parents"). Surprisingly, pulp necrosis after intrusion of primary incisors is not a common finding,[39] and unlike the recommendations for intruded permanent teeth, removal of the pulp is not recommended. Even if the apex of an intruded primary incisor avoids contact with its permanent successor, the permanent tooth may have still been damaged. It could have been affected during the sudden movement of the primary tooth from its original position to its final alignment. This explains the discrepancy found between the low percentage (10% to 20%) of primary incisors pushed toward the developing permanent teeth[39] and the high percentage (38% to 77%) of affected permanent teeth after intrusion of their primary predecessors.[44,68–70] The effect of intrusion of primary incisors on their permanent successors varies from discoloration and dysplasia of the enamel to eruption disturbances and crown dilacerations (Fig. 40.25).[71]

Complications After Avulsion

Several outcomes of early loss of primary incisors have been described in the dental literature.[72] Loss of space can be expected if the injury occurred before eruption of the primary canines and in children with a crowded dentition.[73] If primary incisors are lost before the child masters articulation, speech development may be affected.[74,75] However, articulation becomes normal after eruption of the permanent teeth.[76] The impact to the primary incisor pushes the tooth into the surrounding tissues before the tooth is completely detached from the PDL and damages the permanent successors in 38% to 85% of cases.[77,78] The younger the child is when injured, the higher the prevalence of damage to the permanent teeth.[44] Delayed and ectopic eruption of permanent incisors in cases of avulsion of their primary predecessors have been described and attributed to lack of guidance, development of scar tissue, and deflection of the developing permanent tooth bud by the injured primary incisor.[11]

Injuries to Developing Permanent Teeth

The most damaging sequelae of injuries to primary teeth are their effects on the unerupted developing permanent teeth. Anatomically, the permanent anterior teeth develop close to the apices of primary incisors (see Fig. 40.24). Thus a periapical pathologic process that is caused by necrotic pulps, intrusion injuries, or overinstrumentation of primary root canals can irreversibly damage the permanent teeth. If the injury occurs during the development of the permanent tooth crown, enamel hypoplasia or hypocalcification may occur (Fig. 40.25). These injuries can also alter the path of the developing permanent tooth crown, causing root dilaceration or ectopic eruption. For these reasons, the clinician should plan management of injuries to primary teeth with the ultimate objective of preventing or minimizing damage to the succeeding permanent teeth. Enamel calcification of permanent central incisor crowns is usually completed by age 4 years, so the risk of injury to them is greater in children younger than that.

Soft Tissue Injuries

Injuries to soft tissues frequently accompany dental injuries. Bleeding and swelling that could compromise the airway are primary concerns and severe injuries should be referred to a surgeon for management. Tongue lacerations are common and the literature on their management is largely anecdotal. Although some recommend suturing tongue wounds that do not approximate or that involve the border, a study of tongue lacerations in 28 patients in a children's hospital found no difference in healing

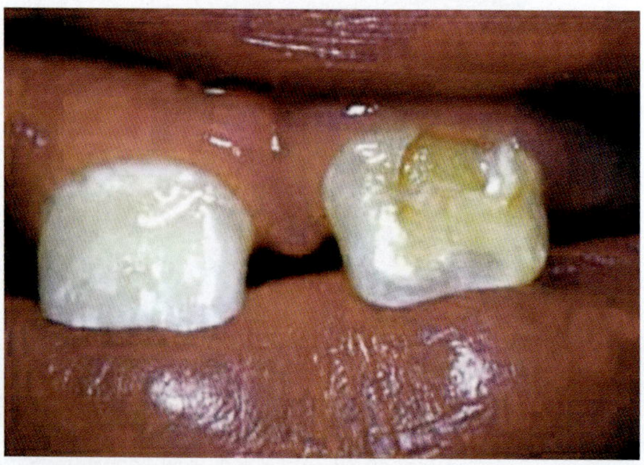

• **Fig. 40.25** Hypoplasia of the patient's maxillary left permanent central incisor as a result of intrusion of a primary incisor.

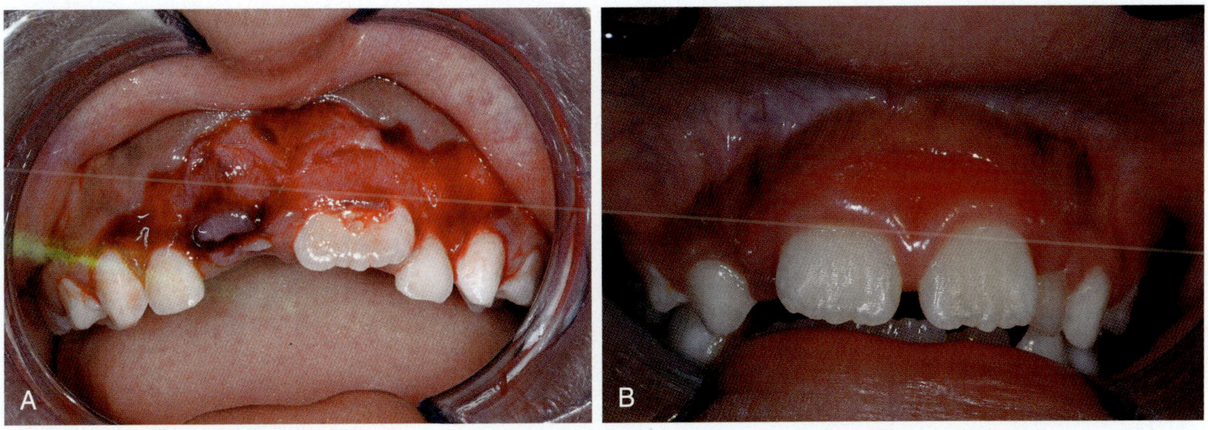

• **Fig. 40.26** (A) Day of injury. The child's attached gingivae was avulsed secondary to a bicycle accident. (B) Four months after injury.

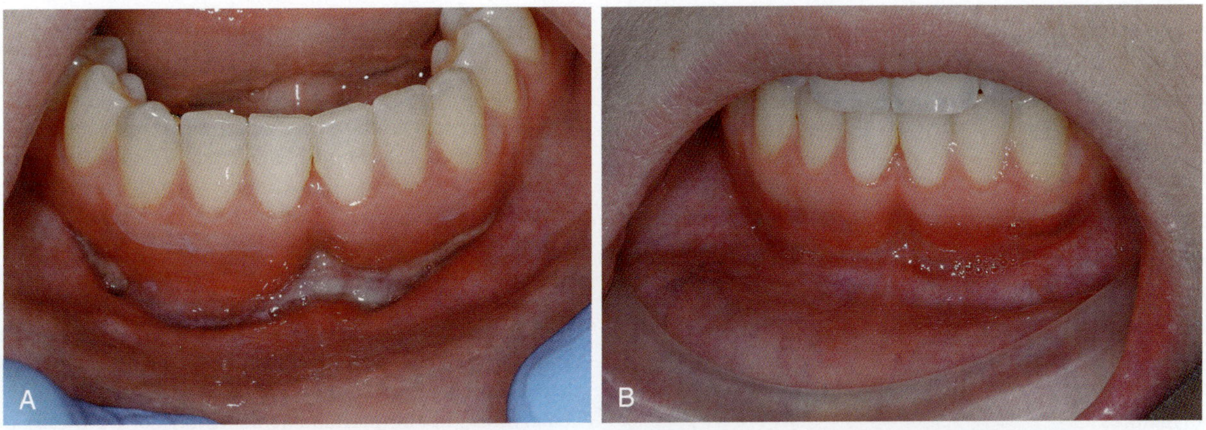

• **Fig. 40.27** (A) Two days after injury. Sulcus laceration extending canine to canine. (B) Ten days after injury.

outcomes whether the tongues were sutured or not.[79] An additional concern is behavior management as a young child may need sedation or general anesthesia to provide treatment.

Tooth fragments imbedded in the lip, as in Fig. 40.9, are particularly problematic. The fragments can be difficult to localize unless superficially positioned, and tissue swelling can compromise their recovery. They can sometimes be removed with thorough saline irrigation, but if this is unsuccessful, the patient should be referred to a surgeon.

Fortunately, intraoral wounds can heal well if undisturbed. Loose flaps of attached gingivae or oral mucosa should be reapproximated with sutures, if possible, but in some cases placing sutures is not possible. Fig. 40.26 demonstrates a case where the child's attached gingivae was totally avulsed secondary to a bicycle accident. The wound was debrided, and, as the periosteum was intact, no treatment other than a 0.12% chlorhexidine twice daily mouthrinse was provided. The wound healed well by secondary intention. Fig. 40.27 illustrates a wound in the sulcus of the lower lip that extended canine to canine. The child presented two days after the injury. No bleeding was occurring, and the wound was well approximated, so no sutures were placed. The child rinsed twice per day with 0.12% chlorhexidine rinse, and the wound healed uneventfully.

Wounds that are contaminated by dirt or debris should be thoroughly debrided. The child's tetanus immunization status should be checked as a booster may be indicated. Systemic antibiotics may also be considered if secondary infection is a concern.

Severe soft tissue injuries such as those caused from (1) biting on electrical cords, (2) thermal burns from ingesting scalding liquid, (3) chemical burns from ingesting cleaning or drain solution, and (4) animal bites should be referred for prompt medical attention and managed in a hospital setting with a multidisciplinary team.

Summary

Injuries to a young child's teeth can have long-lasting effects. Proper management, focusing on diagnosis, treatment, and follow-up care, can minimize long-term consequences. Thus it is important for dentists to stay updated and accessible for urgent care. Flowcharts for managing injuries are included in eFigs. 40.28–40.31, and the website www.dentaltraumaguide.org is recommended for current information on dental injury management.

Visit eBooks.Health.Elsevier.com to see full list of references.

41

Managing Traumatic Injuries in the Young Permanent Dentition

DENNIS J. MCTIGUE AND EHSAN N. AZADANI

CHAPTER OUTLINE

Injuries to the primary dentition are discussed in Chapter 40. Also covered there are the following fundamental areas relevant to managing trauma in children of any age:

- Classification of traumatic injuries to teeth
- Medical and dental history
- Clinical and radiographic examinations
- Common reactions of teeth to trauma
- Soft tissue trauma

This chapter deals with injuries to the young permanent dentition, but the reader is strongly advised to review the fundamental areas just noted in Chapter 40. Frequent reference will be made to them. Additionally, clinical pathways outlining treatment options for all injuries are available online in eFigs. 41.20 to 41.24.

The reader is encouraged to review and use an excellent online resource, "The Dental Trauma Guide" (www.dentaltraumaguide.org), to assist in diagnosing and treating tooth injuries. This guide, developed by Dr. Jens O. Andreasen and sponsored in part by the University Hospital, Copenhagen, and the International Association of Dental Traumatology (IADT),[1] contains updated guidelines on a broad array of injuries and is easy to use.

Etiology and Epidemiology of Trauma in the Young Permanent Dentition

Falls during play account for most injuries to young permanent teeth. Children engaging in contact sports are at greatest risk for dental injury, though the use of mouthguards greatly reduces their frequency (see Chapter 42). In the teenage years, automobile accidents cause a significant number of dental injuries when occupants not wearing seat belts hit the steering wheel or dashboard. As noted in Chapter 40, children with seizure disorders also injure their permanent teeth more frequently. In contrast to the primary dentition, permanent teeth suffer crown fractures more frequently than luxation injuries. The lower crown-root ratio and denser alveolar bone in the permanent dentition contribute to this phenomenon. Maxillary central incisors are again most commonly injured, and protruding incisors are at greatest risk (Fig. 41.1).[2]

Classification of Injuries to Young Permanent Teeth

Classification of tooth fractures and luxation injuries is discussed in Chapter 40 (see Fig. 41.1).

History

The essential elements of the medical and dental history are discussed in Chapter 41. The use of a trauma assessment form to help organize the gathering of historical and clinical data is emphasized (see Fig. 40.8). The potential for child abuse should be considered and followed up per the discussion in Chapter 43. The reader is reminded to determine the status of the child's tetanus prophylaxis and to consult the child's physician if there is any question about its adequacy.

Another issue worthy of review relates to the potential for injury to the central nervous system. Older children are likely to suffer harder blows at play, and thus the dentist should find out if the child lost consciousness or became disoriented or nauseated after the injury. Positive findings indicate immediate medical consultation. As noted in Chapter 40, significant head injuries can lead to symptoms many hours after the initial trauma, and parents should be cautioned to watch for the signs noted previously for

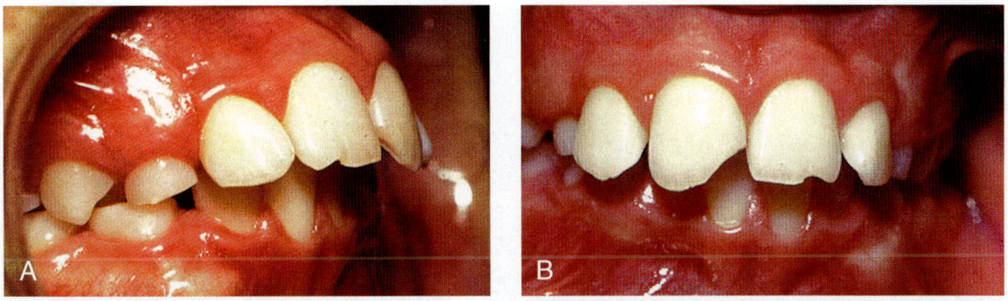

• **Fig. 41.1** (A) Lateral view showing large horizontal overjet. (B) Same patient with fractured central incisors. (From McTigue DJ. Management of orofacial trauma in children. *Pediatr Ann.* 1985;14:125-129.)

24 hours, including waking the child every 2 to 3 hours throughout the night.[3–5]

Clinical Examination

Refer to Chapter 40 for a thorough discussion of the clinical examination. An important difference between the primary and permanent dentition exists in respect to "vitality" or sensibility testing. Whereas it is not routinely performed in the primary dentition, sensibility testing can be a useful diagnostic aid in the permanent dentition. The dentist should be aware that pulp testing might not elicit reliable responses from erupting permanent teeth and from those with open apices. Furthermore, recently traumatized teeth may not respond to any sensibility test for several months. Positive findings immediately after a traumatic injury are thus more valuable for assessing pulp vitality than are negative responses.

Cold testing with agents like difluorodichloromethane or carbon dioxide snow yields the most reliable results,[6] although the thermal shock of the low temperature applied can cause infraction lines in the enamel.[7] Some clinicians prefer electrical vitality testing because it uses a stimulus that can be gradually increased and precisely recorded. Using both cold tests and electric pulp tests provided the best sensitivity and specificity in a group of adult patients.[8]

Pulp tests that use cold or electrical impulse do not actually measure "vitality" because that requires confirmation of uninterrupted blood flow through the pulpal tissue. Instead, these tests measure neural response, which serves as a proxy for vascular health. Laser Doppler flowmetry has potentially great clinical value because this technique directly measures blood flow and does not rely on sensory nerve response.[9] This technique is also painless and is reliable in teeth with immature apices.[10] However, modifications in this instrument's design and a significant reduction in its cost are necessary for it to achieve widespread use. Another noninvasive technique that has potential diagnostic value is pulse oximetry, which measures blood oxygen saturation in the vessels monitored.[11,12] Although there is currently no commercial product available, future technologic advances will enable development of affordable devices that attach to teeth and will give the clinician a better measure of tooth vitality.

Principles of radiographic diagnosis for permanent teeth do not differ from those for primary teeth. A common error made by dentists in diagnosing traumatic injuries is to take an insufficient number of radiographs. Additional views taken from slightly different angles both vertically and horizontally can significantly improve the accuracy of diagnosis.[13]

It is important to note the urgency of follow-up radiographs after injury. Reviewing radiographs at 1 month after injury will detect signs of pulpal necrosis and rapidly progressing (inflammatory) resorption. At 2 months, replacement resorption can be detected.[13]

Cone beam computed tomography (CBCT) enables the clinician to view a three-dimensional image of a dental injury.[14] The increased radiation, complexity, and cost of this procedure, however, contraindicate its use in children for most dentoalveolar injuries. CBCT should be used only when the patient's history and a clinical examination demonstrate that the benefits to the patient outweigh the potential risks. The clinician should use CBCT only when the need for imaging cannot be met by lower dose two-dimensional radiography.

With the technical improvements in cell phone photography and electronic health records, capturing good clinical images of dental injuries is now relatively easy and is recommended. Photographs document the initial injury, follow-up, soft tissue healing, and reeruption of intruded teeth. They are also valuable for insurance and medicolegal issues that might arise. Further, photos forwarded by a parent/caregiver or emergency department medical staff can greatly assist the dentist in triaging an injury and planning immediate care.[13]

Pathologic Sequelae of Traumatized Teeth

Refer to Chapter 40 for a discussion of the pathologic sequelae of traumatized teeth.

Treatment of Traumatic Injuries to the Permanent Dentition

The dentist treating a traumatic injury follows essentially the same principles of gathering historical information and completing a clinical examination, regardless of the child's age. Furthermore, the pathologic sequelae of injuries to teeth are similar for both primary and permanent teeth. However, there are many significant differences in the way that injuries to permanent teeth are treated. As in the primary dentition, a complete diagnostic workup (described in Chapter 40) should precede all treatment. Even though a blow may cause little, if any, obvious injury to a permanent tooth, it may lead to pulp necrosis as a result of disruption of the neurovascular bundle at the apex of the tooth. Posttreatment evaluation is indicated for all traumatic injuries.

Enamel Fractures

In some cases, minor enamel fractures can be smoothed with fine disks. Larger fractures should be restored using an acid-etch/composite resin technique (see Chapter 31 for restorative techniques).

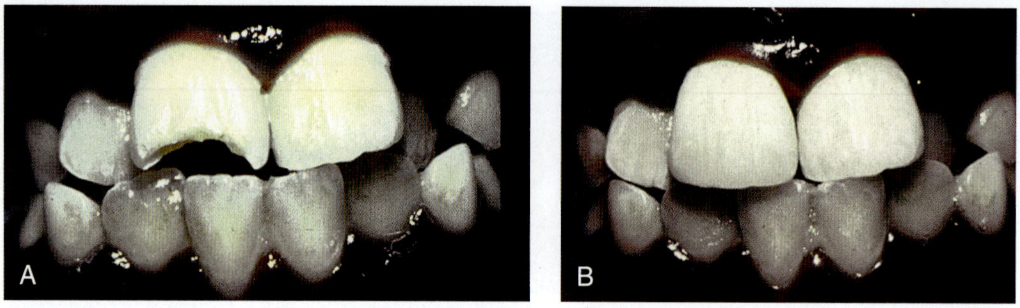

• **Fig. 41.2** A fractured incisor (A) can quickly be restored using an acid-etch/composite resin technique (B).

Enamel and Dentin Fractures

The IADT Guidelines classify dental fractures as either "uncomplicated," meaning there is no pulpal exposure, or "complicated," meaning that the pulp has been exposed. The primary issue in managing fractures that expose dentin is to prevent bacterial irritants from reaching the pulp. Standard care in the past called for covering exposed dentin with calcium hydroxide (CaOH) or glass ionomer cement to seal out oral flora. Sealing exposed dentin with a bonding agent enables the unexposed pulp to form reparative dentin. Some clinicians have then advocated simultaneous acid etching of dentin and enamel, followed by dentin and enamel bonding without placement of CaOH or glass ionomer.[15] However, a review of pulp capping with dentin adhesive systems reported that these systems are not indicated owing to increased inflammatory reactions, delay in pulp healing, and failure of dentin bridge formation.[16] The authors recommend covering the deepest portion of dentin fractures with glass ionomer cement, followed by a dentin-bonding agent (see Chapter 31). The tooth can then be restored with an acid-etch/composite resin technique (Fig. 41.2). If adequate time is not available to restore the tooth completely, an interim covering of resin material (a resin "patch") can temporize the tooth until a final restoration can be placed. If a resin material cannot be placed due to cooperation or isolation issues, a resin-modified glass ionomer temporary coverage is acceptable. Some dentists routinely place such a partial restoration to ensure an appropriate posttreatment evaluation when the patient returns for the final restoration. This is a reasonable strategy, if care is taken to ensure an adequate seal. Another option may be to immediately rebond a fractured segment to the injured tooth. Refer to Chapter 32 for a description of this technique.

Fractures Involving the Pulp

The management of crown fractures that expose the pulp is particularly challenging (Fig. 41.3 See also Fig. 31.8). Pertinent clinical findings that dictate treatment include the following:

1. Vitality of the exposed pulp
2. Degree of root maturation of the fractured tooth
3. Restorability of the fractured crown

The objective of treatment in managing these injuries is to preserve a vital pulp in the entire tooth (see Chapter 33). This allows for physiologic closure of the root apex in immature teeth. It is important to note that root end closure does not signal completion of root maturation. Progressive deposition of dentin normally continues in roots through adolescence, making them stronger and more resistant to traumatic insult. Maintaining a vital pulp in the tooth crown allows the clinician to monitor the tooth's vitality periodically.

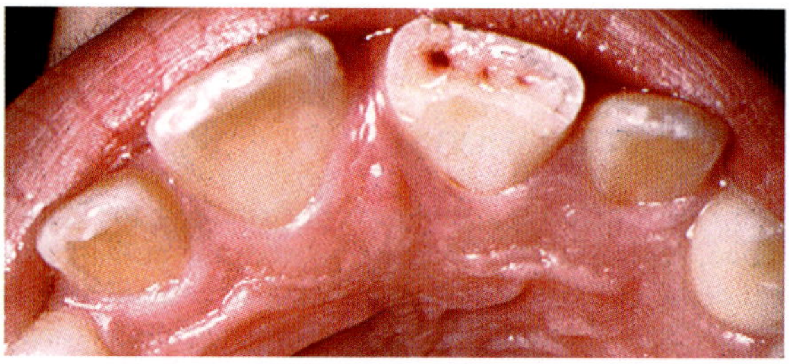

• **Fig. 41.3** Crown fracture exposing the pulp.

For crown fractures with pulpal exposure, three treatment alternatives are available, based on the clinical findings just noted:

1. Pulpotomy
2. Direct pulp cap
3. Pulpectomy

Pulpotomy

The objectives of the pulpotomy technique are to remove only the inflamed pulp tissue and to leave healthy tissue to enhance physiologic maturation of the root. Owing to its significantly higher success rate, pulpotomy is favored over the next potential option, direct pulp cap.

It is difficult to determine clinically how far the inflamed pulp extends. The tooth shown in Fig. 41.4 had been fractured for 4 days with a pulp exposure approximately 3 mm in diameter. The dentist elected to remove all tissue in the pulp chamber, with obvious success. Fig. 41.4B demonstrates complete maturation of the root, including apical closure and dentinal wall thickening as well as a calcific barrier at the amputation site. However, maintaining some pulp tissue in the crown allows the dentist to monitor the vitality of the tooth and thus is preferable when possible.

Cvek noted that in most cases of pulps exposed for more than a few hours, the initial biologic response is pulpal hyperplasia.[17] Inflammation in these cases rarely extends beyond 2 mm. In his study involving 60 teeth with pulps exposed from 1 hour to 90 days, Cvek removed only 2 mm of the pulp and the surrounding dentin. He covered the pulp stumps with CaOH and reported a success rate of 96% (Figs. 41.5 and 41.6). More recently, studies have substantiated the superiority of partial pulpotomy compared with direct pulp cap even for exposures up to 4 mm and performed days after the injury.[18]

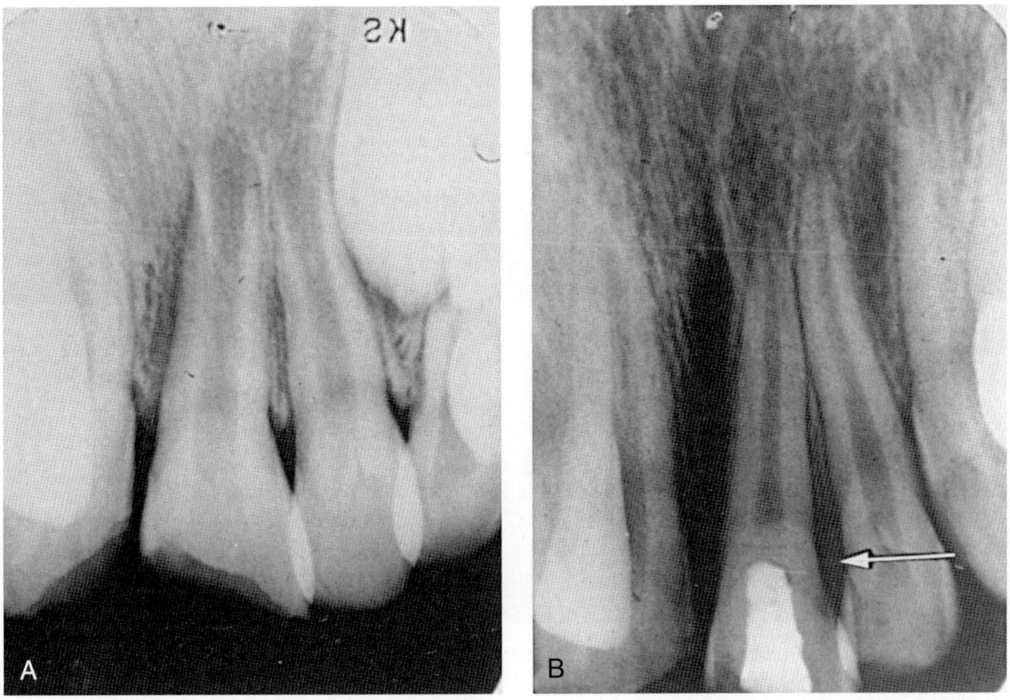

• **Fig. 41.4** (A) Crown fracture exposing the pulp in an immature permanent incisor. Note the open apex and thin dentinal walls in the root. (B) A calcium hydroxide pulpotomy stimulated the formation of a calcific barrier *(arrow)* and enabled the root to mature, demonstrating apical closure and root wall thickening.

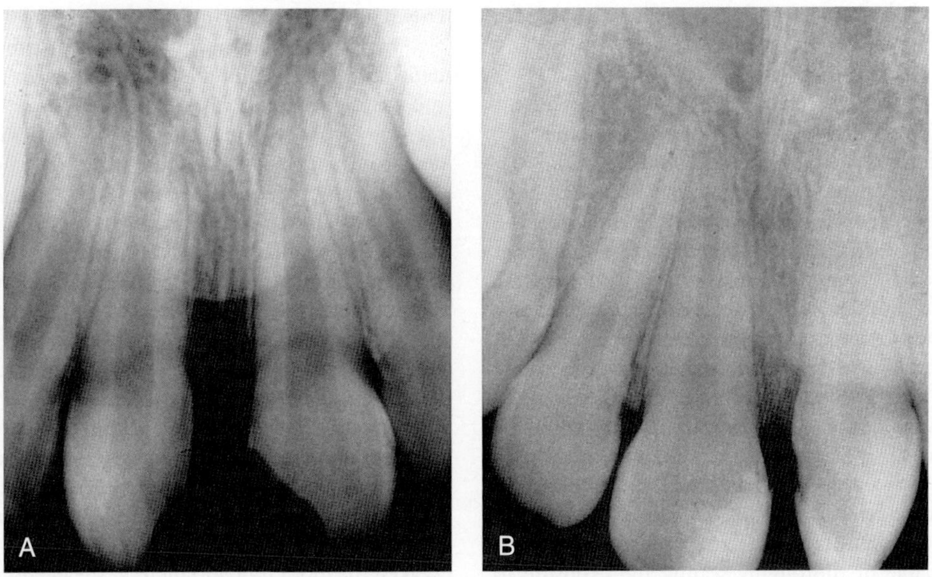

• **Fig. 41.5** (A) Maxillary right permanent central incisor suffered crown fracture with pulp exposure. (B) One-year postoperative radiograph of the same tooth successfully treated with a calcium hydroxide partial pulpotomy. Note completion of root development both apically and laterally.

Absolute isolation to prevent contamination of the pulp with oral bacteria is essential. The inflamed pulp is gently removed to a level approximately 2 mm below the exposure site with a sterile diamond bur at high speed. Copious irrigation is mandatory to avoid pulp injury. The preparation should provide adequate space for the pulp dressing material and a layer of glass ionomer seal. Cleaning the cavity and the pulpal surface using a small cotton pellet and sodium hypochlorite is recommended. Attaining a bacteria-tight coronal seal is essential for the success of this technique. The tooth can then be esthetically restored with composite resin. See also Chapter 33 Case Study: Management of Complicated Crown Fractures in Permanent Teeth details the partial pulpotomy technique.

Mineral trioxide aggregate (MTA) has been shown to perform well in pulpotomies, causing dentinal bridge formation while maintaining normal pulpal histologic features.[19,20] As noted previously, however, its tendency to stain teeth is a clinical concern.[21]

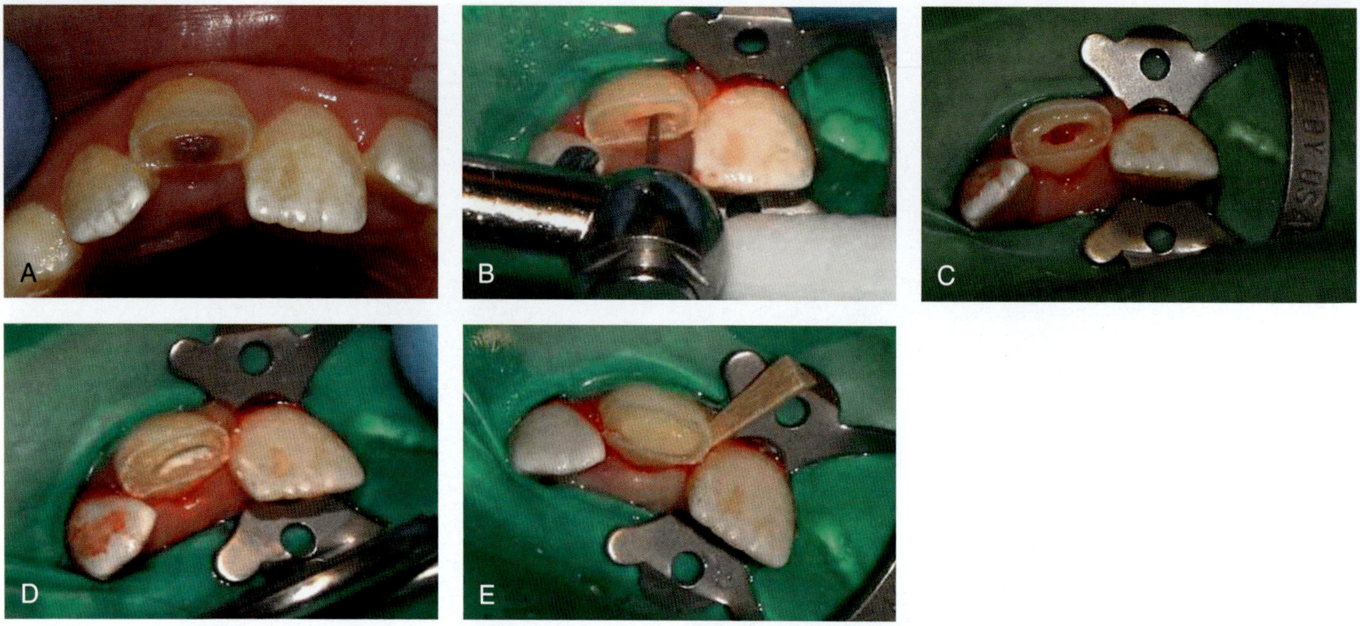

• **Fig. 41.6** Partial Pulpotomy Technique. (A) Complicated crown fracture of the maxillary right central incisor, exposing the pulp. (B) Removing pulp to a depth of 2 mm with sterile diamond bur. (C) Blood clot after pulp amputation. (D) Calcium hydroxide base on pulp stump. (E) Glass ionomer seal. (Courtesy Dr. Ashok Kumar.)

See Chapters 32 and 33 for details on its use. Nonstaining MTA or any nonstaining biocompatible calcium silicate cement designed for direct introduction to live pulpal tissue may be used for this technique.

Direct Pulp Cap

The direct pulp cap is only indicated in exposures that cannot be treated with a pulpotomy. This may be because of the child's behavior or inability to access adequate facilities (such as in a hospital emergency department) or because treatment of other injuries is prioritized over dental care. A direct pulp cap can be completed quickly with less armamentarium than a pulpotomy and can serve as a temporary bandage until a pulpotomy can be completed.

The chances for pulp healing decrease if the tissue is inflamed, has formed a clot, or is contaminated with foreign materials. The objective, then, is to preserve vital pulp tissue that is free of inflammation and physiologically walled off by a calcific barrier.

A rubber dam is applied, and the tooth is gently cleaned with water. Commercially available CaOH paste, MTA, or other nonstaining calcium silicate cement is applied directly to the pulp tissue and to surrounding dentin.[22] It is essential that a restoration be placed that is capable of thoroughly sealing the exposure to prevent further contamination by oral bacteria. As in the management of dentin fractures, it is acceptable to use an acid-etch/composite resin system for an initial restoration. A calcific bridge stimulated by the capping material should be evident radiographically in 2 to 3 months. Although MTA for direct pulp caps has been reported to be as successful as CaOH,[23] significant discoloration of the tooth crown can occur with its use (see Fig. 33.2).[21]

In fractures exposing pulps of immature permanent teeth with incomplete root development, a direct cap is never the treatment of choice. Failure in these cases leads to total pulpal necrosis and a fragile, immature root with thin dentinal walls. As noted earlier, the direct cap can serve as a temporary bandage until a pulpotomy can be performed.

Pulpectomy

A pulpectomy involves complete pulp tissue removal from the crown and root and is indicated when no vital tissue remains. It is also indicated when root maturation is complete, and the permanent restoration requires a post buildup. In the absence of rapidly progressing (inflammatory) root resorption, treatment is to obturate the canal with gutta-percha. The reader is referred to standard endodontic textbooks for more information on this technique.

One of the greatest challenges facing the clinician is the treatment of a nonvital immature permanent tooth with an open apex. See Chapter 33 Nonvital Pulp Treatment for Immature Teeth for more detailed information about various techniques. Physiologic root maturation cannot occur without the presence of vital pulp tissue, apical papilla stem cells, odontoblasts, and the Hertwig epithelial root sheath.[24] Traditional treatment for these cases was an apexification procedure wherein CaOH was carried to the root apex to contact vital tissues directly. The CaOH stimulated the formation of a cementoid barrier against which gutta-percha could subsequently be condensed. Multiple visits over a period of 9 to 18 months were required, however, and the outcome was a shortened root with thin walls (Fig. 41.7).[25] In addition, long-term CaOH therapy may weaken the tooth root and increase the likelihood of root fractures.[26]

An alternative to the CaOH apexification technique for managing devitalized immature incisors is the apical barrier technique using MTA or other biocompatible preparations designed for the purpose of root repair.[27] The material is condensed into the apical area. Gutta-percha is then condensed against the MTA barrier typically followed by warm gutta-percha backfill (Fig. 41.8). Though overall treatment time is greatly reduced, the shortened root and thin walls continue to place the tooth at risk for subsequent cervical root fracture.

Regenerative Endodontics

Iwaya, Hoshino, and others reported a dramatic alternative to apexification of necrotic immature teeth termed revascularization

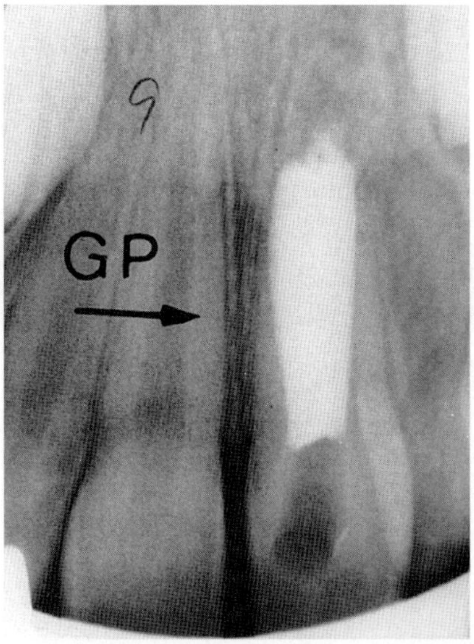

• **Fig. 41.7** An apexification procedure allowed this immature permanent tooth to be obturated successfully with gutta-percha (GP). The root, however, remains fragile and at increased risk of future trauma because no further dentinal wall apposition can occur.

or "regenerative" endodontics.[28–30] These procedures seek to replace damaged dentin, root structures, and pulp cells with live tissues that restore normal physiologic function.[31] The concept is to thoroughly disinfect the root canal system and then stimulate bleeding from the apical papilla to fill the root chamber with a blood clot. A host of growth factors in the area then act on dental stem cells, primarily from the apical papilla, to use the clot as a scaffold and differentiate into healthy cells of the pulp-dentin complex that can complete physiologic root maturation.

The technique (Fig. 41.9) is to first cleanse the canal by extirpating the necrotic pulp followed by copious irrigation with sodium hypochlorite or ethylenediaminetetraacetic acid.[32] Owing to the immature status of the root and thin radicular walls, instrumentation is kept to a minimum and used mainly to agitate the irrigant. The canal space is then dried using sterile paper points. Antibacterial medication or CaOH is carefully placed into the canal up to the cementoenamel junction (CEJ) to avoid discoloration.[29,33] The access cavity is sealed with a sterile cotton pellet and glass ionomer cement.

The patient is scheduled for a follow-up appointment in 3 to 4 weeks. At the follow-up appointment, the area is anesthetized with local anesthetic containing no epinephrine. The antibiotic paste or CaOH is rinsed out, and a sterile endodontic file is placed beyond the apex to initiate bleeding. A clot is allowed to form as close to the CEJ as possible to facilitate root thickening at the tooth cervix. MTA or similar material is then placed against the clot or a collagen barrier, and the final restoration is placed. Root maturation should be apparent radiographically within several months (Fig. 41.10).[34,35]

Regenerative endodontics is still an emerging field, and no evidence-based guidelines are available to inform the clinician about its precise indications or technique. As this treatment may involve several lengthy appointments, its use is limited to young children who are unable to cooperate. Other options such as apexification should be considered in those situations.

Criteria for Success

Criteria to judge success of the techniques used to manage pulpal insult in fractured teeth include the following:

- Completion of root development in immature teeth
- Absence of clinical signs such as pain, mobility, or fistula
- Absence of any radiographic signs of pathologic processes, such as periapical radiolucency of bone or root resorption

Posterior Crown Fractures

Posterior crown fractures in the permanent dentition pose a restorative challenge for the clinician. These fractures usually occur secondary to hard blows to the underside of the chin, and vertical crown fractures may result (Fig. 41.11). Although bonding with posterior composite resins is sometimes possible, full coverage with stainless steel or cast metal crowns is often the only restorative alternative. The reader is reminded to watch for mandibular fractures and cervical spine injuries in these cases.[36]

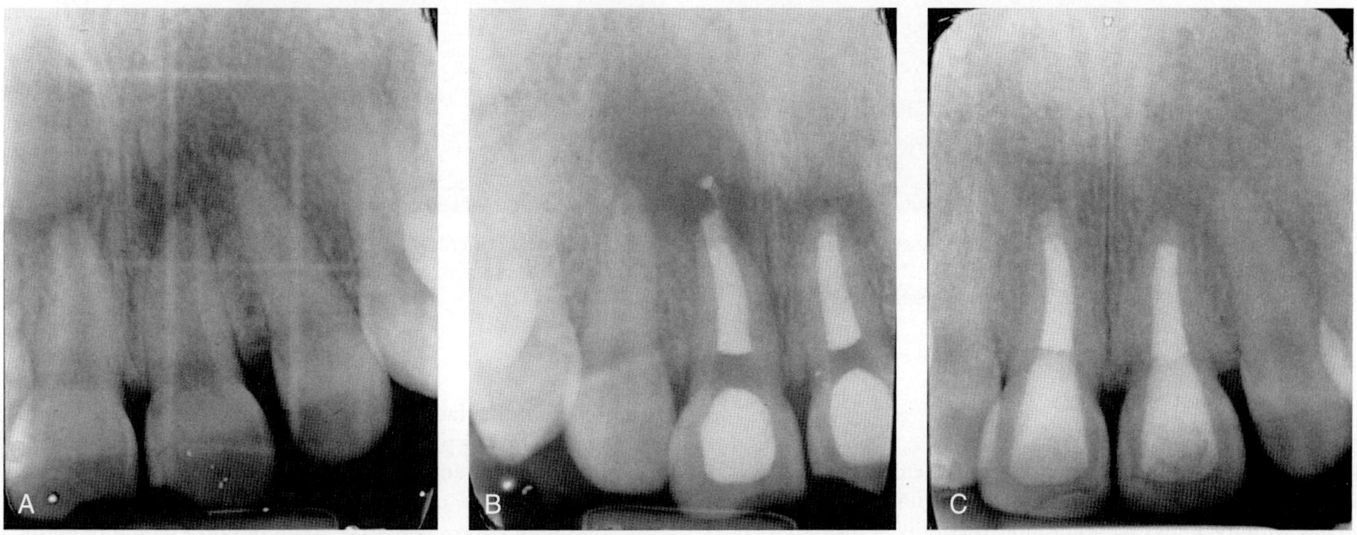

• **Fig. 41.8** Apexification Using Apical Barrier Technique. (A) Preoperative view. (B) Four-week postoperative view. (C) Twenty-seven-month postoperative view.

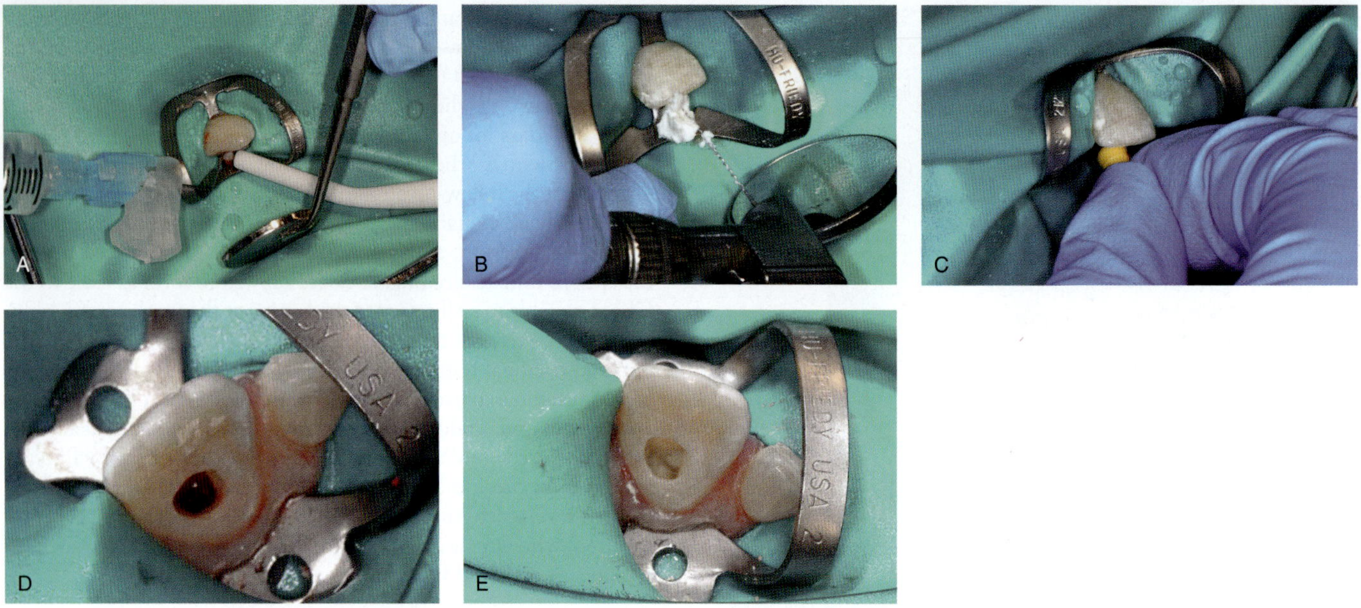

• **Fig. 41.9** Regenerative Endodontic Technique. (A) Copious irrigation of pulp canal with sodium hypochlorite. (B) Spinning triple antibiotic paste. (C) Stimulating bleeding by extending file 2 to 3 mm beyond tooth apex. (D) Blood clot at cervix of tooth. (E) Mineral trioxide aggregate placed on blood clot.

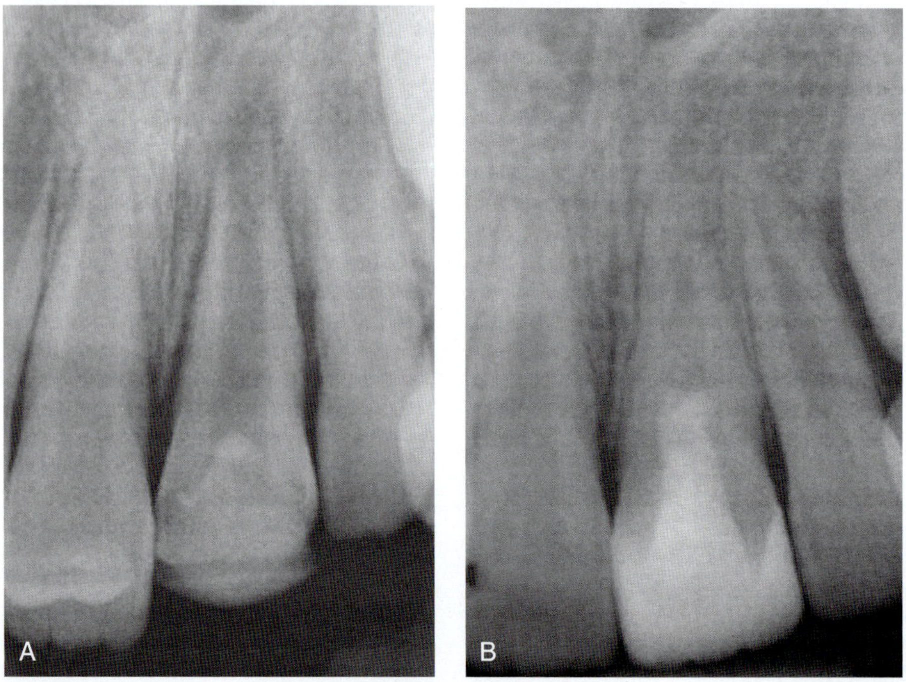

• **Fig. 41.10** Successful Revascularization of Necrotic Immature Permanent Left Maxillary Central Incisor. (A) Preoperative radiograph of immature incisor with complicated crown fracture, open apex, and apical periodontitis. (B) Twenty-seven-month postoperative view. Note apical closure and root wall thickening.

Root Fractures

The prognosis for root fractures is best when the fracture occurs in the apical one-third of the root. The prognosis worsens progressively with fractures that occur more cervically in the root. Bender and Freedland reported that more than 75% of teeth with intraalveolar root fractures maintain their vitality.[37]

A tooth with a fractured root is usually mobile, and its coronal fragment is often displaced. Several baseline radiographs should be taken from various angulations to verify the extent of the fracture. Optimal results are obtained if the coronal fragment is repositioned as soon as possible.[13] The tooth position should be verified radiographically. Accurate repositioning of the tooth enhances the likelihood of both hard tissue healing of the root fracture and pulp

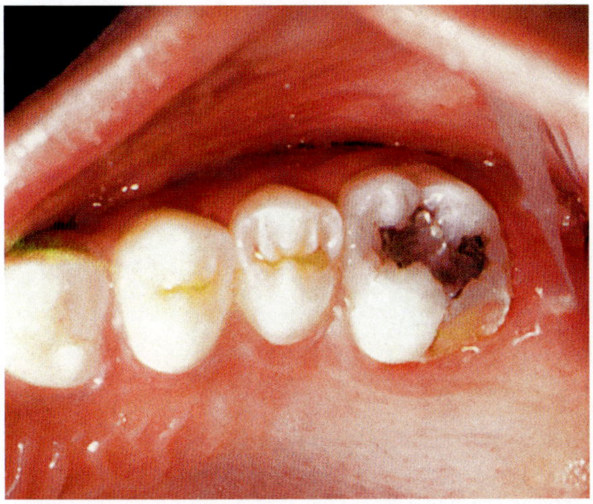

• **Fig. 41.11** A vertical crown fracture of the distolingual cusp of this maxillary molar occurred secondary to a blow to the underside of this child's chin.

healing.[38] Immature teeth with incompletely formed root apices and positive pulp sensitivity at the time of injury are also significantly related to pulp healing and hard tissue repair of the fracture.

Tooth splinting techniques are detailed later in this chapter; however, current evidence indicates that teeth with roots fractured in the apical and middle thirds heal better if splinted for only 3 to 4 weeks with a functional splint that allows for some mobility of the teeth.[13,39] Teeth sustaining cervical third root fractures should be stabilized with a flexible splint for 3 to 4 months.

Root canal therapy should not be initiated until clinical and radiographic signs of necrosis or resorption are apparent. Even in those cases, treatment can often be limited to the coronal fragment because in most instances the apical fragments maintain their vitality. As the coronal fragment lacks apical constriction, a technique similar to MTA apexification should be used to obturate the coronal fragment.

Managing Sequelae to Dental Trauma

In Chapter 40, common reactions of the teeth to trauma, including pulpal necrosis, are described. Three of the most challenging sequelae include pulp canal obliteration (PCO), rapidly progressing (inflammatory) resorption (both external and internal), and replacement resorption. These pathologic processes can occur after crown fractures or luxation injuries.

Pulp Canal Obliteration

PCO is a degenerative pathologic process that ultimately leads to obliteration of the pulp canal (Figs. 41.12 and 41.13B). Andreasen showed that its occurrence depends on the type of luxation injury sustained and the stage of root development.[40] Thus immature teeth with open apices suffering moderate to severe injuries are likely to undergo PCO. It was noted previously that most primary teeth with PCO resorb normally, and thus treatment is usually not indicated. A conservative approach is also recommended for PCO in the permanent teeth. Current evidence indicates that pulp necrosis is an uncommon sequela of PCO, reportedly as low as 1%[40] or as high as 33%.[41] Crown discoloration (yellowing) may occur more frequently due to increased dentin thickness, which makes the crown less translucent. Endodontic procedures can be successfully completed in a great majority of obliterated canals if necessary.[7] The dentist is advised, then, to closely monitor PCO in permanent teeth and to initiate endodontic procedures only in response to periapical changes or for prevention of coronal discoloration in fully mature teeth.

Rapidly Progressing (Inflammatory) Resorption

Rapidly progressing (inflammatory) resorption can occur externally, internally, or both (see Fig. 41.13). It commonly arises after

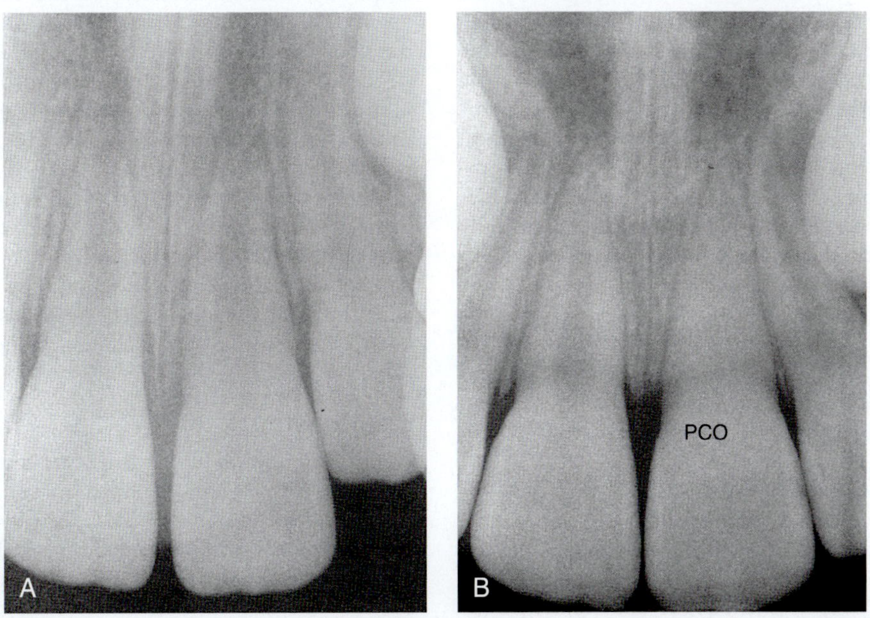

• **Fig. 41.12** (A) Ten-day postoperative view of immature maxillary left central incisor in 7-year-old child that had been extruded and repositioned. (B) Sixteen-month postoperative view demonstrating pulp canal obliteration (PCO).

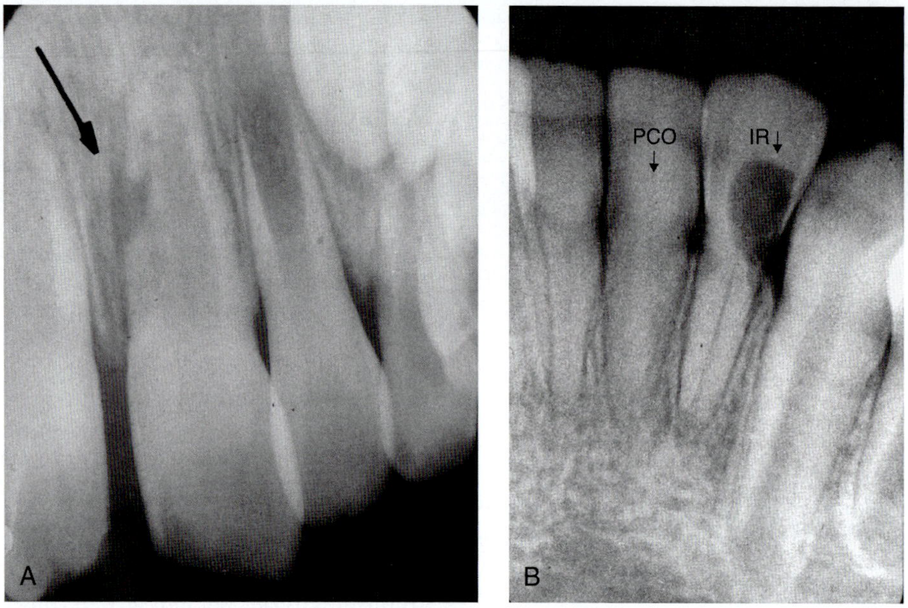

• **Fig. 41.13** (A) External rapidly progressing resorption *(arrow).* (B) Internal resorption (IR) of the lateral incisor; pulp canal obliteration (PCO) of the permanent central incisor. (B, From McTigue DJ. Management of orofacial trauma in children. *Pediatr Ann.* 1985;14:125-129.)

luxation injuries when the periodontal ligament (PDL) is inflamed, and the pulp is necrotic.[42] Odontoclastic activity can occur so rapidly that the teeth are destroyed in a matter of weeks. Rapidly progressing resorption can be prevented by prompt extirpation (within 3 weeks) of the pulp in mature teeth that have suffered luxation injuries with significant tooth displacement. Luxated teeth with open apices should be observed closely, and their pulps should be extirpated at the first sign of pulp necrosis or root resorption. Regenerative endodontic or apical barrier techniques are then indicated to complete treatment.

Immediate management of rapidly progressing resorption is essential. As soon as this process is detected radiographically, the pulp tissue in the tooth is thoroughly extirpated. Copious irrigation with sodium hypochlorite assists in the dissolution of organic debris in the canal. In permanent teeth, CaOH is placed in the canal with a technique identical to that used to induce apexification (see Chapter 33). Here the objective is not to induce apical closure but to create an environment unfavorable for the resorptive process. It is theorized that CaOH has antiseptic properties because of its extreme alkalinity. This medicament apparently percolates through the dentinal tubules to the areas of resorption at the PDL and halts its progress.[42]

CaOH should be retained in the tooth until radiographic signs of healing are apparent. This may take several months, and repeated applications of CaOH may be necessary if the resorption progresses. When radiographs confirm that the process has stopped, gutta-percha is placed as the final filling material.

Replacement Resorption (Ankylosis)

Replacement resorption occurs most commonly after severe luxation injuries like avulsions or intrusions, in which PDL cells are destroyed. Alveolar bone directly contacts cementum on the involved tooth and fuses with it. Then, as the bone undergoes its normal physiologic, osteoclastic, and osteoblastic activity, the root is resorbed or replaced with bone (Fig. 41.14). In young children with rapid bone turnover, roots are completely resorbed in 3 to 4 years. In adults, the process may take up to 10 years. Replacement resorption can be prevented by prompt and appropriate management of luxation injuries.

Treating Luxation Injuries in the Permanent Dentition

The reader is referred to Chapter 40 for the definition of the various types of luxation injuries. Luxation injuries damage the supporting structures of the teeth—that is, the PDL and alveolar bone. In addition, in mature teeth with closed apices, the pulp frequently becomes necrotic. Careful monitoring of the pulp's vitality is essential, and extirpation should be completed if clinical or radiographic signs of necrosis appear. Pulp necrosis occurs less frequently when immature teeth with open apices are luxated, but, as noted earlier, PCO is a common finding in these cases. Thus in luxation injuries the health of both the pulp and the PDL must be considered.

The vitality of the *PDL* is far more important than *pulp* vitality in determining the prognosis of luxated teeth. The primary objective of treatment in these injuries is to maintain PDL vitality. Clinical and radiographic monitoring in the weeks and months after the injury is critical. The reader is referred to the IADT Guidelines' recommended follow-up times for each specific type of injury.[13]

Concussion

Concussion injuries in permanent teeth must be followed closely. Although the prognosis is normally good, pulp necrosis and root resorption have been reported. Generally, no treatment is needed other than monitoring of the pulp vitality for a year. Involved teeth can be carefully taken out of occlusion if the child reports pain.

Subluxation

Pulp necrosis occurs far more commonly in subluxated permanent teeth than in primary teeth, especially in permanent teeth

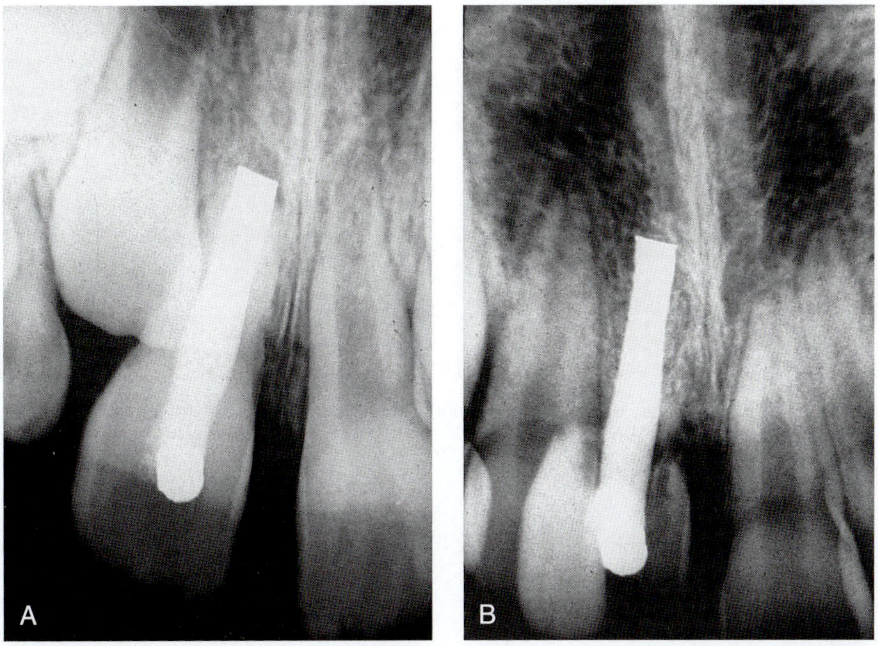

• **Fig. 41.14** (A) A permanent incisor that had been avulsed and stored dry for 3 hours was filled with gutta-percha before reimplantation. (B) Three years later, replacement resorption has completely destroyed the root.

with closed apices. These teeth should be monitored closely with radiographs for at least 1 year, and root canal therapy should be instituted at the first sign of pathologic change. Immature teeth with open apices are less likely to undergo pulpal necrosis. Splinting of subluxated teeth is often not necessary. However, when it is required for patient comfort, splinting should be limited to a maximum of 2 weeks.[13]

Intrusive Luxation

The prognosis for intruded permanent teeth is guarded. These teeth frequently undergo pulpal necrosis, root resorption, and alveolar bone loss. Treatment for intruded teeth is controversial, owing to the lack of research in this area.[43] Guidelines published by the IADT recommend different strategies, depending on the apical development of the intruded tooth.[13]

The treatment of choice for immature teeth is to allow them to reemerge spontaneously. Pulp vitality must be closely monitored. If no movement is noted within 4 weeks, orthodontic repositioning using light forces should be employed (Fig. 41.15).

Mature permanent teeth intruded less than 3 mm should be allowed to reemerge without intervention. If no movement is noted within 8 weeks, they should be repositioned surgically and splinted for 4 weeks or extruded orthodontically before they ankylose. Those teeth intruded beyond 7 mm should be repositioned surgically. For mature teeth intruded between 3 and 7 mm, evidence is scarce to clearly indicate whether orthodontic or surgical repositioning is preferable; however, surgical repositioning is often preferred. Surgical repositioning is favored because it will facilitate the pulp extirpation in intruded teeth that would otherwise be difficult to access. The pulp in mature intruded teeth will likely become necrotic as the blood vessels at the apex of the tooth have undergone ischemia; this will lead to rapidly progressing resorption, so the pulp should be extirpated within 2 weeks after the injury. CaOH should be placed in the root canal using the same technique as described for apexification in Chapter 33, and the CaOH in the canal should be replaced if signs of root resorption persist. Radiographic monitoring of the tooth should occur for at least 1 year.

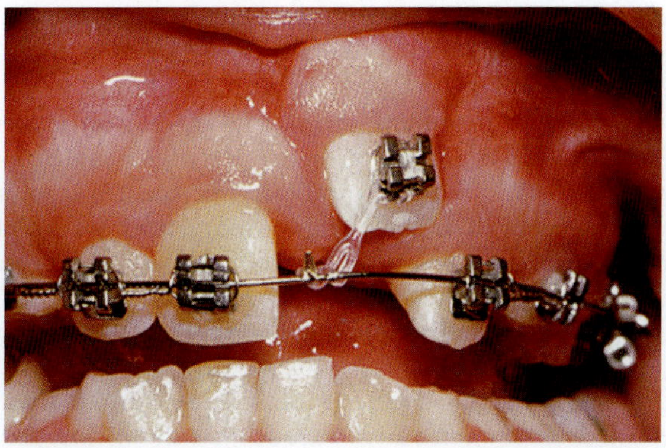

• **Fig. 41.15** Orthodontic repositioning of intruded permanent incisor prevents replacement resorption (ankylosis) and alveolar bone loss.

Extrusion

Extruded permanent teeth (Fig. 41.16A) should be repositioned as soon as possible and splinted for 2 to 4 weeks depending on whether fracture of the marginal bone exists. It normally takes the PDL fibers this period to reanastomose. Extruded permanent teeth with closed apices will undergo pulpal necrosis; therefore root canal therapy should be initiated within 3 weeks. Extruded teeth with open apices have a chance to revascularize and maintain their vitality, so the decision to initiate therapy should be delayed until clinical or radiographic signs indicate necrosis.

Lateral Luxation

Fracture of the marginal bone or alveolar socket wall frequently occurs in lateral luxation injuries and can complicate their management

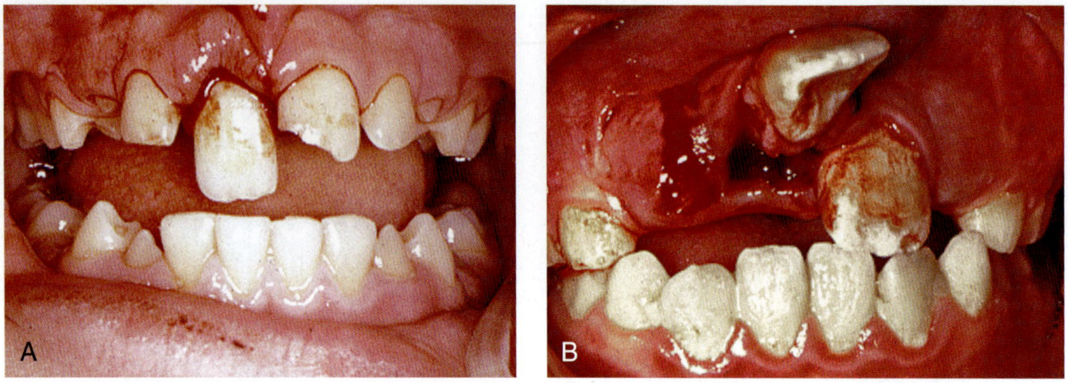

• **Fig. 41.16** (A) Extrusion injury of maxillary right central incisor and crown fracture of maxillary left central incisor. (B) Laterally luxated tooth.

(see Fig. 41.16B). In the most severe cases, PDL and marginal bone loss occur. Treatment is to reposition the teeth and alveolar fragments as soon as possible. A splint should then be applied for 4 weeks or longer, depending on the degree of bone involvement. The authors' current protocol includes prescribing a 0.12% chlorhexidine mouthrinse to assist with hygiene and to minimize gingival inflammation.[1] If the apices are closed, the pulps will likely become necrotic; therefore endodontic therapy should be instituted 2 weeks after the teeth are splinted. Again, teeth with open apices should be monitored until signs of necrosis are evident.

Avulsion

The prognosis for long-term retention of an avulsed permanent tooth worsens the longer the extraoral "dry time" (time tooth is out of its socket).[44] The primary therapeutic concern is to maintain the vitality of PDL fibers, and the longer they are out of the mouth, the worse the prognosis for their survival. It is imperative that the avulsed tooth be immediately replanted by the first capable person, whether that person is a parent, teacher, or sibling (Fig. 41.17).

Owing to a variety of circumstances, it is sometimes not possible to replant a tooth immediately. Research has shown that the best transport medium for avulsed teeth is cell culture media such as ViaSpan (DuPont Merck Pharmaceutical Company, Wilmington, DE) or Hanks Balanced Salt Solution (HBSS; United Biochemicals, Sanborn, NY).[45] ViaSpan is not readily available for clinical use, but HBSS is commercially available as EMT Tooth Saver (Biochrom AG, Berlin, Germany). Use of HBSS significantly increases the likelihood of PDL cell survival for several hours.[46]

The best alternative storage medium if culture media or HBSS is not available is cold milk.[47,48] It is readily available, it is relatively aseptic, and its osmolality is more favorable to maintaining the vitality of the PDL cells than is saline solution or tap water. Cold milk has been shown to maintain the ability of PDL precursor cells to reproduce for twice as long as room temperature milk.[49] Ice should not be added to milk, which would alter its osmolarity (a bag or cup of milk containing the tooth can be put on ice). Though some studies have indicated that storing the tooth in the patient's mouth (saliva) may be favorable toward PDL survival, the danger of an alarmed child swallowing, aspirating, or chewing on the tooth eliminates this option in the authors' opinion. Water is *not* a good transport medium because it is a hypotonic solution and causes PDL cells to swell and rupture. In cases in which the tooth cannot be immediately replanted, with the tooth stored in cold milk, the patient should be taken to the dentist as soon as possible.

Because root resorption is so closely correlated with the extraoral dry time, the dentist should replant the tooth in its socket as soon as possible after the child arrives. Adequate evidence exists, however, to support the immediate placement of the avulsed tooth into HBSS while the patient is brought to the dental office and appropriate informed consent is being obtained from the parent.[6] Soaking the tooth may reduce ankylosis and help debride necrotic cells, foreign bodies, and bacteria. The authors' current protocol is again to prescribe an oral mouthrinse of 0.12% chlorhexidine used empirically to reduce the likelihood of bacterial invasion of the PDL space. Controversy exists regarding the benefit of systemic antibiotics for pulp or periodontal healing.[50–52] Given the evidence that systemic antibiotics can prevent bacterial invasion of the necrotic pulp,[53] the IADT Guidelines recommend a 1-week course of doxycycline for tooth avulsion in patients age 12 or older.[1] The decision to prescribe antibiotics should also be based on other factors such as the presence of soft tissue wounds contaminated by dirt and other debris. Doxycycline is preferred, owing to its antiresorptive properties[54]; however, tetracycline antibiotics are known to stain developing teeth. Therefore penicillin V is the antibiotic of choice for children under 12 years. Oral doxycycline can be prescribed 2.2 mg/kg/dose every 12 hours and penicillin V 25 to 75 mg/kg/day given in divided doses every 6 to 8 hours. Evidence that systemic antibiotics improve the clinical outcomes of avulsed teeth is lacking.

When immature teeth with open apices are avulsed, the ideal treatment objective is healing: spontaneous revascularization of the pulp in addition to maintenance of PDL health. This would enable physiologic maturation of the immature root, including apexogenesis and root wall thickening. The tooth should be splinted for approximately 1 to 2 weeks. See Case Study: Splinting for an Avulsed Tooth. Success in these cases has been reported; therefore dentists should await clinical or radiographic signs of necrosis before initiating regenerative endodontic therapy. When the splint is removed, the dentist may note that the tooth is quite mobile. This mobility is preferable to long-term rigid splinting, because the latter has been correlated with an increased incidence of replacement resorption. The mobility of the tooth physiologically interrupts areas of incipient resorption/ankylosis on the PDL, allowing it to heal normally.

In mature teeth with closed apices, a flexible splint that affords the tooth functional mobility should be applied for 7 to 14 days. One to two weeks after the avulsion injury, the necrotic pulp

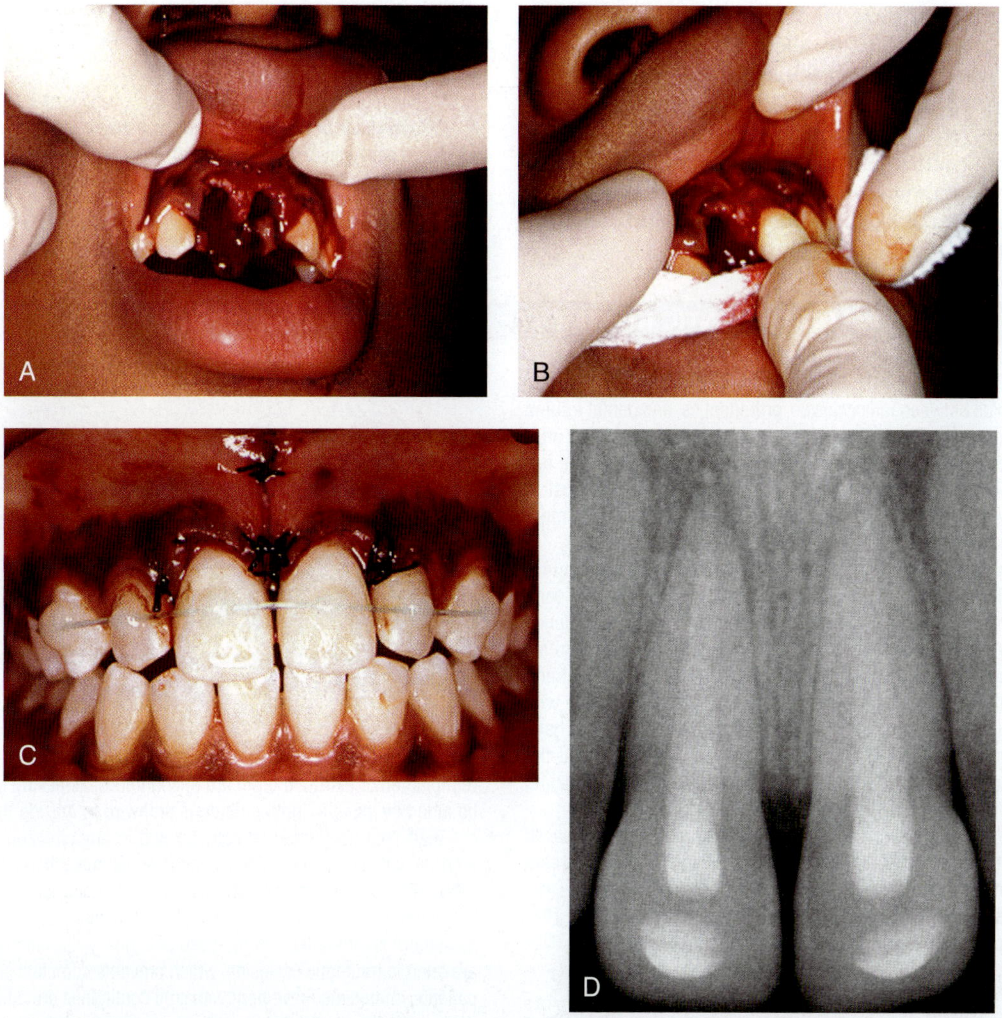

• **Fig. 41.17** (A) Both maxillary permanent central incisors avulsed. (B) Reimplanting avulsed teeth with finger pressure. (C) Esthetic, flexible splint fabricated using 50-pound test monofilament fishing line retained with composite resin. (D) Calcium hydroxide pulpectomies completed to prevent rapidly progressing resorption. (Courtesy Dr. Jeff Hays.)

should be extirpated, and CaOH should be placed to prevent the initiation of rapidly progressing inflammatory root resorption (see Fig. 41.17D). Importantly, root canal therapy should not be performed in the hand before replantation. This extends the extraoral dry period and places the PDL at greater risk to injury as a result of the additional manipulation of the tooth. In cases where the pulp was not removed within 2 to 3 weeks of the replantation, or when rapidly progressing resorption is evident radiographically, the CaOH should be maintained in the tooth until radiographic signs of healing are apparent. The authors' preference is to postpone the gutta-percha obturation until there are no signs of progressive inflammatory root resorption or replacement resorption. As a general recommendation, this typically takes 2 to 4 months for patients after the prepubertal growth spurt and longer for those before the prepubertal growth spurt. The CaOH can then be removed and a gutta-percha obturation completed.

PDL cells on avulsed teeth that have been stored dry for more than 1 hour are necrotic, and these teeth will eventually ankylose and resorb.

In summary, the procedure for replantation of an avulsed tooth after obtaining profound local anesthesia is as follows:

1. Hold the tooth by the crown to prevent damage to the PDL.
2. Gently rinse the tooth with the best solution that is immediately available. Water is acceptable provided the tooth is immediately replanted. No attempt should be made to scrub or sterilize the tooth.
3. Manually replant the tooth in the socket as soon as possible. In cases where resistance is encountered, the socket can be irrigated with normal saline to remove the blood clot.
4. Apply a light, functional splint for 1 to 2 weeks.
5. Complete CaOH pulpectomy after 1 week and then remove splint.

Splinting Technique

Various methods of splinting teeth have been advocated, but it is apparent that the ideal splint should possess the following characteristics:

1. Be passive and not cause trauma
2. Be flexible and allow functional movement of the tooth
3. Allow for vitality testing and endodontic access
4. Be easy to apply and remove

Many splints can meet these criteria, and several good commercial products are available. To allow for flexibility, a light orthodontic arch wire or a 30- to 60-pound test monofilament fishing line can be used (see Fig. 41.17C). After splint application, patients should be given postinjury instructions (Box 41.1). For all traumatic dental injuries, patients should be counseled on the necessity of follow-up appointments to monitor for progressing disease and to improve the likelihood of tooth survival. See Case Study: Splinting for an Avulsed Tooth.

• BOX 41.1 Postinjury Instructions for Patients

- Soft diet for the duration of the splint
- Maintain good oral hygiene
- Chlorhexidine 0.12% mouthrinse for a week
- Avoid activities with risk of dental injury
- Return for follow-up as instructed

PREVENTIVE/INTERCEPTIVE ORTHODONTIC TREATMENT

Henry Fields

There are relationships between malocclusion, orthodontics, and dental trauma patients. Certain types of malocclusions are more prone to trauma, and after trauma, orthodontics can play a role in treatment. The data are clear that patients with protrusive teeth (excess overjet) and incompetent lips are most at risk for traumatic dental injuries (TDIs)—as are children with previous primary dentition TDIs or permanent dentition TDIs before 9 years of age.[1–3]
If this is the case, why not just provide early phase I orthodontic treatment for children with significant class II malocclusion? Information from the two early treatment randomized prospective clinical trials combined with experience from Britain do not make the case based on an analysis of the benefits of treatment.[4] This is especially true if we recognize that most TDIs are enamel and dentin fractures with moderate long-term sequelae compared with those with periodontal type injuries (intrusion, extrusion, avulsion, and luxation) that have significant long-term consequences. It can be reasonably concluded that the benefits of treatment for this latter group can have an impact, but predicting who is most at risk is not easy.

Given this fact, early orthodontic treatment for those who have increased overjet, incompetent lips, and a history of permanent dentition TDI before 9 years old makes some sense if the treatment is limited to retraction of the incisors (not early class II growth modification) and then definitive orthodontics later. This, combined with a mouthguard that is worn consistently, can greatly reduce TDI.

Orthodontic Treatment for Immediate Trauma

There is a place for orthodontics, as mentioned in this chapter, after TDI for patients who have experienced intrusion, avulsion, and lateral luxation injuries. Contemporary thought is that all immature intruded and mature teeth intruded less than 3 mm should have a chance to reerupt for approximately 4 weeks and 8 weeks, respectively.[12] For those with mature roots intruded 3 to 7 mm and for those that do not actively or completely reerupt after observation, orthodontic traction can be useful. Orthodontics as an alternative to surgical repositioning appears to have better supporting tissue outcomes[5] but may be impractical in terms of treatment time and appointments required as the intrusion approaches or exceeds 7 mm. Although there are many methods to extrude teeth, using a light flexible overlay wire like 0.012 or 0.014 NiTi, supported by a heavier base wire (0.016 or 0.018 steel), is relatively simple and effective (Fig. 41.18). Conversely, when avulsed teeth are not completely

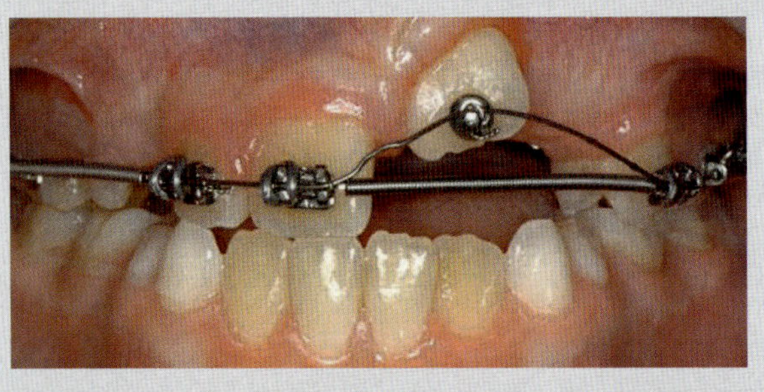

• Fig. 41.18 Extrusion using a base wire and a flexible overlay wire. Remember that the method works by having the overlay wire slide through the brackets, so loose steel ties are recommended. Probably extending the overlay wire through one bracket on either side of the intruded tooth is adequate because the more brackets, the more friction that is incurred and the slower the movement.

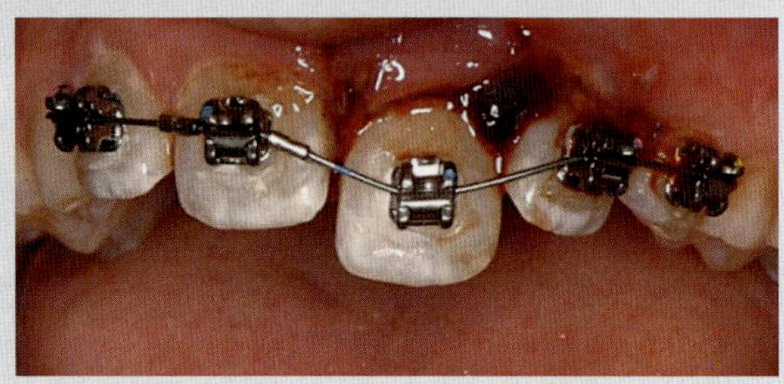

• Fig. 41.19 Intrusion or alignment can sometimes be accomplished by a continuous flexible wire, while monitoring any negative reactive side effects.

reimplanted or extruded teeth are encountered, achieving good positioning can be aided by using a light continuous archwire to intrude them (Fig. 41.19).

Teeth that have been laterally luxated in any direction can be immediately repositioned and splinted. If this cannot be accomplished and they have consolidated in a new position without occlusal interference, ideally waiting for 3 months is recommended, as one would with a transplanted tooth before orthodontic movement is attempted.[6] In the case of lingually displaced maxillary teeth, they are often in traumatic occlusion, which prevents complete jaw closure. For these patients, immediate movement with light continuous orthodontic forces is best to better align the teeth and eliminate the occlusal interferences.

Orthodontic Treatment for Patients With Traumatic Dental Injuries

There is often a question of when to start orthodontic treatment for patients with TDIs. Should treatment begin immediately, or should there be a period of healing before starting orthodontic tooth movement? Current recommendations suggest delaying orthodontic treatment for 3 months for minor dental trauma such as concussion, subluxation, and crown fractures. If the patient sustains major dental trauma (avulsion, root fracture, severe luxation), orthodontic treatment should possibly be delayed for up to 1 year to allow healing and determine the status of the injured teeth.[7]

Patients who have experienced orthodontic treatment and trauma are more at risk for root resorption and pulpal necrosis of the injured teeth than those who have had either orthodontics or trauma alone.[8–10] Those teeth with completed endodontic treatment are usually less prone to root resorption than normal teeth.[11]

Orthodontics can also be helpful after traumatic injury when teeth are missing and spaces need to be closed or teeth repositioned for subsequent restorative treatment. The advent of temporary anchorage devices has altered the possibilities for tooth movement dramatically in these cases.

References

1. Bauss O, Freitag S, Rohling J, et al. Influence of overjet and lip coverage on the prevalence and severity of incisor trauma. *J Orofac Orthop.* 2008;69:402-410.
2. Goettems ML, Brancher LC, da Coasta CT, et al. Does dental trauma in the primary dentition increases the likelihood of trauma in the permanent dentition? A longitudinal study. *Clin Oral Investig.* 2017;21:2415-2420.
3. Glendor U, Koucheki B, Halling A. Risk evaluation and type of treatment of multiple dental trauma episodes to permanent teeth. *Endod Dent Traumatol.* 2000;16:205-210.

PREVENTIVE/INTERCEPTIVE ORTHODONTIC TREATMENT—cont'd

4. Thiruvenkatachari B, Harrison JE, Worthington HV, et al. Orthodontic treatment for prominent upper front teeth (Class II malocclusion) in children. *Cochrane Database Syst Rev.* 2013;(11):CD003452.
5. Andreasen JO, Bakland LK, Andreasen FM. Traumatic intrusion of permanent teeth: part 3—a clinical study of the effect of treatment variables such as treatment delay, method of repositioning, type of splint, length of splinting and antibiotics on 140 teeth. *Dent Traumatol.* 2006;22:99-111.
6. Paulsen HU, Andreasen JO, Schwartz O. Pulp and periodontal healing, root development and root resorption subsequent to transplantation and orthodontic rotation: a long-term study of autotransplanted premolars. *Am J Orthod Dentofacial Orthop.* 1995;108:630-640.
7. Kindelan SA, Day PF, Kindelan JD, et al. Dental trauma: an overview of its influence on the management of orthodontic treatment: part 1. *J Orthod.* 2008;35:68-78.
8. Brin I, Ben-Bassat Y, Heling I, et al. The influence of orthodontic treatment on previously traumatized permanent incisors. *Eur J Orthod.* 1991;13:372-377.
9. Bauss O, Scheafer W, Sadat-Khonsari R, et al. Influence of orthodontic extrusion on pulpal vitality of traumatized maxillary incisors. *J Endod.* 2010;36:203-207.
10. Bauss O, Reohling J, Sadat-Khonsari R, et al. Influence of orthodontic intrusion on pulpal vitality of previously traumatized maxillary permanent incisors. *Am J Orthod Dentofacial Orthop.* 2008;134:12-17.
11. Spurrier SW, Hall SH, Joondeph DR, et al. A comparison of apical root resorption during orthodontic treatment in endodontically treated vital teeth. *Am J Orthod Dentofacial Orthop.* 1990;97:130-134.
12. Bourguignon C, Cohenca N, Lauridsen E, et al; International Association of Dental Traumatology guidelines for the management of traumatic dental injuries: intrusive luxation. *Dent Traumatol.* 2020;36(4):350-364.

Summary

Advances in dental research have greatly improved the ability of dentists to ensure long-term retention of traumatized teeth in children. It is the dentist's responsibility to stay abreast of this new information and to be available to patients who need urgent treatment. eFigs. 41.20 through 41.24 provide flowcharts for management of various types of injuries to permanent teeth. Additionally, as noted in the beginning of this chapter, www.dentaltraumaguide.org is an excellent resource for up-to-date information on the management of dental injuries.

Visit eBooks.Health.Elsevier.com to see full list of references.

42

Sports Dentistry

STEPHEN CRAIG MILLS AND ANDREW SPADINGER

CHAPTER OUTLINE

Introduction

Millions of children and adolescents worldwide engage in sports daily. Regular physical activity offers significant health benefits and should be encouraged. According to the National Youth Sports Strategy, 2020,

> *"The benefits for youth who engage in regular physical activity are clear: they have improved bone health, weight status, cardiorespiratory and muscular fitness, cardio-metabolic health, and cognitive function and a reduced risk of depression. Playing sports can provide additional benefits, including developing competence, confidence, and self-esteem; reducing risk of suicide and suicidal thoughts and tendencies; and improving life skills, such as goal setting, time management, and work ethic."*[1]

The Aspen Institute's *Project Play* reported that in 2022, 61.1% of US children ages 6 to 17 played a team sport at least once, and 37.4% did so regularly. Participation was higher among boys (40.2%) than girls (34.5%), with basketball being the most common sport.[2] The National Federation of State High School Associations (NFHS) noted nearly 8 million high school athletes in the 2022–2023 school year.[3] The Centers for Disease Control and Prevention (CDC) reported that 54.1% of children ages 6 to 17 participated in sports during the previous year.[4]

Despite these benefits, sports can increase the risk of injury, including orofacial trauma. Many of these injuries are preventable. Sports dentistry emerged to manage and prevent such injuries. Its current scope includes overall oral healthcare for athletes, though for most youth, prevention and treatment of injury remain the primary focus.[5]

Definition of Sports Dentistry

Sports dentistry is the branch of dentistry dealing with prevention and treatments of the pathologies and injuries of the oral cavity and the stomatognathic system related to sports practice. The stomatognathic system is the anatomical and functional system comprising the teeth, jaws, associated soft tissues, facial muscles and the temporomandibular joint (TMJ).[5]

Risk of Orofacial Injuries in Sports

The unique question when discussing youth sports participation is whether this results in a greater actual risk of being injured. Incidence reports list dental injuries in sports as a "rare occurrence" compared with other injuries such as overuse injuries; lacerations; contusions; and joint, bone, tendon and ligament injuries.[6] One review showed the incidence of dental injuries was merely 0.4% of all injuries.[7] In contrast, prevalence studies have shown a fairly large percentage of athletes have, in fact, experienced oral injuries over their sporting careers. Two systematic reviews showed rates of 10% to 61% and 7.1% to 71.5% of athletes have experienced a dental injury while participating in sports.[8,9]

Risk factors for dental injuries include similar risk factors to overall trauma such as excess dental overjet and lip incompetence. Males outnumber females in both participation as well as total injuries. The rate of injuries is higher in competition compared with practices. Most injuries occur in so-called "contact sports" such as field hockey, basketball, and baseball.[7]

Dental Trauma in Sports

The treatment of dental trauma is discussed in detail in Chapters 40 and 41, but dental trauma in sports is unique in several ways. The initial assessment of the injury is often handled by nondental personnel such as parents, coaches, school nurses, and athletic trainers. The education of these partners is an important aspect of injury recognition. Athletes, even at a fairly young age, often do not want to leave a contest immediately. The initial evaluation and handling of injuries is therefore of critical importance. The use of information sheets or mobile applications can be useful. The International Association of Dental Trauma offers printable posters and a free dental trauma first aid mobile application.[10] ToothSOS, which was launched in the summer of 2018, has been a significant aid to members of the sports medicine team.[11] Communication with partners and initial responders is also critical. The use of a cell phone photograph for initial triage of injuries is a modern and important resource.

The team dentist is a part of an athletic team's sports medicine group whose role is to ensure the dental health and treatment of the athletes. They are often required to provide treatment at an athletic venue. As such, team dentists carry an emergency kit to provide on-site, game-time treatment when necessary.

The concept of the "team dentist" has been recognized for quite some time and a description of the duties of the team dentist was published in 1991.[12] Most pediatric athletes do not have access to a team dentist, but the overall concept can be useful as a way for any dentist to familiarize themselves with sports dentistry. In addition, there are many youth sports tournaments that need medical coverage for the large number of athletes participating and the potentially large number of injuries that could occur. Orofacial and dental injuries can occur, and dentists are often the best suited to handle such injuries. It is recommended that interested dentists volunteer to take part in these tournaments, but they should also be well equipped to play their role. To be prepared as a field-side provider of emergency dental services, the dentist should have an appropriately well-stocked emergency kit. The basic contents of the kit are described in Box 42.1.

Most articles on dental trauma recommend that all injuries be evaluated immediately and that continuing to play is not advisable.[13] Although this is ideal, players often hesitate to leave a game or match due to a dental injury; thus the sports dentist must differentiate between injuries requiring immediate care and those that can be delayed; these are all decisions that will affect the success of the dental treatment. There are several references that deal with the timing recommended for handling dental emergencies[14,15] (see Chapters 40 and 41). Return to play after injury is important to the athletes in sports. Most dental injuries may not impair the athletes' ability to compete, but the risk of reinjury and subsequent failure to heal is of legitimate concern. It is critical that injuries are either allowed to heal or, at the very least, the injured area is adequately protected with a high-quality piece of protective equipment such as a face shield and/or a mouthguard.

• BOX 42.1 Contents of a Field-Side Dental Emergency Kit

Gloves/masks	Composite/plastic instrument
Curing light	Sutures/scissors
2 × 2 gauze	Mirrors/explorers
Flashlight	Etchant/bonding agent
Local anesthetics	Tongue depressors
Theracal/Vitrebond	Dremel motor/burrs
Needles/syringe	Canned air
Splint materials	
Wire cutters	

Prevention of Dental Injuries in Sports

Face Shields

Dental sports injuries can be effectively prevented or at least lessened in severity with the use of protective devices such as face shields and athletic mouthguards.

Face shields are required in many sports such as American football, youth ice hockey, professional ice hockey goaltenders, and men's lacrosse and are becoming increasingly common for cricket, women's softball, youth baseball, and more. Face shields are attached to helmets of some kind. Historically, in American football, in the 1950s 50% of all injuries were to the face and mouth. The introduction of face shields successfully reduced that number by half.[16]

Face shields can be used for primary prevention, but they are also used commonly to allow for facial and or dental healing after an accident. Retail available or custom-made face shields for soccer, basketball, and other sports after facial injury are now a common sight (Fig. 42.1). These do not need to be attached to a helmet and can be worn directly and separately from a helmet.

Mouthguards

The athletic mouthguard has become the symbol of sports dentistry and is one of the most effective injury prevention devices available to athletes. Athletes have tried to prevent dental injuries in one form or another for quite a while. The athletic mouthguard in the modern style originated in the early 20th century.[17] Mouthguards are now used in many sports both where they are required and where they are a personal choice of the athlete. In the United States the NFHS recommends mandating mouthguards at the high school level in men and women's ice hockey and lacrosse, field hockey, football, and for wrestlers who are wearing fixed orthodontic appliances. The NFHS does not, in and of itself, mandate mouthguards; instead it makes recommendations for individual states to adopt mandates through their own state high school regulatory bodies. Accordingly, it is standard practice that all states follow NFHS guidance for high school sports. Certain other large sports organizations like USA Hockey create their own mandatory rules depending on age groups. At the college level, as of 2024, mouthguards are mandated in several sports by large organizations. The National Collegiate Athletic Association (NCAA) mandates mouthguards in American football, men's and women's lacrosse, and women's field hockey. In contrast, a mandate for NCAA ice hockey athletes, both men and women, was removed in 2016. Boxing is the only sport currently in the United States that requires mouthguards at the professional level.

Mouthguards have been reported to help in the prevention of dental injuries, soft tissue injuries, bone fractures, TMJ injuries, and even concussions. Recently they have also been mentioned in increasing athlete balance, stability, and improving athletic performance.

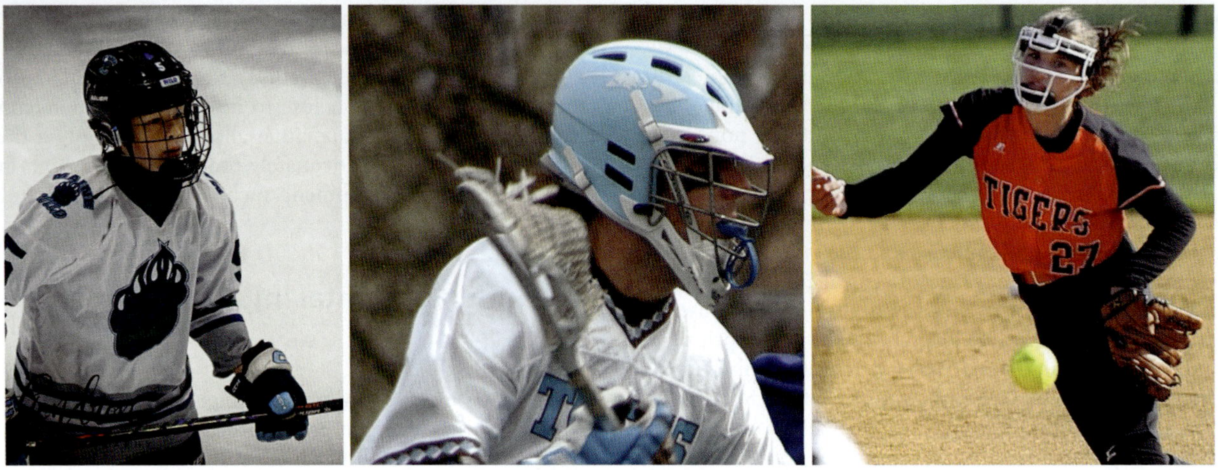

• **Fig. 42.1** Various Forms of Facial Protection Worn by Hockey Players. Full face shields significantly reduce injury risk, with more than a twofold decrease in craniomaxillofacial injuries and a greater than ninefold decrease in dental injuries. (From Cimba MJ, Labe B, Dazen CM, et al. Do mandatory face shields reduce the number of craniomaxillofacial injuries in the National Hockey League? *J Oral Maxillofac Surg*. 2021;79[6]:1313-1318.)

Types of Injuries

Dental Injuries

Properly fitted mouthguards are highly effective at reducing the incidence of dental injuries. One systematic review with meta-analyses (MA) based on 12 cohort trials has reported that the overall risk of orofacial injuries for nonmouthguard users to be 2.3 times that of users. In 11 trials involving self-reported questionnaire outcomes, nonusers were 2.3 times more likely to suffer orofacial injuries.[18]

In another systematic review two MA were performed. The studies used were classified into two groups: those studies that were free of problems or had minor problems (MA1), and studies that were only free of problems (MA2). The MA1 group showed that 73% of mouthguard users had a lower prevalence of dental trauma. The MA2 group demonstrated an 83% lower prevalence of dental trauma. In other words, the injury prevention prevalence was "strong" in the mouthguard wearers versus nonwearers.[9]

Soft Tissue Injuries

Soft tissue injuries have been reported especially among boxers. There are no significant reports demonstrating reductions in soft tissue injuries by wearing mouthguards. Historically professional boxers first used modern style mouthguards to lessen the likelihood of soft tissue injuries leading to mouth bleeding. For a short while mouthguards were actually outlawed in boxing as they were considered to give the wearers an unfair advantage.

Temporomandibular Joint Injuries

Athletic mouthguards are often believed to protect the TMJ, with clenching into full occlusion commonly viewed as offering the greatest protection. A resilient mouthguard can offer a good basis into which an athlete can clench their teeth. There are not many clinical articles supporting this as a protective effect. There is one report that uses a sophisticated biomechanical analysis to show that when the maxillary incisors are struck the impact force is decreased to the condyle and to the disc when the mouthguard is in place.[19] A recent prospective study stated, "The incidence of TMJ pain and clicking in individuals who did not use mouthguards were 81.4% and 82.6%, respectively."[20] Therefore, while the evidence is sparse, it appears the TMJ can benefit by the wearing of a mouthguard.

Bone Injuries

Fractures to the alveolar bone, the mandible, and facial bones are not uncommon in many sports. There is a lack of recent research that demonstrates the ability of a mouthguard to decrease the likelihood of cortical bone fractures. There are two often cited studies using artificial experimental designs. In 1967, Hickey showed that, in cadavers, a mouthguard could decrease mandibular bone deformation when the cadaver was struck on the chin.[21] Takeda et al., in 2004, reproduced this experiment but used an artificial skull set and found a similar decrease in bone deformation.[22] However, clinical in vivo studies are lacking.

Concussions

The ability of an athletic mouthguard to reduce the incidence and severity of traumatic brain injuries (concussions) in sports had its beginnings with a 1964 article by Jack Stenger that chronicled his successful efforts to help a Notre Dame player named Jim Schaff stop having concussions while playing football.[23] This, combined with the article by Hickey in 1967, showed decreased intracranial pressure on cadavers when struck on the mandible while wearing a mouthguard, which led to the acceptance of the idea that *mouthguards can protect against concussions.*[21] These two articles were cited continuously and very routinely for the next several decades.

With time and after several systematic reviews, this belief was questioned. In fact, it became apparent that the literature did not support the idea of mouthguards protecting against concussions. The 2001 Summary and Agreement Statement of the 1st International Symposium on Concussion in Sports held in Vienna stated,

"Although the use of correctly fitting mouthguards can reduce the rate of dental orofacial and mandibular injuries, the evidence that they reduce cerebral injuries is largely theoretical, and clinical evidence for a beneficial effect in reducing concussion rates has not yet been demonstrated scientifically."[24]

Since 2014, however, there has been a return to the belief that mouthguards can play a role in the prevention of concussion or can at least lead to a decrease in incidence. Starting with Winters and DeMont's study in 2014, which showed a small but significant decrease in concussions in high school football[25] and followed by work from the University of Alberta in three separate articles (the most recent of which are cited), this connection is being rekindled.[26,27]

These articles and others have led to the 2022 Amsterdam International Consensus Conference on Concussion in Sport making the statement, "Mouthguards were associated with a 28% reduced concussion rate in ice hockey across all age groups, indicating that mouthguards should be mandated in child and adolescent ice hockey and supported at all levels of play."[28] Although this statement primarily addresses efforts in youth hockey, it is the strongest international positive statement on the connection of mouthguards and sports concussions in many years. Thus it can be inferred that, particularly in youth ice hockey, a mouthguard can effectively serve as a protective measure against concussions.

Mouthguard Types

The Glossary of Prosthetic Terms defined a mouthguard as a removable occlusal device that is useful in reducing mouth injuries and protecting the teeth and surrounding structures from injury.[29] The American National Standards Institute/American Dental Association (ADA) Standards on Dental Care Products (ANSI/ADA SCDP) Specification No. 99 (2013) delineated the following types of mouthguard[30]:

- Type 1: Stock (Fig. 42.2)
- Type 2: Mouth-formed (Fig. 42.3)
  Class 1: Thermoplastic
  Class 2: Chemical setting
- Type 3: Custom (Fig. 42.4)
  Class 1: Vacuum-formed
  Class 2: Model-formed

These types are described in Table 42.1. The most generally acceptable to both athletes and dental professionals are the custom-fitted type. This type provides excellent fit and comfort, does not appreciably interfere with speech or breathing, and can be tailored to the needs of individual athletes who participate in a variety of sports. An excellent reference for a more detailed discussion on the material and physical characteristics of mouthguards, as well as an excellent overview, can be found in Roberts (2023).[31]

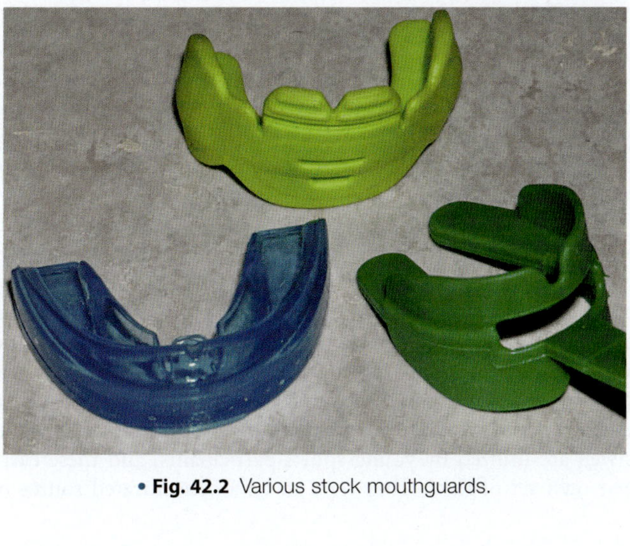

• **Fig. 42.2** Various stock mouthguards.

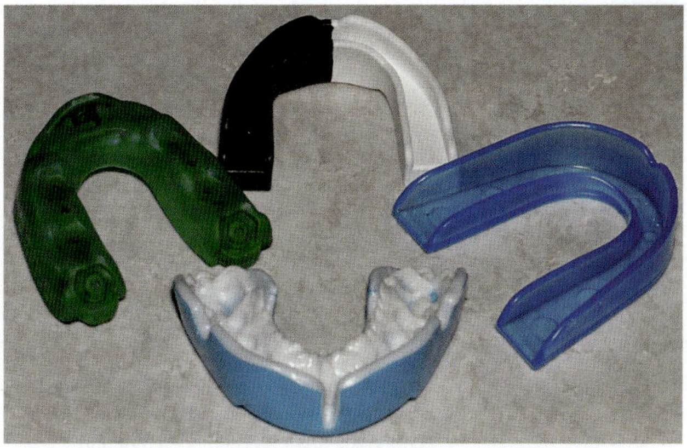

• **Fig. 42.3** Various types of mouth-formed mouthguards.

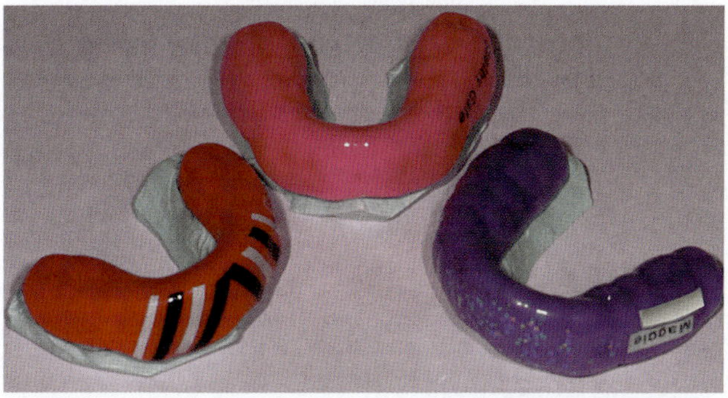

• **Fig. 42.4** Various designs of custom-fitted mouthguards (note the casts they sit on and that they can be customized with colors and design).

History of Mouthguards

The history of the modern mouthguard traditionally starts with a mouthguard made by Philip Wolfe for his friend Ted "Kid" Lewis, a professional boxer and dates to around 1913. Lewis had been suffering from intraoral cuts during his bouts, which led to his losing fights. The mouthguard greatly solved his problem.[17] Mouthguards had been used informally and without fitting for boxing before this and there was a type of mouth protector used in baseball players as early as the 1860s. The use of mouthguards in American football proved to be very successful and this actually catapulted the use of mouthguards into common usage.

The evolution of the modern custom mouthguard began in the 1950s, primarily utilizing latex rubber or with the development of thermoforming techniques in the late 1950s and early 1960s. Dr. Bill Godwin introduced and is largely credited with the idea of vacuum forming mouthguards at the University of Michigan. He used ethylene vinyl acetate (EVA) that he obtained from the automobile industry around Detroit. This material was excellent as it was easily thermoformed and had properties of absorbing and

TABLE 42.1 Summary of Mouthguard Types and Their Advantages and Disadvantages

Stock mouthguard (SMG)	Predetermined sizes No adjustment possible Most inexpensive type available in retail settings Poor fit: easily dislodged; must be clenched on to retain in the mouth; might be difficult to speak or breathe with one in place
Thermoplastic, mouth-formed mouthguard (MFMG) "boil and bite"	Adapted to fit the individual by heating in hot water and molding in the oral cavity using biting and soft tissue pressures Most commonly used type: relatively inexpensive, widely available in retail settings, more comfortable than SMG (improved fit and retention) Poor fit unless properly molded Often difficult to fit over and around existing fixed orthodontic appliances
Custom mouthguard (CMG)	Fabricated for the individual from dental impressions or digital scans, with vacuum forming and heat pressure as well as innovative 3D-printing technologies The most comfortable, the most retentive, and the most protective type of mouthguard Protection can be customized for individual sports Most expensive type

From Abbott PV, Tewari N, O'Connell AC, et al. The International Association of Dental Traumatology (IADT) and the Academy for Sports Dentistry (ASD) guidelines for prevention of traumatic dental injuries: Part 3: mouthguards for the prevention of dental and oral trauma. *Dent Traumatol.* 2024;40 Suppl 1:7-9.

distributing injurious forces to the teeth. Godwin used a commercial vacuum cleaner and heated the material in either boiling water or with a Bunsen burner.[32] Subsequent various vacuum-forming machines that could heat and vacuum the materials were developed. EVA became the standard material upon which the modern custom fitted mouthguard is made.

Around 1962 Dr. A. G. Jacobs invented the heat-fitted mouth-formed mouthguard where an athlete could fit their own mouthguard by first boiling an over-the-counter product in water and then forming it in their own mouth. This concept has become known as the "boil and bite" mouthguard. This introduction made it easy for everyone to access a formed mouthguard without having to be involved with a dentist. The boil and bite industry has grown and become much more sophisticated. However, these products, while improved, continue to be considered bulky to wear and still seem to inhibit easy speech and breathing.[17]

Currently, the standard for excellence in mouthguards is the heat pressure laminated mouthguard (Fig. 42.5). This guard utilizes a special machine that can thermoform and laminate several sheets of material successively over a cast or a three-dimensional (3D)-printed image of an athlete's teeth (Fig. 42.6). It is usually the maxillary arch because most injuries are to the maxillary anterior teeth (except in the case of a mandibular prognathic occlusion). One can utilize this layering technique to create different thicknesses of material where needed, can interpose different material between or upon these layers, and can easily allow for customization such a decorations and identification (see Fig. 42.4; eFig. 42.7).

With advancements in digital technology, custom mouthguards can now be made using intraoral scanners and 3D printing. Digital scans of the dental arches allow for the creation of 3D printed models for thermoforming or direct 3D printing of mouthguards. This technology also enables layering of different materials for enhanced protection. It may soon surpass thermoforming as the preferred method for producing custom-fit mouthguards.[33]

The definition of the "best" mouthguard is increasingly complex due to evolving materials and techniques. Thermoformed guards may use various layered materials, including polymers, silicone, or polyvinylsiloxane, and some incorporate airspaces for added force absorption. In contrast, 3D-printed mouthguards use entirely different materials from traditional EVA-based models. New multilayer designs with diverse material properties are now available. As a result, setting universal standards for thickness, fit, and tooth coverage is no longer feasible. Instead, future standards should focus on the mouthguard's ability to absorb and distribute force across different types and fabrication methods.

Until that time, an adequate mouthguard must have various properties. The Academy for Sports Dentistry has published a policy statement on the ideal mouthguard, which lists the basic properties that must be considered for an adequate mouthguard (Box 42.2).[34]

Future Directions for Sports Dentistry

Sports dentistry is a part of the world of sports medicine for athletes. Dentists must concentrate on the treatment and prevention of dental injuries. However, there is much more that dentistry can give to today's athletes of all ages. Obviously, children and adolescent athletes do not have access to all the benefits of elite athletes. There are several areas that are of particular importance to young players including sports nutrition, eating disorders, the use of sports drinks and energy drinks, and maximizing total oral health and its influence on athletic performance.

Sports Nutrition

The sports nutrition specialist is a regular member of the sports medicine team for athletes at the professional and elite levels. Elite athletes have unique training requirements that lead to specific dietary needs for both energy and performance.[35] Young athletes usually do not have access to these special advisors, but there are some simple aspects of nutrition that can have dental implications. The concept of eating disorders in athletes has been widely studied, especially in sports that are appearance critical (e.g., gymnastics, figure skating) or where weight classes are important (e.g., wrestling). Female athletes are particularly vulnerable to this, and coaches and specialists should foster a positive body image among athletes and pay special attention to the eating behaviors of adolescent athletes.[36,37]

The demands of training can lead to dehydration, and drinking water is critical. Every year a certain number of young athletes suffer severe heat illnesses due to inadequate hydration. The use of sports drinks can combat these catastrophic accidents. However, these drinks are meant for supplementation during training and not necessarily as a good-tasting leisure beverage. Many of these drinks are high in calories, and most are significantly erosive. In general, sports drinks are more erosive than sodas.[38] Energy drinks as well are utilized by young sports participants, and these carry their own set of risks. They tend to be a concentrated source of

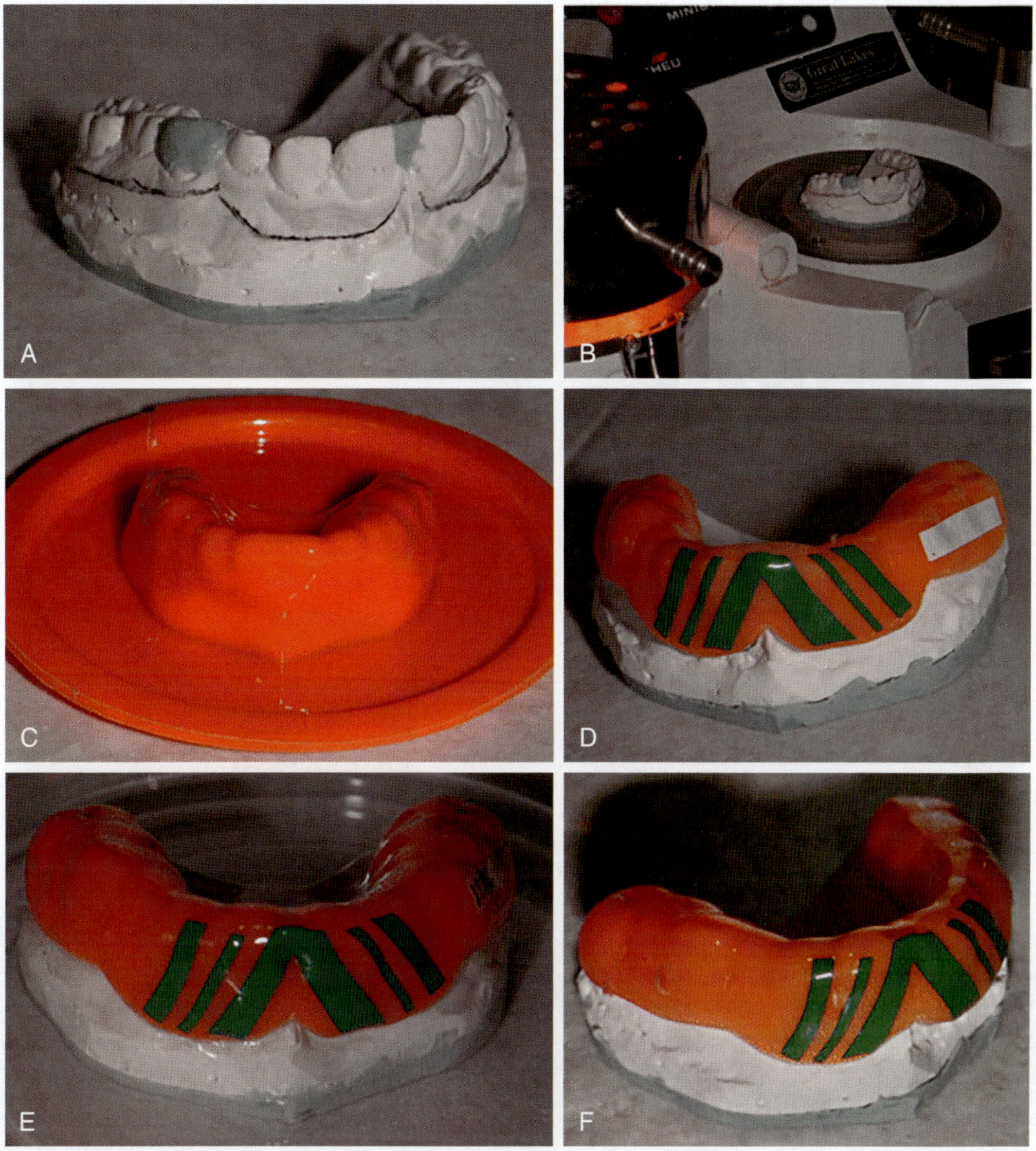

• **Fig. 42.5** (A) Properly trimmed cast. (B) Thermoforming machine heating the first layer. (C) First layer. (D) Trimmed and decorated first layer. (E) Clear second layer laminated on cast. (F) Final trimmed heat pressure laminated mouthguard.

energy with large amounts of sugar. They are even more erosive than sports drinks, and the caffeine and taurine have some concerning cardiac implications as well. Young athletes should be encouraged to use water as the first source of hydration and to use sports drinks only in specific circumstances.

Oral Health as a Part of Total Health and Implications for Athletic Performance

Research indicates a substantial prevalence of oral disease in elite and professional athletes.[39] It has long been known that athletes, especially at the elite level, seem to demonstrate lower oral health than one might expect from those who should try to maximize their overall ability to compete. This surprising finding has led to explorations trying to connect oral health with an athlete's ability to perform at their maximum ability, even for young athletes. Thus the dentist can use the opportunity to educate young athletes on the importance of maintaining oral health as an important aspect of total health.

Intraoral Appliances for Enhanced Athletic Performance

For most pediatric patients, athletic mouthguards are used solely for the reduction of dental and oral injuries. However, at the elite levels, intraoral appliances have been used, in addition to protection, to maximize an athlete's ability to perform. This capability relies largely on the ability to gauge the ideal occlusion or "bite" of an athlete with the use of electromyography or other types of occlusion force modalities. Although research targets the elite athlete, it also highlights the benefits of correctly fitting a mouthguard to one's own occlusion, no matter the age.[40]

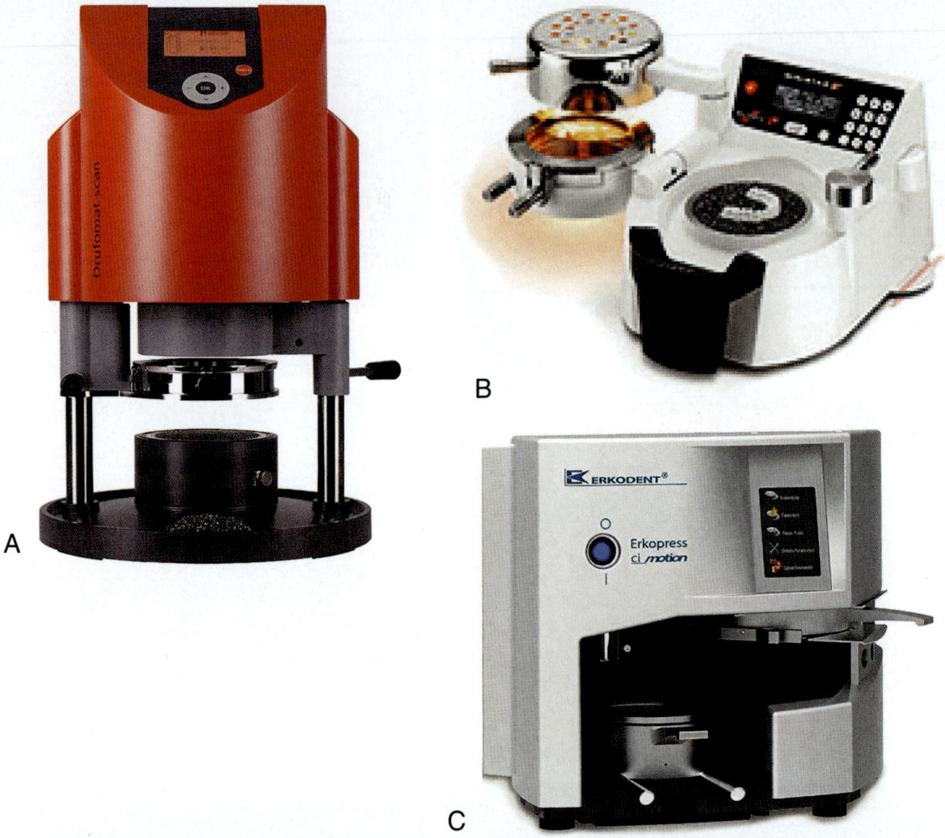

• **Fig. 42.6** Typical Heat Pressure Forming Machines (A, C); B, Thermoforming Machine or Pressure Moulding Machine. (A) Drufomat (Dreve America Corp., Eden Prairie, MN). (B) MINISTAR S® (Photos provided by SCHEU-DENTAL GmbH). (C) Erkodent Erkopress ci motion (Glidewell, Newport Beach, CA).

• BOX 42.2 Ideal Properties of Mouthguards

Fits well, is not easily dislodged, and must be worn correctly.
Absorbs and distributes the forces, which can be injurious to the teeth and the oral structures.
Allows for excellent speech and breathing commensurate with the sport being played.
Covers all the areas that are needed for adequate protection.
Balanced for optimal occlusion.
Provides a definite ability to clench into a firm, locked position to stabilize the temporomandibular joint.
Should not distort athlete's posture which might invite further injury.

Summary

Many children and adolescents participate in sports of all types. Many of these activities put the athletes at risk for orofacial injuries. Pediatric dentists are ideal people to inform young athletes and sports organizations because they are educated and experienced in treating dental trauma. They are ideally situated to educate patient athletes and families about the best ways to prevent injuries, especially with the most effective mouthguards. In addition, subjects such as sports nutrition and how best to maximize oral health to improve athletic performance could be very useful to these young athletes. It is essential that dentists, especially pediatric dentists, be knowledgeable to counsel their patients about the connections of their sporting activities and optimal oral health.

Visit eBooks.Health.Elsevier.com to see full list of references.

43

Abuse, Neglect, Bullying, and Human Trafficking

ANUPAMA R. TATE AND JENNIFER L. CULLY

CHAPTER OUTLINE

Introduction

Child abuse and neglect affects at least one of seven children annually in the United States[1] and can include physical and sexual abuse, which may be evidenced by bite marks, dental neglect, and medical child abuse (MCA). In all 50 states, dental professionals are mandated to report suspected cases of abuse and neglect to child protection agencies or law enforcement agencies. The Centers for Disease Control and Prevention (CDC) defined child maltreatment as "any act or series of acts of commission or omission by a parent or other caregiver that results in harm, potential for harm, or threat of harm to a child."[16]

Ethical and Legal Obligation

The American Dental Association (ADA) has principles of ethics and codes of professional conduct that describe dentists' obligation to become familiar with the signs of abuse and neglect and to report suspected cases of child maltreatment to social service or law enforcement agencies.[7] Dentists should be aware that jurisdictional laws vary in their definitions of abuse and neglect, in their reporting requirements, and the extent to which immunity is granted to good faith reporters; however, their duty is to put the welfare of the child first. Failure to report child abuse can lead to severe consequences including fines or time in prison for the health professional.[8] Beyond the legal obligation to report, not completing this crucial duty can lead to injury or even death of the child.[8]

A known bias among healthcare professionals is the hesitance to report suspected abuse when the family is of similar background to the professional.[3] Dentists should recognize the impact of implicit bias and its influence on diagnosing and reporting child maltreatment.[4–6] Reports or suspicions of abuse or neglect should be made immediately to the local Department of Child and Family Services or other jurisdictions.

Decision Making

The American Academy of Pediatric Dentistry (AAPD) and the American Academy of Pediatrics (AAP) offer resources on the technical aspects of identification, documentation, management, and referral guidance when reporting abuse and neglect.[9,10] When examining a patient and a suspicious lesion or injury is noted, one should attempt to discern more about the history of events through use of open-ended questions. One can consider asking nonthreatening questions to the parent and the patient separately to determine whether discrepancies in the accounts of the injury are reported. In addition to inconsistent histories, delay of treatment can also be a possible indicator of abuse or neglect. The dentist does not have an obligation to investigate or prove abuse or neglect. The suspicion of abuse and/or neglect is enough to warrant a report. The collection of evidence and investigations should be left to trained professionals.

Physical Abuse

In 2021, 49 states, the Commonwealth of Puerto Rico and the District of Columbia reported 588,229 victims of child abuse and neglect. Nationally it is estimated that 3,016,000 children received an investigation response or alternative response to a child maltreatment report and approximately 1820 children die of abuse and neglect on an annual basis. Approximately 70% of these children were younger than age 3.[16,17] Missed recognition and reporting of "sentinel injuries," or minor injuries that may indicate a higher risk of abuse and neglect, in young children is significant; 27.5% of abused infants had a previous minor inflicted injury that had been recognized by a parent or physician but was usually not reported to authorities.[21] The majority of these sentinel injuries involved bruising to the face, forehead, or ear. The TEN-4-FACESp (*T*orso, *E*ar, *N*eck, *F*renulum, *A*ngle of jaw, *C*heeks, *E*yelids, *S*ubconjunctivae in children younger than *4* years, bruising anywhere in infants younger than 5 months, or *p*atterned bruising) rule has been used to aid in identifying bruises of concern for abuse.[22] Lacerations or tears to the oral frena in premobile infants should also be considered potential sentinel injuries and are frequently associated with other findings of serious physical abuse.[21,23,24]

Due in part to exposed placement and complex anatomy, the head and face are more vulnerable to serious injury than other body regions. Craniofacial, head, face, and neck injuries occur in more than half of child abuse cases.[18–21] In a review of 40 cases of child homicides resulting from physical abuse, it was noted that 36 (90%) had orofacial injuries.[25] In children, areas of accidental injury are typically boney protuberances, such as chins, elbows, shins, and knees. Circumferential bruising of upper arms, neck, ears, and bruises in patterns (e.g., belt, handprint) and various stages of healing should induce suspicion of abuse. Oral injuries may be inflicted with instruments such as eating utensils or a bottle during forced feedings, hands, fingers, scalding liquids, or caustic substances resulting in injuries to tongue, lips, buccal mucosa, palate (soft and hard), gingiva, alveolar mucosa, or frenum. This also includes fractured, displaced, or avulsed teeth, or facial bone and jaw fractures. Lips are noted as the most common site for inflicted oral injuries (54%) followed by the oral mucosa, teeth, gingiva, and tongue.[26] Fig. 43.1 depicts an injury to the maxillary frenulum of a toddler. Unintentional or accidental injuries to the mouth are common and should be distinguished from physical abuse by reviewing the history (timing and mechanism of the injury) and ensuring it is consistent with the features of the injury and the child's developmental abilities.

In addition to reporting, consultation with a knowledgeable dentist or child abuse pediatrician may be beneficial. The AAP clinical report "The Evaluation of Suspected Child Physical Abuse" provides additional guidance[10] and, for information about state requirements, contact the AAP state advocacy team (e-mail: stgov@aap.org).

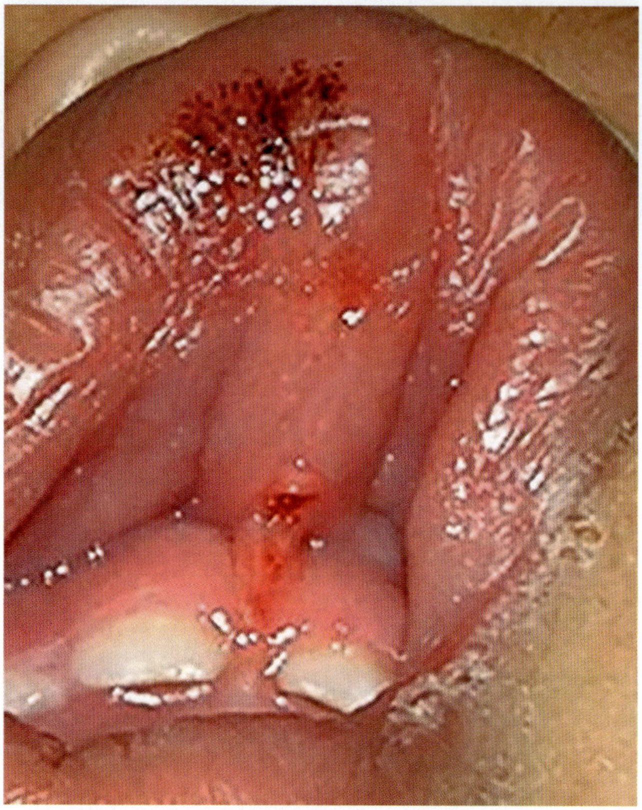

• **Fig. 43.1** Maxillary frenulum injury.

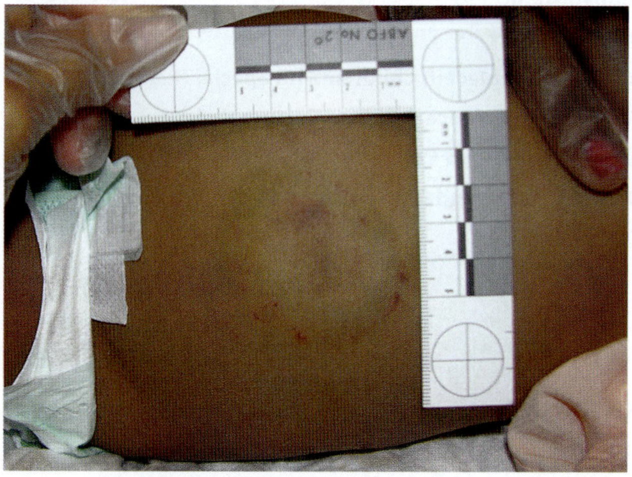

• **Fig. 43.2** Bite marks on young child's abdomen.

Bite Marks on the Skin

Acute or healed bite marks on the skin need to be suspected when ecchymoses, abrasions, or lacerations are found in elliptical, horseshoe-shaped, or ovoid patterns.[41] Bite marks can present with a central ecchymosis on the skin due to the pressure and suction formed by the tongue that is created by closing of the teeth leading to extravascular bleeding (Fig. 43.2). Common locations for bite marks are the cheeks, back, sides, arms, buttocks, and genitalia.[44] Toddlers may bite to express anger or frustration; however, an intercanine distance measuring more than 3 cm is suspicious for an adult human bite.[42] Typically, human bites compress flesh and can cause abrasions, contusions, and lacerations but rarely avulsion of tissue, whereas bites produced by dogs and other carnivorous animals tend to tear flesh.[42]

In cases where abuse is suspected, one should document the bite mark characteristics both with a written description and photographs that utilize a scale marker (e.g., ruler) to show the size of the lesion (see Fig. 43.2). Ideally the pattern, size, contour, color, and evolution of a bite mark can be evaluated by a forensic odontologist in cases of abuse. The American Board of Forensic Odontology (ABFO) guidelines no longer endorse positive identification of a suspect's dentition to a bite mark because bite marks found on human skin are challenging to differentiate due to similarities in dentition, distortion on skin, and time elapsed between the injury and the analysis.[41] Recent investigations have led to questions about the scientific validity, and overapplication of bite mark analysis in legal proceedings.[43] Dentists trained as forensic odontologists can assist dental professionals in the detection and evaluation of bite marks related to physical and sexual abuse.[41] The ABFO (https://abfo.org) provides resources to locate an expert and review the standards and guidelines for evaluating bite marks.

Sexual Abuse

The oral cavity is a frequent site of sexual abuse, and acquisition of sexually transmitted infections (STIs) can occur as a result.[28] In one report, STIs were detected in 11.4% of preadolescents and in 22.9% of adolescents evaluated for sexual abuse.[29] Although physical signs of sexual abuse can be far more difficult to identify, intraoral findings of child sexual abuse can include erythema, petechiae, ulcerations, and condylomas of the lips, palate, tongue, and nasopharynx.[36]

When child sexual abuse is suspected or diagnosed, the case must be reported to child protective services and/or law enforcement agencies for investigation.[32–35] Specialized hospitals and child protection clinics equipped with experienced medical personnel are best suited for collecting specimens, using appropriate tests to support forensic investigations, and maintaining a chain of evidence. Typically testing involves swabbing the buccal mucosa and tongue with a sterile, cotton-tipped applicator. The swab can then be air-dried and packaged appropriately for laboratory analysis.

Vertical and nonsexual transmission of certain pathogens can occur; therefore consultation with an expert is recommended for positive STI tests in infants and prepubertal children. For example, oropharyngeal human papillomavirus (HPV) infections may be transmitted sexually, horizontally through nonsexual contact from a child or caregiver's hand to the genitals or mouth, or vertically from mother to infant during birth.[30,31]

Medical Child Abuse

MCA, previously known as "Munchausen's syndrome by proxy," is a form of child maltreatment in which a caregiver subjects a child to unnecessary and potentially harmful medical care due to the caregiver's exaggeration, falsification, or induction of an illness or medical condition.[37]

There is no typical presentation of MCA. Commonly the fabricated illness involves multiple organ systems resulting in unnecessary medical interventions, diagnostic tests, repeated examinations, surgeries, and/or medications. Apnea, seizures, feeding problems, bleeding, pain, and rashes are frequently reported symptoms. One report described four cases of MCA involving the oral cavity with children ranging from 9 months to 6 years.[38] In one case, an infant presented with mucosal desquamation, drooling, and dysphagia and it was later found to be caused by the caregiver placing an acid-based powder in food and on toys.[38] In another case, there was recurrent mucosal bleeding and ulcerations, which were initially diagnosed as Stevens-Johnson syndrome, and then cicatricial pemphigoid. However, after the child's death from poisoning, it was later determined that the child's oral manifestations were caused by the forced ingestion of toxic cleaning products. In all four of these cases, the perpetrator was the child's mother. Mothers are far more likely to commit MCA, and about half of them have worked in the medical field.[39]

Making an MCA diagnosis can be difficult because the clinical presentation may not match the history provided and caregivers may insist on diagnostic tests, dental treatments, and medical procedures. A thorough review of all available medical and dental records may be needed to discover concerning patterns to make the correct diagnosis.[40] Consultation with a child abuse pediatrician may be helpful when MCA is suspected.

Bullying

In the United States, 28% of students in grades 6 to 12 report they have been bullied and 70% of children have witnessed someone being bullied in the past year.[67] Thirty-three percent of middle school students report being cyberbullied.[67] The CDC notes that bullying may inflict harm or distress on the targeted youth including physical, psychological, social, or educational harm.[67] Worldwide investigators from many countries and cultures have found that children with orofacial or dental abnormalities, or malocclusions, are frequently subjected to bullying.[57–59] A recent study noted untreated dental caries presented as the main oral health predictor of the occurrence of bullying episodes in adolescence.[55] Another study noted that children and adolescents who were bullying victims had a higher frequency of possible awake bruxism as a result of the emotional stress.[54] Lesbian, gay, bisexual, transgender, and questioning (LGBTQ+) teens,[63] overweight children and youth,[64] and children with special healthcare needs[65,66] are at high risk for being bullied for reasons other than orofacial abnormalities. Children who are bullied may suffer serious psychological consequences, including depression and suicidal ideation.[60–62] A recent study found a relatively high experience of self-harm reported by adolescent school children, with many reporting self-harm because of their dentofacial appearance and bullying because of dentofacial features.[56]

Because children with dental abnormalities are at increased risk for bullying, dental professionals should ask their patients about bullying and advocate for antibullying prevention programs in community settings. The AAP and CDC have resources like healthychildren.org and stopbullying.gov, respectively, which offer caregivers educational resources on bullying.[77,78]

Human Trafficking

Human trafficking is a violent crime with over 28 million individuals trafficked worldwide.[79] Human trafficking is a major global child health issue that has substantial medical, psychological, and dental ramifications, and it may be in the form of labor or sex trafficking.[79] Human trafficking occurs when a perpetrator or trafficker takes an action (e.g., recruiting, harboring, providing) and then employs a means of force, fraud, or coercion to compel a victim to provide sexual acts or labor services.[79] This is known as the Action-Means-Purpose model.[79,80] In adults, regardless of the type, trafficking involves force, fraud, or coercion. However, in children under the age of 18 years, force, fraud, or coercion is not necessary to meet the definition of sex trafficking.[79,80] Under federal law, children participating in commercial sexual acts are always considered trafficked.[79] Some examples of sex trafficking include escort services, residential brothels, strip clubs, personal sexual servitude, remote interactive sexual acts (e.g., web-based cameras, texts), and pornography.[84] Sexually explicit photos and videos may also be called "child sexual abuse material" (CSAM) as this term greater encompasses the sexual exploitation of children. These abusive images and videos, often disseminated via technology (i.e., social media, online gaming, email), re-victimize the child each time they are viewed.[85] Some children may engage in "survival sex," which is the exchange of sexual activities for basic necessities such as food, money, or shelter.[79]

Dental professionals may encounter victims who present with infections, injuries, or a variety of other physical or behavioral health conditions.[45,50] Reliable estimates of children experiencing human trafficking are difficult to obtain because of the complicated nature of the definitions of trafficking, underreporting, and failure to recognize trafficking. Although the average age of children who are exploited for sex is 12 years old, children as young as 6 years old are also targeted.[46] Risk factors that increase likelihood of being victims of human trafficking include children who are or have been in foster care,[47] identify as LGBTQ+,[48] who run away from home,[49] or are incarcerated in juvenile detention facilities.[50]

Victims of trafficking often experience physical and sexual violence and may have observable injuries with inconsistent or limited histories. Oral health issues are common with more than half (54%) of trafficked women and adolescents reporting dental problems, most commonly tooth loss and dental pain.[51,52] Dental problems can be especially acute in child trafficked victims who suffer from inadequate nutrition, dental caries, infection, and tooth loss.[53]

Some states require mandatory human trafficking training for dental licensure; however, because human trafficked children may visit the dental healthcare setting, all dental professionals should be aware of human trafficking screening tools and the risk factors for human trafficking to identify children, of all genders, at risk. Safe reporting and timely connection of patients to resources can be lifesaving. Victims of trafficking can text (text "BeFree" or 233733) or call (1-888-373-7888) the US National Human Trafficking Hotline.[79] When reporting suspicion of child abuse related to human trafficking, it is recommended to contact both local authorities and the US National Human Trafficking Hotline. Dental professionals can also have an important impact by advocating for antitrafficking efforts.

Dental Neglect

The AAPD defined dental neglect as the "willful failure of parent or guardian, despite adequate access to care, to seek and follow through with treatment necessary to ensure a level of oral health essential for adequate function and freedom from pain and infection."[69] Dental neglect can be challenging to identify because of the chronic nature of dental caries. One must recognize the influence of social factors on children's oral health including access to care, dental disease, behaviors, and oral health inequalities.[68] It is important to differentiate between caregivers who willfully fail to seek care and those who lack knowledge or awareness or have barriers to care when determining the need to report cases to authorities.

Factors considered necessary for the diagnosis of neglect are as follows[73]:

- Child is harmed or at risk for harm because of lack of dental healthcare.
- Recommended dental care offers significant net benefit to the child.
- Anticipated benefit of the dental treatment is significantly greater than its morbidity so parents would likely choose treatment over nontreatment.
- Parent understands the dental advice given and access to dental care is available but not used.

Failure to seek or obtain proper healthcare may result from challenges in accessing dental care or insurance and factors such as isolation (physical or cultural), transportation difficulty, ignorance, or lack of perceived value of oral health. When recommending and discussing treatment options, it is important to consider a child's social, emotional, and medical ability to undergo treatment as well as the family's cultural and religious differences.[74] If the caregiver fails to obtain care for a child's oral or dental disease after barriers have been addressed, the case warrants reporting to the appropriate child protective services agency.

Abuse and Neglect in Children With Special Healthcare Needs

Child abuse and neglect in children with disabilities is reported in 3% to 10% of the population.[11] The rate of child abuse and neglect is at least three times higher in children with disabilities than in typically developing children. Special attention should be paid to reduce the risk of abuse in these children and youth[12] because patients with chronic illnesses or disabilities sometimes can place higher emotional, physical, economic, and social demands on their caregivers.[13] The financial stress and care and supervision responsibilities of raising a child with disabilities is often high and may contribute significantly to overall family stress leading to an increased risk of abuse and neglect in children with disabilities.[14,15] Similar to physical abuse, neglect is more prevalent in children with disabilities than in children without disabilities.[2] The complex health needs of children with disabilities may result in the failure of the child to receive essential preventive care, medications, and treatments.[71,72] Children with disabilities, who often rely on multiple caregivers, are a vulnerable population who are at increased risk of abuse and neglect and therefore special attention should be paid to reduce this risk in these children and youth.[2]

Teen Dating Violence (Intimate Partner Violence)

It has been estimated that one in four children are exposed to caregiver intimate partner violence (IPV).[81] Children who are exposed to IPV are at higher risk for maltreatment and physical, psychosocial, and psychological effects.[81] IPV is defined as "physical violence, sexual violence, stalking and psychological aggression (including coercive tactics) by a current or former intimate partner."[81] Violence in an adolescent relationship is known as teen dating violence (TDV)[82] or adolescent relationship abuse (ARA).[83] A recent survey from the CDC indicates that in the United States, 1 in 12 high school students have experienced physical dating violence and 1 in 12 have experienced sexual dating violence.[82] Female students and those individuals who identify as LGBTQ+ or who are unsure of their gender identity are at greater risk for TDV.[82] Victims of TDV are more likely to experience depression and anxiety; engage in drugs, alcohol, and tobacco or other unhealthy behaviors; exhibit antisocial behavior such as lying, theft, and bullying; and have suicidal ideation.[82] It is therefore important to support healthy, nonviolent relationships in adolescents to prevent the long-lasting effects on the individual, family, and community.[82]

Adverse Childhood Exposures

Adverse childhood experiences (ACEs) are potentially traumatic events that occur in childhood, which can include, but are not limited to, experiencing violence, abuse, or neglect, or growing up in a household with substance use problems, mental health problems, or

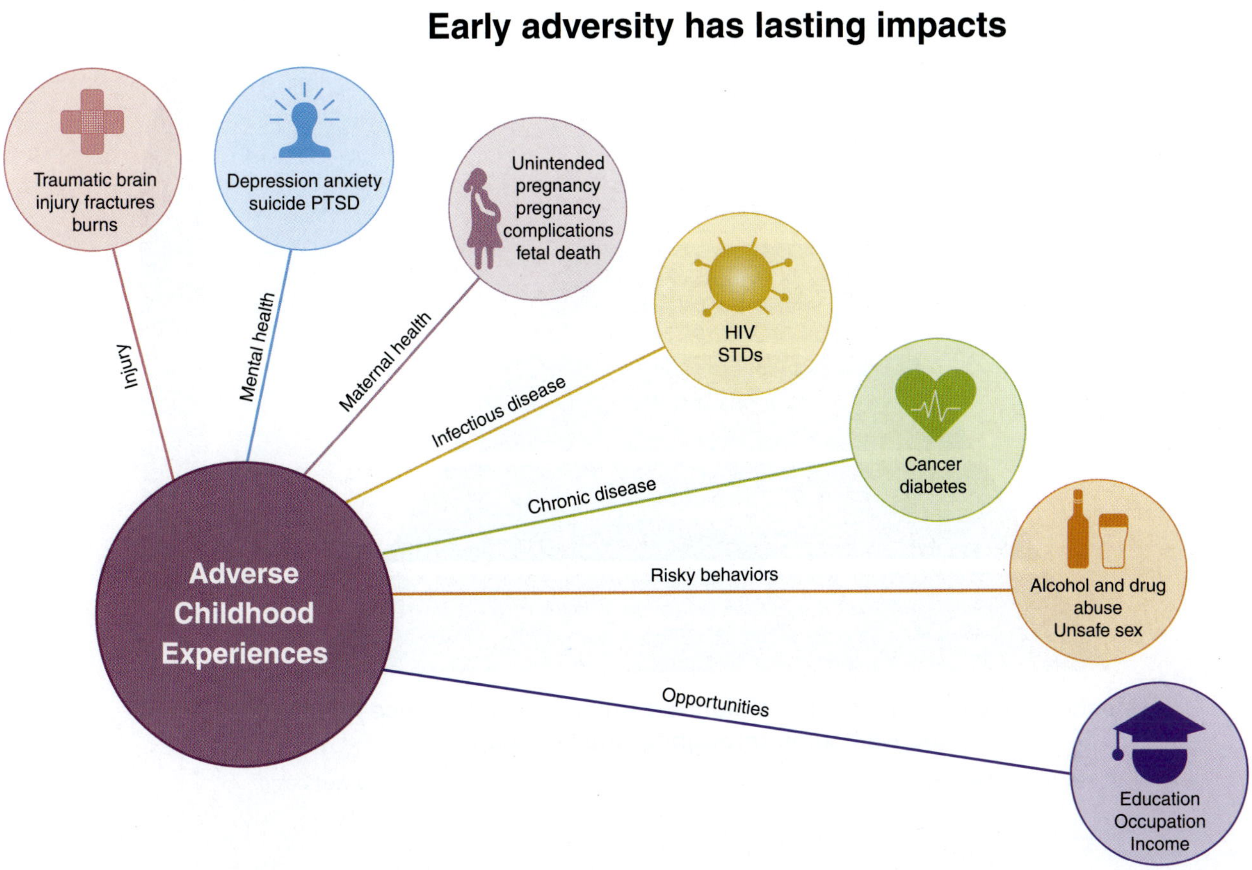

• **Fig. 43.3** Adverse childhood experiences. *PTSD,* Posttraumatic stress disorder; *STD,* sexually transmitted disease. (From www.acestudy.org.)

instability due to parental separation or household members being in jail or prison.[75] Fig. 43.3 shows common ACEs. Children who experience abuse or neglect are at increased risk for poor oral health, including a higher incidence of untreated tooth decay, low priority for oral hygiene, and more missed dental appointments compared with the general population.[70] In the United States, approximately 64% of adults reported they had experienced at least one type of ACE before age 18, and nearly 1 in 6 reported they had experienced four or more types of ACEs.[75]

Toxic stress from ACEs can negatively affect brain development, immune systems, and stress-response systems and can affect children's attention, decision making, and learning. ACEs are linked to lifelong health consequences (Fig. 43.4) for survivors and their families including poor health outcomes, mental illness, and substance misuse as adolescents and adults.[27]

Documentation and Protocols

In cases of child maltreatment, documentation of clinical and behavioral findings in the patient's record is important. One should document what is said with quotes and note, by name, who said it. Documentation should include clinical photos or images and a rationale for treatment or nontreatment. One should document consultation with other healthcare providers and/or reports to Child Protective Services and other agencies. Reports of child maltreatment to local authorities are allowable without parental consent under Health Insurance Portability and Accountability Act regulations. However, in most cases parents should be informed about your concerns. Direct communication like, "I care about your child and in this case the presentation of injury and history are leading me to explore all possible causes and as a mandated reporter I am required to make a report to Child Protective services" can be considered. If the provider is concerned about the child's immediate safety or the safety of office staff, local police should be contacted before the child leaves the office. Having office protocols, including easy access to local child protection websites or phone numbers and discussions with office staff about safety and patient privacy, are important.

Conclusion

Child abuse can result in short- and long-term emotional, physical, and mental health disturbances. It is critical for all dental professionals to appropriately recognize and report all suspected victims of child maltreatment to prevent further escalating injury and or death to the child. Dental professionals can play an important role by increasing community awareness and advocacy of local programs and resources to help prevent child abuse. Ongoing professional education is critical and programs like Prevent Abuse and Neglect through Dental Awareness[76] can help providers remain knowledgeable and familiar with resources to assist reporting child maltreatment.

Visit eBooks.Health.Elsevier.com to see full list of references.

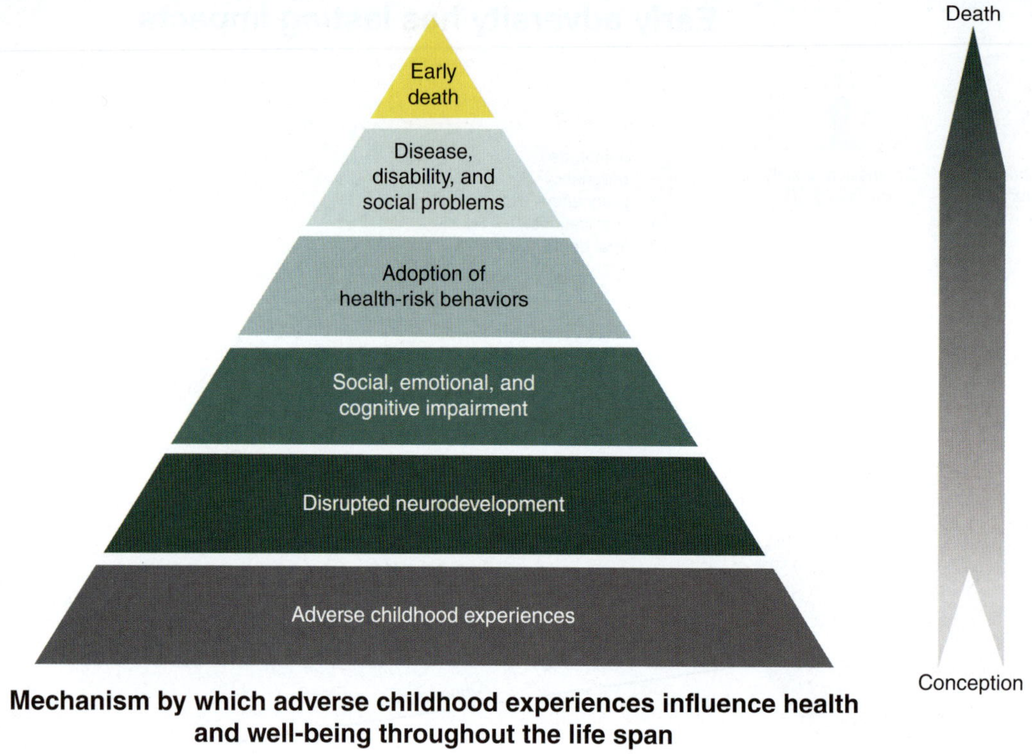

• **Fig. 43.4** Adverse childhood experiences and their effect on health and well-being.

44

Ensuring Accessible Care for All—Dental Public Health

SCOTT B. SCHWARTZ AND M. GENTRY BYRD

CHAPTER OUTLINE

Introduction

One of the primary challenges facing the dental profession is ensuring that all children and adults enjoy the benefits of good oral health. This chapter provides an overview of dental public health and outlines how our profession is responsible for optimizing the oral health of all children through evidence-based public health approaches, at the core of which are education and prevention.

Definition of Dental Public Health

Dental public health is defined as "the science and art of preventing and controlling dental diseases and promoting dental health through organized community efforts."[1] A common misconception about dental public health is that its primary objective is the delivery of dental care to low-income persons. Although this is important, the actual delivery of dental care is only one aspect of dental public health. Based on the core values of public health, the 10 essential public health services serve as a roadmap to guide all stakeholders in public health (Fig. 44.1). Specific activities of dental public health are derived from this model to understand oral health outcomes and includes examples of activities related to children's oral health (Box 44.1).

Over 40% of all infants born are Medicaid eligible, making pediatric public health initiatives paramount to improve health outcomes at the population level.[2] Although nonmodifiable factors like genetic makeup contribute to an individual's risk of disease, dental disease is driven more substantially by upstream, modifiable social determinants of health (SDOH), which are mainly economic and social in nature. A multilevel approach is helpful to understand chronic disease outcomes and is applicable to children's oral health (Fig. 44.2). Studies investigating childhood chronic disease show that geographical location and neighborhood of where a child lives is significant. Interestingly, across the United States, there is considerable state-level variation and regional clustering of oral health outcomes specifically.[3] When comparing state dental policies for children, which show broad variation, and the complexities of which will be discussed later, the majority of states do not adequately provide for basic dental care for children.[4] Strategic early interventions and policies can be better tailored to communities with improved understanding of their unique health disparities and barriers. From a broader health promotion prospective, it may be helpful to view childhood caries as a chronic disease that has risk factors in common with other chronic conditions (for example, childhood obesity), including geography, socioeconomic status, access to healthy food, and access to medical/dental care. A common risk factor approach clusters risk factors of chronic disease together and strives to address fewer determinants at the higher levels of influence; for example, health policy reform and nutrition programs have great potential to impact comprehensive health outcomes, not just oral health.[5] Furthermore, integration of oral health promotion into existing public health programs, primary care settings, and public school programs helps optimize oral health for all children.

Role of the Individual Practitioner

Dental professionals are in a unique position to improve the oral health of their patients and their community. Though treatment of individual patients in an office setting is the cornerstone of pediatric dental practice, it cannot comprehensively address the needs of all children. As with principles of pediatric dental practice, dental public health calls for evidence-based approaches to promote oral health within our communities. It requires awareness of community needs and necessitates

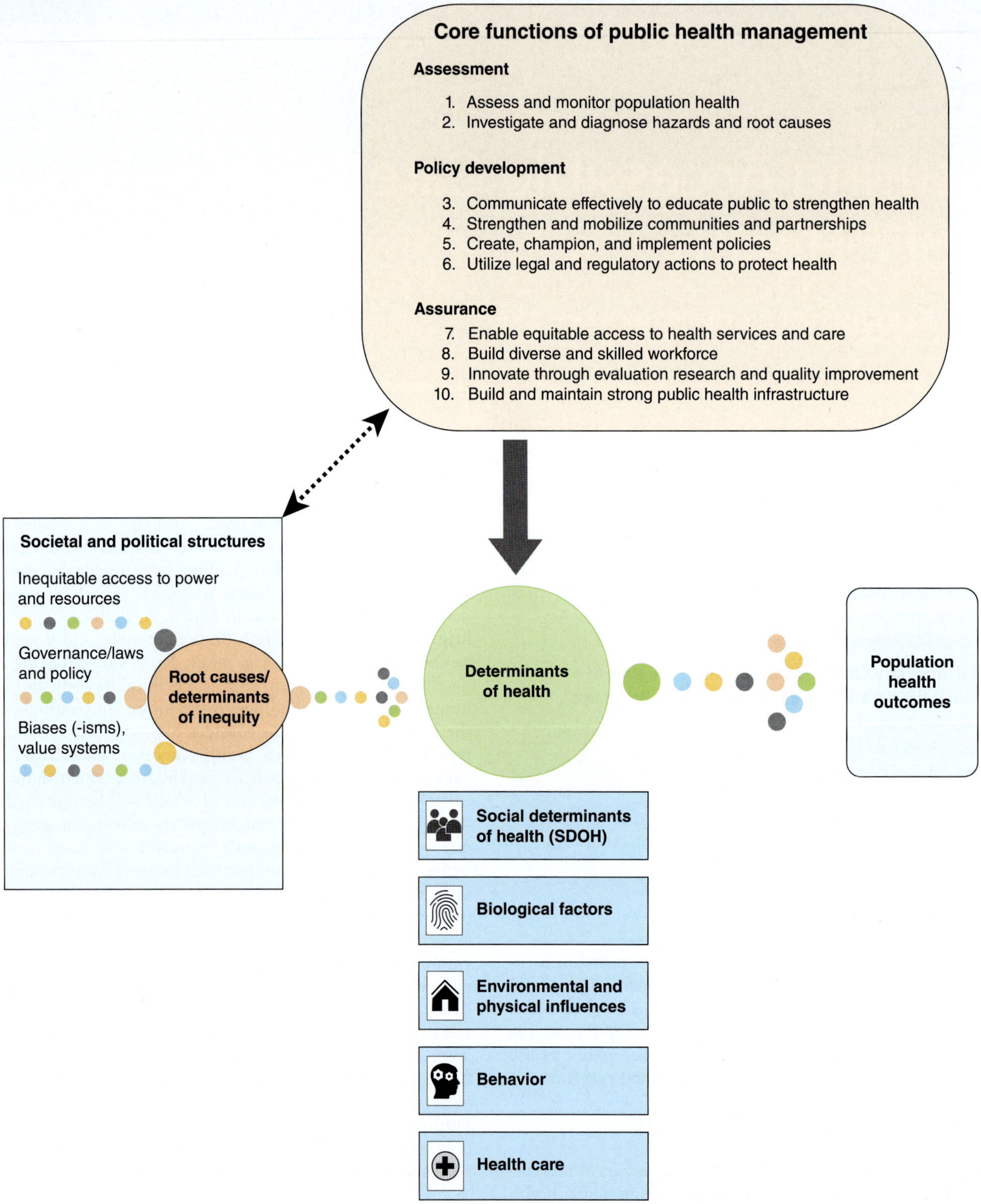

• **Fig. 44.1** Schematic of the core public health functions, 10 Essential Public Health Services, determinants of inequity, and the determinants of health. The core functions of public health altogether focus on improving conditions to promote population health and reduce inequities. The *dashed arrow* illustrates that determinants of inequity can influence public health management and vice versa. (From Perry IA. Assessment, policy development, and assurance: evolving the core functions of public health to address health threats. *AJPM Focus*. 2023;3[1]:100172.)

• BOX 44.1 Examples of Dental Public Health Activities Affecting Children

Assessment

1. Documenting the oral health status of children through epidemiologic surveys
2. Assessing the supply and availability of dentists to meet the needs of children
3. Assessing the status of water fluoridation in communities
4. Assessing the need for dental care for children with special healthcare needs
5. Identifying barriers to dental access
6. Screening children before entering school

Policy Development

1. Developing policies and advocating for legislative action to ensure access to oral health services for low-income, underserved, hard-to-reach, and vulnerable children
2. Developing programs that focus on primary and secondary prevention
3. Developing programs to provide dental care to children with special health needs or without access to adequate dental care
4. Adopting state rules mandating oral health screening for children entering school for the first time

Assurance

1. Encouraging and coordinating efforts to provide oral health education and promotion in schools, clinics, community settings, and other settings
2. Expanding or establishing new dental clinical sites (e.g., Community Health Center expansions)
3. Developing promotional activities by the State Health Agency to meet the oral health needs of a specific target group or community
4. Targeting topical and systemic fluoride programs to areas with nonfluoridated water supplies and high-risk populations
5. Including an oral health component in all school health initiatives
6. Establishing school-based prevention programs and school-based or school-linked dental clinics as components of comprehensive school health
7. Establishing programs to train medical professionals and other health-related workers to recognize oral health problems, including early childhood caries
8. Integrating oral health services into appropriate health, education, and social service programs (e.g., Maternal and Child Health; nutrition; Women, Infants, and Children; health promotion; school health)

Modified from Association of State and Territorial Dental Directors. *Guidelines for State and Territorial Oral Health Programs.* June 2010.

responsibility on the part of the individual practitioner to educate, advocate, and collaborate.

It is important for the individual practitioner to understand that the oral health status and needs of children receiving care in a private practice setting may not represent the status and needs of *all* children in the community. Children with unmet dental needs frequently do not utilize dental care regularly. The challenge for dentists, therefore, is to look beyond the individual dental office and make a broad assessment of their community's needs while assessing their own role in enhancing the oral health of the entire community. The Association of State and Territorial Dental Directors (ASTDD) developed and disseminated a needs assessment model last revised in 2021, which was designed to help communities identify and address their oral health needs. A community-based needs assessment process (Fig. 44.3) will also provide an excellent opportunity to educate a community about the importance of oral health.

In addition to participating in needs assessment activities, practitioners are also the primary advocates for the oral health of children. Engaging in advocacy efforts (local level, state level, and nationally) to promote advances in oral health is a responsibility of all providers, and it can occur at multiple spheres of influence including individual, community, and policy/legislative levels (Fig. 44.4). Providers are often called on to participate in public health activities, including advocating for fluoridation of community water supplies, participating in school and community health promotion activities, advocating for physicians to be reimbursed for the application of fluoride varnish for at-risk children, and advising policymakers regarding dental care programs including Medicaid. Support and guidance for the individual practitioner becoming involved in dental public health activities can be sought from a variety of sources, including the oral health components of state public health agencies, county boards of health, dental/medical societies, and various community boards and organizations. One important issue practitioners often find themselves involved with is enhancing access to dental care for members of their communities. This topic is discussed in the following sections.

Access to Care

Although regular dental care contributes substantially to good oral health for millions of children, a significant number of children and adults face significant challenges receiving the care they need (see "Prevention of Dental Diseases" in Chapter 13). These children are most often from low-income or minority families, and unfortunately these groups tend to experience more oral disease, and with increased severity, than other children.[6,7] The SDOH that contribute to poor oral health outcomes for these children are lack of finances (including lack of third-party coverage), lack of transportation and geographical isolation, language and cultural barriers, and availability of dental providers who accept Medicaid.

Another major factor that limits use of dental services is lack of perceived need for care and low oral health literacy. Although financial, cultural, behavioral, social, and biologic factors are among the major determinants of oral health, literacy skills are hypothesized to contribute to oral health outcomes. Oral health literacy is defined as "the degree to which individuals have the capacity to obtain, process, and understand basic oral health information and services needed to make appropriate health decisions."[8] Individual patient skills, the provider's ability to communicate effectively and accurately, and the informational demands placed on patients by healthcare systems affect health literacy. Low health literacy has been linked to poor health outcomes, lower use of preventive services, increased use of hospital emergency rooms, and higher healthcare costs.[9]

Dental Participation in Medicaid

Historically, financial limitations have been among the most formidable barriers for low-income children in receiving healthcare.

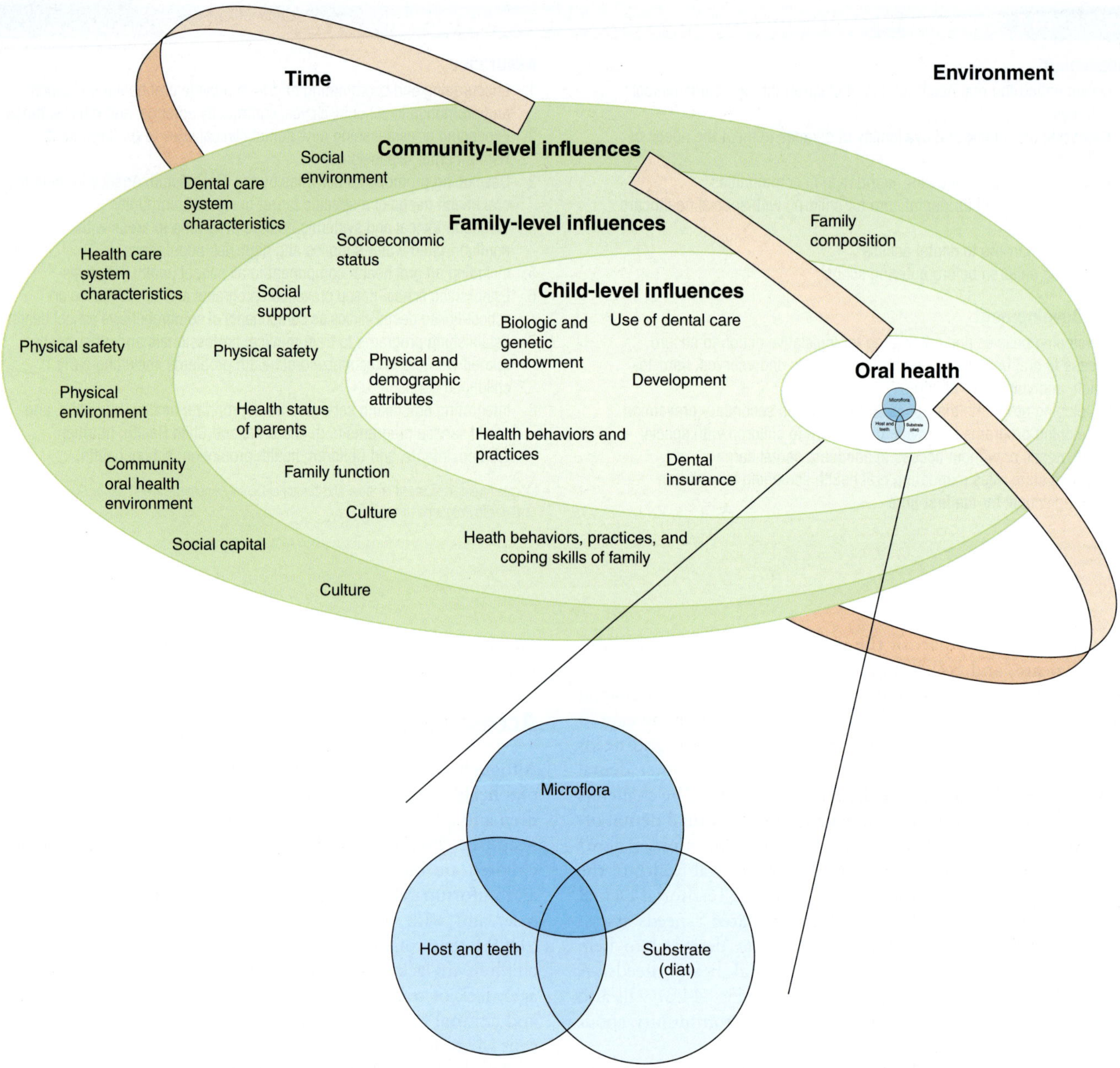

• **Fig. 44.2** Schematic demonstrating the various levels of influence on the oral health of a child. (From Fisher-Owens SA, Gansky SA, Platt LF, et al. Influences on children's oral health: a conceptual model. *Pediatrics.* 120;2007:e510-e520; Adapted from Keyes PH. *Int Dent J.* 1962;12:443-464 and National Committee on Vital and Health Statistics. Shaping a Health Statistics Vision for the 21st Century. Washington, DC: Department of Health and Human Services Data Council, Centers for Disease Control and Prevention, National Center for Health Statistics; 2002.)

In 1965 the federal government attempted to reduce these financial barriers by creating a Medicaid program (Title 19) that pays for medical and dental care for eligible low-income children. Adult dental coverage under Medicaid is optional, and covered services vary widely from state to state. As states look to balance budgets, often comprehensive adult dental Medicaid benefits are affected, either reduced to emergency care only or eliminated entirely. This is unfortunate, as evidence suggests that the oral health status of children can be negatively affected by poor oral health and lack of dental coverage for their caregivers.[10] However, coverage for child dental services is mandatory because of a 1968 amendment to the Medicaid program creating the Early and Periodic Screening, Diagnostic and Treatment (EPSDT) program (US Congress, 1968).[11] The purpose of the EPSDT program is to identify the health problems of children as early as possible and to provide comprehensive preventive and remedial care.

Since 1965, the Medicaid program has been the primary public insurance program for the financing of dental services for low-income children in the United States. In 1997 the State Children's Health Insurance Program (SCHIP) was started to expand public insurance to children in families with incomes too high to qualify for Medicaid but not adequate to purchase private insurance; the program is now simply known as the CHIP program (Centers for Medicare and Medicaid Service [CMS]).[11] In January 2015, the

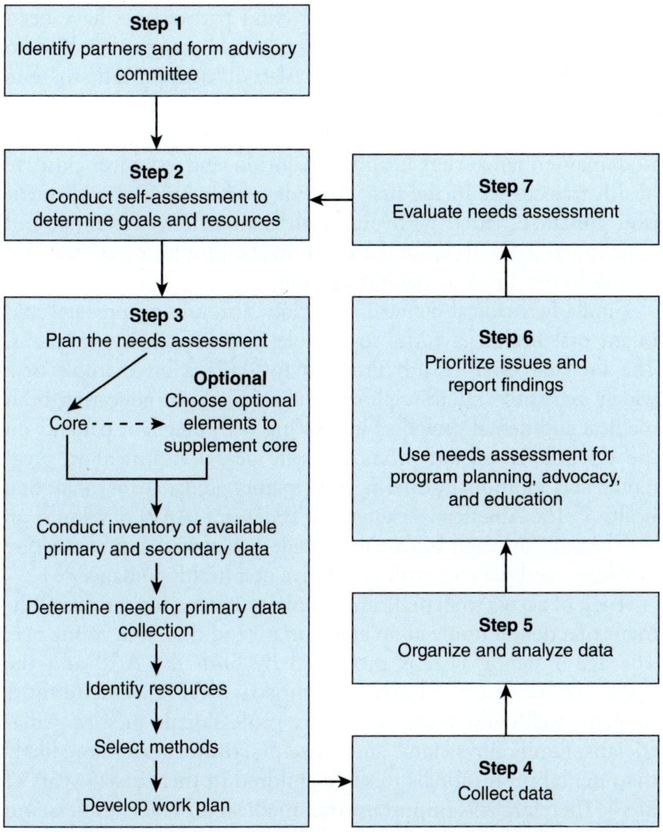

• **Fig. 44.3** Association of State and Territorial Dental Directors Seven-Step Needs Assessment Model. (Redrawn from Association of State and Territorial Dental Directors. *Assessing Oral Health Needs: ASTDD Seven Step Model*. www.astdd.org/docs/astdd-guidelines-for-oral-health-programs.pdf. Revised 2024. Accessed November 18, 2024.)

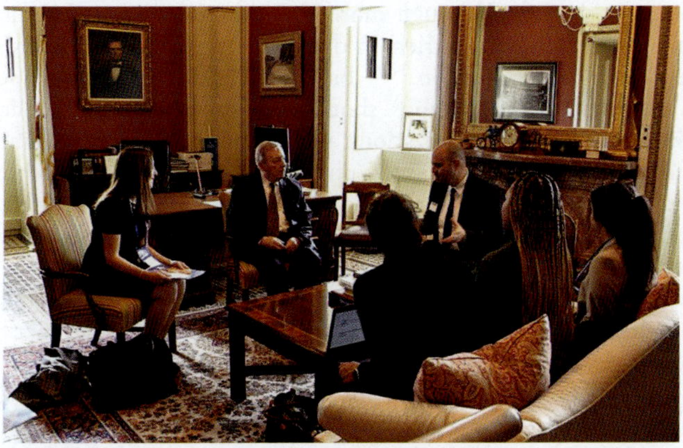

• **Fig. 44.4** Pediatric dentists from Illinois meet with Senator Dick Durbin during the American Academy of Pediatric Dentistry Pediatric Oral Health Advocacy Conference in Washington, DC to discuss issues related to children's oral health.

Affordable Care Act (ACA) required that all children who were up to 133% of the federal poverty level be transitioned from CHIP to Medicaid.[12]

Although Medicaid and CHIP have been successful in improving access to dental services for some, in 1996 a report from the Inspector General of the US Department of Health and Human Services (DHHS) indicated that only 1 in 5 Medicaid-eligible children receive any dental services annually (US Office of the Inspector General, 1996).[13] However, the number of children receiving dental services under Medicaid has grown continuously since the turn of the century. By 2012, almost half of all children under age 20 were reported to receive dental services, compared with 29.3% in 2000; as of 2021 this has reached a plateau, remaining around 50%.[13,14] Interestingly, 41.8% of Medicaid/CHIP enrollees had at least one dental care visit in 2021 compared with 58.7% of children with private insurance.[14]

One of the biggest barriers to dental care is the lack of dentists willing to accept Medicaid-enrolled children. Rates of participation vary by state and by the definition of participation.[15] The most common reason cited by dentists for their lack of participation in Medicaid was the low reimbursement rates.[16] As overhead expenses such as staff and supplies increase, Medicaid reimbursement rates oftentimes stagnate or decrease proportionally to overhead costs, as incremental rate increases are not typically built into state budgets to stay on par with inflation. Even as small as a 10% increase in Medicaid reimbursement has been associated with increased dental provider participation. With the ever-increasing cost of dental education, more expensive education creates further barriers for dental providers to be able to participate in rendering care at a low reimbursement, even if they would prefer to from a values standpoint.[15]

A number of states have increased reimbursement rates to try and improve dentists' acceptance of Medicaid enrollees; however, there are multiple other variables that dictate improved access and utilization.[17] Historically, states found success in raising Medicaid reimbursement rates after being successfully sued because of poor access to dental care; however, a 2015 US Supreme Court Decision *Armstrong et al. v. Exceptional Child Center, Inc. et al.* made it impossible for individual providers to sue a state for low Medicaid reimbursement increases.[18,19] A recent wave of dental Medicaid reimbursement increases in states like Nebraska, Illinois, Missouri, South Dakota, Virginia, and Ohio were the result of grassroots advocacy efforts led by state dental organizations.

Nonfinancial barriers for dentists to participate in Medicaid are also significant. For example, in a study from Iowa, although dentists were more likely to rank low fees as the most important problem, more dentists said that broken appointments were a more important problem in their practice than low reimbursement.[20] Dentists who were less busy and those who ethically feel obligated to advocate for and treat Medicaid enrollees were most likely to be accepting all new Medicaid patients in their practice.[21,22]

The Pediatric Dental Benefit Within the Affordable Care Act

One of the largest changes in healthcare coverage in the history of the United States involved implementation of the Patient Protection and Affordable Care Act by President Barack Obama in 2010. Although private dental benefits for adults were completely absent from the law, a pediatric dental benefit was included.[12]

For adults, states were given the option under the ACA to expand Medicaid, which included dental benefits of some kind in most scenarios. Between 2013 and 2016, there was an increase of 15.5 million people enrolled in Medicaid or CHIP.[23] In states that did not expand Medicaid, children make up a significant portion of Medicaid and CHIP combined. Currently, 41 states have chosen Medicaid expansion and there are 79 million people enrolled in Medicaid or CHIP.[24]

Despite the best of intentions, the ACA lacked an effective pathway to provide comprehensive dental coverage for children due to several loopholes. The law allowed several variations that either eliminated mandated dental coverage for children or provided for a large deductible that made dental coverage available only when large health expenditures had been met by the family.[25]

Federally Qualified Health Centers

As part of his "Great Society" plan to eliminate poverty, President Lyndon Johnson funded eight neighborhood health centers in 1965. This neighborhood health center concept has continued to develop and expand through the years. It has evolved into a nationwide network of roughly 1300 federally qualified health centers (FQHCs), which includes Community Health Centers, Migrant Health Centers, Health Care for the Homeless programs, and public housing primary care programs. The mission of these centers is to increase access to affordable healthcare services for low-income families. FQHCs are located throughout the country in areas with limited access to primary healthcare for a significant portion of the population due to economic, geographical, and/or cultural barriers. FQHCs provide primary and preventive healthcare services including dental care in many centers. In doing so, FQHCs have played a large role in modeling the integration of oral health into primary care.

Fiscal year (FY) 2023 collections for FQHCs were $46 billion, with $4.5 billion from dental services. Program statistics from the 2023 Uniform Data System (UDS) for that same year were as follows[26]:

Total users: 31.3 million
Total patients who received a dental service: 6.4 million
Total dentists: 5362
Total hygienists: 2821
Total dental therapists: 39
Other dental personnel: 12,343

Over the past 5 years, children (<18 years old) have consistently represented almost one-third of patients served.[26] The role of FQHCs in the provision of oral healthcare for individuals who would otherwise not be able to access or afford care has increased over the past decade, and this trend is projected to continue.

Prenatal and Early Childhood Oral Health: The Role of Nondental Professionals and Public Health Programs

The health of an infant begins with the caregiver. Mothers with untreated dental disease have children with a higher likelihood of experiencing caries, and with increased severity.[10] A recent systematic review found that mothers with access to prenatal oral healthcare have reduced early childhood caries incidence in their children.[27] It can be argued that prenatal oral health initiatives offer the most upstream prevention for dental disease onset in early childhood, especially as some pregnant women of low socioeconomic status gain dental coverage through insurance during pregnancy that they may not have otherwise.

Successful integration of oral health activities, including prevention, education, and screening in the prenatal and infancy developmental stage, is occurring in the public health sector, namely through Maternal Child Health clinics and Women, Infants, and Children (WIC) clinics. WIC is a national public health nutrition program in which child participants have been linked to increased participation in dental services that lead to improved oral health outcomes.[28] Also, it is important to note from a nutrition standpoint, the recent inclusion of dietary guidelines focused on the infancy and toddler developmental time period may enhance oral health prevention and establish positive health trajectories in the first 1000 days of life.[29] Optimal nutrition guidance paired with oral health education, screening, and appropriate referrals is fundamental in the promotion of oral and overall health in an at-risk population.

Similarly, medical-dental integration surrounding prenatal and infant oral health gave rise to notable interdisciplinary programs. The Prenatal Oral Health Program (pOHP) is an example of a widely accessible interdisciplinary online platform educating both medical and dental providers interfacing with pregnant patients on the importance of and promoting safe dental treatment in pregnancy, and additionally offering anticipatory guidance for infant oral health.[30] The American Academy of Pediatrics (AAP) developed an oral health campaign toolkit to provide pediatricians, prenatal care providers, and patients with preventive oral health guidance.[31]

Lack of access to dental care is a major barrier for the establishment of a dental home at an appropriate and desirable young age. The age 1 dental visit is promoted by both the AAP and the American Academy of Pediatric Dentistry (AAPD). Due to more frequent well-child visits, healthcare professionals such as pediatricians, family physicians, and nurse practitioners are more likely than dental professionals to serve children in their first 5 years of life.[32] Therefore it is important that medical providers understand their crucial role in alleviating oral health disparities by including oral health as part of their practices.

Policy changes have broadened and facilitated the role of the nondental provider in oral healthcare. In 2014 the US Preventive Services Task Force recommended the application of fluoride varnish by primary care providers.[33] The ACA stipulates insurance coverage for varnish application for children 1 to 5 years old without cost sharing. Although more providers are applying varnish and reporting fewer barriers in doing so, application is inconsistent and barriers remain.[34,35] Barriers include confusion about what pediatric populations should receive varnish, and policy alignment among organizations, which could reduce uncertainty and increase uptake.[36] Given physician provision of preventive oral health services, including fluoride varnish, has been shown to reduce the prevalence of childhood caries, promoting this intervention is crucial.

One primary and consistent barrier to physicians incorporating oral health is lack of knowledge, including a declining number of pediatricians who feel they are able to diagnose dental caries.[6,37–40] The AAP has a section on oral health that publishes routinely updated policies and promotes several educational resources intended for the medical professional, patient, and oral health advocate. Fortunately, pediatricians have expressed fewer barriers to incorporating oral health in practice, leading to increased physician application of fluoride varnish and dental referrals to younger patients.[40] Nevertheless, there is limited uptake of oral examination and caries risk assessment. As a matter of advocating for the children in their community, the individual pediatric dentist should consider providing education and resources to child-focused medical providers in their community.

It is important that medical educators make an effort to include oral health as a required component in both pediatric and family medicine residency programs and offer continuing education programs for all child health professionals. Research has shown that incorporation of infant oral health education in pediatric residency programs can improve oral health knowledge, confidence, and behavior of residents while delivering oral healthcare services.[41,42] The same has been observed in training programs for practicing medical providers.[43–45] Extensive programs in Washington,[43] North Carolina,[44] and California[45] focused on training medical professionals in providing preventive dental services such as counseling, oral screening, risk assessment, fluoride application, and referral. They also addressed issues regarding Medicaid reimbursement for these preventive services. Overall results of these training sessions were positive in terms of increased oral health knowledge, integration of preventive services in the medical offices, and improved accuracy among these professionals in identifying children needing referrals. Survey results from pediatricians who rotated through the University of Iowa's Infant Oral Health Program (IOHP) during their residency are encouraging. These pediatricians, compared with those who graduated before the inclusion of this rotation in their training curriculum, were more knowledgeable about important early childhood caries preventive measures, such as parental brushing and use of smear amount of fluoride toothpaste, for the young child. In addition, these pediatricians were more likely to examine the teeth of children 3 years of age and younger.[46]

Although the medical profession has acted to increase participation of pediatric primary care providers in delivering oral healthcare services for young children, few medical practitioners in isolated areas of the country have assumed this responsibility. More action is required to increase education about preventive oral healthcare in medical schools and residency programs, to make continuing education programs available nationwide, to lobby policymakers about the importance of reimbursement for pediatric oral healthcare services, and to establish more effective collaboration between dentistry and medicine and other stakeholders in public health.

Project Head Start

Head Start is the largest preschool program in the country and serves children from low-income families and children with disabilities. It was established in 1965 and is administered by the DHHS. Head Start is a comprehensive child development program intended to address educational, social, nutritional, medical, and emotional needs of children from birth to age 5 years, pregnant women, and their families.[47] They are child-focused, culturally conscious programs and their overall goal is to increase the school readiness of young children in low-income families. Head Start operates in all 50 states, the District of Columbia, Puerto Rico, Virgin Islands, and Outer Pacific Islands. In addition, it provides child development services to migrant children and families and Indian tribal nations. From 2022 to 2023, nearly 800,000 children were enrolled in any Head Start program with funding approaching $12 billion.[48]

Since its inception, Head Start has grown and been modified significantly. In 1995 the federal government began grant funding Early Head Start programs, serving pregnant women and children up to 3 years old. At the same time, Head Start and Early Head Start began providing services through community childcare centers (Fig. 44.5). Head Start Performance Standards established in 1975 have evolved to increase program efficacy. In 2007 educational standards were aligned with state-level standards and qualifications for educators increased. In 2016 standards were again modified to address historical data and new educational evidence.[47]

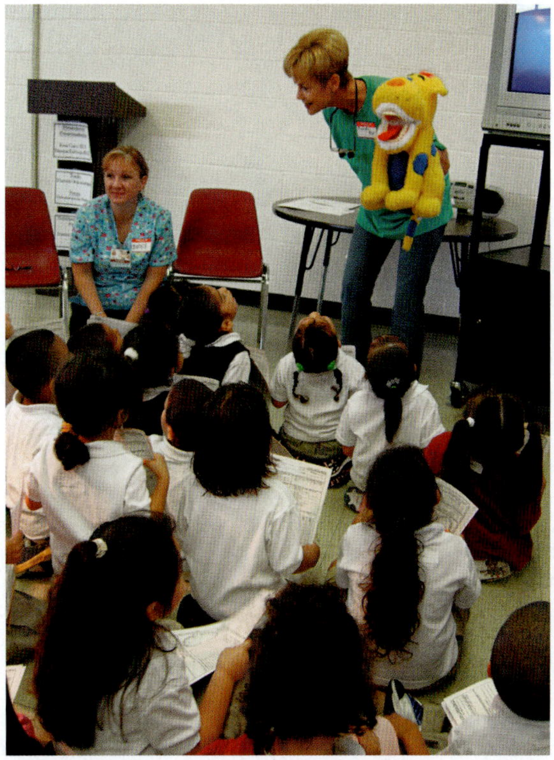

• **Fig. 44.5** Dental hygienists provide education to Head Start children. (From Geurink KV. *Community Oral Health for the Dental Hygienist*. 3rd ed. Saunders; 2012.)

Head Start has historically maintained a strong commitment to the health of children and their families enrolled in its programs. This commitment reflects the documented connection between school readiness and good health, including good oral health. Head Start and Early Head Start have a mandatory dental component requiring all enrolled children to receive a dental examination complete with prophylaxis and follow-up care for necessary restorative treatment. Head Start programs establish and maintain dental records for children enrolled in their program, but the necessary dental treatment is usually provided by dental professionals in the community or within public health clinics. Head Start programs are the payer of last resort for necessary dental treatment for children enrolled in their program who are not eligible for funding from Medicaid or other sources. This unique public-private partnership has been instrumental in helping ensure access to care for low-income preschool children nationwide. One of the stated goals of Head Start is to attempt to link families to an ongoing healthcare system to ensure that the child continues to receive comprehensive healthcare even after leaving the Head Start program.[49] At the beginning of the program year in 2022, 79.9% of children had accessible dental care, rising to 86.2% by 2023.[50]

All Head Start grantees have a health services manager who must ensure that families, staff, and community resources are coordinated for the delivery of quality health services to children. This work includes training families and staff to conduct ongoing observations to spot signs of health problems, including "lift the lip" techniques (Fig. 44.6). The health services manager and staff recruit and build professional relationships with community health and dental professionals to work toward good health for all children.

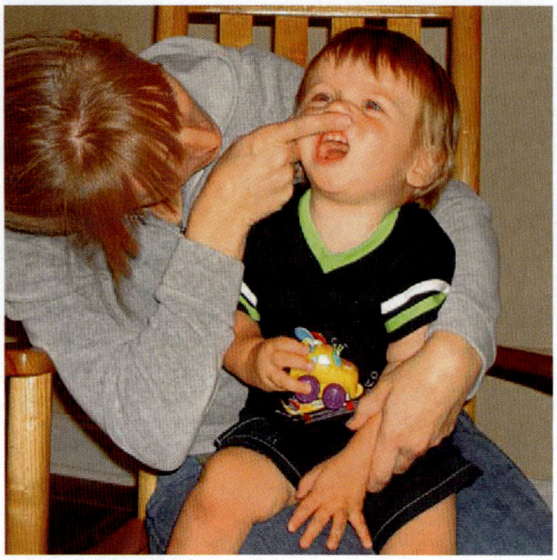

• **Fig. 44.6** Mother uses the "lift the lip" technique to check her child's mouth for decay. (From Bird DL, Robinson DS. *Modern Dental Assisting*. 10th ed. Saunders; 2012.)

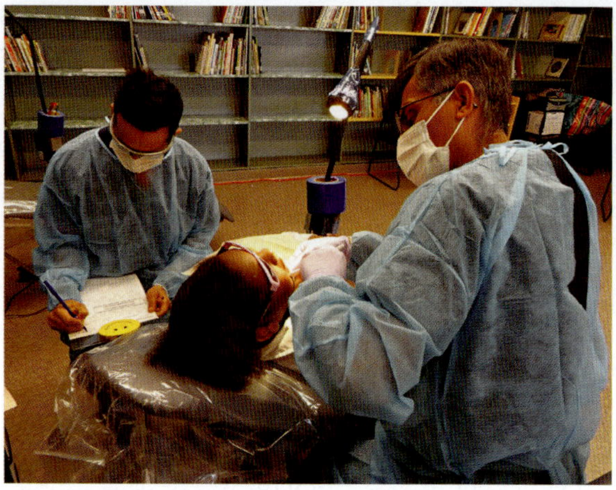

• **Fig. 44.7** Dentists place dental sealants as part of a school-based sealant program. Commonly, through one of these programs, examinations and sealants are provided to children in second through sixth grades.

Special Medicaid Dental Programs

States are encouraged to innovate their Medicaid programs to increase access and utilization among its members, particularly its youngest enrollees. One example is the Access to Baby and Children Dentistry (ABCD) program in Washington State. ABCD is a public-private partnership in which care coordinators help connect families and dental offices, where children under age 6 years can receive additional preventive care, and dentists receive advanced training in pediatric dentistry behavior management techniques and enhanced reimbursements.[51] Preliminary studies have shown that ABCD improved dental care utilization and led to less dental disease.[52,53] Similar programs exist in North Carolina (focusing on medical care providers) and Iowa.[54–56]

School-Based Dental Care

The attainment of school age presents another unique opportunity for enhancing the oral health of children. Schools are a logical site for promoting oral health through educational and prevention[57] programs and delivering dental services to school-aged children because they provide a high concentration of children at the same location.[58] The United States has enjoyed a long tradition of successfully implementing oral health activities in school settings. The Centers for Disease Control and Prevention has established guidelines for school-based dental services through Coordinated School Health programs, which were set up to improve basic health outcomes in school-based settings. Examples of services that can be provided in these settings include oral health education, fluoride mouth rinsing (FMR), sealant placement, oral health screenings and referrals, and comprehensive restorative care.

Health education, including oral health education, has long been considered an important part of school curricula in the United States. Dentists and other dental health professionals often have the opportunity to contribute to these activities by visiting classrooms and participating in health fairs or other special events. Oral health information presented in these forums can generate interest and stimulate changes in knowledge and attitudes. However, it is important for the oral health professional to understand that these changes are commonly short-lived and that desired behavioral changes require regular, long-term follow-up.[59]

Once an important component of a population-health caries risk reduction approach, school-based FMR programs have fluctuated in promotion and use over the past 40 years. Children participating in school-based FMR programs rinse for 1 to 2 minutes daily with 10 mL of a 230 parts per million (ppm) sodium fluoride solution or weekly with a 900 ppm sodium fluoride solution. Mouth rinsing activities are generally supervised by a classroom teacher, a school nurse, or other persons with appropriate training.[60]

A 2016 Cochrane review estimated that routine use of a 230 to 900 ppm fluoride mouth rinse resulted in a 27% reduction in decayed, missing, and filled tooth surfaces in permanent teeth, irrespective of community water fluoridation (CWF) or fluoride toothpaste use. However, the widespread presence of over-the-counter fluoride products, CWF, and existing reductions in caries prevalence raised questions about cost-effectiveness and shifted focus away from this intervention. These programs are most likely to be cost-effective when targeted at schools with additional risk factors along with a lack of water fluoridation (e.g., low-income status, high caries rate, lack of access to primary care).[60]

School sealant programs are an effective, but substantially underused intervention for increasing the prevalence of sealants. Recent evidence continues to support school-based sealant programs as cost-effective and an important method for uptake in high-risk populations.[61,62] Two different models exist, one in which oral health professionals come to schools to evaluate children and refer to participating dentists or another where oral health professionals come to schools and apply sealants after a brief evaluation. Because of the timing of eruption for first permanent molars, second grade is a common age to initiate sealant programs. The majority of sealant programs use a four-handed approach, with each team generally providing sealants to 10 to 15 children a day (Fig. 44.7). The increased use of glass ionomer as a pit-and-fissure sealant has the potential to increase sealant retention and efficacy of these programs, as the material is less technique sensitive and more tolerant of moist conditions compared with resin sealant. Despite their known success, school sealant programs are not widely used. Barriers to increased programming include funding, licensure, state policy guidelines regarding supervision, and Medicaid reimbursement.[63]

CariedAway is a preventive oral health intervention targeting high-risk youth in New York City primary schools utilizing glass ionomer as sealant and restorative material, fluoride varnish application, and silver diamine fluoride (SDF) to control caries. SDF is applied to the posterior dentition only. Evidence demonstrates SDF and varnish worked at least as well as glass ionomer sealants and varnish in caries arrest and prevention.[64] Furthermore, studies demonstrate that despite black staining, oral health quality of life among youth participating in CariedAway is not negatively impacted.[65] Given funding as a major barrier to school sealant programs, the comparatively lower cost of SDF may be a viable alternative.

Oral health screenings are carried out in schools under a number of different circumstances. Often, oral health screenings are provided as part of health fairs or in combination with other community activities. The purpose of these screenings is generally to identify gross problems using minimal equipment, including a penlight and tongue blade. When screenings are performed in conjunction with school sealant programs or as part of surveys gathering oral health data from children, the mirror and explorer examination is often more complete.

School-based oral health screenings generally result in a referral for follow-up care, including area dentists, community health, or school-based clinics. Only rarely are school-based screenings or examinations intended to take the place of complete dental examinations by dentists outside the school. This information should be communicated to parents and guardians as part of the consent process for children who are screened in school-based settings so that they understand the intent of the school-based screening and the limitations of the procedures provided (e.g., no radiographs or definitive treatment).

Comprehensive school-based dental care is not common in the United States, although there are some examples. In Virginia, comprehensive school-based dental programs were first introduced in 1921, with ongoing programs functioning ever since.[66] School-based dental care has been a key feature of the community since 2013 in Cincinnati, Ohio. Now at least five schools have clinics where children attending those schools, and those from area schools, can receive comprehensive care. During the 2018–2019 school year, 84% of students at one school in Cincinnati had an examination and preventive care and 88% of students had all dental needs addressed.[67]

Some localities may utilize a mobile coach or dental van to deliver varying levels of care to students at school. Services offered in this setting may include screening, preventive care, or comprehensive restorative care. Although these mobile clinics may address needs short term, they do not function as a dental home and there is limited evidence to determine the positive impact on the oral health of school children. Despite the efforts both here and abroad, geographical variation in oral health outcomes persist.

School-based dental care can increase both access and use of dental services for children who do not or cannot receive care in the private sector. School-based dental programs, regardless of scope, should be planned carefully to optimize chances for success. The most fundamental aspect of planning involves a careful assessment of the need for school-based dental services and ongoing evaluation of such programs. School-based programs should not attempt to replace services provided in the private sector, nor should they compete for patients who are adequately served by existing resources. A profound piece missing from school-based dental clinics is that parents are not part of the educational component of the visit; in the long term, this is one of the most significant aspects of a preventive dental visit. Experimental intense education efforts fail to improve oral health outcomes in school-based settings compared with outcomes attributable to education through traditional dental services, because parental modeling is the most significant determinant of patient behavior.[68]

Visit eBooks.Health.Elsevier.com to see full list of references.

45

Temporomandibular Disorders

THOMAS R. STARK AND ERIK B. ANDERSON

CHAPTER OUTLINE

Temporomandibular Disorders in Children and Adolescents

The temporomandibular joint (TMJ) is an important structure that allows children and adolescents to engage in intricate jaw activities necessary for daily activities such as eating, speaking, and yawning. Growth and development of the TMJs occurs during childhood and adolescence. Like other joints, the TMJs are susceptible to damage from an injury or a disease process. An appreciation of the anatomical features and common conditions affecting the joint is crucial for diagnosing and managing young patients with temporomandibular disorders (TMDs).

Temporomandibular Joint Anatomy and Function

The TMJ has unique structural and neuroanatomical components that distinguish it from other synovial joints.[1] It is important to appreciate the functional components of the TMJs in order to offer patients contemporary information about the joint's mechanics, healing capacity, and potential sources of pain. Understanding the musculoskeletal and histologic aspects of the joint and surrounding structures allows providers to educate patients about healthy and diseased states.

The structural components of the TMJs include the mandibular condyles, glenoid fossae of the temporal bones, synovial membranes, ligaments, and articular discs. The nerves and vessels supplying the joint and surrounding structures form the neurovascular components. Bony structures are encased in a fibrous capsule, and the articular surfaces of the joint are lined with nonvascular, noncellular fibrocartilage. The TMJs are distinguished from other synovial joints by the presence of fibrocartilage rather than hyaline cartilage, which accounts for their favorable durability and healing capacity.[2] Viscous synovial fluid occupies the joint spaces, providing cushioning and lubrication for the articulating surfaces. Between the condyle and glenoid fossae sits the articular disc, which also cushions the joint and facilitates highly specialized jaw movements. Composed of dense fibrous connective tissue, the discs do not contain nerves or vessels. However, their posterior attachments are highly innervated and vascular. The posterior attachments, ligaments, and bony structures are potential sources of joint pain.[2] Sensory and proprioceptive innervation is supplied to the joint by the trigeminal nerve.

Bony structures of the TMJs are held together and controlled by skeletal muscles. The paired muscles of mastication (masseters, medial pterygoids, and temporalis) elevate the mandible (close the mouth). In contrast, the lateral pterygoids and, to a lesser extent, the digastric muscles depress the jaw (open the mouth). Activation of the inferior lateral pterygoid muscles protrudes the mandible.[2] Masticatory muscles are innervated by the mandibular branch of the trigeminal nerve, and the facial nerve innervates muscles involved in facial expression. Cervical muscles, including the supra and infra hyoids and sternocleidomastoids, stabilize the head during mastication, swallowing, and other complex jaw movements.[3,4] The cervical and spinal accessory nerves innervate cervical muscles. The convergence of upper cervical and trigeminal sensory circuits provides an anatomical basis for the phenomenon of pain referral in the orofacial regions.[5]

A basic understanding of TMJ biomechanics is necessary to understand both TMJ function and dysfunction.[2] Characterized as ginglymoarthrodial joints, the TMJs are capable of rotational (hinging) and translational (gliding) movements in three planes.[6] Within each joint, the glenoid fossa of the temporal bone and mandibular condyle are separated by an articular disk (Fig. 45.1). The articular discs divide the joints into superior and inferior joint spaces. Rotational jaw movements occur in the inferior joint space, and the superior joint space facilitates translational movements.[7] The paired TMJs primarily function in unison. However, the joint can undergo distraction on one side while being simultaneously compressed on the opposite.

Temporomandibular Joint Growth and Development

Initiation and development of the TMJ trails other synovial joints in the body.[8] TMJ components are derived from the first pharyngeal

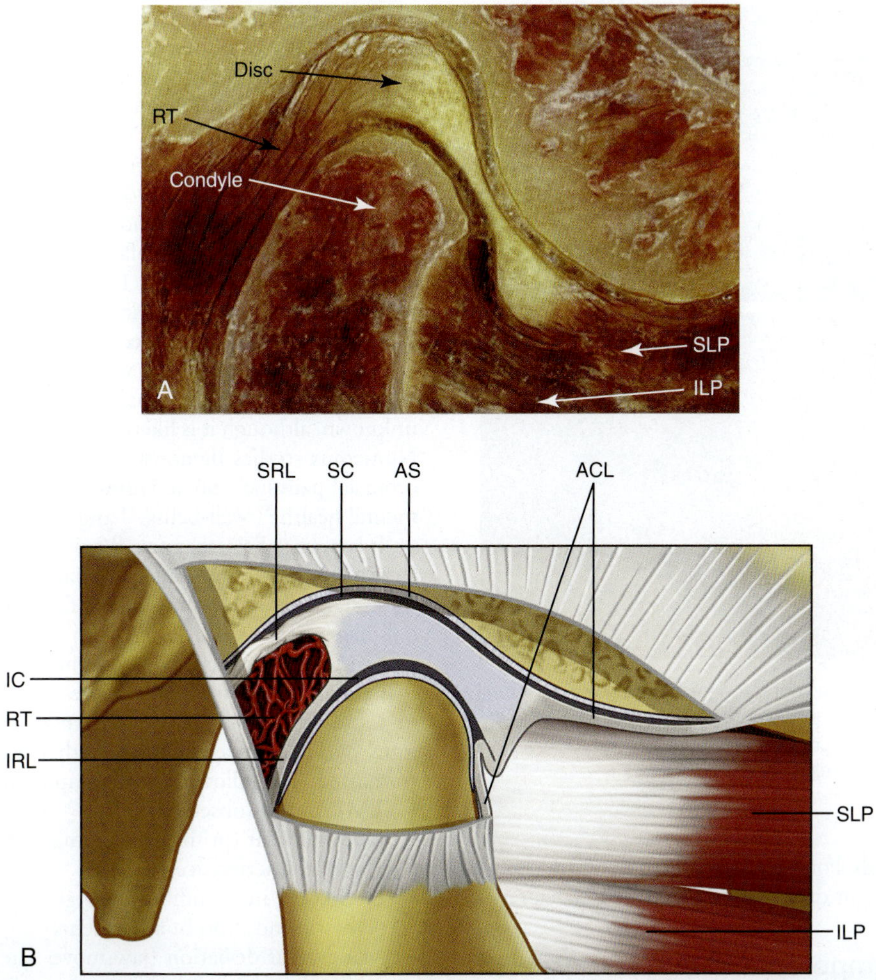

• **Fig. 45.1** Temporomandibular Joint. The diagram depicts a lateral view of the anatomical aspects of the temporomandibular joint including the articular disk interposed between the mandibular condyle and the glenoid fossa of the temporal bone. The articular surface (AS), along with the superior and inferior joint space or cavities (SC and IC) comprise the functional components of the joint. Additional structures of the joint include the anterior capsular ligaments (ACL), superior and inferior retrodiscal lamina (SRL and IRL), and the richly innervated and highly vascular retrodiscal tissue (RT). The lateral pterygoid muscles (ILP and SLP) located anterior to the articular disk are also depicted. (Courtesy (A) Dr. Per-Lennart Westeson, Rochester, NY, (B) Dr. JP Okeson.)

arch, and embryologic development occurs in three stages: blastemic, cavitation, and maturation.[8] The blastemic stage occurs from 7 to 8 weeks in utero. During this time, the organization of the glenoid fossa of the temporal bone and mandibular condyle begins. During weeks 9 to 11 of the cavitation stage, mesenchyme between the condyles and fossae forms the articular discs, and the outlines of the joint spaces become apparent. The inferior joint space vital for rotational movements precedes the development of the superior space. The TMJs continue to develop from 12 weeks until birth during the maturation stage. Highlights of the maturation stage include the formation of the joint's capsules by 17 weeks and cartilage from 19 to 20 weeks.[9] Disturbances in TMJ development can cause hypoplasia and lead to asymmetric malformations (Fig. 45.2).[10] Furthermore, congenital disorders involving the TMJs are frequently accompanied by defects in the mandible and ear due to the proximity to and coordinated development with the TMJs.[9] Craniofacial microsomia, Treacher Collins syndrome, Goldenhar syndrome, and primary condylar aplasia are examples of congenital disorders affecting the TMJs.[10]

The TMJs continue to undergo significant changes from birth through adolescence. Over time, the fossae deepen, the condyle-disc-fossa relationship stabilizes, and ligaments and muscles surrounding the joint become increasingly robust.[11] During the first few years of life, the mandibular condyles are loosely assembled within the shallow mandibular fossae, allowing the jaws to move freely in all three planes.[9] Mandibular growth occurs most rapidly during infancy and early childhood.[12] Growth of the condyles and forces from masticatory muscles are thought to influence joint morphology.[9] The condyles undergo endochondral ossification and grow in a superior and posterior direction, displacing the mandible inferiorly and anteriorly.[11] The bony prominence in the mandibular fossa's anterior section is referred to as the articular eminence. This anatomical feature facilitates the movement of the disc-condyle complex during complex jaw movements. By age 3, the articular eminence is approximately halfway formed, and by age 12, the joint has nearly reached the adult level of maturity. While apposition and resorption guide the fossa's growth and adaptation, remodeling of the mandibular condyles occurs through

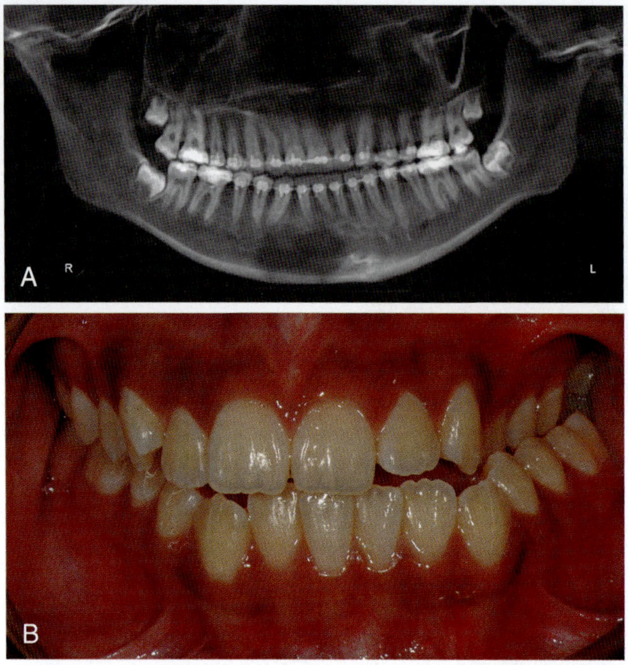

• **Fig. 45.2** (A) The panoramic radiograph demonstrates jaw asymmetry resulting from hypoplasia of the left mandibular condyle. (B) The clinical presentation depicts a posterior crossbite and a mandibular midline deviation due to the hypoplastic mandibular condyle.

secondary cartilage growth. For further information on the postnatal growth and development of the mandible, refer to Chapter 2.

Introduction to Temporomandibular Disorders

TMD refers to a group of painful or nonpainful conditions involving one or both TMJs, the masticatory muscles, or other surrounding structures.[13] Although some patients with a TMD may not require interventions beyond education and reassurance, others may require further evaluation and treatment. Orofacial pain is a general term that includes TMDs and other pain syndromes of the head and neck.[5] Pain and jaw dysfunction are common,[14–16] and children and adolescents may seek treatment for either acute or chronic orofacial pain. Acute pain lasts from days to weeks, but chronic pain may persist for months or even years.[17] As a rule, the longer pain persists, the more challenging it becomes to manage. Long-standing TMDs tend to be resistant to conventional treatment[17]; however, acute TMD pain may resolve spontaneously or with minimal interventions.

Evaluating TMD research can be challenging due to differences in study design, populations, and diagnostic criteria.[18,19] The Diagnostic Criteria for Temporomandibular Disorders (DC-TMD) protocol consists of a structured clinical examination with specific interview questions to aid in identifying individuals with TMDs. It offers a validated, objective methodology for evaluating adult patients with TMDs.[20] The protocol, developed as part of an international consortium, was recently updated to include guidance for pediatric and adolescent patients.[21] The updated protocol provides values and parameters to evaluate patients and classify TMDs into subgroups: (1) myogenous (muscle related) and (2) arthrogenous (joint related). A second portion of the DC-TMD includes the psychological status and pain-related disability that may affect patient outcomes.[22]

TMD prevalence in children and adolescents varies in the literature.[23–25] Epidemiologic studies reveal that TMDs are a sizable public health concern, with up to 7% of the total population requiring treatment.[7] Although uncommon in young children, signs and symptoms of TMDs often present during adolescence.[16,27,28] TMD prevalence ranges from 7.3% to 30.4% in children and adolescents.[27] According to a systematic review, the most common TMD diagnoses in children and adolescents are disk displacement and myofascial pain.[29] Another systematic review found TMJ sounds in 14% of children.[18] TMD symptoms tend to fluctuate with time in children and adolescents[25,30]; however, TMD-related pain becomes more prevalent in adolescence and young adulthood.[30] As with adults, TMDs tend to be more common in females than males.[31] The reason for this disparity is unknown, although it is likely related to hormonal differences.[32–34] Numerous studies demonstrate the negative impact TMDs and orofacial pain have on activities of daily living,[35] quality of life,[36] mental health,[37] well-being,[38] and sleep quality.[39]

It is essential to recognize the wide range of objective and subjective findings commonly associated with TMDs. Uncovering these signs and symptoms helps practitioners establish a differential diagnosis.

Signs are clinically observable findings. They may reflect normal variations or transient changes consistent with normal findings and have no clinical significance. On the other hand, some signs of TMDs may indicate further evaluation or treatment is warranted. The following are examples of signs:

- TMJ sounds (observed)
- Occlusal wear (primary or permanent teeth)
- Occlusal interferences
- Limitation in mandibular range of motion (ROM; $<$32 in pediatric and $<$36 in adolescents)
- Mandibular deviation (jaw moves laterally and returns to the midline) upon opening
- Mandibular deflection (jaw moves laterally toward the right or left side) upon opening
- Tenderness with palpation and/or manipulation

Symptoms are findings based on subjective information gathered from interviewing the patient and caregiver. Most children and adolescents can describe their symptoms. Very young children or patients with medical and intellectual disabilities may not be able to describe their symptoms adequately. The following should be considered when evaluating for TMD symptoms:

- Jaw pain
- Jaw tightness
- Jaw instability
- Jaw dysfunction
- Bite discomfort or feeling of instability
- Oral motor activity (tooth grinding, habitual jaw movements)
- Ear pain
- Neck pain
- Headaches or migraine symptoms (e.g., light sensitivity, nausea, dizziness)

The relationship between signs and symptoms remains unclear. For example, symptoms, such as pain and dysfunction, are not consistently associated with clinical signs such as TMJ sounds or occlusal wear.[40] The clinician is cautioned not to predict a future diagnosis of a severe TMD based on current signs and symptoms. Most cases of TMDs in adolescence are benign and self-limiting, only rarely progressing to a more serious condition.[41] In fact, a prospective study in adolescent females found degenerative changes secondary to TMJ arthritis remained stable over a 30-year period.[42]

• BOX 45.1 Etiologic Factors for Temporomandibular Joint Dysfunction in Children and Adolescents

Inherited

Hemifacial microsomia or other craniofacial anomaly
Juvenile idiopathic arthritis (formerly juvenile rheumatoid arthritis)
Ehlers-Danlos syndrome
Marfan syndrome

Acquired

Behavioral (parafunction, excessive gum chewing)
Infectious (septic arthritis)
Traumatic (injury from sports, accident, abuse)
Iatrogenic (damage from steroid, surgery, irradiation)
Neoplastic (tumors)
Idiopathic (hemifacial atrophy, idiopathic condylar resorption)
Degenerative (osteoarthritis)

No unique model or combination of etiologic factors can accurately predict TMD onset or development.[5] Therefore it is not possible to foresee who will acquire severe TMDs and, more importantly, who will experience a transition from acute to chronic or recurrent pain. Moreover, it is impossible to identify those requiring invasive or advanced treatment.[43] The focus on etiology should be determining and modifying the initiating, predisposing, and perpetuating factors.[5] Initiating factors are related to onset (e.g., trauma, stress); predisposing factors are related to risk (e.g., ligament laxity, jaw asymmetry); and perpetuating factors interfere with recovery (e.g., bruxism, poor sleep). Like other aspects of TMDs, there is considerable individual variability. Indeed, the cause of TMDs in some individuals may be unknown. Degenerative disease, developmental abnormalities, trauma, and other conditions usually have a clear and obvious relationship to TMDs, but other factors, such as malocclusion, have weak or conflicting associations (Box 45.1).

TMJ sounds are related to mechanical or degenerative issues within the joint, and they have been linked to the development of a TMD.[18] Patients often notice TMJ sounds due to the proximity of the TMJs to the auditory canals. Clicking, popping, snapping, scraping, and grinding sounds associated with jaw function can occur in patients of all ages.[25] Although joint sounds in infants and toddlers are rare, they have been reported to occur in 17% to 30% of school-aged children and adolescents.[45] Although TMJ sounds may persist in adulthood, it is not uncommon for TMJ sounds to come and go during childhood.[45]

Disorders of the TMJ can be identified by determining the presence or absence of joint sounds. Patients with TMJ disk displacement with reduction hear a clicking sound when they open their mouths or move the jaw from side to side. The clicking sound occurs as the mandibular condyle momentarily "recaptures" the displaced articular disc.[2] Conversely, patients with TMJ disk displacement without reduction do not hear a clicking sound because their articular discs block translational jaw movements.[44] Providers should suspect disk displacement without reduction in patients with a history of abrupt discontinuation of jaw-clicking sounds and a sudden, significant decrease in mouth opening. Grating or grinding noises signal degeneration of the bony components of the TMJ, as is seen in patients with degenerative joint diseases such as osteoarthritis. Unique condylar anatomy, partial jaw subluxation, and temporary sticking of the disk also account for TMJ sounds.[45]

Etiology of Temporomandibular Disorders

Parafunction, including awake and sleep bruxism, has been implicated in the etiology of TMDs.[46] Sleep bruxism, recently defined through an international consensus, is rhythmic and nonrhythmic masticatory muscle activity that occurs during sleep. It is not a movement disorder in otherwise healthy individuals.[47] Teeth grinding, tapping, and clenching often occur during rhythmic masticatory muscle activity.[48]

Sleep bruxism is an involuntary behavior thought to be driven by psychosocial factors and neurotransmitters in the regions of the brain responsible for motor function.[49] On the other hand, bruxing while awake (diurnal bruxism) is often a habit or voluntary behavior. Other parafunctional activities that may contribute to TMDs include lip biting, cheek biting, and chewing on other tissues or objects. These parafunctional activities may occur alone or in combination.

Bruxism is a common parafunctional activity in children and adolescents. Variations in study design can make it difficult to interpret data related to bruxism.[50] For instance, many studies do not objectively confirm the presence of bruxism with polysomnography or electromyography.[50,51] Furthermore, surveys relying on a parent's report of bruxism are subject to bias.[51,52] Nonetheless, sleep bruxism is reported to occur in approximately 14% to 38% of children and 13% to 22% of adolescents.[49,53] It appears to occur equally in males and females,[54] peaks during childhood, and persists into adulthood in some patients.[55]

Primary sleep bruxism occurs without a known cause, whereas secondary sleep bruxism is related to another factor, such as a medical condition or substance use. Sleep bruxism is highly prevalent in a variety of medical conditions such as gastroesophageal reflux disease,[56] cerebral palsy, Down syndrome, attention-deficit/hyperactivity disorder, autism spectrum disorder, and acute neurologic conditions.[57–59] Sleep bruxism also frequently presents in patients with obstructive sleep apnea.[60] Studies have demonstrated that sleep bruxism in adolescence may be associated with behavioral problems or psychosocial disorders.[59,61] Several medications and substances have been associated with sleep bruxism. For instance, antidepressants such as selective serotonin reuptake inhibitors[62] or stimulants such as methylphenidate, caffeine, and nicotine can lead to sleep bruxism.[63,64]

Surprisingly, sleep bruxism is not consistently associated with TMDs in children and adolescents. On the other hand, awake bruxism has demonstrated an association with TMDs in adolescents.[46] For this reason, a patient's worsening jaw pain during the day may be linked to habitual daytime bruxism. By contrast, if a patient experiences jaw pain upon waking, sleep bruxism should be suspected as a potential etiologic factor.

Malocclusion and orthodontic treatment have been reviewed extensively; however, neither has shown a clear and consistent relationship with TMDs.[65–68] Although occlusal features have been historically identified as risk factors, no single occlusal factor has been isolated as a source for TMDs.[66] In fact, the presence of some occlusal factors, such as nonworking interferences and anterior open bite, may be the result rather than the cause of a TMD.[66] Furthermore, the literature does not support a relationship between malocclusion and signs of a TMD, such as TMJ sounds.[69,70] A majority agree that prophylactic removal of occlusal interferences is contraindicated in patients with a TMD.[2,71] Nevertheless, an unstable occlusion coupled with excessive parafunction may increase the risk of developing a TMD. Although the evidence does not support preventive orthodontic therapy to avoid TMDs,[67,72] a recent systematic review found an association between unilateral TMJ disorders and facial asymmetry.[73] Orthodontic therapy is not a reliable treatment option for managing existing TMDs.[73,74] Although some studies indicate an increased risk of a brief, transient TMD during orthodontic treatment,[75] it does not appear to cause long-standing TMDs in growing patients.[76]

Traumatic injuries to the masticatory system and the differing levels of individual response to injury warrant further consideration, as there is a modest correlation between a history of trauma and TMD development.[77] Falls are common among children, and injuries to the chin or jaw can damage the TMJs.[78] Fractures and other extensive injuries in growing patients can lead to jaw asymmetry.[78] After an acute jaw injury, pain, swelling, decreased mouth opening, or changes in occlusion should alert practitioners of a potential condylar or subcondylar fracture. Fractures can be identified with a panoramic radiograph or more advanced techniques.[78] Referral to an orthodontic specialist should be considered to help prevent or minimize the possibility of jaw and facial asymmetry in the growing patient. Ligaments and other structures can also be damaged after trauma. TMJ ankylosis is a rare but serious manifestation of jaw trauma resulting in the fusion of the mandible to the cranial base or zygoma. The condition is associated with a decreased mandibular ROM and asymmetry in growing children.[79] Additionally, iatrogenic trauma from third molar removal or other dental procedures can cause TMDs.[80]

Some medical conditions may increase a patient's risk of developing a TMD. Systemic diseases such as juvenile idiopathic arthritis (JIA), Ehlers-Danlos syndrome, and Marfan syndrome have been associated with TMDs.[81,82] Congenital conditions, such as hemifacial microsomia and Treacher Collins syndrome, or local structural factors such as hyper- or hypoplasia of the mandibular condyle or a bifid condyle, may also contribute to TMDs.[10,83] Although rare, tumors, cysts, and pseudotumors may also present as TMDs.[84] Another uncommon but well-described localized condition, idiopathic condylar resorption (ICR), may present in pediatric or adolescent patients.

Last, pain in the TMJ region may be referred from another structure.[85] Potential referral sources include pain from the neck,[86] salivary glands,[87] lymph nodes,[88] ears,[89,90] and teeth. Migraine and tension-type headaches commonly occur in adolescent patients and may also present as a TMD.[91,92] In cases of referred pain, symptom improvement or resolution can only occur when the true source of the pain is identified and eliminated.

Diagnosis and Treatment of Temporomandibular Disorders

Clinicians must first establish a problem list and differential diagnosis before providing treatment recommendations for patients with TMDs. The American Academy of Orofacial Pain guidelines provide criteria for categorizing TMDs into two main subgroups: (1) myogenous (muscle related) and (2) arthrogenous (joint related).[7] Painful extracapsular (muscular) TMDs are commonly subdivided into myalgia and myofascial pain conditions. Intracapsular (joint-related) conditions are categorized as inflammatory (capsulitis), disk displacement disorders (reducing and nonreducing), degenerative disorders (osteoarthritis), and subluxation.[7]

A thorough understanding of muscle and joint pain characteristics will aid practitioners in providing an accurate diagnosis.[5] For example, joint-related pain is often localized to a focal area in front of the patient's ear, whereas muscle-related pain may be more diffusely localized and is often bilateral. Identifying whether the patient's chief complaint is primarily muscular or joint related will help guide treatment decisions. For instance, muscle pain may improve with massage, jaw exercises, and heat, whereas joint pain may resolve with antiinflammatory medications, a soft diet, and rest.

Screening Assessment for Temporomandibular Disorders

Screening for TMDs helps practitioners appreciate a patient's baseline jaw function and identify factors related to the overall health of their masticatory system. The patient interview, including a thorough medical, dental, and social history, is a key component of the TMD screening evaluation. During the interview, clinicians should aim to uncover TMD risk factors such as bruxism, past trauma, TMJ sounds, recent occlusal changes, jaw dysfunction, and pain. Inquiring about other chronic pain conditions, such as low back pain, stomach aches, neck pain, or headaches, also provides valuable information because these conditions are frequently associated with TMDs.[93,94] Primary headaches, such as migraine and tension-type headaches, frequently present as pain in the temporal region and may be misinterpreted as a TMD. Patients with pain and concurrent light sensitivity or nausea may suffer from a headache disorder.[94] Identifying stressors and screening for psychological conditions can also be useful because high stress and behavioral health problems have been associated with TMDs in adolescent populations.[95,96]

Comprehensive Assessment for Temporomandibular Disorders

A comprehensive assessment should be performed if a patient presents with a TMD. The patient's symptoms, especially the chief complaint, can help the clinician establish a diagnosis. Patients with a TMD commonly present with reports about pain, muscle tightness, jaw instability, and joint sounds. When conducting the interview, it is recommended to use a systematic approach because symptoms are subjective. The OPQRSTU acronym is a useful tool to help practitioners collect information about the patient's pain complaints (Table 45.1). Identifying the onset, provoking and palliating factors, quality, region, severity, timing, and impact of pain enables providers to objectively assess pain complaints. The history of the pain complaint, as well as past treatments and results of those treatments, should also be obtained.

The clinical examination aims to confirm the information gathered from the interview and reproduce the patient's chief complaint. When performing the musculoskeletal examination, the presence of a parent or chaperone is recommended. Clinical signs such as TMJ sounds, tenderness with palpation, and alterations or limitations in mandibular opening are evaluated during the examination. Providers should also assess posture and identify signs of parafunction like masseter hypertrophy and wear facets on the teeth. Palpation of the TMJs, masticatory structures, and cervical structures helps identify the patient's chief complaint. Furthermore, palpation can identify pathology such as a soft tissue mass or crepitation of the TMJ. The preauricular region may be painful if joint inflammation is present. Conversely, muscles

TABLE 45.1 "OPQRSTU" Tool for Evaluating Pain Symptoms

Onset	When did pain first begin? What was associated with pain initiation? (Trauma, eating, stress)
Provoking and **P**alliating factors	What makes pain worse? (Eating, poor sleep) What makes pain better? (Heat, ice, rest)
Quality	What does pain feel like? (Ache, throb, tight)
Region	Where is the pain? (Point with one finger)
Severity	How intense is the pain? (0–10/10, mild, moderate, severe)
Timing	Is pain intermittent or constant? How long does pain last? When does pain occur? (Time of day, during school, during jaw function, at rest)
U—"You"	How does pain affect the patient? (Interferes with school, activities, sleep)

may also exhibit pain, especially if firm bands of muscle (i.e., trigger points) are appreciated during palpation. Excessive jaw clenching can lead to symptomatic masticatory muscles, and neck pain may be related to poor posture (Fig. 45.3). Functional manipulation of the TMJs and masticatory muscles can provide practitioners with additional information needed to support the patient's diagnosis.

Palpation of the TMJs involves standing directly in front or behind the patient and using the index fingers to apply light, steady pressure. The lateral capsules of the TMJs should be palpated while the patient opens and closes the mouth and moves the mandible from side to side (Fig. 45.4). TMJ palpation helps detect irregular movement of the condyles as well as joint noises or pain. The patient should be asked if it feels the same on both sides or if either side feels sore during palpation. The presence or absence of pain or joint sounds should be documented. Clicking during opening and closing usually indicates a disk displacement with reduction. The grating sensation of crepitus is usually a sign of joint degeneration found in specific conditions such as osteoarthritis or ICR, or a systemic condition such as JIA.

The palpation technique for masticatory muscles is like the technique used for the TMJs (Fig. 45.5). A slight increase in finger pressure is acceptable when palpating muscles. The clinician may appreciate taut bands or discrete nodules within the patient's musculature that are exquisitely painful when pressed. Palpation of these sites may cause the patient's pain to spread within the muscle or even radiate to a distant region (e.g., forehead, temple). Localized muscle pain is referred to as myalgia. However, when a patient's pain spreads or radiates upon palpation, the diagnosis is myofascial pain.

The superior and inferior aspects of the masseter muscles and posterior, middle, and anterior aspects of the temporalis muscles should be palpated. The temporalis tendon may be palpated intraorally by placing the index finger in the vicinity of the insertion of the temporalis muscle on the coronoid process. The lateral pterygoid muscles are best tested by having the patient protrude the mandible against chin resistance, which generally produces pain if the lateral pterygoid is symptomatic (Fig. 45.6). The medial pterygoid muscles are difficult to evaluate because they function in concert with the masseter muscles and require intraoral palpation near the floor of the mouth.

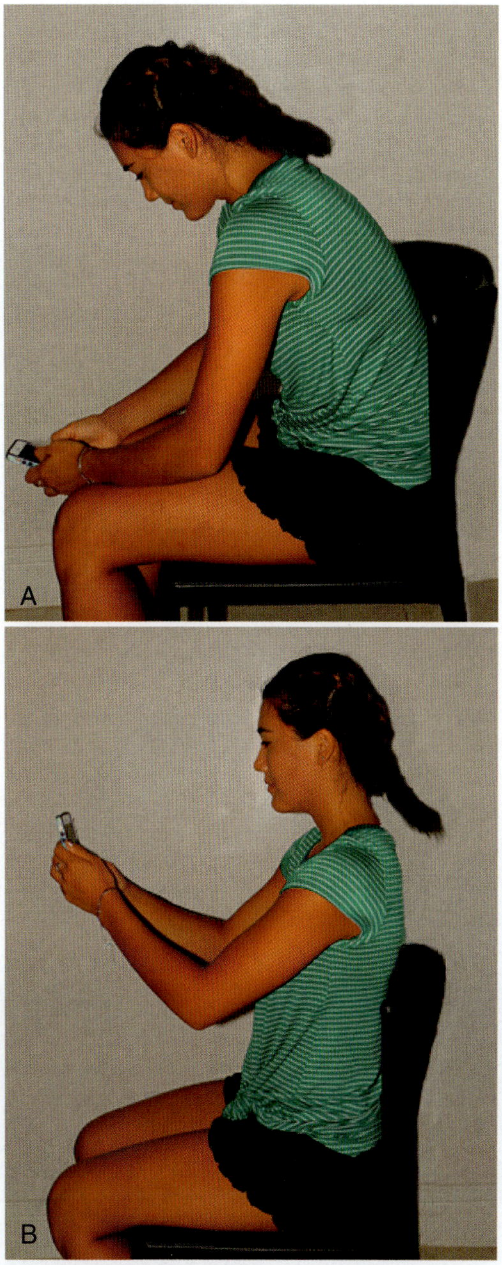

• **Fig. 45.3** (A) Patient demonstrates a forward head posture and rounding of the shoulders while using a mobile device. This posture puts strain on the cervical musculature. (B) Improved head and shoulder posture relieves tension in the cervical muscles.

Cervical muscles are palpated in a similar manner to the masticatory muscles. Muscles, such as the trapezius and sternocleidomastoid, may be palpated directly or by gently gripping the musculature between the thumb and index or middle finger (Fig. 45.7). Some patients may experience orofacial pain caused by pain referral from cervical structures. The patient's "site" and "source" of pain are different.[2] In this case, the patient's orofacial pain complaint cannot improve until the pain in the cervical structures is addressed.

Mandibular function should be assessed, and the ROM should be recorded to determine the patient's relative ability to function

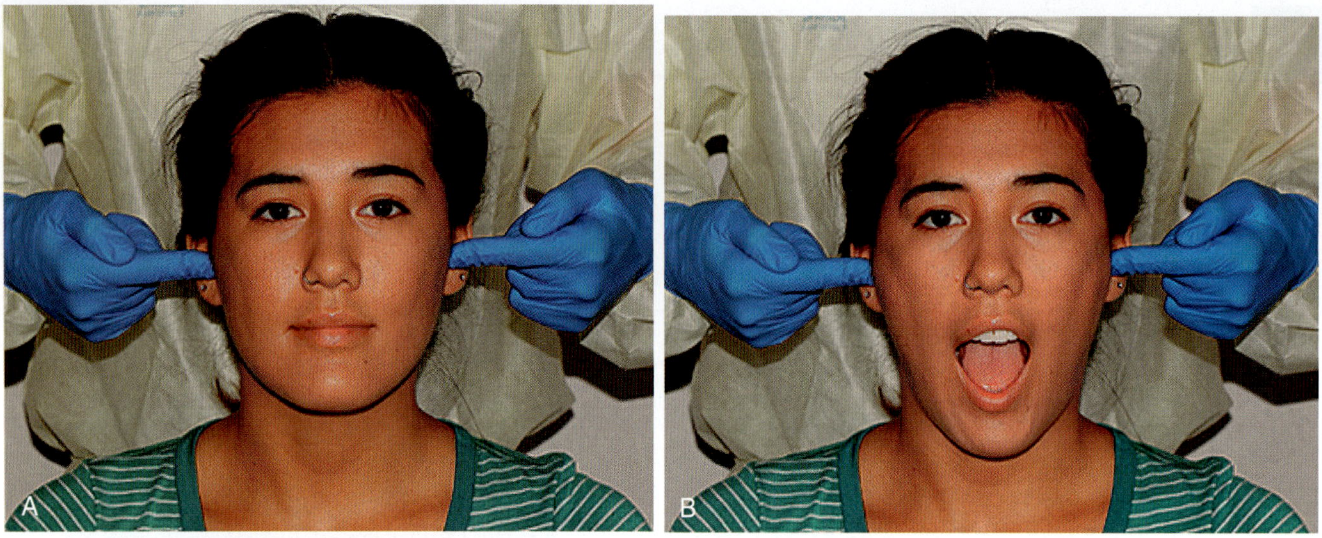

• **Fig. 45.4** (A) Temporomandibular joint palpation during rest. Pain with palpation is a sign of a joint-related problem. (B) The joint is palpated during motion to detect any irregular movement of the condyles as well as joint noises or pain.

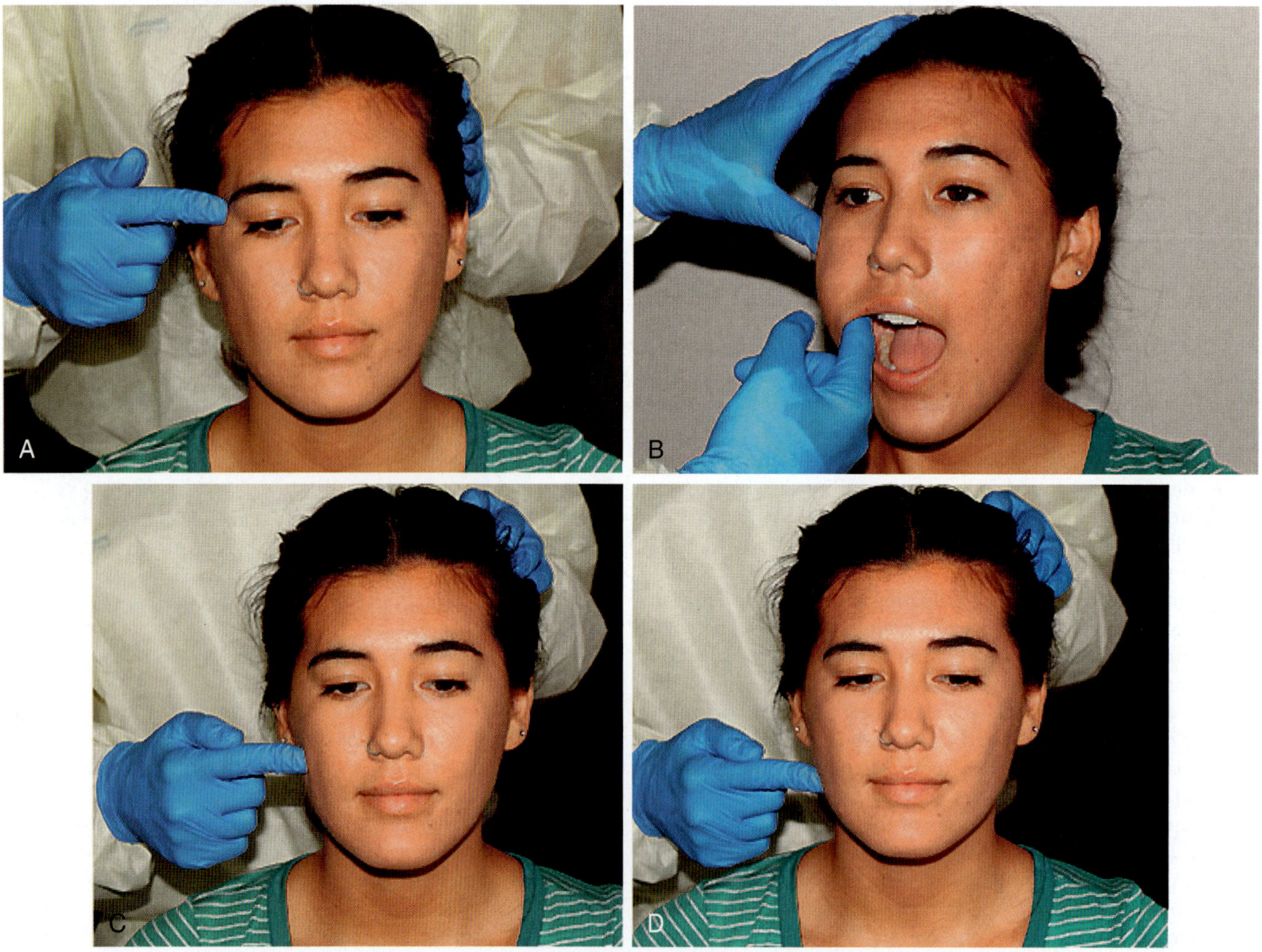

• **Fig. 45.5** A systematic approach to masticatory muscle palpation allows the clinician the ability to identify the areas of muscular involvement. (A) The clinician can start with palpating the temporalis muscle followed by (B) intraoral palpation of the temporalis tendon. After examination of the temporalis muscle, (C) the superior and (D) inferior aspects of the masseter muscle are palpated.

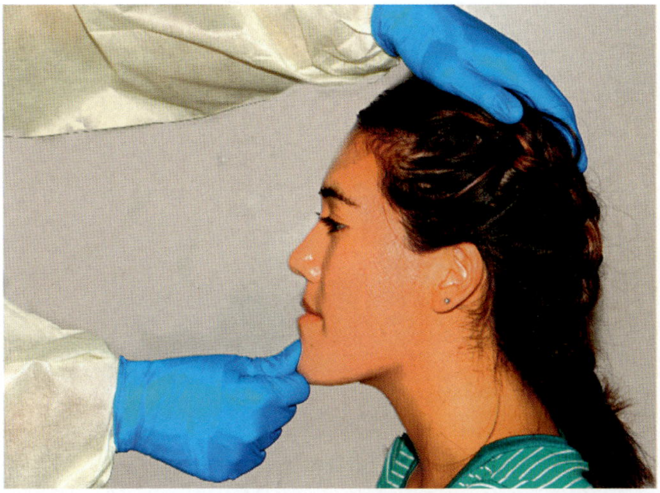

• **Fig. 45.6** The lateral pterygoid muscles can be tested by having the patient protrude the mandible against resistance.

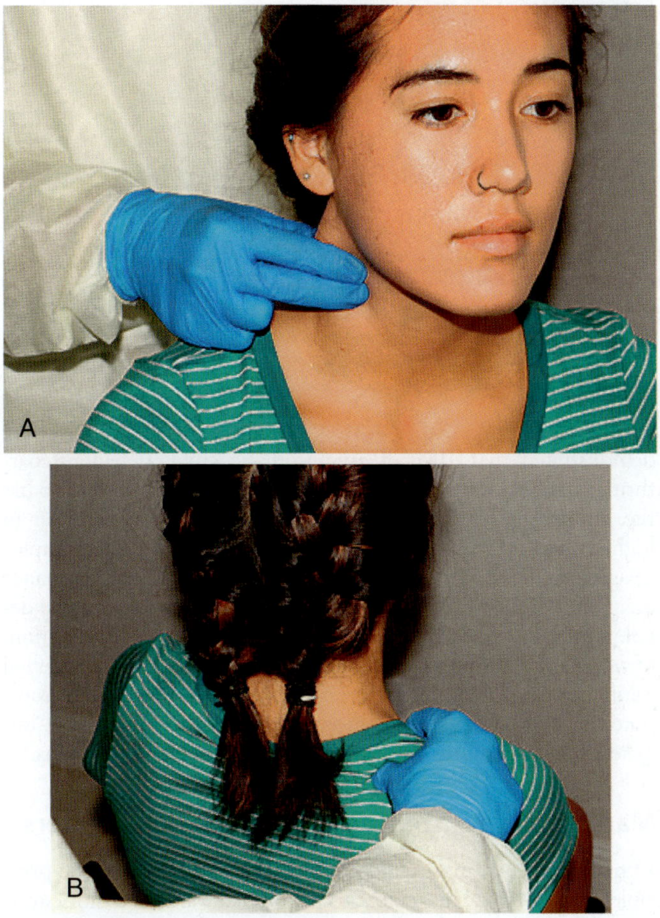

• **Fig. 45.7** Palpate the cervical muscles to determine their contribution to orofacial pain. (A) Palpate the sternocleidomastoid and (B) trapezius muscles using a pincher grasp.

during eating and speaking. Deviation (movement away from midline that returns to midline) or deflection (persistent movement away from midline) may also be observed. Deviations can be caused by either a muscle or TMJ condition. Deflection is commonly associated with disk displacement without reduction or less commonly with another condition that interferes with translational movements such as TMJ ankylosis. In these situations, the jaw deflects toward the affected side. The mandibular ROM can be measured with a millimeter gauge placed between the incisal edges of the upper and lower anterior teeth. The patient's overbite is added to the value to accurately reflect the distance the mandible opens. If the patient has an anterior open bite, this amount is subtracted from the maximal measurement. The same teeth should be measured to provide consistent readings. Passive ROM or assisted opening can be assessed by placing gentle downward mandibular pressure with the thumb and index finger (Fig. 45.8). Muscle pain may limit mandibular ROM. The limited opening can be overcome with a passive maneuver to prop open the mouth. If mouth-opening limitation persists, and firm resistance is encountered during assisted mouth opening, the patient may have a disk displacement without reduction. Mandibular ROM of less than 32 mm is considered limited in school-aged children, and 36 mm is limited in adolescents.[21] A ROM less than 40 mm is considered to be limited mobility in adult patients.[21,96] If a patient has TMJ sounds, practitioners should record the vertical measurement where the joint noises occur. Additionally, lateral movement of the mandible can be recorded to determine if the condyles are translating freely from side to side. The amount of lateral movement is measured in millimeters of change in the maxillary and mandibular dental midlines. Less than 8 mm indicates limited mobility in adults. The amount of protrusive movement can also be recorded, and less than 5 mm is considered limited in adults.[96] To date, no clinical norms have been established in children for lateral or protrusive movements. In summary, alterations in movement may indicate a deviation in form or a disk displacement with reduction. Severely decreased movement may indicate a disk displacement without reduction. Excessive ROM may indicate joint hypermobility, such as that found in connective tissue disorders (e.g., Marfan syndrome, Ehlers-Danlos syndrome).

Psychosocial Assessment

It is critical to build rapport with adolescent patients to gain trust and identify both protective and risk factors. Adolescent patients with TMDs may engage in high-risk behaviors or have significant behavioral health concerns. Providers can conduct a structured psychosocial interview by using the HEADSSS or SSHADESS screening evaluation tool[97] (Box 45.2).

Behavioral health comorbidities, such as depression, anxiety, and posttraumatic stress disorder, can affect TMD recovery and prognosis.[98] Catastrophic thinking, rumination, magnification, and feelings of hopelessness are well-established barriers to recovery from chronic pain.[94] Because psychosocial issues may not be readily discussed with parents or dentists, it is important to refer patients to a provider skilled in treating behavioral health conditions.

Imaging and Temporomandibular Disorders

The role of imaging in TMD diagnosis relies on the basic principles of selection criteria. Imaging should be considered when there is a history of, or the clinician suspects there is, a symptomatic intracapsular (joint) condition. Asymptomatic joint sounds alone do not warrant imaging. A panoramic radiograph is generally regarded as an appropriate screening radiograph. The selection criteria for initial TMJ imaging include the following:

1. Recent trauma or history of progressive pathologic joint condition

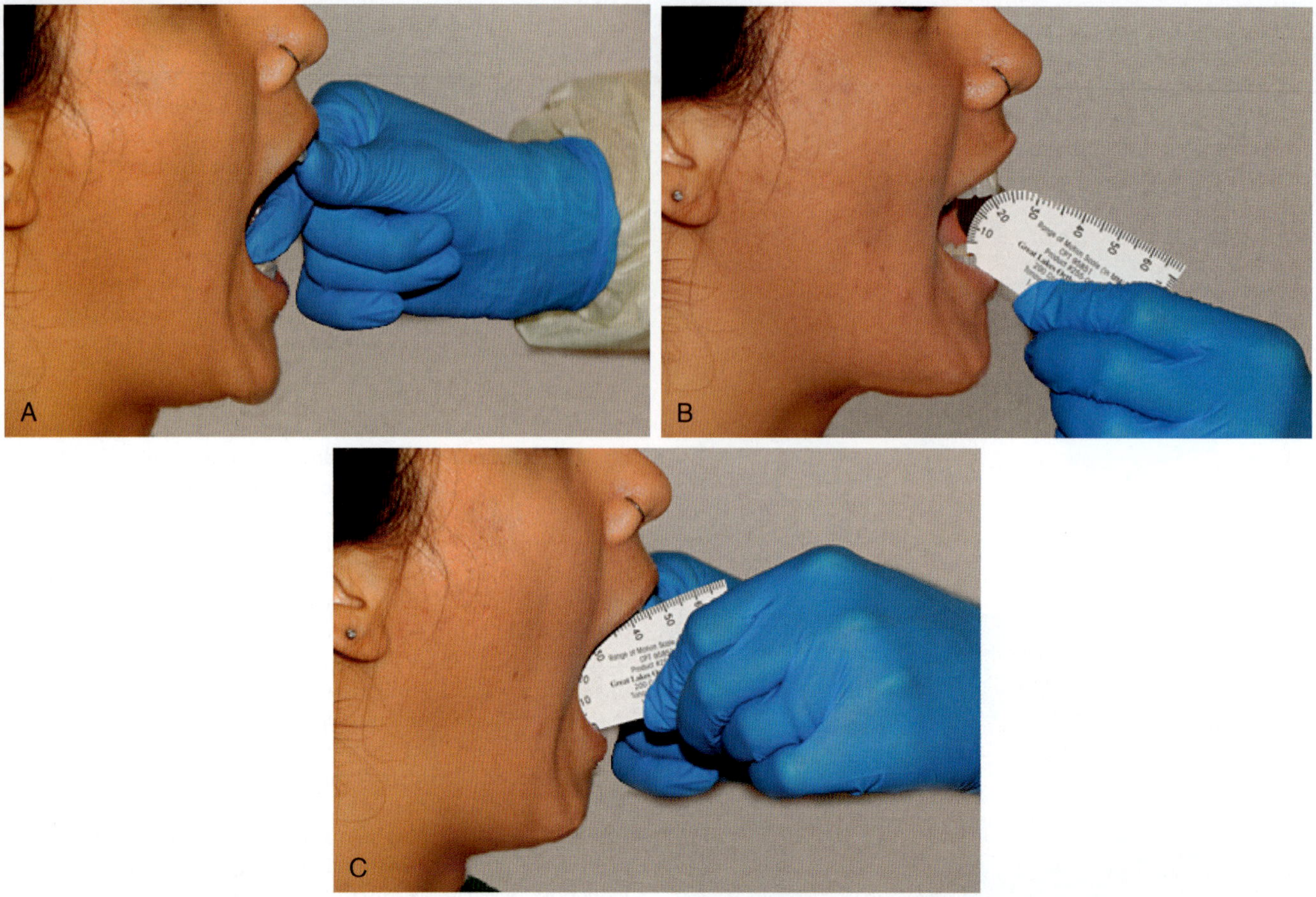

• **Fig. 45.8** (A) In patients with jaw pain, apply slow, steady pressure using the thumb and index finger to assess the maximum assisted or passive mandibular range of motion (ROM). (B) The pain-free mandibular ROM was only 21 mm. (C) Assisted or passive mandibular ROM increased to 43 mm.

• BOX 45.2 Psychosocial Screening Tool for Adolescent Patients

SSHADESS[a]	HEADSSS[b]
Strengths	Home
School	
Home	Activities
Activities	Education/Employment
Drugs and substance use	Drugs
Emotions, eating	Suicidal ideation/Depression
	Sex and Relationships
	Safety and Abuse
Sexuality	
Safety	

[a]From Ginsburg KR, Carlson EC. Resilience in action: an evidence-informed, theoretically driven approach to building strengths in an office-based setting. *Adolesc Med State Art Rev.* 2011;22(3): 458-481, xi. PMID: 22423460.

[b]From Goldenring, John M, Cohen E. Getting into adolescent heads. *Contemp Pediatr.* 1988;5(7): 75-90.

2. Significant dysfunction and alteration in ROM
3. Significant occlusal change (open bite, mandibular shift)

The practitioner is cautioned not to rely solely on imaging, as radiographic changes may be a result of adaptive remodeling.[7] For example, one study of symptomatic and asymptomatic children demonstrated that 10% of asymptomatic children had osteoarthritic changes in the mandibular condyles.[99] TMJ imaging also has the limitations of poor specificity and sensitivity in addition to higher financial costs and radiation burden. When more complex imaging is required, open and closed-mouth magnetic resonance imaging (MRI) is usually chosen for good hard and soft tissue detail. Intravenous contrast may be added to improve visualization; however, asymptomatic pediatric patients often show incidental joint effusions.[99] Computed tomography (CT) or cone beam computed tomography (CBCT) show excellent hard tissue detail but generally require more radiation than conventional radiographs.[100]

Management of Temporomandibular Disorders

Dentists can treat most children and adolescents using basic principles of TMD management. However, advanced treatment is sometimes necessary. For patients with long-standing or recalcitrant orofacial pain, referral to an orofacial pain specialist or another provider with experience managing TMDs should be considered.

Patients with nonpainful TMDs typically do not require treatment. For example, most patients with annoying but nonpainful TMJ sounds can be managed with education and reassurance alone.[2] Providers should focus on the condition's nonprogressive nature. Patients should be advised to avoid habitual jaw-clicking behaviors; there are no interventions supported by research to manage painless TMJ sounds.[101]

Patients with painful TMDs may benefit from targeted education and therapeutic interventions.[2,7] Most importantly, the patient should be advised to avoid activities that cause or increase pain. It is also critical to identify and modify behaviors such as eating tough foods, biting nails, chewing gum, talking or singing excessively, and playing a musical instrument. Daytime jaw clenching should also be addressed and controlled. Additionally, it is recommended to eliminate substances that increase sleep bruxism. Patients should be advised to decrease stress, consume a healthy diet, and get adequate sleep. Conservative interventions, such as warm or cold compresses, jaw exercises, and a brief course of clock-regulated analgesics, are suggested. Additional conservative treatment options, such as breathing techniques, relaxation, and biofeedback training, can be considered to supplement initial treatment strategies.[2,102] Following these recommendations can promote the healing process and often results in symptom resolution.

If bothersome TMD symptoms persist, an occlusal appliance or splint can be offered. Custom-designed, full-coverage, removable splints are generally recommended. Splints are typically used at nighttime and are designed to allow for eruption and positioning of teeth if the patient is in the mixed dentition. Randomized controlled trials in adolescent populations demonstrate that occlusal appliance therapy at night is generally more effective than education or relaxation therapy alone.[26,103]

Although acute TMDs may resolve with little to no interventions, chronic TMDs tend to be more challenging to treat. Over time, patients with chronic pain undergo functional changes in the central nervous system, which affect pain processing. Current evidence supports a biopsychosocial approach to chronic pain management. This approach includes simultaneous management of biologic (pain processing within the central nervous system), psychological (cognitive and emotional aspects factors), and social (family dynamics, socioeconomic status) factors related to the patient's persistent pain.[104,105] Behavioral interventions such as cognitive behavioral therapy are strongly recommended for chronic TMDs.[106]

Pharmacologic management beyond over-the-counter analgesics can be considered depending on the diagnosis. A short course of nonsteroidal antiinflammatory drugs (NSAIDs) that are approved for use in pediatric and adolescent patients may be used to manage acute inflammatory joint pain. If excessive joint swelling leads to a posterior open bite, a more potent antiinflammatory may be considered. More complex pharmacologic management may be indicated in cases of chronic myofascial pain and headaches.[7]

Physical therapy can be helpful in managing a chronic TMD because it is a musculoskeletal condition. Jaw exercises, stretching, and postural exercises have been proven to reduce pain and improve active and passive ROM.[106,107] Jaw exercises, along with splint use, have been shown to be more effective than splints in reducing pain and increasing mouth opening.[103] Ultrasound, transcutaneous electrical nerve stimulation (TENS), and dry needling are examples of additional treatment modalities physical therapists may offer.

Some patients who are resistant to conservative treatments may be evaluated for specialized injections, arthrocentesis, or, in rare cases, TMJ surgery. TMJ arthrocentesis without steroids can be considered for both growing and skeletally mature patients. Injected glucocorticoids are not recommended as first-line therapy in growing children because of the potential for calcifications within the joint or arrested growth.[107,108] Surgical interventions should be considered as a last resort only after all other options have been exhausted.

As with all dental problems, a dentist may determine that referral to another dental specialist is in the patient's best interest. An interdisciplinary approach can be beneficial for some pediatric and adolescent patients with TMDs and orofacial pain.

Idiopathic Condylar Resorption

Idiopathic condylar resorption (ICR), also called progressive condylar resorption, is a pathologic process characterized by progressive resorption of one or both condylar heads with volume loss of the condyles and rami. As condylar height is lost, the mandible can rotate in a clockwise fashion during remodeling, creating an anterior open bite.[109]

There is a strong female predilection with onset typically occurring during adolescence.[110] The etiology of the process is unknown; however, mechanisms may include hormonal changes,[111] biomechanical forces after increased muscular tension, and a history of trauma.[112] It has also been associated with an existing steep mandibular plane angle and class II jaw relationship.[113]

The process may be found incidentally on panoramic imaging and/or the patient may develop mandibular asymmetry or signs and symptoms of TMJ dysfunction. Further imaging can include CBCT and MRI, allowing for better visualization of the hard and soft tissues of the TMJ complexes.[114] Additionally, follow-up imaging can be invaluable in determining if the process is active or arrested.[109] Radiographic findings can include cortical erosions, loss of condylar and ramus volume, and flattening of the condyle[109,114] (Fig. 45.9).

Considered a self-limited process with a duration of 6 months to 2 years, management can range from no treatment to condylar replacement and osteotomy.[113] A comparison with JIA must be mentioned as it presents with a similar demographic overlap in adolescent females. Depending on the subtype of JIA, systemic findings such as cervical spine involvement and laboratory tests to exclude rheumatoid factors can help distinguish from ICR.[109,115]

Visit eBooks.Health.Elsevier.com to see full list of references.

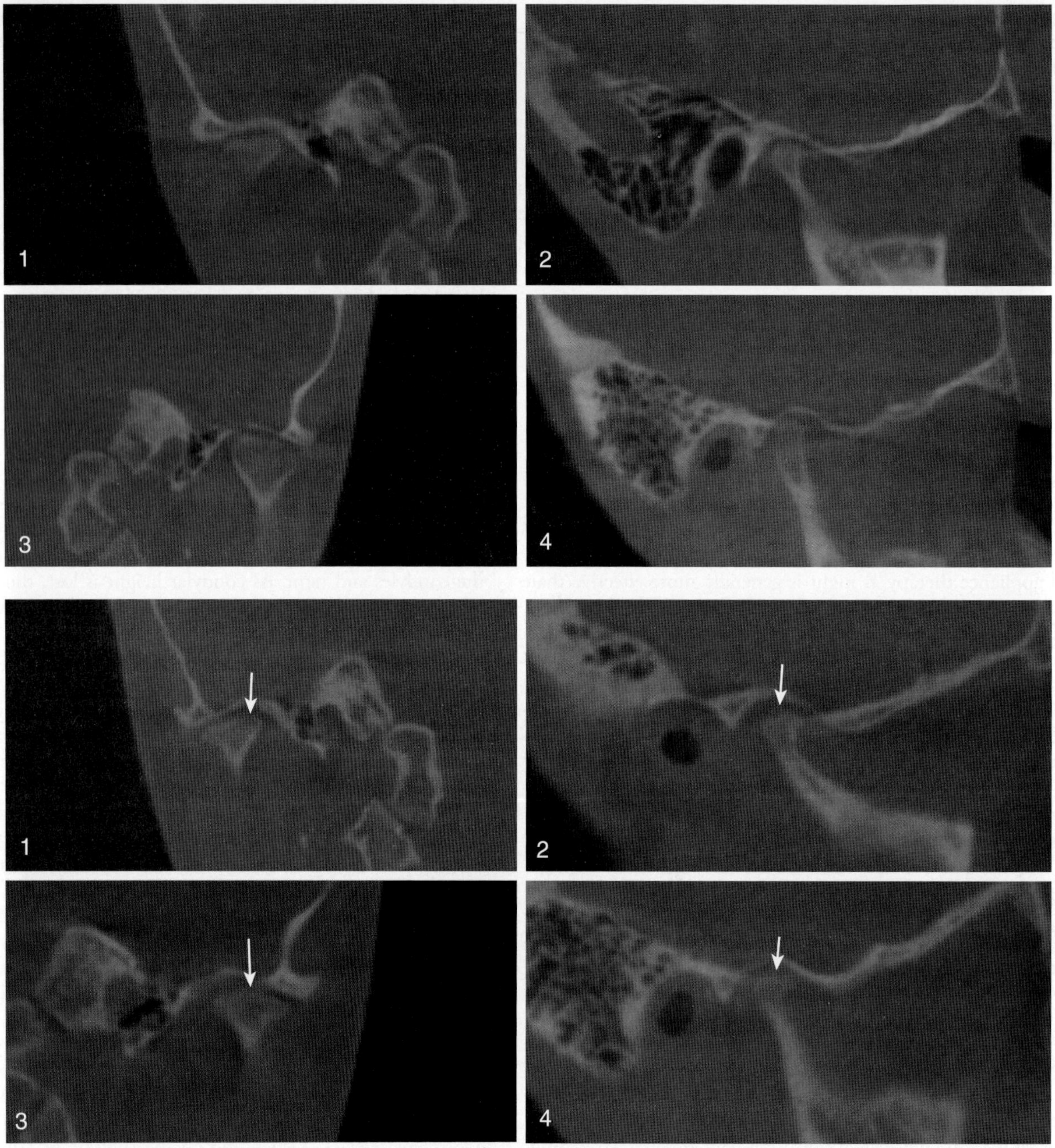

• **Fig. 45.9** (A) Initial cone beam computed tomography (CBCT) imaging shows continuity of the condylar surfaces. (1) Right coronal, (2) right sagittal, (3) left coronal, (4) left sagittal. (B) Ten-month follow-up CBCT demonstrates flattening and erosive changes *(arrows)* on the left condyle and flattening and loss of condylar volume *(arrows)* on the right. (1) Right coronal, (2) right sagittal, (3) left coronal, (4) left sagittal.

46

Management of Missing Teeth in a Growing Patient

MARK VEAZIE, JESSICA Y. LEE, AND JOHN R. CHRISTENSEN

CHAPTER OUTLINE

Introduction and Background

Dental trauma is a significant cause of tooth loss in children and adolescents, particularly during sports or physical activities. The prevalence of traumatic dental injuries varies by age, sex, and geographical location. Globally, studies suggest that the prevalence of dental trauma in permanent teeth ranges from 5% to 12% among children and adolescents.[1] Boys are typically more affected than girls due to greater participation in physical activities. The most common teeth involved in trauma are the maxillary central incisors, which are more vulnerable due to their anterior positioning and prominence.

Congenital absence of one or more teeth, hypodontia, is one of the most common developmental anomalies in the pediatric population. The prevalence of hypodontia in permanent dentition ranges from 6% to 10% globally, with variability based on geographical region and ethnicity.[2] The mandibular second premolars and maxillary lateral incisors are the most frequently missing teeth. Nonsyndromic hypodontia is the most common and accounts for most cases.[3] Studies show that hypodontia is slightly more common in females than in males.[3] Syndromic hypodontia is frequently associated with genetic conditions, including ectodermal dysplasia and cleft lip and palate. In patients with ectodermal dysplasia, the prevalence of missing teeth can be as high as 80% to 90%.

Dental caries is the leading cause of tooth loss in children, particularly in low- and middle-income countries. According to the World Health Organization (WHO), untreated dental caries is the most prevalent health condition globally, affecting approximately 60% to 90% of schoolchildren. In cases of severe dental decay, premature tooth loss is common.

Other dental conditions such as molar-incisor hypomineralization (MIH) can contribute to early loss of teeth. MIH is a developmental condition that affects the enamel of first permanent molars and often permanent incisors. The prevalence of missing permanent teeth in children with MIH is influenced by the severity of hypomineralization, the associated dental caries, and the quality of dental care received. The prevalence of MIH varies across populations but is generally estimated to be between 3.6% and 25% globally.[4] This condition is more commonly seen in children aged 6 to 12, as it affects teeth during their development and eruption. Although MIH itself does not directly cause tooth loss, it can lead to increased risk of extraction, especially when the enamel becomes severely compromised. Affected molars, particularly first permanent molars, may require extraction if they suffer from severe breakdown and restorative treatments fail. The prevalence of missing permanent teeth, specifically first permanent molars, in children with MIH is highly dependent on the severity of the condition and access to dental treatment. Studies indicate that up to 13% of children with MIH may experience extraction of one or more first permanent molars by adolescence, especially in cases of severe MIH.[5]

In children and adolescents, the management of missing permanent teeth can be challenging to manage clinically. Traditionally, the problem of missing teeth in this age group has been addressed with prosthodontic replacement or orthodontic space closure. Removable partial dentures and appliances bear psychosocial implications for the young patient, whereas orthodontic space closure, arguably an age-appropriate solution, can have biomechanical limits in anchorage. Dental implants are not indicated in growing patients due to ankylosis and infraocclusion that precipitate long-term functional and esthetic problems; implants warrant consideration only when skeletal maturity is reached. Ideally, any substitute should adapt with the growth and development in the oral region, restore soft and hard tissues, and have potential for long-term survival.

Diagnosis and Assessment

Diagnosis and assessment are essential in managing patients with missing permanent teeth. Evaluation of many factors will affect treatment options and prognosis in these cases. The evaluation should include clinical and radiographic examinations and a growth assessment. These factors are the most important but should be supplemented with an orthodontic assessment. Sustainable treatment options can be obtained through careful consideration.

The first step in diagnosis is forming treatment objectives. This will guide the direction and extent of treatment. Within the treatment objectives should be the chief complaint of the patient and family. It is not always possible to satisfy the chief complaint, but a review of treatment options will help them make appropriate decisions. The etiology of the missing tooth or teeth is a beginning piece of required information. For instance, genetic causes (e.g., ectodermal dysplasia, cleft lip/palate) may require more extensive considerations compared with other cases. The management of these cases is often beyond the scope of a single practitioner. Most cases benefit from a collaborative, interdisciplinary approach.

Clinical Examination and Records

The goals should be to establish the oral health status (oral hygiene, active carious lesions, etc.), skeletal development, occlusion, and relevant facial characteristics of an individual. These factors should be documented through written and photographic means.

Extraoral:

Extraoral evaluation of a patient is a systematic assessment of facial features and the functional status of the patient.

Intraoral:

Document the current oral health status of the patient.

Records:

Photographic documentation should be obtained that will augment information gathered during the clinical examination. Depending on the given case, additional records may be requested to supplement the analysis and treatment planning (Fig. 46.1).

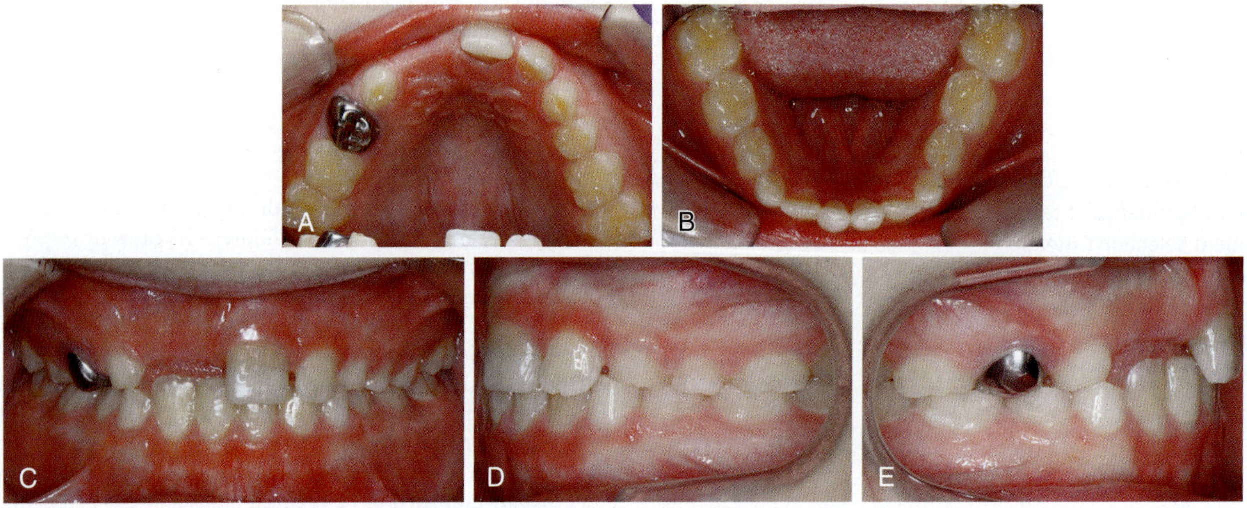

• Fig. 46.1 (A–E) This patient suffered a traumatic dental injury while riding a motorized four-wheel vehicle. The left central incisor was fractured, and the right central and lateral incisors were avulsed and never recovered.

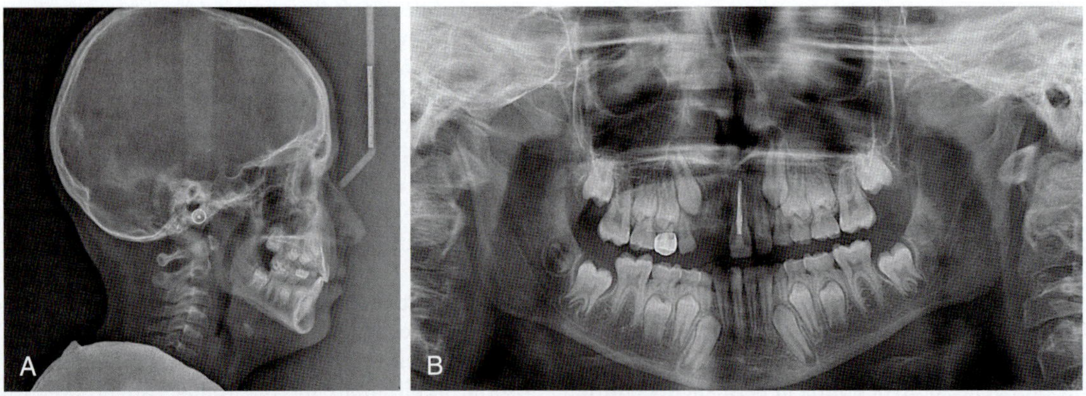

• Fig. 46.2 (A–B) A cephalometric and panoramic film was obtained on the patient described in Fig. 46.1. The radiographs provide information on the skeletal and dental relationships and the status of the primary and permanent teeth.

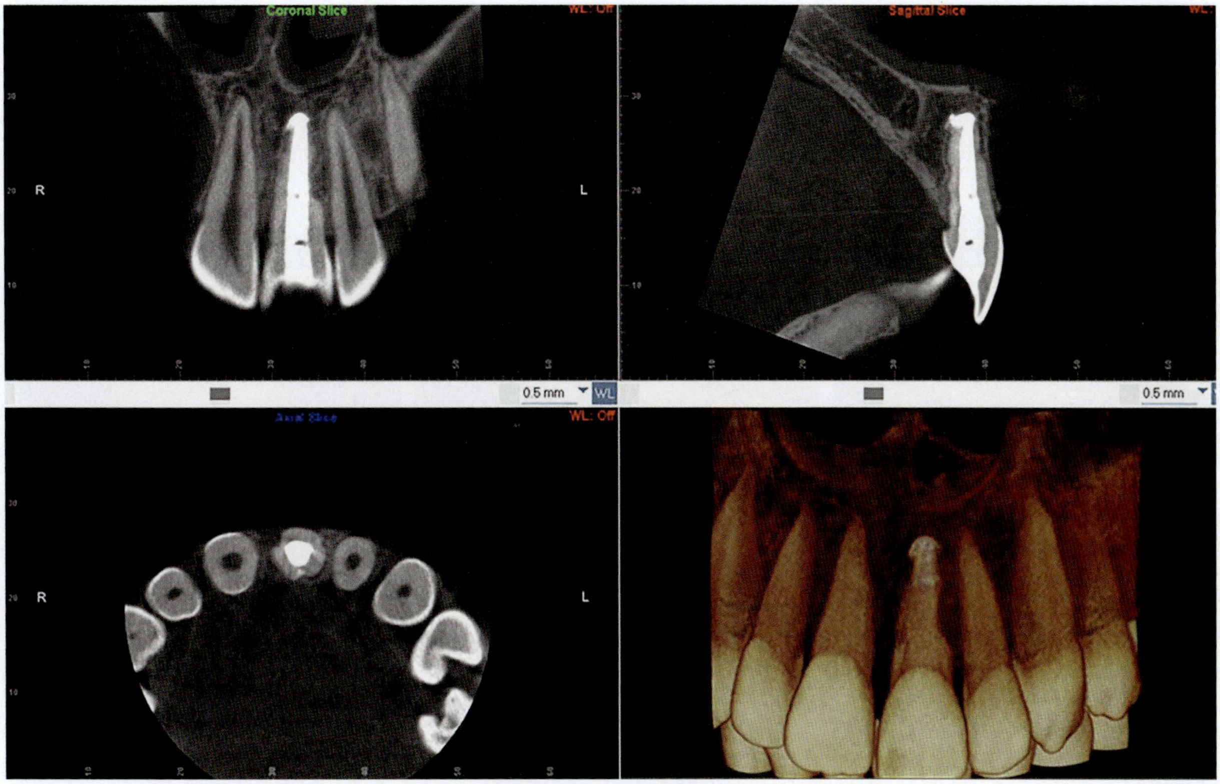

• **Fig. 46.3** This cone-beam computed tomography was obtained to determine the status of an avulsed maxillary left central incisor after endodontic treatment was completed. There are several areas of root resorption apparent that create a questionable prognosis for the tooth.

Extraoral and intraoral photos are obtained after a clinical examination.

The number and type of radiographs are guided by the location and number of missing teeth. Panoramic radiographs assess the developing dentition and identify pathologies (Fig. 46.2).

Cone-beam computed tomography (CBCT) augments traditional radiographs or can substitute for the cephalometric and panoramic radiograph (Fig. 46.3).

Treatment Planning

There are a multitude of factors that affect treatment options. Discussion with the patient and family to determine their interest is an important first step. It is important to determine the compliance and commitment of the family as treatment modalities can be lengthy and complex. Financial costs for each treatment option considered should be given to the family. Extensive treatment options should be discussed in terms of the length of treatment, the number of required visits, and the total financial costs.

Compared with other pediatric dental procedures, treatment options in children with missing permanent teeth require longer treatment times, involve modifications, and require multiple dental specialists to provide optimal outcomes.

Multidisciplinary Collaboration

Treatment planning and delivery of care for children with missing teeth can be cumbersome for a single provider. Collaboration with multiple disciplines can provide an increased number of treatment options and allow for increased success (Fig. 46.4).

Treatment Options

Several treatment options are used to replace teeth with documented and predictable outcomes. Interdisciplinary discussions should be considered to determine the best option, but it should be noted that not every discipline is necessary for every case. A team approach will provide greater breadth and insight into potential solutions for the patient.

Removable Appliances

Removable appliances are an affordable and reliable treatment option for missing teeth. They are often used for missing anterior teeth to restore esthetics and considered in some cases to replace posterior teeth (Fig. 46.5).

Although these are reliable and effective options, removable appliances are seen as temporary solutions. The appliances often require adjustment or fabrication of additional appliances as the patient transitions through the different dentitional phases. In addition, due to their removable nature, appliances are lost or broken. On the other hand, removable appliances can be the most cost-effective way to replace missing teeth until a more permanent solution is determined.

Fixed Appliances

Fixed prosthetic restorations or appliances are another option to replace missing teeth. They are the preferred option for individuals that have finished growth or are in the adult stage of life. They may be considered interim or intermediate-term restoration in the anterior region (Fig. 46.6).

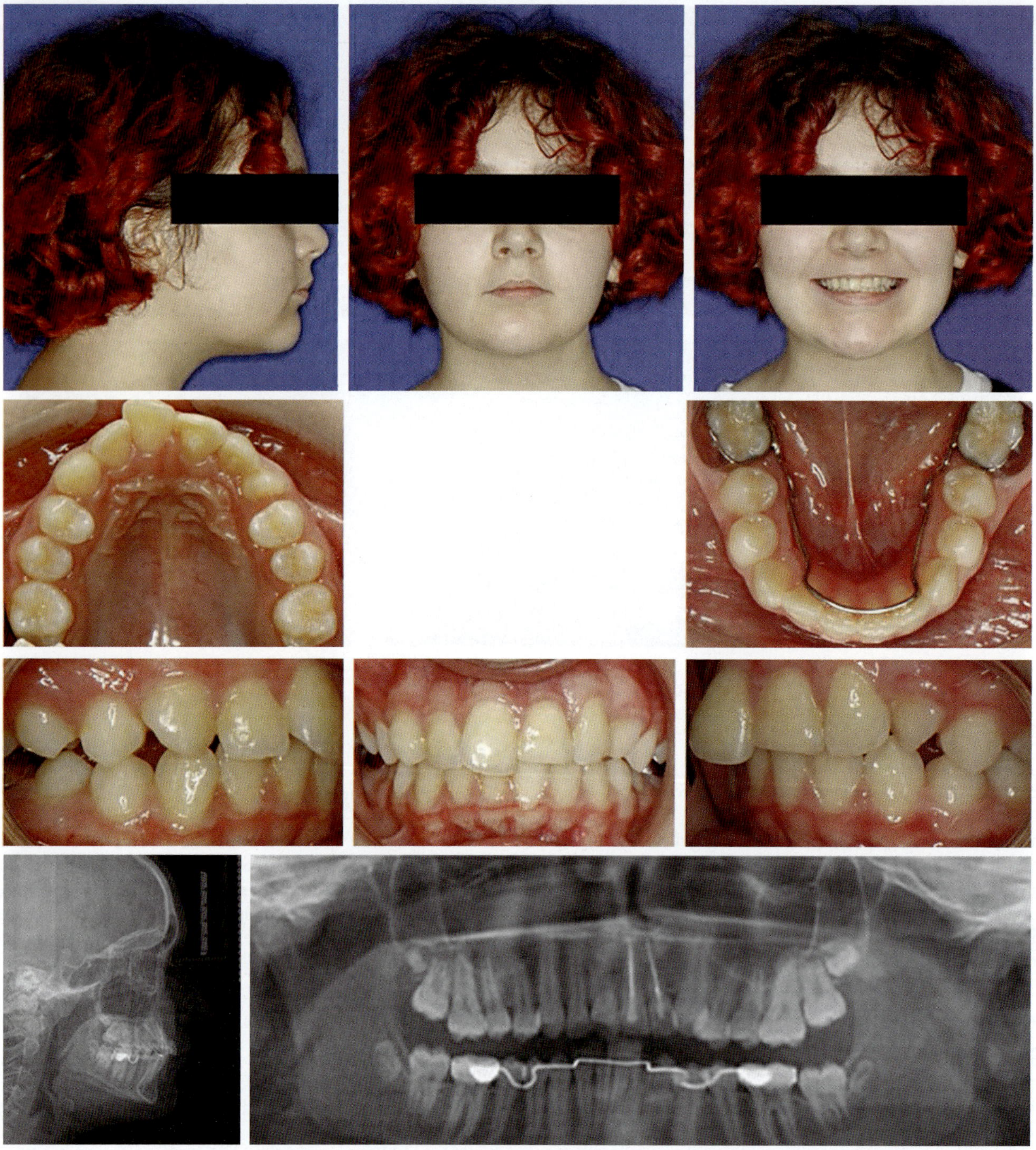

• **Fig. 46.4** Records were obtained and shared with different specialists on the team because the patient has two ankylosed incisors, the maxillary left central and lateral incisors. The team discussed different treatment options such as prosthetic replacement (implants), orthodontic space closure, and dental autotransplantation with the family. Ultimately, dental autotransplantation was chosen.

Dental implants are rarely used in the growing child largely due to the reason the dental implant does not erupt, nor does it produce supporting alveolar tissues (bone and soft tissue). As the face grows, the implant can become more and more infraoccluded. In addition, the anterior maxilla is undergoing a resorptive process as the face ages.[6] The volume of bone decreases with age. The developing vertical bone defect is hard for the patient and the provider to manage. If the practitioner is considering a dental implant, the patient's growth status should be assessed to determine whether this is the appropriate time. It is difficult to determine when a patient has finished growing. The provider can use repeated growth measures such as cephalometric superimpositions and repeated height measures to determine proper timing. Even though growth appears to be finished, change continues throughout life and is difficult to predict.[7,8]

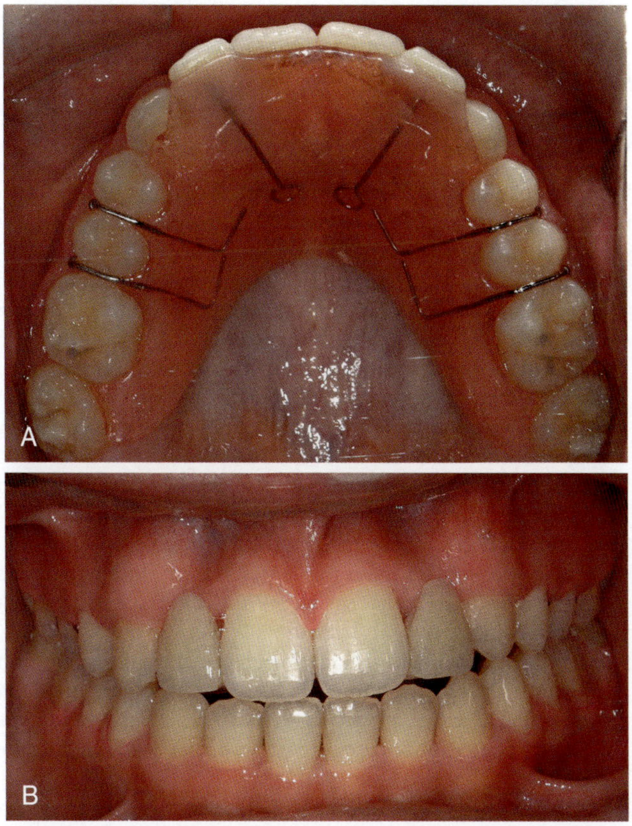

• **Fig. 46.5** (A–B) A removable acrylic appliance with two pontic teeth was used to replace the patient's congenitally missing maxillary lateral incisors. This is an interim prosthesis used while the patient is growing before a permanent prosthesis can be made.

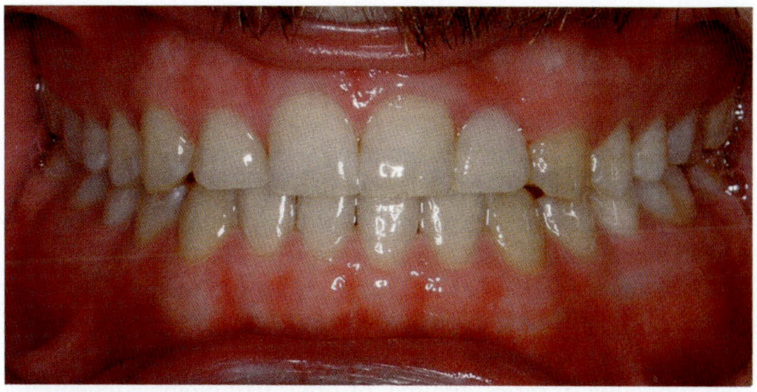

• **Fig. 46.6** A winged bridge was used to replace the congenitally missing maxillary left lateral incisor. Esthetics depend on the amount of remaining alveolar bone in the missing tooth position. In this case, there was adequate bone and a minimal upper lip elevation when smiling.

Orthodontic Space Closure

Orthodontic space closure is a common treatment strategy for addressing missing teeth in growing patients, particularly when tooth agenesis, trauma, or early loss due to caries occur. When managing missing teeth in pediatric and adolescent patients, space closure offers a functional and esthetic solution, with the additional benefit of utilizing the patient's natural dentition. Given that growing patients have active craniofacial growth, treatment planning must accommodate ongoing developmental changes to achieve optimal long-term results.

Maxillary lateral incisor agenesis is a common indication for space closure in growing patients. In these cases, canines are moved into the lateral incisor position (canine substitution). This approach provides a more natural and long-lasting solution.

Canines serve an important role in the dentition as cornerstones of the arch, guiding lateral movements and protecting posterior teeth during occlusal function. Studies have demonstrated that, with proper alignment and reshaping, canines can effectively replace lateral incisors without compromising occlusal function (Fig. 46.7).

Mandibular second premolar agenesis is also common, with a prevalence of about 2% to 5% in the general population.[2] Space closure in this case involves mesial movement of the posterior teeth. Consideration must be given to the potential effect on occlusion, particularly the relationship between the maxillary and mandibular molars. Achieving long-term stability after orthodontic space closure is crucial, especially in growing patients. Proper retention protocols, including fixed retainers or removable appliances, help prevent relapse as the patient continues to grow.

Tooth Autotransplantation

Tooth autotransplantation is defined as the transplantation of a tooth from one site into a different site in the oral cavity of the same individual and may be a good treatment option for children with missing teeth. The transplanted tooth can be fully erupted, partially erupted, or unerupted. It may have complete or partial root formation. The method was outlined by Slagsvold and Bjercke in the 1970s for patients with missing premolars and maxillary incisors.[9] Tooth autotransplantation can involve three distinct scenarios: (1) transplantation of a tooth from one site into a different site (conventional transplantation); (2) surgical repositioning of a tooth within the same site (intraalveolar transplantation); and (3) extraction of a tooth, extraoral treatment, and reimplantation in the same site (intentional reimplantation).[10]

Success rates for tooth autotransplantation vary depending on several factors, including the patient's overall health, the specific tooth involved, the reason for the transplantation, the skill of the surgeon, and the postoperative care provided. Long-term outcomes of autotransplanted teeth have been cited in the literature with impressive longitudinal follow-up spanning up to 41 years.[11] Success and survival rates for tooth autotransplantation are reported to be between 80% to 90% and 68% to 100%, respectfully.[11–13] This is comparable to the survival of tooth implants, which have a reported survival from 73% to 100% at an average of 14 years of follow-up.[14] Two recent publications reported on survival and success rates of more than 95% over 10 years for tooth autotransplantation. One discussed moving 1654 posterior teeth to another posterior tooth position and the other discussed moving 910 posterior teeth to the maxillary anterior region.[15,16]

Common complications that can affect the success rate of autotransplantation include replacement resorption (ankylosis), pulpal necrosis, and root resorption.[10] Although pulpal necrosis is defined as a type of failure, many of these teeth receive endodontic treatment, which has sufficiently high success rates, making the overall outcome for these transplanted teeth favorable with a high overall survival rate. Ankylosis and root resorption are far more significant factors in determining the success or failure of the transplant. Thus far, the longest longitudinal follow-up study of autotransplantation cases that spanned between 17 and 41 years confirmed an average survival rate of 90%.[17]

Beyond long-term outcomes, autotransplantation offers a natural tooth replacement that responds and functions like a natural tooth. In growing patients, transplanted teeth follow the development of the alveolar process and have demonstrated preservation and regeneration of bone in the recipient site. Autotransplantation has shown potential for bone induction and has been attempted in patients with cleft palate involving multiple teeth.[18]

Clinical scenarios where transplantation is applicable include tooth loss due to caries, trauma, or other pathology; congenitally missing teeth; ectopic eruption of canines; surgical uprighting of severely impacted teeth; multiple missing teeth; or combinations of these scenarios. Autotransplantation requires careful patient selection and an interdisciplinary team for appropriate management and success of treatment.

Patient Selection Criteria

Selecting the appropriate patient is critical for the success of tooth autotransplantation. Ideal candidates should meet the following criteria:

- Age: Younger patients (8 to18 years of age) are the most suitable candidates because they have more regenerative potential for healing, including revascularization of the transplanted tooth and continued alveolar bone growth.[17]
- Systemic health: Patients should be in good general health, without conditions that may impair healing, such as diabetes or immune deficiencies. Systemic diseases that negatively affect healing can lower the chances of success.
- Dental and periodontal health: Both the donor and recipient sites should be free from active periodontal disease and infection. Additionally, the recipient site should have adequate soft tissue volume to allow primary closure during the transplantation. An intact and healthy periodontal ligament (PDL) will help generate new bone and soft tissue. Bone grafting is not necessary if primary soft tissue closure can be accomplished.
- Patient compliance: Success relies heavily on the patient to follow postoperative care instructions, maintain good oral hygiene, and attend follow-up appointments.

Donor Tooth Selection

The success of autotransplantation is influenced by the selection of the donor tooth. The ideal characteristics for a donor tooth include the following:

- Stage of root development: Immature teeth with ⅔ to ¾ root development are preferred because they have the highest chance of revascularization and PDL regeneration.[19] These teeth are likely to survive and integrate functionally. Teeth with fully developed roots have a higher risk of pulp necrosis due to the inability to revascularize and ankylosis depending on the difficulty of removal.
- Tooth morphology and size: The size and shape of the donor tooth should match the recipient site as closely as possible. This is especially important in esthetic areas (e.g., anterior teeth) to ensure that the transplanted tooth blends well with adjacent teeth.
- PDL health: Healthy PDL on the donor tooth is essential for successful healing. Trauma to the PDL during extraction or handling can increase the risk of ankylosis or root resorption.

Commonly used donor teeth include premolars (in cases where extractions are already indicated for orthodontic reasons), third molars, and canines.

Recipient Site Preparation

Proper preparation of the recipient site is critical to ensure the survival and successful integration of the transplanted tooth.[20] Key considerations include the following:

- Soft tissue volume: The recipient site should have sufficient keratinized soft tissue so the transplanted tooth can be stabilized with primary closure. The transplanted tooth will begin to develop a long epithelial attachment during the first weeks of healing. If healing is successful, the PDL will begin to replace the missing bone and soft tissues. The tooth can be moved with orthodontic force.
- Space: In cases where the recipient site has been edentulous for a prolonged period, orthodontic or surgical intervention may be needed to ensure adequate space in both a mesiodistal and vertical direction for the transplanted tooth. The surgeon does not want to injure adjacent teeth, and the transplant should stay out of occlusion while healing.
- Healing environment: The recipient site should be free from infection, active periodontal disease, and excessive inflammation. Inflammatory conditions should be treated before the autotransplantation procedure to promote optimal healing conditions.

Tooth autotransplantation is a highly effective treatment option for managing missing teeth in growing children and adolescents (Fig. 46.8).

Dental Implants

Dental implants are an effective and widely used solution for replacing missing teeth in adults. However, their use in children and adolescents requires special consideration due to the dynamic nature of craniofacial growth. Placing implants in growing patients presents unique challenges, as ongoing skeletal development can lead to implant malposition or esthetic issues over time. Dental implants may be indicated for children with missing teeth in select cases, but the decision to place implants in children must be approached cautiously, considering the growth phase and individual craniofacial development. There are specific contraindications for placing dental implants in children due to the risks associated with ongoing craniofacial growth. Dental implants are osseointegrated and do not adapt to changes in the surrounding bone. This can lead to implant misalignment as the jaw grows and neighboring teeth shift in position.[7] Implant placement in children before growth is complete can result in vertical and horizontal discrepancies. Additionally, placing implants in the anterior region before growth is complete can result in esthetic challenges, such as vertical infraocclusion (implant ankylosis), leading to discrepancies in the smile line and visible implant margins as adjacent teeth continue to erupt. The timing of dental implant placement in children is critical to avoid complications related to craniofacial growth. Most clinicians recommend delaying implant placement until craniofacial growth is complete, which typically occurs around 18 to 20 years for males and 16 to 18 years for females.

Before proceeding with dental implant placement in a child or adolescent, a thorough assessment should be carried out to evaluate whether the patient is ready for implant therapy. The growth status of the patient must be assessed carefully, using clinical and

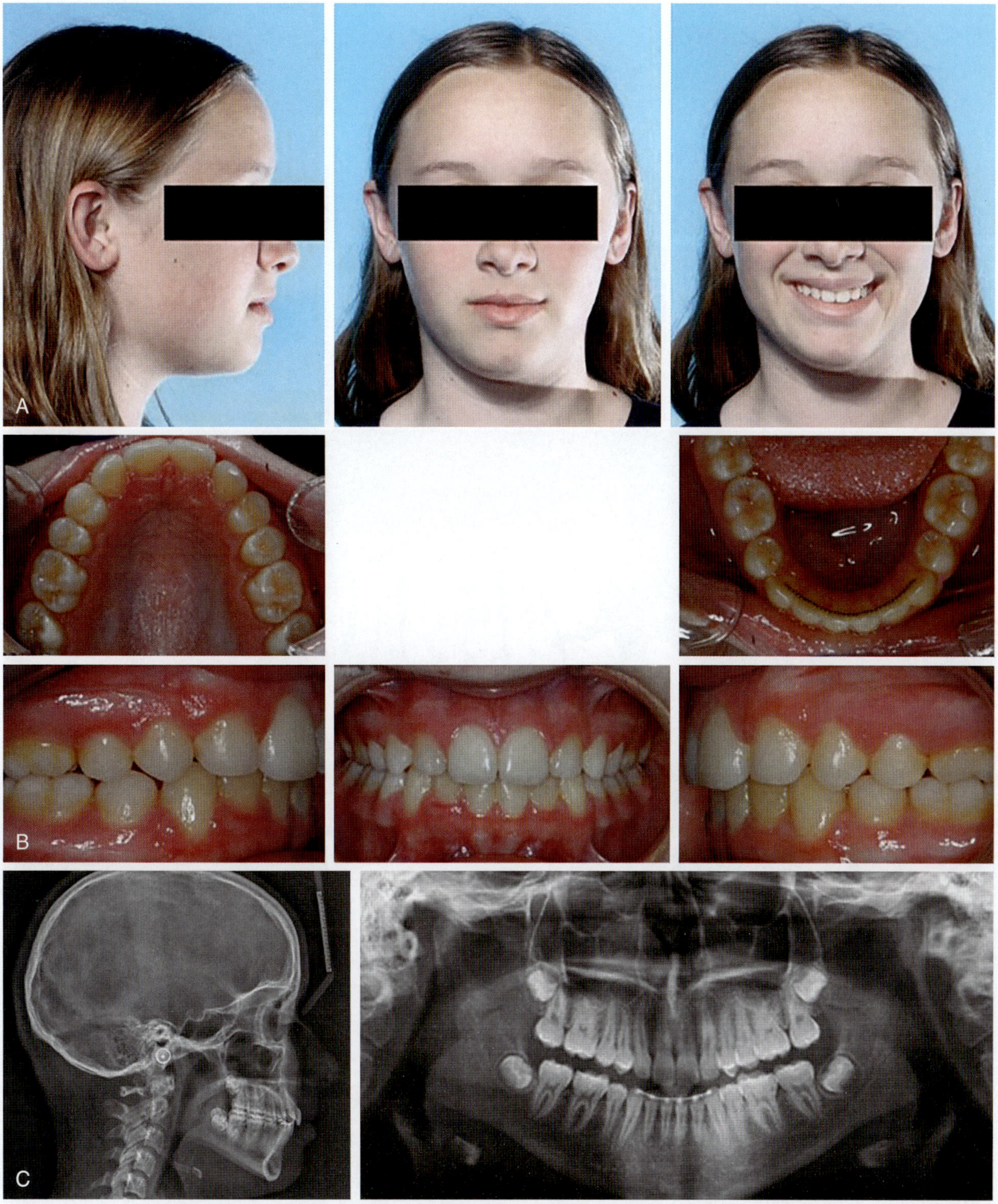

• **Fig. 46.7** The final records show a patient with bilateral substitution of the maxillary lateral incisors with canines. Due to the arch length deficiency, two lower premolars were removed, and the case was treated similar to a four premolar extraction case. The maxillary canines and first premolars were reshaped and restored with composite resin to mimic the lateral incisors and canines.

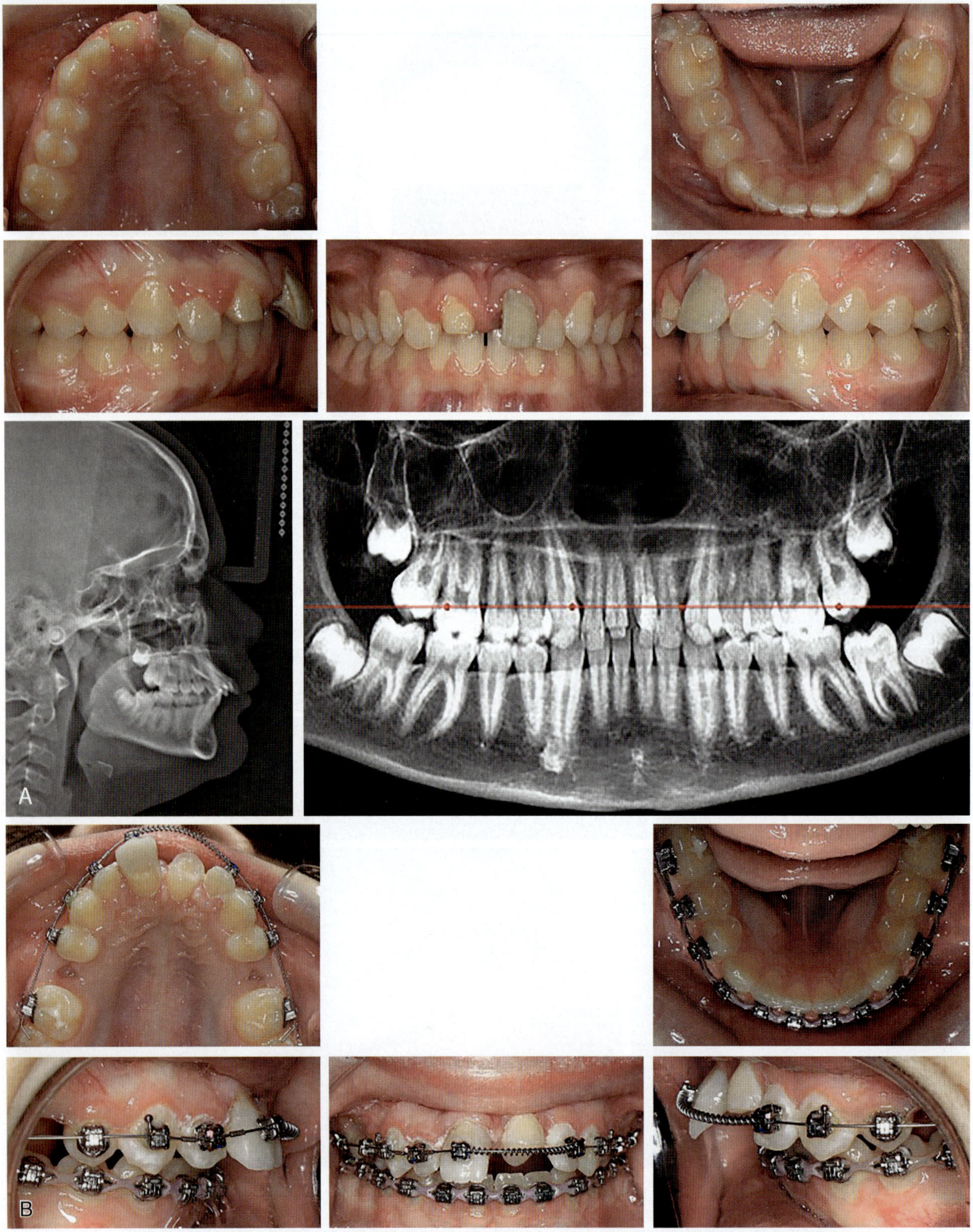

• **Fig. 46.8** (A) This patient sustained a traumatic dental injury two years before the records. Both central incisors were deemed to have a poor long-term prognosis with a fixed prosthetic solution. The family agreed to transplant upper second premolars into the central incisor position due to the maxillary incisor protrusion and class II malocclusion. (B) These photos show the patient after having one of the two transplanted premolars restored with a composite resin to mimic a central incisor.

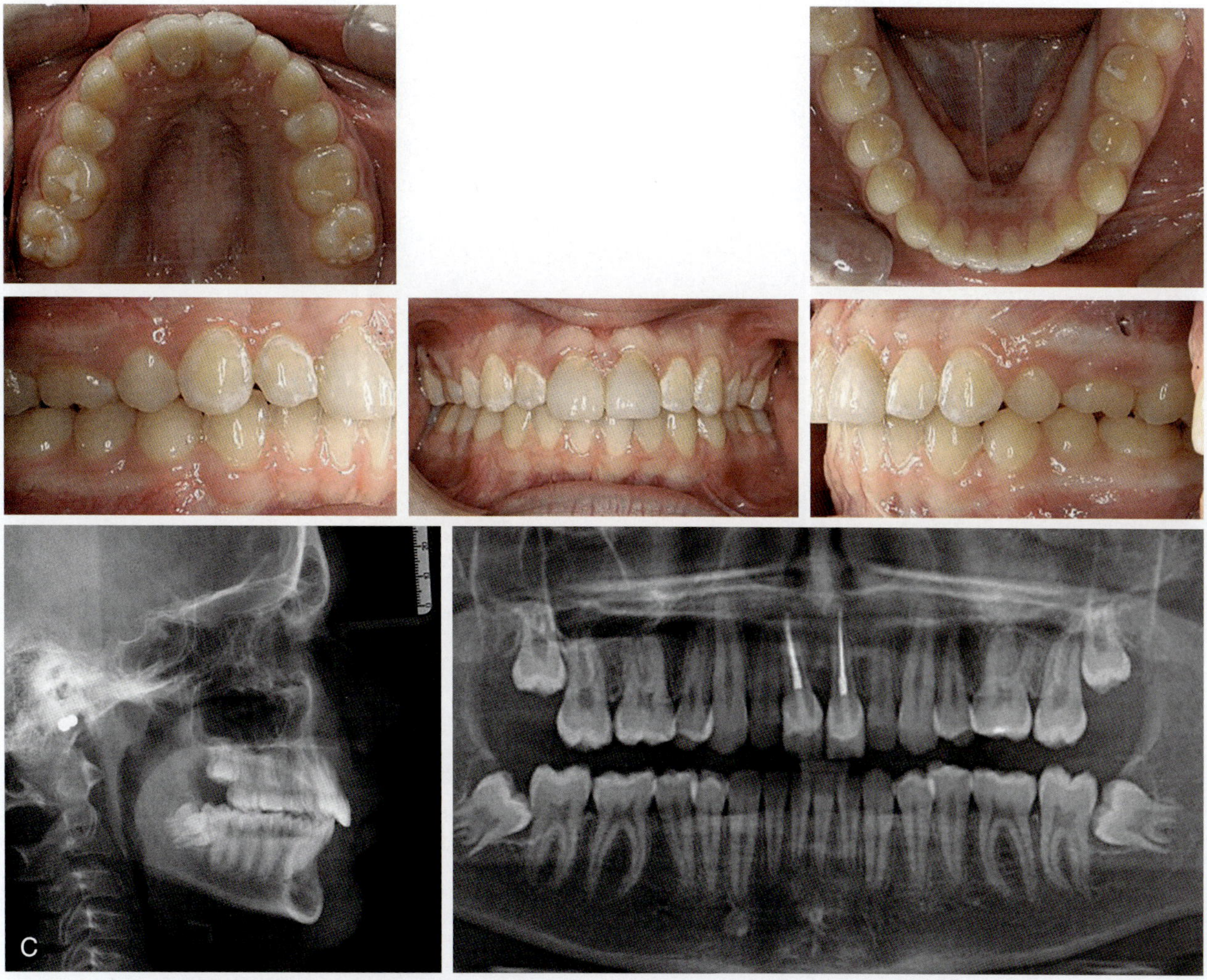

• **Fig. 46.8, cont'd** (C) The final records illustrate a class II molar class I canine relationship with reduced incisor protrusion. The maxillary second premolars were shaped to become were reshaped to become maxillary central incisors.

radiographic methods including serial cephalometric radiographs, hand-wrist radiographs, and clinical assessment.[21]

Dental implants placed in children and adolescents once growth is complete have shown high success rates comparable to those in adults. Studies indicate success rates of over 90% when implants are placed after the cessation of growth.[22] Implants placed in sites with adequate bone volume and density have higher success rates. Sites with insufficient bone may require bone grafting to achieve optimal conditions for implant placement. Modern implant designs with improved surface technology have increased the success rates of implants in pediatric cases, enhancing osseointegration and long-term stability. Proper hygiene and follow-up care are essential to ensure the longevity of dental implants in children.

Extraction of Permanent First Molars

Overview

Permanent first molars are among the first permanent teeth to erupt. Given their early eruption, they are exposed to the most environmental and physical stressors across permanent teeth. Unfortunately, these stressors can lead to significant tooth breakdown. Treatment becomes quite involved with pulpal issues and hard tissue loss and often leads to tooth removal. The primary cause of permanent first molar loss is caries, though other common reasons exist that necessitate their removal.[23,24] These reasons include severe MIH and other qualitative or quantitative enamel defects (Fig. 46.9).[24]

Indications and Prognosis

There are times to consider extraction of permanent first molars. Before making the determination for molar extraction, careful clinical and radiographic examination should be performed. This will help establish the prognosis and restorability of the tooth in question.

Second molar substitution is an ideal way to replace a permanent first molar while minimizing impairments in occlusion and space. Second molar substitution involves the extraction of the permanent first molar at an appropriate age and time that will allow the eruption of the permanent second molar for space

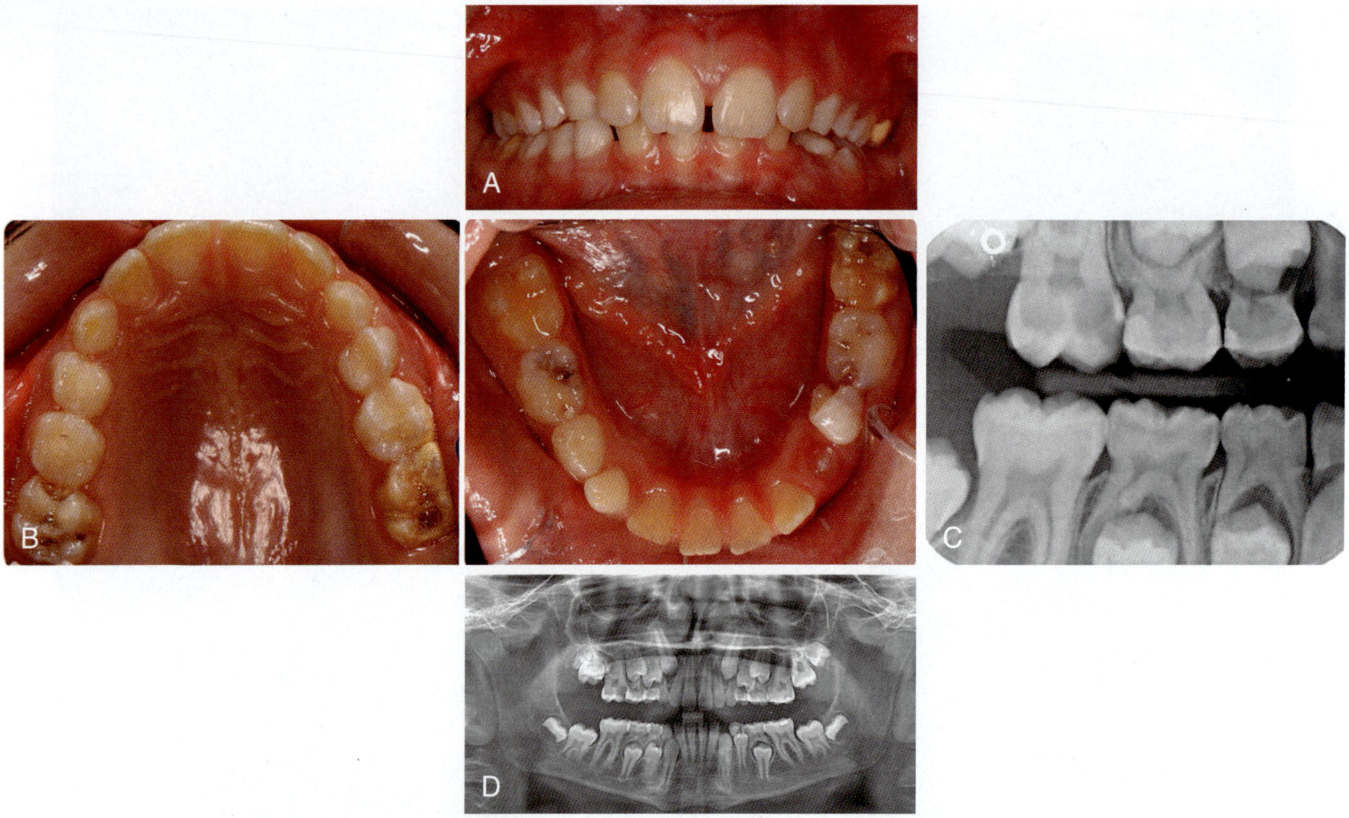

• **Fig. 46.9** (A) A 10 year old male patient with molar incisor hypomineralization (MIH). Note the discoloration of the first permanent molars. (B) The discoloration and physical breakdown of the first permanent molars is apparent in the occlusal view. This demonstrates the variability in severity of MIH affected molars, even within the same patient. (C) Bitewing view of the patient's right side. The image demonstrates the rapid breakdown of tooth structure that occurs with MIH-affected teeth. (D) Panoramic film illustrates the radiographic variability of tooth breakdown in MIH-affected teeth.

closure, optimal molar angulation, and acceptable occlusion. Both arches require careful consideration, but extra attention should be paid to the mandibular arch when considering second molar substitution.[25] This is because the mandibular arch has a significantly lower level of successful substitution compared with the maxillary arch.[25] There are reasons for the decreased success in the mandibular arch, the most significant is the cortical bone thickness.[26]

In general, extraction of permanent first molars should be performed earlier rather than later in the child's dental development. In most cases, early extraction of first molars allows for increased success of second molar substitution. Preferably, the timing of molar substitution occurs well before second molar eruption and early in its development to allow for ideal space closure (Fig. 46.10). Later extractions typically have a decreased chance of space closure and ideal occlusion.[25] The extraction of nonrestorable permanent first molars should always be considered, regardless of age.

Summary

In managing missing teeth in a growing patient, careful diagnosis and assessment serve as the foundation for effective treatment. A thorough clinical examination, imaging, and understanding of the patient's dental history are essential to determining the cause of tooth absence. Growth status is equally critical, as treatment should align with the patient's developmental phase to ensure successful, long-term results.

For many patients, removable and fixed appliances play a role in managing spaces caused by missing teeth. Removable appliances are often preferred for younger patients because they provide flexibility and can be adjusted as growth continues, serving as temporary space maintainers. In contrast, fixed appliances are more stable and are ideal for guiding permanent teeth into their correct positions, especially for patients with less growth potential. The choice between these appliances depends on the individual's age, compliance, and specific dental needs.

Orthodontic space closure is another important approach to eliminate space left by missing teeth. By closing space, orthodontic treatment can enhance stability and streamline future restorative efforts. However, achieving a balanced bite and maintaining facial esthetics remain essential considerations, requiring precise planning and execution.

Tooth autotransplantation offers a unique solution, particularly for young patients. By transplanting a donor tooth within the same mouth, dentists can provide a more natural replacement for missing teeth. Success with autotransplantation depends on careful timing, proper planning, and diligent postoperative care.

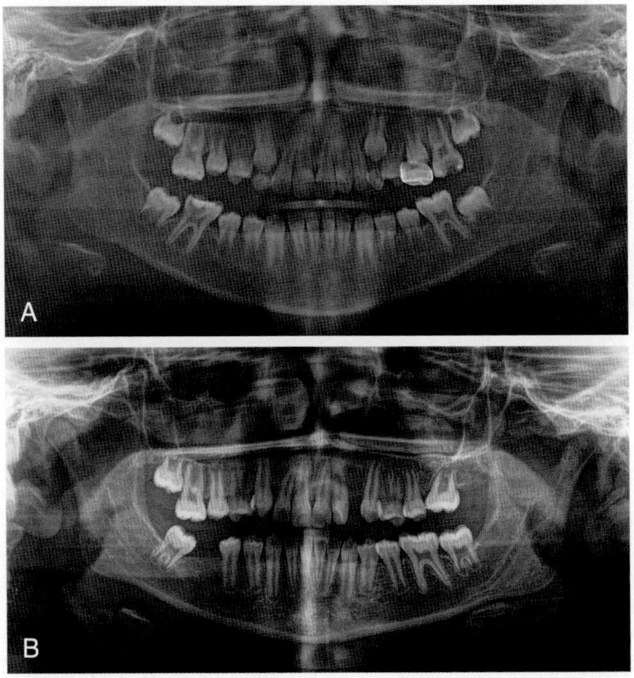

• **Fig. 46.10** (A) Panoramic radiograph of a 9 year old female patient with MIH affecting teeth #14 and #30. Second molar substation was determined to be the best treatment option. Second molars are in appropriate stage of development to attempt molar substitution. (B) Panoramic radiograph of same patient 11 months after the extraction of #14 and #30. There is nearly complete closure of space in the upper left with near ideal tooth angulation. Tooth #31 did not have the same result. Second molar substitution fares better in the maxilla compared to the mandible.

This option is particularly valuable for patients who may not be candidates for implants. Although dental implants are often seen as a definitive solution for select cases, their use in growing patients is limited. Implants are generally deferred until growth is complete, with temporary measures used in the interim to maintain space.

In some cases, extraction of permanent first molars may be necessary when these teeth are severely decayed or compromised. Timing is crucial, as removing first molars can affect the eruption and alignment of neighboring teeth, particularly the second molars. In carefully selected cases, extraction can encourage natural closure of spaces and optimize the alignment of surrounding teeth.

Overall, managing missing teeth in young patients is a multifaceted process that requires aligning treatment strategies with the patient's growth and development. The goal is to provide functional and esthetic solutions that adapt over time, allowing for stable, long-term outcomes tailored to each patient's unique growth pattern.

Visit eBooks.Health.Elsevier.com to see full list of references.

47

Sleep-Disordered Breathing

AUDREY JUNG-SUN YOON AND HEESOO OH

CHAPTER OUTLINE

With increasing recognition of the impact of sleep-related breathing disorders in children, the role of dental professionals in identifying and managing pediatric obstructive sleep apnea (OSA) has become increasingly important. Pediatric dentists, with their specialized expertise in craniofacial growth, airway anatomy, and oral health, are uniquely positioned as frontline healthcare providers in the early detection of OSA. Their ability to screen for risk factors during routine dental visits, coupled with frequent interactions with young patients and their families, provides a valuable opportunity for timely intervention to prevent the significant health consequences associated with untreated OSA.

Sleep-disordered breathing (SDB) comprises a range of breathing disturbances that occur during sleep, including snoring, OSA, central sleep apnea (CSA), and hypoventilation syndromes, essentially encompassing any disruption to normal breathing patterns while asleep.[1] Pediatric obstructive SDB is considered a progressive spectrum, ranging from snoring, upper airway resistance syndrome (UARS), and obstructive sleep apnea syndrome (OSAS) of varying severity, and extending to obesity hypoventilation syndrome (Fig. 47.1). Snoring is the most common manifestation of SDB in children, affecting approximately 7% to 27% of the pediatric population. OSA is defined by recurrent episodes of complete or partial upper airway obstruction during sleep, resulting in reduced or paused airflow despite ongoing respiratory effort and arousals that cause disrupted sleep.[1,2] The prevalence of OSA in children is estimated to range from 1% to 5%, depending on the population studied and the diagnostic criteria used.[1,3,4] The peak prevalence of pediatric OSA typically occurs between 2 and 8 years of age, largely driven by adenotonsillar hypertrophy, the most common etiology of pediatric OSA. However, the childhood obesity epidemic has shifted this pattern, with an increasing number of adolescents also affected. Although adenotonsillar hypertrophy remains a key contributor to airway obstruction in young children, obesity has become a significant factor across all age groups, exacerbating the prevalence of OSA in the pediatric and adolescent populations in the United States.[1,3–7] Untreated SDB may affect cognitive development, behavior, and physical growth. Early intervention is crucial to prevent long-term consequences on learning, social behavior, and cardiovascular health.[1]

Although snoring is the hallmark symptom, other manifestations include mouth breathing, restless sleep, daytime fatigue, behavioral problems, and growth delays. Left untreated, pediatric OSA can lead to serious consequences, including neurocognitive impairment, cardiovascular issues, and adverse effects on facial growth and development.[1,4–7]

In providing collaborative patient-centered care, professional guidelines from organizations such as the American Academy of Pediatrics (AAP), the American Academy of Pediatric Dentistry (AAPD), and the American Academy of Dental Sleep Medicine (AADSM) emphasize the importance of interdisciplinary collaboration in diagnosing and managing pediatric OSA. These guidelines encourage dentists to screen for symptoms of SDB, educate

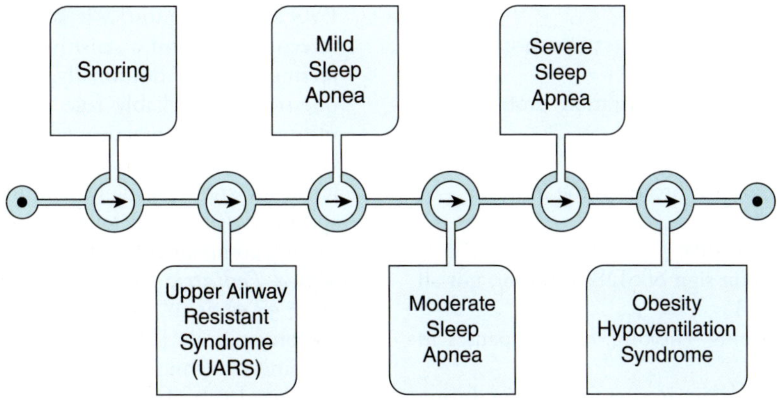

• **Fig. 47.1** Spectrum of Obstructive Sleep-Disordered Breathing. Obstructive sleep-disordered breathing encompasses a spectrum of conditions ranging from primary snoring to more severe disorders such as obstructive sleep apnea.

parents/caregivers about potential risks, and refer at-risk patients for further evaluation and treatment.

Etiology of Pediatric Obstructive Sleep Apnea

The etiology of SDB in children is multifactorial and involves craniofacial development, airway anatomy, and genetic and environmental influences.[2,4] These factors affect airway patency during sleep, often leading to partial or complete obstruction, particularly in those with anatomical or developmental predispositions.[1,4]

Anatomical Factors

Enlarged tonsils and adenoids are a primary cause of upper airway obstruction in younger children, particularly in the supine position during sleep. However, inadequate airway size, insufficient neuromuscular tone of the airway muscles, or both can contribute to the condition. Children with certain craniofacial anomalies, neuromuscular diseases, or hypotonia are at higher risk for developing OSA.[7] A retruded maxilla or mandible or high-arched palate and narrow dental arches can reduce the airway space and are often associated with mouth breathing, which may further affect normal craniofacial growth and increase the risk of SDB.[1,4–8]

Craniofacial Development

Craniofacial development plays a central role in SDB susceptibility in children. At birth, the face is about 40% of adult size, increasing to 65% at 3 years of age, and is only completed after puberty.[5,8] Facial growth is influenced principally by genetic factors, but environmental inputs may also contribute, including the route of breathing.[4,5,8]

Genetic Factors

Genetic predispositions can affect craniofacial structure and muscle tone, affecting airway patency. Children with conditions like Down syndrome, Pierre Robin sequence, or syndromes such as Treacher Collins or Apert syndrome often have underdeveloped jaw structures or characteristic airway narrowing, increasing their risk of OSA.[1,4,7,9] Genetics can also provide insight into the increased risk for OSA in the African American population. Studies, such as one by Buxbaum et al., have shown that genetic factors, independent of body mass index (BMI), contribute to SDB prevalence.[4,5,10] Additionally, a family history of SDB or conditions like obesity and asthma may increase a child's risk.

Environmental Factors

Childhood obesity rates have risen in recent decades, and excess body weight is a recognized risk factor for SDB due to increased fat deposits around the airway, which can contribute to collapse. For every increase in BMI by 1 kg/m^2, the risk of pediatric OSA increases by 12%.[4,11]

Chronic nasal obstruction from allergic rhinitis often leads to mouth breathing, which can alter craniofacial growth and airway size, increasing the risk of OSA.[4] These conditions can worsen SDB symptoms, especially during sleep.

Certain feeding patterns and habits (e.g., prolonged bottle feeding, pacifier use) may affect tongue posture and jaw development, potentially influencing airway structure over time. Breastfeeding has been shown to positively affect proper orofacial muscle development, lowering the risk of development of malocclusion, such as posterior crossbites as well as class II malocclusion, which could contribute to the prevention of pediatric OSA.[4,7] Early screening of infants to assess for tongue or lip tie, breastfeeding practices, which promotes positive development of the orofacial musculature,[12] and elimination of nonnutritive habits such as pacifier or digit sucking, are proper steps in ensuring proper development of the child.[4,13]

Clinical Presentation of Sleep-Disordered Breathing in Children

Pediatric OSA manifests differently from adult OSA, presenting distinct nighttime and daytime symptoms. Screening for pediatric OSA requires a comprehensive approach to identify anatomical, behavioral, and symptomatic indicators of SDB, enabling early referral and interdisciplinary care.[7] Dentists should evaluate children presenting with the following symptoms of pediatric OSA[7]:

- **Daytime symptoms** may include:
  - Behavioral issues: Hyperactivity, irritability, or difficulty focusing, which may be mistaken for attention-deficit/hyperactivity disorder (ADHD)

- Aggressive behavior
- Excessive daytime sleepiness (though less common in children than adults)
- Poor academic performance, concentration problems, or difficulty learning
- Growth problems such as failure to thrive
- Dry mouth, sore throat, or bad breath in the morning
- Morning headache

- **Nighttime symptoms** may include:
  - Snoring: The most common sign of SDB; however, not all snoring children have OSA
  - Pauses in breathing: Gasping, choking, or long pauses in breathing during sleep
  - Restless sleep: Frequent tossing, turning, or moving during the night
  - Difficulty staying asleep, frequent awakenings
  - Mouth breathing: A key indicator of possible airway obstruction
  - Sweating: Children with SDB may sweat excessively during sleep
  - Enuresis (Bedwetting): SDB has been associated with increased rates of bedwetting in children

Screening for Sleep-Disordered Breathing

Medical and Family History Review

Pediatric dentists should review the patient's medical history for factors associated with SDB. Key indicators include chronic allergies, asthma, recurrent ear or throat infections, and a family history of sleep apnea or SDB. Additional risk factors such as obesity, premature birth, and certain syndromic conditions should also be considered, as they may increase the likelihood of SDB.

Cognitive, Behavioral, and Developmental Assessment

Children with SDB often exhibit symptoms that overlap with those of ADHD, such as hyperactivity, irritability, and difficulty concentrating. Although these symptoms may mimic ADHD, they are sometimes rooted in the effects of SDB.[2] In addition, growth and physical development should be carefully evaluated, as signs of delayed growth or failure to thrive can indicate disrupted sleep and insufficient oxygenation during critical developmental stages. Obesity is the second most common cause of pediatric OSA, preceded only by adenoid and tonsillar hypertrophy. Obesity, a significant contributing factor, is clinically defined as a BMI exceeding the 95th percentile for age and sex, based on standardized growth curves. This underscores the importance of addressing obesity and anatomical factors when managing and treating SDB in children.[1,4,9]

Screening Tools and Questionnaires

Pediatric Sleep Questionnaire (PSQ) (Fig. 47.2)[14,15] is a validated and widely used tool with a sensitivity of 0.81 and a specificity of 0.87 within the general pediatric population. The PSQ is structured into four subscores: breathing, behavior, sleepiness, and other domains. If the total number of "Yes" responses are more than 8 or a total score exceeding 0.33—indicating that more than 33% of the questions are answered positively—there is a high likelihood of SDB.[16] Although the PSQ is not diagnostic, it is recognized as an effective initial screening tool and a sensitive questionnaires available for detecting SDB.[16] Additionally, negative responses to certain key questions can reliably rule out the condition, enhancing its utility in clinical practice.[1,17]

OSA-18 (Fig. 47.3) is a validated tool designed to assess the quality of life and SDB daily symptoms in children. It has higher specificity (0.73) but lower sensitivity (0.56) than PSQ, making it a complementary tool.[18]

Modified Pediatric Epworth Sleepiness Scale (ESS-CHAD)[19] (Fig. 47.4) is an adapted version of the original Epworth Sleepiness Scale (ESS), tailored specifically to assess daytime sleepiness in children and adolescents. It is designed for children aged 6 to 16, and it evaluates daytime sleepiness levels and can prompt further investigation if abnormal scores are observed. Janssen et al. reported that ESS-CHAD is a reliable and internally valid measure of daytime sleepiness in adolescents 12 to 18 years old.[20]

The overall performance of questionnaire tools seems to support their use more as a screening than a diagnostic tool.[1] These screening survey tools can guide initial assessment and are valuable for baseline measurements.[16]

Clinical Oral and Craniofacial Examination

Mallampati and Tonsils: The Mallampati classification, Friedman tongue classification, and Brodsky tonsil size scale are useful tools for assessing airway obstruction risk (Figs. 47.5 and 47.6).[21–24] Tonsillar hypertrophy that obstructs more than 50% of the airway requires further evaluation.[1,4,6,22,24] A meta-analysis by Friedman et al. demonstrated a significant correlation between tonsillar hypertrophy and the severity of OSA.[22]

Palatal Structure and Dental Arches: Evaluate for high-arched palates or narrow dental arches, which may contribute to airway restriction. Narrow arches may also indicate a habit of mouth breathing.[4,6,23–27] Palatal height and arch width is difficult to accurately diagnose but should be noted.

Jaw Size and Position[7]: Evaluate for retrognathia or micrognathia (receded or small jaw) that can contribute to airway constriction. Subtle radiographic findings, such as inferior positioning of the hyoid bone and reduced mandibular or maxillary length, may also indicate airway compromise. Jaw growth should be regularly monitored in growing patients, as interventions may be considered if structural concerns persist.[4,6,23–27]

Tongue Posture and Function: Evaluate tongue tie, low tongue posture, or restricted tongue movement. Abnormal tongue posture or habits like tongue thrusting may affect airway patency and craniofacial development.[24–27]

Breathing Habits: Identify whether the child primarily breathes through the mouth. Chronic mouth breathing is often linked to nasal obstruction and can contribute to abnormal jaw and facial development. Nasal resistance measured by using rhinometry had high sensitivity and specificity for predicting polysomnographic OSAS.[1,28]

Tooth Wear: A high frequency of OSA has been observed in dental patients exhibiting significant tooth wear, including abrasion, attrition, erosion, and abfraction. Research indicates a positive correlation between severe bruxism and more pronounced OSA symptoms. Bruxism, often linked to sleep disturbances and airway obstruction, may serve as an indicator for underlying SDB and should prompt further evaluation for OSA.[4]

Pediatric Sleep Questionnaire

(Screening)

Name of the child:________________________ Date of birth:__________

Person completing this form: ______________________________

Date that you are completing the questionnaire: ____________

Instructions: Please answer the questions about how your child **IN THE PAST MONTH.** Circle the correct response or *print* your answers in the space provided. "Y" means "yes," "N" means "no," and "DK" means "don't know." For this questionnaire, the word "usually" means "more than half the time" or "on more than half the nights."

Please answer the following questions as they pertain to your child in the past month.

		YES	NO	Don't Know
1.	**While sleeping, does your child:**			
	Snore more than half the time?	Y	N	DK
	Always snore?	Y	N	DK
	Snore loudly?	Y	N	DK
	Have "heavy" or loud breathing?	Y	N	DK
	Have trouble breathing, or struggle to breath?	Y	N	DK
2.	**Have you ever seen your child stop breathing during the night?**	Y	N	DK
3.	**Does your child:**			
	Tend to breathe through the mouth during the day?	Y	N	DK
	Have a dry mouth on waking up in the morning?	Y	N	DK
	Occasionally wet the bed?	Y	N	DK
4.	**Does your child:**			
	Wake up feeling unrefreshed in the morning?	Y	N	DK
	Have a problem with sleepiness during the day?	Y	N	DK
5.	**Has a teacher or other supervisor commented that your child appears sleepy during the day?**	Y	N	DK
6.	**Is it hard to wake your child up in the morning?**	Y	N	DK
7.	**Does your child wake up with headaches in the morning?**	Y	N	DK
8.	**Did your child stop growing at a normal rate at any time since birth?**	Y	N	DK
9.	**Is your child overweight?**	Y	N	DK
10.	**This child often:**			
	Does not seem to listen when spoken to directly	Y	N	DK
	Has difficulty organizing tasks and activities	Y	N	DK
	Is easily distracted by extraneous stimuli	Y	N	DK
	Fidgets with hands or feet, or squirms in seat	Y	N	DK
	Is "on the go" or often acts as if "driven by a motor"	Y	N	DK
	Interrupts or intrudes on others (eg butts into conversations or games)	Y	N	DK

• **Fig. 47.2** Pediatric Sleep Questionnaire (PSQ). PSQ is the most popular pediatric sleep screening questionnaire. If the total number of "Yes" responses are more than 8, it may indicate a problem with a sleep-related breathing disorder.

Functional Airway Evaluation Screening Tool (FAirEST-6)[29]: FAirEST-6 (Fig. 47.7) is a clinical tool designed for dentists and healthcare providers to assess the functional aspects of airway health and identify potential risks associated with SDB in children.[23,30] Six red flags for pediatric SDB include mouth breathing, mentalis strain, tonsil hypertrophy, ankyloglossia, dental wear, and narrow palate. By examining these key components, FAirEST-6 aids pediatric dentists and other healthcare providers in identifying potential airway dysfunctions and risks associated with SDB. This tool supports early detection and intervention, promoting multidisciplinary collaboration for treatments such as myofunctional therapy, orthodontics, or ear, nose, and throat (ENT) referrals.

ID#: _ _ _ _ _ _ _ _ Name Code: _ _ _ _ DOV: _ _ - _ _ _ - _ _ _ _
d d m m m y y y y

OSA-18 Quality of Life Survey

Evaluation of Sleep-Disordered Breathing

Instructions: For each question below, please fill in the circle that best describes how often each symptom or problem has occurred during the past *4 weeks* (or since the last survey, if sooner). Thank you.

	None of the time	Hardly any of the time	A little of the time	Some of the time	A good bit of the time	Most of the time	All of the time
<u>SLEEP DISTURBANCE</u>							
During the past *4 weeks*, how often has your child had…							
…loud snoring?	①	②	③	④	⑤	⑥	⑦
…breath holding spells or pauses in breathing at night?	①	②	③	④	⑤	⑥	⑦
…choking or gasping sounds while asleep?	①	②	③	④	⑤	⑥	⑦
…restless sleep or frequent awakenings from sleep?	①	②	③	④	⑤	⑥	⑦
<u>PHYSICAL SUFFERING</u>							
During the past *4 weeks*, how often has your child had…							
…mouth breathing because of nasal obstruction?	①	②	③	④	⑤	⑥	⑦
…frequent colds or upper respiratory infections?	①	②	③	④	⑤	⑥	⑦
…nasal discharge or runny nose?	①	②	③	④	⑤	⑥	⑦
…difficulty in swallowing foods?	①	②	③	④	⑤	⑥	⑦
<u>EMOTIONAL DISTRESS</u>							
During the past *4 weeks*, how often has your child had…							
…mood swings or temper tantrums?	①	②	③	④	⑤	⑥	⑦
…aggressive or hyperactive behavior?	①	②	③	④	⑤	⑥	⑦
…discipline problems?	①	②	③	④	⑤	⑥	⑦
<u>DAYTIME PROBLEMS</u>							
During the past *4 weeks*, how often has your child had…							
…excessive daytime drowsiness or sleepiness?	①	②	③	④	⑤	⑥	⑦
…poor attention span or concentration?	①	②	③	④	⑤	⑥	⑦
…difficulty getting out of bed in the morning?	①	②	③	④	⑤	⑥	⑦
<u>CAREGIVER CONCERNS</u>							
During the past *4 weeks*, how often have the above problems…							
…caused you to worry about your child's general health?	①	②	③	④	⑤	⑥	⑦
…created concern that your child is not getting enough air?	①	②	③	④	⑤	⑥	⑦
…interfered with your ability to perform daily activities?	①	②	③	④	⑤	⑥	⑦
…made you frustrated?	①	②	③	④	⑤	⑥	⑦

OVERALL, HOW WOULD YOU RATE YOUR CHILD'S QUALITY OF LIFE AS A RESULT OF THE ABOVE PROBLEMS?

(Circle one number)

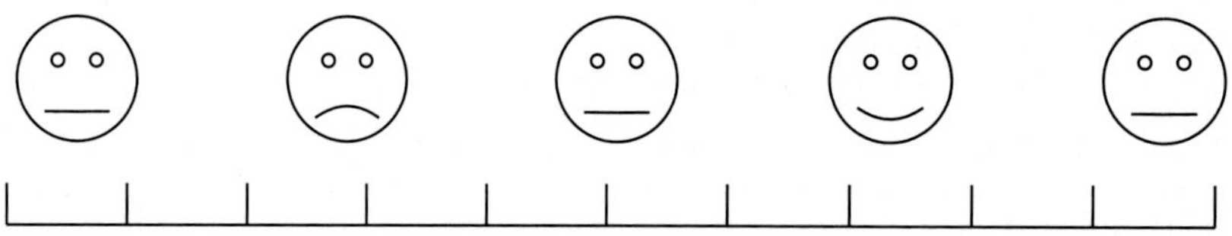

0 1 2 3 4 5 6 7 8 9 10

Worst Possible Quality-of-Life | Half-way Between Worst and Best | Best Possible Quality-of-Life

• **Fig. 47.3** OSA-18. The OSA-18 Questionnaire is used in pediatric populations to evaluate how obstructive sleep apnea symptoms affect various aspects of daily functioning.

PEDIATRIC EPWORTH SLEEPINESS SCALE (ESS)

How likely is your child to doze off or fall asleep in the following situations, in contrast to feeling just tired? This refers to their usual way of life in recent times. Even if they have not done some of these things recently try to imagine how it would have affected them.

Use the following scale to choose the most appropriate number for each situation:

0 = Would never doze or sleep
1 = Slight chance of dozing or sleeping
2 = Moderate change of dozing or sleeping
3 = High chance of dozing or sleeping

_____ 1. Sitting and reading
_____ 2. Watching TV
_____ 3. Sitting inactive in a public place
_____ 4. Being a passenger in a motor vehicle without a break
_____ 5. Lying down in the afternoon when circumstances permit
_____ 6. Sitting and talking to someone
_____ 7. Sitting quietly after lunch
_____ 8. Doing homework or taking a test

Total score __________

A total score of 10 or more indicates that your child is sleepy. Please discuss this questionnaire with your child's health care provider.

• **Fig. 47.4** Modified Pediatric Epworth Sleepiness Scale (ESS-CHAD). ESS-CHAD is a modified version of the original Epworth Sleepiness Scale to assess daytime sleepiness in children and adolescents.

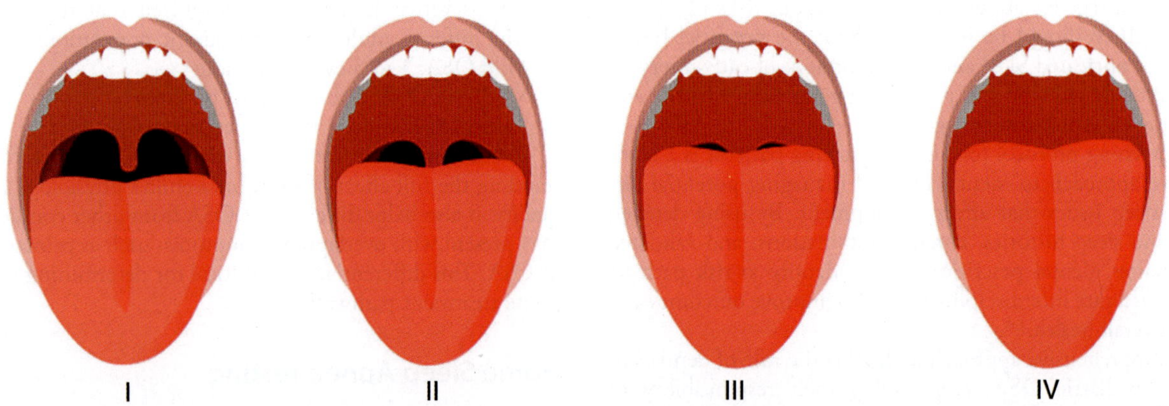

• **Fig. 47.5** Modified Mallampati Grade. Class I: Faucial/tonsillar pillars, uvula, and soft palate are all visible. Class II: Partial visibility of the faucial/tonsillar pillars, uvula, and soft palate. Class III: Base of the uvula, soft and hard palate visible. Class IV: Only hard palate is visible. (Mallampati Score Visual Contributed by Jmarchn. Creative Commons.)

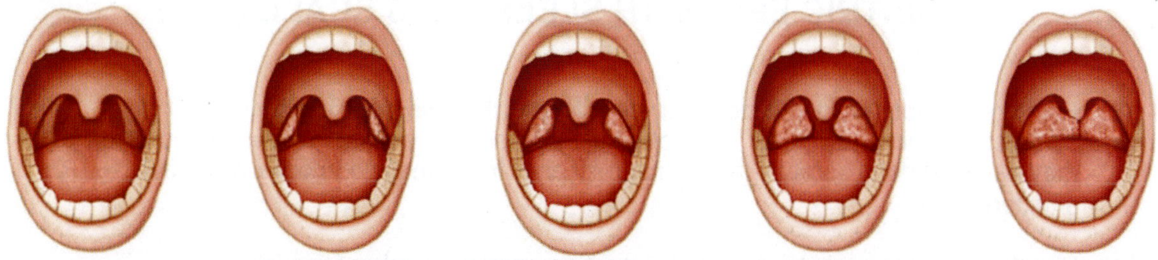

• **Fig. 47.6** Brodsky Tonsil Grading Scale Grades. Clinical grading of tonsil size: grade 0, tonsils limited to the tonsillar fossa; grade 1, tonsils occupying up to 25% of the space between the anterior pillars in the oropharynx; grade 2, tonsils occupying 25% to 50% of the space between the anterior pillars; grade 3, tonsils occupying 50% to 75% of the space between the anterior pillars; grade 4, tonsils occupying 75% to 100% of the space between the anterior pillars.

Interdisciplinary Collaboration and Referrals

Referral to Sleep Physician or ENT: For children exhibiting multiple SDB risk factors or symptoms, a referral to a pediatric sleep physician or an ENT specialist is recommended for a comprehensive evaluation. This may include polysomnography (PSG) or further imaging if warranted.[4,7,9]

Orthodontic Consultation: In cases where craniofacial development suggests a narrow airway or malocclusion, consider early orthodontic evaluation. Interventions like maxillary expansion may be beneficial in alleviating mild to moderate SDB symptoms and promoting healthy airway development.[4,5,9,24,27] The orthodontist should discuss the orthodontic findings with a pediatric sleep physician or ENT physician before beginning treatment for SDB alone and inform the parent that the treatment may not provide definitive relief.

Collaboration With Pediatricians: Regular communication with the child's pediatrician ensures a coordinated approach to treatment and monitoring, especially if SDB overlaps with other health conditions.

Educate Parents and Caregivers: Raising awareness among parents and caregivers about the symptoms and risks of SDB is crucial. They should be informed about the potential health effects of untreated SDB and the importance of early intervention. Provide guidance on promoting good sleep hygiene and avoiding environmental triggers.

The screening protocol for SDB in growing patients is a comprehensive approach to identifying and managing potential airway and sleep issues that affect development. By using detailed medical and sleep histories, clinical examinations, and validated questionnaires, dental practitioners can identify at-risk patients early and facilitate interdisciplinary care to improve outcomes and enhance overall health.[1,4]

This comprehensive approach highlights the role of dentists in managing pediatric OSA, emphasizing their responsibility to screen, assess, and collaborate with medical professionals in delivering optimal care.

Diagnostic Tool for Pediatric Obstructive Sleep Apnea

Although pediatric dentists play a pivotal role in identifying children at risk for OSA, definitive diagnosis requires specialized tools and expertise beyond the scope of dental practice. These diagnostic methods provide a clear understanding of the presence and severity of OSA, guiding targeted interventions. Among these tools, PSG stands as the gold standard, supported by emerging technologies and adjunctive diagnostic approaches that expand the possibilities for accurate and accessible assessments.

Polysomnography

PSG (Fig. 47.8), commonly referred to as a sleep study, is the most reliable and comprehensive diagnostic tool for pediatric OSA. Conducted in a controlled sleep laboratory, PSG monitors and records multiple physiologic parameters during sleep, offering a detailed picture of the child's breathing and sleep patterns. It captures key data points such as respiratory effort, oxygen saturation levels, the frequency and duration of apneic and hypopneic events, and disruptions in sleep architecture.[1]

One of the critical metrics derived from PSG is the apnea-hypopnea index (AHI), which quantifies the number of apneas (complete cessation of airflow) and hypopneas (partial reduction in airflow) per hour of sleep.[31] The AHI score provides a measure of OSA severity. It should be recognized that the measures of severity differ in adults and the pediatric population:

- Mild OSA: 1 to 5 events per hour
- Moderate OSA: 5 to 10 events per hour
- Severe OSA: Greater than 10 events per hour

PSG's comprehensive nature makes it invaluable for understanding the full effect of OSA on a child's physiology and sleep quality. It also helps differentiate OSA from other conditions that may present with overlapping symptoms, such as primary snoring or CSA. This differentiation is critical for determining the appropriate treatment pathway.

Home Sleep Apnea Testing

For older children, especially those in resource-limited settings, home sleep apnea testing (HSAT; Fig. 47.8) may be considered. HSAT uses portable devices to record data such as oxygen saturation, airflow, and respiratory effort while the child sleeps at home. This approach offers several advantages, including convenience, lower cost, and the ability to assess sleep in a more natural environment.[32]

However, HSAT has limitations, particularly in the pediatric population. It is generally less sensitive and may fail to capture the subtle nuances of pediatric OSA, such as partial upper airway

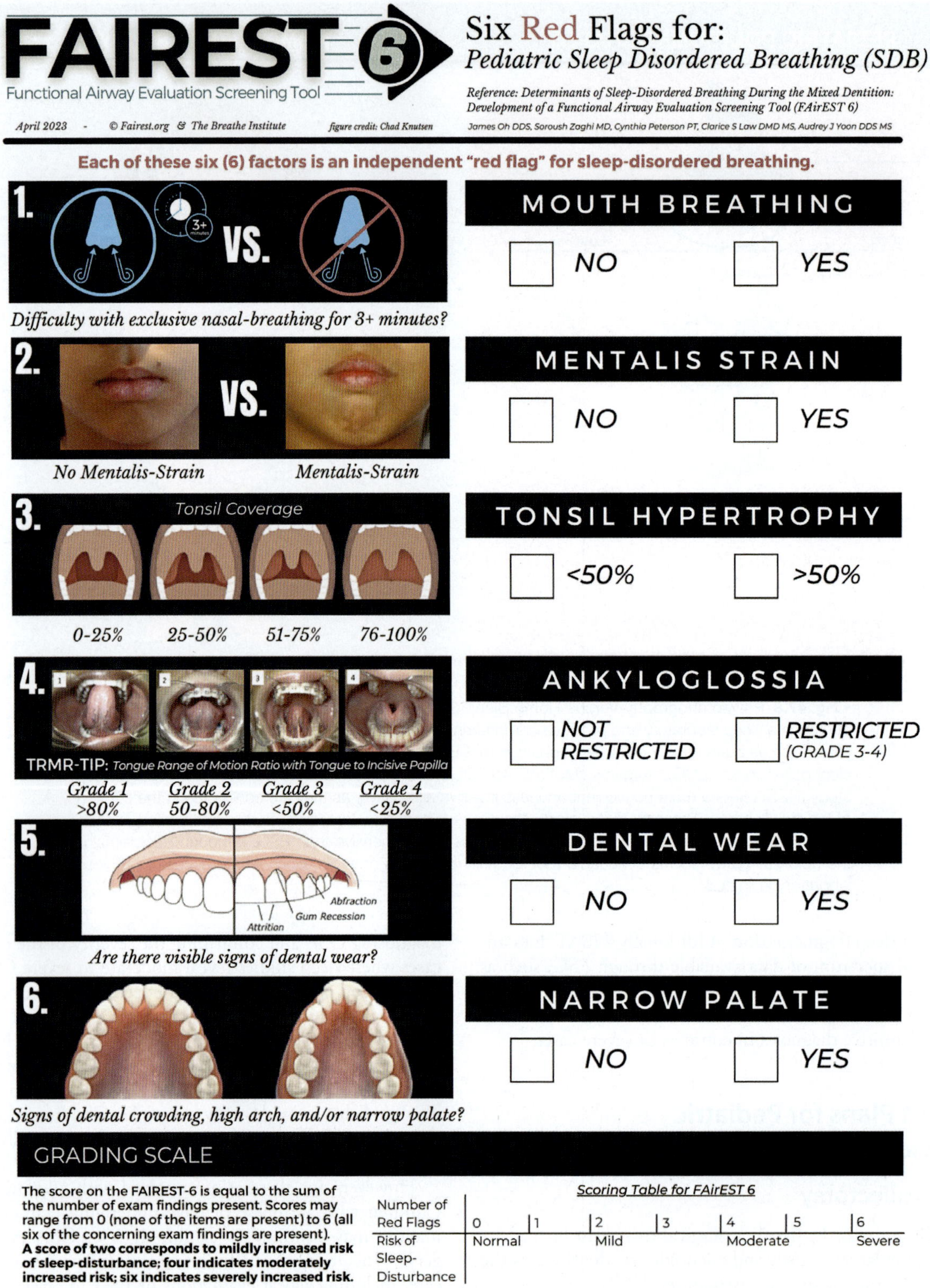

• **Fig. 47.7** The Functional Airway Evaluation Screening Tool (FAirEST-6). FAirEST-6 is a systematic clinical tool designed to assess six critical aspects of airway health and function in children.

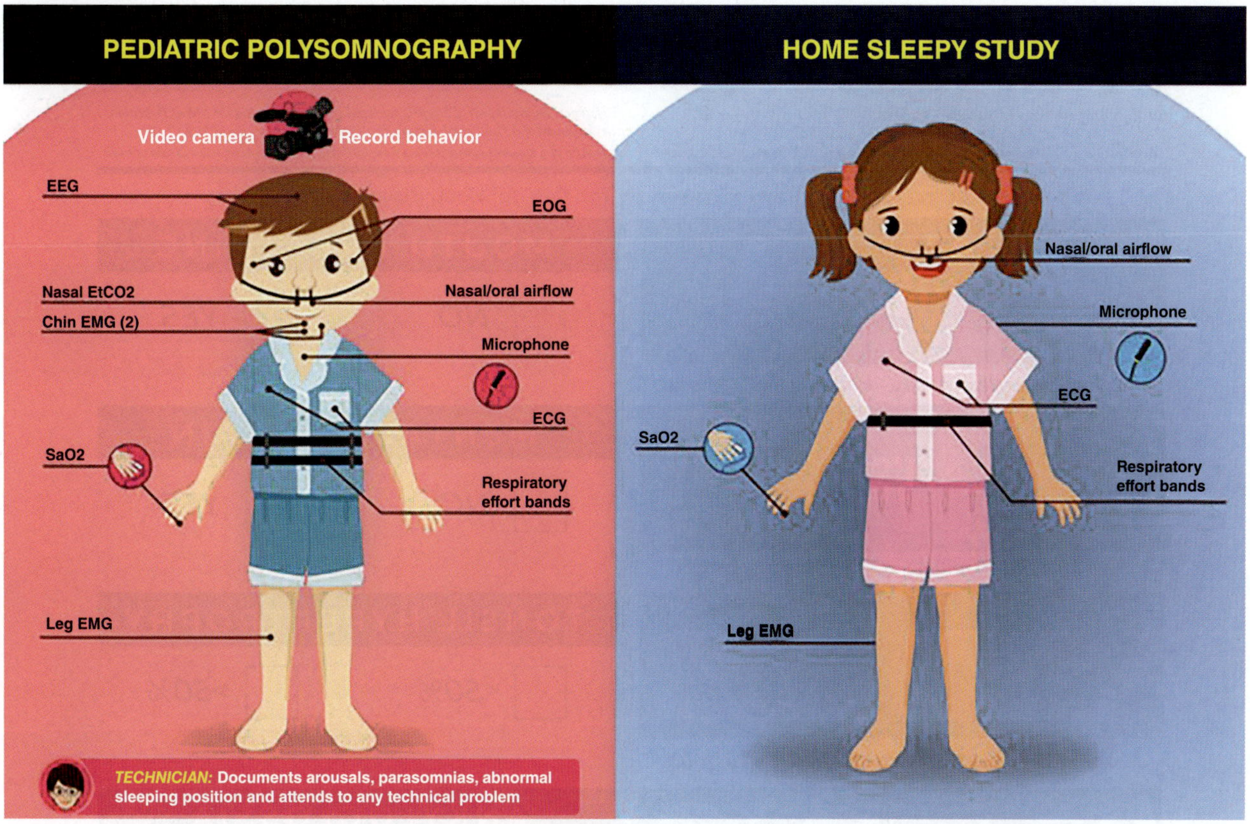

• **Fig. 47.8** Polysomnography Versus Home Sleep Study in Children. Polysomnography (PSG) is conducted in a sleep laboratory and provides comprehensive data by monitoring multiple physiologic parameters such as brain activity electroencephalogram (EEG), muscle tone electromyogram (EMG), heart rate electrocardiogram (ECG), oxygen saturation, respiratory effort, airflow, and body movements. Home sleep study (HSS) offers a more convenient and less invasive alternative, as they are conducted in the comfort of the child's home. These studies typically focus on fewer parameters, such as respiratory effort, airflow, oxygen saturation, and heart rate, making them less comprehensive than PSG. Although PSG remains the gold standard, HSS is a valuable tool for initial screening or in situations where access to a sleep laboratory is limited.

obstructions or sleep fragmentation. Additionally, HSAT does not provide the full spectrum of data available through PSG, such as sleep stage analysis. As a result, HSAT is typically reserved for older children or as a preliminary screening tool, with PSG still required for definitive diagnosis in complex or severe cases.

Treatment Plans for Pediatric Sleep-Disordered Breathing[1]

Adenotonsillectomy

Adenotonsillectomy is the first-line surgical treatment for pediatric SDB when enlarged tonsils and adenoids are identified as the primary contributors to airway obstruction.[1,33]

The most common reason for recommending adenotonsillectomy is the presence of enlarged tonsils and adenoids, which can significantly narrow the upper airway. This narrowing often manifests as persistent snoring, restless sleep, or pauses in breathing during sleep—hallmark symptoms of SDB.

Children who exhibit these symptoms, particularly when they interfere with daily functioning, are candidates for the procedure. Although clinical evaluation often provides sufficient evidence of adenotonsillar hypertrophy, PSG remains the gold standard for diagnosing OSA and confirming the severity of the condition. In cases where sleep studies reveal moderate to severe OSA, surgical intervention is typically the most effective course of action.[34]

The procedure is relatively straightforward and involves the removal of the tonsils and adenoids to clear the airway. The effects of the surgery are often immediate, with parents noticing significant improvements in their child's breathing, sleep quality, and daytime behavior within days to weeks. Children who previously struggled with restless sleep or snoring may finally experience uninterrupted, restorative sleep.

However, not all cases are resolved with adenotonsillectomy. Children who are obese or have underlying craniofacial abnormalities may continue to exhibit signs of OSA even after surgery.[34] This residual risk underscores the importance of follow-up care, including repeat evaluations or PSG to assess the effectiveness of the surgery and determine whether further interventions are needed.

Medical Management

Allergy Management

Allergies can significantly contribute to SDB by causing chronic nasal congestion and inflammation, both of which increase airway resistance and promote mouth breathing. Managing these allergies

is a critical aspect of treating SDB, particularly in children with environmental or seasonal sensitivities.[35,36]

The use of corticosteroids and leukotriene antagonists has shown effectiveness in the treatment of OSA. Corticosteroids reduce nasal inflammation, and antihistamines target the histamine-mediated allergic response.[37,38]

Several studies of intranasal steroids showed a moderate improvement in patients who had mild OSAS. However, significant residual OSAS remained in most of the studies.[38,39]

Weight Management

Obesity is a growing concern in pediatric SDB. Weight management plays a role in the prevention and treatment of SDB in children, particularly in those with obesity-related SDB. Excess weight contributes to airway obstruction through several mechanisms, including increased fat deposits around the upper airway, reduced lung volume, and systemic inflammation, which exacerbates airway resistance and collapse during sleep. Along with many other health-related benefits, achieving weight loss and increasing exercise seem to be beneficial for OSAS and should be recommended along with other interventions for OSAS in obese children and adolescents.[1]

Parents play a vital role in this process, as dietary changes and exercise routines are most successful when implemented as family-wide initiatives. Although weight loss may take time, even modest reductions in body weight can significantly improve airway function and reduce the severity of SDB.[40,41]

Positive Airway Pressure Therapy

For children with moderate to severe OSA, or those whose symptoms persist despite other treatments, continuous positive airway pressure (CPAP) therapy has been shown to be effective.[42] This treatment involves wearing a mask connected to a CPAP machine, which delivers pressurized air to keep the airway open during sleep.

Although highly effective, CPAP can be challenging for pediatric patients, as many children find the mask uncomfortable or the noise of the machine disruptive. Success with CPAP often depends on parental involvement and careful customization of the mask and pressure settings.[43]

Prolonged use of CPAP may affect craniofacial growth in children. Long-term use of CPAP in children/adolescence can exert external pressure on the midface, potentially leading to midfacial hypoplasia, nasal obstruction, and dental malocclusions, such as class III skeletal patterns. Therefore monitoring craniofacial changes during CPAP use is essential.[44]

Orthodontic and Dentofacial Interventions

Rapid Maxillary Expansion

Rapid maxillary expansion, or RME, is an orthodontic treatment used to widen the upper jaw and nasal passages. This technique is particularly beneficial for children with a high-arched or narrow palate, which can restrict nasal airflow and exacerbate SDB symptoms.[45,46]

The process involves using a palatal expander, a device custom-fitted to the child's mouth. Over a series of weeks, gentle pressure is applied to gradually separate the midpalatal suture, increasing the width of the maxilla. This expansion not only creates more room in the oral cavity but also enlarges the nasal airway, reducing resistance to breathing.[47]

Parents and clinicians often report a noticeable reduction in snoring and mouth breathing after RME. Scientific studies have shown that RME can lower the AHI, a measure of the severity of sleep apnea.[48] The best outcomes are achieved when the procedure is performed during early or mixed dentition stages, as the palatal suture becomes less malleable with age.

Maxillary Protraction

Maxillary protraction, an effective treatment for maxillary deficiency, has gained attention as a noninvasive approach for addressing SDB in pediatric patients. Techniques like rapid palatal expansion (RPE) with facemask therapy are commonly used to increase transverse maxillary dimensions and advance the maxilla anteriorly, which helps enlarge the nasopharyngeal airway and reduce upper airway resistance. A systematic review and meta-analysis evaluated the effects of maxillary protraction, with or without RPE, on airway dimensions. The study concluded that such interventions significantly increase nasopharyngeal airway dimensions in children with class III malocclusion, potentially alleviating SDB symptoms.[49]

For older children or those with more mature craniofacial structures, approaches like miniscrew-assisted rapid palatal expansion (MARPE) and skeletal anchorage devices, including Bollard plates, provide controlled skeletal changes to further optimize airway outcomes. A preliminary report using bone-anchored maxillary protraction showed the effectiveness of maxillary protraction in treating pediatric OSA, demonstrating improved AHI and OSA symptoms. The outcomes were dependent on the age of treatment initiation and patient compliance.[50]

Mandibular Advancement Appliances

Mandibular advancement devices are another orthodontic option, particularly suited for children with retrognathia—a condition where the lower jaw is set back compared with the upper jaw. These devices work by repositioning the mandible forward, which opens the airway and prevents collapse during sleep.[51]

Although effective, these appliances are best used in older children who have reached the mixed or permanent dentition stages but before the end of pubertal peak, as they rely on stable teeth for anchorage. They are a noninvasive alternative to surgical approaches and can be particularly beneficial in cases of mild to moderate OSA.[52] Regular follow-ups are essential to adjust the device as the child grows, ensuring sustained benefits.

Myofunctional Therapy

Myofunctional therapy is an often overlooked yet effective treatment for pediatric SDB. This noninvasive approach involves a series of exercises designed to strengthen the muscles of the tongue, lips, and oropharynx. Although it is not a standalone solution for all children, it serves as a complement to orthodontic or surgical interventions, reducing the risk of relapse and enhancing overall outcomes. By improving muscle tone and coordination, myofunctional therapy can address underlying functional issues such as poor tongue posture, mouth breathing, and improper swallowing patterns.[53,54]

For instance, children who habitually breathe through their mouths may develop a forward head posture or narrow palate, both of which can contribute to SDB. Myofunctional therapy retrains these habits, encouraging nasal breathing and proper oral posture. Myofunctional therapy does not have evidence-based support to be used alone and should be considered as an adjunct therapy.

Growth Modification Techniques and Proposed Guidelines for Sleep-Disordered Breathing in Children

Growth modification is a tool in managing SDB in children, as it leverages periods of active craniofacial growth to address structural issues contributing to airway obstruction. Maxillary expansion or functional appliances are designed to stimulate maxillary and mandibular growth and enhance airway dimensions.

In 2023, Yoon et al. proposed a multidisciplinary protocol for growth modification tailored to craniofacial phenotyping (Table 47.1).[27]

This framework outlines a detailed approach for orthodontic interventions aimed at promoting growth modification in children with SDB. The protocol highlights the critical role of collaboration among pediatric sleep medicine specialists to design individualized treatment plans focused on enhancing upper airway health.

Preschool Stage (Infancy to 5 Years: Primary Dentition)

During this stage of development, the growth and remodeling of cranial bones are shaped by genetic influences and functional activities such as breathing, chewing, and swallowing. These functional activities play a role in the development of craniofacial structures and the upper airway.[55] The cranial base acts as a foundational structure that integrates growth within the nasal and oral cavities. Although its length and flexion are primarily genetically determined, factors like breathing patterns and head posture also significantly affect its development.[56]

During this stage, focus should be on promoting nasal breathing and addressing mouth breathing to support healthy craniofacial growth. Nasal obstructions and low tongue posture can disrupt critical functions and hinder facial development.[55,57] Encouraging nasal respiration and eliminating harmful habits such as thumb sucking and tongue thrusting are essential at this age. For children with airway obstruction caused by enlarged adenoids or tonsils, adenotonsillectomy may be necessary, particularly in cases of OSA between the ages of 3 and 7. Additionally, improving tongue mobility and managing allergies can enhance upper airway function and craniofacial development.

Growth modification during this stage often involves maxillary expansion and advancement to improve nasal airflow by creating adequate space.[47] Myofunctional therapy can play a role in enhancing speech, swallowing patterns, and tongue posture.[53]

Early Childhood (Ages 6 to 9: Early Mixed Dentition)

During early childhood, significant growth occurs in the nasal cavity as the nasomaxillary complex continues to develop, with notable forward growth of the maxilla. Concurrently, the mandible undergoes shape changes, including a reduction in the gonial angle and forward and downward movement of the hyoid bone.[58] The tongue also increases in size and strength, and swallowing function reaches full maturity during this period.

TABLE 47.1 A Multidisciplinary Craniofacial Growth Modification Roadmap for Children With Sleep-Disordered Breathing: ***This outlines a comprehensive framework for orthodontic growth modification in children with sleep-disordered breathing, emphasizing interdisciplinary collaboration among pediatric sleep medicine practitioners.***

	Preschool primary dentition	School early mixed dentition	School late mixed dentition	Adolescence permanent dentition	Post-adolescence
Age	0–5	6–9	10–11	12–15	16–18
Cranial base	Nasal breathing nasal expansion postural correction				
Nasomaxillary complex		Nasomaxillary AP growth midfacial advancement	TAD anchored orthopedic for midfacial advancement		
	Slow/semi rapid maxillary expansion	Conventional semi rapid/rapid maxillary expansion (transverse)		TAD assisted maxillary expansion (MARPE)	
Mandible	Unlock deep overbite and overjet to grow mandible functional appliance (controversial) control vertical growth for favorable Mn Growth		Peak Mn. Growth Stimulate Mandible A-P Growth Consider TAD to change growth direction	TAD for mandibular autorotation	
Lymphoid	Adenotonsillectomy (enlarged tonsil peak at age 3–7, adenoid age 10)				Lingual tonsillectomy
Functional	Myofunctional therapy (nasal breathing, proper tongue posture, chewing, swallowing, address parafunctions)				

A-P, anteroposterior; *AP,* anteroposterior; *MARPE,* miniscrew-assisted rapid palatal expansion; *Mn,* mandible; *TAD,* temporary anchorage device.

Orthodontic treatments in early childhood focus on supporting nasomaxillary development and addressing craniofacial growth patterns. RPE is commonly used to widen the maxillary arch,[48] and reverse-pull headgear (facemask therapy) can assist in advancing the midface. Correcting malocclusions, such as deep overbites and reverse overjet, is crucial for promoting balanced craniofacial growth. Myofunctional therapy is particularly valuable at this stage, helping establish nasal breathing habits and prevent potential developmental issues. For children with significantly enlarged lymphoid tissues obstructing the upper airway, adenotonsillectomy may be necessary to restore airflow and support healthy overall growth.

Middle Childhood (Ages 10 to 11: Late Mixed Dentition)

During middle childhood, the nasomaxillary complex continues its forward and downward growth, leading to further expansion of the nasal cavity and increased interdigitation of the midpalatal suture. This stage is also characterized by significant mandibular growth, with vertical development evident in both the maxilla and mandible.[58]

As lymphoid tissues naturally shrink with age, the tongue reaches its full size, moving forward and downward while gaining strength. These changes, along with continued palate development and dentition changes, contribute to the near-complete maturation of swallowing function.

Orthodontic interventions at this stage often address transverse discrepancies using RPE. For cases requiring enhanced forward growth of the nasomaxillary complex, treatments may include MARPE or temporary anchorage devices (TADs) combined with facemask therapy to get more skeletal forward growth.[59] Functional appliances, such as class II correctors, are frequently used to promote mandibular growth, facilitating optimal craniofacial development during this critical period.[52]

Adolescence (Ages 12 to 15: Permanent Dentition)

Adolescence is characterized by ongoing vertical growth of the nasomaxillary complex. During this period, girls typically experience steady increases in mandibular length and ramus height, and boys often reach their peak mandibular growth between ages 13 and 15. This stage also sees substantial vertical development of the mandible, which can lead to counterclockwise rotation of the lower jaw.[58]

As lymphatic tissues, such as the tonsils and adenoids, naturally diminish in size, swallowing function reaches full maturity, supported by further development of tongue strength. As skeletal growth approaches completion, orthodontic treatments during adolescence become particularly effective when bone-anchored mini screws (TADs) are used[60]; TADs offer enhanced predictability and stability for skeletal corrections at this stage.[59] MARPE and/or miniplates are commonly employed to address transverse discrepancies and promote midface advancement in patients with SDB. The use of class II correctors or functional appliances in orthodontics remains a topic of debate, particularly regarding their ability to stimulate mandibular growth. TADs are frequently used to facilitate favorable mandibular autorotation, which can help reduce symptoms associated with SDB. There seems to be more craniofacial remodeling than tooth-related dental compensation.

Postadolescence (Ages 16 to 18: Permanent Dentition)

In postadolescence, skeletal growth is nearly complete, with only minor residual changes occurring in the mandible. The forward and downward movement of the hyoid bone continues, influenced by mandibular positioning and the vertical growth of the cervical vertebrae. Tongue strength also gradually increases during this period. However, hypertrophy of the lingual tonsils, which may develop after puberty, can lead to retroglossal airway obstruction, contributing to OSA, particularly in individuals with craniofacial abnormalities or obesity.[61]

Treatment strategies for individuals with fully mature skeletal structures often prioritize direct skeletal modifications. TAD-supported palatal expanders are also useful in managing high-arched and narrow palates, and transverse skeletal discrepancies.[62] TADs can play a role in facilitating mandibular autorotation, helping optimize airway dimensions.

For patients with pronounced retroglossal obstruction, lingual tonsillectomy combined with myofunctional therapy can enhance airway patency.[63] In more severe or complex cases, orthognathic surgery, particularly maxillomandibular advancement (MMA), is recommended once skeletal growth is complete. MMA has proven to be highly effective in significantly increasing upper airway volume, providing substantial improvement for patients with OSA.[64] As previously discussed, surgical intervention should be part of an interdisciplinary approach if the sole goal is airway patency. In many cases, improvements in occlusion and facial esthetics also improve airway issues.

Conclusion

Pediatric dentists play a role in the early detection, screening, and managing of SDB. Through incorporating routine screenings into regular dental checkups, implementing orthodontic treatments when needed, and collaborating with a multidisciplinary team of specialists, pediatric dentists can enhance the care and outcomes for children experiencing SDB.

Visit eBooks.Health.Elsevier.com to see full list of references.

48

Tethered Oral Tissues

ALLEGRA NOTTOLI AND ANNA H. MESSNER

CHAPTER OUTLINE

Definitions and Terminology

The term "tethered oral tissues" refers to conditions in which oral frenula (e.g., lingual, labial, or buccal) restrict oral movement and may include normal anatomical variation or pathologic presentation with limitations to function. This may include effects on breastfeeding, speech, and dentition throughout the life course.

A frenulum (plural: frenula; also referred to interchangeably as a frenum, with the plural frena) is a mucosal membranous fold that connects two anatomical structures to each other. Within the oral cavity, there are several different frenula (Fig. 48.1). The intraoral frenula include the following: the lingual frenulum, the labial frenula, and the buccal frenula. The lingual frenulum connects the ventral surface of the tongue to the floor of the mouth. The labial frenula connect the lips to the alveolar mucosa around the central incisors. This includes the maxillary labial frenulum and the mandibular labial frenulum. The maxillary labial frenulum connects the upper lip to the alveolar mucosa of the maxillary central incisors, and the mandibular labial frenulum connects the lower lip to the alveolar mucosa of the mandibular central incisors. These labial frenula provide stability to the lips. The buccal frenula connect the cheeks (buccal mucosa) to the alveolar mucosa of the posterior teeth, both in the maxilla and the mandible. There are typically four buccal frenula, which, when combined with the aforementioned labial and lingual frenula, result in a total of seven frenula commonly present intraorally.[1] These buccal frenula, along with the buccinator muscle, work to keep the bolus of food between the teeth during mastication and swallowing.[2]

Recent anatomical research has provided a more comprehensive and detailed understanding of the structural complexities of the lingual frenulum. Rather than a simple band of mucosa, Mills et al. have described the lingual frenulum as a dynamic fold consisting of a layer of fascia underneath the layer of oral mucosa.[3] With movement of the tongue, part of the genioglossus muscle as well as lingual nerve branches may also be included in this fold. Variants in the layers included in an individual's lingual frenulum can lead to variations in appearance, particularly in opacity. Lingual frenula can present along a spectrum of opacity, in which a translucent frenulum indicates solely mucosa, and an opaque frenulum includes mucosa, fascia, and occasionally the genioglossus muscle.[4]

Ankyloglossia, as defined by the clinical consensus statement released by the American Academy of Otolaryngology—Head and Neck Surgery (AAO-HNS), is a "condition of limited tongue mobility caused by a restrictive lingual frenulum."[2] Some practitioners have been utilizing the terms "anterior" and "posterior" ankyloglossia. The AAO-HNS acknowledged that the term "anterior" ankyloglossia is more recently being used to describe a lingual frenulum that extends close to or reaches the tip of the tongue, thereby restricting mobility of the tongue.[2] For many practitioners who do not use this terminology, they use the term "ankyloglossia" as an equivalent to "anterior ankyloglossia." The term "posterior tongue tie" is controversial, and there is no consensus regarding the definition or existence of "posterior tongue tie" or "posterior ankyloglossia."[2] Based on the anatomical findings that the lingual frenulum does not connect to the posterior

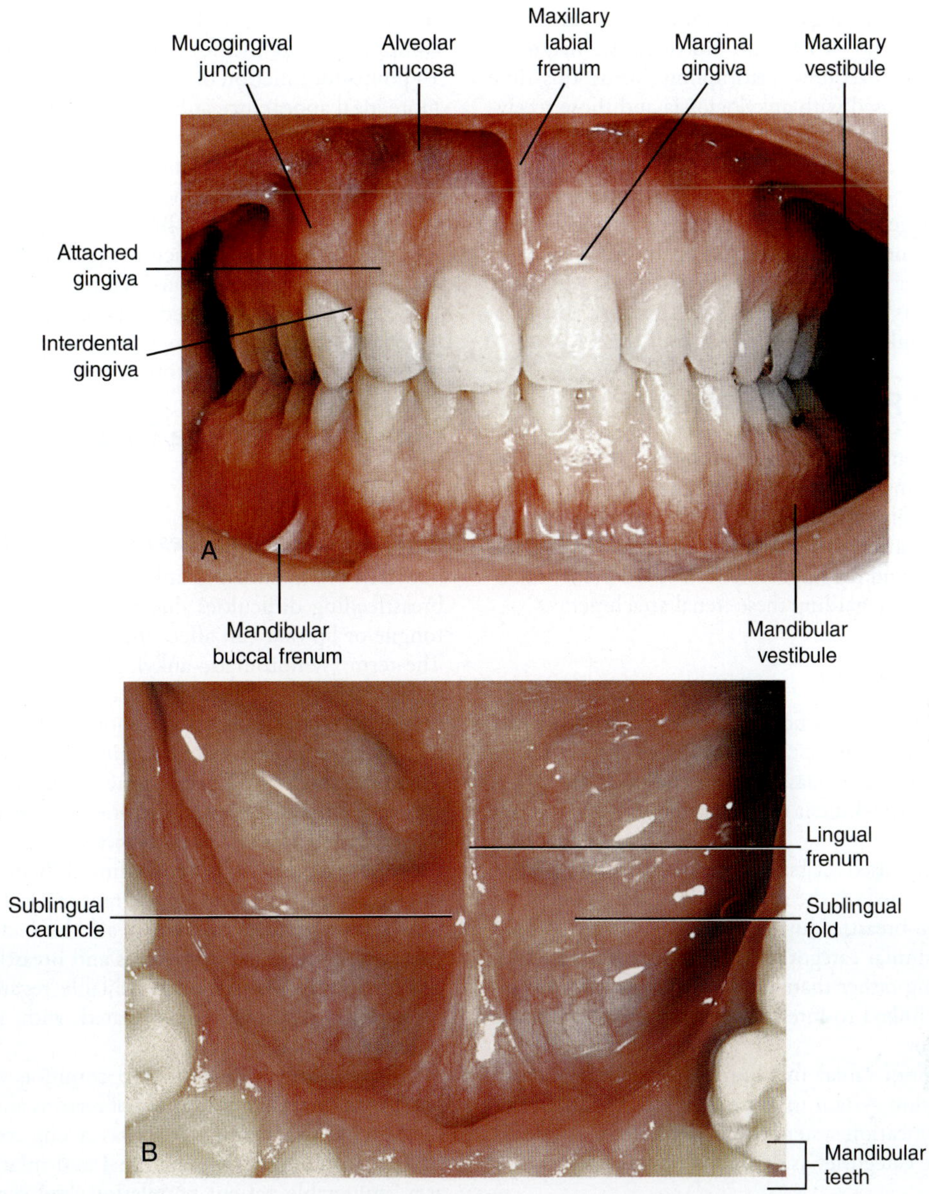

• **Fig. 48.1** (A) View of vestibule including labial and buccal frena. (A, From Liebgott B. *The Anatomical Basis of Dentistry*. 3rd ed. Mosby; 2011.) (B) View of the floor of the mouth including lingual frenum. (B, Courtesy Margaret J. Fehrenbach, RDH, MS, and from Fehrenbach MJ, Herring SW. *Illustrated Anatomy of the Head and Neck*. 6th ed. Saunders; 2021.)

tongue or tongue base, Mills et al. contend that the term "posterior tongue tie" is anatomically incorrect and should be discontinued.[3]

The terms "lip tie" and "cheek tie" refer to the tethering or tightness of the labial and buccal frenula, respectively. "Upper lip tie," referring to the maxillary labial frenulum, does not have a consistent definition.[2] The term "cheek tie" or "buccal tie" is used to describe a perceived tightness of the buccal frenula; however, there are no established criteria to assess the presence or degree of restriction associated with these frenula.[2]

Surgical treatments of frenula include three distinct procedures: frenotomy, frenuloplasty, and frenectomy, though they have often been inappropriately used interchangeably. It is important to understand and distinguish between these surgical procedures, as they have different indications, methods, and potential complications. Frenotomy is the simple incision of the frenulum. Frenuloplasty includes both incision of the frenulum and rearrangement of the tissue. Frenectomy is the excision and removal of the frenulum.

Epidemiology

The diagnosis of ankyloglossia has risen markedly over the past two decades. Frequency of ankyloglossia has been reported to be as high as 10.7%, varying based on study population and diagnostic criteria, with most frequent findings to be around 3% to 5%.[5–11] Between 1997 and 2012, patient discharge data revealed a nearly tenfold increase in the number of children in the United States diagnosed with ankyloglossia, accompanied by a comparable rise in frenotomy procedures.[12] Diagnosis and frenotomy continued to double from 2012 to 2016, with a 110.4% increase in inpatient diagnoses of ankyloglossia.[13] Similar trends have been reported between 2004 and 2019, with ankyloglossia diagnoses and lingual frenotomy procedures quadrupling during this time period.[14] Children diagnosed with ankyloglossia and those receiving frenotomy procedures are more frequently male, non-Hispanic White, privately insured, and from families with higher parental income and education.[12–14] Several potential explanations for this increase have been suggested, including increased incidence, improved accuracy of diagnosis, and the possibility of overdiagnosis.[4] In older children, lower incidence has been reported, with incidence of 2.8% at 6 years[15] and 2.02% at 7 to 12 years.[6] This pattern may suggest that ankyloglossia improves over time.

Classification of Frenal Attachments

Classification of frenal attachments is important in communicating and describing varying attachments of frenula and is often used in discussions surrounding diagnosis and treatment planning. As such, common classification systems are presented for both the maxillary labial frenum and the lingual frenum to aid in identification and communication regarding these frenal attachments.

Maxillary Labial Frenum

One of the most common classifications used to categorize the maxillary labial frenum is that described by Placek Mirko, sometimes referred to as the Placek classification.[16] This classification describes four types of attachment of the maxillary labial frenum (Box 48.1, Fig. 48.2).

Another commonly used classification system comes from Kotlow, with grading based on the appearance of the frenum and suggested influence on breastfeeding (Box 48.2).[17] This classification system presents similar categories to the Placek classification, with numerical grading rather than descriptive categories and severity of the grading linked to interference with breastfeeding as proposed by the author.

The Stanford superior labial frenulum classification aims to simplify the classification system to improve intra- and interrater reliability.[18] This classification system combines Kotlow's grades II and III to create three categories as described in Box 48.3.

Lingual Frenum

The majority of classifications for the lingual frenum are in relation to ankyloglossia. A commonly used classification system for the lingual frenum is the Coryllos classification, which describes the frenum without addressing function or ankyloglossia (Box 48.4, Fig. 48.3).[19]

Assessment tools that include function as well as anatomy include the Hazelbaker Assessment Tool for Lingual Frenulum Function (HATLFF)[20] and the Bristol Tongue Assessment Tool (BTAT).[21] The HATLFF is the most complex assessment system, comprising 10 points for appearance of the lingual frenulum and 14 points for function of the tongue, with higher scores indicating more ideal appearance and function. The BTAT was developed to apply similar assessment criteria as the HATLFF, but with a focus on greater ease and efficiency of use. The BTAT is scored from 0 to 8, with higher scores indicating higher severity of ankyloglossia. The Tongue-Tie and Breastfed Babies (TABBY) assessment tool was developed as a picture version of the BTAT in order to aid in assessment and consistency, as depicted in Fig. 48.4.[22] Although frequently utilized, these assessment tools have not been validated, and there is no consensus regarding the most ideal assessment tool for evaluating ankyloglossia.[2]

• BOX 48.1 Placek Classification of Maxillary Labial Frenum Attachments

Mucosal: attachment of frenal fibers into the mucogingival junction
Gingival: attachment of frenal fibers within the attached gingiva
Papillary: attachment of frenal fibers extending into the interdental papilla
Papillary penetrating: frenal fibers crossing the alveolar process and extending up to the palatine papilla

Conception to Age Three

Breastfeeding

Breastfeeding Difficulties and Tethered Oral Tissues

Tethered oral tissues and ankyloglossia have been associated with breastfeeding difficulties due to the restricted movement of the tongue or lip that can affect the infant's ability to latch and feed. The term "symptomatic ankyloglossia" refers to a restrictive lingual frenulum that leads to breastfeeding difficulties that persist despite lactation support. The most common symptoms reported with symptomatic ankyloglossia include maternal nipple pain and poor latching.[8,11,23] Though some infants with ankyloglossia may experience breastfeeding difficulties, many are able to feed without issue.[24,25] Lip tie, or a restrictive maxillary frenum, has also been associated with infant feeding difficulties, but this relationship is unclear based on the current level of evidence.[17,26] Buccal ties, or restrictive buccal frenula, are also included in the discourse surrounding tethered oral tissues and breastfeeding, though there is significantly less evidence available regarding buccal ties and breastfeeding difficulties compared with restrictive lingual or maxillary frenula.

Breastfeeding difficulties are common among dyads in the postpartum period for a variety of reasons and can be taxing to the mother. For this reason, there was strong consensus that it is important to recognize the maternal and infant breastfeeding dyad as a "vulnerable patient population, and care should be taken to ensure adequate support services, education and counseling, and shared decision making."[2] Although ankyloglossia can be associated with poor latching and nipple pain as well as inadequate weight gain and dehydration, these symptoms can also be associated with other etiologies, and not all infants with ankyloglossia have difficulties breastfeeding. For these reasons, it is important to perform a thorough evaluation, consider differential diagnoses and etiologies, and review treatment and management options. A multidisciplinary team approach including team members such as pediatricians, otolaryngologists, lactation professionals, and dentists is advised for the best interest of the breastfeeding dyad.

Evaluation

Thorough evaluation of breastfeeding history and clinical presentation are important for diagnosis of symptomatic ankyloglossia, but inconsistencies among diagnostic criteria can present challenges for consistency across providers and disciplines. The most recent clinical report released by the American Academy of Pediatrics (AAP) presents an ankyloglossia algorithm (Fig. 48.5) along with important aspects of the history and physical examination to review when considering a diagnosis of ankyloglossia.[4] These

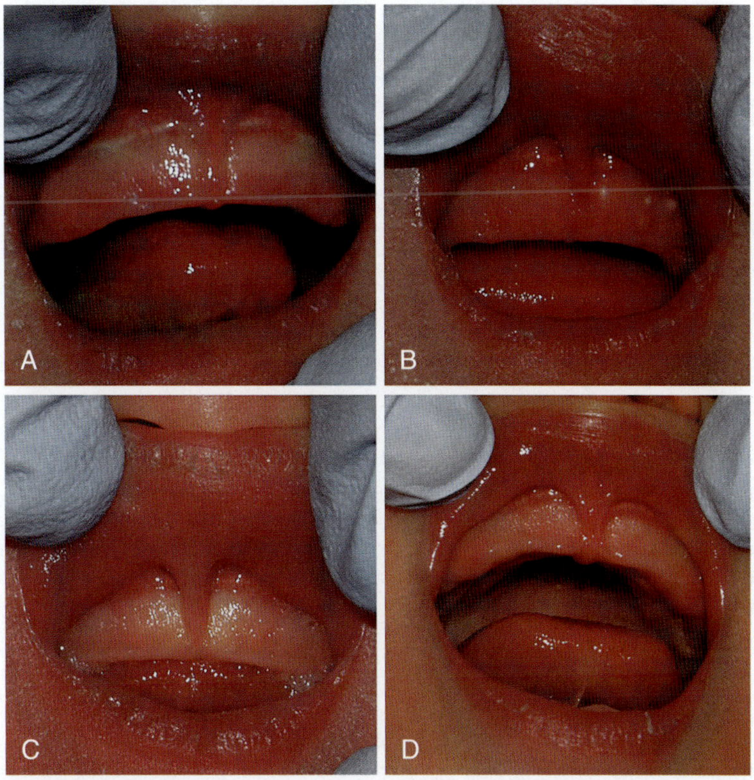

• **Fig. 48.2** Placek Classification of Maxillary Labial Frenum Attachments. (A) Mucosal, (B) gingival, (C) papillary, (D) papillary penetrating.

• BOX 48.2 Kotlow Classification of Maxillary Labial Frenum Attachments

Grade I: "normal" frenum with minimal mucosal attachment
Grade II: insertion of the frenum above the teeth, attaching primarily into gingival tissue
Grade III: insertion of the frenum between the central incisors, just in front of the anterior papilla
Grade IV: insertion of the frenum attaching to the papilla and extending to the hard palate

• BOX 48.3 Stanford Superior Labial Frenulum Classification

Type 1: insertion of the frenulum is near the mucogingival junction
Type 2: insertion of the frenulum is along the mid attached gingiva
Type 3: insertion of the frenulum is along the inferior margin at the alveolar papilla, and can continue to the posterior surface

• BOX 48.4 Coryllos Classification of "Tongue Ties"

Type 1: attachment of the frenum from the tip of the tongue to in front of the alveolar ridge
Type 2: attachment of the frenum from 2–4 mm behind the tip of the tongue to on or just behind the alveolar ridge
Type 3: attachment of the frenum from the midtongue to the middle of the floor of the mouth
Type 4: attachment of the frenum against the base of the tongue

include the following: review of the prenatal course and maternal history and characteristics, infant feeding history, visual inspection of the head and neck, atypical craniofacial features, tongue movement and suck reflex, appearance of the frenulum, and assessment of milk transfer and weight gain.[4] The AAO-HNS consensus statement advised a similar list of factors for evaluation of an infant referred for ankyloglossia,[2] and a combined list of factors from these two resources is summarized in Box 48.5. Although several assessment and scoring tools for ankyloglossia have been proposed, including the HATLFF[20] and the BTAT[21] described previously, none have been validated. For this reason, especially in considering the recent rise in ankyloglossia diagnoses and frenotomies, there is a need for standardized and validated diagnostic tools for symptomatic ankyloglossia.

Evaluation of the maxillary labial frenum in the context of breastfeeding has been proposed based on its appearance and attachment.[16–18] Although these classification systems provide terminology to describe differing appearances of the maxillary frenum, there is not a clear relationship between the grade of the maxillary frenum and comfort or challenge with breastfeeding or other clinical symptoms.[26,27] As such, appearance of the frenum alone is not an indication for intervention. It is suggested that an aberrant or restrictive maxillary labial frenum may affect breastfeeding by preventing the creation of an airtight seal around the breast through flanging of the lips.[1] If this is the case, evaluation of the role of the maxillary labial frenum in breastfeeding should focus on functional movements including flexibility and flanging of the upper lip rather than solely attachment. Flanging of the lips is thought to help with breastfeeding, but it is not mandatory.[28]

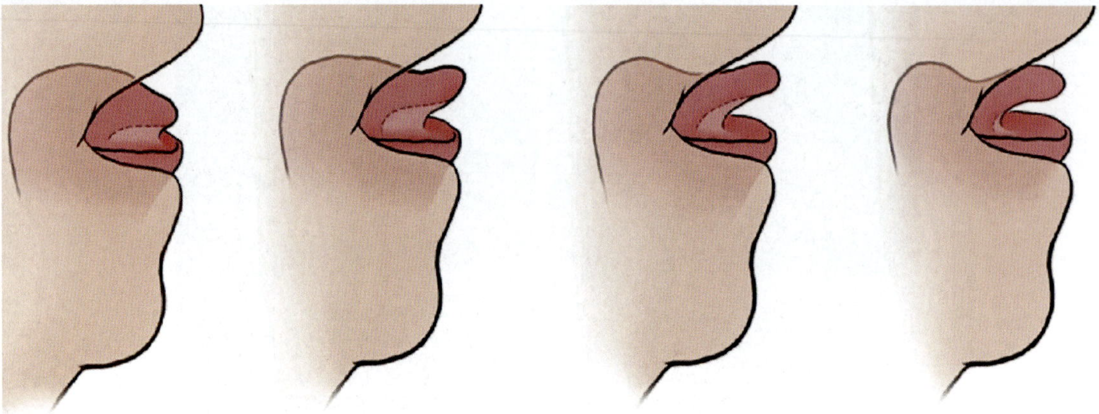

Type I Type II Type III Type IV

• **Fig. 48.3** Coryllos classification Type I: thin and elastic frenulum; attaches the tip of the tongue to the alveolar ridge, and the tongue forms a heart shape. Type II: thin and elastic frenulum; 2 to 4 mm behind the tongue tip, attaches by the alveolar ridge. Type III: thick, fibrous, and nonelastic frenulum; attaches midtongue to the floor of the mouth. Type IV: the frenulum is not seen, but felt, with fibrous or submucosal thick and shiny attachment from the base of the tongue to the floor of the mouth.

TABBY Tongue Assessment Tool

	0	1	2	SCORE
What does the tongue-tip look like?	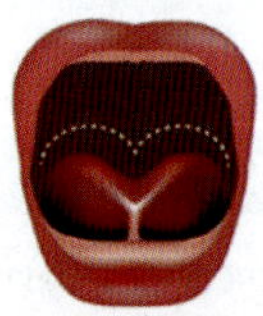	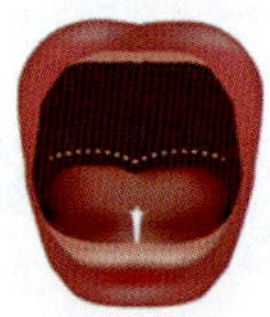	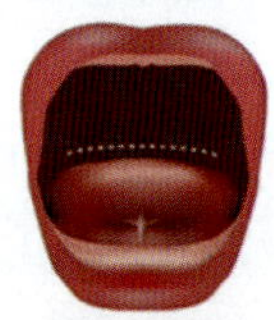	
Where it is fixed to the gum?	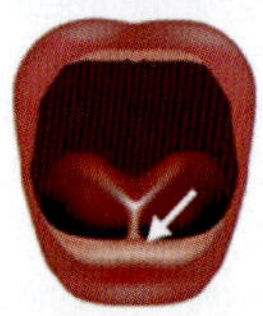	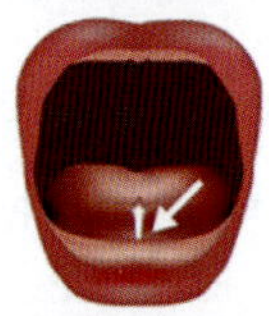	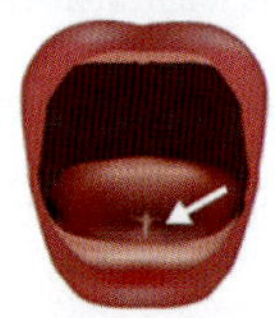	
How high can it lift (wide open mouth)?	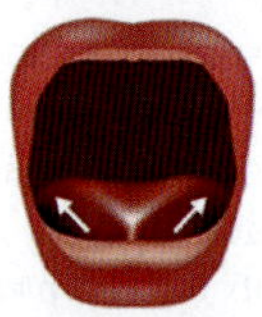	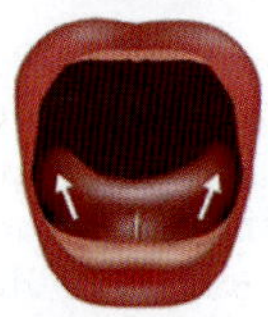	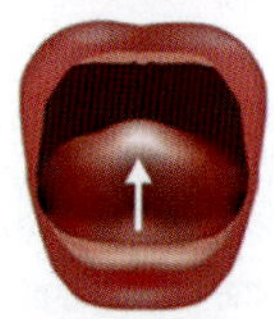	
How far can it stick out?	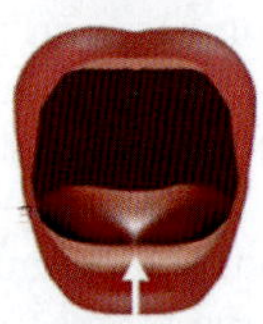	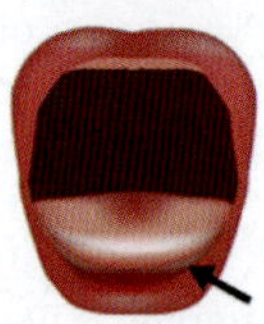	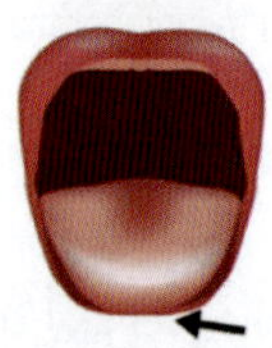	

• **Fig. 48.4** Tongue-Tie and Breastfed Babies (TABBY) assessment tool.

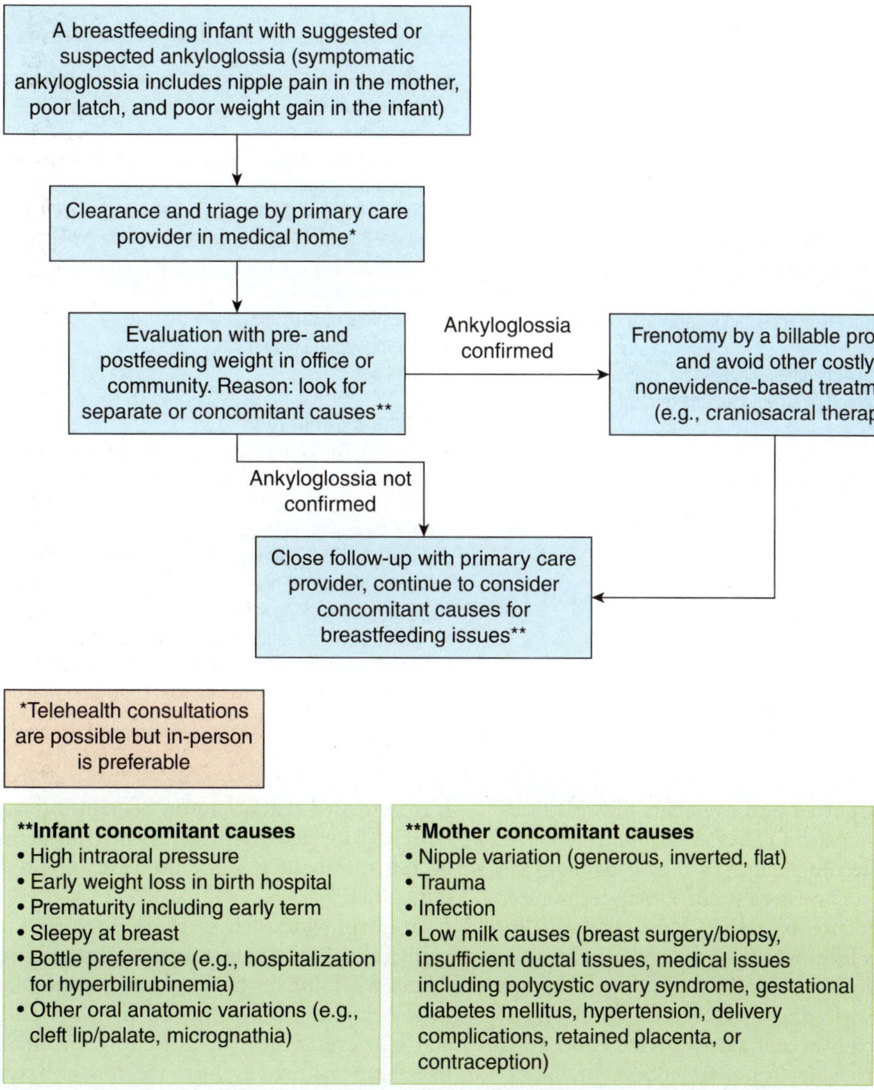

• **Fig. 48.5** Ankyloglossia algorithm.

There are currently no validated methods of assessment of the maxillary labial frenum in the context of breastfeeding, which may contribute to overdiagnosis of lip ties in some communities. Though restrictive buccal frena have also been suggested to have an effect on breastfeeding, there are currently no criteria with which to evaluate restriction of buccal frena.

Management/Treatment

The determination of treatment for breastfeeding difficulties should again be done in the context of a multidisciplinary team with thorough counseling and informed consent for the family. Nonsurgical treatment options for tethered oral tissues and breastfeeding difficulties may include observation and monitoring, lactation consultation, or speech-language pathology consultation. Lactation professionals work closely with the breastfeeding dyad to evaluate and improve the process of breastfeeding for the mother and infant. Lactation consultants can provide normal noninvasive lactation interventions that may improve breastfeeding difficulties but should be able to identify infants for whom these interventions have not improved their feeding and refer to appropriate providers for additional treatment options. If families decide to pursue surgical options for treatment, lactation consultants can also be helpful in working with the dyad to establish a good latch after the procedure.

Surgical treatment may be a good option for infants with ankyloglossia or other tethered oral tissues who are having challenges with breastfeeding. As with any surgical procedure, informed consent must be obtained, in which the risks, benefits, and alternatives are thoroughly discussed. A recent systematic review and meta-analysis by Cordray et al. found significant improvement in breastfeeding self-efficacy, maternal pain, infant latch, and infant reflux after frenotomy in symptomatic breastfeeding dyads with feeding difficulties and ankyloglossia.[29] The included studies lacked long-term follow-up, with the longest follow-up period being only 1 month. Thus it is difficult to draw any conclusions about long-term benefits. There was also significant heterogeneity regarding evaluation and diagnosis techniques, in addition to outcome measures, making it difficult to compare due to inconsistent methodology. Previous systematic reviews with stricter inclusion criteria have had similar challenges regarding the quality of available and included studies.[30,31] Francis et al. reported that based on a small body of evidence, frenotomy may

• BOX 48.5 Factors for Evaluation and Assessment of Symptomatic Ankyloglossia in Infants

History
- Intrapartum and postpartum medications
- Breast surgeries
- Family history
- Lactation/breastfeeding history
  - Previous breastfeeding experience
  - Frequency and length of breastfeeding sessions
  - Use of formula supplementation or pumping
  - Utilization of lactation support
  - Abnormal features of infant feeding (coughing, choking, color change, early tiring, bilious emesis)
  - Description of breastfeeding difficulties (nipple pain, nipple trauma, long feeding times, difficulty latching or staying attached to the breast)

Maternal Factors
- Common discomfort during first few weeks of breastfeeding
- Breast and nipple anatomy
- Poor positioning or support at breast
- Maternal milk supply
- Breast infection

Infant Factors
- Prematurity
- Abnormal palatal, mandibular, or maxillary development (craniofacial abnormalities)
- Neurologic disorders
- Cardiovascular disorders (e.g., congenital heart disease)
- Metabolic disorders
- Endocrine disorders (e.g., congenital adrenal hyperplasia)
- Nasal obstruction (e.g., choanal atresia, piriform aperture stenosis)
- Upper airway obstruction (e.g., bilateral vocal cord paralysis, laryngomalacia)
- Intestinal obstruction
- Laryngopharyngeal reflux
- Infection

Physical Examination
- Examination of the tongue, maxilla, mandible, palate
- Appearance and palpation of frenula
  - Tongue extension over alveolar ridge
  - Tongue lift midway to palate
  - Heart-shaped tongue when extended
- Assessment of tongue movement and coordination
- Testing of sucking reflex
- Assessment for signs of airway obstruction
- Assessment of milk transfer (pre- and postfeeding weights, feeding session observation, weight gain compared with growth standards)

be associated with mother-reported improvements in breastfeeding and potentially in nipple pain. O'Shea et al. found that frenotomy reduced the breastfeeding mother's nipple pain in the short term but did not find a consistent positive long-term effect on breastfeeding.[31] The evidence base lacks large, high-quality randomized controlled trials from which to draw conclusions regarding the benefits, especially long-term, of frenotomy for symptomatic ankyloglossia in breastfeeding dyads. Given the potential benefits of frenotomy and the overall safety of the procedure, lingual frenotomy can be a viable treatment option for infants experiencing symptomatic ankyloglossia as part of a team approach to management. If families choose to pursue surgical treatment, published studies tend to advocate for early frenotomy, including infants less than 1 month of age in consideration of abandonment of breastfeeding that may occur if breastfeeding issues are not resolved in a timely manner.[2,32] Lingual frenotomy in an infant is depicted in Fig. 48.6.

Surgical treatments of the maxillary labial frenum ("lip tie") as well as buccal frena ("buccal tie") have also been of recent interest as it relates to breastfeeding. Surgical release of the maxillary labial frenum has been reported to be effective in improving breastfeeding difficulties in infants, though the available studies are significantly limited methodologically. Existing studies lack large sample sizes, long-term follow-up, proper control groups, and consistent definitions of lip ties. Systematic review of the literature found no randomized controlled trials investigating the relationship between the maxillary labial frenum or maxillary frenotomy and breastfeeding outcomes and concluded a poor level of evidence for routine release in infants with breastfeeding difficulties.[33] Given the normal presence of the maxillary labial frenum, inconsistent definitions, and unclear relationship to breastfeeding difficulties, the AAO-HNS panel was unable to reach consensus regarding surgical intervention for upper lip ties.[2] There was consensus, however, that it is being overdiagnosed in some communities.[2] It is suggested that attention be paid to breastfeeding education, especially for new mothers, before considering surgical treatment of the maxillary frenum in neonates presenting with feeding difficulties.[27]

Some providers have recently advocated for surgical treatment of buccal ties in conjunction with the release of other tethered oral tissues when infants present with breastfeeding issues. Frenotomy or frenectomy of these buccal frenula would likely not improve and may even hinder breastfeeding for infants. Though attempts have been made to evaluate the role of buccal ties and buccal tie release regarding breastfeeding,[34,35] they have significant limitations and there are no high-quality observational or experimental studies. Given the lack of evidence regarding the role of restrictive buccal frenula in breastfeeding difficulties or the impact of surgical treatment of these frenula, the AAO-HNS reached consensus that recommends against the release of buccal frenula.[2]

Though surgical treatment of tethered oral tissues in infants is generally safe and well tolerated, there are some contraindications to surgical intervention, and families should understand the risks of the procedure. Relative contraindications to frenotomy in infants include mandibular retrognathia or micrognathia, neuromuscular disorders or hypotonia, and coagulation or bleeding disorders. An important possible outcome after frenotomy that should be discussed with the family is failure to see improvement in breastfeeding or relief of nipple pain. Rarer potential complications include reattachment of the frenum, bleeding, infection, airway obstruction, damage to salivary or other floor-of-the-mouth structures such as the lingual nerve, cyst formation, oral aversion, and scarring.[1,2]

Oral Hygiene and Caries Risk

Tethered oral tissues, particularly a restrictive maxillary labial frenum, have been hypothesized to affect oral hygiene and increase

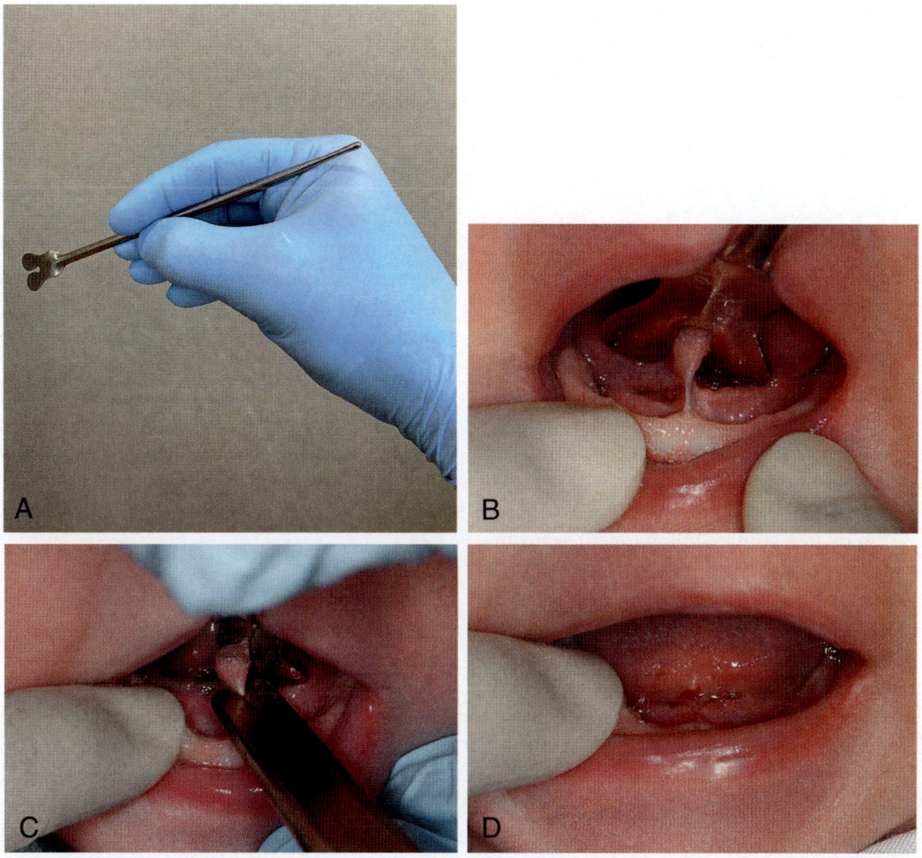

• **Fig. 48.6** Lingual frenotomy. (A) A Brodie probe is useful in retracting the tongue and protecting the floor of the mouth. (B) The tongue is retracted with the Brodie probe. (C) An incision is made in the frenum with blunt-ended dissecting scissors. (D) Immediate post-op following incision.

the risk of developing carious lesions. Limited lip mobility caused by a restrictive frenum may lead to the retention of breast milk, liquids, and food in the vestibule and on the facial surface of the maxillary incisors, thereby increasing the risk of dental decay. Additionally, a restrictive frenal attachment may also pose a challenge to self-cleansing through saliva or tongue clearance, as well as complicate toothbrushing. Reports of an association between tethered oral tissues and dental caries are limited,[36] though anticipatory guidance regarding oral hygiene practices targeting areas such as the cervical third and vestibule near a restrictive frenulum may be warranted.[1]

Surgical Intervention for Prevention

Given the recent increase in parental concern for the relationship between tethered oral tissues and issues such as breastfeeding, speech, airway, and esthetics such as diastemas, there has also been interest in surgical treatment of frenal attachments to prevent these issues. There is no sufficient evidence to recommend surgical intervention for prevention of any of these concerns. The AAO-HNS consensus statement reached consensus that it is not necessary to perform a lingual frenotomy in an infant with little or no restriction in tongue mobility to prevent a future feeding or speech disorder and that maxillary labial frenotomy in infants or children in the primary dentition will not prevent a maxillary diastema.[2] The AAP clinical report agreed that frenotomy to prevent future speech issues or obstructive sleep apnea is not evidence based.[4]

The Primary Dentition Years: Three to Six Years

Speech Development

Speech Issues and Tethered Oral Tissues

Tethered oral tissues have also become a point of discussion in regard to speech and speech development. Ankyloglossia has the potential to affect speech by restricting tongue movements that are required to produce and articulate certain sounds. The sounds most frequently affected include lingual and sibilant sounds as well as rolling an R.[37,38] Articulation difficulties have been reported for sounds such as */s/, /z/, /t/, /d/, /l/, /sh/, /ch/, /th/,* and */dg/*.[1] Though articulation issues can be associated with ankyloglossia, they are a very normal part of speech development in preschool children, which must be considered in context. Sounds associated with typical speech development are described in Box 48.6.

Although there have been associations reported between ankyloglossia and speech articulation issues, the evidence base has

• BOX 48.6 Typical Speech Development Milestones

1–3 years: early sounds (p, m, h, w, b, d, n)
2–4 years: middle sounds (k, g, t, f, y)
4–5 years: later sounds (l, j, r, sh, ch, s, v, z, th)

limitations. Speech as reported by parents is used in several studies, but this measure is subjective and tends to be less accurate compared with analyses by speech-language pathologists. When formally assessed by a speech-language pathologist, the majority of children referred for speech concerns related to ankyloglossia were found to have speech errors appropriate for their age and development.[39] The literature is also limited regarding study design, with many observational and smaller experimental studies and limited control groups. Much of the literature is also focused on surgical intervention, with few studies following speech outcomes for nonsurgical interventions or no intervention. Despite the limitations in the evidence, potential effects of ankyloglossia on speech articulation are recognized by various specialties and should be considered for patients and families. Although ankyloglossia may have an association with articulation issues, it has not been shown to cause speech delays, which may in fact be caused by a developmental delay rather than an anatomical issue.

Evaluation of Speech in Patients With Tethered Oral Tissues

Though ankyloglossia does not typically affect speech,[2,38] many patients with ankyloglossia may experience articulation challenges, as assessed by caregivers as well as speech-language pathologists. Most children can compensate for any movement restrictions related to a tight frenulum and have intelligible speech, but a subset of children may benefit from speech evaluation and treatment. There are no currently standardized or validated methods for evaluating the lingual frenulum and its role in speech production. Although tongue mobility is hypothesized to be a key factor in the relationship between ankyloglossia and speech, preoperative measurements of tongue mobility and protrusion do not accurately or reliably predict speech or articulation difficulties.[37] If speech difficulties are observed or if families report a concern about a child's speech, recommendation should be made for the family to see a speech-language pathologist. Consultation with a speech-language pathologist will aid in the evaluation of the patient's speech as well as help identify potential contributing factors and recommendations for management.

Management/Treatment

After evaluation by a speech-language pathologist, treatment options such as speech therapy and/or surgical treatment may be recommended. First-line treatment for speech issues, including those potentially related to tethered oral tissues, is typically speech therapy. Speech therapy can help children learn how to better form and articulate sounds and make adaptations accordingly. Few studies exist comparing surgical and nonsurgical treatment (e.g., speech therapy) of speech issues in patients with ankyloglossia, but caregiver perception of speech has been reported to be comparable between the two groups.[40]

Surgical treatment of tethered oral tissues may be recommended to improve tongue mobility and potentially speech. Although surgical treatment of the frenulum has been shown to improve tongue mobility, speech and articulation may or may not improve.[37,41] Regarding surgical intervention and timing, a randomized controlled trial found that there was no significant difference in tongue mobility, speech production, and intelligibility between the surgical and nonsurgical groups among the 2 to <3 years of age group, but did see significant improvements in the surgical intervention groups for those 3 to 5 years old.[42] Additional evidence found no significant difference in tongue mobility or speech in young children with or without intervention for ankyloglossia in infancy.[41] Given these findings, surgical intervention for ankyloglossia as it relates to speech issues may be delayed until at least 3 years of age and must consider growth and time for development of speech skills and adaptations. Despite some studies reporting improvements in speech after surgical intervention, there is still insufficient evidence, especially of high quality, to conclude that surgical treatment of tethered oral tissues improves speech and articulation.

Airway and Breathing Considerations

Recent concerns have been raised that a short or restrictive lingual frenulum may contribute to symptoms of sleep-disordered breathing and obstructive sleep apnea (OSA). The proposed mechanism postulates that the tight frenulum results in low tongue posture and restricted tongue elevation, thereby hindering maxillary expansion and resulting in a narrow maxillary arch.[43] Although there may be some association with a palatal transverse deficiency and obstructive sleep apnea, there is currently no evidence that suggests a causal relationship between ankyloglossia or a short lingual frenulum and OSA.[2] In fact, anterior attachment of the lingual frenulum can help prevent posterior collapse of the tongue, raising the concern that surgical release of the frenulum could potentially worsen OSA, especially for those at high risk for obstruction.[44–46] There is currently insufficient evidence to support an association between OSA and tethered oral tissues, and although pediatric dentists can play a role in screening for and providing adjunctive treatments for OSA, comprehensive management of sleep-disordered breathing and OSA in pediatric patients should be coordinated by a sleep specialist.

The Transitional Years: Six to Twelve Years

Maxillary Labial Frenum and Midline Diastema

As permanent teeth erupt, a common concern is the midline diastema. Diastemas may pose orthodontic, esthetic, and/or psychological challenges for the pediatric patient. In the conversation surrounding midline diastemas, a tethered or tight maxillary labial frenum has been proposed as a potential contributing factor. Consequently, there is ongoing discussion surrounding the use of surgical intervention on the maxillary labial frenum for treatment or prevention of midline diastemas. This discussion encompasses both the question of whether surgical intervention is beneficial regarding midline diastemas as well as the optimal timing of such intervention.

A midline diastema may be caused by several different factors including normal growth or variation, missing or supernumerary teeth, improper fusion of the premaxilla, undersized maxillary anterior teeth, or an enlarged or malpositioned maxillary labial frenum.[47] As such, it is important to identify the etiology of the midline diastema to recommend the most appropriate treatment. A midline diastema is a very common and normal finding for children in the mixed dentition stage before eruption of the permanent canines. With eruption of the permanent canines, the majority of diastemas will close spontaneously. Given this normal trajectory of diastema closure with permanent canine eruption, it is not recommended to intervene regarding the midline diastema before this stage.[1]

If a midline diastema persists after eruption of the permanent canines, it may be caused by any of the several factors described earlier. As such, it is important to thoroughly evaluate the patient to determine the most likely etiology. In cases where the maxillary midline diastema is associated with the maxillary labial frenum, the frenum is typically of the papillary or papillary penetrating type.[48] If the frenum is found to be the most likely cause, discussion should be had with the patient and the family to determine whether the midline diastema is a concern for them, and if so, what treatment options may be available. Midline diastemas are more common in certain ethnic populations and therefore may be more culturally desired or accepted in some communities than in others. If the patient and family decide that they would prefer to have the diastema closed, this may be accomplished with dental restorations, orthodontics, surgical intervention, or a combination of these methods.

In cases where maxillary labial frena are contributing to a midline diastema, orthodontic space closure and surgical intervention are commonly recommended treatment modalities. Pediatric dentists and orthodontists generally agree that surgical intervention for the maxillary labial frenum should be delayed until after the permanent canines are erupted and after orthodontic closure of the space.[49] This recommendation is consistent with the normal trajectory of spontaneous closure of the maxillary midline diastema with eruption of the permanent canines and the tendency for the maxillary labial frenum to migrate apically with age. At this stage, the preferred surgical treatment is generally frenectomy, though frenotomy or frenuloplasty may also be considered. The majority of published literature reports frenectomy for the maxillary labial frenum associated with midline diastema. Concomitant orthodontic treatment and frenectomy have more predictable success than frenectomy alone for cases with a prominent maxillary labial frenum and midline diastema.[48] Regarding the relative timing of these interventions, rationale has been presented for surgical intervention both before and after orthodontic space closure. Although some contend that a low attachment of the maxillary labial frenum may hinder space closure, many orthodontists and pediatric dentists prefer to delay frenectomy until after space closure, as scar tissue from early surgical intervention can impede space closure. Although surgical treatment of the maxillary labial frenum is suggested to reduce the risk of diastema relapse, proper retention planning remains essential to minimize the likelihood of relapse. An example of management of the maxillary labial frenum and midline diastema is depicted in Fig. 48.7.

Frenula and Orthodontic Treatment

Frenula and tethered oral tissues can have a role in orthodontic treatment and should be evaluated and considered in orthodontic treatment planning. As discussed in the earlier section, a hyperplastic or papillary-penetrating maxillary labial frenum may contribute to a midline diastema. The lingual frenum can also contribute to a lower diastema as well as tooth rotations because of the tight attachment (Fig. 48.8). Frenal attachments, especially those that are hypertrophic or attached nearer to the free gingival margin, may also contribute to gingival recession and decreased periodontal attachment (Fig. 48.9). Areas of tension at the gingival margin or recession due to aberrant frenal attachments should be identified, and consultation with a periodontal specialist should be considered to discuss and coordinate treatment and timing if indicated. Treatment may include gingival grafting along with repositioning of the frenum (see Chapter 21). Abnormal frenal attachments may also pose a challenge to space closure and should be identified during orthodontic examination before treatment planning.

Social/Mechanical Issues

For older children and adolescents, tethered oral tissues may present issues related to social and mechanical factors. Some of these issues identified in the AAO-HNS consensus statement included difficulty licking, difficulty keeping teeth clean, diastema, and sense of social embarrassment.[2] Consensus was reached that some older children with social/mechanical issues related to ankyloglossia will experience improved quality of life after frenotomy/frenuloplasty, though there is a lack of high-quality evidence to support these statements.[2] A systematic review of studies analyzing treatment of ankyloglossia for reasons other than breastfeeding found a small number of low-quality studies analyzing social outcomes related to ankyloglossia.[50] Findings included significantly improved ability to self-cleanse teeth using the tongue, lick outside of lips, and eat ice cream in patients treated for ankyloglossia compared with untreated participants as well as improved tongue mobility.[50] Although evidence on social and mechanical issues related to tethered oral tissues in older children, as well as the effects of surgical intervention, is limited, older children and their families may still express concern about these issues.

Surgical Intervention

Definitions

Surgical treatments of frenula include three distinct procedures: frenotomy, frenuloplasty, and frenectomy. It is important to understand and distinguish between these surgical procedures, as they have different indications, methods, and potential complications. Frenotomy is the simple incision of the frenulum. Frenuloplasty includes both incision of the frenulum and rearrangement of the tissue. Frenectomy is the excision and removal of the frenulum.

Surgical Technique

Surgical intervention can be performed using a variety of techniques, including scissors, scalpel, and laser. The most common technique for frenotomy, particularly in infants, is scissor clipping of the frenulum, which does not usually require anesthetic or sutures for newborns. Topical anesthetic with benzocaine is not recommended for infants due to risk of methemoglobinemia. Injected local anesthetic agents are also not recommended for infants, though oral sucrose has been recommended to decrease pain response in infants undergoing painful procedures such as frenotomy.[2,51] Frenotomies may also be performed using a soft tissue laser. Frenuloplasty is performed traditionally with a scalpel, and frenectomy procedures may be accomplished with a scalpel or laser. For more details regarding the steps of these surgical techniques, please refer to Chapter 29.

The use of laser for frenotomies, frenectomies, and other soft tissue surgical procedures is becoming increasingly popular, especially

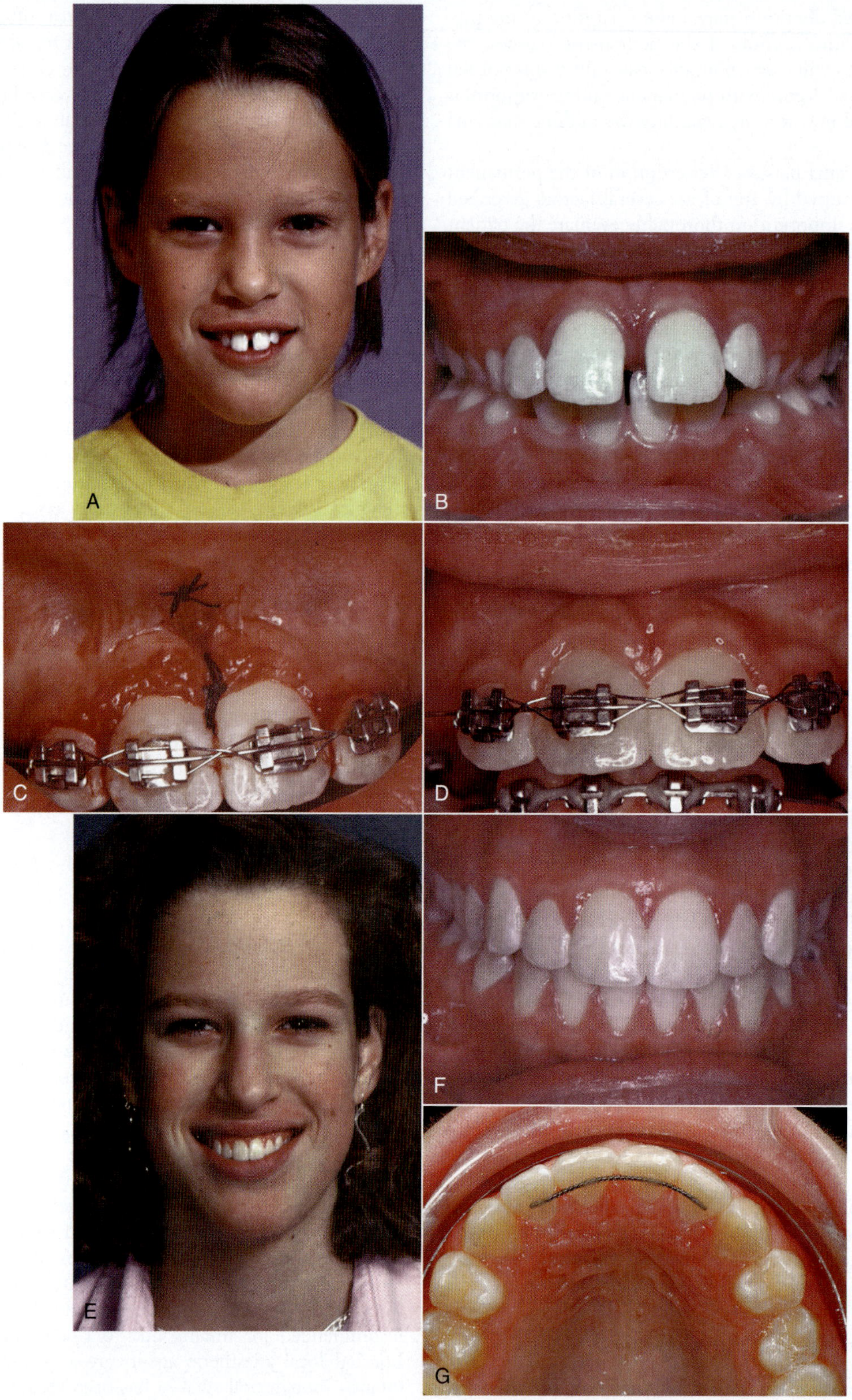

• **Fig. 48.7** Management of a Maxillary Midline Diastema. (A) Facial appearance showing the protruding maxillary incisors caught on the lower lip. (B) Intraoral view before treatment. (C) Teeth aligned and held tightly together with a figure-of-eight wire ligature before frenectomy. (D) Appearance immediately after frenectomy with the conservative technique advocated by Edwards in which a simple incision is used to allow access to the interdental area, the fibrous connection to the bone is removed, and the frenal attachment is sutured at a higher level. (E) Facial appearance 2 years after completion of treatment. (F) Intraoral view 2 years after treatment. (G) Bonded retainer, made with 1.75-mil steel twist wire. It is important for the retainer wire to be flexible enough to allow some displacement of the incisors in function; a rigid wire is much more likely to break loose.

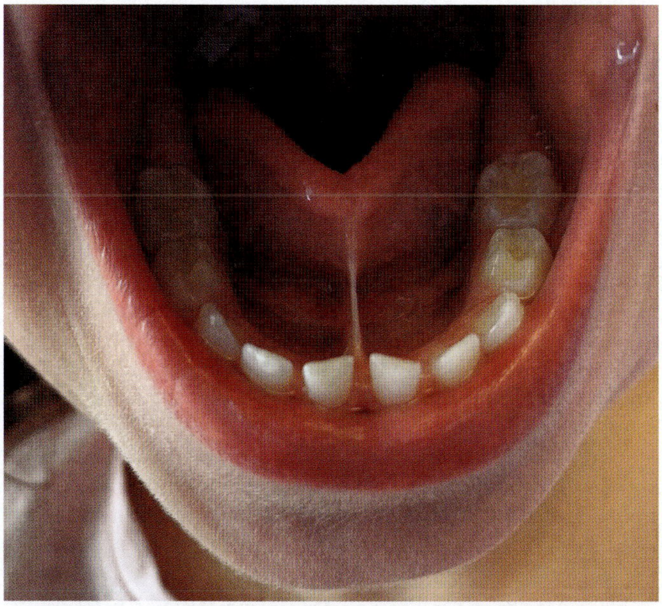

• **Fig. 48.8** Tight lingual frenum contributing to diastema between lower central incisors and mesial rotation toward the attachment.

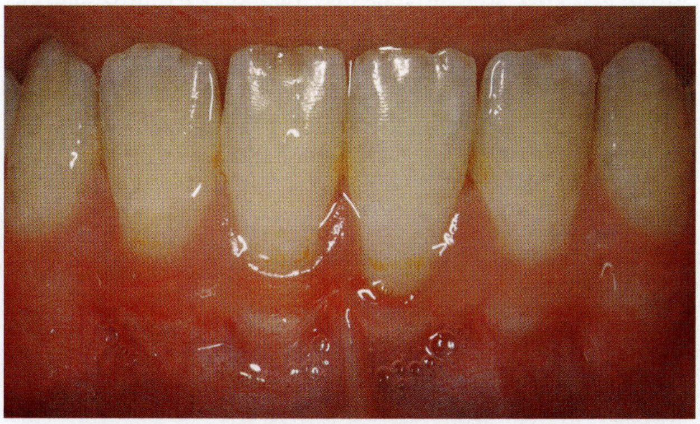

• **Fig. 48.9** Frenal Position Contributing to Periodontal Disease. Patients with high frenum positioning and thin biotype are more likely to develop gingival recession. Plaque control may be more difficult for patients with this condition. Treatment normally requires frenectomy and/or soft tissue grafting. (Courtesy Dr. Jonathan Reside.)

among dentists. This may be because of the reported benefits of decreased operative time, minimal bleeding, lack of need for sutures, reduced intra- and postoperative pain, and fewer postoperative complications.[1] Among various dental specialties, lasers were preferred by pediatric dentists and orthodontists, whereas oral surgeons tended to favor scalpels or scissors.[49] This preference is likely attributable to the varying clinical training and comfort, with surgeons being more comfortable with traditional cold techniques utilizing blades, while other specialties favor the minimal bleeding and suture-free advantages of laser techniques. Though lasers are increasing in popularity, there is currently insufficient evidence to support claims of superiority of laser frenotomy compared with other techniques.[2]

Postsurgical Care

After surgery to the frenulum, patients and families should be advised regarding management of bleeding, use of over-the-counter analgesics, oral hygiene, and soft diet. The use of a dressing with antibiotics is not indicated or necessary.[1] In recent years, some groups have advocated for postoperative stretching and other exercises, based on the rationale that these activities may prevent reattachment or scar tissue formation and provide neuromuscular reeducation to promote improved range of motion and movement patterns.[52] Survey of members of the American Society of Pediatric Otolaryngology found that 38% of respondents recommended massaging/stretching the wound, but a specific standard recommendation was not identified.[53] No significant difference was found between massage and nonmassage groups regarding improvement in breastfeeding or recurrence after frenotomy.[54] The AAO-HNS reached consensus that there is no evidence to support a standard postprocedure care regimen, such as stretching, massaging, or manual elevation of the tongue, after frenotomy for ankyloglossia.[2] Additionally, the AAP clinical report does not recommend stretching exercises involving repeated opening of the wound to prevent reattachment, further stating that they may cause oral aversion.[4]

Complications

Frenotomy is generally regarded as a safe procedure with minimal risks. It is important, however, to understand and prepare for potential complications. The most reported complications include tissue reattachment and excessive bleeding. Especially when considering frenotomy in infants and the risk of bleeding, it is important to verify the history of vitamin K injection.[4] Some additional reported complications after frenotomy include poor feeding, infection, scarring, formation of a mucus retention cyst, hematoma formation, hypovolemic shock, apnea, airway obstruction, and Ludwig angina.[1,44,55] Given the proximity of the lingual frenulum to structures in the floor of the mouth, surgery may result in damage to the lingual nerve and therefore result in numbness or paresthesia. Providers performing surgical procedures to address tethered oral tissues should be aware of potential complications and discuss the risks with patients and families as part of informed consent.

Special Considerations: Craniofacial Anomalies, Syndromic and Nonsyndromic Conditions

Special consideration must be made for patients with craniofacial anomalies and other conditions. Abnormal or absent frenal attachments have been associated with several genetic and congenital conditions. Additionally, interventions for some craniofacial anomalies may result in abnormal or altered tethered oral tissues.

Conditions Associated With Abnormal Frenal Attachments

Agenesis of intraoral frena, particularly of the mandibular labial and lingual frena, is associated with Ehlers-Danlos syndrome (EDS).[56] Although not pathognomonic for EDS, this finding can be utilized to identify infants at risk of the disorder before presentation of additional, more characteristic clinical findings. A congenitally absent mandibular labial frenum may also suggest the possibility of infantile hypertrophic pyloric stenosis (IHPS). Hypoplastic or absent mandibular frena are commonly seen in patients with IHPS, making this clinical presentation a potential tool to aid in diagnosis of the condition.[56] Absence or malformation of the maxillary labial frenum is seen in most patients with holoprosencephaly, as the sequence affects structures of the midline.

The finding of a bifid maxillary labial frenum has been described with Pallister W syndrome (a.k.a. W syndrome); however, due to the rarity of this disorder and the limited number of documented cases, the link between this finding and the condition is not definitive. The bifid maxillary labial frenum is likely associated with the characteristic central clefting of the palate or upper lip observed in Pallister W syndrome.[56]

Patients with Ellis–van Creveld syndrome commonly present with hyperplastic frena, both in the maxilla and the mandible (Fig. 48.10). Multiple hyperplastic frena can also be associated with oral-facial-digital syndrome, particularly in females (Fig. 48.11). Pallister-Hall syndrome includes multiple oral manifestations including abnormal supernumerary frena. Patients with Opitz C syndrome present with similar abnormal frena, including multiple supernumerary attached buccal frena.[56]

Ankyloglossia has also been associated with several syndromes and congenital conditions including Opitz syndrome (a.k.a. oculo-genital-laryngeal syndrome and BBB/G compound syndrome), Beckwith-Wiedemann syndrome, oral-facial-digital syndrome, Simpson-Golabi-Behmel syndrome, and X-linked cleft palate. Patients with generalized recessive dystrophic epidermolysis bullosa experience severe oral manifestations including obliteration of the vestibule and ankyloglossia, with continuous blister formation and scarring.[57]

A rare finding in patients with complex craniofacial anomalies is ankyloglossia superior syndrome, of which glossopalatine ankylosis is the predominant feature.[58] Glossopalatine ankylosis (or ankyloglossia superior) describes the adherence of the tongue to the hard palate, which is typically treated surgically (Fig. 48.12). Ankyloglossia superior syndrome is when glossopalatine ankylosis is found alongside other abnormalities including cleft palate, microglossia, limb deformities, and gastrointestinal malformations.[58,59] Ankyloglossia superior has been associated with several craniofacial conditions and syndromes, including Hanhart syndrome, Charlie M syndrome, aglossia-adactylia, and more recently, Moebius syndrome.[59]

Given the association of abnormal frenal attachments with various syndromic and nonsyndromic conditions, providers may utilize certain frenal abnormalities as a diagnostic adjunct alongside other criteria.

Tethered Oral Tissues in Patients With Cleft Lip and Palate

Patients with cleft lip and palate may also present with abnormalities of frenal attachments that vary on an individual basis. Depending on the location of the cleft site, the attachment of the

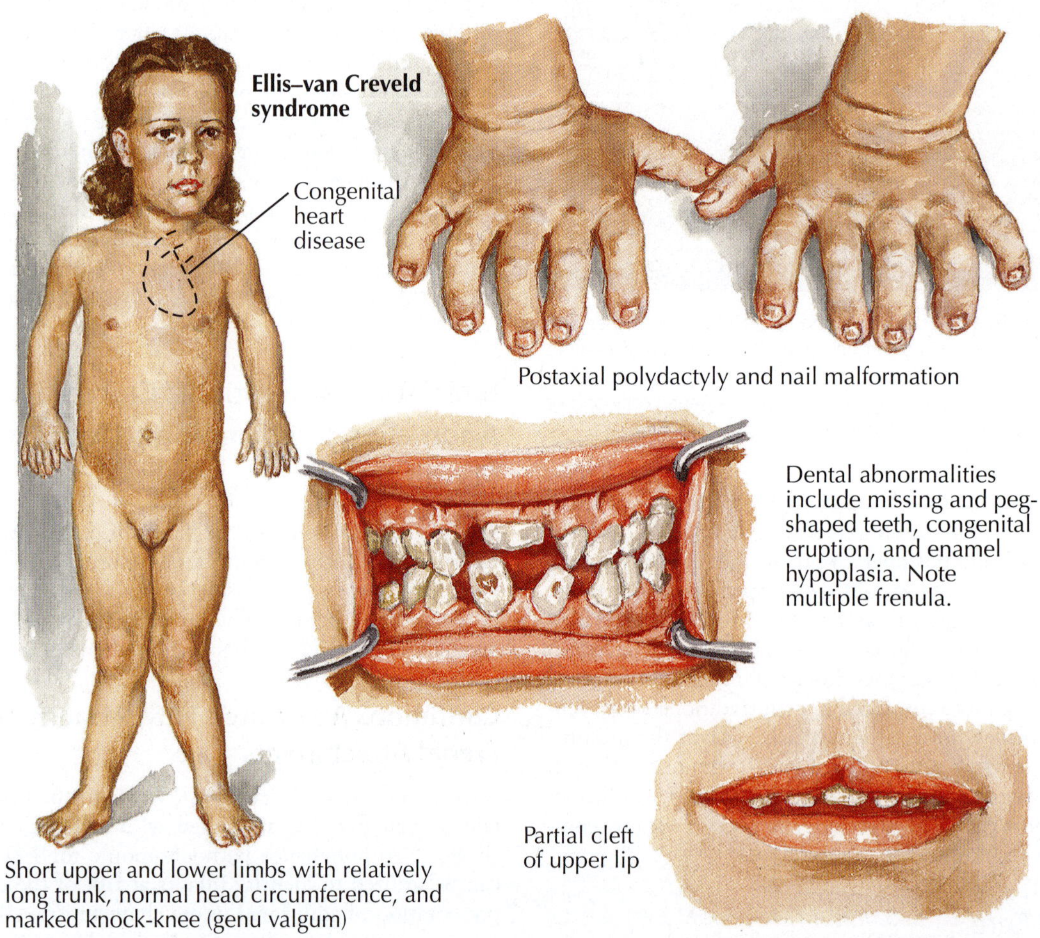

• **Fig. 48.10** Characteristic features of chondroectodermal dysplasia (Ellis–van Creveld syndrome) including multiple oral frenula.

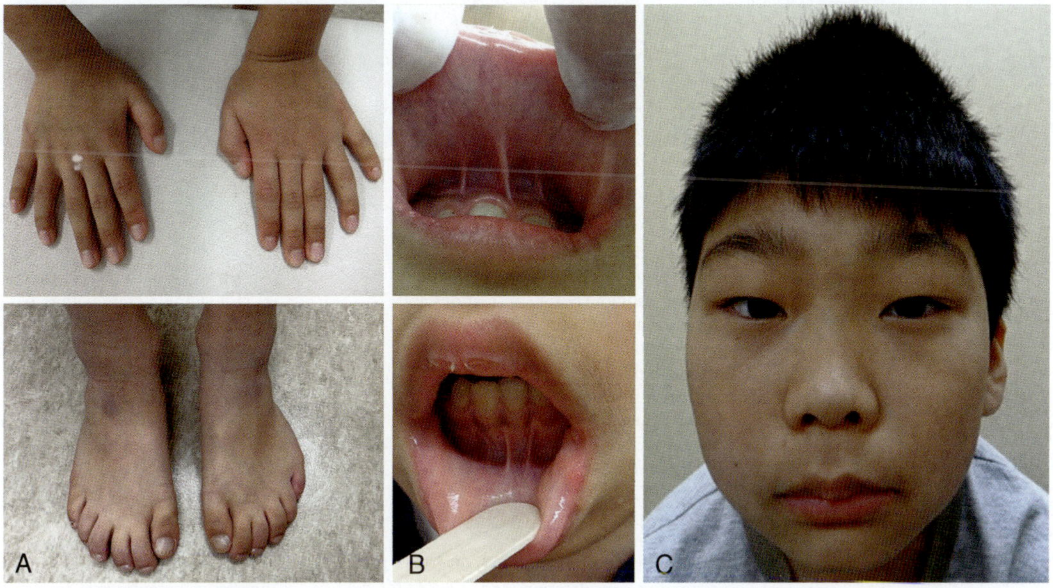

• **Fig. 48.11** Characteristic oro-facial-digital syndrome features of a 13-year-old patient with a PRKACB variant. (A) Note the bilateral postaxial-polydactyly of both fingers *(top)* and toes *(bottom)*. (B) Note the multiple oral frenula. (C) Note the long face, short columella, and hypertelorism.

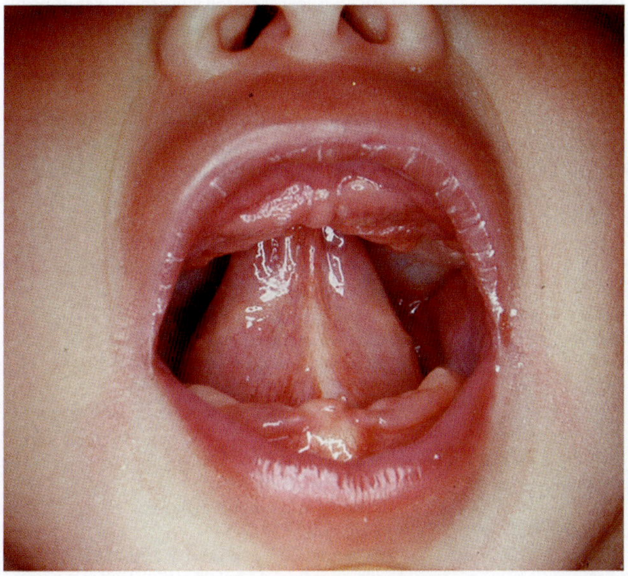

• **Fig. 48.12** Glossopalatine ankylosis at birth in a patient with Hanhart syndrome.

frenulum may be altered. Additionally, surgical interventions for cleft lip, alveolus, and palate may require alteration of the frenal attachments. Providers should identify any abnormalities in these soft tissue attachments, monitor their condition and the surrounding teeth and periodontium, and instruct patients and families regarding oral hygiene techniques. Depending on the condition of these attachments, special care may need to be taken to lift the tissues away from the teeth to cleanse them properly and prevent decay and periodontal disease. Scar tissue may also be present due to previous surgeries, leading to stricter attachments, which can present challenges to access hygiene. These areas may also be more challenging to anesthetize. For patients with cleft lip and palate, providers should evaluate the status of intraoral soft tissue attachments and instruct patients and families accordingly.

Visit eBooks.Health.Elsevier.com to see full list of references.

Index

B

C

J

K

L

P

U

V

W

X

Y

Z